Clinical Pharmacy and Therapeutics

For Churchill Livingstone

Commissioning Editor Laurence Hunter
Production Controller Debra Barrie
Sales Promotion Executive Marion Pollock

Clinical Pharmacy and Therapeutics

Edited by

Roger Walker BPharm PhD MRPharmS

Senior Lecturer in Clinical Pharmacy, Welsh School of Pharmacy,
University of Wales, Cardiff; Honorary Pharmacist, University Hospital of Wales, Cardiff

Clive Edwards BPharm PhD MRPharmS

Senior Lecturer in Clinical Pharmacy, Wolfson Unit of Clinical
Pharmacology, University of Newcastle upon Tyne; Honorary Pharmacist, Royal
Victoria Infirmary, Newcastle upon Tyne

CHURCHILL LIVINGSTONE
EDINBURGH LONDON MADRID MELBOURNE NEW YORK AND TOKYO 1994

CHURCHILL LIVINGSTONE
Medical Division of Longman Group UK Limited

Distributed in the United States of America by Churchill
Livingstone Inc., 650 Avenue of the Americas, New York,
N.Y. 10011, and by associated companies, branches and
representatives throughout the world.

First published 1994

ISBN 0 443 04553 4

British Library Cataloguing in Publication Data
A catalogue record for this book is available from the British
Library.

Library of Congress Cataloging in Publication Data
Clinical pharmacy and therapeutics/edited by Roger Walker, Clive
   Edwards.
      p.   cm.
      Includes index.
      ISBN 0-443-04553-4
      1. Chemotherapy. 2. Pharmacology. 3. Therapeutics. 4. Pharmacy.
   I. Walker, Roger, Ph. D. II. Edwards, Clive, Ph. D.
      [DNLM: 1. Pharmacology, Clinical. 2. Drug Therapy.   WB 330 C641
   1994]
   RM262.C5   1994
   615.5'8--dc20
   DNLM/DLC
   for Library of Congress   93-20832

The
publisher's
policy is to use
**paper manufactured
from sustainable forests**

Produced by Longman Singapore Publishers (Pte) Ltd.
Printed in Singapore

Contents

Preface

The aim of this textbook is to help pharmacy students, pharmacists and other health care workers understand clinical disorders and promote the safe, appropriate and effective use of drug therapy. In order to relate theory to practice the chapters in Section 3 have a variety of case studies at the end to encourage the application of the therapeutic principles contained within.

Clinical Pharmacy and Therapeutics has been written by pharmacists and clinicians and reflects the close working relationship between the two professions. We believe that this is the first textbook of clinical pharmacy written by such a combination of practitioners from within the UK. The mix of authors and their depth of knowledge provide a comprehensive overview of medical, therapeutic and patient-related issues.

Historically clinical pharmacy has been seen as the domain of those working in the hospital sector. As the gap between the primary and secondary health sectors diminishes and shared care becomes established, it is apparent that community pharmacists should derive much benefit from the clinical and therapeutic information contained within these covers.

The authors have made every effort to ensure that the information contained within each chapter was correct at the time of writing. However, it remains the responsibility of the reader to check the doses given, evaluate the appropriateness of opinions presented, ensure drugs are used within the remit of their licensed indications and take cognizance of new developments in therapeutics. But then, after all, that is what a clinical pharmacist routinely does.

Cardiff and Newcastle   R. W.
1994   C. E.

Acknowledgements

We are indebted to all the authors who have contributed to this textbook for their hard work and ability to meet the deadlines imposed. The help of many unnamed colleagues and typists is also acknowledged as is the assistance given to us by the staff at Churchill Livingstone.

On a personal note, may we thank all our colleagues and the students who have participated in our undergraduate or postgraduate courses in clinical pharmacy at universities in Newcastle, Sunderland and Cardiff. They gave us the inspiration and motivation to produce this book.

Finally, we would like to acknowledge the patience and support of our families and the endurance and understanding of our wives, Ann and Joy. Without their support this textbook would never have been complete.

R. W.
C. E.

Contributors

Christopher Acomb BSc MPharm MRPharmS
MCPP
Clinical Pharmacy Services Manager, Bradford
Hospitals NHS Trust, West Yorkshire, UK

Rosalind Anderson BSc (Pharm) MRPharmS
Pharmaceutical Adviser, Tameside FHSA,
Hyde, Cheshire, UK

C. Heather Ashton DM FRCP
Professor of Clinical Psychopharmacology and
Honorary Consultant Clinical Pharmacologist,
University of Newcastle upon Tyne, Newcastle
upon Tyne, UK

Paul J. Baker BSc MSc MRPharmS MCPP
Clinical Services Pharmacist, Birmingham
Heartlands Hospital, Birmingham, UK

Catrin E. Barker BSc MRPharmS DipClinPharm
Senior Clinical Pharmacist, Department of
Pharmacy, Royal Liverpool Children's NHS
Trust , Alder Hey Hospital, Liverpool, UK

D. Nicholas Bateman BSc MD FRCP
Consultant Physician, Freeman Hospital; Reader
in Therapeutics, University of Newcastle upon
Tyne, Newcastle upon Tyne, UK

Linda Beeley MA FRCP
Consultant Clinical Pharmacologist, Queen
Elizabeth Hospital, Birmingham, UK

Adrian J. Bint MBChB FRCPath
Consultant Microbiologist, Royal Victoria
Infirmary, Newcastle upon Tyne, UK

Peter N. Bramley BSc MBChB MRCP
Senior Registrar in Gastroenterology,
Department of Gastroenterology and Liver
Services, Aberdeen Royal Infirmary, Aberdeen,
UK

David Branford BPharm MRPharmS MCPP
Unit Pharmacist, Glenfrith Unit, Leicester;
Principal Lecturer, De Montfort University,
Leicester, UK

Mark Campbell BSc MRPharmS
Drug Use Review Manager, Northern Regional
Drug and Therapeutics Centre, Newcastle upon
Tyne, UK

Judith A. Cantrill BSc MSc MRPharmS
Clinical Senior Lecturer, Department of
Pharmacy, University of Manchester,
Manchester, UK

J. Edmond Charlton FRCA
Consultant in Pain Management and
Anaesthesia, Royal Victoria Infirmary,
Newcastle upon Tyne, UK

Christine M. Clark BSc MRPharmS
Director of Pharmacy, University of Manchester
Department of Pharmacy, Hope Hospital,
Manchester, UK

Soraya Dhillon BPharm PhD MRPharmS
Regional Development Pharmacist, North East
Thames RHA; Course Director, Diploma/MSc
Pharmacy Practice, The School of Pharmacy,
University of London, London, UK

Clive Edwards BPharm PhD MRPharmS
Senior Lecturer in Clinical Pharmacy, Wolfson
Unit of Clinical Pharmacology, University of
Newcastle upon Tyne; Honorary Pharmacist,
Royal Victoria Infirmary, Newcastle upon Tyne,
UK

Brian K. Evans BPharm PhD MRPharmS
Chief Administrative Pharmaceutical Officer,
South Glamorgan Health Authority, Temple of
Peace and Health; Research Pharmacist,
Gastroenterology Unit, University Hospital of
Wales, Cardiff, UK

Raymond W. Fitzpatrick BSc (Pharm) PhD
MRPharmS
Director of Pharmacy, The North Staffordshire
Hospital, Stoke on Trent; Senior Lecturer,
Department of Pharmacy Policy and Practice,
Keele University, Staffordshire, UK

Kevin P. Gibbs BPharm DipClinPharm
MRPharmS
Clinical Pharmacy Manager, Pharmacy
Department, Queen Alexandra Hospital,
Portsmouth, UK

F. Kate Gould MB BS MRCPath
Consultant Microbiologist, Freeman Hospital,
Newcastle upon Tyne, UK

Emma M. Graham-Clarke BPharm MPhil
MRPharmS
Senior Clinical Pharmacist, Dudley Road
Hospital; Clinical Fellow, University of Aston,
Birmingham, UK

James W. Gray MBChB MRCP MRCPath
Lecturer in Medical Microbiology, University of
Newcastle upon Tyne, Newcastle upon Tyne, UK

A. Harper BSc MSc
Principal Pharmacist, Royal United Hospital,
Bath, UK

Brian S. Hebron BPharm PhD MRPharmS
Principal Pharmacist, Dudley Road Hospital;
Senior Clinical Fellow, University of Aston,
Birmingham, UK

Peter Hudgson FRCP FRACP
Consultant Neurologist and Senior Lecturer in
Neurology, Regional Neurosciences Centre,

Newcastle General Hospital, Newcastle upon
Tyne, UK

Stephen A. Hudson BPharm MPharm
MRPharmS
Clinical Pharmacy Director, Department of
Pharmaceutical Sciences and School of
Pharmacy, University of Strathclyde, Glasgow;
Principal Pharmacist, Western General Hospital,
Edinburgh, UK

Harry R. Ingham MBChB FRCPath Dip Bact
Consultant Microbiologist, Regional Public
Health Laboratory, Institute of Pathology,
General Hospital, Newcastle upon Tyne, UK

Elizabeth A. Kay BPharm MSc MRPharmS
MCPP
Director of Clinical Pharmacy, United Leeds
Teaching Hospitals NHS Trust, Leeds, UK

Niall P. Keaney MB BSc PhD FRCP
Consultant Physician in Respiratory Medicine
and Clinical Pharmacology, Royal Infirmary;
Divisional General Manager, City Hospitals,
Sunderland, UK

Stephen M. Kelsey BSc MRCP
Senior Registrar, Department of Haematology,
Royal London Hospital, London, UK

Stuart J. Knight Dip Pharm (NZ) MRPharmS
Staff Pharmacist, HIV and Genitourinary
Medicine, Charing Cross Hospital, London,
UK

Anne Lee BSc MPhil MRPharmS
Drug Information Services Manager, Regional
Drug and Therapeutics Centre, Wolfson Unit,
Newcastle upon Tyne, UK

David K. Luscombe BPharm PhD CBiol FIBiol
FRPharmS
Professor of Clinical Pharmacy, Welsh School of
Pharmacy, University of Wales, Cardiff, UK

Mary C. Maclean BSc MRPharmS
Oncology Pharmacist, Royal London Hospital,
London, UK

Pamela Magee BSc MSc MRPharmS
Principal Clinical Pharmacist, Queen Elizabeth
Medical Centre, Birmingham, UK

Margaret Malone BSc MSc PhD MRPharmS MCPP
Associate Professor in Pharmacy Practice, Albany College of Pharmacy, Albany, USA

Janet M. Marks DM FRCP
Emeritus Consultant Dermatologist, Royal Victoria Infirmary, Newcastle upon Tyne, UK

Philip J. Marsh BSc MB ChB MRCPath
Senior Registrar in Microbiology, Royal Victorial Infirmary, Newcastle upon Tyne, UK

Margaret Nicolson MSc MRPharmS
Principal Pharmacist, Christie Hospital NHS Trust; Honorary Clinical Lecturer, University of Manchester, Manchester, UK

Anthony J. Nunn BPharm MRPharmS
Director of Pharmacy, Royal Liverpool Children's NHS Trust, Alder Hey Hospital, Liverpool, UK

Stephen J. Pedler MB MRCPath
Consultant Microbiologist, Department of Microbiology, Royal Victoria Infirmary, Newcastle upon Tyne, UK

Jane C. Portlock BPharm PhD MRPharmS
Primary Education Consultant and Honorary Senior Lecturer, School of Pharmacy, Portsmouth University; Local Tutor for Centre for Pharmacy Postgraduate Education, Portsmouth, UK

J. Peter Pratt BSc (Pharm) MRPharmS
Chief Pharmacist, Community and Priority Care Services, Middlewood Hospital, Sheffield; Honorary Tutor, Department of Psychiatry, University of Sheffield; Honorary Tutor, School of Pharmacy, Bradford University, Bradford, UK

Michael D. Rawlins BSc MD FRCP (Lond & Edin) FRPM
Professor of Clinical Pharmacology, University of Newcastle upon Tyne, Newcastle upon Tyne, UK

Philip A. Routledge MD FRCP
Professor of Clinical Pharmacology, University of Wales College of Medicine, Cardiff, UK

Josemir W. A. R. Sander MD
Associate Specialist in Neurology, National Hospital, Chalfont St Peter; Clinical Research Fellow, Institute of Neurology, London, UK

David K. Scott PhD MRPharmS
Principal Pharmacist (Clinical Training), Oxford Regional Health Authority, Oxford, UK

Hilary F. Scott BSc MPhil MRPharmS
Pharmaceutical Adviser, Essex Family Health Services Authority, Clacton-on-Sea, Essex; Previously Research Pharmacist, Birmingham and Midland Eye Hospital, Birmingham, West Midlands

Hamasaraj G. M. Shetty BSc MRCP (UK)
Lecturer in Clinical Pharmacology and Therapeutics and Honorary Senior Registrar in General and Geriatric Medicine, University of Wales, College of Medicine, Cardiff, UK

Carol A. Stevens BSc DipClinPharm MRPharmS
Principal Pharmacist, The Royal London Hospital, London, UK

Ivan H. Stockley BPharm PhD FRPharmS
Special Lecturer, Department of Physiology and Pharmacology, University of Nottingham Medical School, Nottingham, UK

Lucy Titcomb BSc MRPharmS MCPP
Principal Pharmacist, Birmingham and Midland Eye Hospital, Birmingham, UK

Seán C. Turner BPharm MRPharmS
Clinical Pharmacist, Department of Pharmacy, Royal Liverpool Children's NHS Trust, Alder Hey Hospital, Liverpool, UK

Roger Walker BPharm PhD MRPharmS
Senior Lecturer in Clinical Pharmacy, Welsh School of Pharmacy, University of Wales, Cardiff; Honorary Pharmacist, University Hospital of Wales, Cardiff, UK

Martin P. Ward Platt MD MRCP
Consultant Paediatrician (Neonatal Medicine), Royal Victoria Infirmary, Newcastle upon Tyne, UK

Pamela S. Warrington MSc MRPharmS
Deputy Chief Pharmacist, Scottish Office Home
and Health Department, Edinburgh, UK

Peter Watson BSc MBChB MRCP (UK) DMRD
Consultant Physician in Genito-Urinary
Medicine, Newcastle General Hospital; Clinical
Lecturer, Department of Medicine, University of
Newcastle upon Tyne, Newcastle upon Tyne, UK

Ken Woodhouse MD FRCP
Professor of Geriatric Medicine, University of
Wales College of Medicine, Cardiff, UK

Cheryl M. Way BPharm MRPharmS
Unit Pharmacy Manager, Cardiff Royal
Infirmary, Cardiff, UK

Robert D. Swallow BPharm MRPharmS
Principal Pharmacist, Clinical Teaching and
Hepatology, St James's University Hospital,
Leeds; Honorary Lecturer in Continuing
Professional Education; Honorary Lecturer in
Medicine, The University of Leeds, Leeds, UK

SECTION ONE

GENERAL

Chapter 1

Practical pharmacokinetics

R. Fitzpatrick

Clinical pharmacokinetics may be defined as the study of the time course of the absorption, distribution, metabolism and excretion of drugs and their corresponding pharmacological response. In practice, pharmacokinetics makes it possible to model what may happen to a drug after it has been administered to a patient. Clearly, this science may be applied to a wide range of clinical situations, hence the term clinical pharmacokinetics.

General applications

Knowledge of pharmacokinetics is useful in appreciating when maximal response is likely to occur after the start of a therapeutic regimen. By knowing the half-life of a drug, the time to reach steady state may be estimated (Fig 1.1) and thus when maximal therapeutic response is likely to occur, irrespective of whether drug level monitoring is needed.

The same type of information can be used to determine whether a loading dose of a drug is necessary, since drugs with longer half-lives are more likely to require loading doses for acute treatment.

Clinical pharmacokinetics can be useful in determining dosage alteration in renal failure if the fraction excreted unchanged (Fe value) is known. This parameter can be found in most pharmacology textbooks.

An understanding of the pharmacokinetics of absorption may also be useful in evaluating the

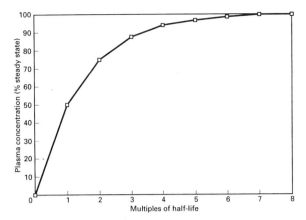

Fig. 1.1 Time to steady state.

appropriateness of particular formulations of a drug in a patient.

Application to therapeutic drug monitoring (TDM)

The application of clinical pharmacokinetics is usually associated with TDM and its subsequent utilization. There are various levels of sophistication for this type of application.

Knowledge of the distribution time and an understanding of the concept of steady state can facilitate determination of appropriate sampling times.

For most drugs which undergo first order elimination, a linear relationship exists between dose and concentration which can be used for dose adjustment purposes. However, if the clearance of the drug changes as the concentration changes (e.g. phenytoin), then this must be known in order to avoid inappropriate dose adjustments.

It has been demonstrated that by applying pharmacokinetic principles to the interpretation of TDM data, the utilization of the service is improved.

More sophisticated use of pharmacokinetics involves the use of population pharmacokinetic data to produce initial dosage guidelines, e.g., nomograms for digoxin and gentamicin. Population pharmacokinetic data have also been used to produce specific blood level predictions.

It is essential for pharmacists to have an understanding of pharmacokinetics if they are to be involved in complex dosage individualization using steady state blood levels or using test dose blood level data.

Given the wide range of clinical situations in which pharmacokinetics can be applied, pharmacists must have a good understanding of the subject and how to apply it in order to improve their contribution to patient care.

BASIC CONCEPTS
Volume of distribution

Apparent volume of distribution may be defined as the size of a compartment which will account for the total amount of drug in the body if it were present in the same concentration as in plasma. This means that it is the apparent volume of fluid in the body which results in the measured concentration of drug in plasma for a known amount of drug given, i.e.:

$$\text{Plasma concentration (Cp)} = \frac{\text{Amount of drug in body (Ab)}}{\text{Apparent volume of distribution (Vd)}}$$

This relationship assumes that the drug is evenly distributed throughout the body in the same concentration as in the plasma. However, this is not the case in practice, since many drugs are present in different concentrations in various parts of the body. Thus, some drugs such as digoxin have a very large apparent volume of distribution. This concept is better explained in Figure 1.2.

Apparent volume of distribution (Vd) may be used to determine the plasma concentration (Cp) after an intravenous loading dose:

$$Cp = \frac{\text{Loading dose}}{Vd} \qquad (1)$$

Conversely, if the desired concentration is known, the loading dose may be determined:

$$\text{Loading dose} = \text{Desired Cp} \times Vd \qquad (2)$$

In the previous discussion, it has been as-

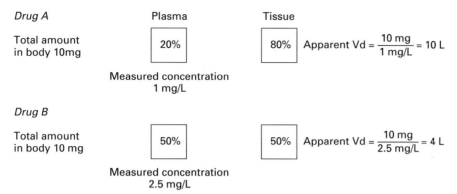

Fig. 1.2 Distribution: more of drug A is distributed in the tissue compartment resulting in a higher apparent volume of distribution than drug B, where more remains in the plasma.

sumed that after a given dose a drug is instantaneously distributed between the various tissues and plasma. In practice this is seldom the case. Although a drug may be distributed into many tissues, it is reasonable for practical purposes to generalize by referring to tissue as if it were a single entity or compartment. Thus, the body may be described in pharmacokinetic terms as if it were divided into two compartments; the plasma and the tissues.

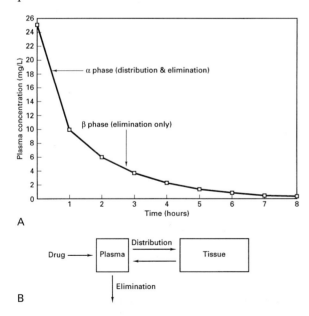

Fig. 1.3 (A) Two compartment model showing two phases in the plasma concentration/time profile. (B) Representation of a two compartment model showing distribution of drug between plasma and tissue compartments.

Figure 1.3 depicts the disposition of a drug immediately after administration and relates this to the plasma concentration/time graph.

Initially, the plasma concentration falls rapidly, due to distribution and elimination (α phase). However, when an equilibrium is reached between the plasma and tissue (i.e. distribution is complete) the change in plasma concentration is due to elimination from the plasma (β phase) and the plasma concentration falls at a slower rate. The drug is said to follow a two compartment model. However, if distribution is completed quickly (within minutes), then the α phase is not seen and the drug is said to follow a one compartment model.

The practical implications of a two compartment model are that any sampling for serum concentration monitoring purposes should be carried out after distribution is complete, and intravenous bolus doses should be given slowly to avoid transient side effects due to high peak concentrations.

Elimination

Drugs may be eliminated from the body by a number of routes. The primary routes are metabolism (usually in the liver) into an inactive compound, excretion of the unchanged drug in the kidneys, or a combination of both.

The main pharmacokinetic parameter describing elimination is clearance (Cl). This is defined as the volume of plasma completely emptied of drug per unit time. For example, if the concentration of a drug in a patient is 1 g/L and the clearance is 1 L/hour, then the rate of elimination will be 1 g/hour.

Thus, a relationship exists:

$$\text{Rate of elimination} = Cl \times Cp \qquad (3)$$

Total body elimination is the sum of the metabolic rate of elimination and the renal rate of elimination. Therefore:

$$\text{Total body clearance} = Cl \text{ (metabolic)} + Cl \text{ (renal)}$$

Thus, if the fraction eliminated by the renal route is known (Fe), then the effect of renal impairment on total body clearance can be estimated.

For most drugs clearance is constant. Therefore, it is clear from equation (3) that as the plasma concentration changes so will the rate of elimination. However, when the rate of administration is equal to the rate of elimination, the plasma concentration is constant (Cp_{ss}) and the drug is said to be at steady state. At steady state:

$$\text{Rate in} = \text{Rate out.}$$

At the beginning of a dosage regimen the plasma concentration is low. Therefore, the rate of elimination is less than the rate of administration, and accumulation occurs until steady state is reached (Fig. 1.1).

$$\text{Rate of administration} = \text{Rate of elimination}$$
$$= Cl \times Cp_{ss} \qquad (4)$$

It is clear from equation (3) that as the plasma concentration falls (for example on stopping treatment or after a single dose) the rate of elimination also falls. Therefore, the plasma concentration time graph follows a non-linear curve characteristic of this type of *first order* elimination (Fig. 1.4). This is profoundly different from a constant rate of elimination irrespective of plasma concentration, which is typical of *zero order* elimination.

For drugs undergoing first order elimination, there are two other useful pharmacokinetic parameters in addition to volume of distribution and clearance. These are elimination rate constant and elimination half-life.

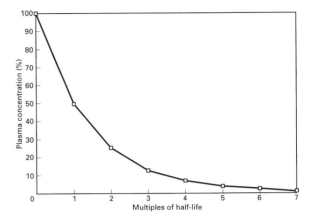

Fig. 1.4 First order elimination.

Elimination rate constant (k_e) is the fraction of the amount of drug in the body eliminated per unit time. For example, if the body contains 100 mg of a drug and 10% is eliminated per unit time, then $k_e = 0.1$. In the first unit of time, 0.1×100 mg or 10 mg is eliminated, leaving 90 mg. In the second unit of time, 0.1×90 mg or 9 mg is eliminated, leaving 81 mg. Elimination continues in this manner. Therefore:

$$\text{Rate of elimination} = k_e \times \text{Amount of drug in body (Ab)} \qquad (5)$$

Combining equations (3) and (5):

$$Cl \times Cp = k_e \times Ab$$

and since:

$$Cp = \frac{Ab}{Vd}$$

then:

$$Cl \times \frac{Ab}{Vd} = k_e \times Ab$$

Therefore: $\quad Cl = k_e \times Vd \qquad (6)$

Elimination half-life ($t_{1/2}$) is the time it takes for the plasma concentration to decay by half. In five half-lives the plasma concentration will fall to approximately zero (Fig. 1.4).

The equation which is described in Figure 1.4 is:

$$Cp_2 = Cp_1 \times e^{-k_e \times t} \qquad (7)$$

Where Cp_1 and Cp_2 are plasma concentrations and t is time.

If half-life is substituted for time in equation (7), Cp_2 must be half of Cp_1.

Therefore:

$$0.5 \times Cp_1 = Cp_1 \times e^{-k_e \times t_{1/2}}$$
$$0.5 = e^{-k_e \times t_{1/2}}$$
$$\ln(0.5) = -k_e \times t_{1/2}$$
$$-0.693 = -k_e \times t_{1/2}$$
$$t_{1/2} = \frac{0.693}{k_e} \qquad (8)$$

There are two ways of determining k_e, either by estimating half-life and applying equation (8) or by substituting two plasma concentrations in equation (7) and applying natural logarithms.

$$\ln Cp_2 = \ln Cp_1 - (k_e \times t)$$
$$k_e \times t = \ln Cp_1 - \ln Cp_2$$
$$k_e = \frac{\ln Cp_1 - \ln Cp_2}{t}$$

In the same way as it takes approximately five half-lives for the plasma concentration to decay to zero after a single dose, it takes approximately five half-lives for a drug to accumulate to steady state on repeated dosing or during constant infusion (Fig. 1.1).

This graph may be described by the equation:

$$Cp_t = Cp_{ss} (1 - e^{-k_e \times t}) \qquad (9)$$

Where Cp_t = plasma concentration at time t after the start of the infusion. Thus (if the appropriate pharmacokinetic parameters are known), it is possible to estimate the plasma concentration any time after a single dose or the start of a dosage regimen.

Absorption

In the preceding sections, the intravenous route has been discussed and with this route all of the administered drug is absorbed. However, if a drug is administered by any other route it must be absorbed into the bloodstream. This process may or may not be 100% efficient.

The fraction of the administered dose which is absorbed into the bloodstream is bioavailability (F). Thus, for oral administration, the dose or rate of administration must be multiplied by F.

In addition to bioavailability, the other useful pharmacokinetic parameter is the absorption rate constant (k_a). This term is the fraction of the dose remaining, which is absorbed per unit of time. It is the converse of k_e, which describes the fraction eliminated per unit time. Thus, the absorption rate constant (k_a) is a quantitative measure of how quickly a formulation is absorbed. This is useful when comparing different formulations, particularly slow-release preparations. It is related to absorption half-life in the same way as k_e is related to elimination half-life.

Dosing regimens

From the preceding sections, it is possible to derive equations which can be applied in clinical practice.

From equation (1) we can determine the change in plasma concentration ΔCp immediately after a single dose:

$$\Delta Cp = \frac{S \times F \times Dose}{Vd} \qquad (10)$$

Where S = salt factor, which is the fraction of active drug when the dose is administered as a salt (e.g. aminophylline is 80% theophylline, therefore S = 0.8).

Conversely, to determine a loading dose:

$$Loading\ dose = \frac{Desired\ change\ in\ Cp \times Vd}{S \times F} \qquad (11)$$

At steady state, it is possible to determine maintenance dose or steady state plasma concentrations from a modified equation (4):

$$Rate\ in = \frac{S \times F \times Dose}{T} = Cl \times Average\ Cp_{ss} \qquad (12)$$

where T = dosing interval.

Peak and trough levels

For oral dosing and constant intravenous infusions, it is usually adequate to use the term average steady state plasma concentration (average

Cp_{ss}). However, for some intravenous bolus injections it is sometimes necessary to determine peak and trough levels (e.g. gentamicin).

At steady state, the change in concentration due to the administration of an intravenous dose will be equal to the change in concentration due to elimination over one dose interval.

$$\Delta Cp = \frac{S \times F \times Dose}{Vd} = Cp_{max} - Cp_{min}$$

Within one dosing interval the maximum plasma concentration ($Cp_{ss\ max}$) will decay to the minimum plasma concentration ($Cp_{ss\ min}$) as in any first order process.

Substituting $Cp_{ss\ max}$ for Cp_1 and $Cp_{ss\ min}$ for Cp_2 in equation (7):

$$Cp_{ss\ min}\ Cp_{ss\ max} \times e^{-k_e \times t}$$

where t = dosing interval.

If this is substituted into the preceding equation:

$$\frac{S \times F \times Dose}{V} = Cp_{ss\ max} - Cp_{ss\ max} \times e^{-k_e \times t}$$

Therefore:

$$Cp_{ss\ max} = \frac{S \times F \times Dose}{Vd\ [1 - e^{-k_e \times t}]} \qquad (13)$$

$$Cp_{ss\ min} = \frac{S \times F \times Dose}{Vd\ [1 - e^{-k_e \times t}]} \times e^{-k_e \times t} \qquad (14)$$

Interpretation of drug concentration data

The availability of the technology to measure the concentration of a drug in serum should not be the reason for monitoring. There are a number of criteria which should be fulfilled before therapeutic drug monitoring is undertaken:

• low therapeutic index
• good concentration–response relationship
• no easily measurable physiological parameter.

In the absence of these criteria being fulfilled, the only other justification for undertaking TDM is to monitor compliance or to confirm toxicity.

In the preceding sections, the time to steady state has been discussed. When TDM is carried out as an aid to dose adjustment, the concentration should be at steady state. Therefore, approximately five half-lives should elapse before sampling after initiation or changing a maintenance regimen. The only exception to this rule is when toxicity is suspected.

When steady state has been reached, it is important to sample at the correct time. It is clear from the discussion above that this should be done when distribution is complete.

Under most circumstances, providing the preceding criteria are observed, adjusting the dose of a drug is relatively simple, since a linear relationship exists between dose and concentration if a drug follows first order elimination (Fig. 1.5A).

Although most drugs follow first order elimination, when a drug is eliminated by the liver it is possible for the metabolic pathway to become saturated, since it is an enzymatic system. Thus initially the elimination is first order, but once saturation of the system occurs, elimination becomes zero order. This results in the characteristic dose/concentration graph of Figure 1.5B. For the majority of drugs eliminated by the liver, this effect is not seen at normal therapeutic doses and only occurs at very high supratherapeutic levels, which is why the kinetics of some drugs in overdose is different from normal. However, one important exception is phenytoin, where saturation of the enzymatic pathway occurs at

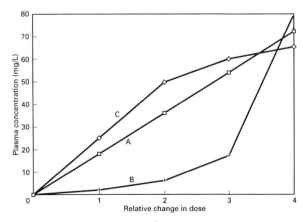

Fig. 1.5 Dose/concentration relationships: (A) first order elimination; (B) capacity limited clearance; (C) increasing clearance.

therapeutic doses. This will be dealt with in the section on phenytoin.

The only other situation where first order elimination is not seen is where clearance increases as the serum concentration increases (Fig. 1.5C). Under normal circumstances, the plasma protein sites available to a drug far outnumber the capacity of the drug to fill those binding sites. Therefore, the proportion of the total concentration of drug which is protein bound is constant. However, this situation is not seen in one or two instances (e.g. valproate and disopyramide). For these particular drugs, as the concentration increases the plasma protein binding sites become saturated, thus the ratio of unbound drug to bound drug increases.

The elimination of these drugs increases disproportionately to the total concentration, since this is dependent on the unbound concentration.

Wherever TDM is carried out, a therapeutic range is usually used as a guide to the optimum concentration. The limits of these ranges should not be taken as absolute. Some patients may respond to levels above or below these ranges, whereas others may experience toxic effects within the so-called therapeutic range. These ranges are only adjuncts to dose determination, which should always be done in the light of clinical response.

CLINICAL APPLICATIONS

Estimation of creatinine clearance

Since many drugs are renally excreted, and the most practical marker of renal function is creatinine clearance, it is often necessary to estimate this in order to undertake dosage adjustment in renal impairment. The usual method is to undertake a 24–hour urine collection coupled with a serum creatinine measurement. The laboratory then estimates the patient's creatinine clearance. The formula used to determine creatinine clearance is based upon the pharmacokinetic principles in equation (4).

Rate of elimination is calculated from the measurement of total amount of creatinine contained in the 24-hour urine sample divided by 24, i.e.:

$$\frac{\text{Amount of creatinine}}{24} = \text{Rate of excretion (mg/h)}$$

Using this rate of excretion and substituting the measured serum creatinine for Cp_{ss} in equation (4) the creatinine clearance can be calculated.

However, there are practical difficulties with this method. The whole process is cumbersome and there is an inevitable delay in obtaining a result. The biggest problem is the inaccuracy of the 24-hour urine collection.

An alternative approach is to estimate the rate of production of creatinine (i.e. rate in) instead of the rate of elimination (rate out). Clearly this has advantages, since it does not involve 24-hour urine collections and requires only a single measure of serum creatinine. There are data in the literature relating creatinine production to age, weight and sex, since the primary source of creatinine is the breakdown of muscle.

Thus, equations have been produced which are rearrangements of equation (4), i.e.:

$$\text{Creatinine clearance} = \frac{\text{Rate of production}}{Cp_{ss}}$$

Rate of production is replaced by a formula which estimates this from physiological parameters of age, weight and sex.

It has been shown that the equation produced by Cockcroft & Gault appears to be the most satisfactory. A modified version using SI units is shown below:

Creatinine clearance for females (ml/min)

$$= \frac{F \times (140 - \text{Age (yr)}) \times \text{Weight (kg)}}{\text{Serum creatinine } (\mu mol/L)}$$

where F = 1.04 (females) or 1.23 (males).

Digoxin

Action and uses

Digoxin is the most widely used of the digitalis glycosides. Its primary actions on the heart are those of increasing the force of contraction and decreasing conduction through the AV node.

Historically, it has been used in the treatment of heart failure, although alternative agents are now frequently used. Currently, its main role is in the treatment of atrial fibrillation. Measurement of heart rate is the primary method of monitoring its clinical effect, but knowledge of the drug's pharmacokinetics can be helpful in predicting a patient's dosage requirements.

Serum concentration/response relationship

- < 0.5 microgram/L – no clinical effect
- 0.7 microgram/L – some positive inotropic and conduction blocking effect
- 0.8–2 microgram/L – optimum therapeutic range
- 2–2.5 microgram/L – increased risk of toxicity, although tolerated in some patients
- > 2.5 microgram/L – GI, CVS and CNS toxicity.

Distribution

Digoxin is widely distributed and extensively bound in varying degrees to tissues throughout the body. This results in a high apparent volume of distribution. The population average is 7.3 L/kg (lean body weight). However, since distribution is altered in patients with renal impairment, a more accurate estimate in these patients is given by:

$$Vd = 3.8 \times \text{Lean BWt} + (3.1 \times \text{Creatinine clearance in ml/min})$$

A two compartment model best describes digoxin disposition (Fig.1.3) with a distribution time of 6 to 8 hours. Clinical effects are seen earlier after intravenous doses, since the myocardium has a high blood perfusion and affinity for digoxin. Sampling for TDM must be done no sooner than 6 hours post-dose, otherwise an erroneous result will be obtained.

Elimination

Digoxin is eliminated primarily by renal excretion of unchanged drug (60 to 80%), but some

hepatic metabolism occurs (20 to 40%). The population average value for digoxin clearance is:

Digoxin clearance (ml/min)
= 0.8 × BWt + (Creatinine clearance in ml/min)

However, in patients with severe congestive heart failure, hepatic metabolism is markedly reduced together with a slight reduction in renal excretion.

In CHF:

Digoxin clearance (ml/min)
= 0.33 × BWt + (0.9 × Creatinine clearance)

Lean body weight should be used in these equations.

Absorption

Digoxin is poorly absorbed from the gastrointestinal tract and dissolution time affects the overall bioavailability. The two oral formulations of digoxin have different bioavailabilities:

F (tabs) = 0.65, F (liquid) = 0.8

Practical implications

Using population averages it is possible to predict serum concentrations from specific dosages, particularly since the time to steady state is long. Population values are only averages and individuals may vary. In addition, a number of diseases and drugs affect digoxin disposition.

As can be seen from the preceding discussion, congestive heart failure, hepatic and renal disease all decrease the elimination of digoxin. In addition, hypothyroidism increases the concentration (decreased metabolism and renal excretion) and increases the sensitivity of the heart to digoxin. Hyperthyroidism has the opposite effect. Hypokalaemia, hypercalcaemia, hypomagnesaemia and hypoxia all increase the sensitivity of the heart to digoxin. There are numerous drug interactions reported of varying clinical significance. The usual cause is either altered absorption or clearance.

Theophylline

Theophylline is an alkaloid related to caffeine. It has a variety of clinical effects including mild diuresis, CNS stimulation, cerebrovascular vasodilatation, increased cardiac output and bronchodilatation. It is the latter which is the major therapeutic effect of theophylline. Theophylline does have some serious toxic effects. However, there is a good serum concentration/response relationship.

Serum concentration/response relationship

- < 5 mg/L – no bronchodilatation[1]
- 5–10 mg/L – some bronchodilatation
- 10–20 mg/L – optimum bronchodilatation, minimum side effects
- 20–30 mg/L – increased incidence of nausea, vomiting[2] and cardiac arrhythmias
- > 30 mg/L – cardiac arrhythmias, seizures.

Distribution

Theophylline is extensively distributed throughout the body, with a population average volume of distribution of 0.48 L/kg.

It does not distribute very well into fat, and estimations should be based on lean body weight. A two compartment model best describes theophylline disposition, with a distribution time of approximately 40 minutes.

Elimination

Elimination is a first order process primarily by hepatic metabolism to relatively inactive metabolites.

The population average for theophylline clearance = 0.04 L/h/kg. Theophylline clearance is affected by a number of diseases/drugs/pollutants. Therefore, where there is cirrhosis, conges-

tive heart failure (with hepatomegaly) or severe respiratory obstruction ($FEV_1 < 1$ L), this value should be multiplied by 0.5., 0.4 and 0.8 respectively. Conversely, patients who smoke (defined as > 10 cigarettes per day) metabolize theophylline more quickly and the normal value for clearance should be multiplied by 1.6. Concurrent cimetidine, erythromycin or ciprofloxacin therapy all decrease metabolism by 50%.

Neonates metabolize theophylline differently, with 50% being converted to caffeine. Therefore, when it is used to treat neonatal apnoea of prematurity, a lower 'therapeutic range' is used (usually 5 to 10 mg/L), since caffeine contributes to the therapeutic response.

Product formulation

Aminophylline (the ethylenediamine salt of theophylline) is only 80% theophylline. Therefore, the salt factor (S) is 0.8. Most SR preparations show good bioavailability but not all SR preparations are the same. The absorption rate constant (k_a) provides a good guide to slow-release characteristics. Generally, the lower the k_a value the better the slow-release capabilities.

Practical implications

Intravenous bolus doses of aminophylline need to be given slowly (preferably by short infusion) to avoid side effects due to transiently high blood levels during the distribution phase. Oral doses with slow-release preparations can be estimated using population average pharmacokinetic values and titrated proportionately according to blood levels and clinical response. In most circumstances, slow-release preparations may be assumed to provide 12 hours' cover. However, more marked peaks and troughs are seen with fast metabolizers (smokers and children). In these cases, the slow-release preparation with the lowest k_a value may be used twice daily (e.g. Theo-Dur k_a = 0.18 or Uniphyllin k_a = 0.22). Alternatively, thrice daily dosage is required if a standard (k_a 0.3 to 0.4) slow-release product is used (e.g. Phyllocontin k_a = 0.37 or Nuelin SA k_a = 0.33).

---

[1] Some patients exhibit a clinical effect at these levels. This may be due to bronchodilatation or some other mechanism of action – perhaps an anti-inflammatory effect.
[2] Nausea and vomiting can also occur in the 'therapeutic range'.

Gentamicin

Clinical use

The spectrum of activity of gentamicin is similar to other aminoglycosides but its most significant activity is against *Psuedomonas aeruginosa*. It is still regarded by many as first choice for this type of infection.

Therapeutic range

Gentamicin has a low therapeutic index, producing dose-related side effects of nephro- and ototoxicity. The use of blood level monitoring to aid dose adjustment is essential if these toxic effects which appear to be related to peak and trough serum levels are to be avoided. It is generally accepted that the peak level (drawn 1 hour post-dose after an intravenous bolus or intramuscular injection) should not exceed 12 mg/L and the trough level (drawn immediately predose) should not exceed 2 mg/L.

Distribution

Gentamicin is relatively polar and distributes primarily into extracellular fluid. Thus, the apparent volume of distribution is only 0.25 L/kg. Gentamicin follows a two compartment model with distribution being complete within 1 hour.

Elimination

Elimination is by renal excretion of the unchanged drug. Gentamicin clearance is approximately equal to creatinine clearance.

Practical implications

Since the therapeutic range is based on peak (1 hour post-dose to allow for distribution) and trough (predose) concentrations, it is necessary to be able to predict these from any given dosage regimen. Initial dosage may be based on the patient's physiological parameters.

Gentamicin clearance may be determined from creatinine clearance. Volume of distribution may be determined from lean body weight. Elimination constant k_e may then be estimated from equation (6).

By substituting this value and the desired peak and trough levels into equation (7), the optimum dosage interval can be determined (add on 1 hour to this value to account for sampling time). Using this value (or the nearest practical value) and the desired trough value substituted into equation (14), it is possible to determine the appropriate dose.

Dosage changes for gentamicin are not as straightforward as for theophylline or digoxin, since increasing the dose will increase the peak and trough levels proportionately. If this is not desired, then use of pharmacokinetic equations is necessary. By substituting the measured peak and trough levels and the time between them into equation (7), it is possible to determine k_e (and half-life from equation (8) if required). To find the volume of distribution it is necessary to know the Cp_{max} immediately after the dose (time zero), not the 1-hour value which is measured.

To obtain this, equation (7) may be used, this time solving for Cp_1. Subtracting the trough level from Cp_{max} at time zero the volume of distribution may be determined from equation (10). Using these actual values for k_e and Vd, a new dose and dose interval can be determined as before.

Lithium

Lithium is effective in the treatment of acute mania and in the prophylaxis of manic depression. The mechanism of action is not fully understood, but it is thought that it may substitute for sodium or potassium in the CNS. Lithium is toxic, producing dose-dependent and dose-independent side effects. Thus, TDM is essential in assisting in the management of the dosage.

Dose-dependent effects

The serum concentration/response relationship derived on the basis of the 12-hour standardized lithium level (measured 12 hours after the evening dose of lithium) is shown below:

- < 0.4 mmol/L – little therapeutic effect
- 0.4–1.0 mmol/L – optimum range for prophylaxis
- 0.8–1.2 mmol/L – optimum range for acute mania
- 1.2–1.5 mmol/L – causes possible renal impairment
- 1.5–3.0 mmol/L – causes renal impairment, ataxia, weakness, drowsiness, thirst, diarrhoea
- 3.0–5.0 mmol/L – confusion, spasticity, dehydration, convulsions, coma, death.

(Levels > 3.5 mmol/L are regarded as a medical emergency.)

Dose-independent effects

These include tremor, hypothyroidism (approximately 10% of patients on chronic therapy), nephrogenic diabetes insipidus, gastrointestinal upset, loss in bone density, weight gain (approximately 20% of patients gain more than 10 kg) and lethargy.

Distribution

Lithium is unevenly distributed throughout the body, with a volume of distribution approximately 0.5 to 1 L/kg. Lithium follows a two compartment model (Fig. 1.3) with a distribution time of 8 hours (hence, 12-hour sampling criterion).

Elimination

Lithium is excreted unchanged by the kidneys. Lithium clearance is approximately 20% of the creatinine clearance, since there is extensive reabsorption in the renal tubules.

In addition to changes in renal function, dehydration, diuretics (particularly thiazides), ACE inhibitors and NSAIDs (except aspirin and sulindac) all decrease lithium clearance.

Conversely, aminophylline and sodium loading increase lithium clearance.

Notwithstanding the above factors, there is a wide interindividual variation in clearance, and lithium half-life in the population varies between 8 and 35 hours with an average of approximately 18 hours. Lithium clearance shows a diurnal variation, being slower at night than during the day.

Practical implications

Since lithium excretion is a first order process, changes in dosage result in a proportional change in blood levels. Because of the long distribution phase, blood samples should be drawn 12 hours after the evening dose, since this will represent the slowest excretion rate. Population pharmacokinetic data (particularly volume of distribution) cannot be relied upon to make initial dosage predictions although renal function may give an approximate guide to clearance. Blood level measurements are reported in SI units. Therefore, it is useful to know the conversion factors for the various salts. 100 mg of lithium carbonate is equivalent to 2.7 mmol of lithium ion, whereas 100 mg of lithium citrate is equivalent to only 1.1 mmol of lithium ion.

Phenytoin

Phenytoin is used in the treatment of primary and secondary generalized tonic–clonic epilepsy. It is associated with dose-independent side effects which include hirsutism, acne, coarsening of facial features, gingival hyperplasia, hypocalcaemia and folic acid deficiency. However, the more serious side effects of phenytoin are concentration related.

Serum concentration/response relationship

- < 5 mg/L – generally no therapeutic effect
- 5–10 mg/L – some anticonvulsant action
- 10–20 mg/L – optimum concentration for anticonvulsant effect
- 20–30 mg/L – nystagmus, blurred vision
- > 30 mg/L – ataxia, dysarthria, drowsiness, coma.

Distribution

Phenytoin follows a two compartment model with a distribution time of 30 to 60 minutes. The apparent volume of distribution is 1 L/kg.

Elimination

Phenytoin is metabolized by the liver, which is the main organ of elimination. However, this metabolic route can be saturated at normal therapeutic doses. This results in the characteristic dose/concentration curve in Figure 1.5B. Therefore, instead of the usual first order pharmacokinetic model, a Michaelis–Menten enzyme model is more appropriate.

Using this model, the daily dosage of phenytoin can be described by:

$$\frac{S \times F \times Dose}{T} = \frac{V_{max} \times Cp_{ss}}{K_m + Cp_{ss}} \quad (15)$$

K_m is the plasma concentration at which metabolism proceeds at half maximal rate. The population average for this is 6 mg/L, although this value varies greatly with age and race.

V_{max} is the maximum rate of metabolism of phenytoin and is more predictable at approximately 7 mg/kg/day.

Elimination half-life

Since clearance changes with blood concentration, half-life also changes. The usual reported value is 22 hours, but this increases as concentration increases. It is difficult to predict when steady state will be reached but, as a rule of thumb, 1 to 2 weeks should be allowed to elapse before sampling after a dosage change.

In overdose, it can be assumed that metabolism of the drug is occurring at the maximum rate of V_{max}. Therefore, the decline in plasma concentration is linear (zero order) at approximately 7 mg/L/day.

Practical applications

Since the dose/concentration relationship is non-linear, changes in dose do not result in proportional changes in plasma concentration (Fig. 1.5B). Using the Michaelis–Menten model, if the plasma concentration is known at one dosage, then V_{max} may be assumed since this is the more predictable parameter and K_m calculated. The revised values of K_m can then be used to estimate the new dosage required to produce a desired concentration. Alternatively, a nomogram may be used to assist in dose adjustments.

Care is needed when interpreting TDM data and making dosage adjustments when phenytoin is given concurrently with other anticonvulsants, since these affect distribution and metabolism of phenytoin. Since phenytoin is approximately 90% protein bound, hypoalbuminaemia and renal failure will affect this, and care is needed when estimating doses in these clinical situations.

The oral formulations of phenytoin show good bioavailability. However, tablets and capsules contain the sodium salt (S = 0.9), whereas the suspension is phenytoin base (S = 1). Intramuscular phenytoin is slowly and unpredictably absorbed, due to crystallization in the muscle tissue and is, therefore, not recommended.

Carbamazepine

Carbamazepine is used to treat generalized tonic–clonic and complex partial seizures. There are a number of dose-independent side effects, including various dermatological reactions and, more rarely, aplastic anaemia and Stevens–Johnson syndrome. However, the more common side effects are concentration related.

Serum concentration/response relationship

- < 4 mg/L – little therapeutic benefit
- 4–12 mg/L – optimum therapeutic range for monotherapy
- > 9 mg/L – possible side effects of nystagmus, diplopia, drowsiness and ataxia, particularly if patients are on other anticonvulsant therapy
- > 12 mg/L – side effects common, even on monotherapy.

Distribution

Carbamazepine is distributed widely in various organs, with the highest concentration found in liver and kidneys. Carbamazepine is 70 to 80% protein bound and shows a wide variation in population average apparent volume of distribution (0.8 to 1.9 L/kg). This wide variation is thought to be due to variations in absorption (since there is no parenteral form) and protein binding.

Elimination

Carbamazepine is eliminated almost exclusively by metabolism, with less than 2% being excreted unchanged in the urine. Elimination is a first order process, but carbamazepine induces its own metabolism. Thus, at the beginning of therapy, clearance is 0.01 to 0.03 L/h/kg rising to 0.05 to 0.1 L/h/kg on chronic therapy. Autoinduction begins in the first few days of commencing therapy and is maximal at 2 to 4 weeks.

Since clearance changes with time so does half-life, with reported values as long as 35 hours after a single dose decreasing to 5 to 7 hours on regular dosing.

Absorption

Absorption after oral administration is slow with peak concentrations being reached from 2 to 24 hours post-dose (average 6 hours). Absorption is incomplete, with bioavailability estimated at approximately 80% (F = 0.8).

Practical implications

Use of pharmacokinetic equations is limited, due to the autoinduction effect. However, there are a number of important practical points. Blood samples should not be drawn before steady state, which will not be achieved until 2 to 4 weeks after starting therapy or 3 to 4 days after subsequent dose adjustments. When sampling, the trough level should be measured because of the variable absorption pattern. Complex calculations are not helpful, but as a rule of thumb

each 100 mg dose will increase the plasma concentration at steady state by approximately 1 mg/L in adults. A number of other drugs (including phenytoin) when given concurrently will affect carbamazepine metabolism and subsequent blood levels.

Phenobarbitone

Phenobarbitone is effective in the treatment of generalized tonic–clonic and complex partial seizures. It is also useful in the treatment of febrile seizures.

Serum concentration/response relationship

- < 15 mg/L – little therapeutic effect
- 15–40 mg/L – optimum range
- 40–50 mg/L – sedation, confusion (elderly), although may be tolerated by some patients
- > 60 mg/L – serious toxic effect of ataxia, lethargy, stupor, coma.

The sedation which commonly manifests early on in therapy becomes less with continued therapy.

Distribution

Phenobarbitone readily distributes into most body tissues and is 50% protein bound. The population average volume of distribution is 0.7 to 1 L/kg.

Elimination

Phenobarbitone is primarily (80%) metabolized by the liver, with approximately 20% being excreted unchanged in the urine. Elimination is a first order process, but is relatively slow with a population average clearance of approximately 0.004 L/h/kg. However, as with theophylline, clearance in children is increased. In the case of phenobarbitone, the adult clearance value is doubled in children. Applying equations (6) and (8) to these population values gives an estimate of half-life in the order of 5 days. This is much shorter in children and longer in the elderly.

Practical application

In view of the long half-life, single daily dosage is possible with phenobarbitone. Samples for therapeutic monitoring may be drawn any time during a dose interval, since concentration fluctuation between doses is minimal. However, the patient should be at steady state, which takes 2 to 4 weeks (1 to 2 weeks in children). The pharmacokinetics of phenobarbitone may be altered by liver and (less markedly) renal disease. They are not affected by the concurrent administration of other anticonvulsants.

Primidone

Like phenobarbitone, primidone is effective in the treatment of generalized tonic–clonic and partial seizures. Much of primidone's anticonvulsant activity is due to the metabolites, phenobarbitone and phenylethylmalonamide. Therefore, primidone serum concentrations are only useful to confirm transient toxicity. Toxic manifestations such as sedation, nausea and ataxia are seen at concentrations greater than 15 mg/L. Plasma concentration should be drawn approximately 3 hours post-dose, which corresponds to peak concentration.

Phenylethylmalonamide assays are not available routinely, although this metabolite probably contributes to anticonvulsant activity. Measurement of phenobarbitone levels is of limited value, since conversion of primidone to phenobarbitone is variable between individuals. However, phenobarbitone levels may be helpful in dosage selection, where seizures are not adequately controlled despite regular dosage or where there is suspected toxicity.

Valproic acid

Valproic acid has a broad spectrum of anticonvulsant activity, being useful in generalized absence, generalized tonic–clonic and partial seizures.

Serum concentration/response relationship

There is no clear concentration/response relationship for valproic acid, although a range of 50 to 100 mg/L is often quoted as being optimal. Levels exceeding this range do not confer any additional therapeutic benefits. Although there is no clear relationship between serum levels and toxic effects, the rare hepatotoxicity associated with valproic acid appears to be related to very high levels of > 150 mg/L.

Distribution

Valproic acid is extensively bound to plasma protein (90 to 95%). Unlike other drugs, valproic acid can saturate protein-binding sites at concentrations greater than 50 mg/L, thus altering the free fraction of drug. Thus, the apparent volume of distribution varies from 0.1 to 0.5 L/kg.

Elimination

Elimination of valproic acid is almost entirely by hepatic metabolism, with less than 5% being eliminated by the kidneys.

As a result of the saturation of protein-binding sites and the subsequent increase in free fraction of the drug, clearance of the drug increases at higher concentrations. Thus, there is a non-linear change in plasma concentration with dose, as shown in Figure 1.5C.

Practical implications

In view of the lack of a clear concentration response relationship and the variable pharmacokinetics, there are limited indications for the measurement of valproic acid levels. In most cases, dosage should be based on clinical response. However, in a few cases where seizures are not controlled at high dosage, a serum level may be helpful in confirming treatment failure. If monitoring is to be undertaken, levels should be drawn at steady state (2 to 3 days). A trough sample will be the most useful, since wide fluctuations of blood levels may occur during a dose interval.

Cyclosporin

Cyclosporin is a neutral lipophilic cyclic ende-capeptide extracted from the fungus *Tolypocladium inflatum gams*. It is a potent immunosuppressive agent which is used principally to reduce graft rejection after kidney, heart, heart–lung, liver, pancreas and bone marrow transplants. The drug has a low therapeutic index, with a number of toxic effects including nephrotoxicity, hepatotoxicity, gastrointestinal intolerance, hypertrichosis and neurological problems. Efficacy in reducing graft rejection as well as the main toxic effect of nephro- and hepatotoxicity appear to be concentration related.

Serum concentration/response relationship

With all drugs that are monitored the 'therapeutic range' is a window with limits which are not absolute. It is even more difficult to define a therapeutic range for cyclosporin, since there are a number of influencing factors. Firstly, the measured concentration varies depending on sampling matrix (i.e. whole blood, plasma or serum). Secondly, it depends on whether the assay is specific for cyclosporin alone or nonspecific to include metabolites. A target concentration range of 200 to 400 microgram/L is generally accepted for the immediate postoperative phase following renal transplants. Levels below the lower limit of this window are associated with an increased incidence of graft rejection. Levels above the upper limit are associated with an increased incidence of nephrotoxicity and hepatotoxicity, although an upper limit of 800 microgram/L has also been suggested. This target range can be reduced to 100 to 200 microgram/L, 3 to 6 months post-transplant. These target ranges are based on assays specific for cyclosporin parent compound.

Distribution

Cyclosporin is highly lipophilic and is distributed widely throughout the body with a volume of distribution of 4 to 8 L/kg. There is variable distribution of cyclosporin within blood, since whole blood concentration is approximately twice plasma concentration. Within plasma, cyclosporin is 98% protein bound.

Elimination

Cyclosporin is eliminated primarily by hepatic metabolism, with wide interindividual variation in clearance (0.1 to 2 L/h/kg). In children these values are approximately 40% higher, with a resulting increased dosage requirement on an mg/kg basis. In elderly patients or patients with hepatic impairment a lower clearance rate has been observed.

Practical implications

In addition to the wide interpatient variability in distribution and elimination kinetic parameters, cyclosporin absorption is variable and incomplete (F = 0.2 to 0.5 in normal subjects). In transplant patients this variation in bioavailability is even greater and bioavailability increases during the first few months after transplant. Furthermore, a number of drugs are known to interact with cyclosporin. All these factors suggest that therapeutic drug monitoring will assist in optimum dose selection. However, use of population averages in dose prediction is of little benefit, due to wide interpatient variation. Sampling matrix should be whole blood, since there is variable distribution of cyclosporin between blood and serum. Samples should represent trough levels and be drawn at steady state, which is achieved 2 to 3 days after initiating or changing dosage (average half-life is 9 hours). Cyclosporin concentration monitoring should be undertaken every 2 to 3 days in the immediate postoperative phase until the patient's clinical condition is stable. Thereafter, monitoring can be undertaken every 1 to 2 months.

Summary pharmacokinetic data for all the drugs discussed is contained in Table 1.1.

Table 1.1 Summary of pharmacokinetic data*

Drug	Range	Vd (L/kg)	Cl (L/h/kg)	Half-life (h)
Digoxin	0.8–2.0 microgram/L 1–2.6 nmol/L	7. 3	See text	36
Theophylline	10–20 mg/L 55–110 micromol/L	0.48	0.04	8
Gentamicin	Pk 5–12 mg/L, Tr < 2 mg/L	0.25	$1 \times CrCl$	2
Lithium	0.4–0.8 mmol/L	0.5–1	$0.2 \times CrCl$	18
Phenytoin	10–20 mg/L 40–80 micromol/L	1	$K_m = 6$ mg/L $V_{max} = 7$ mg/kg/day	
Carbamazepine	4–12 mg/L 17–50 micromol/L	0.8–1.9	0.05–1	
Phenobarbitone	15–40 mg/L 65–172 micromol/L	0.7–1	0.004	120
Primidone	< 15 mg/L < 69 micromol/L	0.6		
Valproate	< 100 mg/L < 693 micromol/L			
Cyclosporin	200–400 microgram/L			9

* Note: estimates based on average patient. See text for variability.

CASE STUDIES

CASE 1.1

Mrs L. A. is a 26-year-old lady who is taking drug X, a new anticonvulsant, in a dosage of 100 mg three times daily. The drug has a low therapeutic index and accurate dosage is essential. The drug has a half-life of approximately 8 hours and Fe value = 0.7. Although the current dose is satisfactory, Mrs L. A.'s renal function deteriorates to half normal over a few days.

Q Calculate the most appropriate new dosage required to maintain seizure control, in view of decreased renal function.

CASE 1.2

Mr H. D. is a 62-year-old, 63 kg, male asthmatic who is commenced on Nuelin SA on 1st May at a dose of 500 mg 12 hourly (6.00 a.m. and 6.00 p.m.). On 4th May his 6.00 p.m. dose was omitted, as was his 6.00 a.m. dose on 5th May. As his condition worsened, it was decided to commence him on intravenous therapy on 5th May.

Q1 Will the patient be at steady state by the time his first dose is omitted?

Q2 Using population values, estimate plasma theophylline concentration at 10.00 a.m. on 5th May.

Q3 Calculate the loading dose of intravenous aminophylline required to raise the patient's theophylline level to 15 mg/L.

Q4 Estimate the infusion rate necessary to maintain this. Assume 100% bioavailability and 12 hours of theophylline release with the SR product.

CASE 1.3

M. A. is a 74-year-old, 60 kg man who has a *Pseudomonas* infection. He has been started on intravenous gentamicin 80 mg, 8-hourly (bolus doses). However, his serum creatinine is raised at 220 micromol/L and the doctor is worried about toxicity.

The pharmacist is asked to advise on what levels this dosage is likely to produce.

Q1 Estimate k_e, Vd and Cl from population data.

Q2 Predict steady state peak and trough levels likely to be achieved with 80 mg, 8-hourly.

Q3 The actual levels at steady state are:

- Peak (1 hour post-dose) 9.5 mg/L
- Trough (immediately predose) 5.7 mg/L.

Recalculate the patient's pharmacokinetic parameters and new dosage regimen to achieve a peak of 7 to 10 mg/L and a trough of less than 2 mg/L.

CASE 1.4

Mrs B. D. is a 60-year-old, 55 kg lady who is diagnosed as having generalized tonic–clonic seizures. The doctor wishes to prescribe phenytoin.

Q1 On the basis of population data, calculate a possible dosage regimen. A dosage of 350 mg at night is actually commenced. 3 weeks later the patient is admitted to hospital, confused and with an unsteady gait. A blood sample on the day of admission showed a phenytoin level at 36 mg/L.

Q2 How long should therapy be withheld before recommencing phenytoin?

Q3 Calculate a new maintenance dose in the light of the available blood level data.

ANSWERS TO CASE STUDIES

CASE 1.1

A Firstly, calculate the effect of change in renal function on total body clearance. Since (Cl total) = Cl (met) + Cl (renal), the fraction of normal clearance is $(0.3) + (0.7 \times 50\%) = 0.65$. Therefore, total daily dosage = 300 mg $\times$ 0.65 = 200 mg. Cl and k_e are related and change proportionately, k_e = 0.65 $\times$ Normal. Therefore, half-life = 1/0.65 $\times$ Normal = 1.5 $\times$ 8 = 12 hours. Therefore, the 200 mg is best given in two divided doses. The new regimen which will maintain control is 100 mg twice daily.

CASE 1.2

A1 On the basis of population averages Cl = 2.52 L/h, Vd = 30.24 L. Using equation (6), k_e = 0.083 h^{-1}, and equation (8), $t_{\frac{1}{2}}$ = 8.3 hours. Therefore, the patient will be at steady state after 2 days of therapy.

A2 Substituting these parameters into equation (12), the steady state plasma concentration = 16.5 mg/L. The 6.00 a.m. dose on 4th May will last for 12 hours, therefore, concentration will begin to fall after 6.00 p.m. on 4th May for 16 hours until 10.00 a.m. on 5th May. Substituting the steady state estimate and k_e into equation (7), Cp at 10.00 a.m. = 4.37 mg/L (or 16 hours is approximately 2 $\times$ half-life, therefore, Cp = 25% of 16.5 mg/L = 4.1 mg/L).

A3 Change in plasma concentration needed = 10.63 mg/L. Using equation (11) loading dose needed = 401 mg. (F = 1; S = 0.8 for aminophylline.)

A4 Substituting desired state concentration into equation (12) the infusion rate required is 47.25 mg/h. (F = 1; S = 0.8 for aminophylline.)

CASE 1.3

A1 Using the Cockcroft & Gault equation, creatinine clearance = 22.14 ml/min. Therefore, gentamicin clearance = 1.33 L/h. From population data Vd = 15.6 L.
Using equation (6), k_e = 0.085 h^{-1}. and equation (8), $t_{\frac{1}{2}}$ = 8.12 hours.

A2 Substituting these parameters into equation (13), $Cp_{ss\ max}$ = 10.39 mg/L. Substituting this estimated $Cp_{ss\ max}$ in equation (7), peak at 1 hour post-dose = 9.54 mg/L and trough = 5.26 mg/L.

A3 Substituting the actual levels into equation (7), k_e = 0.073 h^{-1} and, from equation (8), $t_{\frac{1}{2}}$ = 9.5 hours. Substituting this k_e in equation (7) and taking trough level for CP_2 and dose interval for t, $Cp_{ss\ max}$ = 10.22 mg/L. Therefore, the change in plasma concentration immediately after a dose is 10.22 – 5.7 = 4.52 mg/L. Substituting this into equation (10), Vd = 17.54 L. Substituting the desired peak and trough levels of 8 mg/L and 1.5 mg/L into equation (7), the time for this fall in concentration will be 23 hours. Since peak is measured 1 hour post-dose, a satisfactory practical dose interval will be 24 hours. Substituting the actual k_e, Vd, the desired trough level and dose interval of 24 hours into equation (14) results in an estimated dose of 125 mg. Therefore, a dose of 125 mg every 24 hours should produce the desired peak and trough levels.

CASE 1.4

A1 K_m estimate = 6 mg/L. V_{max} estimate = 385 mg/day. Substituting these into equation (15) with a desired plasma concentration of 15 mg/L, the estimated dose is 305 mg daily.

A2 Since at the maximal rate of metabolism, elimination is zero order and concentration decline is approximately 7 mg/L/day, therapy should be withheld for 2 days.

A3 Substituting the estimated V_{max}, the previous dose and the measured plasma concentration into equation (15), gives a revised estimate of K_m = 6.7 mg/L. Resubstituting back into the equation for a desired plasma concentration of 15 mg/L results in a new dosage of 300 mg/day.

BIBLIOGRAPHY

Amdisen A, Lithium. In: Evans W E, Shentag J J, Jusko W J. (eds) Applied pharmacokinetics. Spokane: Applied Therapeutics 1983, 586–617

Gugler R, Unruh G E. Clinical pharmacokinetics of valproic acid. Clinical Pharmacokinetics 1980; 5: 67–83

Hvidberg E F, Dam M. Clinical pharmacokinetics of anticonvulsants. Clinical Pharmacokinetics 1976; 1: 161–188

Jermain D M, Crismon M L, Martin E S. Population pharmacokinetics of lithium. Clinical Pharmacy 1991; 10(5): 376–381

Luke D R, Halstenson C E, Opsahl J A, Matzke G R. Validity of creatinine clearance estimates in the assessment of renal function. Clinical Pharmacology and Therapeutics 1990; 48: 503–508

MacKichan J J, Kutt H. Carbamazepine: therapeutic use and serum concentration monitoring. In: Taylor W J, Finn A L (eds) Individualising drug therapy: practical applications of therapeutic drug monitoring. New York: Gross, Towsend, Frank 1981

Michalko K J, Blain L. An evaluation of a clinical pharmacokinetic service for serum digoxin levels. Therapeutic Drug Monitoring 1987; 9: 311–319

Rambeck B, Boenigk H E, Dunlop A, Mullen P W, Wadsworth J, Richens A. Predicting phenytoin dose: a revised nomogram. Therapeutic Drug Monitoring 1980; 1: 325–354

Tserng K, King K C, Takieddine F N. Theophylline metabolism in premature infants. Clinical Pharmacology and Therapeutics 1981; 29: 594–600

Wilensky A J, Friel P N, Levy R H, Comfort C P, Kaluzny S P. Kinetics of phenobarbital in normal subjects and epileptic patients. European Journal of Clinical Pharmacology 1982; 23: 87–92

Vozeh S, Uematsu T, Aarons L, Matre P, Landolt H, Gratzl O. Intravenous phenytoin loading in patients after neuro-surgery and in status epilepticus: a population pharmacokinetic study. Clinical Pharmacokinetics 1988; 14(2): 122–128

Winter M E. Basic clinical pharmacokinetics, 2nd edn. Vancouver, Washington: Applied Therapeutics, 1990

Chapter 2

Drug interactions

A. Lee   I. H. Stockley

An awareness of the problems that may arise due to drug interactions is vital for the practising pharmacist. The problem of drug interactions was recognized as long ago as 1895, when Oliver & Schaefer noted that an adrenal extract could cause arrhythmias in a dog anaesthetized with chloroform. Today, with the increasing complexity of therapeutic agents available, and widespread polypharmacy, the potential for drug interactions is enormous. However, although many thousands of reports of adverse drug interactions have appeared in the biomedical literature, only a relatively small number are clinically significant. Thus, the importance of drug interactions to the clinical pharmacist today primarily involves knowing or predicting those occasions when a potential drug interaction is likely to have clinically significant consequences, and, if so, the steps which may be taken to avoid them, or alternative treatments which may be preferable. In order to predict the possible consequences of the co-administration of two or more drugs it is essential for the pharmacist to have a practical knowledge of the pharmacological mechanisms involved in drug interactions, an awareness of those drugs which are associated with the greatest risk of interaction, and of the most vulnerable patient groups. This chapter will review the basic mechanisms and properties of interactions between drugs, giving clinically important examples in each case. Due to constraints on space, interactions will not be discussed in depth. However, the most common adverse drug interactions associated with individual drug groups will be tabulated in the relevant chapters.

DEFINITION

A drug interaction has been defined as the modification of a drug's effect by prior or concomitant administration of another drug. However, an alternative has been proposed which states that a drug interaction has occurred when the pharmacological effect of two or more drugs given together is not just a direct function of their individual effects. Likewise, the effect of a drug may be modified by food, smoking, alcohol or environmental pollutants, but these interactions will not be discussed here. Where a therapeutic combination leads to an unexpected change or complication in the condition of the patient, such an interaction would be described as clinically significant. There are many drug interactions which result in beneficial rather than adverse effects, e.g. the administration of carbidopa, an extracerebral dopadecarboxylase inhibitor, together with levodopa to prevent its peripheral degradation to dopamine. Interactions of a pharmaceutical or physicochemical nature may occur when two or more drugs are mixed prior to administration. These interactions, which are better described as pharmaceutical incompatibilities, are outwith the scope of this chapter and have been discussed in detail elsewhere (see Bibliography). This chapter will concentrate on drug–drug interactions occurring within the body which have the potential to affect adversely patient care.

EPIDEMIOLOGY

A number of studies, with many important differences in design and methodology, have attempted to estimate the incidence of drug interactions. Estimates range from 2.2 to 30% in studies carried out in hospital inpatients, and from 9.2 to 70.3% in patients in the community. Many investigators based their conclusions on potential drug interactions and failed to consider whether patients actually experienced symptoms that could be attributed to them. On the basis of available data it is not possible accurately to define the incidence of clinically significant drug interactions, but it is likely that the figure is quite low (less than 1%).

Drugs most likely to be involved in adverse drug interactions

A small number of widely used drugs are implicated consistently in drug interactions, and these are shown in Table 2.1. They are usually potent therapeutic agents with a narrow therapeutic index, where a small increase in plasma concentration may produce toxicity, e.g. theophylline, lithium and digoxin, or drugs with which a small decrease in plasma concentration may result in loss of therapeutic effect, e.g. carbamazepine and cyclosporin.

Susceptible patients

The probability of a drug interaction increases with the number of drugs received by a patient, and at least one study has documented an exponential increase in the incidence of adverse drug interactions in relation to the number of drugs given. Drug interactions are more likely to occur in specific patient groups, including the elderly, critically ill patients, and those undergoing complicated surgical procedures. These patients often have impaired organ function, which may affect the elimination of drugs from the body, thus increasing the likelihood of drug interactions. Patients with chronic conditions such as diabetes, asthma or epilepsy may face exacerbations of their clinical problems by an adverse

Table 2.1 Drugs commonly involved in drug interactions

Digoxin
Lithium
Warfarin
Theophylline
Cyclosporin
Oral contraceptives
Phenytoin
Monoamine oxidase inhibitors

interaction which would have minor consequences for another patient. The elderly are undoubtedly the group at greatest risk of drug interactions.

MECHANISMS OF DRUG INTERACTIONS

Drug interactions are conventionally discussed according to the mechanisms involved. There are some situations where drugs interact by unique mechanisms, but, on the whole, certain mechanisms of interaction are encountered time and again. These mechanisms may be conveniently divided into those involving the pharmacokinetics of a drug and those affecting the pharmacodynamic response to it. In general, the effects of pharmacodynamic interactions are more predictable. Some drug interactions are known to be due to a combination of more than one mechanism.

Pharmacokinetic interactions

Pharmacokinetic interactions may occur by a number of mechanisms whereby one drug alters the absorption, distribution, metabolism or elimination of another drug. Due to marked interindividual variability in these processes, such interactions may be expected but their ex-

tent cannot easily be predicted. In general, serious clinical consequences are unlikely, although some interactions are demonstrated in most patients receiving a potentially interacting combination (e.g. ketoconazole and cyclosporin).

Absorption

The absorption of orally administered drugs from the gastrointestinal tract is complex and variable, making drug interactions of this type difficult to predict. It is important to recognize that the majority of these interactions result in changes in absorption rate, although in some instances the extent of absorption is affected. For the most part, the absorption rate is usually unimportant provided the total amount of drug absorbed is not markedly affected. However, delayed absorption can be clinically significant where the drug affected has a short half-life, or where it is important to achieve high plasma concentrations rapidly, as may be the case with analgesics or hypnotics. Most drug interactions in this category result in decreased rather than increased absorption, and many can be avoided if an interval of 2 to 3 hours is allowed between the administration of the interacting drugs. Some important absorption interactions are shown in Table 2.2.

Drug binding in the gastrointestinal tract. Certain drugs react directly within the gastro-

Table 2.2 Some clinically significant drug–drug absorption interactions		
Drug affected	Interacting drugs	Effect of interaction
Digoxin Thyroxine Warfarin	Cholestyramine	Reduced absorption due to binding/ complexation in the gut
Tetracyclines Ciprofloxacin and other quinolones	Antacids (i.e. containing aluminium, magnesium) Iron salts	Reduced absorption due to formation of a chelate complex within the gut
Bisphosphonates	Antacids Calcium salts	Reduced absorption due to chelation
Digoxin	Metoclopramide	Reduced absorption due to increased gut motility
Digoxin	Propantheline	Increased absorption due to decreased gut motility

intestinal tract to form chelates and complexes which are not readily absorbed. The drugs most commonly implicated in this type of interaction include tetracycline, and the quinolone antibiotics which can complex with iron, and antacids containing calcium, magnesium and aluminium. Tetracyclines may chelate with divalent or trivalent metal cations to form insoluble complexes, which may result in greatly reduced serum tetracycline concentrations. Such interactions are well documented and clearly may be clinically important when they arise, but they are easily avoided. Activated charcoal acts as an adsorbent agent within the gut, and this property is used to therapeutic advantage in the management of poisoning, but inevitably it can affect the absorption of drugs given in therapeutic doses. Antacids can adsorb a considerable number of drugs, but they can affect the absorption of co-administered agents in a variety of other ways. Cholestyramine and related anion exchange resins bind cholesterol metabolites and bile acids in the intestinal lumen preventing their reabsorption, and thus lower total cholesterol. Such agents may also bind a wide variety of acidic drugs such as digoxin, thyroxine and warfarin, likewise preventing their absorption. Colestipol appears less likely than cholestyramine to interact by this mechanism.

Changes in gastrointestinal pH. The absorption of many drugs may be affected by alterations in gastrointestinal pH, although there are few examples of interactions of this nature which have clinically significant consequences. For example, the alkalinizing effects of antacids on the gastrointestinal tract are transient and the effects of an interaction may be minimized by leaving an interval of 2 to 3 hours between the antacid and the potentially interacting drug. The subject of drug interactions with antacids has recently been reviewed and the authors conclude that probably the only interactions of clinical relevance are those which involve metal ion chelation or formation of insoluble salts. H_2-antagonists inhibit gastric acid production, which may alter the rate of gastric emptying, and hence the rate of drug absorption. However, studies of this mechanism have produced inconsistent

results, and a recent review concluded that such effects are unlikely to be clinically relevant.

Antacids, H_2-antagonists and probably omeprazole, by increasing gastric pH, may markedly reduce the bioavailability of drugs such as ketoconazole which require an acidic medium for adequate absorption.

Drug effects on the gastrointestinal flora. Bacterial flora predominate in the large bowel, and are present in much smaller numbers in the stomach and small bowel. Thus drugs which are well absorbed from the small bowel are less likely to be affected by changes in gut flora. In a small proportion of patients a substantial amount of digoxin is inactivated by intestinal bacteria, and the introduction of a broad-spectrum antibiotic such as erythromycin may lead to substantially increased plasma digoxin concentrations.

Changes in bacterial flora are also thought to be involved in the interaction between oral contraceptives and broad-spectrum antibiotics. This interaction has been widely reported in the literature, despite the fact that clinical pharmacokinetic studies with broad-spectrum antibiotics have failed to substantiate such an interaction. There is good evidence that ethinyloestradiol undergoes enterohepatic recirculation. Ethinyloestradiol conjugates are excreted in the bile, then hydrolysed by bacteria in the colon to liberate unchanged oestrogen which is then reabsorbed into the portal circulation. Diminished bacterial flora may result in decreased oestrogen levels, with an increased risk of contraceptive failure. It has been suggested that certain individuals may be particularly at risk of this interaction, although it is recognized that the mechanism has not been fully elucidated.

Effects on gastrointestinal motility. The small intestine is the major site of absorption for most orally administered drugs; thus gastric emptying is an important determinant of absorption rate. Drugs which slow gastric emptying may delay and attenuate the speed with which other drugs are absorbed. Anticholinergic agents, opiates and tricyclic antidepressants reduce gastrointestinal motility and delay gastric emptying, which usually results in an increased time taken to achieve peak plasma concentrations, although in some cases it may also result in reduced bioavailability of the affected agent. Other drugs with anticholinergic activity which might influence gastrointestinal motility include antihistamines and phenothiazines.

Metoclopramide, on the other hand, is known to increase the rate of gastric emptying and has been shown to accelerate the absorption of certain drugs including paracetamol, diazepam, propranolol and lithium. Absorption may be diminished from the stomach, but accelerated from the small bowel. Cisapride also enhances the absorption of diazepam and ethanol from the small intestine. In general, although there are a number of such interactions leading to changes in the absorption rate of drugs, there are few examples of changes in extent of absorption as a result of this mechanism.

Distribution

Once absorbed a drug is distributed to its site of action, and during this process it may interact with other drugs. In practice the main mechanism behind these interactions is protein-binding displacement, although the clinical significance of such interactions has been greatly overemphasized.

A drug displacement interaction is defined as a reduction in extent of plasma protein binding of one drug caused by the presence of another drug, resulting in an increased free or unbound fraction of the displaced drug. Only unbound drug molecules are pharmacologically active. Therefore such interactions are likely to be of clinical importance where the affected drug is highly protein bound, so that a relatively small decrease in its bound fraction will result in a large percentage increase in its unbound fraction. Albumin is the principal plasma protein to which acidic drugs such as warfarin are bound, while basic drugs are generally bound to alpha$_1$-acid glycoprotein. Although a large number of drug interactions which are believed to result from this mechanism are cited in the literature, the role of protein binding as a cause of clinically important interactions has recently been questioned and it is now recognized that, for most

drugs, displacement from protein-binding sites is accompanied by a compensatory increase in metabolism and/or excretion, which ensures that the new steady state free concentration is similar to that present before the displacing drug was added. That is, the total drug concentration falls to accommodate the rise in free fraction, with minimal alteration in pharmacological effect. Thus it is likely that most protein-binding displacement drug interactions are of doubtful clinical importance, despite the fact that many textbooks suggest otherwise. Perhaps the most widely quoted example is the potentiation of warfarin's anticoagulant effect by non-steroidal anti-inflammatory drugs (NSAIDs), which was first described in 1959. Further reports of this effect appeared in the scientific literature over the following years, together with an in vitro study showing that phenylbutazone displaced warfarin from protein-binding sites. It was then assumed that any NSAID would enhance the anticoagulant effect of warfarin. However, the interaction between warfarin and phenylbutazone has now been shown to be primarily due to a stereoselective inhibition of the metabolism of warfarin. Warfarin is available as a racemic mixture of two enantiomers, R warfarin and S warfarin; and of the two the S enantiomer is five times more potent as an anticoagulant. Phenylbutazone inhibits the metabolism of the more potent S warfarin and induces that of the less potent R warfarin, resulting in a greater proportion of the more potent enantiomer in plasma, and increased anticoagulant effects. It is now clear that the majority of NSAIDs do not interact with warfarin or other anticoagulants, although azapropazone, phenylbutazone and oxyphenbutazone do have such an effect. In each case the mechanism is predominantly inhibition of drug metabolism, although protein binding displacement may be involved. There are few, if any, examples of clinically important interactions which are entirely due to protein-binding displacement.

Drug metabolism

Most clinically important interactions involve the

effect of one drug on the metabolism of another. Metabolism refers to the process by which drugs are biochemically modified to facilitate their degradation and subsequent removal from the body. The most important site of drug metabolism is the liver, although other organs such as the kidneys, lung, gut, skin and placenta are involved. Drug metabolism consists of phase I reactions such as oxidation, hydrolysis and reduction and phase II reactions, which primarily involve conjugation of the drug with substances such as glucuronic acid, and sulphuric acid. Most lipophilic drugs are eliminated by oxidation in the liver. Phase I metabolism generally involves the hepatic cytochrome P450 enzyme system or 'microsomal mixed function oxidases', which are the most important enzymes involved in drug metabolism. Each P450 is encoded by a separate gene, and it is estimated that there may be as many as 200 different P450 genes in humans. The importance of these enzymes for drug interactions is that enzyme inducers and inhibitors may preferentially affect certain isoenzymes of cytochrome P450, and consequently may only affect the metabolism of selected drugs. For example, omeprazole has the potential to inhibit the metabolism of drugs metabolized to a great extent by the cytochrome P450 enzyme subfamily IIC (e.g. diazepam, phenytoin), but not of those metabolized by subfamilies IA (e.g. theophylline), IID (e.g. propranolol) and IIIA (e.g. cyclosporin, lignocaine). The therapeutic implications of enzyme induction and enzyme inhibition will depend largely on the relative biological activity of the drug and its metabolites. In most cases the metabolites are less active than the parent drug, and consequently the action of the affected drug is usually potentiated by enzyme inhibition and reduced by enzyme induction.

Enzyme induction. Enzyme induction primarily affects phase I metabolism, although some phase II reactions may also be affected. The most powerful enzyme inducers in clinical use are the antibiotic rifampicin and antiepileptic agents such as barbiturates, phenytoin and carbamazepine, the latter being able to induce its own metabolism (autoinduction). Other drugs with enzyme-inducing properties include grise-ofulvin and dichloralphenazone. Cigarette smoking and chronic alcohol use can also induce drug-metabolizing enzymes. The enzyme inducers encountered most commonly in clinical practice are shown in Table 2.3. Since the process of enzyme induction requires new protein synthesis, the maximum effect is usually not seen for 2 to 3 weeks after starting an enzyme-inducing agent, and, similarly, the effects may take several weeks to dissipate when the inducing agent is stopped. Rifampicin, however, which has a fairly short half-life, is known to induce enzymes more rapidly than inducers with longer half-lives, and the effect also has a correspondingly rapid offset. This may be especially important where rifampicin is given as a short course in the prophylaxis of meningococcal meningitis in women taking the oral contraceptive pill. Enzyme induction usually results in a decreased therapeutic response to the affected drug, except perhaps in the case of drugs with active metabolites. The effects of enzyme induction vary considerably between patients, and are dependent upon age, genetic factors, concurrent drug treatment and disease state. There is evidence that the enzyme-induction process is dose dependent, although some drugs may induce enzymes at all doses. It is not normally possible to predict the effects of a particular enzyme inducer in a given patient, due to the differences between potentially affected drugs and the interindividual variability in effects.

Enzyme inhibition. Enzyme inhibition is an extremely common mechanism behind the interaction of two drugs. Such interactions often result in exaggerated and prolonged responses with an increased risk of toxicity. Most inhibitory

Table 2.3 Enzyme inducers in common use
Barbiturates
Carbamazepine
Dichloralphenazone
Ethanol (chronic)
Griseofulvin
Phenytoin
Primidone
Rifampicin
Tobacco smoke

interactions involve the hepatic mono-oxygenase enzymes (i.e. mixed function oxidases). A number of drugs have the capacity to inhibit these enzymes, usually by competitive binding to cytochrome P450 to form a stable complex which prevents access of other agents to the P450 enzyme system. The drugs most commonly implicated in interactions due to enzyme inhibition are shown in Table 2.4. Enzyme inhibition appears to be a dose-related phenomenon. Inhibition of metabolism of the affected drug begins as soon as sufficient concentrations of the inhibitor appear in the liver, and the effects are usually maximal when the new steady state plasma concentration is achieved. Thus, potentiation of pharmacological effects can occur very quickly for drugs with a short half-life, but takes much longer for those with a long elimination half-life. The clinical significance of this type of interaction depends on various factors, including dosage (of both drugs), alterations in pharmacokinetic properties of the affected drug, such as a prolonged half-life, and patient characteristics such as disease state. Interactions of this type are again most likely to affect drugs with a narrow therapeutic range, such as theophylline. For example, the introduction of an enzyme inhibitor such as ciprofloxacin or cimetidine in a patient taking chronic theophylline could result in a doubling of plasma concentration. The ability to inhibit drug metabolism may be related to specific chemical structures. For example, a number of known enzyme inhibitors contain an imidazole ring, including cimetidine, ketoconazole, itraconazole, metronidazole and omeprazole.

Table 2.4 Enzyme inhibitors in common use	
Allopurinol	Isoniazid
Amiodarone	Itraconazole
Azapropazone	Ketoconazole
Chloramphenicol	Metronidazole
Cimetidine	Omeprazole
Ciprofloxacin	Oral contraceptives
Diltiazem	Phenylbutazone
Disulfiram	Propoxyphene
Enoxacin	Sulphonamides
Erythromycin	Valproate
Ethanol (acute)	Verapamil

Elimination interactions

Most interactions involving elimination or excretion occur in the kidneys. Relatively few drugs are sufficiently water soluble to rely on renal excretion without requiring prior metabolism in the liver. A change in glomerular filtration rate, tubular secretion or urinary pH can alter the elimination of some drugs. Interference with renal excretion is the mechanism behind some drug interactions involving digoxin and lithium. Concomitant administration of quinidine, amiodarone, diltiazem and verapamil can bring about a large increase in steady state serum digoxin concentrations primarily due to inhibition of its renal and non-renal clearance. Thiazide diuretics, and to a lesser extent loop diuretics, reduce the excretion of lithium by increasing its reabsorption from the proximal tubules. This interaction has resulted in serious lithium toxicity, and lithium doses should be reduced in any patient requiring diuretic therapy. In addition, both angiotensin converting enzyme (ACE) inhibitors and non-steroidal anti-inflammatory drugs (NSAIDs) can impair lithium excretion leading to toxicity.

Pharmacodynamic interactions

Pharmacodynamic interactions are those where the effects of one drug are changed by the presence of another drug at its site of action. In some cases the interaction is due to direct effects at the receptor, but more often it is due either to an interplay of receptor effects or combined interference with biochemical or physiological mechanisms. Interactions of this type are much less easily classified than those due to pharmacokinetic changes.

Antagonistic interactions

It is to be expected that a drug with an agonist action at a particular receptor type will interact with antagonists at that receptor. For example, the bronchodilator action of a selective beta$_2$-adrenoreceptor agonist such as salbutamol will be antagonized by beta-adrenoreceptor antagonists. In patients with peptic ulceration, spironol-actone antagonizes the mineralocorticoid effects of carbenoxolone through an effect at the aldos-terone receptor. Carbenoxolone also antagonizes competitively the renal electrolyte handling effects of spironolactone.

Additive or synergistic interactions

If two drugs which have the same pharmacologi-cal effect are given together, the effects may be additive. There are numerous examples of such effects, but the most common is probably exces-sive drowsiness where more than one drug with central nervous system depressant effects are taken concurrently. Another example is the increased risk of bleeding in anticoagulated patients taking salicylates. Such effects are not strictly speaking drug interactions, although in practice additive toxicity of more than one drug is a common cause of adverse drug reactions.

Interactions due to changes in drug transport mechanisms

The antihypertensive effects of adrenergic neu-rone blocking drugs such as guanethidine, bethanidine and debrisoquine are prevented or reversed by tricyclic antidepressants, though these antihypertensives are now seldom used. The pharmacological action of the adrenergic neurone blockers appears to depend on their uptake into the neurone in the same way as nor-adrenaline and other biogenic amines enter nerve terminals, known as uptake 1. Tricyclic anti-depressants, and several other drugs including phenothiazines, butyrophenones and indirectly acting sympathomimetics, block the transport mechanism localized in the cell membrane, and thus prevent competitively the access of the adrenergic neurone blockers to the noradrenaline storage sites.

Interactions due to disturbances in fluid and electrolyte balance

Drugs which decrease plasma potassium con-centrations may alter the therapeutic effects of cardiac glycosides such as digoxin as well as other antiarrhythmic drugs. The risks of digoxin cardiotoxicity are enhanced by hypokalaemia. Similarly, hypokalaemia increases the risks of ventricular arrhythmias associated with anti-arrhythmic agents such as procainamide, quini-dine and amiodarone. Angiotensin converting enzyme inhibitors have a potassium-sparing effect, such that the concurrent use of potassium supplements or potassium-sparing diuretics may lead to dangerous hyperkalaemia.

Indirect pharmacodynamic interactions

As stated previously, there are many indirect pharmacodynamic interactions, and several of those with potential clinical significance will be briefly discussed. The use of beta-adrenoreceptor antagonists in patients taking insulin or oral hypoglycaemics can produce hypoglycaemia. Propranolol is known to reduce glycogen break-down and delay the rise in blood glucose after hypoglycaemia, while cardioselective beta-adrenoreceptor antagonists are generally devoid of such effects. In addition, the recognition of hypoglycaemia by a patient may be impaired by beta-adrenoreceptor antagonists because of the absence of the usual warning symptoms which are mediated by the sympathetic ner-vous system. Cardioselective beta-adrenoreceptor blockers are preferred if it is necessary for a diabetic patient to take a beta-adrenoreceptor antagonist.

Non-steroidal anti-inflammatory drugs (NSAIDs) and antihypertensives. Drug inter-actions with NSAIDs are frequently reported, as they are among the most widely used drugs. The majority of these interactions are due to pharmacokinetic mechanisms, and many are clinically insignificant. Clinically important in-teractions are known to occur with loop diuretics and antihypertensive agents. Indomethacin and other NSAIDs reduce renal sodium excretion and inhibit the increase in renal prostaglandins that accompanies administration of frusemide. Sulindac, which apparently spares renal prosta-glandins, has been reported not to interact with loop diuretics in this way. In addition, the anti-hypertensive efficacy of ACE inhibitors and beta-adrenoreceptor blockers may be reduced in patients taking concurrent NSAIDs as a result of this mechanism.

Monoamine oxidase inhibitors (MAOIs). Monoamine oxidase inhibitors (MAOIs) are a group of antidepressants which act by inhibiting the monoamine oxidase enzymes. These enzymes are involved in the breakdown of catecholamines and indolethylamines (e.g. serotonin/5HT, histamine), and are located in nerve endings, the liver and the gut. Administration of a sympathomimetic amine, such as phenylpropanolamine, or dietary tyramine, to a patient taking an MAOI will lead to the release of accumulated noradrenaline from storage sites, producing a syndrome of sympathetic overactivity characterized by severe hypertension, headache, excitement, delirium, hyperpyrexia and cardiac arrhythmias; subarachnoid haemorrhages and death have resulted. As the MAOIs produce an irreversible enzyme inhibition, the possibility of an interaction may persist for up to 20 days after the last dose is taken. Termination of the drug's effect depends on synthesis of further enzyme.

MAOIs and tricyclic antidepressants. Although the exact mechanism of this interaction is not understood, it is likely to be due to the combined inhibition of catecholamine reuptake by tricyclic antidepressants and the interference with catecholamine metabolism by MAOIs. It is now recognized that the combination of these drugs may be used under careful psychiatric supervision if certain precautions are observed. Clomipramine and imipramine are the tricyclic antidepressants which have been implicated in these interactions most often; this is thought to reflect their relative selectivity for 5HT. Thus, newer antidepressants which act by selective inhibition of 5HT reuptake, such as fluvoxamine, fluoxetine, paroxetine and sertraline, are likely to be especially dangerous in combination with MAOIs, and the concurrent use of these agents should be avoided. The combination of fluoxetine and MAOIs has already been reported to cause several fatalities. This selective 5HT reuptake inhibitor has a very long-acting active metabolite, norfluoxetine, and consequently an interval of 5 weeks is recommended between fluoxetine discontinuation and institution of MAOI therapy.

The combination of MAOIs with pethidine has resulted in serious reactions characterized by hypertension, rigidity, sweating and excitation, and several deaths have been reported. Other opiates have generally not been associated with these effects. The underlying mechanism has not been established, although increased CNS levels of 5HT have been suggested as the cause. However, a recent case report has described a serious adverse reaction believed to be due to an interaction between pethidine and selegiline, a selective MAO-B inhibitor. Since 5HT is not a substrate of MAO-B, this casts some doubts on the theory of enhanced central serotonergic activity as the cause of the interaction.

CONCLUSIONS

There is no doubt that drug interactions can be an important clinical problem. The published literature on the subject is huge, and it is impossible to memorize all those of potential clinical significance. However, as this chapter has shown, an understanding of the drugs at risk, the most common mechanisms, and the most vulnerable patients, will help minimize the effects of adverse drug interactions on patient care.

BIBLIOGRAPHY

Brosen K. Recent developments in hepatic drug oxidation. Implications for clinical pharmacokinetics. Clinical Pharmacokinetics 1990; 18(3): 220–239

Hansten P D, Horn J R. Drug interactions and updates. Lea & Febiger 1990

McInnes G T, Brodie M J. Drug interactions that matter: a critical reappraisal. Drugs 1988; 36: 83–110

MacKichan J J. Protein binding drug displacement interactions: fact or fiction? Clinical Pharmacokinetics 1989; 16: 65–73

Orme M L'E. Drug interactions of clinical importance. In: Davies D M (ed) Textbook of adverse drug reactions, 4th edn. Oxford University Press 1991

Stockley I H. Drug interactions: a source book of adverse interactions, their mechanisms, clinical importance and management, 2nd edn. Blackwell Scientific Publications 1991

Trissel L A. Handbook on injectable drugs. 6th edn. American Society of Hospital Pharmacists 1990

Welling P G. Interactions affecting drug absorption. Clinical Pharmacokinetics 1984; 9: 404–434

Chapter 3

Adverse drug reactions

A. Lee   M. D. Rawlins

The problem of adverse drug reactions as a significant cause of morbidity and mortality has been recognized since the earliest times. As early as 400 BC Hippocrates warned about the dangers of drugs, recommending that they should never be prescribed unless the patient had been thoroughly examined. In 1785 when William Withering described the benefits of digitalis he also described the vomiting, alteration of vision, bradycardia, convulsions and death it could cause. Subsequently, the great therapeutic advances of the twentieth century have been accompanied by a growing awareness of the problems of adverse reactions to medicines among both health care professionals and consumers. It is essential that the practising pharmacist has a knowledge of the adverse effects of drugs, including their predictability and reversibility, their frequency and severity, their predisposing factors and recognition, their relationship to dosage and duration of treatment, and their prevention. There is a voluminous worldwide literature on adverse drug reactions, including several comprehensive textbooks devoted to the subject, and this chapter only represents an introduction to the subject. It concentrates on the epidemiology, mechanisms and classification of adverse drug reactions, important predisposing factors, and how adverse reactions are identified and evaluated.

DEFINITION AND CLASSIFICATION

An adverse drug reaction has been defined by

the World Health Organization as 'any response to a drug which is noxious, unintended and occurs at doses used in man for prophylaxis, diagnosis or therapy'. There are several ways of classifying adverse reactions, but the simplest is to separate them into Types A and B, as proposed by Rawlins & Thompson in 1977 (Table 3.1). Type A reactions are qualitatively normal but *augmented* responses to drugs, such as bradycardia with a beta-adrenoreceptor blocker or hypoglycaemia with a sulphonylurea. Many Type A reactions are due to a property of the drug which is unrelated to its primary therapeutic effect, such as galactorrhoea with domperidone and dry mouth with phenothiazines. Type A reactions are usually predictable from the pharmacology of a drug, they are generally dose dependent and although they are relatively common they do not generally cause serious illness. Most Type A reactions resolve when the dose is reduced and because they are relatively common they are usually identified before a drug has been marketed.

Some Type A adverse reactions have a long latency. Examples include teratogenicity, chloroquine retinopathy, and delayed effects such as the vaginal clear-cell adenocarcinoma which may occur in the daughters of women who received diethylstilboestrol during pregnancy.

Type B reactions, in contrast, are *bizarre* effects that are unpredictable on the basis of a drug's known pharmacology. Examples include haemolysis with methyldopa, or thrombocytopenia with angiotensin converting enzyme inhibitors. Type B reactions are generally unrelated to dosage and, although comparatively rare, they often cause serious illness and death. Type B reactions account for many drug withdrawals from the market, such as the Guillain–Barré syndrome induced by zimeldine. Continuous post-marketing surveillance ('pharmacovigilance') is often required before many Type B reactions can be identified. They are generally due to hypersensitivity, or an 'idiosyncratic' mechanism. However, as knowledge increases, the ability to predict Type B responses should increase accordingly.

EPIDEMIOLOGY

Many studies have attempted to determine the incidence, or frequency, of adverse drug reactions both in hospital and in the community. The estimates of incidence observed in these studies vary widely and these probably reflect differences in the methods used to detect and report adverse drug reactions. It is also apparent that a higher yield of adverse reactions is found when investigators undertake both detection and monitoring themselves, rather than relying on others to notify them of potential cases. Another possible cause of variation is that no standard definition of an adverse drug reaction has been used throughout these studies.

Most studies have found that around 5% of hospital admissions are attributable to adverse drug reactions; that 10 to 20% of patients will experience an adverse reaction during their stay in hospital; and that, as a result, the length of stay may be increased in up to 50% of these patients. Drug-related deaths have been reported to occur in 0.1% of medical inpatients and in 0.02% of surgical patients. In general practice the incidence of adverse reactions is reported to be around 2%, although studies in hospital outpatients have suggested that the incidence of adverse drug reactions may be as high as 30%.

Despite the problems involved in accurately determining the incidence of adverse drug reactions, it is generally accepted that they increase hospital admission rates, increase morbidity and

Table 3.1 Comparison between Type A and Type B adverse drug reactions		
	A (augmented response)	B (bizarre response)
Pharmacologically predictable	Yes	No
Dose-dependent	Yes	No
Incidence	High	Low
Morbidity	High	Low
Mortality	Low	High
Management	Dosage adjustment often appropriate	Stop

mortality, and thus significantly increase health care costs. A further problem is the fact that drug-induced disease is rarely specific and almost invariably mimics naturally occurring disease. Few adverse drug reactions are associated with diagnostic clinical or laboratory findings which demarcate them from the features of a spontaneous disease. Moreover, many of the subjective effects frequently attributed to drugs (such as headache, nausea and dizziness) occur commonly in otherwise healthy individuals taking no medication and in patients taking a placebo.

PREDISPOSING FACTORS

Multiple drug therapy

It has been shown consistently that the incidence of adverse reactions increases exponentially with the number of drugs taken, indicating that the effects of multiple drug use are not simply additive. A number of factors may contribute to this disproportionate rise. High prescribing rates are associated with severity of illness, and severely ill patients may be predisposed to certain adverse drug reactions. Symptomatology in such patients may be erroneously attributed to adverse drug reactions. Drug interactions may also play a part.

Age

Some, though not all, studies have found that the elderly suffer from more adverse reactions than younger patients. It is difficult to determine whether the elderly are more susceptible to adverse reactions or whether this reflects increased drug exposure. Inappropriate and unnecessary drug treatment is certainly one cause of adverse reactions in this patient group. Changes in drug pharmacokinetics due to an age-related decline in organ function, and changes in drug distribution and metabolism, may predispose elderly patients to adverse drug reactions. For example, the half-life of diazepam increases linearly, from 20 hours at 20 years of age to 90 hours in those over 80 years, partly because of an increase in the volume of distribution.

The risk of adverse drug reactions is also increased in the neonate, especially when premature, because some of the enzymes involved in drug metabolism and elimination are poorly developed. The most hazardous drugs include morphine, barbiturates, sulphonamides, vitamin K analogues and chloramphenicol. The newborn also have an increased sensitivity to morphine and its derivatives which is thought to be due to poorly developed glucuronidation and the inefficiency of the immature blood–brain barrier, resulting in severe respiratory depression. Sulphonamides and vitamin K analogues may induce, or aggravate, kernicterus. Neonates are unable to metabolize chloramphenicol effectively and accumulation may occur giving rise to the 'grey baby' syndrome. Acute extrapyramidal reactions with metoclopramide and neuroleptic drugs are more common in younger adults, and this may be due to changes in dopamine receptor function.

Gender

Many adverse drug reactions seem to be more common in women than in men, although the reasons for this difference are unknown. Women are reputed to be more susceptible to the toxic effects of digoxin, heparin and captopril. Chloramphenicol-induced aplastic anaemia is twice as common in women than in men, and phenylbutazone-induced agranulocytosis is three times as common.

Intercurrent disease

Clearly patients with underlying renal or liver disease have an increased risk of adverse drug reactions due to drugs which are eliminated by these organs. There are, however, other disease states which may predispose to adverse reactions, such as the increased incidence of the adverse effects of co-trimoxazole in AIDS patients.

Race and genetic polymorphism

Race and genetic polymorphism may account for

alterations in the handling of drugs and their end-organ effects. Many reactions which were previously described as idiosyncratic have now been shown to have a clearly defined genetic basis.

MECHANISMS OF TYPE A ADVERSE DRUG REACTIONS

The individual response to drugs shows great variation. This is manifest either as different doses being required to produce the pharmacological effect, or different responses to a defined dose. Such interindividual variation is the basis of Type A adverse reactions. Dose-related adverse reactions may occur because of variations in the pharmaceutical, pharmacokinetic, or pharmacodynamic properties of a drug, and are often due to the underlying disease state or pharmacogenetic characteristics of the patient. In some individuals combinations of these causes may be responsible.

Pharmaceutical causes

Adverse reactions can occur due to pharmaceutical aspects of a dosage form either because of alterations in the quantity of drug present, or in its release characteristics. The release of active drug from a pharmaceutical preparation is dependent on various formulation factors including particle size, and the nature and quantity of excipients used. In addition, release rates and formulation characteristics may determine local gastrointestinal toxicity. In 1983 a rate-controlled preparation of indomethacin (Osmosin) was withdrawn following the receipt of a significant number of reports of gastrointestinal bleeding and haemorrhage. This was probably due to the irritant effects of a very high concentration of the active ingredient on a localized area of intestinal mucosa. As a result of stringent requirements laid down by drug regulatory authorities which limit the content of active drug in relation to the stated dose, adverse effects due to variability in the quantity of drug present are extremely unusual in developed countries.

Pharmacokinetic causes

Quantitative alterations in the absorption, distribution, metabolism, and elimination of drugs may lead to alterations in the concentration of a drug at its site of action with corresponding changes in its pharmacological effects. Such alterations may produce either an exaggerated response or therapeutic failure.

Absorption

Differences in both the rate and extent of drug absorption may cause adverse effects. Factors which can influence the extent of absorption of a drug include dosage, pharmaceutical factors, gastrointestinal tract motility, the absorptive capacity of the gastrointestinal mucosa, and 'first-pass' metabolism in the liver and gut wall before it reaches the systemic circulation. The rate of absorption of orally administered drugs is largely determined by the rate of gastric emptying, which is influenced by factors including the nature of the gastric contents, disease and concomitant drugs. The majority of adverse reactions resulting from changes in drug absorption are reduced therapeutic efficacy or therapeutic failure.

Distribution

The distribution of drugs to various tissues and organs is dependent on factors which include regional blood flow, plasma protein and tissue binding. Changes in how a drug is distributed may, theoretically, predispose to adverse effects although the clinical importance of such mechanisms is unclear.

Elimination

Generally drugs are excreted in the urine or bile, or metabolized by the liver to yield metabolites which are then excreted by the kidneys. Changes in drug elimination rates are probably the most important cause of Type A adverse drug reactions. Reduced elimination leads to drug accumulation, with potential toxicity due to increased plasma and tissue levels. Conversely, enhanced elimination leads to reduced plasma and tissue drug levels, with potential therapeutic failure.

Renal excretion

Impaired glomerular filtration leads to reduced elimination of drugs which undergo renal excretion. Individuals with reduced glomerular filtration (such as patients with intrinsic renal disease, the elderly and neonates) are liable to develop Type A adverse reactions to 'normal' therapeutic doses of drugs which are mainly excreted by the kidney. Some of the most potentially toxic drugs in this respect are digoxin, angiotensin converting enzyme inhibitors, aminoglycoside antibiotics, some class I antiarrhythmic agents (disopyramide, flecainide), and many cytotoxic agents. The occurrence of these adverse drug reactions may be minimized by adjusting the dosage given to individual patients on the basis of their renal function.

Drug metabolism

Lipid-soluble agents are frequently metabolized to water-soluble compounds which then undergo excretion by the kidney. Metabolism occurs predominantly in the liver, although the kidney, lungs, skin and gut also have some metabolizing capacity. In man, drug metabolism can be divided into two phases. Phase I reactions (oxidation, reduction or hydrolysis) expose, or add, functionally reactive groups. Phase II reactions (sulphation, glucuronidation, acetylation or methylation) involve conjugation of the drug at a reactive site produced during phase I. Drugs that possess reactive groups undergo phase II reactions only. Others are sufficiently water-soluble after phase I metabolism to be eliminated by renal excretion.

Interindividual differences or alterations in the rate at which drugs are metabolized result in corresponding variations in elimination rates. Reduced rates of metabolism may lead to drug accumulation and an increased risk of Type A adverse drug reactions, while enhanced rates of metabolism may result in therapeutic failure.

There is wide interindividual variation in some routes of metabolism, even among normal individuals, because of genetic and environmental influences. This particularly applies to oxidation, hydrolysis and acetylation.

Microsomal oxidation

Drug oxidation occurs mainly in the smooth endoplasmic reticulum of the liver by the cytochrome P450 enzyme system. There are multiple cytochrome P450 isoenzymes in man that differ in the specificity of the reactions they catalyse. Many common drugs are substrates for microsomal oxidation including tricyclic antidepressants, antiepileptics, oral anticoagulants, benzodiazepines, phenothiazines, and some antiarrhythmic agents.

Drug oxidation rates are subject to very wide variation between normal individuals. As a result, some individuals will develop toxic concentrations after normal therapeutic doses of drugs such as phenytoin and nortriptyline. These individual variations in rates of microsomal oxidation are due to genetic, biological and environmental factors. Some drugs show a genetic polymorphism for microsomal oxidation, of which the 4-hydroxylation of debrisoquine is probably the best known. Poor metabolizers have defective oxidation and develop severe postural hypotension after small single doses. Approximately 90% of Caucasians are extensive metabolizers and 10% are poor metabolizers. Poor metabolizers of debrisoquine are poor metabolizers of other drugs including nortriptyline, flecainide, metoclopramide, and timolol. In general, they appear to be particularly susceptible to Type A adverse reactions. The abnormality is due to the defective expression of the cytochrome P450 IID6 isoenzyme. Three other genetic defects involving P450 isoenzymes have been described, involving the oxidation of tolbutamide, mephenytoin and carbocysteine, although that with tolbutamide requires confirmation. Despite the fact that genetic polymorphisms are likely to account for much of the individual variability in rates of microsomal oxidation, it is clear that environmental influences such as dietary constituents and environmental pollutants are also involved. Furthermore, rates of microsomal oxidation may be altered at the extremes of life. In general, oxidized drugs have a longer half-life in babies than in adults. In the elderly, rates of microsomal oxidation of many drugs appear to decline as the likelihood of susceptibility to type A adverse reactions rises. Studies have failed to demonstrate an age-related decline in the activities, or affinities, of drug-metabolizing enzymes in the fit elderly. There is, however, a marked reduction in liver mass and liver blood flow with increasing age, which appears to account for the overall reduced hepatic metabolism of drugs. Changes in enzyme activities may be of greater importance with ageing in the presence of disease or frailty.

The potential effects of enzyme induction and inhibition on other drugs are discussed in the chapter on drug interactions.

Hydrolysis

Suxamethonium apnoea is the best-known example of an alteration in drug response due to individual variation in drug hydrolysis. The neuromuscular blocking effects of suxamethonium are usually short lived, as the drug is rapidly inactivated in plasma by hydrolysis. The hydrolysis is catalysed by plasma pseudocholinesterase which exists in several different genetically determined forms. Individuals homozygous for the atypical gene (about 1 in 2500 of the UK population) may develop prolonged neuromuscular blockade. Suxamethonium apnoea may also be somewhat prolonged in individuals who are heterozygous for the gene (i.e. who possess both the usual and the atypical gene). The frequency of the atypical genes shows marked racial variation. The frequency of the low affinity enzyme gene is low in Africans and Japanese, high in Iraqi and Iranian jews, and intermediate in Caucasians. Phenotypic studies of patients who develop prolonged neuromuscular blockade after suxamethonium do not always, however, reveal recognizable genetic abnormalities. Liver and renal disease, malnutrition, other drugs, and occupational exposure to organo-

phosphorus insecticides, can also influence the activity of plasma cholinesterase. Atypical resistance to suxamethonium has also been described in association with a form of cholinesterase that has an activity three times that found in normal individuals.

Acetylation

A number of drugs are metabolized by acetylation. These include dapsone, isoniazid, hydralazine, phenelzine, procainamide and many sulphonamides (including sulphamethoxazole and sulphapyridine). The rate of acetylation is under genetic control and shows a polymorphism, such that individuals may be phenotyped as either 'slow' or 'rapid' acetylators. The variability is due to differences in the activity of the liver enzyme N-acetyltransferase. Slow acetylators are homozygous for the autosomal recessive gene whilst fast acetylators are either heterozygous, or homozygous for the dominant gene. In the UK about half the population are rapid acetylators, but there are considerable racial differences. The incidence of rapid acetylation is highest amongst the Japanese and Eskimos and lowest in certain African tribes.

Slow acetylators are at increased risk of developing Type A adverse reactions. Thus, isoniazid-induced peripheral neuropathy, the haematological adverse effects of dapsone, and the adverse effects of sulphapyridine are more likely to occur in these individuals.

Pharmacodynamic causes

Although many Type A adverse drug reactions have a pharmacokinetic basis, some are due to enhanced sensitivity of target organs or tissues. It is also likely that pharmacokinetic and pharmacodynamic adverse reactions may result from a combination of these mechanisms.

Many drugs exert their pharmacological action by combining with specific receptors either on cell membranes, or within the cytoplasm or nucleus. Specific receptors appear to be protein molecules and some, though not all, are enzymes. The target organs of different individuals might respond differently to drugs which act through specific receptors, if there are qualitative or quantitative differences in receptors between individuals. There is, indeed, emerging evidence of interindividual variation in receptor sensitivity and the existence of polymorphisms in muscarinic receptors has recently been described.

MECHANISMS OF TYPE B ADVERSE DRUG REACTIONS

Type B reactions are inexplicable in terms of the normal pharmacology of the drug. The cause may be pharmaceutical or pharmacokinetic, or may lie in target organ response. Many adverse drug reactions in this category have come to be known as 'idiosyncratic' reactions which, until recently, have tended to form a dustbin for those adverse drug reactions that could not be classified under any other heading. This situation is now changing slowly as their underlying mechanisms are becoming clear.

Pharmaceutical causes

Pharmaceutical causes of Type B adverse reactions may occur due to decomposition of the active constituents, the effects of pharmaceutical excipients (i.e. colourings, preservatives and antioxidants), or the actions of synthetic by-products of the active constituents. In most cases the administration of a decomposed drug will result in therapeutic failure, but in some cases the decomposition product may be toxic and potentially lethal. Adverse reactions have resulted from the incorporation of clearly toxic substances such as diethylene glycol (which caused 105 deaths in the USA in 1937 when it was used as a solvent in sulphanilamide elixir); the use of certain excipients in susceptible patient groups, such as asthmatics or very low birthweight neonates; and the alteration of an excipient mixture resulting in changes in the bioavailability of drugs such as digoxin and phenytoin. An example is the recently recognized, potentially fatal syndrome of eosinophilia and myalgia associated with L-tryptophan, which is likely to be due to a contaminant. A number of adverse reactions due to pharmaceutical excipients are recognized. Regulatory authorities have largely prevented the introduction of toxic excipients, and most problems can be avoided. The subject of adverse reactions to pharmaceutical excipients has recently been reviewed (see Bibliography).

Pharmacokinetic causes

Abnormalities of absorption, distribution, metabolism or elimination may give rise to Type B adverse effects in certain individuals. Some teratogenic and 'idiosyncratic' effects of drugs may be due to deficiencies in certain detoxification mechanisms. For example, it has been suggested that fetuses deficient in microsomal epoxide hydrolase are likely be at increased risk of the teratogenic effects of phenytoin, and that patients who have previously experienced adverse reactions to carbamazepine are also deficient in the same enzyme.

Pharmacodynamic causes

Qualitative differences in the response to drugs may be considered as genetic or immunological. There are a number of situations where genetic abnormalities may lead to abnormal and unpredictable responses to drugs.

Erythrocyte glucose 6-phosphate dehydrogenase (G6PD) deficiency

Glucose-6-phosphate dehydrogenase is an enzyme required for the stability of red blood cells. Individuals with a sex-linked inherited deficiency in this enzyme are particularly susceptible to haemolysis due to oxidant drugs such as primaquine, sulphonamides and sulphones, and nitrofurantoin. There are more than 80 distinct variants of G6PD but not all are associated with drug-induced haemolysis. The frequency of the enzyme deficiency also varies widely between and within various populations. In the African type G6PD (A$^-$) activity is 8 to 20% of normal, and only red cells over 50 days old have insufficient enzyme to protect them from oxidant drugs.

The Mediterranean type, on the other hand, is characterized by severe enzyme deficiency (0 to 4% enzyme activity) even in young cells. Haemolysis in patients with the African type is usually mild, while in patients with the Mediterranean type it is severe and potentially fatal. Many drugs have been associated with haemolysis in G6PD deficiency, but the severity of the reaction varies between drugs and also depends on the type of enzyme deficiency. It is now recognized that infections are probably the most common precipitant of haemolysis in G6PD-deficient individuals, and that many drugs have been unfairly accused of causing haemolysis. Some published lists of drugs to be avoided in G6PD deficiency include drugs with either no haemolytic potential or only a trivial one in the common forms of G6PD deficiency, e.g. paracetamol. The number of currently available medicines with proven haemolytic potential in G6PD-deficient individuals is relatively small; primaquine is probably the best-known example. In the common African type of deficiency, G6PD (A⁻), daily administration of 30 mg of primaquine leads to haemolysis beginning after 2 to 3 days. There is no reliable in vitro test of a drug's haemolytic potential in G6PD deficiency and it varies with the severity of the enzyme deficiency, with other factors affecting the metabolism of the drug in that individual, with co-existent stresses such as infection and with the dose of the drug that is administered. Drugs and other agents that should be avoided in G6PD deficiency are shown in Table 3.2.

Hereditary methaemoglobinaemias

An inherited deficiency of methaemoglobin

Table 3.2 Drugs and other agents to be avoided in G6PD deficiency
Doxorubicin
Methylene blue
Nitrofurantoin
Nalidixic acid
Primaquine
Sulphamethoxazole
Sulphasalazine

reductase in erythrocytes renders affected individuals susceptible to the development of methaemoglobinaemia and cyanosis in response to oxidant drugs. Thus, any of the drugs listed in Table 3.2 may cause this effect.

Porphyrias

The porphyrias are a heterogeneous group of inherited disorders of haem biosynthesis. The disorders are transmitted as autosomal dominants, with the exception of the rare congenital porphyria, which is recessive. The effects of drugs are of most importance in patients with acute porphyrias, in whom certain commonly prescribed agents may precipitate life-threatening attacks. Other trigger factors include alcohol, infection, reduced caloric intake, hormonal changes and pregnancy. In the acute porphyrias, patients develop abdominal and neuropsychiatric disturbances, and they excrete in their urine excessive amounts of the porphyrin precursors 5-aminolaevulinic acid (ALA) and porphobilinogen. A number of drugs may induce excess porphyrin synthesis. However, it is extremely difficult to predict whether or not a drug may cause problems in patients with porphyria and the only factors shown to be clearly linked with porphyrinogenicity are lipid solubility and membrane fluidization (i.e. the ability to disrupt the phospholipid bilayer of the cell membrane). A number of commonly used drugs induce ALA synthase in the liver, but there is wide variation between porphyric patients in their sensitivity to drugs which may trigger attacks. Thus, whereas a single dose of a drug may be sufficient to trigger an acute attack in one patient, another may require a number of relatively large doses of the same drug to produce any clinically significant effect. Comprehensive lists of drugs which are known to be unsafe and drugs which are thought to be safe for use in acute porphyria are available (see Bibliography).

Malignant hyperthermia

Malignant hyperthermia is a rare but potentially fatal condition in which there is a rapid rise in body temperature (at least 2°C an hour) occurring without obvious cause after administration of anaesthetics or muscle relaxants. The condition usually follows the administration of an inhalational general anaesthetic, often halothane, in combination with suxamethonium. In addition to the temperature rise, the syndrome is characterized by stiffness of skeletal muscles, hyperventilation, acidosis, hyperkalaemia, and signs of increased activity of the sympathetic nervous system. It is likely that the condition is triggered by an abnormal calcium-induced release of intracellular ionized calcium, which may be due to an inherited defect of cellular membranes. The condition is associated with a 60 to 70% mortality rate.

Glucocorticoid glaucoma

In genetically predisposed individuals glucocorticoids can cause a rise in intraocular pressure leading to blindness. Development of increased intraocular pressure appears to be correlated with dosage, and may persist for several months after stopping steroid treatment. It is important to remember that this complication may arise in patients treated with glucocorticoid eye drops.

Cholestatic jaundice induced by oral contraceptives

Oral contraceptives are known to cause jaundice in some women, especially during the first month of medication, which recovers rapidly on discontinuation of treatment. Available evidence suggests that a genetic component is important for the development of the reaction. The under-

lying mechanism for this reaction is unclear, but it is likely that oestrogen-induced changes in the composition of membrane lipids are involved.

Immunological reasons for abnormal response

A few drugs (e.g. peptides of foreign origin such as streptokinase) are immunogenic and may cause immunological reactions in their own right. Most immunological adverse reactions, however, are idiosyncratic. Examples are shown in Table 3.3. Increased susceptibility to some immunological reactions is seen in atopic patients, and in association with certain human histocompatability antigens.

DETECTION AND MONITORING OF ADVERSE DRUG REACTIONS

By the time a drug is marketed it will usually have been given to an average of 1500 people, and it is likely that clinical trials will only have picked up the most common ADRs. It is unlikely that Type B reactions, with an incidence of 1 in 500 or less, will have been identified by the time a drug becomes available for widespread use. It is only after much wider use that rare reactions, or those which occur predominantly in certain subgroups within the population, such as the elderly, are detected; and it is therefore essential to monitor safety once a drug has been marketed. The methods which are used more commonly in post-marketing surveillance are described below.

Case reports

The publication of single case reports, or case

Table 3.3 Immunological mechanisms of adverse drug reactions (according to Coombs & Gell classification, 1968)			
Immunological reaction	Immunological mechanism	Clinical manifestation	Drugs
Type I	IgE mediated	Anaphylaxis	Penicillin
Type II	Humoral cytotoxic	Haemolysis	Methyldopa
Type III	Humoral immune-complex (IgM, IgG) mediated	Serum sickness Acute glomerulonephritis Systemic lupus erythematosus	Streptokinase Hydralazine
Type IV	Cell-mediated injury	Morbilliform skin eruptions	Amoxycillin

series, of adverse drug reactions in the medical literature is an important means of detecting new and serious reactions, particularly Type B reactions. Case reports have, in the past, been vital in alerting the professions to several serious adverse reactions, such as the oculomucocutaneous syndrome associated with practolol, and halothane-induced hepatitis. In recent years, published single case reports have probably been of lessening importance with the emergence of formalized spontaneous reporting systems.

Cohort studies

Cohort studies are prospective studies which study the fate of a large group of patients taking a particular drug. The best studies compare adverse event rates in groups of patients taking the drug of intent, with a comparative group. Cohort studies include ad hoc investigations set up to investigate specific problems (e.g. the Royal College of General Practitioners' oral contraceptive study), studies sponsored by pharmaceutical companies, prescription event monitoring (PEM), and a variety of record linkage schemes.

Case-control studies

Case-control studies compare drug usage in a group of patients with a particular disease with use amongst a matched control group who are similar in potentially confounding factors, but who do not have the disease. The prevalence of drug taking is then compared between the groups, and a significant excess of drug takers in the disease group may be evidence of an association with the drug. This is a useful retrospective method which can provide valuable information on the incidence of Type B reactions and the association between drugs and disease. Examples of associations which have been established by case-control studies are Reye's syndrome and aspirin, and the relationship between maternal diethylstilboestrol ingestion and vaginal adenocarcinoma in female offspring. The case-control method is an effective means for confirming whether or not a drug causes a given reaction once a suspicion has been raised. It is not capable

of detecting previously unsuspected adverse reactions.

Spontaneous reporting schemes

The thalidomide tragedy led to the institution, in many countries, of national schemes for the voluntary collection of adverse drug reaction reports, of which the Committee on Safety of Medicines (CSM) adverse reactions reporting scheme is one. The CSM's scheme has now been operating for more than 25 years and has received over 300 000 reports of suspected adverse reactions. Doctors are asked to report all suspected *serious* adverse reactions, and *all* suspected reactions to newer products (marked with an inverted black triangle symbol in product information and in the British National Formulary). Spontaneous reporting schemes cannot provide estimates of risk because the true number of cases is invariably underestimated, and the denominator is not known. However, the CSM's spontaneous reporting scheme has been shown to provide valuable early warnings or signals of possible adverse drug reactions, and to enable the study of factors associated with them. The Committee on Safety of Medicines' spontaneous reporting scheme, the 'yellow card scheme', is available for all doctors and for all drugs; it is capable of detecting both rare and common reactions; and it is relatively inexpensive to operate. It is unfortunate that there is still considerable under-reporting of reactions, and it is likely that less than 10% of serious adverse reactions are notified. Reports should be made despite uncertainty about a causal relationship, irrespective of whether or not the reaction is well recognized, and regardless of other drugs having been given concurrently.

IDENTIFICATION OF ADVERSE DRUG REACTIONS

The establishment of a causal relationship between a specific drug and a clinical event is a fundamental problem in adverse drug reaction assessment. Firstly, adverse drug reactions frequently mimic other diseases and, secondly, many of the symptoms attributed to adverse drug reactions occur commonly in healthy individuals who are not taking any medication. Clinicians may thus fail to recognize the features of an adverse drug reaction because they do not fit into a clearly defined pattern. There is some evidence that patients themselves are capable of correctly distinguishing probable adverse drug reactions from other types of adverse clinical event. When a patient is prescribed a new drug, he should also be given information on possible adverse drug reactions including how to recognize them, and what to do if one occurs. For example, patients taking warfarin should know that if they notice unusual bruising, or black stools, they should seek medical help at once. Patients taking new products should be asked to report any unexpected symptoms which develop whilst taking the drug or within a month or so of its discontinuation.

When a suspected adverse reaction has occurred, it may be helpful to try to assess whether it is definitely, probably or possibly due to the drug. This process, known as causality assessment, is fraught with difficulties, although some decision on the likelihood that a drug caused a particular reaction is usually taken, perhaps subconsciously in some cases. Various systematic approaches, or algorithms, have been developed in an attempt to rationalize causality assessment of adverse reactions, but these are of limited value.

Factors taken into account when assessing the likelihood of an adverse drug reaction

Where an adverse drug reaction is suspected a full history, particularly details of other drugs taken by the patient, and including over-the-counter and herbal medicines, is important. The patient should be asked about the nature and timing of the symptom or event, and whether such effects have occurred in the past. The temporal relationship of a suspected adverse drug reaction is important. It is relatively easy to recognize an adverse reaction that occurs soon after drug administration and an event predating prescription is clearly unlikely to be drug related. Once more than a few weeks have elapsed, however, the association between the drug and the

event is more difficult. This is well illustrated by the practolol syndrome. There are very few cases where it is certain that a given drug caused a particular reaction in a specific patient, even though the drug is known to cause the reaction in some recipients. Unlike other conditions in medicine, adverse drug reactions rarely produce characteristic physical signs and laboratory investigations. It is reassuring to find that an adverse reaction resolves once a drug is stopped, but this may take time. Occasionally the adverse reaction is irreversible, as in tardive dyskinesia which may actually deteriorate when the offending drug is withdrawn. Rechallenge sometimes occurs inadvertently but is only rarely justified clinically to confirm a diagnosis. Positive rechallenge is often taken as proof of a causal relationship, but this may not always be the case, particularly where the suspected reaction is subjective in nature, such as headache. A *suspicion* that a drug has caused an adverse reaction is all that is necessary for a report to be submitted to the CSM; it is not necessary to have a confirmed diagnosis.

Delayed adverse effects of drugs

A number of adverse effects may only become apparent after long-term treatment, such as the relatively harmless melanin deposits in the lens and cornea that are seen after years of phenothiazine treatment, and which should be distinguished from pigmentary retinopathy, a dose-related adverse effect occurring within several months of initiation of treatment. Other examples include the development of vaginal carcinoma in the daughters of women given stilboestrol during pregnancy for the treatment of threatened abortion, and immunosuppressives and chemotherapeutic agents which can induce malignancies that may not be apparent until years after treatment has been given.

Adverse effects associated with drug withdrawal

Some drugs cause symptoms when treatment is stopped abruptly, for example the benzodiazepine withdrawal syndrome, rebound hypertension following discontinuation of antihypertensives such as clonidine, and the acute adrenal insufficiency that may be precipitated by the abrupt withdrawal of corticosteroids. These are all Type A reactions.

CONCLUSION

Adverse drug reactions are an inevitable risk associated with the use of modern medicines. However, careful attention to dosage, taking into account factors such as age and renal function, will minimize the risk of Type A reactions in many patients. Genetic status should be taken into account in the few cases where this is appropriate, and it is now possible to genotype individuals, using recombinant DNA methods, for some of the known polymorphisms. The pharmacist is well placed to assist in the prevention, detection and monitoring of adverse drug reactions, and this role should be further strengthened in the future.

BIBLIOGRAPHY

Chaplin S. Genetically determined differences in susceptibility to adverse drug reactions. Adverse Drug Reaction and Acute Poisoning Review 1984; 4: 211–236

D'Arcy P F, Griffin J P. Iatrogenic Diseases, 3rd edn. Oxford: Oxford Medical Publications 1986

Davies D M. Textbook of Adverse Drug Reactions, 4th edn. Oxford: Oxford Medical Publications 1991

Dukes M N G. Meyler's side effects of drugs, 11th edn. Amsterdam Elsevier Science Publishers 1988

Golightly L K, Smolinske S S, Bennett M L, Sutherland III E W, Rumack B H. Pharmaceutical excipients: adverse effects associated with inactive ingredients in drug products (Part I). Medical Toxicology 1988; 3: 128–165

Golightly L K, Smolinske S S, Bennett M L, Sutherland III E W, Rumack B H. Pharmaceutical excipients: adverse effects associated with inactive ingredients in drug products (Part II). Medical Toxicology 1988; 3: 209–240

Chapter 4

Laboratory data

R. Walker   C. Edwards

This chapter will consider the common biochemical and haematological tests which are of clinical and diagnostic importance. For convenience each individual test will be dealt with under a separate heading. In reality a disturbance of one parameter cannot be considered in isolation without referral to the pattern of other tests within the group.

It is usual for a reference range to be quoted for each individual test (see Table 4.1). This range is based on the assumption that 95% of the population are normal and spans the 2.5 to 97.5 percentile. The 'normal' range must always be used with caution since it takes little account of an individual's age, sex, weight, height, time since last meal, muscle mass or disease state,

Table 4.1 Biochemical data: typical normal adult reference values (SI units) measured in serum	
Laboratory test	Reference range
Albumin	35–55 g/L
Bilirubin	
Total	< 17 µmol/L
Conjugated (direct)	< 4 µmol/L
Calcium	2.20–2.55 mmol/L
Creatinine	50–120 µmol/L
Glucose	
Fasting	3.3–6.7 mmol/L
Non-fasting	< 10.0 mmol/L
Osmolality	282–295 mOsm/kg
Potassium	3.5–5.0 mmol/L
Sodium	135–145 mmol/L
Urea	3.0–6.5 mmol/L
Uric acid	0.15–0.47 mmol/L

many of which can influence the value obtained. Reference ranges are valuable guides but must not be used as sole indicators of health and disease. A single test value can rarely be interpreted. A series of values are usually required to ensure clinical relevance and eliminate erroneous values caused by spoiled specimens or interference from diagnostic or therapeutic procedures.

Further specific information on the clinical and therapeutic relevance of each test may be obtained by referral to the relevant chapter within this textbook.

BIOCHEMICAL DATA

Sodium and water balance

Sodium and water metabolism are closely interrelated both physiologically and clinically, and play a major role in determining the osmolality of serum.

Water constitutes approximately 60% of body weight in men and 55% in women. Approximately two-thirds of the water is found in the intracellular fluid (ICF) and one-third in the extracellular fluid (ECF). Of the extracellular fluid, 75% is found within interstitial fluid and 25% within serum (see Fig. 4.1).

Water, in general, permeates freely between the ICF and ECF and its movement is determined by the osmotic content of each compartment. The compartment with the higher osmotic concentration determines that water moves in that direction. The osmotic content of the two compartments is, in general, the same, i.e. they are isotonic. The kidneys are an exception to the rule.

The osmolality of the ECF is largely determined by sodium and its associated anions, chloride and bicarbonate. Glucose and urea have a lesser, but nevertheless important role in determining ECF osmolality. Protein (especially albumin) makes only a small (0.5%) contribution to the osmolality of the ECF but is a major factor in determining water distribution between the two compartments. The contribution of proteins to the osmotic pressure of serum is known as the colloid osmotic pressure or oncotic pressure.

The major contributor to the osmolality of the ICF is potassium.

The amount of water taken in and lost by the body depends on intake, diet, activity and the environment. Over a given period of time the intake of water is normally equal to that lost (Table 4.2). The minimum daily intake necessary to maintain balance is approximately 1100 ml. Of this, 500 ml is required for normal excretion of waste products whilst the remaining volume is lost via the skin (sweating), lungs (breathing) and gastrointestinal tract (faeces). Water can be readily lost from the body via the kidneys (renal tubular disorders; diabetes insipidus; increased osmotic load due to diabetes mellitus), lungs (e.g. hyperventilation), or gut (e.g. diarrhoea).

In a healthy subject the major factor controlling water balance is thirst.

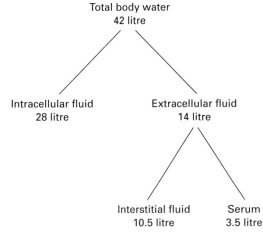

Fig. 4.1 Approximate distribution of water in a 70 kg man.

Table 4.2 Typical daily water balance for a healthy 70 kg adult			
	Input (ml)		Output (ml)
Oral fluids	1400	Urine	1500
		Lung	400
Food	700	Skin	400
Metabolic oxidation	400	Faeces	200
Total	2500		2500

Water depletion

Water depletion will occur if intake is inadequate or loss excessive. The excessive loss of water is unusual except in diabetes insipidus or following the overenthusiastic use of diuretics.

Water can only be lost from the ECF. Patients will have a raised serum sodium (hypernatraemia), with a slight elevation of serum protein concentration and haematocrit. Severe water depletion may induce cerebral dehydration and circulatory failure.

Once the underlying cause for the water depletion has been identified, water should be given orally, or by nasogastric tube. Intravenous 5% dextrose or hypotonic saline, if there is sodium loss, may also be effective. Two-thirds of the deficit should be corrected in 24 hours and the remainder in the following 24 hours.

Water excess

Water excess is usually associated with an impairment of water excretion such as that caused by the inappropriate secretion of antidiuretic hormone (ADH) or renal failure. Excess intake is rarely a cause since the healthy adult kidney can excrete water at a rate of up to about 2 ml/minute. Patients affected usually present with signs consistent with cerebral overhydration, although if of gradual onset over several days they may be asymptomatic. Hyponatraemia is usually present.

Water and ECF osmolality

If the body water content changes independently of the amount of solute, osmolality will be altered (normal range 282 to 295 mOsm/kg of water). A loss of water from the ECF will increase its osmolality and result in the movement of water from the ICF to ECF. This increase in ECF osmolality will stimulate the hypothalamic thirst centres to promote a desire to drink whilst also stimulating the release of ADH. The ADH increases the permeability of the renal collecting ducts to water, and promotes water reabsorption with consequent concentration of urine.

If the osmolality of the ECF falls, there is no desire to drink and no secretion of ADH. Consequently a dilute urine is produced which helps restore ECF osmolality to normal.

The ADH secretion is also stimulated by angiotensin II, arterial and venous baroreceptors, volume receptors, stress (including pain) and exercise and drugs such as morphine, nicotine, chlorpropamide, tolbutamide, carbamazepine and vincristine. If serum volume decreases by more than 10% the hypovolaemia stimulates ADH release and overrides control based on osmolality.

Sodium distribution

The body of an average 70 kg man contains approximately 3000 mmol of sodium. 70% of this sodium is freely exchangeable whilst the remainder is complexed in bone. Most of the exchangeable sodium is extracellular, and results in a normal serum range of 135 to 145 mmol/L. In contrast, the ICF concentration of sodium is only 4 to 10 mmol/L.

Each day approximately 1000 mmol of sodium is secreted into the gut and 25 000 mmol filtered by the kidney. The bulk of this is recovered by reabsorption from the gut and renal tubules. It should be clear therefore that partial failure of homeostatic control can potentially have disastrous sequelae.

Sodium and ECF volume

The ECF volume is dependent upon total body sodium since sodium is almost entirely restricted to the ECF, and water intake and loss are regulated to maintain a constant concentration of sodium in the ECF compartment.

Sodium balance is maintained by renal excretion. Normally, 70% of filtered sodium is actively reabsorbed in the proximal convoluted tubule, with further reabsorption in the loop of Henle. Less than 5% of the filtered sodium load reaches the distal convoluted tubule where aldosterone can stimulate further sodium reabsorption.

Other factors such as natriuretic peptide hormone can also control sodium reabsorption. This hormone is secreted by the cardiac atria in response to atrial stretch following a rise in atrial pressure following, say, volume expansion. It is natriuretic (increases sodium excretion in urine) and amongst other actions reduces aldosterone concentration.

Sodium depletion

Inadequate oral intake of sodium is rarely the cause of sodium depletion although inappropriate parenteral treatment may occasionally be implicated. Sodium depletion is usually the consequence of excessive loss in either isotonic or hypotonic fluid which results in a decrease in ECF volume. The normal response of the body to the associated hypovolaemia includes an increase in aldosterone secretion (which stimulates renal sodium reabsorption) and an increase in ADH secretion if ECF volume depletion is severe.

The serum sodium level can give an indication of depletion, but it must be borne in mind that the serum sodium may be:

- increased, e.g. where there is sodium and water loss but with predominant water loss as occurs in excessive sweating
- normal, e.g. where there is isotonic sodium and water loss as occurs from burns or a haemorrhage, or
- decreased, e.g. sodium loss with water retention as would occur if an isotonic sodium depletion was treated with a low sodium solution.

Sodium excess

Sodium excess can be due to increased intake or decreased excretion. Excessive intake is not a common cause although iatrogenic hypernatraemia, associated with the inappropriate use of hypertonic saline occurs frequently.

Sodium excess is usually due to impaired excretion. It may also be caused by a primary mineralocorticoid excess, e.g. Cushing's syndrome or Conn's syndrome, but is often due to a secondary aldosteronism associated with, for example, congestive cardiac failure, nephrotic syndrome, hepatic cirrhosis with ascites, or renal artery stenosis.

Hypernatraemia

Hypernatraemia is much less common than hyponatraemia. The possible causes of hypernatraemia include water depletion, combined sodium and water depletion with predominant water loss, or sodium excess. Of these possible causes excess body sodium is the least common cause.

Drug-induced hypernatraemia is often the result of a nephrogenic diabetes insipidus-like syndrome whereby the renal tubules are unresponsive to ADH. In such a situation the affected patient presents with polyuria, polydipsia or dehydration. Lithium, demeclocycline and phenytoin are the most common causative agents.

The diabetes-insipidus-like syndrome with lithium has been reported after only 2 weeks of therapy. The syndrome is usually reversible on discontinuation. Whilst affected, however, many patients are unresponsive to exogenous ADH.

Demeclocycline can also cause nephrogenic diabetes insipidus. As with lithium the diabetes insipidus is unresponsive to exogenous ADH. Demeclocycline is often the drug of choice in the management of patients with the syndrome of inappropriate ADH secretion (SIADH).

Phenytoin generally has a less pronounced effect on urinary volume than lithium and demeclocycline and does not cause nephrogenic diabetes insipidus. Phenytoin inhibits ADH secretion at the level of the central nervous system.

Hypernatraemia can be caused by a number of other drugs (Table 4.3) and by a variety of mechanisms. For example, hypernatraemia secondary to sodium retention is known to occur with corticosteroids whilst the administration of sodium-containing drugs parenterally in high doses also has the potential to cause hypernatraemia.

Table 4.3 Examples of drugs known to cause hypernatraemia
ACTH
Anabolic steroids
Androgens
Carbenicillin
Carbenoxalone
Clonidine
Corticosteroids
Diazoxide
Oestrogens
Lactulose
Liquorice
Methoxyflurane
Methyldopa
Oral contraceptives
Oxyphenbutazone
Phenylbutazone
Sodium bicarbonate

Table 4.4 Examples of drugs known to cause hyponatraemia
Aminoglutethimide
Amitriptyline
Ammonium chloride
Amphotericin
Captopril
Carbamazepine
Chlorpropamide
Cisplatin
Clofibrate
Cyclophosphamide
Diuretics
acetazolamide
amiloride
chlorthalidone
ethacrynic acid
frusemide
metolazone
mannitol
spironolactone
thiazides
triamterine
Heparin
Imipramine
Indomethacin
Lithium
Miconazole
Non-steroidal anti-inflammatory agents
Opiates
Tolbutamide
Vasopressin
Vincristine

Hyponatraemia

Following from the discussion above, a decrease in serum sodium can be the result of sodium loss, water retention in excess of sodium, or a combination of both factors. A number of drugs have also been implicated as causing hyponatraemia (Table 4.4).

The inappropriate secretion of ADH is the mechanism underlying many drug-induced hyponatraemias. In this syndrome the drug may augment the action of endogenous ADH, (e.g. chlorpropamide), increase the release of ADH (e.g. carbamazepine), or have a direct ADH-like action on the kidney (e.g. oxytocin). Hyponatraemia can also be induced by mechanisms different from those described above. Whilst lithium is useful in treating SIADH, paradoxically in some patients it damages the kidney and results in a failure to conserve sodium. Likewise the natriuretic action of diuretics can predispose to hyponatraemia.

There are also a variety of disorders which can also cause hyponatraemia (Table 4.5).

Potassium

The total amount of potassium in the body, like sodium, is 3000 mmol. About 10% of the body potassium is bound in red blood cells, bone and brain tissue and is not exchangeable. The remaining 90% of total body potassium is free and exchangeable with the vast majority having an intracellular location. Only 2% of the exchangeable total body potassium is in the ECF, the compartment from where the serum concentration is sampled and measured. Consequently, the measurement of serum potassium is not an accurate index of total body potassium, but together with the clinical status of a patient it permits a sound practical assessment of potassium homeostasis.

The serum potassium concentration is controlled mainly by the kidney with the gastrointestinal tract normally having a minor role. The potassium filtered in the kidney is almost completely reabsorbed in the proximal tubule. Potassium secretion is largely a passive process in response to the need to maintain membrane potential

Table 4.5 Common causes of hyponatraemia
Primary ADH-dependent
Ectopic secreting tumours
carcinoma bronchus
carcinoma prostate
Respiratory system
pneumonia
tuberculosis
asthma
Central nervous system
tumours
encephalitis
stroke
epilepsy
Drugs
Secondary ADH-dependent
Hypotension
Nausea/vomiting
Endocrine
hypocortisolism
hypothyroidism
ADH-independent
Renal failure
Impaired renal perfusion
cardiac failure
hepatic failure
nephrotic syndrome
Diuretics

neutrality associated with active reabsorption of sodium in the distal convoluted tubule and collecting duct. The extent of potassium secretion is determined by a number of factors including:

- the amount of sodium available for exchange in the distal convoluted tubule and collecting duct
- the availability of hydrogen and potassium ions for exchange in the distal convoluted tubule or collecting duct
- the ability of the distal convoluted tubule or collecting duct to secrete hydrogen ions
- the concentration of aldosterone
- tubular fluid flow rate.

As described above, both potassium and hydrogen can neutralize the membrane potential generated by active sodium reabsorption and consequently there is a close relationship between potassium and hydrogen ion homeostasis. In acidosis, hydrogen ions are normally secreted in preference to potassium, i.e. hyperkalaemia is

often associated with acidosis (except in renal tubular acidosis), and in alkalosis fewer hydrogen ions will be present and potassium is excreted, i.e. hypokalaemia is often associated with alkalosis.

The normal daily dietary intake of potassium is of the order of 60 to 200 mmol which is more than adequate to replace that lost from the body. It is unusual for a deficiency of normal intake to account for hypokalaemia. A transcellular movement of potassium into cells, loss from the gut or excretion in the urine are the main causes of hypokalaemia.

Hypokalaemia

Transcellular movement into cells. The shift of potassium from the serum compartment of the ECF into cells accounts for the hypokalaemia reported following intravenous, or less frequently, nebulized administration of beta-adrenoreceptor agonists such as salbutamol. Parenteral insulin also causes a shift of potassium into cells and is used for this purpose in the management of patients with hyperkalaemia.

Loss from the gastrointestinal tract. Although potassium is secreted in gastric juice much of this, together with potassium ingested in the diet, is reabsorbed in the small intestine. Stools normally contain some potassium, but in a patient with chronic diarrhoea or a fistula considerable amounts of potassium may be lost and precipitate hypokalaemia. Likewise, the abuse of laxatives increases gastrointestinal potassium loss and may precipitate hypokalaemia. Analogous to the situation with diarrhoea, the potassium secreted in gastric juice may be lost following persistent vomiting and can also contribute to hypokalaemia.

Loss from the kidneys. Mineralocorticoid excess, whether it be primary or secondary aldosteronism or Cushing's syndrome, can all increase urinary potassium loss and cause hypokalaemia. Likewise increased excretion of potassium secondary to renal tubular damage has been reported. In particular, the use of nephrotoxic antibiotics such as gentamicin has been implicated as a causative factor in hypokalaemia.

The central regulatory role of aldosterone-stimulated potassium–sodium exchange in the distal convoluted tubule and collecting duct is a site for the action of many drug-induced hypokalaemias. Glucocorticoids mimic aldosterone and can therefore increase potassium loss. Similarly, the glycyrrhizinic acid component of liquorice has an aldosterone-like effect and has been implicated as causing muscle weakness secondary to hypokalaemia. Carbenoxolone is a drug which can be used in the treatment of ulcers and has a similar structure to glycyrrhizinic acid. It too has been reported to cause hypokalaemia.

The presentation of large amounts of non-reabsorbable anions to the renal tubule demands the excretion of equivalent amounts of cations. Cations are provided in the form of potassium and hydrogen ions which are lost from the body and can therefore contribute to hypokalaemia. In the past such anionic loads have been associated with high dose parenteral sodium penicillin, or the administration of carbenicillin.

Finally, perhaps the most commonly used groups of drugs which can cause hypokalaemia are thiazide and loop diuretics. Both groups of drugs increase the amount of sodium delivered and available for reabsorption at the distal convoluted tubule and collecting duct. Consequently, this will increase the amount of potassium excreted from the kidneys. Some of the drugs known to cause hypokalaemia are shown in Table 4.6.

Clinical features. The patient with hypokalaemia may be asymptomatic. However, the symptoms most commonly present include muscle weakness, hypotonia, paralytic ileus, depression and confusion. Arrhythmias may occur with typical changes on the electrocardiogram (ECG) of ST depression, T wave depression/inversion and prolonged P–R interval. Rarely there may be impaired renal concentrating ability with polyuria and polydipsia.

Hyperkalaemia

Hyperkalaemia may arise due to excessive intake, decreased elimination or shift of potassium from cells to the ECF. It is rare for excessive oral

Table 4.6 Examples of drugs known to cause hypokalaemia

Adrenocorticoids
Alcohol
Amphotericin B
Azlocillin
Carbenicillin
Carbonic anhydrase inhibitors
Corticotrophin
Diuretics
  loop
   thiazide
Insulin
Laxatives
Mezlocillin
Piperacillin
Salicylates
Ticarcillin
Ticarcillin + clavulanate
Urea
Vitamin B_{12}
Vitamin D

intake to be the cause of hyperkalaemia. The inappropriate use of parenteral infusions containing potassium is probably the most likely (iatrogenic) cause of excessive intake. Hyperkalaemia is a common problem in patients with renal failure due to their inability to excrete a potassium load.

The use of potassium-sparing diuretics such as amiloride, triamterene, spironolactone together with angiotensin converting enzyme inhibitors, which decrease aldosterone secretion and thus reduce renal potassium loss, are a recognized cause of hyperkalaemia particularly in the elderly. Mineralocorticoid deficiency states such as Addison's disease where there is a deficiency of aldosterone also decrease renal potassium loss and contribute to hyperkalaemia.

The majority of body potassium is intracellular. Severe tissue damage, catabolic states or impairment of the energy-dependent sodium pump, as occurs in hypoxia or diabetic keto-acidosis, may result in hyperkalaemia due to potassium moving into and sodium moving out of cells. Table 4.7 gives examples of some drugs known to cause hyperkalaemia.

Clinical features. Hyperkalaemia can be asymptomatic but fatal. An elevated potassium has many effects on the heart; notably the resting membrane potential is lowered and the action

Table 4.7 Examples of drugs known to cause hyperkalaemia

Angiotensin converting enzyme inhibitors
Non-steroidal anti-inflammatory agents
Beta-adrenoreceptor blocking agents
Cyclosporin
Digoxin (in acute overdose)
Diuretics, potassium sparing
Heparin
Penicillins, potassium containing
Potassium supplements
Succinylcholine chloride

potential shortened. Characteristic changes of the ECG precede ventricular fibrillation and cardiac arrest.

In emergency management of a patient with hyperkalaemia intravenous calcium gluconate (or chloride) at a dose of 10 ml of 10% solution is given intravenously over 1 minute. This does not reduce the potassium concentration but antagonizes the effect of hyperkalaemia on cardiac tissue. Immediately thereafter glucose 50 g with 20 units of soluble insulin by intravenous infusion will lower serum potassium levels within 30 minutes by increasing the shift of potassium into cells. In less urgent cases 10 units of soluble insulin may be added to 1 L of 10% glucose.

If acidosis is present 40 ml of 8.4% bicarbonate (40 mmol) may be injected over 5 minutes as an alternative to glucose and insulin.

The long-term management of hyperkalaemia may involve the use of oral or rectal polystyrene sulphonate resins which remove potassium from the body.

Calcium

The body of an average man contains about 1 kg of calcium. 99% of this is bound to bone. Only about 0.0005% of body calcium is found in the serum. Calcium is present in serum bound mainly to the albumin component of protein (46%), complexed with citrate and phosphate (7%), and as free ions (47%). Only the free ions of calcium are physiologically active.

The serum calcium level is often determined by measuring total calcium, i.e. that which is free and bound. Although the measurement of ionized calcium is becoming more widely available, it does not offer a clear advantage over total calcium.

In alkalosis the hydrogen ions dissociate from albumin, and calcium binding to albumin increases together with an increase in complex formation. If the concentration of ionized calcium falls sufficiently clinical symptoms of hypocalcaemia may occur despite the total serum calcium concentration being unchanged. The reverse effect, i.e. increased ionized calcium occurs in acidosis.

Changes in serum albumin also affect the total serum calcium concentration independently of the ionized concentration. A variety of equations are available to correct the calcium concentration. A commonly used formula is shown in Figure 4.2. Caution must be taken when using such a formula in the presence of disturbed blood hydrogen ion concentrations.

Hypercalcaemia

Hypercalcaemia may be caused by a variety of disorders such as malignant disease, hyperparathyroidism, thyrotoxicosis, vitamin D intoxication, renal transplantation and acromegaly.

Thiazide diuretics, lithium, tamoxifen and calcium carbonate are examples of some of the drugs commonly implicated in causing hypercalcaemia.

Hypocalcaemia

Hypocalcaemia can be caused by a variety of disorders including vitamin D deficiency, disorders of vitamin D metabolism, hypoparathyroidism and acute pancreatitis.

For albumin < 40 g/L

Corrected calcium = [Ca] + 0.02 × (40 − [alb]) mmol/L

For albumin > 45 g/L

Corrected calcium = [Ca] − 0.02 ([alb] − 45) mmol/L

Fig. 4.2 Formula for correction of total plasma calcium concentration for changes in albumin concentration: albumin concentration = [alb] (albumin units = g/L); calcium concentration = [Ca] (total calcium units = mmol/L).

Anticonvulsant drugs such as phenytoin and phenobarbitone, aminoglycosides (e.g. gentamicin or amikacin), phosphate enemas and magnesium sulphate have all been implicated in causing hypocalcaemia.

Creatinine

The serum creatinine concentration of an individual is largely determined by its rate of production, rate of renal excretion and volume of distribution. It is frequently used to evaluate the renal function of an individual.

Creatinine is produced at a fairly constant rate from creatine and creatine phosphate in muscle. Daily production is constant, is a function of muscle mass and declines with age from 24 mg/kg/day in a healthy 25-year-old to 9 mg/kg/day in a 95-year-old. Creatinine undergoes complete glomerular filtration with little reabsorption by the renal tubules. Its clearance is therefore usually a good indicator of the glomerular filtration rate (GFR). As a general rule, and only at steady state, if the serum creatinine doubles this equates to a 50% reduction in the GFR and consequently renal function. Serum creatinine can be transiently elevated following meat ingestion (but less so than urea) or strenuous exercise. Individuals with a high muscle bulk produce more creatinine and therefore have a higher serum creatinine compared to an otherwise identical but less muscular individual.

The value for creatinine clearance is higher than the true GFR due to the active tubular secretion of creatinine. In a patient with a normal GFR this is of little significance. In an individual where the GFR is low (<10 ml/minute) the tubular secretion may make a significant contribution to creatinine elimination and overestimate the GFR. In this type of patient the breakdown of creatinine in the gut can also become a significant source of elimination.

Urea

The catabolism of dietary and endogenous amino acids in the body produces large amounts of ammonia. Ammonia is toxic and its concentration is kept very low by conversion in the liver to urea. Urea is eliminated in urine and represents the major route of nitrogen excretion. The urea is filtered from the blood at the renal glomerulus and undergoes significant tubular reabsorption. This tubular reabsorption is pronounced at low rates of urine flow. Moreover, urea levels vary widely with diet, rate of protein metabolism, liver production and the GFR. A high protein intake from the diet or following haemorrhage in the gut and consequent absorption of the protein from the blood may produce slightly elevated serum urea levels (up to 10 mmol/L). Urea concentrations of more than 10 mmol/L are usually due to renal disease or decreased renal blood flow following shock or dehydration. As with serum creatinine levels, serum urea levels do not begin to increase until the GFR has fallen by 50% or more.

Serum urea concentrations are often used as an index of renal glomerular function, although the serum creatinine provides a more accurate assessment. The production of urea is increased, as outlined above, by high protein intake, in hypercatabolic states or following a gastrointestinal bleed. Production is decreased in situations where there is a low protein intake and in some patients with liver disease. It is therefore essential that a change in urea should not be used to implicate a change in renal function without exploring possible extrarenal influences on the serum concentration of urea.

Albumin

Albumin is a protein synthesized in the liver. It has a half-life of about 20 days and comprises some 60% of total serum protein. The albumin in the body is mainly (60%) located in the interstitial compartment of the ECF. The remainder is located in the smaller, but relatively impermeable serum compartment, where it is present at a higher concentration than in the interstitial compartment. The concentration in the serum is important in maintaining serum volume since it accounts for approximately 80% of serum colloid osmotic pressure. A significant reduction in serum albumin concentration often results in oedema.

Albumin has an important role in binding, amongst others, calcium, bilirubin and many drugs. A reduction in serum albumin may increase free levels of agents which are normally bound and adverse effects may result if the 'free' entity is not rapidly cleared from the body.

A low serum albumin may occur in patients with chronic liver dysfunction due to impaired synthesis, or in malnutrition states where there is an inadequate supply of amino acids to maintain albumin production. Often the total body albumin concentration is appropriate although a low serum albumin level is measured. This may result from a dilutional hypoalbuminaemia or following a shift of albumin from serum to interstitial fluid. Dilutional hypoalbuminaemia may occur following parenteral infusion of excess protein-free fluid, or in fluid retention states such as pregnancy. The movement of albumin from serum into interstitial fluid is often associated with increased capillary permeability in postoperative patients or those with septicaemia. A shift of protein is known to occur physiologically when moving from lying down to the upright position. This can account for an increase in serum albumin of up to 10 g/L and contribute to the variation in serum concentration of highly bound drugs subjected to therapeutic drug monitoring.

Other causes of hypoalbuminaemia include catabolic states associated with a variety of illnesses, and increased loss of albumin from the body either from a damaged kidney as occurs in the nephrotic syndrome where it is lost in the urine; via the skin following burns or a skin disorder such as psoriasis; or from the intestinal wall in a protein-losing enteropathy.

An increase in serum albumin is rare and may be iatrogenic (e.g. inappropriate infusion of albumin) or the result of dehydration or shock.

Bilirubin

At the end of their life, red blood cells are broken down by the reticuloendothelial system mainly in the spleen. The haemoglobin molecules which are subsequently liberated are split into globin and haem. The globin enters the general protein pool, the iron in haem is reutilized and the re-maining tetrapyrrole ring of haem is degraded to bilirubin. This accounts for 80% of the formed bilirubin with myoglobin and the cytochromes largely contributing the remaining 20%.

The bilirubin in serum is usually classified as being unconjugated or conjugated. Unconjugated bilirubin is insoluble in water, soluble in fat and transported in the blood bound to albumin. This bound bilirubin is taken up by hepatocytes in the liver in a process involving specific carrier proteins. The bilirubin is transported to the smooth endoplasmic reticulum where it undergoes conjugation mainly with glucuronic acid. The conjugated bilirubin is water soluble and secreted into the gut in bile. In the gut it is broken down by bacteria into urobilinogen, a colourless compound, which is subsequently oxidized in the colon to urobilin, a brown pigment excreted in the stools. Some of the urobilinogen is absorbed and most is subsequently re-excreted in bile (enterohepatic circulation). A small amount is absorbed into the systemic circulation and excreted in urine where it too may be oxidized to the brown pigment urobilin.

The liver produces 300 mg of bilirubin each day. However, because the mature liver can metabolize and excrete up to 3 g daily, serum bilirubin concentrations are not a sensitive test of liver function.

The bilirubin in serum is normally unconjugated, bound to protein, not filtered by the glomeruli and does not normally appear in the urine. Bilirubin in the urine (bilirubinuria) usually reflects an increase in serum concentration of conjugated bilirubin and indicates an underlying pathological disorder.

An elevation of serum bilirubin concentration above 50 μmol/L (i.e. approximately 2.5 times the normal upper limit) will reveal itself as jaundice. The classical yellow discoloration of the skin and sclerae seen in this particular disorder is due to bilirubin deposition and is a feature of liver disease. Elevated bilirubin levels can be caused by increased production of bilirubin (e.g. haemolysis, ineffective erythropoiesis), impaired transport into hepatocytes (e.g. interference with bilirubin uptake by drugs such as rifampicin, hepatitis), decreased excretion (e.g. drugs such as rifampicin and methyltestosterone, intrahepatic obstruction due to cirrhosis, tumours etc.) or a combination of the above factors.

Glucose

The serum glucose concentration is largely determined by the balance of glucose moving into and leaving the extracellular compartment. In a healthy adult this movement is capable of maintaining serum levels below 10 mmol/L regardless of the intake of meals of varying carbohydrate content.

The renal tubules have the capacity to reabsorb all the glucose from the glomerular filtrate. Consequently, little unchanged glucose is normally lost from the body. Glucose in the urine (glycosuria) is normally only present when the concentration in serum exceeds 10 mmol/L at which it is said to exceed its renal threshold.

Normal ranges for serum glucose concentrations are often quoted as fasting (3.3 to 6.7 mmol/L) or non-fasting (<10.0 mmol/L) glucose concentration ranges. Fasting blood glucose levels are generally of greater diagnostic value. Blood glucose levels which exceed the upper normal values indicate impaired glucose tolerance. Other signs and symptoms if present, notably those attributable to an osmotic diuresis, will permit the diagnosis of diabetes mellitus to be made.

Uric acid

Uric acid is the end product of purine metabolism. The purines, which are used for nucleic acid synthesis, may be produced by the breakdown of nucleic acid from ingested meat or synthesized within the body.

Monosodium urate is the form in which uric acid usually exists at the normal pH of body fluids. The term urate is used to represent any salt of uric acid.

Two main factors contribute to elevated serum uric acid levels: an increased rate of formation and reduced excretion. Uric acid is poorly soluble and an elevation in serum concentration may readily result in deposition, as monosodium urate, in tissues or joints. Deposition usually precipitates an acute attack of gouty arthritis.

The aim of treatment is to reduce the concentration of uric acid and prevent further attacks of gout. Low serum uric acid levels appear to be of no clinical significance.

Enzymes

Throughout the body there are a wide variety of enzymes which can be measured and provide valuable diagnostic information (Table 4.8).

Many enzymes are located within cells and are only present in blood in very small amounts as a consequence of normal cell turnover. When a cell is damaged increased amounts of the intracellular enzymes are released into the blood. Other factors can also elevate blood enzyme levels. Typical examples include increased cell turnover, cell proliferation of neoplasia, increased enzyme synthesis, obstruction to secretion and decreased clearance.

It is important to remember that the assay of 'serum enzymes' is a measurement of catalytic activity and not actual enzyme concentration. Activity can vary depending on assay conditions and consequently the reference range between laboratories may vary widely.

Whilst the measurement of enzymes may be very specific, the enzymes themselves may not be specific to a particular tissue or cell. Many enzymes arise in more than one tissue and an increase in the serum activity of one enzyme can represent damage to any one of the tissues which contain the enzyme. In practice this problem may be circumvented because some tissues contain two or more enzymes in different proportions which are released on damage. For example, alanine and aspartate transaminase both occur

Table 4.8 Enzyme data: typical normal adult reference values (conventional units) in serum	
Laboratory test	Reference range
Acid phosphatase	0.5–11 units/L
Alanine transaminase	0–35 units/L
Alkaline phosphatase	25–100 units/L
Aspartate transaminase	0–35 units/L
Creatine kinase	0–105 units/L
Gamma-glutamyl transpeptidase	0–40 units/L
Lactate dehydrogenase	50–190 units/L

in cardiac muscle and liver cells but their site of origin can often be differentiated because there is more alanine transaminase in the liver than the heart. In those situations where it is not possible to look at the relative ratio of enzymes it is often possible to differentiate the same enzyme from different tissues. Such enzymes often have the same catalytic activity but differ in some other measurable property and are referred to as isoenzymes.

The measured activity of an enzyme will be dependent upon the time it was sampled relative to its time of release from the cell. If a sample is drawn too early after a particular insult to a tissue there may be no detectable enzyme activity. If it is drawn too late the enzyme may be cleared from the blood and no activity detected.

Alkaline phosphatase

Alkaline phosphatases are a group of enzymes present in most tissues. Their exact metabolic function is unclear although they are thought to play an important role in the calcification of bone. They are present in high concentrations in the liver, bone (osteoblasts), intestinal wall and placenta. Each site of origin produces a specific isoenzyme of alkaline phosphatase.

Physiological increases in serum alkaline phosphatase activity occur in pregnancy due to release of the placental isoenzyme and during periods of growth in children and adolescents when the bone isoenzyme is released.

Pathological increases in serum alkaline phosphatase of bone origin may arise in disorders such as osteomalacia and rickets, Paget's disease of bone, bone tumours, renal bone disease, osteomyelitis and healing fractures. Disorders of the liver which may elevate alkaline phosphatase include intra- or extrahepatic cholestasis, space-occupying lesions (e.g. tumour, abscess) and hepatitis. Inflammatory bowel disease may elevate the level of intestinal alkaline phosphatase.

Acid phosphatase

Acid phosphatase is present in the prostate, liver, erythrocytes, platelets and bone. It is found in high concentrations in the prostate gland and its serum concentration is elevated in some patients with cancer of the prostate. However, its role in the diagnosis of this disorder is limited since serum activity is only elevated in about 20% of patients with a tumour solely of the gland. In patients who have cancer of the prostate with metastases the serum level is raised in some 80% of patients. It is therefore of greater clinical value in this latter situation where it can be used to monitor treatment.

The measurement of acid phosphatase will probably decline in the future since a prostate-specific antigen (PSA) can now be measured and used diagnostically to detect cancer of the prostate, and associated metastasis.

Transaminases

The two transaminases of diagnostic use are aspartate transaminase (AST; also known as serum glutamate-oxaloacetate transaminase, SGOT) and alanine transaminase (ALT; also known as serum glutamate-pyruvate transaminase, SGPT). The two enzymes are found in many body tissues with aspartate transaminase being generally found in the lower concentration. The exception to this rule is the liver where they are present in equivalent amounts. There are no tissue-specific isoenzymes of aspartate transaminase.

Serum aspartate transaminase levels are increased in a variety of disorders including acute hepatitis and liver necrosis, crush injuries, severe tissue hypoxaemia, myocardial infarction, surgery, trauma, muscle disease, cholestasis, chronic hepatitis and pancreatitis. Alanine transaminase is elevated to a similar extent in the disorders listed which involve the liver and to a lesser extent, if at all, in the other disorders.

Gamma-glutamyl transpeptidase

Gamma-glutamyl transpeptidase (GGT; also known as gamma-glutamyl transferase) is present in high concentrations in the liver, kidney and pancreas where it is found within the endoplasmic reticulum of cells. It is a sensitive indicator of hepatobiliary disease but is of little value in differentiating a cholestatic disorder from hepatocellular disease. It can also be elevated in alcoholic liver disease, hepatitis, cirrhosis, pancreatitis and congestive cardiac failure.

Serum levels of gamma-glutamyl transpeptidase activity can be raised in the absence of disease. This situation arises when an increase in enzyme production occurs within cells with the enzyme being subsequently released into serum as part of normal cell turnover. Drugs which cause enzyme induction such as phenytoin, phenobarbitone and rifampicin have this effect and patients so treated will have elevated levels of gamma-glutamyl transpeptidase.

Serum gamma-glutamyl transpeptidase activity is usually raised in an individual with alcoholic liver disease. However, it can also be raised in heavy drinkers of alcohol who do not have liver damage, due to enzyme induction. Its activity can remain elevated for up to 4 weeks after stopping alcohol intake.

Lactate dehydrogenase

Lactate dehydrogenase (LD) has five isoenzymes (LD_1 to LD_5). Total lactate dehydrogenase activity is rarely measured because of the lack of tissue specificity. The enzyme is widely distributed throughout the body with high concentrations being found in heart muscle, skeletal muscle, liver, kidney, brain and erythrocytes. Levels of activity are elevated following damage to the liver, skeletal muscle and kidneys in patients with lymphoma, and in both megaloblastic and haemolytic anaemias. Elevation of LD_1 and LD_2 occurs after myocardial infarction, renal infarction or megaloblastic anaemia; LD_2 and LD_3 are elevated in acute leukaemia; LD_3 is often elevated when there is a malignancy of many tissues; and LD_5 is elevated after damage to liver or skeletal muscle.

Lactate dehydrogenase isoenzyme LD_1 is often measured following a suspected myocardial infarction. This isoenzyme shows greater catalytic activity with α-hydroxybutyrate as a substrate compared to the other isoenzymes and this substrate is used for its measurement in the laboratory. Consequently it is often referred to as α-hydroxybutyrate dehydrogenase (HBD).

Following a myocardial infarction peak serum levels are achieved after 2 to 3 days after which they decline over 7 or more days.

Creatine kinase

Creatine kinase (CK) is present in relatively high concentrations in heart muscle, skeletal muscle and the brain in addition to being present in smooth muscle and other tissues. Levels are markedly increased following shock and circulatory failure, myocardial infarction and muscular dystrophies. Less marked increases have been reported following muscle injury, surgery, physical exercise, muscle cramp, epileptic fit, intramuscular injection and hypothyroidism.

Creatine kinase has two protein subunits, M and B, which combine to form three isoenzymes, BB, MM and MB. BB is found in high concentrations in the brain, thyroid and some smooth muscle tissue. Little of this enzyme is present in the serum even following damage to the brain. The enzyme found in serum of normal subjects is the MM isoenzyme which originates from skeletal muscle.

Cardiac tissue contains more of the MB isoenzyme than skeletal muscle. Following a myocardial infarction there is a characteristic increase in serum creatine kinase activity. It is often unnecessary to measure activity of the MB isoenzyme unless there is a possibility of a contribution of creatinine kinase from another source. Such a situation may arise in an individual with a suspected myocardial infarction which occurs after exercise, trauma or an intramuscular injection.

HAEMATOLOGY DATA

The haematology profile is an essential part of the investigation of all hospital inpatients and not just those with primary haematological disease.

Typical measurements reported in a haematology screen with their normal values are shown in Table 4.9, whilst a list of the common descriptive terms used in haematology are presented in Table 4.10.

Table 4.9 Haematology data: typical normal adult reference values

	Normal range
Haemoglobin (Hb)	13.5–18.0 g/dl males
	12.0–16.0 g/dl females
Red blood cell count (RBC)	$4.5–6.5 \times 10^{12}$/L males
	$4.0–6.0 \times 10^{12}$/L females
Reticulocyte count	0.5–1.5% of erythrocytes
Packed cell volume (PCV)	0.4–0.54 males
	0.37–0.49 females
Mean cell volume (MCV)	80–100 fl
Mean cell haemoglobin (MCH)	27–32 pg
Mean cell haemoglobin concentration (MCHC)	31–36 g/dl
White cell count (leucocytes)	$3.5–11.0 \times 10^9$/L
Differential white cell count:	
Neutrophils (30–75%)	$1.5–7.5 \times 10^9$/L
Lymphocytes (5–15%)	$1.0–4.0 \times 10^9$/L
Monocytes (2–10%)	$0.2–0.8 \times 10^9$/L
Basophils (<1%)	$< 0.1 \times 10^9$/L
Eosinophils (1–6%)	$0.04–0.4 \times 10^9$/L
Platelets	$150–400 \times 10^9$/L
Erythrocyte sedimentation rate (ESR)	< 10 mm/hour
Serum iron	12–30 µmol/L
Total iron binding capacity (TIBC)	45–70 µmol/L
Serum ferritin	24–300 µcg/L males
	15–300 µcg/L females

Table 4.10 Descriptive terms in common use in haematology

Anisocytosis	Abnormal variation in cell size (usually refers to RBCs), e.g. red cells in iron deficiency anaemia
Agranulocytosis	Lack of granulocytes (principally neutrophils)
Aplastic	Depression of synthesis of all cell types in bone marrow (as in aplastic anaemia)
Basophilia	Increased number of basophils
Hypochromic	MCHC low, red cells appear pale microscopically
Leucocytosis	Increased white cell count
Leucopenia	Reduced white cell count
Macrocytic	Large cells
Microcytic	Small cells
Neutropenia	Reduced neutrophil count
Neutrophilia	Increased neutrophil count
Normochromic	MCHC normal; red cells appear normally pigmented
Pancytopenia	Decreased number of all cell types: it is synonymous with aplastic anaemia
Poikilocytosis	Abnormal variation in cell shape, e.g. some red cells appear pear shaped in macrocytic anaemias
Polychromasia, polychromatic	Many reticulocytes present
Thrombocytopenia	Lack of platelets

Red blood cell count (RBC)

Red blood cells are produced in the bone marrow by the process of erythropoiesis. One of the major stimulants of this process is erythropoietin, produced mainly in the kidney. Immature erythroblasts develop into mature erythrocytes which are then released into the circulation.

Erythroblasts → normoblasts → reticulocytes → erythrocytes
(nucleated)　　(non-nucleated)

Normally only mature, non-nucleated erythrocytes are seen in the peripheral blood.

The lifespan of a mature red cell is usually about 120 days. If this is shortened, as for instance in haemolysis, the circulating mass of red cells is reduced and with it the supply of oxygen to tissues is decreased. In these circumstances, red cell production is enhanced in healthy bone marrow by an increased output of erythropoietin. Red cells are destroyed either by rupturing within the circulation or by removal by the reticuloendothelial system such as the spleen and liver.

The most common cause of a low RBC is anaemia. Some of the different types of anaemia may be identified by measurement and microscopic examination of the red blood cells, since cells may be microcytic (e.g. iron deficiency anaemia) or macrocytic (e.g. in folic acid and vitamin B_{12} deficiency anaemias).

A high RBC (erythrocytosis or polycythaemia) indicates increased production by the bone marrow and may occur as a physiological response to hypoxia, as in chronic airways disease, or as a carcinoma of red cells such as polycythaemia rubra vera.

Reticulocytes

Reticulocytes are the earliest non-nucleated red cells. They owe their name to the fine net-like appearance of their cytoplasm which can be seen, after appropriate staining, under the microscope and contains fine threads of RNA in a reticular network. Reticulocytes normally represent between 0.5 and 1.5% of the total RBC and do not feature significantly in a normal blood profile. However, increased production (reticulocytosis) can be detected in times of rapid red cell regeneration as occurs in response to haemorrhage or haemolysis. At such times the reticulocyte count may reach 40% of the RBC. The reticulocyte count may be useful in assessing the marrow's response to iron, folate or vitamin B_{12} therapy. The count peaks at about 7 to 10 days after starting such therapy and then subsides.

Mean cell volume (MCV)

The mean cell volume is the average volume of a single red cell. It is measured in femtolitres (10^{-15} litres). Terms such as microcytic and macrocytic are descriptive of a low and high MCV, respectively. They are useful in the process of identification of various types of anaemias such as iron deficiency (microcytic) and megaloblastic (macrocytic) anaemias.

Packed cell volume (PCV) (haematocrit)

The PCV or haematocrit is the volume of red cells in 100 ml of whole blood. It can be measured by centrifuging a capillary tube of blood and then expressing the volume of red cells packed in the bottom as a percentage of the total volume. It is reported as a fraction of unity or as a percentage, e.g. 0.45 or 45%. PCV is calculated nowadays as the product of MCV and RBC. PCV often reflects the RBC and will therefore be decreased in any sort of anaemia, in haemorrhage or haemolysis. It will be raised in polycythaemia and pregnancy. It may however be altered irrespective of RBC, when the size of the red cell is abnormal as in macrocytosis and microcytosis.

Mean cell haemoglobin (MCH)

MCH is the average weight of haemoglobin contained in a red cell. It is measured in picograms (10^{-12} gram) and is calculated from the relationship:

$$MCH = \frac{Haemoglobin}{RBC}$$

MCH is dependent on the size of the red cells as well as the concentration of haemoglobin in the cells. Thus it is usually low in iron deficiency anaemia when there is microcytosis and there is less haemoglobin in each cell, but it may be raised in macrocytic anaemia.

Mean cell haemoglobin concentration (MCHC)

MCHC is a measure of the average concentration of haemoglobin in 100 ml of red cells. It is usually expressed as grams/decilitre but may be reported as a percentage. MCHC will be reported low in conditions of reduced haemoglobin synthesis, such as iron deficiency anaemia. In contrast, in macrocytic anaemias MCHC may be normal or only slightly reduced, because the large red cells may contain more haemoglobin, thus giving a concentration approximating that of normal cells. MCHC can be raised in severe prolonged dehydration. If MCHC is low, the descriptive term hypochromic may be used (for example a hypochromic anaemia) whereas normochromic describes a normal MCHC.

Haemoglobin

The haemoglobin concentration in males is normally greater than in females, reflecting in part the higher RBC in men. Lower concentrations in women are due at least in part to menstrual loss.

Haemoglobin is measured to detect anaemia and this is its most common application.

In some relatively rare genetic diseases, the haemoglobinopathies, alterations in the structure of the haemoglobin molecule can be detected by electrophoresis. Abnormal haemoglobins which can be detected in this manner include HbS (sickle haemoglobin in sickle cell disease) and HbA_2 found in β-thalassaemia carriers.

Platelets (thrombocytes)

Platelets are formed in the bone marrow. A marked reduction in platelet number (thrombocytopenia) may reflect either a depressed synthesis in the marrow or destruction of formed platelets.

Platelets are normally present in the circulation for 8 to 12 days, a useful fact when evaluating a possible drug-induced thrombocytopenia, since recovery should be fairly swift when the offending agent is withdrawn.

A small decrease in the platelet count may be seen in pregnancy and following viral infections. Severe thrombocytopenia may result in spontaneous bleeding. A reduced platelet count is also found in disseminated intravascular coagulation which manifests clinically as severe haemorrhages particularly in the skin and results in rapid consumption of clotting factors and platelets.

An increased platelet count (thrombocytosis) occurs in malignancy, inflammatory disease and in response to blood loss.

Erythrocyte sedimentation rate (ESR)

The ESR is a measure of the settling rate of red cells in a sample of anticoagulated blood, over a period of 1 hour, in a cylindrical tube.

In health the normal value is less than 10 mm/hour. The Westergren method, performed under standardized conditions, is commonly used in haematology laboratories. The ESR is strongly correlated with the ability of red cells to aggregate into orderly stacks or rouleaux. In disease, the most common cause of a high ESR is an increased protein level in the blood, such as the increase in acute phase proteins seen in inflammatory disease. Proteins are thought to affect the repellent surface charges on red cells and cause them to aggregate into rouleaux and hence the sedimentation rate increases. Although some conditions may cause a low ESR, the test is principally used to monitor inflammatory disease. ESR may be raised in the active phase of rheumatoid arthritis, inflammatory bowel disease, malignant disease and infection. ESR is non-specific and therefore of little diagnostic value, but serial tests are helpful in following the progress of disease and its response to treatment.

White blood cell count (WBC)

White cells (leukocytes) are comprised of two types of cell – the granulocytes and the agranular cells. They are made up of various types of cells (Fig. 4.3) with different functions and it is logical to consider them separately. A haematology profile often reports a total white cell count and a differential count, the latter separating the composition of white cells into the various types.

Neutrophils

Neutrophils or polymorphonucleocytes (PMNs) are the most abundant white cell. They have a phagocytic function, with many enzymes contained in the lysosomal granules. They are formed in the bone marrow from the stem cells which form myoblasts and these develop through a number of stages into the neutrophil with a multiple-segmented nucleus. Neutrophils constitute approximately 40 to 70% of circulating white cells in normal healthy blood. Their circulating life is 10 to 20 days. The neutrophil count increases in the presence of infection, tissue

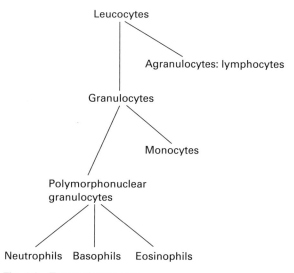

Fig. 4.3 Types of white cells.

damage (e.g. infarction) and inflammation (e.g. rheumatoid arthritis, acute gout). Neutropenia, also described as agranulocytosis in its severest forms, is associated with malignancy and drug toxicity, but also may occur in viral infections such as influenza, infectious mononucleosis and hepatitis.

Basophils

Basophils normally constitute a small proportion of the white cell count. Their function is poorly understood but basophilia occurs in various malignant and pre-malignant disorders such as leukaemia and myelofibrosis.

Eosinophils

Eosinophils represent normally less than 6% of the white cells. Their function appears to be concerned with inactivation of mediators released from mast cells, and eosinophilia is therefore apparent in many allergic conditions such as asthma, hay fever and drug sensitivity reactions as well as some malignant diseases.

Monocytes

Monocytes are macrophages. Their number increases in some infections such as typhoid, subacute bacterial endocarditis, infectious mononucleosis and tuberculosis.

Lymphocytes

Lymphocytes are the second most abundant white cells after neutrophils in the circulating blood, but the majority of them are found in the spleen and other lymphatic tissue. They are formed in the bone marrow (B-lymphocytes) and the thymus (T-lymphocytes). An increase in lymphocyte numbers occurs particularly in viral infections such as rubella, mumps, infectious hepatitis and infectious mononucleosis.

Other blood tests

Monitoring anticoagulant therapy

Blood clotting in the body is mediated through a cascade of coagulation factors which can be split into an extrinsic and an intrinsic element. The extrinsic and intrinsic pathways can be evaluated in the laboratory by the prothrombin time (PT) and the activated partial thromboplastin time (APTT).

Extrinsic pathway. In vivo, phospholipoproteins and organelle membranes from damaged tissue cells enter the blood. These phospholipids or tissue factors are normally extrinsic to the circulation but when released into the blood they activate various coagulation factors which constitute the so-called extrinsic pathway. Factor VII binds to these lipids and is activated to Factor VIIa. This in turn activates Factor X to Xa in the presence of calcium ions.

$$\text{VII} + Ca^{2+} + \text{Tissue factor} \longrightarrow \text{VIIa} \longrightarrow \text{X}$$

Intrinsic pathway. The intrinsic system depends on substances normally present in blood for its activation. The intrinsic mechanism is initiated by activation of factor XII to XIIa. This activation occurs in vivo by adsorption on to negatively charged surfaces such as subendothelial collagen (exposed by injury to blood vessels) or, in vitro, by adsorption on to surfaces such as glass or kaolin. Surface adsorption activates factor XII by exposing an active enzyme site. Factor XIIa then activates XI and so on.

Foreign surface $\longrightarrow$ XII $\longrightarrow$ XIIa $\longrightarrow$ XI $\longrightarrow$ XIa
contact $\qquad \longrightarrow$ IX+Ca^{2+} $\longrightarrow$ IXa (+VII+Ca^{2+} + PF3)
$\qquad \longrightarrow$ X

(PF3 is platelet factor 3, a phospholipid which has a partial thromboplastic action.)

Common pathway. The extrinsic and intrinsic pathways converge at the level of Factor X, from which there is a common pathway whereby thrombin and fibrin are eventually formed, leading to formation of a fibrin clot.

One stage prothrombin time (PT)

The prothrombin time (PT) is a test used to measure the clotting time of plasma in the presence of tissue extract (thromboplastin) and indicates the overall efficiency of the extrinsic system. It is used to monitor warfarin therapy (warfarin inhibits the formation of factors II, VII,

IX and X). The test involves adding extrinsic thromboplastin (a phospholipid extract of mammalian tissue, e.g. brain) to citrated plasma and adding calcium to clot the mixture. The time to form the fibrin clot is recorded. Control blood has a PT of 12 to 15 seconds.

The results of the test are commonly expressed as a ratio of the PT time of the patient compared with that of the normal control. This is known as the international normalized ratio, (INR; previously the British comparative ratio, BCR).

$$INR = \frac{Patient's\ PT}{Control\ PT}$$

The desirable ratio varies according to the indication for the anticoagulant, and the limits chosen vary from centre to centre. Patients with atrial fibrillation can be treated at an INR of 1.7 to 2.5, whereas those with recurrent deep vein thrombosis and pulmonary embolisms require an INR of 3 to 4.5.

The most common use of the PT and INR is to monitor oral anticoagulant therapy, but it can also be used to assess liver function.

Thrombotest

This test measures the function of the extrinsic system but has largely been replaced by the PT and INR in the United Kingdom. Results are expressed as a percentage (normal control = 100%). With increasing anticoagulation, the percentage falls and the desired therapeutic end point is about 10 to 15%.

Activated partial thromboplastin time (APTT)

The APTT is used to assess the intrinsic pathway and is the most common method for monitoring heparin therapy.

A thromboplastic reagent (a preparation of phospholipid extracted from an animal or vegetable source) acts as a substitute for platelet phospholipids. The reagent is added to an activator such as activated silicone. If the activator is kaolin, the test may be referred to as the PTTK (partial thromboplastin time kaolin) or the KCCT (kaolin cephalin clotting time). Cephalin is a brain extract supplying the thromboplastin.

The mixture of thromboplastin and activator is mixed with citrated plasma to which calcium is added and the time for the mixture to clot is recorded. The normal range is 30 to 40 seconds. The desirable APTT for optimal heparin therapy is between 1½ and 2½ times the normal range.

Coombs' test

Coombs' reagent is a mixture of antihuman immunoglobulin antibody and anticomplement antibody. When added to washed red blood cells, it will detect antibody or complement on the cell surface and cause agglutination of the red cells. The test is positive (i.e. agglutination occurs) in cases of autoimmune anaemia.

Serum iron, iron binding capacity and ferritin

Iron circulating in the serum is bound to transferrin. It leaves the serum pool and enters the bone marrow where it becomes incorporated into haemoglobin in developing red cells. Serum iron levels are extremely labile and fluctuate throughout the day. In normal adults the total iron binding capacity (TIBC) is about one-third saturated with iron.

Serum iron is decreased in iron deficiency anaemia after iron stores have been depleted, in chronic inflammatory disease and in malignancy. Serum TIBC is low in infection but is increased in iron deficiency anaemia.

Measurement of serum ferritin is a useful method of estimating iron stores. Serum ferritin concentration is directly related to the available storage iron in the body. The serum ferritin level falls below the normal range in iron deficiency anaemia and its measurement provides a useful monitor for repletion of iron stores after iron therapy.

BIBLIOGRAPHY

O'Connor N, Bunch C. Laboratory diagnosis in haematology. Medicine International 1991; 96: 3984–3989
Tietz N W (ed). Clinical guide to laboratory tests, 2nd edn. London: W B Saunders, 1990
Zilva J F, Pannall P R, Mayne P D (eds). Clinical chemistry in diagnosis and treatment, 5th edn. London: Edward Arnold, 1988

Chapter 5

Parenteral nutrition

M. Malone

The safe infusion of nutritional substrates by the central intravenous route was not developed until the late 1960s. Since then progress has been made in establishing intravenous nutritional requirements under normal circumstances and also during different types of illness. Recently efforts have been concentrated on the development of new substrates and of improved infusion methods and devices. The provision of nutritional support by the intravenous route is now commonplace in hospitals and may also be continued on a long-term basis at home.

Parenteral nutrition is expensive, complex and can be associated with life-threatening complications. The use of parenteral nutrition is usually therefore restricted to situations where the gastrointestinal tract is non-functional or inaccessible. The term intestinal failure has been used to describe this situation and, like renal failure, it may be acute or chronic. The principal indications for TPN are shown in Table 5.1.

Specially formulated nutrients can be delivered directly into the gastrointestinal tract, and this is referred to as enteral nutrition. This may be administered by mouth or by tube feeding either nasoenteric or via an enterostomy. Enteral nutrition has the advantage of being more physiological, less complicated and about 10% of the cost of TPN. The principal indications for enteral nutrition are shown in Table 5.2. Many others exist but can be summarized as those patients who fail to maintain their nutritional status and require artificial support preferably

Table 5.1 Principal indications for total parenteral nutrition in adult patients

Preoperative	Malnourished patient > 10% recent weight loss
Postoperative complications	Sepsis, fistulae, ileus or gastrointestinal stasis
Short bowel syndrome	Post-infarction of bowel, trauma
Gastrointestinal disease	Crohn's disease, ulcerative colitis, pancreatitis, radiation enteritis, malabsorption
Major trauma	Burns, accidents, intensive care patients, acute renal failure

Table 5.2 Principal indications for enteral nutrition

Upper gastrointestinal disorders	Neoplasm, trauma, fractures of head and neck
Lower gastrointestinal disorders	Malabsorption states for a variety of causes
Post-trauma	Intensive care patients, burns, coma

via the enteral route unless it is non-functional, when the intravenous route should be used.

COMPONENTS OF A TPN REGIMEN

An intravenous nutritional regimen aims to supply all the nutrients that would be consumed or considered essential in a normal diet. Each regimen is individually tailored to meet the requirements of a particular patient. It will be designed to contain the correct amounts of water, protein, carbohydrate, fat, electrolytes, trace elements and vitamins. The feeding regimen is designed to account for baseline requirements and any abnormal losses or additional requirements due to the disease process. Some of these will be discussed later.

Taking each of the components in turn:

Water

Water is the principal component of the human body and accounts for more than 50% of total body weight.

The maintenance or baseline requirements for the volume of fluid required can be estimated using the formula shown below:

$$\text{ml/day} = 1500 \text{ ml} + 20 \times (\text{body weight} - 20 \text{ kg})$$

For example, for a 70 kg man:

$$\text{Fluid requirement} = 1500 + 20 \times (70 - 20)$$
$$= 2500 \text{ ml/24 h}$$

Alternatively an estimate of requirements can be made by assuming a baseline requirement of 30 to 35 ml/kg, i.e. $70 \times 35 = 2450$ ml.

It should be stressed that these are estimated requirements and that the actual requirement will be tailored to the individual during the initial course of feeding.

The estimated fluid requirement is based on loss of 1500 ml in urine, 200 ml in faeces, 400 ml via sweating and 400 ml from the lungs. That lost via sweating and from the lungs is termed insensible loss. A small volume, approximately 200 to 400 ml is produced by catabolism or breakdown and utilization of body metabolic stores.

The baseline requirements for water will be affected by a number of factors:

Fever. Allow 10 to 15% of water extra for each °C of body temperature above normal. This is to account for increased insensible loss during sweating and from the lungs during hyperventilation.

Increased anabolism. Initially when converting a patient from a starved to an anabolic state more water will be required to provide for new cells.

High environmental temperature. This will increase fluid requirements.

Humidity. High humidity will decrease fluid requirements and low humidity will increase them.

Abnormal losses from the gastrointestinal tract. Losses of fluid, for example as vomit, stoma losses or diarrhoea, all increase requirements.

Abnormal loss from the skin. This occurs particularly when the epithelial layer is lost or damaged, e.g. in burns patients or from an open wound.

Drug therapy. Parenteral administration of

drugs may contribute significantly to fluid intake and will need to be accounted for in the overall total requirement.

Cardiac failure. Impairment of cardiac function may limit the electrolytes and volume of fluid which would ideally be administered.

Renal failure. An inability to excrete water and electrolytes effectively will alter the fluid requirements of the patient and may compromise the nutrient intake depending on the degree of impairment.

Protein

Protein is administered in the form of L-amino acids. Of the 20 amino acids required for protein synthesis, 8 are considered to be essential because they cannot be synthesized in the body. Some amino acids are semi-essential in that their requirements exceed supply in specific cases, e.g. histidine is essential in infants whilst cysteine, tyrosine and taurine may be essential in neonates. The remaining amino acids are considered non-essential.

The amount of protein required depends on the clinical situation and the degree of malnutrition. Protein requirements are usually prescribed in grams of nitrogen (1 g nitrogen = 6.25 g protein). Most commercial solutions specify the strength in grams of nitrogen per litre. Many solutions are available and vary in their amino acid content and also other components they contain, such as electrolytes, glucose and antioxidants.

The protein requirements can be estimated using the values given in Table 5.3.

An additional 2 to 4 g of nitrogen per litre

of fistula output may be required. Patients who have been starved may also have increased requirements.

When nutrition is being administered the individual requirements can be tailored on the basis of nitrogen excretion in the urine, faeces and any abnormal losses. The amount that is then given is the total amount lost plus 2 to 3 g per 24 hours.

Calorie requirements

The resting energy expenditure is estimated to be 30 to 35 kcal/kg per 24 hours. This is affected by injury and sepsis and varies throughout the course of the illness. The calorie:nitrogen ratio may vary between 200:1 in hypermetabolic patients to 100:1 in non-catabolic individuals.

Many nomograms and equations have been developed to estimate energy expenditure.

Carbohydrate

Carbohydrate is usually provided in the form of dextrose. Other sources have been used in the past but have been less effective and are associated with greater metabolic problems. The calorie content and osmolality of commonly used dextrose solutions are shown in Table 5.4.

The concentrated solutions are hypertonic and of low pH (pH 3 to 5) and are therefore irritant to vessel walls. They should be administered via a central venous line directly into the fast flowing blood in the right atrium to dilute the solution as rapidly as possible.

Table 5.3 Daily nitrogen requirements in adult patients with altered metabolic states	
Patient's metabolic state	Nitrogen requirement g/kg/24 h
Basal	0.15
Catabolic	0.2
Hypercatabolic (burns/severe trauma)	0.3

Table 5.4 The energy and osmolality values of dextrose solutions		
Dextrose solution concentration (w/v)	Energy kcal/L	Osmolality mOsm/kg
5%	190	278
10%	380	555
20%	760	1110
50%	1900	2775
70%	2660	3885
Useful information: 1 g anhydrous dextrose provides 3.8 kcal; plasma osmolality 282–295 mOsm/kg		

Fat

Fat is required for the provision of essential fatty acids and as a vehicle for fat-soluble vitamins. In addition it is useful as a calorie source (9 kcal/g). A biochemical deficiency state may occur after 4 weeks of TPN in patients who are not given fat. It has been suggested that 500 ml of 10% fat emulsion infused per week is sufficient to prevent deficiency.

Fat emulsions available in the UK are based on soya bean oils. They are either long-chain triglyceride (LCT) or mixed LCT and medium-chain triglyceride (MCT) emulsions. Some commercially available preparations are shown in Table 5.5. Fat emulsions are useful as they provide a high calorie source in a low volume. They are isotonic with plasma and can be given through peripheral vessels without causing major damage.

Electrolytes

The daily i.v. requirement of each of the electrolytes commonly monitored, common sources and purpose of each are shown in Table 5.6. Electrolyte requirements may vary in the first week of TPN but usually become stable as the clinical condition of the patient stabilizes. Alterations in requirements due to abnormal losses or excretion will be discussed later.

Trace elements

Trace elements can also be called micronutrients as they are essential yet required in very small quantities. Many trace elements are involved as cofactors in enzyme systems. Deficiency of most trace elements is uncommon in TPN of less than 3 months' duration unless the patient was previously severely malnourished. This applies to all except zinc which may become deficient much earlier in treatment particularly in patients with diarrhoea or high output fistulae, as each litre lost contains 12 to 17 mg of zinc. Zinc deficiency may cause diarrhoea, alopecia and a distinctive skin rash.

The common trace elements, their source, deficiency state and daily i.v. requirement are shown in Table 5.7. They are usually added routinely in standard quantities to TPN regimens and supplemented with individual elements as necessary.

Vitamins

Vitamins can be divided into those which are fat soluble and those which are water soluble. Fat-soluble vitamins are stored in the body and are unlikely to become depleted in the short term. Water-soluble vitamins which are excreted renally are not stored to a large extent.

Deficiency syndromes associated with particular vitamins are shown in Table 5.8, along with the recommended intake per 24 hours and examples of commercially available preparations.

METHODS OF DELIVERY

Ideally all the nutrients to be administered intravenously for a 24-hour period should be mixed together in a single container. These commonly contain up to 3 litres of fluid but other sizes are available. These are aseptically prepared in the pharmacy or purchased from commercial production units. Where this system is unavailable or impractical due to rapidly changing requirements, the separate components are infused individually from bottles. This latter system is more likely to become contaminated by bacteria

Table 5.5 Fat emulsions used in total parenteral nutrition			
Solution	kcal/L	kJ/L	Content/L
Intralipid 10%	1100	4600	Fractionated soya oil 100 g Glycerol 22.5 g
Intralipid 20%	2000	8400	Fractionated soya oil 200 g Glycerol 22.5 g
Lipofundin MCT/LCT 10%	1054	4430	Soya oil 50 g MCT 50 g
Lipofundin MCT/LCT 20%	1904	8000	Soya oil 100 g MCT 100 g
Lipofundin S 10%	1064	4470	Soya oil 100 g
Lipofundin S 20%	2029	8520	Soya oil 200 g

Table 5.6 Electrolyte requirements and purpose

Electrolyte	Principal function	Daily intravenous requirement	Symptoms of deficiency	Symptoms of excess	Common sources
Sodium	Main extracellular cation Regulation of water balance Neuromuscular contractility	1–2 mmol/kg	Weakness, lethargy, confusion, convulsions, appetite, nausea and vomiting	Lethargy, coma, convulsions, muscle, rigidity, thirst	Sodium chloride Sodium acetate Sodium phosphate
Potassium	Main intracellular cation Regulation of acid–base balance Neuromuscular contractility	1–2 mmol/kg	Muscle weakness, ileus, arrhythmias, alkalosis	Muscle weakness, paraesthesia, bradycardia, nausea and vomiting	Potassium chloride Potassium phosphate
Magnesium	Cofactor for enzyme systems Neuromuscular contractility	0.1–0.2 mmol/kg	Lethargy, cramps, tetany, paraesthesia, arrhythmias, neuromuscular excitability, hypokalaemia, hypocalcaemia	Decreased muscular activity, lethargy, respiratory depression	Magnesium sulphate Magnesium chloride
Calcium	Mineralization: bones + teeth Neuromuscular contractility	0.1–0.15 mmol/kg	Paraesthesia, tetany, fitting, confusion, arrhythmias	Nausea, anorexia, lethargy, muscle weakness, confusion	Calcium gluconate Calcium chloride
Phosphate	Main intracellular anion Acid–base balance Energy	0.5–0.7 mmol/kg	Weakness, tingling	Non-specific effects on calcium balance	Phosphate salts of sodium & potassium, hydrogen
Chloride	Main extracellular anion Acid–base balance	1–2 mmol/kg	Alkalosis	Acidosis	Chloride salts of above cations

Table 5.7 Trace element requirements

Element	Daily i.v. requirement	Deficiency	Commercially available source
Zinc	50–100 micromoles	Poor wound healing + growth, alopecia, infertility, poor resistance to infection	Zinc sulphate, Additrace, Addamel
Manganese	7 micromoles	? Vit K deficiency	Nutracel, Addamel, Additrace, Manganese chloride
Copper	5 micromoles	Bone marrow function	Copper sulphate, Additrace, Addamel
Iron	50 micromoles	Anaemia	Additrace, Addamel
Chromium	1 micromole	Glucose intolerance	Additrace, Chromium chloride
Molybdenum	200 nanomoles	Arrhythmias + night blindness	Additrace
Selenium	400 nanomoles	Cardiomyopathy, muscle pain	Sodium selenite, Additrace

Table 5.8 Vitamin requirements

Vitamin	Unit	i.v. daily requirement	Purpose	Deficiency syndrome	Commercial i.v. source
Water-soluble					
Thiamine B$_1$	mg	1.4 or 0.5 mg/ 1000 kcal	Coenzyme in carbohydrate metabolism	Cardiomyopathy, neuropathy, encephalopathy	Multibionta, Parentrovite, Solivito
Riboflavine B$_2$	mg	2.1	Component of flavin coenzymes	Cheilosis, angular stomatitis	As above
Pyridoxine B$_6$	mg	2.1	Coenzyme in transamination	Glossitis, cheilosis, dermatitis	As above
Cobalamin B$_{12}$	microgram	2.0	Coenzyme: amino acid and DNA synthesis	Anaemia, neuropathy	Hydroxo- and cyanocobalamin injection
Niacin	mg	7 mg/1000 kcal	Constituent of nicotinamide adenine dinucleotide	Pellagra	As above
Biotin	microgram	350	Coenzyme in carboxylation	Alopecia, dermatitis	Solivito
Pantothenic acid	mg	14	Coenzyme A		Multibionta, Solivito
Ascorbic acid	mg	35	Collagen synthesis, capillary maintenance	Weakness, bleeding of nails and gums	As B$_1$
Folic acid	mg	2	Coenzyme	Anaemia	Folic acid injection, Solivito
Fat-soluble					
Calciferol D	i.u.	100	Calcium and phosphate metabolism	Rickets, Osteomalacia	Vitlipid, calciferol injection
Phytomenadione K	microgram	140	Clotting factors	Prolonged bleeding, bruising	Vitlipid, vitamin K injection
Retinol A	i.u.	3300	Retinal pigments	Night blindness	Multibionta, Vitlipid
Tocopherol acetate E	i.u.	30	Antioxidant	Haemolysis	Intralipid, Multibionta

during repeated connections and disconnections between containers in a non-sterile, ward environment. It is time consuming for the nursing staff to monitor and ensure that the regimen is being infused according to the prescription. Where small volume additives have to be made, this increases the risk of contamination, incompatibility and of items being accidentally omitted from the regimen, due to its complexity.

To avoid the risk of infusion rates varying during the specified administration time or the risk of a large volume being infused unnoticed, pumps or regulator giving sets are used. These ensure accurate and safe delivery of the nutrients.

Many pumps and devices are available. All are costly, often up to several thousand pounds per pump. Administration sets are also expensive and usually compatible only with a particular type of pump and are used on a once-only basis.

Solutions are infused directly into the venous system by either:

- the central venous route
- the peripheral venous route.

The central route requires placement of a silicone catheter (Fig. 5.1). The catheter remains in place for the duration of therapy assuming no problems arise. Peripheral cannulae are usually only suitable for a period of up to 48 hours and feeding via this route is not generally recommended if duration is likely to be greater than 7 days.

The maintenance and care of a central venous catheter requires strict adherence to aseptic protocols to avoid infection due to microbial contamination of the line or exit site. Occasion-

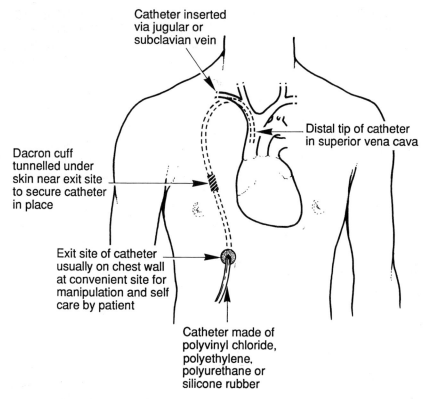

Fig. 5.1 Central venous catheter.

Labels in figure:

Catheter inserted via jugular or subclavian vein

Distal tip of catheter in superior vena cava

Dacron cuff tunnelled under skin near exit site to secure catheter in place

Exit site of catheter usually on chest wall at convenient site for manipulation and self care by patient

Catheter made of polyvinyl chloride, polyethylene, polyurethane or silicone rubber

ally an indwelling system or portacath may be used. In this system a reservoir with a self-sealing rubber diaphragm is attached to a central venous catheter and is implanted underneath the skin, usually on the chest wall. The implanted reservoir is accessed by piercing through the skin with a J-shaped needle connected to the infusion apparatus. This has the advantage of not having the catheter on the skin surface and reduces the inconvenience to the patient, but is not ideal if daily access is required.

FORMULATION

Stability

Total parenteral nutrition solutions are extremely complex. When kept separately from other components they are stable and usually have a shelf life of several years. The majority of stability problems occur when the solutions are mixed together in a single container.

Amino acids

Amino acids are very stable even when mixed with other components. Often they are packed and sealed under nitrogen as they oxidize on exposure to air. Oxygen will leach through plastic on storage and the mixture darkens. This process is accelerated by light.

Fat emulsions

Incompatibilities with fat emulsions cause the majority of formulation problems. Factors affecting lipid stability include:

- pH – increased pH results in increased stability
- nature of amino acid solution
- electrolyte content
- total composition of the mixture.

The lipid emulsion is particularly destabilized by the presence of divalent and trivalent cations.

Davis proposed a formula to calculate a critical aggregation number to assess the cumulative effects of electrolytes on emulsion stability.

If a, b and c = concentration in mmol/L of mono-, di- and trivalent ions, and x = critical aggregation number above which flocculation will occur, then if:

$$x < a + 62b + 770c$$

the mixture will be unstable and the ionic concentration needs to be altered.

Vitamins

Vitamin A is unstable in light. If the bag is not protected with an outer wrapper or does not contain a lipid emulsion, which also provides protection against light, then estimates suggest that only 10% of the vitamin A which is added will be available at the time of infusion. Losses are reduced to about 50% if protection is employed. Artificial light has no effect and so minimal losses occur during the filling process.

Thiamine (B_1) is the most rapidly reduced vitamin. Sodium metabisulphite and amino acids increase the degradation rate.

Ascorbic acid (vitamin C) is the most rapidly oxidized vitamin. The rate of oxidation depends upon:

- the amount of dissolved oxygen in the solution
- the pH (rate increased as pH decreases)
- the presence of trace metals such as copper.

Ascorbic acid oxidizes to dehydroascorbic acid which is metabolically active but which is rapidly degraded to 2,3-diketogulonic acid and then to oxalic acid. The latter may cause oxalate stones.

Many TPN formulations are stable for up to 90 days unless vitamins are added. Once vitamins are added most authorities would advocate infusion within 24 hours.

Nutritional solutions were originally thought to be ideal bacterial and fungal growth media. In practice, the osmolality is generally too high to support favourable growth conditions. Lipid emulsions, however, have been demonstrated to support microbial growth as efficiently as nutrient broth. To reduce the risk of introducing contaminants, solutions are prepared using sterile aseptic technique. The final 3-litre mixed bag cannot be sterilized by an end sterilization method.

Bags which have been prepared are usually stored between 2 and 8°C until they are required. Growth of common contaminants such as *Staphylococcus* species, *Escherichia coli* and *Pseudomonas aeruginosa* is prevented at low temperatures but the organisms remain viable and growth rates will increase as the solution is warmed to room temperature prior to infusion.

Several types of plastics are available for production of TPN bags. Problems arose initially when fat emulsions were added to the usual polyvinyl chloride (PVC) bags as phthallate salts were leached from the plastic into the solution. Bags made from ethyl vinyl acetate (EVA) are usually used for mixtures containing fat emulsions as this contains non-phthallate plasticizers.

Standard formulations

Whilst the needs of individual patients can be met using finely tailored regimens, up to 80% of patients will be managed using standard regimens. These are based on the average-sized patient and adjusted to meet a normal, moderately elevated or a highly elevated nutritional requirement. Within this framework hospitals often 'offer' a series of 8 to 10 standard formulations. Of these half will contain fat to provide 40 to 60% of the calorie source and the rest will use dextrose only. Tailoring of regimens for specific needs is reserved for particular patient groups which will be discussed later.

The prescribing and administration of TPN is made simple by the use of a standard prescription sheet (Fig. 5.2). These usually specify the nutritional requirement for a 24-hour period, infusion details and the components to be supplied.

ASSESSMENT AND MONITORING
Assessment

Assessment of patients requiring nutritional support can be broadly divided into 2 types:

Patient: _____ Ward: _____

Consultant: _____ Unit number: _____

Regimen	Units	R1	R2	R3	R4	Additional requirements
Nitrogen	g	9	9	14	14	
Non nitrogen	Kcal	1850	2220	1850	2220	
Potassium	mmol	60	60	60	60	
Sodium	mmol	148	148	148	148	
Calcium	mmol	7.5	7.5	7.5	7.5	
Magnesium	mmol	14	14	14	14	
Phosphate	mmol	30	30	30	30	
Zinc	micromoles	40	40	40	40	
Multibionta	ml	10	10	10	10	
Heparin	units	9000	9000	9000	9000	
Volume	ml	3000	3000	3000	3000	
						Frequency

M | T | W | Th | F | S | Su

Fat requirements

Intralipid 500ml: 10% ☐ 20% ☐ +Vitlipid adults 10ml

Frequency: | M | T | W | Th | F | S | Su |

Folic acid: 15mg ☐ Tuesday ☐ Friday

Date initiated: _____ Medical Officer: _____

Date discontinued: _____ Pharmacist: _____

Fig. 5.2 Example of standard total parenteral prescription.

- clinical
- biochemical.

Clinical assessment

One of the best measures of clinical assessment is the well-being of the patient. It also includes simple measures such as height and weight. This allows the calculation of an ideal body weight and may help determine the goal for therapy. Weight may be misleading as there are two types of malnutrition, protein–calorie depletion (marasmus) or protein depletion (kwashiorkor). The first is the typical skeletal patient who looks malnourished. The second type may appear obese and well nourished even though they have depleted skeletal muscle reserves. Malnutrition may also present as a mixture of both types. Weight is a difficult parameter to follow in the short term (< 4 weeks) as most weight changes in this period are due to alterations in fluid balance. In the longer term, weight will represent changes in body stores of fat and protein.

The estimation of body fat and muscle stores can be made using anthropometric techniques. These use a calliper type of device to measure:

- mid-arm muscle circumference (MAMC) which assesses muscle stores
- triceps skinfold thickness (TSF) which assesses fat reserves.

MAMC = Arm circumference − [0.314 × Triceps skinfold thickness (mm)]

Malnutrition is indicated if the value is:

- < 230 mm in men, or
- < 220 mm in women.

Triceps skinfold thickness is said to suggest malnutrition if it is:

- < 10 mm in men, or
- < 13 mm in women.

The problem with these techniques is the wide variation between operators taking the measurements. Trends may be useful in monitoring a patient, ideally by the same observer.

Other methods which are used as a research tool include: muscle function testing; subcutaneous allergy testing and response to stimuli, e.g. using *Candida albicans*; total lymphocyte count of less than $1.2 \times 10^9/L$; plasma amino acid profiles; or 3-methylhistidine excretion, a non-recyclable metabolite of muscle protein breakdown.

Biochemical assessment

Most hospitals would formally or informally perform a battery of tests which can be described as a nutritional screen. This would form the basis of an initial assessment and be repeated at intervals during the course of therapy as appropriate.

A nutritional screen would include:

Electrolytes – Na$^+$, K$^+$, Cl^{-1} Urea Creatinine Glucose	checked daily initially and then at decreased frequency depending on the stability of requirements
Albumin Total protein Bilirubin Liver enzymes – AST, ALT, Alk Phos Calcium Phosphate Full blood count Prothrombin time	checked initially and then once or twice/week as required
Nitrogen balance	checked twice/week
Fluid balance	checked daily
Urinary electrolytes	checked as necessary.

If nutrition is likely to last longer than 2 weeks or the patient is severely malnourished:

Iron Iron-binding capacity Folate and red cell folate B$_{12}$ Copper Zinc Magnesium	checked initially and then every 2 weeks thereafter or less often depending on requirements.

If nutrition is going to be long term (> 3 months):

Selenium
Manganese   } checked every
Chromium   3 months.
Vitamins

Monitoring therapy

Electrolytes

It is important when monitoring TPN therapy to avoid interpreting isolated electrolyte values. It is more useful, where possible, to look at trends, and to check unusual or unexpected results prior to taking action.

Serum electrolytes (Na^+, K^+), urea, creatinine and glucose are often checked daily in the first few days of therapy and then the frequency is decreased as appropriate to the stability of the requirements. If patients are critically ill then electrolytes may be checked 2 or 3 times in a 24-hour period.

With all tests the frequency of monitoring will depend upon the patient being treated and the nature and stability of his/her requirements.

Common serum electrolyte abnormalities which may occur are shown in Table 5.9.

Serum calcium usually remains stable and is not required if TPN is for less than 2 weeks, as adequate amounts are mobilized from bone. Hypercalcaemia is usually associated with renal impairment or malignancy.

Magnesium depletion is common where gastrointestinal losses are high, e.g. via stomas, fistulae or diarrhoea.

Protein and liver enzymes

Albumin has a long half-life of up to 21 days and is affected by fluid balance and sepsis as well as malnutrition, so it is not a very sensitive nutritional indicator.

Liver function tests commonly rise during TPN. This has been suggested to be associated with a number of causes including excessive

Table 5.9 Common causes of serum electrolyte abnormalities associated with TPN therapy

Electrolyte	Excess	Depletion
Sodium	Excessive administration Dehydration = water depletion rather than excess Na^+	Intake too low Urine [Na^+] < 20 mmol/L Fluid overload Urine [Na^+] > 20 mmol/L
Potassium	Haemolysis of sample Excessive administration Renal impairment Acidosis – K^+ moves from the cells into extracellular fluid (ECF) Trauma and tissue damage	Inadequate intake Excessive loss – GI loss Diuretics Alkalosis – K^+ moves into cells from ECF Glucose – K^+ moves into cells regulated by insulin Liver failure
Urea	Dehydration Excessive protein catabolism Renal impairment	Overhydration Protein depleted
Creatinine	Renal impairment	Reduced skeletal muscle mass
Phosphate	Excessive administration Renal impairment Acidosis Tissue damage Alkalosis	Inadequate intake Symptoms when PO_4^{2-} < 0.15 mmol/L Increased loss Glucose based TPN
Chloride	Excessive administration Hypernatraemia Metabolic acidosis Respiratory alkalosis	Inadequate intake Hyponatraemia Metabolic alkalosis Respiratory acidosis

glucose administration and may be reduced by lowering the calorie load or by cyclical feeding, e.g. over 12 to 18 hours instead of a continuous 24 hour infusion.

Haematological monitoring

A full blood count including haemoglobin, white cell count and mean cell volume is used to assess anaemia and signs of infection or immuno-suppression. The mean cell volume may indicate the type of anaemia present and this will be confirmed by assessing the body stores of iron, B_{12} and folate.

Assessment of trace elements and vitamins

Generally this is not required unless TPN is going to be for longer than 3 months, as the body stores of trace elements are usually sufficient for this period of time. Zinc may become depleted particularly where there are high gastrointestinal losses and may be associated with poor wound healing and infection.

PATIENTS WITH SPECIFIC REQUIREMENTS

In addition to the general assessment, monitoring and provision of TPN, there are some clinical conditions which require particular attention. By anticipating potential problems and meeting the specific nutritional requirements which have been identified, many difficulties can be avoided.

Starvation

After 24 hours of starvation glycogen stores are depleted. During the following 5 to 7 days the body uses protein as a calorie source (gluconeogenesis) and also mobilizes fatty acids. The ketone bodies produced are used by the brain instead of glucose. There is progressive muscle wasting including the respiratory muscles which may lead to increased susceptibility to chest infections and difficulty in weaning patients from ventilators.

If nutritional support is instituted using a calorie:nitrogen ratio of 150:1 and a nitrogen input of around 0.2 g nitrogen/kg per 24 hours, the effects of starvation will be quickly reversed.

Sepsis and injury

Septicaemia is due to the presence of actively dividing organisms in the blood and the subsequent release of toxins. Changes in energy and protein metabolism occur in two phases. There is an initial ebb phase where the metabolic rate does not become elevated and glucose ceases to be used as a calorie source which leads to hyperglycaemia. This is followed by a prolonged flow phase when the metabolic rate is increased and there is general catabolism of damaged and uninjured tissue. During this time there is an increased rate of fat oxidation relative to that of carbohydrate. The ability to oxidize exogenous carbohydrate once it is provided depends upon the severity of the condition. Severely septic or injured patients continue to metabolize fat. Less severely ill patients seem to metabolize glucose at a higher rate than normal. The effect of this in terms of providing parenteral nutrition is that at least 50% of the calorie requirements should be met using fat. However, concern remains regarding the effect of lipid emulsions on neutrophil function. This may be overcome by using MCT emulsions.

The type of protein solutions required is still a subject for debate. In particular, solutions enriched with branched chain amino acids have a theoretical advantage in replacing skeletal muscle. Some potentially important amino acids, cysteine, tyrosine and glutamine are omitted from standard solutions due to reduced solubility or instability. These may now be incorporated by using di- or tripeptides.

Respiratory impairment

This category applies to any patient with respiratory difficulties and includes those who are mechanically ventilated, who have a postoperative chest infection and those with chronic respiratory disease. These patients have difficulty in excreting carbon dioxide from the lungs, leading to its retention and respiratory acidosis.

This would be compensated in normal individuals by the retention of bicarbonate but this may not be available in sufficient quantities in patients receiving TPN. Patients who are given a high chloride load may be prone to developing hyperchloraemic metabolic acidosis and therefore it may be worthwhile considering giving salts as acetate rather than chloride. Bicarbonate cannot be added to the TPN mixture as it dramatically affects the pH of the solution which may compromise the stability of the other components.

Patients with known respiratory problems or severe respiratory distress should receive 50 to 60% of their kcal requirements as fat. Fat oxidation in the body produces less carbon dioxide per kcal than the metabolism of dextrose.

However, not all the calories can be given as fat, as incomplete metabolism may lead to the accumulation of intermediate metabolites resulting in ketoacidosis.

Cardiac failure

These patients require TPN in:

- a low volume
- with careful electrolyte monitoring, particularly sodium, potassium and magnesium.

Some problems can be avoided by using high strength amino acid solutions, e.g. 17 to 18 g nitrogen per litre, to attain a reasonable intake within a small volume. Using fat to provide 40 to 50% of the calorie requirement will also allow provision of adequate calories in a smaller volume. Accurate estimation of calorie requirements is worthwhile when fluid volume restriction is a prime concern to avoid excessive supplementation using up valuable volume. Careful monitoring of electrolytes is required especially in patients receiving diuretics, ACE inhibitors or digoxin. As these patients are often elderly, glucose tolerance may be reduced and it is important to check blood and urinary glucose to avoid an osmotic diuresis leading to dehydration and further metabolic problems.

Renal failure

The two main problems here are (a) volume restriction and (b) biochemical disturbances. In the normal individual the kidneys play a major role in water and electrolyte homeostasis. Impairment of renal function reduces this ability to fine tune the electrolyte balance. Fluid volume may again be restricted by using high strength amino acid solutions, lipid emulsions and, where necessary, high concentration dextrose solutions, with insulin as required. Accurate fluid balance is essential. Nitrogen balance is also closely regulated with all input and output being accurately charted and measured. Frequent monitoring of serum electrolytes is required. Specialist amino acid solutions are available which contain essential amino acids only. These may have a beneficial effect in patients with acute renal failure but have not been shown to be of value in chronic renal failure. The place in therapy of these solutions is still unclear. In general, patients of this type should receive a high calorie, low protein intake. The use of keto analogues of essential amino acids has yet to be established.

Hepatic failure

The main area of debate here has been the use of branched chain amino acid (BCAA) enriched solutions. These include leucine, isoleucine and valine which together provide 40% of the minimum daily requirements for essential amino acids in man. They have several roles:

- substrates for anabolic protein synthesis
- peripheral (skeletal muscle) calorie substrates
- regulators of protein metabolism
- in the normalization of neurotransmitters.

BCAA have been shown to be of value in restoring plasma amino acid profiles to normal and in improving nitrogen balance. Patients with liver disease have difficulty in handling phenylalanine, methionine and tryptophan. It has been proposed that this may lead to the generation of false transmitters which may play a role in the development of encephalopathy. However, the place of BCAAs in therapy is still widely debated. In general, patients are given a low protein intake of around 20 g of protein per day which can be increased if it is tolerated. It is not recommended to give fat emulsions in severe liver failure. Glucose can be given with careful monitoring for hyperglycaemia and hypokalaemia. Increased amounts of vitamins may also be required.

Patients with gastrointestinal losses

Patients with high gastrointestinal losses via stomas, fistulae, diarrhoea or from open wounds have to be carefully monitored for fluid and electrolyte balance. The most common electrolytes to become depleted are sodium, potassium, magnesium and bicarbonate. Table 5.10 shows the electrolyte content of different intestinal secretions.

Diabetic patients

Patients with diabetes are managed using standard regimens with up to 50% of the calorie requirement being given as fat. Patients with pancreatic disturbance, e.g. pancreatic abscess, also require careful blood glucose monitoring. They can be given lipid emulsions provided their clearance is monitored and the infusion does not produce hyperlipidaemia.

Long-term TPN

In some patients TPN may be required for a prolonged period. It may be required lifelong for a small number of individuals who have no remaining or functional gut. This could arise following small bowel infarction, intestinal obstruction due to a knotting and twisting of the bowel (volvulus) or extensive resection of the gut due to inflammatory bowel disease. In these patients very few have no enteral intake at all, so there is scope for the absorption of limited amounts of nutrients via the gastrointestinal tract. Some will eat normally or supplement their diet with specialized enteral formulations to be discussed later. This allows the frequency of TPN to be reduced from a daily basis to three to five times per week. Careful assessment of requirements is needed to ensure that there is not prolonged over- or underfeeding. In the short term this would be hardly noticed but will have a cumulative effect over a long period. Attention to the less common trace elements is important.

Reports of anaemia due to copper deficiency and cardiomyopathy and myositis due to selenium deficiency have been documented following prolonged TPN with solutions free of these elements. Patients who are ambulant and can be trained in the aseptic technique required for care of their central venous catheter are discharged home. They usually infuse their nutritional solution from a 3-litre bag via a pump. This allows them to be free of infusion devices during the day such that they can return to a relatively normal lifestyle. Many have returned to work or full-time education, whilst continuing with their home TPN (HPN). A national registry and support group exists for all patients requiring intensive nutritional support of this type.

ENTERAL NUTRITION

Enteral nutrition is cheaper, safer and more physiological than intravenous nutrition. It is the best alternative for patients requiring nutritional support which can be delivered safely into the gastrointestinal tract. The enteral feeding tube can be placed such that the distal portion reaches a particular part of the gastrointestinal tract, the position being checked by X-ray screening.

Enteral nutrition can be delivered by several routes:

Table 5.10 Electrolyte content of gastrointestinal secretions				
Fluid type	Na$^+$ (mmol/L)	K$^+$ (mmol/L)	HCO$_3^-$ (mmol/L)	Cl^{-1} (mmol/L)
Gastric	20–80	5–20	—	100–150
Biliary	120–140	5–15	30–50	80–120
Pancreatic	120–140	5–15	70–110	40–80
Small bowel	120–140	5–15	20–40	90–130

- by mouth – limited by palatability and appetite
- by nasogastric tube ⎫
- by nasoduodenal tube ⎬ limited by discomfort and tissue damage by tubes in the long term, there is less problem with newly developed silk tubes
- by nasojejunal tube ⎭
- by feeding gastrostomy or jejunostomy – long-term feeding only.

Infusion of nutrients can be by bolus or by drip. The drip method is preferred. A pump is useful to regulate the osmoles administered per unit time which helps limit diarrhoea. The infusion may be continuous over 24 hours or intermittent, e.g. overnight, as with TPN.

There are a number of reported drug interactions with enteral feeds. Common practice is to administer drugs as crushed tablets or in liquid formulations through the enteral feeding tube. Drug interactions should be suspected where a desired or predicted effect is not observed. Common interactions are shown in Table 5.11. Where possible administering drugs via this route should be avoided as they may bind to the plastic of the tube altering bioavailability. Crushing tablets will cause problems if they have specialized release mechanisms, e.g. enteric coating or sustained-release preparations.

Table 5.11 Common drug interactions with enteral feeds

Drug	Nutrient	Interaction
Anticoagulants	Vitamin K	Decreased efficacy of anticoagulant
Antibiotics	Vitamin k	Decreased absorption
Biguanides	Protein Carbohydrate ⎫	Decreased absorption or loss
Cholestyramine	Fat Fat-soluble vitamins ⎫	Decreased absorption
Aluminium antacids	Phosphate	Binding
Anticonvulsants	Folic acid	Decreased absorption

Table 5.12 Enteral feeds

Type of feed	Indication
Whole protein (polymeric)	Suitable for patients without malabsorption difficulties Vary in composition in terms of nitrogen: kcal ratio, fat content and type; electrolytes, trace elements and vitamins Least expensive Palatable, wide range of flavours
Predigested feeds (elemental diets)	Contain protein as oligopeptides or amino acids Suitable for patients with short bowel syndrome, those with severe pancreatic or mucosal malabsorption in whom proteolysis may be impaired; may be used in Crohn's disease to induce remission Approximately three times more expensive than whole protein Unpalatable
Disease-specific diets	Developed for renal, liver, sepsis and respiratory disease, modified on same principles as for TPN modified formulations
Modular diets	Single components designed for patients with a specific deficiency to correct overall intake Includes medium chain triglycerides and vitamins

Problems may arise with crushed tablet material occluding the catheter.

There are a wide variety of enteral feeds available. Most hospitals should stock a high and a low protein feed, a low sodium and a high electrolyte feed and a predigested feed.

Some novel substrates, glutamine, the ornithine salt of α-ketoglutaric acid (OKGA), medium chain triglycerides and polyunsaturated fatty acids are available. They may have a role in maintaining the integrity of the gastrointestinal tract directly or indirectly by moderating the effect of sepsis or trauma on gastrointestinal permeability.

The use of starter regimens, by increasing the concentration of the feed over several days is no longer advocated. Studies have shown that gastrointestinal problems are related to the rate of delivery of the nutrients rather than the concentration.

The types and the indication for use of enteral feeds available are shown in Table 5.12. Feeds are designed to provide all the nutrients required but may require supplementation with vitamins and trace elements if feeding is to be continued for longer than 4 weeks.

Monitoring of progress whilst receiving enteral nutritional support is similar to that previously discussed, though the frequency may be less intensive. Complications of enteral nutrition can be divided into 3 main groups (Table 5.13).

CASE STUDIES

CASE 5.1

A 58-year-old surgical patient of good nutritional status and weighing 69 kg is admitted for an elective oesophagectomy for a previously diagnosed severe motility disorder. He will be nil by mouth for at least 10 days. The house officer has been told to start TPN in this patient 24 hours postoperatively and requests your help in prescribing the regimen.

Q1 What further information would you require before making a decision?

Q2 Calculate the patient's nutritional requirements for his initial prescription on the basis of the information supplied.

Table 5.13 Complications of enteral nutrition		
Category	Problem	Solution
Tube related	Misplacement	Careful insertion technique
		Checked by X-ray if necessary
	Blockage	Flush regularly during day
	Unwanted removal	Secure with tape
Diet related	Nausea	Less problem with infusion methods
	Vomiting	Diarrhoea may be caused by bacterial overgrowth
	Diarrhoea	or patients on antibiotics
	Cramps	Use antidiarrhoeals as necessary
	Bloating	Decrease rate of infusion
	Pulmonary aspiration	Elevate head of bed
	Regurgitation	Use metoclopramide to increase gastric emptying
	Drug interactions	See Table 5.11
Metabolic	Hyperglycaemia	
	Hyperkalaemia	
	Hypokalaemia	
	Hypophosphataemia	Correct composition of feed and monitor as appropriate
	Hypomagnesaemia	
	Hypozincaemia	

CASE 5.2

Mr C. D., a 32-year-old male with a 10-year history of Crohn's disease was admitted as an emergency to the gastroenterology medical unit. He had a laparotomy 2 years ago which included terminal ileal resection.

His weight on admission was 50.0 kg

PC: Severe acute attack
     Diarrhoea +++ 1 litre/day

O/E: Blood } in stool
     Mucus }
     Pale
     Thin
     Temp. 38.4°C
     Tachycardia

Plan: 1. Bloods: nutritional screen
      2. Central line insertion
      3. Start TPN

Results

		(Normal range)
Hb	8.8 g/dl	(13.5–18)
WCC	12.6×10^9/L	(3.5–11)
Plts	627×10^9/L	(150–400)
ESR	85 mm/h	(<10)
Na$^+$	132 mmol/L	(135–145)
K$^+$	3.0 mmol/L	(3.5–5.0)
Urea	8.6 mmol/L	(3.0–6.5)
Creatinine	80 µmol/L	(50–120)
Albumin	28 g/L	(35–55)
Glucose	5.3 mmol/L	(Non-fasting < 10 mmol/L)
In. phosphate	1.12 mmol/L	(0.8–1.6)
Awaited:	Cu, Zn, Mg	

Q1 Identify the factors which will affect the estimated nutritional requirements of the patient.

Q2 Calculate the nutritional requirements for the first 24-hour period.

Q3 Using the solutions of your choice, convert the requirements identified in Question 2 to the actual volumes of solutions you would recommend for the patient.

ANSWERS TO CASE STUDIES

CASE 5.1

A1 In order to assess a patient's nutritional requirements you need to know the following details:

- Age
- Sex
- Weight – ideal body weight; is maintenance/ repletion required?

- Nutritional status – malnourished, well nourished
- Disease state – normal requirements or catabolic.
- Review of systems:
    renal function – affects volume, protein and electrolyte requirements
    liver function – severe impairment affects protein requirements
    cardiac function – affects volume and electrolyte requirements
    pancreatic function – affects glucose handling
    respiratory function – affects choice of calorie substrate
    gastrointestinal function – abnormal losses need to be assessed and accounted for
    signs of infection – pyrexia, tachycardia.
- Goals and likely duration of therapy
- Central line inserted?
- Other i.v. fluids or drugs.

The patient in Case 5.1 has the following details:

- Review of systems – nothing abnormal diagnosed (NAD)
- Likely duration of therapy – 2 weeks
- Central line inserted at time of laparotomy
- No peripheral lines.

A2 Calculation of nutritional requirements:

Volume
= 1500 ml – 20 × (69 + 20)
= 2480 ml/24 h
or
69 kg × 35 ml/kg = 2415 ml/24 h
therefore 2.5 to 3 litres is adequate.

Calorie requirements
Based upon 30 to 35 kcals/kg
Previously well nourished
Resting energy expenditure = 30 × 69
= 2070 kcal/24 h
(+ 20% = 2484 kcal/24 h)

Calorie source
Dextrose only or
Dextrose and fat depending on local preferences.

Protein requirements
Basal = 0.15 g nitrogen/kg/24 h
       = 10.35 g nitrogen/24 h

Electrolytes
Na$^+$	1–2 mmol/kg	= 69–138 mmol/24 h
K$^+$	1–2 mmol/kg	= 69–138 mmol/24 h
PO$_4^{2-}$	0.5–0.7 mmol/kg	= 35–48 mmol/24 h
Ca^{2+}	0.1–0.15 mmol/kg	= 6.9–10.4 mmol/24 h
Mg^{2+}	0.1–0.2 mmol/kg	= 6.9–13.8 mmol/24 h
Trace elements	} standard amounts	
Vitamins	}	

Using the range of commercial solutions available a 3-litre bag or bottle regimen can be prepared. Final amounts of each component should be rounded up or down to convenient quantities to measure.

CASE 5.2

A1 The patient in Case 5.2 has the following details:

- Age = 32 years
- Sex = male
- Weight = 50 kg, ideal body weight = 70 kg
- Nutritional status
  = poor
  = long-standing malabsorption
  = anaemic, ? B_{12} deficiency also (terminal ileal resection)
- Review of systems:
  renal function
  liver function
  cardiac function   } Nothing abnormal diagnosed
  pancreatic function
  respiratory function
  gastrointestinal function – diarrhoea 1 litre/24 h (estimated content: Na^+ 120–140 mmol/L; K^+ 5–15 mmol/L (Table 5.10)
  Signs of infection – 38.4°C pyrexial and tachycardia, increased fluid requirements by 10%
- Goals and duration of therapy = 2–4 weeks
- Central line inserted in theatre.

A2 Calculation of nutritional requirements:

Volume:
Volume = 1500 mmol + 20 × (50 – 20)
         = 2100 ml/24 h
or   35 ml/kg/24 h
         = 1750 ml/24 h
+   1 litre for diarrhoea
+   10% for °C temperature rise
         = 3100 + 310
         = 3410 ml/24 h
or   = 2750 + 275
         = 3025 ml/24 h
therefore between 3 and 3.5 litres should be adequate.

Calorie requirements:
Resting daily energy expenditure based upon 35 kcals/kg = 1750 kcal/24 h
(+20% = 2100 kcal)
or 150 kcal:1 g nitrogen
= 1500–2100 kcal/24 h

Protein requirements
Catabolic = 0.2 g nitrogen/kg/24 h
           = 0.2 × 50 = 10 g nitrogen/24 h

This may be greater and should be monitored using nitrogen balance studies to tailor requirements. As the patient is previously malnourished an additional 2 to 4 g of nitrogen/24 h may be given to replete his muscle stores.
   Therefore total nitrogen intake should be between 10 and 14 g/24 h initially.

Electrolyte requirements (mmol/24 h)

			Gastrointestinal loss
Na^+	1–2 mmol/kg	= 50–100 + 150 mmol
K^+	1–2 mmol/kg	= 50–100 + 15 mmol
PO_4^{2-}	0.5–0.7 mmol/kg	= 25–35 mmol
Ca^{2+}	0.1–0.15 mmol/kg	= 5–7.5 mmol
Mg^{2+}	0.1–0.2 mmol/kg	= 5–10 + 5–10 mmol

A3 From the solutions you have selected you should be able to list how the requirements are being met, in the following format:

Amino acid	14 g nitrogen/L	= 1000 ml
Intralipid 20% w/v	1000 kcal	= 500 ml
Dextrose 40% w/v	800 kcal	= 500 ml
Dextrose 20% w/v	400 kcal	= 500 ml

Provides: 2500 ml
          2200 kcal
          14 g nitrogen

   Electrolytes should be added as required, 500 ml of sodium chloride 0.9% w/v should be used to increase the volume to 3000 ml. This will provide 75 mmol of sodium and chloride. Most amino acid solutions contain electrolytes. Individual electrolytes can be added separately. Trace elements and vitamins should be added in standard quantities. Increased zinc and magnesium will be required to account for that lost in the gastrointestinal fluid.
   Zinc losses can be estimated using Wolman's formula:

$$Zinc (mg/24 h) = 2 + 17.1a + 12.2b$$

where, a = mass (kg) of stool or ileostomy output in a patient with intact small bowel;
       b = mass (kg) of small bowel fluid loss via fistula/stoma; and 2 = urinary loss.

BIBLIOGRAPHY

Driscoll D F, Blackburn G L. Total parenteral nutrition 1990. Drugs 1990; 40: 346–363

Frayn K N. Fuel metabolism during sepsis and injury. Intensive Therapy and Clinical Monitoring 1987; 174–180

Grimble G K, Payne-James J J, Rees R G, Silk D B A. TPN: Novel energy substrates. Intensive Therapy and Clinical Monitoring 1989; 108–113

Grimble G K, Payne-James J J, Rees R G, Silk D B A. Total parenteral nutrition: Novel nitrogen substrates. Intensive Therapy and Clinical Monitoring 1989; 92–98

Grimble G, Paynes-James J J, Rees R, Silk D B A. Enteral nutrition: Novel substrates. Intensive Therapy and Clinical Monitoring 1989; 51–56

Mirtallo J M, Taeho O. A key to the literature of total parenteral nutrition: Update 1987. Drug Intelligence Clinical Pharmacy 1987; 21: 594–606

Nutrition. Medicine International 1990; 82: 3364–3411

Paynes-James J J, Silk D B A. Enteral nutrition: Background indications and management. Bailliere's Clinical Gastroenterology 1988; 2: 815–847

Phillips G D, Odgers C L. Parenteral and enteral nutrition: A practical guide, 3rd edn. Edinburgh: Churchill Livingstone 1986

Shenkin A. Essential trace elements during intravenous nutrition. Intensive Therapy and Clinical Monitoring 1987; 38–47

LIFE STAGES

Chapter 6

Neonates

M. P. Ward Platt

The neonatal period is the first month after birth, irrespective of the time in pregnancy at which birth takes place. The normal length of human pregnancy lies between 37 and 42 completed weeks, and any baby born outside this is preterm or post-term respectively. Babies born weighing less than 2500 g are called low birth weight, those less than 1500 g very low birth weight, and those less than 1000 g extremely low birth weight.

DEMOGRAPHY

Babies weighing less than 1000 g are often identified as a group at particular risk. The earliest in pregnancy at which newborn babies can sometimes survive is 23 to 24 weeks' gestation, but conventionally any baby born at less than 32 weeks is regarded as being at high risk. There is increasing recognition that it is the gestation at birth rather than the birth weight which is of more practical and prognostic value.

Because of in-utero transfer of high risk babies for delivery at hospitals capable of providing neonatal respiratory support, the proportion of preterm and low birth weight babies seen in such units is greater than in smaller maternity units in peripheral hospitals. Depending on the population and the nature of the hospital, between 6 and 10% of all live born babies will weigh less than 2500 g, and around 2% will be less than 1500 g; in a population as a whole, just over 1% of all babies born will receive respiratory support, usually for respiratory distress syndrome of the newborn.

DRUG DISPOSITION

An important and unique source of drug absorption available up till birth is the placenta. Maternal drugs pass to the fetus and back again before birth, but at delivery, any drugs present in the neonatal circulation cannot readily be eliminated. Important examples include opiates given for maternal pain relief and benzodiazepines given for maternal eclampsia or pre-eclampsia.

Drug absorption by the enteral route is erratic in the newborn baby of any gestation, and unavailable in the ill baby who frequently has a sympathetic ileus. Thus it is usual to give many drugs by the intravenous route to ensure maximum bioavailability. Some drugs, such as paraldehyde and diazepam (for neonatal seizures) and paracetamol (for simple analgesia), can successfully be administered by the rectal route. In the very preterm baby of 28 weeks' gestation or less, the skin is extremely thin and a poor barrier to water loss; consequently it is also permeable to substances in contact with it. This may be a useful property, but is dangerous to the baby if there is prolonged skin contact with alcohol (as in chlorhexidine in 70% methylated spirit), which as well as causing a severe chemical burn can result in systemic methyl alcohol poisoning. The intramuscular route is normally avoided (see 'Principles and goals of therapy', below).

Drugs are distributed within a baby's body as a function of their lipid and aqueous solubility, as at any other time of life. The main difference in the neonate is that the size of the body water pool under renal control is related not to the baby's surface area but to body weight; furthermore, absolute glomerular filtration rate increases logarithmically with post-conceptional age irrespective of the length of a baby's gestation. Extracellular fluid is highest at birth and falls due to the postnatal diuresis over the first 48 hours of postnatal life. Also, the amount of adipose tissue can vary substantially. Any baby

born more than 10 weeks early, and babies of any gestation which have suffered intra-uterine growth retardation, may have very limited reserves of body fat; conversely the infant of a poorly controlled diabetic mother may have a substantial fat layer. Protein binding in the plasma is influenced by the amount of albumin available, and this in turn is related to gestation, with albumin values found 12 weeks prior to term being only two-thirds of adult concentrations.

The metabolic fate of drugs in the newborn is not qualitatively different from that in the older child, e.g. hydroxylation, oxidation and conjugation to sulphate or glucuronide. It is the efficiency with which these processes are carried out that distinguishes the baby from the older person. In addition to the immaturity of the metabolic pathways for drug disposal, drug metabolism is also affected by the physiological hyperbilirubinaemia of the newborn. The bilirubin competes both for enzyme binding sites and for glucuronate and may thus affect drug metabolism for as long as unconjugated hyperbilirubinaemia and jaundice persist.

The relative immaturity of hepatic and renal function results in correspondingly slow elimination of most drugs from the neonate. This is not necessarily a disadvantage, so long as due account is taken of the slow elimination and dose intervals are modified accordingly. It may even be a useful property, as with phenobarbitone which when given as a 'loading' dose (20 mg/kg) will remain in circulation for days in useful therapeutic quantities, often avoiding the need for further doses. On the other hand, drugs such as gentamicin and vancomycin, which have a relatively narrow therapeutic index, must be given far less frequently and plasma drug levels must be assayed in order to avoid toxicity.

There has been little study of pharmacodynamics in the term or preterm neonate. Most clinicians work on the assumption that the kinetics of drug behaviour are so different in this group of patients that the pharmacodynamic properties must follow the same pattern. In practice the most important pharmacodynamic effect is probably that of the behaviour of opiates derived from the mother in labour. Pethidine and diamorphine are the opiates most likely to cause significant respiratory depression in the neonate. Such respiratory depression is treated with naloxone, and a special neonatal preparation (20 microgram/ml) is available. However, after birth the opiates and their metabolites have a long plasma half-life in the baby whereas the naloxone is rapidly eliminated, though its initial effect may be dramatic. The initial result can give a false sense of security with the baby who will become narcosed later, after transfer to the postnatal ward. To prevent such late onset narcosis many paediatricians use adult naloxone (400 microgram/ml, given as 0.5 ml intramuscularly) instead.

COMMON CLINICAL DISORDERS
Respiratory distress syndrome (RDS)

Among preterm babies the most commonly encountered disorder is the respiratory distress syndrome of the newborn, also called hyaline membrane disease from the histopathological appearances at autopsy. The root cause of this disease is immaturity of the lungs, and specifically the lack of pulmonary surfactant which is necessary to maintain airway patency by reducing the surface tension of alveolar water. The condition is rare in babies born close to term and becomes increasingly likely the more preterm a birth takes place. Clinically the condition is manifested by obvious respiratory distress with nasal flaring, rib recession, tachypnoea, and a requirement for oxygen therapy. A relatively big baby born around 6 to 8 weeks premature may need no more than oxygen therapy to overcome the condition, which becomes worse over the first 2 days, reaches a plateau, and then gradually improves. Smaller, more premature and more severely affected babies commonly go into respiratory failure and require mechanical ventilation, which for the last 20 years has been the only, though highly successful, therapy for respiratory failure.

Some babies require high inspired concentrations of oxygen (up to 100%) for days on end during this time; in such pharmacological concentrations the therapeutic index becomes an important issue. Fortunately, pulmonary oxygen toxicity is not a problem to the neonate in the way it is to the adult (though it may have an aetiological role in the production of bronchopulmonary dysplasia, see below); the chief concern is the damage that prolonged arterial hyperoxia can do to the retina, giving rise to retinopathy of prematurity.

Mechanical ventilation is not a comfortable experience for adults and children, but it has taken a long time to appreciate that this may also be true for premature babies. Paralysing agents such as pancuronium are frequently (but not invariably) employed in neonates receiving ventilation but these do no more than prevent the baby from moving, and have no effect on consciousness. Pancuronium is most frequently used, and has the advantage over shorter acting agents that it wears off slowly so the baby is not suddenly destabilized. In recent years the deleterious effects of pain in the newborn have been highlighted. It has now become common practice to use morphine on an 'as needed' basis to provide narcosis and analgesia, whether or not the baby is paralysed, thereby to reduce the distress of neonatal intensive care. However, morphine has a long elimination half-life (over 12 hours on average), and if allowed to accumulate may cause seizures.

RDS caused by surfactant deficiency may effectively be ameliorated by the antenatal administration of steroids to the mother. This approach has been shown to reduce mortality by up to 40% among the infants of mothers so treated; unfortunately it is not possible to identify and treat all mothers whose babies could benefit. The main advantage of maternal steroid therapy accrues to those babies of less than 32 weeks' gestation who are most at risk of death and disability from RDS. It is necessary to give a 48-hour course of betamethasone or dexamethasone (e.g. 6 doses of 6 mg each), and to repeat it after a week if delivery has not taken place but remains likely.

The recent introduction of various exogenous

surfactants – either artificial, or derived from pig or calf – has opened the first new window of therapy for surfactant deficiency since the invention of mechanical ventilation for babies. There is no longer any debate as to whether these surfactants work, but it is not entirely clear how the different preparations compare with one another, and whether surfactant should be given prophylactically or withheld until it is clear that the child has RDS. At least for bovine surfactant there is a clear advantage for prophylactic use in babies born at least 14 weeks preterm.

All the exogenous surfactants are expensive, while antenatal steroids are very cheap; but performing appropriate cost–benefit analyses is very difficult and heavily dependent upon assumptions about product costs. Nevertheless such an approach has been attempted and it has been suggested that a combined approach with antenatal steroids and surfactant would reduce the cost per survivor but, for babies of less than 31 weeks' gestation, increase overall costs because of the increased number of survivors.

Patent ductus arteriosus (PDA)

Two major complications of RDS with important pharmaceutical implications are the development of a clinically significant patent ductus arteriosus and chronic lung scarring (bronchopulmonary dysplasia, BPD). PDA can be a problem in the recovery phase of RDS and usually manifests itself as a secondary increase in respiratory distress and/or ventilatory requirement, an increasing oxygen requirement, wide pulse pressure, and sometimes a characteristic cardiac murmur. Clinical suspicion can be confirmed using echocardiography. About one-third of all babies with birth weights less than 1000 g will develop signs of PDA, but not all PDAs are haemodynamically significant. Where it is deemed clinically necessary to intervene there are two options: medical treatment with indomethacin; and surgical ligation. Indomethacin is usually given intravenously in the UK, but can be given enterally (and always is in those countries where the intravenous preparation is not licensed) although absorption is unpredictable. When given intravenously there is a tran-

sient peak in plasma concentration associated with acute cerebral and mesenteric vasoconstriction. Other side effects include a short term rise in plasma creatinine and gastric haemorrhage; these unwanted features are probably dose related, and a recent randomized controlled trial showed that a low dose, prolonged course (0.1 mg/kg daily for 6 days) was as effective, and produced fewer side effects, than the same total dose given as 0.2 mg/kg, 12-hourly for 3 doses. There is no evidence that there is any advantage to prophylactic administration of indomethacin in babies less than 1000 g, and no randomized controlled trial of efficacy between enteral and intravenous administration. Given the short duration of the course of indomethacin for this purpose, measurement of circulating drug concentrations is of little value. Failure to achieve duct closure after one or more attempts with indomethacin may necessitate surgical ligation.

Bronchopulmonary dysplasia (BPD)

Bronchopulmonary dysplasia is seen most frequently in very immature babies who have undergone prolonged respiratory support. It is characterized by prolonged dependency on oxygen or mechanical ventilation and typical appearances on the chest X-ray, and used to be defined as oxygen dependency lasting over 28 days. The inadequacy of this definition has been highlighted by the fact that most babies born more than 12 weeks early require oxygen for 28 days or more, but seldom require it for more than 8 weeks. A more useful functional and epidemiological definition of established (as opposed to transient) BPD is oxygen dependency at 36 weeks postmenstrual age in a baby born before 32 weeks gestation. The onset of BPD is related to gestation severity of RDS (and whether ventilation caused pulmonary interstitial emphysema), infection, occurrence of PDA, and possibly the use of lipid in parenteral nutrition solutions. Conversely, the efficacy of treatment for BPD is related to how early it is started in relation to a baby's real age and to the progression from acute RDS to early chronic lung disease.

There is now no doubt that dexamethasone can reduce the severity of early lung scarring following ventilation for RDS (and hence prevent BPD becoming established), and that its effectiveness is greatest when it is used relatively early in the course of BPD. A current recommendation is that if there is no progress in reduction of ventilator dependency by 2 weeks of age, in the absence of other factors such as active infection, that dexamethasone should be given as follows: 0.5 mg/kg/day for 3 days, followed by 0.3 mg/kg/day for 3 days, followed by 0.1 mg/kg/day for at least 2 weeks.

Established BPD not severe enough to warrant mechanical ventilation is treated with oxygen, either as increased ambient oxygen delivered in the incubator or through a head box, or through nasal cannulae if the baby is in a cot. Enough oxygen must be used to maintain an oxygen saturation high enough to prevent a further rise in pulmonary artery pressure, while avoiding chronic low grade hyperoxia which could cause retinopathy of prematurity. The elevated pulmonary arterial blood pressure which invariably accompanies BPD can give rise to congestive cardiac failure which is treated with diuretics. Sometimes frusemide is used, but this can cause hypercalcuria and renal calcification; a preferable combination is that of a thiazide with spironolactone. Either of these has the additional advantage of improving lung compliance, and thus reducing energy expenditure on breathing, and treating the systemic hypertension which can also occur.

Infection

Infection is a constant hazard in any intensive care situation, but as local ecology is unique to each unit no blanket recommendations can easily be made for antibiotic policy. Important pathogens are coagulase-negative staphylococci, group B beta-haemolytic streptococci, *Staphylococcus aureus*, and a variety of occasional Gram-negative organisms. Superficial candidal infection is common in all babies, and systemic candidal infection is a risk particularly in babies receiving prolonged courses of broad spectrum antibiotics. In general, it is wise to use narrow-spectrum

agents and short courses of antibiotics whenever possible, and to discontinue 'blind' treatment quickly (e.g. after 48 hours) if confirmatory evidence of bacterial infection is not forthcoming. Pneumonia (especially in ventilated babies) and septicaemia are the two most common serious infections; meningitis, though less rare than in later life, is still a rare event. The other major disease in which infection plays an important part is necrotizing enterocolitis (NEC).

It is usual to commence antibiotic therapy prophylactically whenever preterm labour is unexplained, where there has been prolonged rupture of the fetal membranes prior to delivery, and where the baby is very premature; but local policies vary according to local experience. A standard combination for such early treatment is penicillin and an aminoglycoside, to cover group B streptococci and Gram-negative pathogens, and this may be stopped after 48 hours if cultures prove negative. Blind treatment commencing when a baby is more than 48 hours old commonly uses flucloxacillin and an aminoglycoside. The newer cephalosporins such as cefotaxime and ceftazidime have been heavily promoted for use in the blind treatment of neonatal infection on the grounds of lower toxicity (compared to aminoglycosides) and no requirement for monitoring plasma concentrations; though undoubtedly a useful alternative to chloramphenicol for the treatment of meningitis, the existence of multiply resistant coagulase-negative staphylococci means that in many units vancomycin has to be used frequently in preference to these agents. Furthermore, many courses of blind treatment are short (around 48 hours) because they are discontinued in the light of changing clinical circumstances; there is seldom any need to monitor aminoglycoside levels in this situation, so the use of cephalosporins does not necessarily have an advantage in terms of cost.

Necrotizing enterocolitis (NEC)

Necrotizing enterocolitis is a much feared complication of neonatal intensive care, and can arise in any baby. However, it most commonly occurs in babies already ill for other reasons and is especially associated with smallness for gestational age, birth asphyxia, and PDA. Since many sick babies have multiple problems it has been difficult to disentangle causal associations from spurious links to conditions which occur anyway in ill infants, such as the need for blood transfusion. There is general agreement that the pathophysiology is related to damage to the gut mucosa, in turn due to hypotension and/or hypoxia, coupled with the presence of appropriate organisms in the gut, and that these organisms invade the gut wall to give rise to the clinical condition. It almost never arises in a baby which has never been fed.

A baby who becomes ill with NEC may present acutely with a major collapse, with septicaemia, hypotension, respiratory failure and renal failure; or more slowly with abdominal distension, intolerance of feeds and characteristic brown gastric aspirates, and blood in the stool. A fulminant course does not always develop in this latter situation. The immediate treatment is circulatory support if necessary, antibiotics, and discontinuation of enteral feeds. If radiology shows evidence of perforation, many units attempt surgery to remove the affected portion of gut; otherwise medical treatment is normally the rule.

Antibiotics include Gram-positive and Gram-negative cover, and metronidazole for anaerobes. This is the only situation in which metronidazole is used, and as with other drugs in the neonate, it behaves very differently in term babies compared with adults and children, having an elimination half-life of over 20 hours and a tendency to accumulate. In preterm infants it behaves differently again, having an elimination half-life of up to 109 hours, partly due to failure of hepatic hydroxylation in infants born before 35 weeks' gestation. There is probably a case to be made for monitoring plasma levels of this drug, but in practice this is seldom done.

Haemorrhagic disease of the newborn

The most usual routine intervention in the healthy neonate is that of the administration of vitamin K as prophylaxis for haemorrhagic disease of the newborn. Traditionally this has taken place by giving an intramuscular injection of phytomenadione 1 mg (0.5 ml) either to every newborn baby, or selectively to babies who have met other criteria such as instrumental delivery, preterm birth, etc. The purpose is to provide prophylactic protection against haemorrhagic disease of the newborn, which predominantly affects breast-fed babies as these get very little vitamin K in maternal milk. Formula-fed infants get adequate amounts in their feed, and have a gut flora which generates vitamin K also. The difficulty with such 'routine' intramuscular injections is that explicit assent from the parents should be required prior to an invasive and non-therapeutic intervention, but it commonly is not obtained. Furthermore, muscle bulk is small in the newborn (and particularly the preterm) and other structures such as the sciatic nerve can be hit even if the intention is to give the injection into the lateral thigh.

Recently, concern has emerged that the neonatal administration of vitamin K may be associated with an increased incidence of childhood malignancy. Since early haemorrhagic disease is usually caused by maternal anticonvulsant medication it is still reasonable to give intramuscular vitamin K to these babies. Late disease only occurs in association with breast feeding, fat malabsorption, and cholestasis; these babies should receive intermittent oral supplementation.

Apnoea

Apnoea is the absence of breathing. Babies (and adults) normally have respiratory pauses, but preterm babies in particular are prone to prolonged pauses in respiration (over 20 seconds) which can be associated with significant falls in arterial oxygenation. Apnoea often has both primary and obstructive components, is often accompanied by bradycardia, and requires treatment to prevent life-threatening episodes of arterial desaturation leading to convulsions and brain damage. While for some conditions, such as RDS, the treatment goals are clear cut, for apnoea of prematurity this is not so because it may be difficult to abolish episodes of apnoea and bradycardia altogether. However, they may be greatly reduced in frequency and severity by the administration of methylxanthines such as aminophylline or caffeine. Of the two, caffeine appears to be as effective as theophylline and aminophylline (and these two are in any case partly metabolized to caffeine) but has a wider therapeutic index and there is rarely need to measure plasma concentrations. A decision then has to be taken on how long to continue treatment: in practice many clinicians withdraw respiratory stimulants when the baby is around 34 weeks postmenstrual age, after which time most babies will have achieved an adequate degree of cardiorespiratory stability and no longer need even the most basic forms of monitoring device.

Seizures

A second important area where treatment goals are uncertain is that of neonatal seizures, particularly those resulting from hypoxic ischaemic encephalopathy (HIE). HIE may result from birth asphyxia or from an antepartum insult, and can be graded on a clinical basis according to its severity. In the more severe cases, convulsions occur within 24 hours of birth and continue for 2 to 3 days after which they spontaneously resolve, and the baby passes though a phase of hypertonia before becoming hypotonic. Less severely affected babies quickly return to neurological normality. The therapeutic dilemma lies in the degree of aggression with which convulsions should be treated, since all conventional anticonvulsants are relatively ineffective in reducing electrocerebral activity even if they reduce the clinical manifestations of seizure, and the convulsions tend naturally to cease after 2 or 3 days. Furthermore, there is no clear evidence that strenuous attempts to gain control of seizures have any effect on the subsequent developmental prognosis of the child. On the other hand, seizures which compromise respiratory function should be treated to prevent serious falls in arterial oxygen tension; babies with frequent or continuous seizure activity are difficult to nurse and cause great distress to their parents. Thus, in practice, it is usual to try to suppress the clinical manifestation of seizure activity, and phenobarbitone remains the most commonly used first line treatment. Where a decision is taken to keep a baby on anticonvulsant medication, therapeutic drug monitoring provides helpful information and will need to be repeated from time to time during follow-up.

PRINCIPLES AND GOALS OF THERAPY

The ultimate aim of neonatal care, at all levels, is to maximize disability-free survival and identify treatable conditions which would otherwise compromise growth or development. The treatment of most newborn babies is routine and preventive, and emergency intervention is needed only in a select few; these approaches are completely different and must be considered separately. Even for babies born preterm this means anticipating potential problems and avoiding as far as possible the complications of intensive care.

Effects of rapid growth

The growth of a premature baby, once the need for intensive care has passed, can be very rapid indeed if the child is being fed with 200 ml/kg/day of high calorie formula modified for use with low birth weight infants; indeed most babies born at 27 weeks (and weighing around 1 kg) can be expected to double their birth weights by the time they are 8 weeks old. Since the dose of all medications is calculated on the basis of body weight, constant review of dose is necessary to maintain efficacy, particularly for drugs which may be given for weeks on end, such as respiratory stimulants, diuretics and anticonvulsants. Conversely, all that is necessary to gradually wean a baby from a medication is to hold the dose constant so that the baby gradually 'grows out' of the drug. This practice is frequently used with diuretic medication in BPD, the need for which becomes less as the baby's somatic growth reduces the proportion of damaged lung in favour of healthy tissue.

Therapeutic drug monitoring

The assay of plasma concentrations of various drugs has a place in neonatal medicine, particularly where the therapeutic index of a drug is narrow. It is thus routine to assay levels of antibiotics such as aminoglycosides and vancomycin, usually as a peak and a trough. More rarely it may be necessary to assay minimal inhibitory or bactericidal concentrations of antibiotics in blood or cerebrospinal fluid if serious infections are being treated, but constraints on sampling limit the frequency with which this may be undertaken. Interpretation of plasma concentrations of chloramphenicol is problematic as active metabolites are not included, and safer antibiotics such as ceftazidime and cefotaxime are now replacing chloramphenicol.

Theophylline and aminophylline are handled unpredictably and assay of plasma concentrations is a useful guide to therapy; since a baby may be on such medication for several weeks, assays need to be repeated regularly (probably weekly, for convenience). The use of caffeine, which has a much wider therapeutic index, obviates the need for routine measurement of levels, although it may still be necessary to measure blood levels if a normal dose appears to be ineffective. Where phenobarbitone or other anticonvulsants are given long term, intermittent measurement of plasma levels can be a useful guide to increasing the dose as with methyl xanthines. Digoxin is rarely used in this age group but regular assay of plasma concentrations is of obvious importance. All of these drugs have a long half-life so it is most important that drug concentrations are not measured too early, or too frequently, so that inappropriate changes in dose do not get made before a steady state is reached.

Avoiding harm

There are very few situations in which intramuscular injections are required in the neonate, and because of the lack of muscle bulk it is advisable to avoid them if at all possible. However, it is not always easy to establish intra-venous access, and it may be necessary to use the intramuscular route instead.

As for patients of any age, the minimal necessary intervention should be the rule. For sick preterm infants ventilated for respiratory failure, handling of any kind is a destabilizing influence. Even opening the doors of an incubator causes the interior temperature to fall in all but the newest incubators. It is therefore good practice to minimize the frequency of drug administration and to try to coordinate the doses of different medications.

Timescale of clinical changes

The clinical condition of any baby can change with extraordinary rapidity and it is usual to have to institute treatment very quickly. For example, the decision to start antibiotics is almost invariably on the grounds of clinical suspicion backed up if necessary by indirect laboratory evidence; therapy can be discontinued if it becomes clear that the clinical picture was accounted for by other factors, and confirmation of bacterial infection does not materialize. Thus whether the antibiotic was required is often a question with only a retrospective answer. For the sick preterm infant this model applies to a wide range of interventions. It is seldom possible to wait a few hours for the availability of a drug, and this has obvious implications for the quality of support required of a pharmacy for a neonatal service.

THE PATIENT AND THE PARENT

It is all too easy to take a 'veterinary' approach to neonatal medicine, on the grounds that premature infants cannot communicate their needs and can be treated, especially while receiving intensive care, as little more than a physiological preparation. Such an approach to therapy is fundamentally flawed, for two reasons. First, even when receiving intensive care, any infant who is not either paralysed or very heavily sedated does in fact respond with a wealth of cues and non-verbal communication to their current needs. Monitors therefore do not replace clinical skills, but provide supplementary information and advance warning of problems. Even the most premature babies show individual characteristics, which emphasizes that individualized care is as important in this age group as in any other. Indeed, coordination of care with the rhythms of the baby rather than the rigid routines of the unit has been shown to be beneficial.

Involvement of parents in every aspect of care is a necessary goal in neonatal clinical practice, and care within a special care baby nursery is increasingly regarded as a partnership between professionals and parents rather than the province of professionals alone. Routine administration of oral medication is thus an act in which parents may be expected to participate, and for those whose baby has to be discharged home still requiring continuous oxygen, the parent will rapidly obtain complete control, with support from the hospital and the primary health care team. Increasing numbers of babies, who survive very premature birth, but whose respiratory state requires continued support after discharge, present an increasing therapeutic challenge for the future.

BIBLIOGRAPHY

Albersheim S G, Solimano A J, Sharma A K, Smyth J A, Rotschild A, Wood B J et al. Randomised double blind controlled trial of long term diuretic therapy for bronchopulmonary dysplasia. Journal of Paediatrics 1989; 115: 615–620

Anand K J S, Hickey P R. Pain and its effects in the human neonate and fetus. New England Journal of Medicine 1987; 317: 1321–1329

Morley C J. Surfactant treatment for premature babies – a review of clinical trials. Archives of Disease in Childhood 1991; 66: 445–450

Mugford M, Piercy J, Chalmers I. Cost implications of different approaches to the prevention of respiratory distress syndrome. Archives of Disease in Childhood 1991; 66: 757–764

Rennie J M, Cooke R W I. Prolonged low dose indomethacin for persistent ductus arteriosus of prematurity. Archives of Disease in Childhood 1991; 66: 55–58

Ruggins N R, Milner A D. Site of upper airway obstruction in preterm infants with problematical apnoea. Archives of Disease in Childhood 1991; 66: 787–792

Rutter N. Drug absorption through the skin: a mixed blessing. Archives of Disease in Childhood 1987; 62: 220–221

Scanlon J E M, Chin K C, Morgan M E I et al. Caffeine or theophylline for neonatal apnoea? Archives of Disease in Childhood 1992; 67: 425–428

Volpe J J. Neonatal seizures: current concepts and revised classification. Pediatrics 1989; 83: 422–428

Chapter 7

Paediatrics

C. E. Barker   A. J. Nunn   S. C. Turner

'Paediatrics' is the branch of medicine dealing with the development, diseases and disorders of children. For many purposes it is common to subdivide childhood into the following periods:

- neonate — the first 30 days of life
- infant — from 1 month to 1 year
- child — from 1 year to 12 years
- adolescent – from 12 years to 16 years.

Infancy and childhood is a period of rapid growth and development. The various organs, body systems and enzymes that handle drugs develop at different rates and present a challenge to those who specialize in paediatrics, since drug dosage, formulation, response to drugs and adverse reactions vary throughout childhood. Compared to adult medicine, drug use in paediatrics is not extensively researched and the range of licensed drugs in appropriate dosage forms is limited.

This chapter explores some of the disorders of children together with their treatment which are different to those seen in adults.

DEMOGRAPHY

In 1989 11.5 million of the UK population were less than 16 years of age. Mid-year population projections for this age group in 1991 and 1996 are 11.7 and 12.5 million respectively.

Despite a decline of 38% in the neonatal mortality rate between 1980 and 1989, the decline in infant mortality rate is much less. Between 1 month and 1 year of age, deaths have decreased by only

16%. Sudden infant deaths and deaths from respiratory diseases account for more than half of post-neonatal deaths.

The five main causes of death in those under 15 years of age are road vehicle accidents, congenital abnormalities, diseases of the CNS and sense organs, other causes of poisoning and injury (apart from road vehicle accidents) and malignant neoplasms of lymphatic and haematopoietic tissue.

DRUG DISPOSITION

Pharmacokinetic factors

An understanding of the variability in drug disposition is essential if children are to receive rational and appropriate drug therapy. For convenience the factors that affect drug disposition will be dealt with separately. However, when treating a patient all the factors have a dynamic relationship and none should be considered in isolation.

Absorption

Oral absorption. The absorption process of oral preparations may be influenced by factors such as gastric and intestinal transit time, gastric and intestinal pH and gastrointestinal contents. Posture, disease states and therapeutic interventions such as nasogastric aspiration or drug therapy can also affect the absorption process.

It is not until the second year of life that gastric acid output increases and is comparable on a per kg basis to that observed in adults. In addition gastric emptying time only approaches adult values at about 6 months of age.

Few studies have reported specifically on the absorption process in older infants or children. The bioavailability of sulphonamides, digoxin and phenobarbitone has been studied in infants and children of a wide age distribution. Despite the different physicochemical properties of the drugs, a similar bioavailability pattern was observed in each case. The rate of absorption was correlated with age, being much slower in neonates than in older infants and children. This data suggests that in older infants and children orally administered drugs will be absorbed at a rate and extent similar to that in healthy adults. Changes in the absorption rate would appear to be of minor importance when compared to the age-related differences of drug distribution and excretion.

Intramuscular absorption. Absorption in infants and children after intramuscular (i.m.) injection is noticeably faster than in the neonatal period, since muscle blood flow is increased. On a practical note, i.m. administration is very painful. The route should not be used for the convenience of staff if alternative routes of administration are available.

Topical absorption. Recent advances in transdermal drug delivery systems have led to an increased use of this route of administration. Percutaneous absorption which is inversely related to the thickness of the stratum corneum and directly related to skin hydration, is generally much greater in the newborn and young infant than in the adult.

Rectal absorption. The rectal route of administration is generally less favoured in the UK than in other European countries. It can be useful in patients who are vomiting, or in infants or children reluctant or unable to take oral medication. The mechanism of rectal absorption is probably similar to that of the upper part of the gastrointestinal tract, despite differences in pH, surface area and fluid content. Although some products, such as theophylline, are erratically absorbed from the rectum, the rapid onset of action of other preparations can be invaluable, e.g. rectal diazepam solution produces a rapid cessation of seizures in epilepsy and can be easily administered by parents in an emergency.

Distribution

A number of factors that determine drug distribution within the body are subject to change with age. These include vascular perfusion, body composition, tissue binding characteristics and the extent of plasma protein binding.

As a percentage of total body weight the total body water and extracellular fluid volume decrease with age (Table 7.1). Thus, for water-soluble drugs such as aminoglycosides, larger doses on a mg/kg body weight basis are required in the neonate than in the older child to achieve similar plasma concentrations (e.g. 3 mg/kg/dose of gentamicin in neonates compared to 2.5 mg/kg/dose in older children).

Protein binding. Despite normal blood pH, free fatty acid and bilirubin levels in infants, binding to plasma proteins is reduced as a result of low concentrations of both globulins and albumin. It has been suggested that binding values comparable with those seen in adults are reached within the third year of life for acidic drugs, whereas for basic drugs adult values are not reached until between 7 and 12 years of life. The clinical significance of this reduction in infants and older children is minimal. The influence of disease states on plasma protein binding is more important.

Drug metabolism

At birth the majority of the enzyme systems responsible for drug metabolism are either absent or present in considerably reduced amounts compared to adult values, and evidence indicates that the various systems do not mature at the same time. This reduced capacity for metabolic degradation at birth is followed by a dramatic increase in the metabolic rate in the older infant and young child. In the 1 to 9 years age group in particular, metabolic clearance of drugs is shown to be greater than in adults; as exemplified by theophylline, phenytoin and carbamazepine. Thus to achieve plasma concentrations similar to those observed in adults, children in this age group may require a higher dosage

Table 7.1 Extracellular fluid volume and total body water as a percentage of body weight

Age	Total body water	Extracellular fluid
Preterm neonate	85%	50%
Term neonate	75%	45%
3 months	75%	30%
1 year	60%	25%
Adult	60%	20%

Table 7.2 Theophylline dosage in children older than 1 year

Age	Dosage (mg/kg/day)
1–9 years	24
9–12 years	20
12–16 years	18
Adult	13

than adults on a mg/kg body weight basis (Table 7.2).

Renal excretion

The anatomical and functional immaturity of the kidneys at birth limit renal excretory capacity. Below 3 to 6 months of age the glomerular filtration rate is lower than that of adults, but may be partially compensated by a relatively greater reduction in tubular reabsorption. Tubular function matures later than the filtration process. Generally the complete maturation of glomerular and tubular function is reached only towards 6 to 8 months of age. After 8 months of age the renal excretion of drugs is comparable with that observed in older children and adults.

Changes in renal clearance of digoxin provide a good example of the maturation of renal function. Digoxin half-lives are reported to range from 20 to 70 hours in term babies less than 2 months of age, and decrease dramatically over the next 16 months falling to 12 to 42 hours in infants between 2 and 18 months of age. Maturation of the renal secretory process is thought to be partly responsible.

Other factors

In addition to age-related changes in drug disposition, nutritional status and disease states can influence drug handling. High plasma clearance of antibiotics such as penicillins and aminoglycosides has been demonstrated in children with cystic fibrosis; increased elimination of frusemide has been reported in children with nephrotic syndrome whilst prolonged elimination of frusemide has been reported in infants with congestive cardiac failure. Altered protein binding has been demonstrated in hepatic disease, nephrotic syndrome, malnutrition and cardiac failure.

DRUG THERAPY IN CHILDREN

Dosage

Children should not be treated as mini-adults, yet paediatric dosages are often extrapolated from the usual adult dose. Rather than calculate the proportion of the adult dose it is preferable to consult a textbook or vade mecum in which paediatric doses are quoted and have been confirmed by clinical experience. Many different formulae based on weight and age have been developed for estimating a child's dose from the adult value. Whilst age, weight and height are the easiest parameters to measure, the changing requirement for drug dosage during childhood corresponds most closely with changes in body surface area (BSA). Nomograms which allow surface area to be easily derived are available.

There are practical problems in using the surface area method for prescribing; accurate height and weight may be difficult to obtain in a sick child and manufacturers rarely provide dosage information on a surface area basis. The surface area formula for children has been used to produce the percentage method, giving the percentage of adult dose required at various ages and weights (Table 7.3).

Table 7.3 Percentage of adult dose required at various ages and weights			
Age	Mean weight for age		Percent of adult dose
	lb	kg	
Newborn (full term)	7.7	3.5	12.5
2 months	10	4.5	15
4 months	14	6.5	20
1 year	22	10	25
3 years	33	15	33.3
7 years	50	23	50
10 years	66	30	60
12 years	86	39	75
14 years	110	50	80
16 years	128	58	90
Adult	150	68	100

In selecting a method of dosage calculation the therapeutic index of the drug should be considered. For agents with a narrow therapeutic index, e.g. cytotoxic agents, where recommendations are quoted in per m^2, dosing must be based on the calculated surface area. However for drugs with a high therapeutic index, e.g. penicillin, single doses may be quoted for a wide age range. Between these two extremes, doses are quoted in mg/kg, and this is the most widely used method of calculation. Whichever method is used, the resulting dosage should be modified according to response and adverse effects.

It is important to note that none of the available methods of dosage calculation account for the change in dosage interval which may be required because of age-related changes in drug clearance. Where possible the use of therapeutic drug monitoring to confirm the appropriateness of a dosage is recommended.

Choice of preparation

The choice of preparation and its formulation will be affected by the intended route of administration, the age of the child, availability of preparations, other concomitant therapy and possibly underlying disease states.

Oral route

The oral route is usually the most convenient, but in an uncooperative child it can be the least reliable. Safe and effective drug therapy requires accurate administration, yet the 5 ml spoon is a difficult means of administering liquid medicines. Use of the oral syringe can overcome this problem and avoid the need for dilution of preparations with syrup.

In general, liquid preparations are more suitable for children of less than 5 years of age, although many quite young children can cope with solid dose formulations. Some commercially available products contain excipients such as alcohol, propylene glycol and dyes which may cause adverse effects or be inappropriate for use in children with particular disease states. The osmolality and tonicity of preparations may be important; necrotizing enterocolitis (a disorder seen in the neonatal period) has been associated with high osmolality infant feeding formulae and pharmaceutical preparations. Sugar-free preparations may be necessary in the diabetic child or be desirable in other children for the prevention of dental caries. It is, however, important to be aware of the potential problems associated with substitutes for sucrose. The artificial sweetening agent aspartame, used in some preparations, should be used with caution in children with phenylketonuria because of its phenylalanine content. Other carbohydrates such as sorbitol and glycerol may not contribute to dental caries but produce diarrhoea if large doses are given. In these instances a specially formulated preparation may be preferable.

Injection solutions can sometimes be administered orally although their concentration and pH must be considered together with the presence of unsuitable excipients. Powders may be prepared and used as an alternative. However, lactose is a common diluent in powders and caution must be exercised in children with lactose intolerance as a result of an inborn error of metabolism, or temporarily following gastrointestinal diseases or gut surgery.

Parents must be discouraged from adding the dose of medicine to an infant's feed. Quite apart from potential interactions which may arise with milk feeds, if the entire feed is not taken a proportion of the dose will be lost. It is also important to advise parents when it is not appropriate to crush solid dosage forms (e.g. sustained-release preparations).

Rectal route

Although the rectal route can be useful, it is limited by the range of products available and the dosage inflexibility associated with rectal preparations.

When oral and rectal routes are inappropriate the parenteral route may be necessary.

Parenteral route

Because it is painful, the intramuscular route of administration should be avoided in children.

However, intravenous administration is not without its problems. In infants and children the direct administration of intravenous fluids from the main infusion container is associated with the risk of inadvertent fluid overload. A paediatric administration set, incorporating a graduated volumetric chamber with a maximum capacity of 150 ml should always be used. Although primarily a safety device, the volume within the burette can be readily adjusted allowing its use for intermittent drug administration and avoiding the need for a 'piggy back system'. Use of a volumetric infusion device to control the flow rate is also strongly recommended.

Parenteral products are associated with particular problems in paediatric therapy. The concentration of many proprietary products makes measurement of the small doses required very difficult and can lead to inaccuracies. Reconstitution of powder injections in accordance with manufacturers' directions usually makes no allowance for the displacement volume of the powder itself. Underdosing may occur as a result, since the final volume will be greater than expected and the concentration less than expected.

Dilution of parenteral preparations for infusion often presents problems in paediatrics. In fluid-restricted or very young infants, the volume of diluted drug can exceed the daily fluid requirement. Often stability data on concentrated solutions is lacking, and in this situation it may be necessary to manipulate other therapy to accommodate the treatment or even consider alternative treatment options.

The slow infusion rates often necessary in paediatrics may influence drug therapy. The greater the distance between the administration port and the distal end of the delivery system, and the slower the flow rate, the longer the time required for the drug to be delivered to the patient. In very young infants and children it may take several hours for the drug to reach the patient. This is an important consideration if dosage adjustments are being made in response to serum level monitoring. Bolus injections should always be given as close to the patient as possible.

The trapping of a drug solution at the injection port creates further problems for drug administration. When dose volumes are small the trapped fluid may represent a considerable proportion of the intended dose. Ensuring that drugs are flushed into the main infusion line after administration via an injection port can help to minimize the problem. Flushing volumes can add a significant amount to the daily fluid intake and it may be important to record the volume of flushing solutions used in patients susceptible to fluid overload.

Analogous to oral preparations, excipients may be present in parenteral formulations and associated with adverse effects. Benzyl alcohol, polysorbates and propylene glycol are commonly used agents which may induce a range of adverse effects in children including metabolic acidosis, altered serum osmolality, CNS depression, respiratory depression, cardiac arrhythmias and seizures. Knowledge of the products that contain these ingredients may influence drug selection.

Pulmonary route

The use of aerosol inhalers presents particular problems for children because of the coordina-

tion required. The availability of breath-activated devices and spacer devices has greatly improved the situation. Appropriate inhalational devices for particular age groups are shown in Figure 7.1.

A basic clinical checklist for paediatric drug therapy is shown in Table 7.4.

RENAL DISEASE
Chronic renal insufficiency

The most frequent causes of chronic renal insufficiency in children are glomerulonephritis, urologic abnormalities, hypoplastic kidneys and hereditary nephropathies. It is currently estimated that 1.5 to 3 per million of the world population under the age of 16 years develop end-stage renal disease.

The management of chronic renal failure in children is based on similar principles to that in adults. Additional problems which may arise in children include growth failure and developmental delay.

Both cognitive and motor development dysfunction have been reported in infants with

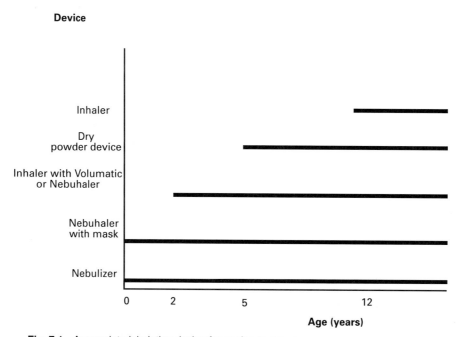

Fig. 7.1 Appropriate inhalation device for each age group.

Table 7.4 Factors to be considered when selecting a drug dosage regimen or route of administration for a paediatric patient

Factor	Comment
1. Age/weight/surface area	Is the weight close to that expected for age? If not, confirm weight difference.
2. Dose	Is the dose appropriate for weight/age/disease state?
3. Dose interval	Is the dosage interval influenced by the child's waking day? If so is this important? Consider preparations with a narrow therapeutic index, e.g. theophylline.
4. Route of administration	Is the route appropriate for the age/disease state?
5. Preparation	Is the preparation or administration device suitable for the age/disease state?
6. Formulation	Is the formulation suitable for paediatric use? Consider excipients/concentration osmolarity.
7. Intravenous preparations	Consider displacement volumes and dilution volumes in relation to daily fluid requirement.
8. Pharmacokinetics	Is the normal pharmacokinetic profile altered in children?
9. Interactions	Consider drug interactions with milk feeds.
10. Adverse effect profile	Are there any long term adverse effects, e.g. effects on growth?
11. Counselling and compliance aids	Use whenever possible, e.g. oral syringes, whistles for Intal spinhaler.
12. Legal considerations	Is the drug licensed for the indication? If not, is the prescriber aware of this?

chronic renal insufficiency, and it has been suggested that the immature brain may be vulnerable to uraemia.

Anaemia, anorexia, protein malnutrition, fluid, electrolyte and acid–base imbalance have been implicated in growth retardation associated with chronic renal failure, and correction of these factors allows catch-up growth in some cases. Growth hormone treatment appears to increase the rate of growth in children with renal disease, but has no effect on height score for bone age, suggesting that final height may not be altered. For this reason, and because of concern about possible adverse effects such as deterioration in renal function, adverse effects on carbohydrate metabolism, and possible links with leukaemia which may be associated with growth hormone treatment the treatment has not been routinely adopted.

Assessment of renal function

Several formulae and nomograms for calculating creatinine clearance and estimating renal function in adults are available, but these cannot be extrapolated to the paediatric population.

Use of the equation suggested by Traub & Johnson provides a simple estimate of creatinine clearance for those between the age of 1 to 18 years:

$$\text{Creatinine clearance (ml/min/1.73m}^2) = \frac{42 \times \text{Height}}{\text{Serum creatinine}}$$

where height is in centimetres, and serum creatinine is in micromoles per litre.

Nephrotic syndrome

The commonest histological form of the nephrotic syndrome which occurs in children is minimal change disease. It rarely occurs in the first year of life and is generally responsive to corticosteroid therapy. In most cases minimal change disease occurs in children aged 2 to 6 years and is idiopathic or primary. Important secondary causes include infection (e.g. hepatitis B), drugs (e.g. penicillamine, non-steroidal anti-inflammatory agents) or diseases (e.g. Henoch–Schoenlein purpura).

Acute renal failure, increased risk of infection, thrombosis and hyperlipidaemia may all occur as features of the disease.

A brief outline of the management of nephrotic syndrome is shown in Table 7.5.

Some children may respond to lower doses of corticosteroids than those suggested. In addition, some centres advocate that longer-term therapy may be of more benefit in preventing relapse. The median time of response is towards the second week of therapy.

Table 7.5   Management of nephrotic syndrome in children

1. Treat symptomatic hypovolaemia and oedema with plasma or salt poor albumin (1 g albumin/kg), followed by 1–2 mg/kg of frusemide 30 minutes later.

2. Prednisolone (60 mg/m^2/day). Discontinue over 6–8 weeks once response is achieved (i.e. urine is protein free on three consecutive days).

3. Frequently relapsing/steroid dependent patients: consider alternate day prednisolone therapy 0.5 mg/kg/alternate day for up to 6 months and review.

4. Non-responsive patients: consider cyclophosphamide 2–3 mg/kg/day or chlorambucil 0.2 mg/kg/day (levamisole and cyclosporin may also be alternatives).

Children receiving maintenance treatment with steroids should have careful growth records maintained, so that the risks of continued therapy can be more readily assessed.

In general children with nephrotic syndrome should be encouraged to maintain as normal an activity level as possible. They should receive a diet with a caloric intake appropriate for age although a restricted intake may be needed in children gaining too much weight on steroids.

Hyperlipidaemia is a common feature of the disease and may increase the risk of atherosclerosis. The role of lipid-lowering agents in children is unclear, primarily because of unanswered questions over their long-term safety.

Haemolytic uraemic syndrome

Haemolytic uraemic syndrome (HUS) is characterized by acute haemolytic anaemia, thrombocytopenia and acute renal failure. Characteristically the disease affects infants and young children of 6 months to 8 years. Endemic outbreaks occur in spring and summer. The aetiology of HUS is uncertain; however, strains of verocytotoxin-producing *Esch. coli* have been implicated in the classical disease. Typically a prodromal illness of fever and diarrhoea (often bloody) is followed by the development of thrombocytopenia, anaemia and oliguria. A much rarer form of HUS has no obvious gastrointestinal prodrome but may present with neurological abnormalities secondary to CNS vascular disease. Prognosis in these patients is much worse.

Treatment for this self-limiting disorder remains primarily supportive. A conservative approach to therapy and early peritoneal dialysis is sufficient.

During the early stages of the disease attention should be paid to volume status and hypovolaemia should be corrected. Hypokalaemia (secondary to diarrhoea) should not be treated in the presence of renal failure if the serum potassium concentration exceeds 3 mmol/L. Hyperkalaemia secondary to haemolysis and renal failure can be treated with calcium resonium 1 g/kg (orally or rectally, maximum 40 g) or insulin, glucose and bicarbonate therapy. These interventions are only temporary and dialysis is indicated for uncontrolled hyperkalaemia.

Oedema should be managed with fluid restriction and high doses of frusemide of up to 5 mg/kg may be necessary. Sodium bicarbonate (1 to 2 mmol/kg/day) is used to control acidosis secondary to renal insufficiency, but patients with prolonged severe acidosis require dialysis. Neurological symptoms and severe catabolism are also indications for dialysis.

Peritoneal dialysis is the dialysis of choice. It is easier to perform in small children and allows for continuous control of the patient's volume, electrolyte and metabolic status without the wide fluctuations of haemodialysis. Hourly dialysis cycles of 30 to 50 ml/kg are generally employed and therapy is often required for 2 to 3 weeks. A continuous daily rise in platelet count is the earliest sign of recovery, the anaemia is slower to resolve.

Up to 95% of patients survive an episode of HUS, and return of normal renal function can be anticipated in 90%. A small number of patients develop mild renal function abnormalities, hypertension or occasionally chronic progressive renal failure.

Enuresis

Childhood enuresis describes the inappropriate

voiding of urine by a child who has reached the age at which satisfactory control of micturition is expected. The term should only be used in children older than 5 years of age. Genetic factors, disease states such as diabetes mellitus and renal failure, and bladder capacity predispose to enuresis.

Treatment includes conditioning therapy such as enuresis alarms, bladder training to increase the size of the bladder, awakening and encouraging the child to empty the bladder late at night (e.g. 11 p.m.) and drug therapy.

Drugs with anticholinergic effects, such as imipramine (2 mg/kg; maximum 25 mg < 7 years, 50 mg 7 to 11 years) propantheline (1 to 2 mg/kg/day) and oxybutynin (1.25 to 2.5 mg twice a day) are the most commonly used pharmacologic agents. The final dose should be administered half to 1 hour before bedtime.

CARDIOLOGY

Paediatric cardiology is predominantly concerned with congenital heart defects (CHD). A ratio of about 100 CHD patients to 1 with acquired heart disease is seen.

Congenital heart defects

CHD is the commonest of all congenital defects with an incidence of 8/1000 live births. Of these approximately:

- 1/3 will present as critically ill within 1 year
- 1/3 will become ill later in life
- 1/3 will have no significant problems.

There are a large number of different defects but eight common lesions account for about 80% of all CHDs and include:

- ventricular septal defect – a hole between the ventricles
- patent ductus arteriosus – persistence of the ductus arteriosus which connects the aorta and pulmonary artery in the fetal circulation and diverts blood from the lungs to the descending aorta; it normally closes within 10 to 15 hours of birth

- atrial septal defect – a hole between the atria
- tetralogy of Fallot – a ventricular septal defect and a pulmonary stenosis
- pulmonary stenosis – narrowing of the pulmonary valve opening, reducing blood flow to the pulmonary artery
- coarctation of the aorta – a narrowing of the aorta
- aortic stenosis – narrowing of the aortic valve opening, obstructing blood flow from the left ventricle to the aorta
- Transposition of the great arteries – the aorta and pulmonary artery are transposed to arise from the right and left ventricle respectively.

The cause of the lesion is unknown in over 90% of cases. However, some factors are known, for example CHD affects 40% of patients with Down's syndrome. Approximately 60% of children with CHD will require some form of surgery.

Acquired heart disease

Acquired heart disease in children is a rare presentation which may arise secondary to:

- Kawasaki disease
- bacterial or viral myocarditis
- acute rheumatic fever
- anthracycline toxicity.

The signs and symptoms of presentation vary widely according to the nature of the underlying condition. A number of patients present with signs of heart failure and common features such as heart murmurs, cyanosis, breathlessness, palpitations, failure to thrive, syncope, dizziness, fatigue and squatting. Chest pain and sudden collapse are uncommon presentations in children.

Arrhythmias

Arrhythmias may occur in children with structurally normal hearts. Some of these will show ahnormalities on electrocardiography, for example the Wolff–Parkinson–White syndrome. Arrhythmias may occur in association with CHD but an increasing number are now seen after cardiac surgery. Drug-induced arrhythmias may also occur.

Drug treatment

Doses of drugs used in paediatric cardiology require experience in their application and are not presented here. Readers are referred to the bibliography for further information.

PAEDIATRIC RESPIRATORY DISEASE

Asthma

Asthma affects more than 10% of children and may occur at any age, although symptoms commonly arise before 4 to 5 years of age.

Common clinical features of childhood asthma include wheeze, a chronic, dry nocturnal cough and episodes of spasmodic croup. Exclusion of diseases such as cystic fibrosis, inhaled foreign body and infectious bronchiolitis, which may present with similar symptoms in young children, is important. Children over 5 years of age can cooperate with pulmonary function tests and these can be used as an aid to diagnosis and assessment of response.

As in adults, intermittent beta$_2$ adrenoreceptor agonists are the first line therapeutic agents. They are less likely to produce immediate benefit in wheezy infants less than 6 months of age and here the use of oral xanthines and nebulized ipratropium should be considered. The use of inhaled beta$_2$-agonists on a regular basis has been implicated as a contributory factor in asthma morbidity and deaths. Although a cause and effect relationship has not been established, if such therapy is required more than three times per week prophylaxis with sodium cromoglycate should be initiated. Inhaled steroids are reserved for children with more severe symptoms. Low doses (400 microgram/day of beclomethasone or budesonide) are usually effective, but in more severe disease the use of higher doses may be warranted. The potential for adrenal and growth suppression exists in children inhaling doses as low as 400 to 600 microgram daily of either beclomethasone or budesonide. However, in very severe disease the potential dangers of uncontrolled asthma are far greater than the adverse effects of therapy. If oral steroids are required in very severe disease, they should be given as alternate-day therapy where possible.

The use of regular inhaled beta$_2$-agonist therapy may be considered in children receiving moderate doses of inhaled steroids, in whom asthma is still not controlled. Similarly addition of inhaled ipratropium at this point may be helpful.

Xanthine preparations may be helpful in the prophylaxis of severe asthma in children receiving moderate doses of steroids. The altered pharmacokinetics of xanthines in children, in addition to concern about their adverse effects on behaviour and their potential for interaction have now led to their use as third line agents.

Acute asthma

Severe attacks of asthma may be precipitated by a number of factors including non-compliance with medication, stress and infection. Once an attack has failed to respond to the standard home treatment, medical attention should be sought. A nebulized beta$_2$-agonist (salbutamol or terbutaline) should be administered if the patient does not have a home nebulizer. Failure to respond to the nebulized dose or relapse within 4 hours of a dose would indicate need for referral to hospital. A suggested algorithm for managing acute asthma is described in Table 7.6.

Sudden infant death syndrome (SIDS)

The sudden infant death syndrome (SIDS) is now the commonest cause of death between 28 days and 12 months of age; however, the pathogenesis of the disorder is still unclear. Much interest has centred on the role of viral illness and upper airway obstruction in SIDS, but more recently identified risk factors which may be important include parental smoking, sleeping position and overinsulation in the infant. Mothers are now advised not to smoke and to avoid placing their child in the prone sleeping position.

The role of drug therapy in SIDS or 'near miss' incidents has also been addressed. The phenothiazines, trimeprazine and promethazine and the antispasmodic agent dicyclomine have re-

Table 7.6 A strategy for managing acute asthma	
1. Oxygen	
2. Nebulized salbutamol	
6 months – 1 year	1 mg
1–7 years	2.5 mg
> 7 years	5 mg
usually 3- to 4-hourly: maximum 2-hourly	
3. Oral prednisolone	
6 months – 1 year	10 mg/day
1–5 years	20 mg/day
5–10 years	30 mg/day
> 10 years	40 mg/day
for 3 days minimum	
If the child is unresponsive to nebulized therapy, deteriorates between nebulized treatment, is vomiting or dehydrated, change to i.v. therapy.	
4. Intravenous therapy	
Aminophylline	Loading dose 6–9 mg/kg* over 30 minutes Maintenance dose 1–9 years 1.2 mg/kg/hour > 9 years 0.75 mg/kg/hour
* If theophylline therapy has been administered in the previous 24 hours, a reduced loading dose of 3 mg/kg should be given or a serum level obtained.	
Hydrocortisone	4 mg/kg stat dose then 2–4 mg/kg every 6 hours

Table 7.7 Relative incidence of various childhood cancers shown as percentage of all childhood cancers	
Disease	Incidence (%)
Leukaemia ALL	27
Leukaemia AML	7
Brain tumour	22
Wilms' tumour	6
Neuroblastoma	6
Retinoblastoma	3
Hepatoblastoma	1
Non-Hodgkin's lymphoma	4
Hodgkin's lymphoma	7
Bone sarcoma	5
Soft tissue sarcoma	6
Others	6

Reference: Stiller C A, Bunch K J. Trends in survival for childhood cancer in Britain – diagnosed 1971–85. British Journal of Cancer 1990; 62: 806–815

ceived particular attention. Although no formal cause and effect relationship between SIDS and drug administration has been confirmed, use of these agents is contra-indicated in young infants.

PAEDIATRIC CANCERS

Paediatric malignancy represents less than 1% of all cancers; however, 1 in 600 children in the UK are affected by cancer, and 1200 new cases are diagnosed each year. The spectrum of malignancy in children is very different from that of adults. Acute lymphoblastic leukaemia (ALL) and acute myeloid leukemia (AML) account for approximately one-third of childhood cancers, while brain tumours account for just over one-fifth. Relative incidence of childhood cancers is shown in Table 7.7.

Major advances in chemotherapy in addition to the development of techniques such as bone marrow transplantation have helped to produce a marked improvement in the prognosis of childhood cancer, and more than 50% of all children with cancer can now be cured. The improved survival rate is also attributed to the development of centres specializing in paediatric oncology and the implementation of controlled clinical trials of therapy, directed by the Medical Research Council (MRC) and the United Kingdom Children's Cancer Study Group (UKCCSG). By assigning patients to different treatment options the clinical trials aim to answer one main question, which may relate to dosage or timing of particular therapies. Analysis of the data on completion of the trial is used as a basis for future protocols.

The advantages of such improvements in therapy would be lost, if it were not for similar advances in supportive therapy. Bone marrow growth factors can reduce the length and severity of chemotherapy-induced neutropenia; new antibiotics have reduced the number of severe infections; new antiemetic agents have helped to reduce some of the more distressing side effects of therapy, and permanent intravenous access devices have removed the need for repeated venepuncture.

With improved treatment and survival of childhood cancers an increased awareness of long-term effects of therapy is important. Endocrine dysfunction, infertility, cardiovascular disease, psychological effects and secondary tumours are some of the potential problems. Thus in designing new protocols a balance between minimizing long-term effects and not jeopardizing treatment success must be achieved.

In general, dosages quoted in protocols are based on surface area. Many treatment protocols last for several years and, as a result of growth, children will show a marked change in surface area, over the period of treatment, when compared with adults. Recalculation of dosages at each treatment stage is necessary to ensure that children are not underdosed. Side effect profiles of drugs may differ between children and adults. For example, children are more susceptible than adults to the extrapyramidal effects of the antiemetic agent metoclopramide. Manufacturers' recommendations for the preparation and dilution of cytotoxic agents for intravenous administration may exceed the fluid tolerance of very young children. Intervention may be necessary to avoid the complications of fluid overload, whilst still considering the toxicities and stabilities of the drug. Use of a checklist as an aide mémoire can be helpful (Table 7.8).

INFLAMMATORY DISORDERS

Juvenile rheumatoid arthritis (Still's disease)

Arthritis in children, unlike in adults, is uncommon but is a significant cause of disability or handicap. Prognosis is generally good with many children requiring only non-steroidal anti-inflammatory drugs (NSAIDs). However, for children more severely affected, treatment regimens may involve potentially toxic drugs such as corticosteroids, gold salts and cytotoxics. Many of the drugs used in adult arthritis are not licensed for use in children.

Juvenile chronic arthritis by definition has an onset under the age of 16 years, affects one or more joints for more than 3 months and excludes other disease with some of the same features, for example psoriatic arthritis, SLE and infection. Pauciarticular (involving four joints or less) on-

Table 7.8 Clinical oncology checklist (reproduced by permission of Butterworth-Heinemann from Siddall S 1988 Chemotherapy: problems and precautions. In: Oakhill A (ed) The supportive care of the child with cancer.)

1. Check the current weight and surface area.
2. Is the oncology treatment part of a protocol and, if so, have all the drugs required been prescribed?
3. Is a test dose necessary?
4. Is the route of administration appropriate and safe, and is extravasation likely? Are staff familiar with reconstitution, administration and extravasation policies?
5. Is the drug compatible with prescribed i.v. fluids – will it be administered before its expiry?
6. Are you aware of possible side effects and problems with drug treatment?
7. Are other drugs or fluids required to counteract toxicity?
8. Has the patient had previous adverse reaction to chemotherapy?
9. Have antiemetics been prescribed and is the time of administration correct?
10. Monitor blood counts and electrolytes. Identify the cause of changes in electrolytes.
11. Has the patient any pre-existing problems, e.g. hypertension, hepatic or renal impairment.?
12. Are prophylactic antibiotics required?
13. Will other drugs prescribed affect the toxicity of any cytotoxics?

set is most common with polyarticular (beginning in the large joints but often involving smaller joints of the hands and feet) and systemic (fever, rash, lymphadenopathy, minimal joint symptoms) onset less common. Laboratory findings associated with rheumatoid arthritis may be present, such as elevated WBC, ESR, ANA, rheumatoid factor.

Depending on the type of onset and the course of the disease approximately 50% of children will respond to a regimen of NSAIDs, physical therapy and attention to their particular psychosocial and educational needs.

NSAIDs currently licensed for use in children include:

- aspirin – associated with Reye's syndrome (although rarely reported in children treated for chronic arthritis) and gastrointestinal effects. High doses are required and plasma level monitoring should be conducted
- ibuprofen
- naproxen (probably first choice for potency,

twice daily dosing, well tolerated and range of presentations – tablets, suspension and suppositories)
- diclofenac (suppositories and modified release tablet)
- mefenamic acid
- piroxicam (dispersible tablets and suppositories)
- tolmetin.

Severe disease may require the use of corticosteroids as potent anti-inflammatory agents. The lowest dose required to bring relief should be used and withdrawn using a reducing dose schedule. Patients should be counselled to carry a 'steroid card'. Administration of doses on alternate days will reduce the adverse effect of corticosteroids on growth.

Other drugs may be used in an attempt to modify the course of juvenile chronic arthritis. Agents such as gold salts, chloroquine, hydroxychloroquine, penicillamine and cytotoxic agents such as azathioprine and chlorambucil have considerable potential for toxicity so careful risk: benefit analysis must be carried out. If used, their dosage must be calculated or titrated carefully and monitoring for the early signs of toxicity instituted.

Recently the use of high dose intravenous immunoglobulins has received considerable attention although use for this purpose is unlicensed. Patients who have previously required steroids for disease control may be able to reduce or even discontinue them following infusions of 2 g/kg at monthly intervals.

Kawasaki disease

Kawasaki disease or acute febrile mucocutaneous lymph node syndrome, is a relatively common childhood illness occurring in epidemics every 3 years. Children aged 6 months to 5 years are predominantly affected with a peak incidence at 9 to 11 months. An infection is the likely cause but so far a causative organism has not been isolated.

Clinical features of the illness include self-limited febrile illness, polymorphous rash, cervical lymphadenopathy, bilateral conjunctival injection, mucous membrane changes (injected pharynx; dry, cracked lips; strawberry tongue), and peripheral extremity changes (oedema; erythema; peeling skin).

A vasculitis affects many blood vessels including those of the coronary circulation, immunological changes are present, there is a leucocytosis and thrombocytosis. Fever may be unresponsive to antibiotics.

Of concern is the association of Kawasaki disease with subsequent coronary artery aneurysms, coronary thrombosis and myocardial infarction. Treatment and monitoring is vigorous to prevent, or at least provide early detection of, these potentially fatal cardiac effects.

The long-term prognosis for children with cardiac abnormalities is not yet known; of particular concern is the question of whether they will have an increased risk of myocardial infarction in later life.

Treatment is aimed at reducing the risk of coronary artery disease and involves the use of high dose intravenous immunoglobulins (2 g/kg given once over 8 hours) and antiplatelet therapy with aspirin (30 to 100 mg/kg/day in the acute phase decreasing to 5 mg/kg/day once fever has reduced) and dipyridamole (5 to 10 mg/kg/day).

BIBLIOGRAPHY

Athreya B H, Cassidy J T. Current status of the medical treatment of children with juvenile rheumatoid arthritis. Rheumatic Disease Clinics of North America 1991; 17(4): 871–889
Barltrop D, Brueton M J. Paediatric therapeutics. Oxford: Butterworth-Heinemann 1991
Gellis S, Kagan B. Current paediatric therapy 13. Philadelphia: W B Saunders, 1990
Griffiths I D, Craft A W. Management of juvenile chronic arthritis. Hospital Update 1988; April: 1372–1384
Hanna J D, Foreman J W, Chan J C M. Chronic renal insufficiency in infants and children. Clinical Paediatrics 1991; 30(6): 365–384
Jordan S C, Scott O. Heart disease in paediatrics. 3rd edn. London: Butterworths 1989
Leff R D, Roberts R J. Problems in drug therapy for paediatric patients. American Journal of Hospital Pharmacy 1987; 44: 865–870
Levin M, Tizard E J, Dilon M J. Kawasaki disease: recent advances. Archives of Disease in Childhood 1991; 66: 1369–1374

Royal Liverpool Children's Hospital. Therapeutic guidelines. Liverpool: Royal Liverpool Children's NHS Trust 1992

Siddall S J. Chemotherapy: problems and precautions. In: Oakhill A (ed). The supportive care of the child with cancer. Butterworth 1988

Stewart F, Hampton E M. Effect of maturation on drug disposition in paediatric patients. Clinical Pharmacy 1987; 6: 548–564

Warner J O, et al. Management of asthma: a consensus statement. Archives of Disease in Childhood 1989; 64: 1065–1079

Warner J O, et al. Asthma: a follow up statement from an international paediatric asthma consensus group. Archives of Disease in Childhood 1992; 67: 240–248

Wilson J T. Drug disposition in infancy and childhood (Seminar in Print). Clinical Pharmacokinetics 1989; 17 (suppl. 1): 1–173

Useful dosage reference sources in paediatrics

Insley J. A paediatric vade-mecum. 12th edn. London: Edward Arnold, 1990

Lewisham and North Southwark Health Authority. Paediatric formulary. 2nd edn. London: Lewisham and North Southwark Health Authority 1990

Royal Liverpool Children's Hospital. Alder Hey book of children's doses. 5th edn. Liverpool: Royal Liverpool Children's NHS Trust 1990

Royal Liverpool Children's Hospital. Cardiac unit book of children's doses. 2nd edn. Liverpool: Royal Liverpool Children's NHS Trust 1991

Chapter 8

Geriatrics

H. Shetty   K. Woodhouse

There has been a steady increase in the number of elderly people, i.e. those over 65 years of age, in most western countries since the beginning of this century. In the UK the population has risen from 4.8% in 1901 to 15.2% in 1981, and the elderly now form about 18% of the population. Moreover, the proportion of those over 75 years has increased even more significantly in the western countries. In the UK the proportion of the 'elderly' population who were over 75 years rose from 29% in 1900 to 38% in 1970, and is projected to reach 44% by the year 2000.

The elderly have multiple and often chronic diseases. It is not surprising therefore that they are the major consumers of drugs. In 1979 one-third of National Health Service (NHS) prescriptions in the UK were for elderly people. In most developed countries the elderly now account for 25 to 40% of drug expenditure.

A recent survey of 778 elderly people in the UK showed that 70% had been on prescribed medication and 40% had taken one or more prescribed drugs within the previous 24 hours; 32% were taking cardiovascular drugs, and the other therapeutic categories used in decreasing order of frequency were central nervous system (24%), musculoskeletal system (10%), gastrointestinal system (8%) and respiratory system (7%). The most commonly used drugs were diuretics; analgesics; hypnotics, sedatives, anxiolytics; antirheumatic drugs and beta-adrenoreceptor blockers.

Institutionalized patients tend to be on larger

numbers of drugs compared with patients in the community. One study has shown that patients in long-term care facilities are likely to be receiving on average, eight drugs. Psychotropic drugs are used widely in nursing or residential homes.

PHARMACOKINETICS

Ageing results in many physiological changes (Table 8.1) which could theoretically affect absorption, first-pass metabolism, protein binding, distribution and elimination of drugs.

Absorption

There is a delay in gastric emptying, reduction in gastric acid output and splanchnic blood flow with ageing. These changes do not significantly affect the absorption of the majority of drugs. Although the rate of absorption of some drugs such as digoxin may be slower, the overall absorption is similar to that in the young.

First-pass metabolism

After absorption, drugs are transported via the portal circulation to the liver, where many lipid-soluble agents are metabolized extensively (more than 90 to 95%). This results in a marked reduction in systemic bioavailability. Obviously, even minor reductions in first-pass metabolism can result in a significant increase in the bioavailability of such drugs.

Impaired first-pass metabolism has been demonstrated in the elderly for several drugs, including chlormethiazole, labetalol, nifedipine,

nitrates, propranolol and verapamil. The clinical effects of some of these (e.g. the hypotensive effect of nifedipine) may be significantly enhanced in the elderly. In frail hospitalized elderly patients, i.e. those with chronic debilitating diseases, the reduction in pre-systemic elimination is even more marked.

Distribution

Table 8.2 lists the age-related physiological changes which may affect drug distribution. Increased body fat in the elderly results in an increased volume of distribution for fat-soluble compounds such as chlormethiazole, diazepam, desmethyl-diazepam and thiopentone. On the other hand, reduction in body water results in a decrease in the distribution volume of water-soluble drugs such as cimetidine, digoxin and ethanol.

Acidic drugs tend to bind to plasma albumin; basic drugs to alpha$_1$-acid glycoprotein. Plasma albumin levels decline with age and, therefore, the free fraction of acidic drugs such as cimetidine, frusemide and warfarin will increase. Plasma alpha$_1$-acid glycoprotein levels may remain unchanged or may rise slightly with ageing, and this may result in minimal reductions in free fractions of basic drugs such as lignocaine. Disease-related perturbations in the level of this glycoprotein are probably more important than age per se.

The age-related changes in distribution and protein binding are probably of significance only in the acute administration of drugs, because at steady state, the plasma concentration of a drug is determined primarily by free drug clearance by liver and kidneys rather than by distribution volume or protein binding.

Table 8.1 Age-related changes in the gastrointestinal tract, liver and kidneys

Reduced gastric acid secretion
Decreased gastrointestinal motility
Reduced total surface area of absorption
Reduced splanchnic blood flow
Reduced liver size
Reduced liver blood flow
Reduced glomerular filtration
Reduced renal tubular function

Table 8.2 Age-related changes in body composition

Reduced lean body mass
Reduced total body water
Increased total body fat
Lower serum albumin
Alpha$_1$-acid glycoprotein unchanged or slightly raised

Renal clearance

Although there is considerable inter-individual variability in renal function in the elderly, in general, glomerular filtration rate declines, as do effective renal plasma flow, and renal tubular function. Because of the marked variability in renal function in the elderly, the dosages of predominantly renally excreted drugs should be individualized. Reduction in dosages of drugs with a low therapeutic index, e.g. digoxin, amino-glycosides, may be necessary. Dosage adjustments may not be necessary for drugs with a wide therapeutic index, e.g. penicillins.

Hepatic clearance

Hepatic clearance (Cl_H) of a drug is dependent on hepatic blood flow (Q) and the steady state extraction ratio (E) as can be seen in the following formula:

$$Cl_H = Q \times \frac{Ca - Cv}{Ca} = Q \times E$$

where Ca and Cv are arterial and venous concentrations of the drug respectively. It is obvious from the above formula that when E approaches unity, Cl_H will be proportional to and limited by Q. Drugs which are cleared by this mechanism have a rapid rate of metabolism, and the rate of extraction by the liver is very high. The rate-limiting step as mentioned earlier is hepatic blood flow and therefore drugs cleared by this mechanism are called 'flow limited'. On the other hand, when E is small, Cl_H will vary according to the hepatic uptake and enzyme activity, and will be relatively independent of hepatic blood flow. The drugs which are cleared by this mechanism are termed 'capacity limited'.

Hepatic extraction is dependent upon liver size, liver blood flow, uptake into hepatocytes, and affinity and activity of hepatic enzymes. Liver size falls with ageing and there is a decrease in hepatic mass of between 20 and 40% between the third and tenth decade. Hepatic blood flow falls equally with declining liver size. Although it is recognised that the microsomal mono-oxygenase enzyme systems are significantly reduced in ageing male rodents, recent evidence suggests that it is not the case in ageing humans. Conjugation reactions have been reported to be unaffected in the elderly by some investigators, but a small decline with increasing age has been described by others.

Impaired clearance of many hepatically eliminated drugs has been demonstrated in the elderly. Morphological changes rather than impaired enzymatic activity appear to be the main cause of impaired elimination of these drugs. In frail debilitated elderly patients, however, the activities of drug-metabolizing enzymes such as plasma esterases and hepatic glucuronyl transferases may well be impaired.

PHARMACODYNAMICS

Molecular and cellular changes that occur with ageing may alter the response to drugs in the elderly. There is, however, limited information about these alterations because of the technical difficulties and ethical problems involved in measuring them. It is not surprising therefore that there is relatively little information about the effect of age on pharmacodynamics.

Changes in pharmacodynamics in the elderly may be considered under two headings:

- those that are due to a reduction in homeostatic reserve
- those that are secondary to changes in specific receptor and target sites.

Reduced homeostatic reserve

Orthostatic circulatory responses

In normal elderly subjects there is blunting of the reflex tachycardia that occurs in young subjects on standing or in response to vasodilatation. Structural changes in the vascular tree that occur with ageing are believed to contribute to this observation, although the exact mechanism is unclear. Antihypertensive drugs, drugs with alpha-receptor blocking effects (e.g. tricyclic antidepressants, phenothiazines, some butyrophenones), drugs which decrease sympathetic outflow from the central nervous system (e.g.

barbiturates, benzodiazepines, antihistamines and morphine), and antiparkinsonian drugs (e.g. levodopa, bromocriptine) are therefore more likely to produce hypotension in the elderly.

Postural control

Postural stability is normally achieved by static reflexes which involve sustained contraction of the musculature and phasic reflexes which are dynamic, short term and involve transient corrective movements. With ageing, the frequency and amplitude of corrective movements increase, and an age-related reduction in dopamine (D_2) receptors in the striatum has been suggested as the probable cause. Drugs which increase postural sway, e.g. hypnotics and tranquillizers, have been shown to be associated with the occurrence of falls in the elderly.

Thermoregulation

There is an increased prevalence of impaired thermoregulatory mechanisms in the elderly, although it is not universal. Accidental hypothermia can occur in the elderly with drugs which produce sedation, impaired subjective awareness of temperature, decreased mobility and muscular activity, and vasodilatation. Commonly implicated drugs include phenothiazones, benzodiazepines, tricyclic antidepressants, opioids, and alcohol on its own or with other drugs.

Cognitive function

Ageing is associated with marked structural and neurochemical changes in the central nervous system. Cholinergic transmission is linked with normal cognitive function, and in the elderly the activity of choline acetyl transferase, a marker enzyme for acetylcholine, is reduced in some areas of the cortex and limbic system. Several drugs cause confusion in the elderly. Anticholinergics, hypnotics, H_2-antagonists and beta-adrenoreceptor blockers are common examples.

Visceral muscle function

Constipation is a common problem in the elderly as there is a decline in gastrointestinal motility with ageing. Anticholinergic drugs, tricyclic antidepressants and antihistamines are more likely to cause constipation or ileus in the elderly. Anticholinergic drugs may cause urinary retention in elderly men, especially those who have prostatic hypertrophy. Bladder instability is common in the elderly and urethral dysfunction more prevalent in elderly women. Loop diuretics may cause incontinence in such patients.

Changes in specific receptors and target sites

Many drugs exert their effect via specific receptors. Response to such drugs may be altered by the number (density) of receptors, the affinity of the receptor, post-receptor events within cells resulting in impaired enzyme activation and signal amplification or altered response of the target tissue itself. Ageing is associated with some of these changes.

Alpha-adrenoreceptors

Alpha$_2$-adrenoreceptor responsiveness appears to be reduced with ageing whilst alpha$_1$-adrenoreceptor responsiveness appears to be unaffected.

Beta-adrenoreceptors

Beta-adrenoreceptor function declines with ageing. It is recognized that the chronotropic response to isoprenaline infusion is less marked in the elderly. Propranolol therapy in the elderly produces less beta-adrenoreceptor blocking effects than in the young. In isolated lymphocytes, studies of cyclic AMP production have shown that on beta-adrenoreceptor stimulation, the dose–response curve is shifted to the right, and the maximal response is blunted.

An age-related reduction in beta-adrenoreceptor density has been shown in animal adipocytes, erythrocytes and brain, and also in human lymphocytes in one study, although this has not been confirmed by other investigators. As maximal response occurs on stimulation of only 0.2% of beta-adrenoreceptors, a reduction in the number by itself is unlikely to account for age-related changes. Some studies have shown a reduction in high-affinity binding sites with ageing, in the absence of change in total receptor numbers, and others have suggested that there may be impairment of post-receptor transduction mechanisms with ageing which may account for reduced beta-adrenoreceptor function.

Cholinergic system

The effect of ageing on cholinergic mechanisms is less well known. Atropine produces less tachycardia in elderly humans than in the young. It has been shown in ageing rats that the hippocampal pyramidal cell sensitivity to acetylcholine is reduced. The clinical significance of this observation is unclear.

Benzodiazepines

The elderly are more sensitive to benzodiazepines than the young, and the mechanism of this increased sensitivity is not known. No difference in the affinity or number of benzodiazepine-binding sites has been observed in animal studies. Habituation to benzodiazepines occurs to the same extent in the elderly as in the young.

Warfarin

The elderly are more sensitive to warfarin. This phenomenon may be due to age-related changes in pharmacodynamic factors. The exact mechanism is unknown.

Digoxin

The elderly appear to be more sensitive to the adverse effects of digoxin, but not to the cardiac effects.

COMMON CLINICAL DISORDERS

A comprehensive discussion of the management of all chronic diseases is beyond the scope of this chapter – some are dealt with elsewhere in this book. This section deals in detail only with the most important 'geriatric' diseases – other conditions are mentioned primarily to highlight areas where the elderly differ from the young, or where modifications of drug therapy are necessary.

Dementia

Dementia is characterized by a gradual deterioration of intellectual capacities. Alzheimer's disease and multi-infarct dementia are the most important diseases of cognitive dysfunction in the elderly. Alzheimer's disease (AD) has a gradual onset and it progresses slowly. Forgetfulness is the major initial symptom. The patient has difficulty in dressing and other activities of daily living. He or she tends to get lost in his/her own environment. Eventually the social graces are lost.

Multi-infarct dementia (MID) is the second most important cause of dementia. It usually occurs in patients in their 60s and 70s and is more common in those with a previous history of hypertension or stroke. Abrupt onset and stepwise progression of dementia is characteristic of MID. Mood changes and emotional lability are common. There may be focal neurological deficit. A number of drugs and other conditions cause confusion in the elderly and their effects may be mistaken for dementia. These are listed in Table 8.3.

Table 8.3   Causes of confusion in the elderly
Drugs
Antiparkinsonian drugs
Barbiturates
Benzodiazepines
Cimetidine
Diuretics
Hypoglycaemic agents
Monoamine oxidase inhibitors
Opioids
Steroids
Tricyclic antidepressants
Conditions
Hypothyroidism
Vitamin B_{12} deficiency
Chronic subdural haematoma
Normal pressure hydrocephalus
Alcoholism

In patients with AD, damage to the cholinergic neurones connecting subcortical nuclei to cerebral cortex has been consistently observed. Postsynaptic muscarinic cholinergic receptors are usually not affected, but ascending noradrenergic and serotonergic pathways are damaged, especially in younger patients. Based on these abnormalities, several drugs have been investigated for the treatment of AD. Lecithin, which increases acetylcholine concentrations in the brain, 4-aminopyridine, piracetam, oxitacetam and pramiracetam, all of which stimulate acetylcholine release, have been tried, but have produced no or unimpressive improvements in cognitive function. Anticholinesterases block the breakdown of acetylcholine and enhance cholinergic transmission. Tetrahydro-aminoacridine (THA, which is a longer-acting anticholinesterase) showed promise in non-blinded clinical studies. A controlled clinical trial, however, did not show any benefit, but the design of this trial has been criticized. Abnormalities of liver enzymes with THA was noted in both studies. The centrally acting direct muscarinic agonist arecoline and the partial muscarinic agonist RS86 have also been shown to produce minimal improvements in cognitive function. Selegiline, which is a selective monoamine oxidase B inhibitor, has been reported to improve mood and cognitive function in approximately 50% of 17 patients given 10 mg/day. This effect is thought to be secondary to its antidepressant action. Vasodilators such as co-dergocrine may, however, enhance the alertness and mood in apathetic patients. At present, therefore, there is no proven, effective drug therapy for AD.

There have been few studies on the management of multi-infarct dementia, although at least one report has shown that the progression of the illness may be delayed by aspirin therapy.

Parkinsonism

Parkinsonism is a relatively common disease of the elderly with a prevalence between 50 and 150 per 100 000. It is characterized by resting tremors, muscular rigidity and bradykinesia (slowness of initiating and carrying out voluntary movements). The patients have a mask-like face, monotonous voice and walk with a stoop and a slow shuffling gait. Treatment of Parkinsonism is covered in Chapter 29.

The elderly are more susceptible than younger patients to some of the adverse effects of antiparkinsonian drugs. Because of the age-related decline in orthostatic circulatory responses, postural hypotension is more likely to occur in elderly patients with levodopa therapy. The elderly are more likely to have severe cardiac disease and levodopa preparations should be used with caution in such patients because of the risk of serious ventricular dysrhythmias. Psychiatric adverse effects such as confusion, depression, hallucinations and paranoia occur with dopamine agonists and levodopa preparations. These adverse effects may persist for several months after discontinuation of the offending drug and may result in misdiagnosis, e.g. of Alzheimer's disease, in the elderly. Bromocriptine and other ergot derivatives should be avoided in elderly patients with severe peripheral arterial disease as they may cause peripheral ischaemia. 'Drug holidays', e.g. discontinuation of drugs for 2 days per week, may reduce the incidence of adverse effects of antiparkinsonian drugs, but their role is questionable.

Stroke

Stroke, due to cerebral embolism, thrombosis or haemorrhage is an important cause of disability in the elderly. The value of drug therapy in primary and secondary prevention, and the treatment of acute stroke have been investigated in several studies.

Primary prevention

A number of large studies has examined the efficacy of aspirin in preventing stroke. They have found no benefit in taking aspirin to prevent stroke in healthy people.

Treatment of acute ischaemic stroke

At present there is no effective treatment for acute ischaemic stroke. Anticoagulation, intravenous infusion of colloids, and high dose steroids have all been shown to be of no significant benefit. Use of hyperosmolar agents has been disappointing, although intravenous glycerol has been shown to have some effect on survival in one study.

Secondary prevention

Aspirin in doses of 300 mg/day has been shown to reduce the reoccurrence of non-fatal strokes. This is likely to be secondary to its antiplatelet effect. Addition of dipyridamole to aspirin does not appear to enhance the protective effect against strokes. Sulphinpyrazone is less effective, more expensive and more toxic than aspirin. Ticlopidine, a new antiplatelet drug, is as effective as aspirin in preventing strokes, but causes reversible neutropenia in 3% and diarrhoea in 20% of patients.

Atrial fibrillation and stroke

Atrial fibrillation unrelated to valvular heart disease occurs in 2 to 5% of people over 60 years of age. It is associated with a fivefold increase in the risk of ischaemic stroke. The risk of stroke increases with age. 15% of all strokes are associated with atrial fibrillation and it has been shown that 36% of patients with 'lone' atrial fibrillation have evidence of previous 'silent infarcts'. About 50 to 75% of strokes in patients with atrial fibrillation are secondary to cardiogenic emboli.

In patients with rheumatic heart disease and atrial fibrillation, the use of anticoagulant therapy has been generally accepted for many years. However, the use in non-rheumatic atrial fibrillation to prevent stroke has previously been controversial. Recent studies have shown that long-term low dose anticoagulant therapy (INR 1.5 to 2.7) with warfarin is indeed safe and beneficial in these patients and reduces the risk of stroke significantly.

Osteoporosis

Osteoporosis is a common metabolic bone disease characterized by a reduction in bone mass per unit volume, particularly affecting post-menopausal females. It is an important cause of morbidity in the elderly. The most important complication of osteoporosis is fracture of the hip. 37 600 people aged over 65 years in the UK had a fracture of hip in 1985; 82% of these were women and 83% of these in turn were over 75 years old. Other complications of osteoporosis include fracture of vertebrae, wrists and humerus.

As the complications of osteoporosis have enormous economic implications, and also because there is no effective and safe long-term treatment for this condition, preventive measures are extremely important. In the elderly, regular exercise such as walking is the safest and the best method of prevention. Regular exercise has been shown to halve the risk of hip fractures. Women should be encouraged to stop smoking before menopause as this has been shown to reduce the risk of hip fracture by 25%. Vitamin D and calcium supplementation are not beneficial unless there is a deficiency of these. Hormone replacement therapy with oestrogen is very effective in the prevention of osteoporosis if given in the immediate postmenopausal period, but is less suitable for elderly females as it is not generally beneficial if started more than 10 years after the menopause. Calcitonin inhibits osteoclasts and decreases the rate of bone resorption, reduces bone blood flow and may have central analgesic actions. It is effective in all age groups and is particularly useful for treatment of compression fractures of vertebrae. It is costly and has to be given parenterally. It should not be given for more than 3 to 6 months at a time to avoid its inhibitory effects on bone resorption and formation, which usually disappear after 2 to 4 weeks. Antibodies do develop against calcitonin, but they do not affect its efficacy. Fluorides and anabolic steroids are the other drugs used for treatment of osteoporosis. They are generally ineffective, have unpleasant side effects and therefore are not widely used.

More recently, intermittent administration of diphosphonates (e.g. disodium etidronate, disodium pamidronate) have been used and have shown some promise in slowing bone loss and reducing fracture rates.

Arthritis

Osteoarthrosis, gout, pseudogout, rheumatoid arthritis and septic arthritis are the important joint diseases in the elderly. Treatment of these conditions is similar to that in the young. Non-steroidal anti-inflammatory drugs (NSAIDs) should be avoided, if possible, in patients with osteoarthrosis. Total hip and knee replacements should be considered in patients with severe arthritis affecting these joints.

Hypertension

Hypertension is an important risk factor for cardiovascular and cerebrovascular disease in the elderly. The incidence of myocardial infarction is two and a half times higher, and that of cerebrovascular accidents twice as high in elderly hypertensive patients compared with non-hypertensive subjects. Elevated systolic blood pressure is the single most important risk factor for cardiovascular disease and more predictive of stroke than diastolic blood pressure.

There is evidence that treatment of both systolic and diastolic blood pressure in the elderly is benefical. One large study (EWPHE) has shown reductions in cardiovascular mortality, cerebrovascular events, and mortality associated with cerebrovascular accidents in treated elderly patients with hypertension. The treatment did not reduce the total mortality significantly. A recent study (SHEP), which used low dose chlorthalidone to treat isolated systolic hypertension (systolic blood pressure 160 mmHg or more with diastolic blood pressure less than 95 mmHg), showed a 36% reduction in the incidence of stroke, with a 5-year benefit of 30 events per 1000 patients. It also showed a reduction in the incidence of major cardiovascular events with a 5-year absolute benefit of 55 events per 1000 patients. In addition, this study reported that antihypertensive therapy was beneficial even in patients over the age of 80 years. However, some other studies have shown that treatment of hypertension in patients of this age group may not be beneficial, and may indeed be harmful.

Treatment of hypertension

Non-pharmacological methods. In patients with asymptomatic mild hypertension non-pharmacological treatment is the method of choice. Weight reduction to within 15% of desirable weight, restriction of salt intake to 4 to 6 g/day, regular aerobic exercise such as walking, restriction of ethanol consumption and stopping smoking are the recommended modes of therapy.

Pharmacological treatment:

Thiazide diuretics. Thiazides lower peripheral resistance and do not significantly affect cardiac output or renal blood flow. They are effective, cheap, well tolerated and have also been shown to reduce the risk of hip fracture in elderly women by 30%. They can be used in combination with other antihypertensive drugs. Adverse effects include mild elevation of creatinine, glucose, uric acid and serum cholesterol as well as hypokalaemia. They should be used in low doses as higher doses only increase the incidence of adverse effects without increasing their efficacy.

Beta-adrenoreceptor blockers. Although theoretically the beta-adrenoreceptor blockers are expected to be less effective in the elderly, they have been shown to be as effective as the diuretics in clinical studies. Water-soluble beta-adrenoreceptor blockers such as atenolol may cause less adverse effects in the elderly.

Calcium antagonists. Calcium antagonists act as vasodilators. Verapamil and to some extent diltiazem decrease cardiac output. These drugs do not have significant effect on lipids or the central nervous system. They may be more effective in the elderly and particularly in the treatment of isolated systolic hypertension. Adverse effects include headache, oedema and postural hypotension. Verapamil may cause conduction disturbances and decrease cardiac output.

Angiotensin converting enzyme (ACE) inhibitors. ACE inhibitors and other vasodilators used for treatment of hypertension are discussed elsewhere. The ACE inhibitors should be used with care in the elderly, who are more likely to have underlying atherosclerotic renovascular disease and to develop renal failure. Excessive hypotension is also more likely to occur in the elderly.

Myocardial infarction

The diagnosis of myocardial infarction in the elderly may be difficult in some patients because of an atypical presentation. In the majority of patients chest pain and dyspnoea are the common presenting symptoms. Confusion may be a presenting factor in up to 20% of patients over 85 years of age. The diagnosis is made on the basis of history, serial electrocardiograms and cardiac enzyme estimations.

The principles of management of myocardial infarction in the elderly are similar to those in the young. Thrombolytic therapy has been shown to be safe and effective in elderly patients.

Cardiac failure

In addition to the typical features of cardiac failure, i.e. exertional dyspnoea, oedema, orthopnoea and paroxysmal nocturnal dyspnoea (PND), elderly patients may present with atypical symptoms. These include confusion due to poor cerebral circulation, vomiting and abdominal pain due to gastrointestinal and hepatic congestion, or insomnia due to PND. Dyspnoea may not be a predominant symptom in an elderly patient with arthritis and immobility. Treatment of cardiac failure depends on the underlying cause and is similar to that in the young. Diuretics, ACE inhibitors, nitrates and digoxin are the important drugs used in the treatment of cardiac failure in the elderly. ACE inhibitors are valuable recent additions for the treatment of cardiac failure and have been shown to reduce mortality in patients with moderate to severe heart failure.

Urinary incontinence

Urinary incontinence in the elderly may be of three main types:

- *stress incontinence* generally due to weakening of pelvic musculature
- *overflow incontinence* due to prostatic hypertrophy in men, urethral stricture, or atony of the bladder secondary to autonomic neuropathy
- *detrusor instability* due to bladder wall disease

or infection. The bladder contracts before it is full and it is the most common cause of incontinence in the elderly.

The first two types of incontinence are not amenable to drug therapy. Some patients with detrusor instability respond to oxybutynin, which has anticholinergic properties and a direct effect on smooth muscle. It should be started in low doses and the dose should be increased gradually. Propantheline, an anticholinergic drug, is also used for treatment of urinary frequency, but adverse effects such as dry mouth, blurred vision and precipitation of glaucoma, particularly in the elderly, limit its use. Terodiline, a secondary amine with anticholinergic and calcium antagonist activity, which had been in clinical use since 1986 for treatment of urinary incontinence, was withdrawn from the market in 1991 because of serious cardiac dysrhythmias. In the long term, many patients with detrusor instability require catheterization.

Constipation

The age-related decline in gastrointestinal motility and treatment with drugs which decrease gastrointestinal motility predispose the elderly to constipation. Decreased mobility, wasting of pelvic muscles and a low intake of solids and liquids are other contributory factors. Faecal impaction may occur with severe constipation which in turn may cause subacute intestinal obstruction, abdominal pain, spurious diarrhoea and faecal incontinence. Adequate intake of dietary fibres, regular bowel habits and use of bulking agents such as bran or ispaghula husk in some cases help to prevent constipation. When constipation is associated with a loaded rectum, a stimulant laxative, e.g. senna, bisacodyl, may be given. Frail, ill elderly patients with a full rectum may have atonic bowels which will not respond to bulking agents or softening agents, and in such cases a stimulant is more effective. A stool softening agent, e.g. docusate sodium is effective when stools are hard and dry. For severe faecal impaction a phosphate enema may be needed. Long-term use of stimulant laxatives leading to abuse and atonic bowel musculature should be discouraged in the elderly.

Peptic ulcer

There is some evidence that non-steroidal anti-inflammatory drug therapy may be associated with an increased risk of death from peptic ulcer in the elderly.

The elderly with peptic ulcer may present with atypical features, such as confusion, making the diagnosis difficult. The treatment of peptic ulcer in the elderly is similar to that in the young although cimetidine may precipitate confusion more frequently in the elderly. *Helicobacter pylori* infection is common and, as with the younger patient, responds well to appropriate antibiotics and colloidal bismuth.

PRINCIPLES AND GOALS OF DRUG THERAPY IN THE ELDERLY

A thorough knowledge of the pharmacokinetic and pharmacodynamic factors discussed is essential for optimal drug therapy in the elderly. In addition, some general principles based on common sense, if followed, may result in even better use of drugs in the elderly.

Avoid unnecessary drug therapy

Before commencing drug therapy it is important to ask the questions: Is it really necessary? Is there an alternative method of treatment? In patients with mild hypertension, for example, it may be perfectly justified to try non-drug therapies which are of proven efficacy. Similarly, unnecessary use of hypnotics should be avoided. Simple measures such as emptying the bladder before going to bed to avoid having to get up, avoidance of stimulant drugs in the evenings or night, moving the patient to a dark, quiet room may be all that is needed.

Effect of treatment on quality of life

The aim of treatment in elderly patients is not just to prolong life, but to improve the quality of life. To achieve this, the correct choice of treatment is essential. In a 70-year-old lady with severe osteoarthrosis of the hip, for example, total hip replacement is the treatment of choice rather than prescribing non-steroidal anti-inflammatory drugs with all their attendant adverse effects.

Treat the cause rather than the symptom

Symptomatic treatment without specific diagnosis is not only bad practice, but also can be potentially dangerous. A patient presenting with 'indigestion' may in fact be suffering from angina and, therefore, treatment with H_2-blockers or antacids is clearly inappropriate. When a patient presents with a symptom every attempt should be made to establish the cause of the symptom and specific treatment, if available, should then be given.

Drug history

A drug history should be obtained in all elderly patients. This will ensure the patient is not prescribed a drug or drugs to which they may be allergic, or the same drug or group of drugs to which they have previously not responded. It will also aid the avoidance of potentially serious drug interactions.

Concomitant medical illness

Concurrent medical disorders must always be taken into account. Cardiac failure, renal impairment and hepatic dysfunction are particularly common in the elderly and may increase the risk of adverse effects of drugs.

Choosing the drug

Once it is decided that a patient requires drug therapy, it is important to choose the drug which is likely to be the most efficacious and which is least likely to produce adverse effects. It is also necessary to take into consideration coexisting medical conditions. For example, it is inappropriate to commence diuretic therapy to treat mild hypertension in an elderly male with prostatic hypertrophy. A calcium antagonist is more appropriate in this situation.

Dose titration

In general, elderly patients require relatively smaller doses of all drugs compared to young adults. It is recognized that the majority of adverse drug reactions in the elderly are dose related and potentially preventable. It is therefore rational to start with the smallest possible dose of a given drug in the least number of doses and then gradually increase both, if necessary. Dose titration should obviously take into consideration age-related pharmacokinetic and pharmacodynamic alterations which may affect the response to the chosen drug.

Choosing the right dosage form

Most elderly patients find it easy to swallow syrups, or suspensions or effervescent tablets rather than large tablets or capsules.

Packaging and labelling

Many elderly patients with arthritis find it difficult to open 'child resistant' containers. Medicines should be dispensed in easy to open containers which are clearly labelled using large print.

Good record keeping

Information about a patient's current and previous drug therapy, alcohol consumption, smoking and driving habits may help in choosing appropriate drug therapy when the treatment needs to be altered. It will help to reduce costly duplications and will also identify and help to avoid dangerous drug interactions.

Regular supervision and review of treatment

A recent survey in the UK showed that 59% of prescriptions to the elderly had been given for more than 2 years, 32% for more than 5 years and 16% for more than 10 years. 88% of all prescriptions given to the elderly were repeat prescriptions. 40% had not been discussed with the doctor for at least 6 months, especially prescriptions for hypnotics and anxiolytics. 31% of prescriptions were considered pharmacologically questionable, and 4% showed duplication of drugs. It is obvious that there is a need for regular and critical review of all prescriptions, especially when long-term therapy is required.

Adverse drug reactions

It is recognized that adverse drug reactions (ADRs) occur more frequently in the elderly. A multicentre study in the UK in 1980 showed that ADRs were the only cause of admission in 2.8% of 1998 admissions to 42 units of geriatric medicine. It also showed that ADRs were contributory to a further 7.7% of admissions. On the basis of this study it can be estimated that up to 15 000 geriatric admissions per annum in the UK are at least partly due to an ADR. Obviously, this has enormous economic implications.

The elderly are more susceptible to ADRs for a number of reasons. They are usually on multiple drugs which in itself can account for the increased incidence of ADRs. It is however recognized that ADRs tend to be more severe in the elderly and gastrointestinal and haematological ADRs are more common than would be expected from prescribing figures alone. Age-related pharmacokinetic and pharmacodynamic alterations and impaired homeostatic mechanisms are the other factors which predispose the elderly to ADRs by making them more sensitive to the pharmacological effects of the drugs. Not surprisingly, up to 80% of ADRs in the elderly are dose dependent and therefore predictable.

Compliance

Although it is commonly believed that the elderly are poor compliers with their drug therapy, there is no clear evidence to support this. Studies in Northern Ireland and continental Europe have shown that the elderly are as compliant with their drug therapy as the young, provided that they do not have confounding disease. Cognitive impairment, which is not uncommon in old age, multiple drug therapy and complicated drug regimens may impair compliance in the elderly.

Poor compliance may result in treatment failure. The degree of compliance required varies depending on the disease being treated. For treatment of a simple urinary tract infection, a single dose of an antibiotic may be all that is required and, therefore, compliance is not important. On the other hand, compliance of 90% or more is required for successful treatment of epilepsy or difficult hypertension.

Various methods have been used to improve compliance. These include prescription diaries, special packaging, training by pharmacists, and counselling.

BIBLIOGRAPHY

Amery A, Birkenhager W, Brixko R, Bulpitt C, Clement D, Deruyttere M et al. Efficacy of antihypertensive drug treatment according to age, sex, blood pressure, and previous cardiovascular disease in patients over the age of 60. Lancet 1986; ii: 589–592

Bayer A J, Chadha J S, Farag R R, Pathy M S J. Changing presentation of myocardial infarction with increasing old age. Journal of the American Geriatrics Society 1986; 34: 263–266

Byyny R L. Hypertension in the elderly. In: Laragh J H, Brenner B M (eds) Hypertension: pathophysiology, diagnosis and management. New York: Raven Press, 1990; 1869–1887

Cartwright A, Smith C. Elderly people, their medicine and their doctors. London: Routledge, 1988

Editorial. Osteoporosis: prevention and treatment. Drug and Therapeutics Bulletin 1989; 27: 1–4

Editorial. Drugs for Alzheimer's disease. Drug and Therapeutics Bulletin 1990; 28: 42–44

Editorial. Treatment for stroke? Lancet 1991; 337: 1129–1131

Final report on the aspirin component of the ongoing physicians health study. New England Journal of Medicine 1989; 321: 129–135

Griffin M R, Ray W A, Schaffner W. Non-steroidal anti-inflammatory drug use and death from peptic ulcer in elderly persons. Annals of Internal Medicine 1988; 109: 359–363

Hamerman D (ed). Rheumatic disorders. Clinics in Geriatric Medicine 1988; 4: 241–470

Kallman H. Constipation in the elderly. American Family Physician 1983; 27: 179–184

Katzman R. Alzheimer's disease. New England Journal of Medicine 1986; 314: 964–973

Klawans H L. Emerging strategies in Parkinson's disease. Neurology 1990; 40 (suppl. 3): 1–76

Lamy P P (ed). Clinical pharmacology. Clinics in Geriatric Medicine 1990; 6: 229–457

Law M R, Wald N J, Meade T W. Strategies for prevention of osteoporosis and hip fracture. British Medical Journal 1991; 303: 453–459

MacLennan W J. The ageing society. British Journal of Hospital Medicine 1988; 39: 112–120

Nolan L, O'Malley K. Adverse drug reactions in the elderly. British Journal of Hospital Medicine 1989; 41: 446–457

SHEP Cooperative Research Group. Prevention of stroke by antihypertensive drug treatment in older persons with isolated systolic hypertension: Final results of the Systolic Hypertension in the Elderly Program (SHEP). JAMA 1991; 265: 3255–3264

Swift C G. Pharmacodynamics: Changes in homeostatic mechanisms, receptor and target organ sensitivity in the elderly. British Medical Bulletin 1990; 46: 36–52

The Boston Area Anticoagulation Trial for Atrial Fibrillation Investigators. The effect of low-dose warfarin on the risk of stroke in patients with non-rheumatic atrial fibrillation. New England Journal of Medicine 1990; 323: 1505–1511

Tregaskis B F, Stevenson I H. Pharmacokinetics in old age. British Medical Bulletin 1990; 46: 9–21

Turpie I D, Skelly J. Urinary incontinence: current overview of a prevalent problem. Geriatrics 1989; 44: 32–38

Wilcock G K. Alzheimer's disease – current issues. Quarterly Journal of Medicine 1988; New Series 66: 117–124

Williamson J, Chopin J M. Adverse reactions to prescribed drugs in the elderly. A multicentre investigation. Age and Ageing 1980; 9: 73–80

Wittry M D, Thornton T A, Chaitman B R. Safe use of thrombolysis in the elderly. Geriatrics 1989; 44: 28–36

Woodhouse K W, James O F W. Hepatic drug metabolism and ageing. British Medical Bulletin 1990; 46: 22–35

Wrenn K. Faecal impaction. New England Journal of Medicine 1989; 321: 658–662

UK-TIA Study Group. United Kingdom transient ischaemic attack (UK-TIA) aspirin trial: interim results. British Medical Journal 1988; 296: 316–320

Vestal R E. Drug use in the elderly: a review of problems and special considerations. Drugs 1978; 16: 358–382

THERAPEUTICS

Chapter 9

Peptic ulcer disease

C. M Clark

Peptic ulcer disease (PUD) is the term used to describe a heterogeneous group of conditions in which there is ulceration of the oesophagus, stomach or duodenum. This is apparently associated with some local disturbance of the physiological equilibrium. Although it was once thought that excess acid secretion was the major aetiological factor, in recent years understanding has broadened considerably.

EPIDEMIOLOGY

In Great Britain PUD is a significant cause of morbidity and mortality. Since 1970 the death rate from this cause has been increasing and in Great Britain in 1989 it accounted for 4500 deaths. PUD affects 5 to 15% of the adult population at some time during their lives. The prevalence of active disease is 1 to 2%.

Duodenal ulcers are approximately three times more common than gastric ulcers and men are more commonly affected than women. However, this picture may be changing as PUD is becoming more common amongst women. Deaths in people over the age of 75 years account for much of the observed increase in mortality and this is thought to be associated with the widespread use of non-steroidal anti-inflammatory drugs in this age group. The disease is uncommon amongst children and juveniles. About 2% of gastric ulcers are malignant whereas duodenal ulcers are never cancerous.

AETIOLOGY

No single cause for PUD has been found but several contributory factors have been identified.

The time-honoured dictum 'no acid, no ulcer' is still broadly correct although gastroduodenal ulceration in the absence of acid is known to occur in some situations. The mucosa of the upper gastrointestinal tract is protected from autodigestion by means of a complex series of physical and chemical mechanisms which are known collectively as the 'mucosal barrier'. These include; gastric mucus, gastric bicarbonate secretion, rapid regeneration of mucosal cells, high local blood flow and local prostaglandin activity (see Table 9.1). A number of factors have been identified which can disrupt one or more of these mechanisms thereby allowing acid/peptic attack to start. These are summarized below. Many peptic ulcers heal spontaneously but the process is not well understood.

Acid and pepsin

Increased acid secretion may play an important role in some patients and the high levels of gastric acid secretion seen in patients with gastrin-secreting tumours (Zollinger–Ellison syndrome) are invariably associated with ulceration. However, acid secretion in the general population varies greatly and, although duodenal ulcer patients tend to secrete more acid than controls, they are not sufficiently different from healthy individuals for this to be a useful prognostic tool. By the same token, gastric ulcer patients tend to secrete less acid than healthy controls. There is a diurnal variation in acid secretion and it may be that disturbances to this pattern which result in prolonged exposure of the mucosa to the acid/pepsin mixture are more important than absolute quantities of acid.

Acid and pepsinogen are secreted by the parietal cells and chief cells respectively, which lie in glands in the stomach lining. Pepsinogen is converted to the active enzyme, pepsin, in the presence of acid and the resulting mixture is highly proteolytic.

Cigarette smoking

Cigarette smoking is clearly associated with a higher incidence of PUD although the underlying mechanisms are uncertain.

Helicobacter pylori

Approximately 80% of PUD patients are infected with this organism. It lives deep in the gastric mucus, adherent to the mucosal cells, mainly in the gastric antrum. It causes an acute gastritis and a reduction in mucus production. This combination may predispose to gastric and duodenal ulcer formation. It is, however, possible to have asymptomatic *Helicobacter pylori* infection.

Non-steroidal anti-inflammatory drugs

All NSAIDs bring about disruption of the mucosal barrier and may cause transient inflammation, erosions or bleeding. NSAID use has increased the frequency with which PUD presents in the population as a whole, but some groups, e.g. the elderly and those with a history of PUD, are clearly at higher risk than others.

Other factors

Alcohol, particularly in high concentrations, causes mucosal damage independently of acid. Bile reflux may play a role in some patients, particularly if the pyloric sphincter is incompetent or if the patient has undergone a partial gastrectomy. Inheritance and blood group 'O' may play a modest role whilst diet is unlikely to be important. Acute physical stress is clearly

Table 9.1 Factors which influence the integrity of the gastroduodenal mucosa	
Aggressive	Defensive
Acid	Gastric mucus
Pepsin	Bicarbonate secretion
Helicobacter pylori	Rapid cell turnover
Refluxed bile salts	High blood flow

linked with acute ulceration but the role of psychological stress is speculative.

Gastro-oesophageal reflux

Gastro-oesophageal reflux occurs when the lower oesophageal sphincter is incompetent. It may be compounded by inadequate clearing of the oesophagus due to a motility defect. Refluxed stomach contents contain acid and possibly bile salts which can rapidly damage the unprotected oesophageal mucosa.

Reflux can be precipitated or aggravated by drugs which relax the lower oesophageal sphincter, such as peppermint or progestogens, or by an increase in intra-abdominal pressure as a result of tight clothing or posture.

PATHOPHYSIOLOGY

Superficial damage to the gastroduodenal mucosa occurs within minutes of exposure to an irritant; however, if the irritant is removed, the natural repair mechanisms are such that all traces of damage may disappear within a matter of hours. If the original cause of damage persists then an acute ulcer may form. Damage to the mucosa may heal within days; however, it may progress and produce a chronic ulcer. The factors which control this process are not clear. A chronic ulcer penetrates more deeply and involves disruption of the submucosa and muscle layers. The ulcer forms a crater with sloughing material in its base. It may be surrounded by inflamed and swollen tissue. If a blood vessel has been eroded by the ulcer process then there may be a blood clot in the crater.

When a chronic ulcer eventually heals there may be extensive scarring which may cause further problems such as pyloric stenosis.

NATURAL HISTORY

PUD is a chronic, relapsing condition which may persist for many years. Some studies have shown relapse rates amongst duodenal ulcer patients as high as 80% in the first 12 months.

Untreated gastric ulcers have a lower and slower recurrence rate but are associated with a higher rate of complications than duodenal ulcers.

CLINICAL MANIFESTATIONS

Patients with PUD usually complain of intermittent epigastric or abdominal pain. It is often described as a gnawing or burning pain but cramping pains and generalized abdominal discomfort also feature. Typically, gastric ulcer patients complain of pain over the epigastrium which is precipitated by eating. Duodenal ulcer patients experience pain which is relieved by food, but often disturbs them at night. Pain may be relieved by vomiting. In practice it is often not possible to distinguish between the two types of ulcer on the basis of history alone and it is more important to identify serious prognostic features such as frequent nausea and vomiting, weight loss and episodes of haematemesis or melaena.

Reflux oesophagitis presents as an episodic, retrosternal burning pain which may be confused with the pain of angina. It commonly occurs after large meals, on lying down or bending over. Other features of the condition include regurgitation and dysphagia.

It is important to realize that all forms of PUD may be asymptomatic so that episodes of bleeding or perforation may occur without warning. Furthermore, ulcers are often diagnosed after a patient has presented with symptoms associated with anaemia such as chronic tiredness or cardiac failure.

INVESTIGATIONS

Initial investigations may include full blood count and faecal occult bloods. Evidence of anaemia or gastrointestinal blood loss will prompt more detailed investigations.

Fibreoptic endoscopy is the definitive diagnostic technique in PUD as it allows direct visualization of the lesion and will differentiate between ulcers and non-ulcer dyspepsia. It also facilitates early biopsy of potentially malignant gastric ulcers and allows biopsy for detection of *Helicobacter pylori.*

Barium contrast radiography is an alternative if endoscopy is not available and is the preferred method for patients with advanced ischaemic heart disease or chronic obstructive airways disease. However, if a gastric ulcer is identified radiologically, it should always be followed up endoscopically to exclude malignancy. Other, supplementary investigations may be required to confirm rarer diagnoses, e.g. plasma gastrin levels may be required to confirm a diagnosis of Zollinger–Ellison syndrome.

In gastro-oesophageal reflux disease oesophageal manometry and luminal pH measurements may be undertaken to establish a diagnosis of lower oesophageal sphincter incompetence.

TREATMENT

There is no cure for PUD. The aims of treatment are to relieve symptoms; promote healing; prevent complications and, by means of maintenance therapy, to prevent recurrence. The relief of symptoms, such as pain and vomiting, is an important element of treatment.

The complications of PUD are serious and potentially fatal. They include haemorrhage, perforation, penetration and pyloric stenosis. Blood loss may be chronic and lead to the development of anaemia of the iron deficiency type or it may be acute and severe if the ulcer process has eroded an artery. Deaths from PUD are due to bleeding or perforation. Perforation may give rise to leakage of gastric contents with consequent peritonitis. Penetration of the ulcer process into adjacent organs can cause other pathologies such as pancreatitis. Finally, pyloric stenosis which occurs as a result of extensive scarring, may cause impaired gastric emptying.

Medical treatment of gastro-oesophageal reflux is used to relieve the symptoms of pain and regurgitation. The most serious complication of reflux disease is oesophageal stricture formation, again caused by extensive scarring, with consequent dysphagia. Such strictures often require repeated surgical dilatation. Gastro-oesophageal

reflux has also been shown to aggravate asthma in susceptible individuals.

Drug treatment

A number of drugs including antacids, selective antimuscarinics, histamine (H_2) antagonists, bismuth chelate, sucralfate, prostaglandins and omeprazole have been shown to heal peptic ulcers (see Table 9.2). They work by a variety of mechanisms which all serve to influence the balance between 'aggressive' (acid, pepsin, *Helicobacter pylori*) and 'defensive' (mucus, bicarbonate, cell turnover) factors in the upper gastrointestinal tract (see Table 9.1). They are all able to achieve a healing rate of 80 to 90% over a period of 4 to 8 weeks, compared with a placebo healing rate of up to 50% over the same period. Although gastric ulcers heal more slowly than duodenal ulcers the treatment is essentially the same.

Anticholinergics and antacids are little used today for ulcer healing because of their disadvantageous side effect profiles. As yet, the only available prostaglandin (misoprostol) and proton pump inhibitor (omeprazole) are limited to closely defined indications. Thus, the choice effectively lies between H_2 antagonists, of which four are available, bismuth chelate and sucralfate. The drugs and their dosage regimens are shown in Table 9.3. The generally accepted view is that a single agent should be used in preference to combinations. This does not preclude the use of antacids for symptomatic relief.

The choice of agent depends on the safety and convenience of the product and the stage of the treatment. Three general therapeutic situations can be defined, namely, first line treatment, second line treatment for treated but unhealed ulcers and maintenance treatment to prevent

Table 9.2 Ulcer healing drugs	
Antisecretory agents	Mucosal protective agents
H_2 antagonists	Sucralfate
Omeprazole	Bismuth chelate
Misoprostol	Prostaglandins (low dose)
Pirenzepine	Antacids

Table 9.3 Drugs for treating peptic ulcer		
Drug	Ulcer healing dosage	Maintenance dosage
Cimetidine	400–600 mg b.d.	400 mg o.n.
Ranitidine	150 mg b.d.	150 mg o.n.
	300 mg o.n.	
Famotidine	40 mg o.n.	20 mg o.n.
Nizatidine	300 mg o.n.	150 mg o.n.
Bismuth	120 mg q.d.s.	—
chelate	240 mg b.d.	
Sucralfate	1 g q.d.s.	1 g b.d.
	2 g b.d.	2 g o.n.
Omeprazole	20–40 mg o.d.	10–20 mg o.d.*
Antacids	400 mmol neutralizing capacity q.d.s.	—
Misoprostol†	200 microgram q.d.s.	200 microgram b.d.–q.d.s.

* 10 mg presentation not available; 20 mg daily dose licensed for maintenance treatment of reflux oesophagitis.
† Only licensed for prophylaxis and treatment of NSAID-induced ulcers.
Key: o.d. – once daily; o.n. – at night; b.d. – twice daily; q.d.s. – four times daily

recurrence. A relapsed ulcer will usually respond to the same treatment as was given originally.

Once an ulcer has been diagnosed treatment with an H_2 antagonist should be started. The minimum of 4 weeks' treatment should be given, even if symptomatic relief occurs earlier. This is essential to ensure that the ulcer heals completely. If symptoms persist after this time then treatment should be continued for a further 4 weeks. A small percentage of ulcers will remain unhealed after 2 months' treatment. The options at this stage are; a further 4 weeks' treatment at the same dose, treatment with an increased dose of the same agent, or a change to a different type of agent, e.g. a mucosal protective agent or proton pump inhibitor (see Fig. 9.1).

There is no controversy about the need for immediate treatment of a peptic ulcer; however, the question of maintenance treatment has been widely debated. It is necessary to balance the risks of treatment against the risks of ulcer recurrence. There is general agreement that those at high risk of recurrence and complications should receive maintenance treatment. High-risk patients include the elderly, smokers, patients taking NSAIDs, those with frequently relapsing disease, those with a history of complications and those with serious chronic concomitant disease.

Maintenance treatment may take the form of intermittent, 'on-demand' or continuous treatment. Intermittent courses of full-dose treatment under medical supervision is not a very satisfactory long-term option as it guarantees prompt treatment rather than preventing recurrence. 'On-demand' treatment is essentially the same except it is controlled by the patient. In practice many patients regulate their own dosage but, because symptomatic relief with H_2 antagonists precedes ulcer healing, there is always the danger that treatment periods will be too short. Continuous maintenance treatment with a single, nightly dose of H_2 antagonist is effective in keeping over 95% of duodenal ulcer patients ulcer free.

The principles of the treatment of reflux oesophagitis are summarized in Table 9.4.

Antacids are widely used and those containing alginates are particularly effective. Alginic acid forms a viscous raft on top of the stomach contents and this acts as a barrier against acid/ peptic reflux. The most logical approach to the management of reflux disease is the use of prokinetic drugs to increase lower oesophageal sphincter (LOS) pressure and improve gastric and oesophageal clearance. The muscarinic agent, bethanechol, is effective but its use is limited by side effects such as abdominal cramps, diarrhoea and urinary frequency.

Metoclopramide and domperidone work by suppressing dopaminergic activity in gastrointestinal smooth muscle and thereby allowing muscarinic effects to predominate. They are moderately effective, but again, their use is limited by side effects. Cisapride acts by facilitating acetyl choline release at nerve endings in gastrointestinal smooth muscle. It is the most effective drug in this group and may be combined with H_2 antagonists for greater benefit. It is given in a four-times-daily regimen and some patients experience abdominal cramps or diarrhoea. The reduction of gastric acid remains the best-established approach to the treatment

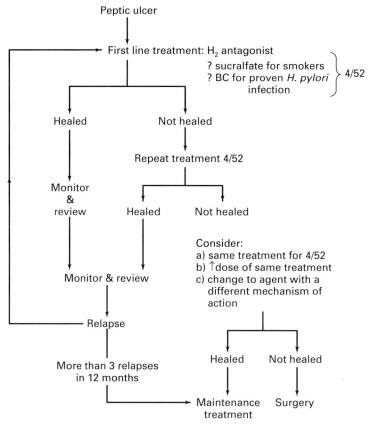

BC – bismuth chelate

Fig. 9.1 Scheme for peptic ulcer treatment.

of reflux disease. H$_2$ antagonists are effective in 40% of patients and omeprazole is effective in most cases. Patients may need up to 8 weeks' treatment and relapse is common. Main-

tenance treatment with either an H$_2$ antagonist or omeprazole is appropriate for severe cases.

Monitoring ulcer treatment

Monitoring ulcer treatment includes surveillance of therapeutic and toxic responses to drug treatment. The therapeutic response is measured mainly by a reduction in symptoms although this index must be used with care as symptoms are frequently alleviated before healing is complete. Confusingly, peptic ulcer symptoms may also manifest in the absence of an active ulcer. Repeat endoscopies offer a definitive index of therapeutic effect but this is not always possible or desirable.

Plasma levels of the antisecretory drugs bear no consistent relationship with the extent of

Table 9.4 Principles of drug treatment for reflux oesophagitis	
Mechanism	Drug
↑ lower oesophageal sphincter pressure ↑ oesophageal clearance ↑ gastric clearance	Bethanechol Metoclopramide Domperidone Cisapride
↓ acid secretion	H$_2$ antagonists, omeprazole
Prevent acid reflux	Antacids/alginate combined products

acid inhibition and so there is no clinical value in their measurement.

Patients should be reviewed regularly for toxic responses, particularly if they have additional risk factors such as impaired renal function or are taking drugs which may interact (see Tables 9.5 & 9.7).

Histamine receptor (H₂) antagonists

The H_2 antagonists are all structural analogues of histamine. They competitively block the histamine receptors in gastric parietal cells, thereby preventing acid secretion. Pepsinogen requires acid for conversion to pepsin and so when acid output is reduced pepsin generation is, in turn, also reduced.

Four products are currently available, namely, cimetidine, ranitidine, famotidine and nizatidine. Although the newer products are generally more potent than cimetidine, there are many similarities between them as a group (see Table 9.6) All

Table 9.5 Adverse reactions to drugs used in the treatment of peptic ulcer and reflux oesophagitis

Drug	Adverse reactions	
	Common	Rare
Cimetidine Ranitidine Famotidine Nizatidine	Diarrhoea Headaches	Nephritis Hepatitis Premature ventricular contractions Bradycardia Tachycardia Mental confusion*
Bismuth chelate	Blackening of tongue, teeth & stools Bismuth absorption	
Sucralfate	Constipation Aluminium absorption	Headaches Nausea
Omeprazole	Gastrointestinal effects Diarrhoea Constipation Nausea Abdominal colic	Skin rashes ↑ serum ALT ↑ serum AST CNS effects Leucopenia
Misoprostol	Dose-related diarrhoea Abdominal pain, nausea and vomiting, flatulence Gynaecological disorders: spotting, cramps, menstrual disorders	
Antacids: Mg-based Al-based	Diarrhoea Constipation	Magnesium absorption Aluminium absorption
Bethanechol	Abdominal cramps Diarrhoea Urinary frequency Blurred vision	
Metoclopramide	Extrapyramidal effects Diarrhoea	
Domperidone		Hyperprolactinaemia
Cisapride		Diarrhoea Abdominal cramps

* CNS disturbances, including mental confusion, occur more frequently with parenteral than with oral cimetidine but are also reported with ranitidine. The incidence is approximately 1%.

Table 9.6 Comparison of H$_2$ antagonists

	Cimetidine	Ranitidine	Famotidine	Nizatidine
Bioavailability	60%	50%	43%	98%
t$_{1/2}$ β	2 h	2–3 h	3 h	1.3 h
Non-renal clearance	70%	30% i.v. 70% oral	30%	40%
Duration of action	5–6 h	9–10 h	12 h	11 h

except nizatidine have an elimination half-life of approximately 3 hours; however, famotidine appears to have the longest duration of action. All are eliminated to a significant extent via the kidneys and all require dosage reduction in renal failure. They all effectively suppress daytime and nocturnal acid secretion but they do not cause total achlorhydria. Ulcer treatment is effective if the intragastric pH is raised to approximately 3. Raising the pH above this value does not improve the rate of healing. In fact, the duration of acid suppression appears to be more important than the extent. The evening dose of an H$_2$ antagonist is particularly important, especially for duodenal ulcer patients. During the daytime gastric acid is buffered for long periods by food but during the night this is not the case and the intragastric pH may fall below 2 for several hours. This has important implications for patient education.

Adverse drug reactions. Experience with cimetidine and ranitidine suggests that the H$_2$ antagonists are a remarkably safe group of drugs. The risk of any adverse reaction is below 3% and serious adverse reactions account for less than 1% (Table 9.5).

Serious potential problems with these drugs are still theoretical; an increased risk of gastric cancer as a result of increased bacterial formation of carcinogens was postulated but not substantiated.

Intrinsic factor secretion is suppressed and so there is a theoretical risk of pernicious anaemia with long-term treatment. Again, this has not turned out to be a problem in practice.

Drug interactions. Much has been made of the drug interactions with cimetidine; however, many have only been demonstrated in vitro and are of doubtful clinical significance (Table 9.7).

Cimetidine inhibits the activity of cytochrome P450 and consequently retards oxidative metabolism of a number of drugs. This is potentially significant for drugs with a narrow therapeutic index. The clearance of theophylline is reduced to about 40% of normal and raised plasma levels occur as a result. Phenytoin metabolism is reduced and toxicity is theoretically possible. The metabolism of a number of benzodiazepines, including diazepam, flurazepam, and triazolam, is impaired and levels are raised.

The interaction with warfarin has frequently been cited as a justification to change to an alternative H$_2$ antagonist; however, careful investigation has shown that this interaction is complex. The metabolism of R-warfarin is affected to a greater degree than that of S-warfarin. As the S enantiomer is the more potent, the pharmacodynamic effects of the interaction may be modest although the plasma levels may be raised. Current opinion suggests that warfarin may safely be used with cimetidine in a once-daily dosage with appropriate monitoring. Other H$_2$ antagonists should be used in patients who are difficult to stabilize on warfarin or for whom frequent monitoring is not feasible.

Bismuth chelate

Bismuth has been included in antacid mixtures for many decades but fell from favour because of its neurotoxicity. Bismuth chelate is a relatively safe form of bismuth which has ulcer-healing properties comparable to those of H$_2$ antagonists. Its mode of action is not well understood but it is thought to have diverse cytoprotective effects. It is also toxic to *Helicobacter pylori*. The relapse rate of duodenal ulcers after bismuth chelate treatment is slower than that seen after H$_2$ antagonists, although this only holds true for the first 12 months. This pattern may be due to elimination of *Helicobacter pylori* during treatment and subsequent reinfection.

Bismuth chelate alone only eliminates the infecting organism in 30% of cases. When given in combination with antibiotics this figure rises to 80%. A 28-day course of bismuth chelate, at a dose of 120 mg, four times daily, combined with

Table 9.7 Clinically important drug interactions with peptic ulcer treatment (adapted from Lauritsen, Laursen & Rask-Madsen 1990 and Gugler & Allgayer 1990)

Drug	Interaction and effect		Mechanism
Cimetidine	Ketoconazole Indomethacin Chlorpromazine	↓ effect	↓ absorption
	Lignocaine Phenytoin Procainamide Theophylline Warfarin	↑ effect	↓ clearance
Ranitidine	Theophylline	↑ effect	↓ clearance*
Famotidine	Theophylline	↑ effect	↓ clearance*
Nizatidine	—	—	—
Bismuth chelate	Iron Calcium Tetracycline	↓ effect	↓ absorption
Sucralfate	Warfarin	↓ effect	↓ absorption
Antacids	Tetracyclines Quinolones Captopril	↓ effect ↓ effect ↓ effect	↓ absorption by 90% ↓ absorption 50–90% ↓ bioavailability – ↓ solubility in ↓ pH
	H₂ antagonists		↓ bioavailability if large doses (> 50 mmol) taken together

* Clinical significance uncertain.

a 7-day course of amoxycillin and metronidazole is recommended.

Bismuth chelate should probably only be given as first line treatment if *Helicobacter pylori* infection is demonstrated. It is not suitable for maintenance treatment in view of the risk of bismuth toxicity. An 8-week minimum washout period is recommended between courses to minimize the possibility of bismuth accumulation. Bismuth chelate is available in liquid and tablet forms, both of which may be given in a twice- or four-times-daily regimen (Table 9.3).

Adverse drug reactions. A certain amount of bismuth is absorbed from bismuth chelate and urinary bismuth excretion may be raised for several weeks after a course of treatment. Bismuth accumulation is more likely in patients with impaired renal function.

Sucralfate

Sucralfate is the aluminium salt of sucrose octa-

sulphate. Although it is a weak antacid this is not its principal mode of action in PUD. It has mucosal protective effects including stimulation of bicarbonate and mucus secretion and stimulation of mucosal prostanoids. In acid it forms a gel which adheres to the ulcer surface and may afford some physical protection and it is capable of adsorbing bile salts. It also prevents alcoholic mucosal injury. These activities appear to reside in the entire molecular complex and are not due to the aluminium ions alone.

It is of interest that cigarette smoking does not delay healing with sucralfate and so this may be a more appropriate first line treatment for smokers. It is effective, in a reduced dose, for maintenance treatment but concerns about long-term aluminium toxicity may rule this out.

Adverse drug reactions. Constipation appears to be the most common problem with sucralfate and this is thought to be related to the aluminium content. About 3 to 5% of a dose is absorbed and therefore there is a risk of aluminium toxicity with long-term treatment. This risk will be correspondingly greater in patients with renal impairment.

Antacids

Traditionally antacids have been used for symptomatic relief. Recent studies have shown that antacids, in the appropriate dosage, can promote healing as effectively as H_2 antagonists. Initially it appeared that large volumes of liquid antacids were necessary for healing but tablet forms have proved to be equally effective and more convenient. The principal mechanism of action was always presumed to be neutralization of acid but recent work suggests that aluminium-containing antacids have other effects which involve cytoprotective activity mediated by mucosal prostaglandins. In future there may be greater use of antacids for ulcer healing but at present their use is confined to symptomatic relief.

The choice of antacid lies between aluminium- and magnesium-based products, although many proprietary products are combinations of the two. Calcium-based products are unsuitable as calcium stimulates acid secretion. Sodium-bicarbonate-containing antacids are unsuitable for regular use because they deliver a high sodium load and generate large quantities of carbon dioxide. It should be noted that magnesium trisilicate mixture contains a large amount of sodium bicarbonate. Some products contain other agents such as dimethicone or alginates. Gaviscon, for example, contains sodium alginate with a mixture of antacids. It is effective in the management of reflux oesophagitis but does not contain sufficient antacid to be useful in duodenal or gastric ulcer treatment.

Adverse drug reactions. Aluminium-based antacids cause constipation and magnesium-based products cause diarrhoea. When combination products are used, diarrhoea tends to predominate as a side effect. Although these are termed 'non-absorbable', a proportion of aluminium and magnesium is absorbed and the potential for toxicity exists, particularly with coexistent renal failure.

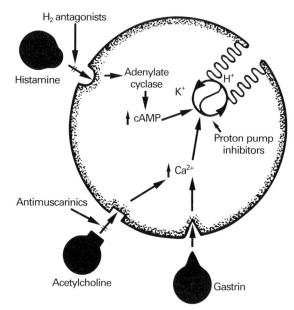

Fig. 9.2 Mechanisms for control of acid secretion in the parietal cell, showing sites of drug action.

Table 9.8 Omeprazole profile	
Bioavailability	35% ($\uparrow$ to 60% on regular dosing)
Half-life	0.5–1.5 h (omeprazole) 0.5–3 h (metabolites)
Non-renal clearance	Approx. 100% hepatic metabolism
Duration of action	24–72 h (depends on regeneration of H^+/K^+ ATPase)

Omeprazole

Omeprazole is a benzimidazole derivative and the most potent antisecretory agent yet available. It irreversibly binds to H^+/K^+ ATPase in gastric parietal cells and thereby blocks the final common step in gastric acid secretion (Fig. 9.2). It produces a long-lasting, dose-dependent suppression of acid secretion. The effect of a single dose may persist for more than 24 hours and regular treatment with doses of 40 mg daily can produce complete achlorhydria. Table 9.8 summarizes the pharmacokinetic profile.

Omeprazole is unstable in acid and is presented in enteric-coated granules in capsules.

Omeprazole heals duodenal ulcers in 2 weeks

and provides rapid symptomatic relief. The usual course of treatment is 20 mg daily, before breakfast, for 4 weeks in duodenal ulceration and for 8 weeks in gastric ulceration. Maintenance treatment with a dose of 10 mg daily has been suggested but has not yet gained acceptance. At present omeprazole is considered to be unsuitable for maintenance treatment in view of the dangers of long periods of achlorhydria. This may be mitigated by the use of 'weekend therapy', that is, dosing for 3 days out of every 7.

Long-term, continuous treatment has been used safely in patients with Zollinger–Ellison syndrome.

Adverse drug reactions. In general omeprazole appears to be well tolerated and the most commonly reported side effects are gastrointestinal symptoms including diarrhoea, constipation, nausea and abdominal colic.

Drug interactions. Like other substituted imidazoles, omeprazole inhibits cytochrome P450 activity in a dose-dependent manner. The clinical consequences of this appear to be mild, if evident at all, at conventional therapeutic doses.

Prostaglandins

Misoprostol is the only product in this class which is currently available. The development of orally active prostaglandins followed the observation that prostaglandins were involved in cytoprotective activity. They have not fulfilled their original promise and it is now clear that their ulcer-healing activity is only expressed when they are given in antisecretory doses. At present the only place for misoprostol is in the prevention of non-steroidal anti-inflammatory drug (NSAID) induced gastric ulcers. Evidence for prevention of duodenal ulcers is awaited. Even in this situation they should be used selectively in high-risk patients such as those over the age of 60 years, those with a history of gastric ulcer or gastric bleeding, those with a history of melaena, cigarette smokers, those with rheumatoid arthritis and those with severe concomitant disease. It is only in these sub-groups that the benefits of treatment outweigh the risks.

Misoprostol is given in a dosage of 200 micrograms four times daily for prophylaxis of NSAID-induced ulcers. Treatment should be discontinued if NSAID treatment ceases.

Adverse drug reactions. Adverse reactions to misoprostol fall mainly into two groups, namely gastrointestinal and gynaecological. These arise directly as a result of prostaglandin effects on other organ systems. Diarrhoea is the most common side effect, and occurs in up to 38% of patients.

THE PATIENT

Lifestyle

Food may be associated with a worsening or improvement in symptoms. Some patients find that certain foods or spices exacerbate their symptoms. Bland diets were recommended in the past but they are of doubtful value. In general, patients should be advised to eat normally and avoid any foods which upset them. Evening snacks are best avoided to prevent stimulation of nocturnal acid secretion.

Smoking delays healing in patients treated with H_2 antagonists. It is also strongly related to ulcer recurrence. Those who smoke fewer than 9 cigarettes a day have relapse rates similar to non-smokers, but those who smoke more than 30 a day are four or five times more likely to relapse in a given time period. The best option is for the patient to give up smoking but if this is not achievable then the use of sucralfate should be considered.

Moderate alcohol consumption is unlikely to have any adverse effects in ulcer patients. Heavy drinking is associated with gastritis and mucosal damage. Any alcohol-induced damage is made worse by concomitant ingestion of aspirin or other NSAID.

In addition to these measures there are a number of specific measures which help patients with reflux oesophagitis. Obese patients should be advised to lose weight and all patients should be advised to avoid tight clothing, in particular, tight waistbands. Elevation of the head of the bed is helpful and this can be done with ordinary house bricks. The use of additional pillows does not achieve the same thing and is generally not beneficial. Smoking, alcohol, caffeine, chocolate and peppermint all reduce lower oesophageal sphincter pressure and should be avoided if possible.

Compliance with drug treatment

Non-compliance with the prescribed regimen is likely to be a major problem amongst peptic ulcer patients as several of the available treatments (including antacids) will provide symptomatic relief before ulcer healing is complete. Maintenance treatment may continue for several years and, in the absence of symptoms, may lead to poor compliance.

For each individual an acceptable, workable regimen should be devised and the importance of the duration of treatment explained. For most patients it should be possible to find a once- or twice-daily dosing schedule for acute treatment and a once-daily regimen for maintenance treatment. The importance of the night-time dose should be emphasized, especially for duodenal ulcer patients. If maintenance treatment has been prescribed after a series of rapid relapses there should be little difficulty in explaining the necessity for continuous rather than 'on-demand' treatment.

There are no particular problems with taking H_2 antagonists and both cimetidine and ranitidine are available in liquid forms (cimetidine syrup, ranitidine dispersible tablets) for patients who cannot swallow tablets.

Bismuth chelate has to be taken four times a day and patients are advised to avoid concurrent intake of milk, food and antacids. This is because the drug is believed to combine preferentially with these products and therefore to be less effective. Twice-daily dosing should be discouraged as it is less effective in eliminating *Helicobacter pylori*. Bismuth chelate is available as liquid and tablets. The liquid has a disagreeable ammoniacal smell and it blackens the tongue.

For this reason the tablets are to be preferred although the liquid can be taken through a straw if absolutely unavoidable. Like iron preparations, bismuth preparations blacken the stools and patients should be warned appropriately.

Sucralfate may be taken on a twice- or four-times-daily basis and should be taken about 30 minutes before food. This is to allow formation of the ulcer-adherent gel which probably contributes to its effectiveness. The drug may adhere to protein in food and efficacy will be reduced unless taken on an empty stomach. As it works best in an acid environment, co-administration of antacids should be avoided. In view of its potential to adsorb other drugs, patients should be advised to leave a gap of 2 hours before taking other medication.

Omeprazole is generally taken on a once-daily basis. Ambulant patients need little encouragement to take it because it produces prompt relief of symptoms. The capsule contains enteric-coated granules and, in very sick patients, it may be necessary to open the capsule and give the dose with 1.4% sodium bicarbonate to ensure availability. There is no liquid form of omeprazole. The drug itself is hygroscopic and the capsule must be stored in a suitable container with a dessicant.

Misoprostol is usually taken at a dose of 200 micrograms four times daily, with or after food. If minor side effects are troublesome the dose may be reduced to 100 micrograms q.d.s. This drug should not be used in pregnant women and women of child-bearing potential should be warned appropriately.

Concurrent treatment

Over-the-counter treatment

Many patients will use antacids for symptomatic relief and it is useful when taking a drug history to document exactly how much is used and in what way. Patients should be advised to use whichever product suits them best. Expensive products are not necessarily superior to cheaper products and recommendations should be made bearing in mind the common side effects of the available agents. Antacids can be most effective when given between meals and at night when acid is not buffered by food in the stomach.

PUD patients should be advised to avoid OTC aspirin, ibuprofen or benorylate. It is more helpful to provide positive information whenever possible and a list of acceptable paracetamol or paracetamol-based products will be more useful than a list of banned items. In view of the number of confusing brand names available patients should be advised to consult the pharmacist, if in any doubt when selecting an analgesic.

Prescription treatment

Patients who are stabilized on cimetidine in combination with warfarin, theophylline, phenytoin or diazepam should be advised not to stop or change their cimetidine dosage without medical supervision. If possible the reasons for this should be explained.

Iron treatment may be necessary in PUD patients to replace loss due to chronic gastrointestinal bleeding. Although treatment may continue for many weeks or months and be mildly inconvenient, the improvement in well-being which accompanies a normal haemoglobin level justifies the effort. Iron preparations should be taken with food to minimize gastric discomfort. They can cause either constipation or diarrhoea which should be managed appropriately.

Several drugs cause relaxation of the lower oesophageal sphincter and may aggravate reflux disease. These include nitrates, theophylline, calcium channel blockers, anticholinergics, beta-adrenergic agonists and alpha-adrenergic antagonists. Peppermint-flavoured antacids may also be unsuitable for this reason.

Socioeconomic aspects of PUD treatment

The costs of PUD to the community are considerable. In Great Britain in 1988, PUD accounted for 38 000 hospital admissions at a cost of ap-

proximately £49 million. The costs and risks of medical treatment compare favourably with surgery for initial treatment of uncomplicated disease and maintenance treatment has a major economic impact. Maintenance treatment reduces the need for repeated hospitalization and investigation in addition to reducing absenteeism arising from chronic ill health. It also undoubtedly improves quality of life.

CASE STUDIES

CASE 9.1

A 28-year-old male patient is admitted with a diagnosis of deep vein thrombosis and pulmonary embolism. He is prescribed intravenous heparin and given a loading dose of warfarin. He has a history of a chronic gastric ulcer for which he takes cimetidine. When interviewed he explains that he takes the cimetidine when he has symptoms which usually amounts to treatment for 3 weeks out every 4.

Q Should he continue with cimetidine or change to another H_2 antagonist?

CASE 9.2

Mrs A. F. is 69 years old and has a previous history of gastric ulceration, but has had no symptoms for 15 years. She has recently been prescribed regular diclofenac for arthritis in her hands. She arrives with a prescription for misoprostol.

Q What advice should she be given?

CASE 9.3

Mr A. D. is 46 years old and has developed active symptoms of his duodenal ulcer each winter for the past 3 years. Each time the ulcer has healed completely on a 4-week course of cimetidine and he has been symptom free in between the acute episodes.

Q Should he be given maintenance treatment?

CASE 9.4

Mr C. E. is a 48-year-old patient who has received an 8-week course of ranitidine for a duodenal ulcer. He continues to complain of symptoms and a repeat endoscopy reveals a large, unhealed ulcer. He is a non-smoker.

Q What treatment strategy would you recommend?

CASE 9.5

Mrs F. G. is a 45-year-old female who presents with a duodenal ulcer for the third time within 15 months. Examination has shown the presence of *Helicobacter pylori*.

Q What treatment strategy would you recommend?

ANSWERS TO CASE STUDIES

CASE 9.1

A Cimetidine is reported to interact with warfarin by delaying its metabolism; however, this interaction is complex and is often clinically unimportant. Two views of the situation suggest that no change is necessary; the arguments are as follows. Firstly, the delayed metabolism gives rise to no problems providing the dose of cimetidine remains regular and constant. Therefore the prescription for cimetidine should remain and the patient should be advised to take it regularly. Secondly, since the metabolism of the less active enantiomer is preferentially delayed, plasma levels of warfarin will rise, but often with little clinical effect and therefore a change in prescription is not always necessary.

It is not necessary to change this prescription but the patient should be closely monitored for anticoagulant control. He should also be advised to take cimetidine regularly as long as he is taking anticoagulants to minimize the possibility of severe gastric bleeding from an ulcer site.

CASE 9.2

A Misoprostol is licensed for prophylaxis and treatment of NSAID-induced ulcers. It is not appropriate for all patients who are receiving NSAIDs and should be reserved for those who are at high risk of developing an ulcer. A patient is in the high-risk category if he or she meets one or more of the following criteria:

- over 60 years of age
- a history of gastric ulcer or bleeding
- a history of melaena
- cigarette smoker
- has rheumatoid arthritis
- has severe concomitant disease.

This patient satisfies three of the criteria and therefore the prescription for misoprostol is appropriate.

She should be advised to take the tablets four times a day, after meals and at bedtime, with food. She should be warned about the possibility of diarrhoea and vaginal bleeding and encouraged to report these to her doctor if they occur. The purpose of the treatment should be explained and she should also be advised to discontinue treatment if NSAID treatment ceases.

CASE 9.3

A This patient suffers from a duodenal ulcer which recurs on a seasonal basis. Opinion is divided on the issue of maintenance treatment with some believing it should be standard practice and others believing it should be restricted to high-risk subgroups. In practice, it is only achievable for good compliers. Nevertheless, it is an established means of preventing ulcer recurrence and, in view of the safety of the available drugs, it should be recommended whenever possible. If this patient is a non-smoker he should be offered maintenance treatment with an H_2 antagonist. If he is a smoker then sucralfate may be a more effective agent. He should, of course, be advised to give up smoking.

CASE 9.4

A This patient has made little or no response to conventional, first line treatment. The options at this stage are either to increase the dose of the present treatment or to change to a different agent. In view of the fact that this treatment has had little impact on the ulcer or the symptoms, an alternative should be selected. Omeprazole would be a suitable choice as it is licensed for use in this situation and provides prompt symptomatic relief and rapid healing.

Omeprazole should be given in a dose of 20 mg daily, before breakfast, for 2 to 4 weeks. This is likely to heal the ulcer but will have no influence on relapse rate. In due course the patient may be a candidate for maintenance treatment, in which case an H_2 antagonist should be the first choice. Omeprazole is not licensed for maintenance treatment, although it is used successfully, long term in patients with Zollinger–Ellison syndrome. Alternate-day or 'weekend' treatment might be considered.

CASE 9.5

A *Helicobacter pylori* is associated with relapse of duodenal ulcers and its elimination prevents early relapse. *Helicobacter pylori* can effectively be eliminated using a combination of bismuth chelate, amoxicillin and metronidazole. The bismuth chelate should be given for a 28-day course but only 7 days' treatment with amoxicillin and metronidazole are needed.

BIBLIOGRAPHY

Adams M H, Ostrosky J D, Kirkwood C F. Therapeutic evaluation of omeprazole. Clinical Pharmacy 1988; 7: 725–745

Bianchi-Porro G, Parente F. Long term treatment of duodenal ulcer: a review of management options. Drugs 1991; 41: 38–51

Das A F, Freston J W, Jacobs J, Fox M A, Morton R E. An evaluation of safety in 37252 patients treated with cimetidine or ranitidine. Internal Medicine 1990; 11: 3–14

Grant S M, Langtry H D, Brogden R N. Ranitidine: an updated review of its pharmacodynamic and pharmacokinetic properties and therapeutic use in peptic ulcer disease and other allied diseases. Drugs 1989; 37: 801–870

Gugler R, Allgayer H. Effects of antacids on the clinical pharmacokinetics of drugs: an update. Clinical Pharmacokinetics 1990; 18: 210–219

Langtry H D, Grant S M, Goa K L. Famotidine: an updated review of its pharmacodynamic and pharmacokinetic properties, and therapeutic use in peptic ulcer disease and other allied diseases. Drugs 1989; 38: 551–590

Lauritsen K, Laursen L S, Rask-Madsen J. Clinical pharmacokinetics of drugs used in the treatment of gastro-intestinal diseases, (Part I). Clinical Pharmacokinetics 1990; 19: 11–31

Lauritsen K, Laursen L S, Rask-Madsen J. Clinical pharmacokinetics of drugs used in the treatment of gastrointestinal diseases, (Part II). Clinical Pharmacokinetics 1990; 19: 94–125

Penston J G, Wormsley K G. Histamine H_2 antagonists versus prostaglandins in the treatment of peptic ulcer disease. Drugs 1989; 37: 391–401

Piper D W. Peptic ulceration. Baillieres Clinical Gastroenterology: International practice and research 1988; Jul 2(3)

Price A H, Brogden R N. Nizatidine: a preliminary review of its pharmacodynamic and pharmacokinetic properties and therapeutic use in peptic ulcer disease. Drugs 1988; 36: 521–539

Siepler J K, Mowers R M, Trudeau W L. Selecting drug therapy for patients with duodenal ulcers. Clinical Pharmacy 1990; 9: 463–467

Chapter 10

Inflammatory bowel disease

B. K. Evans

Crohn's disease and ulcerative colitis are chronic inflammatory conditions of the gut, characterized by periods of remission and relapse over many years. Although quite distinct pathologically, the treatment, including drug therapy, is often very similar.

CROHN'S DISEASE

Crohn's disease takes its name from one of the three physicians who first described the disease in 1932. Crohn's disease may affect any part of the gastrointestinal tract from the lips to the anal margin, but ileocolonic disease remains the commonest presentation. The disease produces considerable morbidity, the cause remains unknown and current treatment is palliative not curative.

EPIDEMIOLOGY

Crohn's disease is very common in northern Europe and North America. It is occurring more frequently in southern Europe but is relatively uncommon in other areas of the world. The highest prevalence is in Scandinavia and Britain (26 to 75 per 100 000 population).

The incidence of Crohn's disease has risen during the last two decades, a rise which cannot solely be attributed to an increased differential diagnosis from ulcerative colitis. The condition is marginally more common in females and most commonly diagnosed in young patients between the ages of 15 and 40 years.

AETIOLOGY

Until recently investigations centred around the role of immunological mechanisms as a causative factor in Crohn's disease but all have been inconclusive.

Immunology

Normal humoral immune responses are seen in patients with Crohn's disease although a defect in cell-mediated immune function may exist due to malnutrition. Improvement in nutritional status will often improve the immune response.

Genetic factors

A consistent genetic association has not been established although 10% of patients have a first degree relative with the disease whilst siblings are affected 30 times more often than the general population. Recent evidence confirms a tenfold familial risk for Crohn's disease and ulcerative colitis. Ankylosing spondylitis sufferers have a ninefold greater prevalence of Crohn's disease. It remains unclear whether Crohn's sufferers are more likely to develop atopic disease, although they are often from families with a history of atopic conditions.

Diet

Dietary intake has centred around milk, fibre and sugar. The role of fibre and milk consumption in Crohn's patients has not been clearly established although some work has confirmed a high refined carbohydrate intake by sufferers compared with controls.

Patients with Crohn's disease are more likely to be smokers than are controls, with the association being stronger for smoking habit prior to disease onset than current smoking habit. The risk of developing the disease increases in women who use oral contraceptives.

Infective agents

Pathological similarities between Crohn's disease and tuberculosis have focused attention on mycobacteria species but no consistent evidence is available. Crohn's disease sufferers have higher faecal counts of anaerobic Gram-negative bacteria and Gram-negative bacteria of the *eubacterium* and *peptostreptococcus* subspecies but the implications of this are unclear.

PATHOPHYSIOLOGY

Ileocolonic disease accounts for 60% of all cases of Crohn's disease with only 20% having colonic involvement and the remainder having ileal or proximal small bowel disease.

Chronic inflammation of the bowel wall, often associated with granulomas and deep fissuring ulceration is common. Patches of defined inflamed areas appear interdispersed by normal bowel. The relationship between pathological and clinical features is shown in Table 10.1.

CLINICAL MANIFESTATIONS

The major clinical features presented depend on the site, extent and severity of disease.

Patients complain of ill health, lassitude and recurrent fever. Clinical features of intestinal involvement are abdominal pain, nausea, diarrhoea, anorexia, and abdominal tenderness. Quite

Table 10.1 Relationship between pathological and clinical features (reproduced by permission of Blackwell Scientific Publications from Misiewicz J J, Pounder R E, Venables C W (eds) 1987 Diseases of the gut and pancreas)

Pathological features	Clinical features
1. Thickened bowel wall Submucosal fibrosis Narrow lumen and strictures	1. Obstructive symptoms Proximal bowel distension
2. Transmural fissures Serosal inflammation	2. Adhesions Inflammatory masses Abscesses Fistulae to adherent bowel, skin or other organs

often weight loss is the most striking feature as a consequence of anorexia. Considering the chronic inflammatory nature of the condition, it is surprising that initial presentation may take the form of a complicated fulminant colitis or be relatively benign.

Terminal ileal disease causes localized abdominal pain associated with a palpable tender mass whilst some patients with extensive disease present with only weight loss. Children affected before puberty may suffer retarded growth and sexual development.

Anal and rectal pathology is the basis for diagnosis. Anal features frequently occur with ileocolonic disease but not with isolated small bowel involvement. The most distressing aspect is sepsis from secondary abscesses and perianal fistulae. Despite anal involvement the rectal mucosa is often unaffected except in severe cases when the mucosa appears thickened.

Intestinal obstruction due to a simple stricture is probably the most common complication in Crohn's disease. Resolution can occur spontaneously but severe attacks can require surgery. Perforation producing an abscess can be seen in patients with very active disease. In colonic disease rectal bleeding of the inflamed mucosa is likely, gradually causing iron deficiency anaemia. During active disease intra-abdominal abscesses discharge their contents through fistulae which sometimes open to the skin and may also penetrate the bladder and vaginal wall, causing recurrent infections.

There appears to be an increased risk of gastro-intestinal malignancy but this remains unproven. Systemic illnesses may accompany the condition and these are shown in Figure 10.1.

INVESTIGATIONS

Clinical, radiological and pathological investigations will confirm diagnosis and recurrent

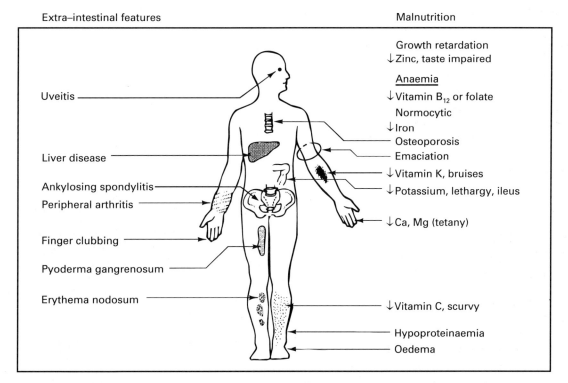

Extra–intestinal features

Malnutrition

Uveitis

Liver disease

Ankylosing spondylitis

Peripheral arthritis

Finger clubbing

Pyoderma gangrenosum

Erythema nodosum

Growth retardation
↓Zinc, taste impaired

Anaemia
↓Vitamin B_{12} or folate
Normocytic
↓Iron
Osteoporosis
Emaciation
↓Vitamin K, bruises
↓Potassium, lethargy, ileus

↓Ca, Mg (tetany)

↓Vitamin C, scurvy

Hypoproteinaemia
Oedema

Fig. 10.1 Some of the extra-intestinal illnesses and features of malnutrition found in patients with Crohn's disease. (Reproduced by permission of Blackwell Scientific Publications from Misiewicz J J, Pounder R E, Venables C W (eds) 1987 Diseases of the gut and pancreas.)

disease. Colonoscopy helps to assess the extent of disease and the nature of colonic strictures and polyps.

Radiology

Upper bowel radiology is performed using a conventional barium meal followed through the intestine, whilst a double contrast barium enema is used in the colon. Narrowed segments of bowel with ulcerated mucosa are commonly seen in the small intestine, with proximal dilatation. Duodenal strictures may cause gastric dilatation and delayed gastric emptying. Distinguishing features include the appearance of aphthoid ulcers, lesions with predominantly right-sided involvement, strictures and fissures.

Histology

Histology confirms the diagnosis and prevents certain small bowel and colonic lesions being wrongly labelled Crohn's disease. Initial diagnosis is frequently established following rectal biopsies, identifying the presence of granulomas, patchy mucosal inflammation, well-preserved goblet cells and few crypt abscesses. This contrasts with the uniformly heavy lymphocytic infiltration of the mucosa in ulcerative colitis (Fig. 10.2). Biopsies taken during treatment provide a useful indication of patient response.

CLINICAL ASSESSMENT

A practical clinical index is valuable in assessing disease activity, response to medical treatment, and in evaluating surgical intervention. A suitable index would include general well-being, abdominal pain, diarrhoea, presence of an abdominal mass and intestinal or systemic complications.

Because abdominal pain and diarrhoea may be unrelated to disease activity the index should be supplemented with laboratory parameters such as serum orosomucoids, C-reactive protein and faecal α_1-antitrypsin concentrations. Alternatively erythrocyte sedimentation rate, albumin concentration and platelet count are helpful.

Malnutrition is often a major problem and assessment of a patient's nutritional status using a mid-arm circumference is important in terms of the treatment programme.

ULCERATIVE COLITIS

Ulcerative colitis is a chronic relapsing inflammatory disorder affecting colonic and rectal mucosa. Its origin and cause remain unclear. The first definitive description was made in 1909 and in certain aspects it resembles Crohn's disease.

If ulcerative colitis affects only the rectal mucosa it is termed proctitis, if it involves the rectum and the sigmoid colon it is known as

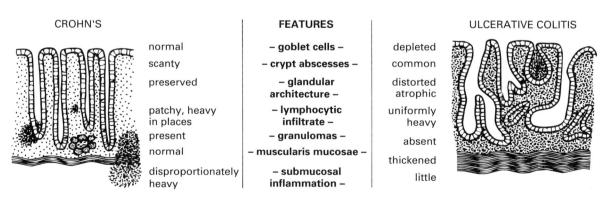

CROHN'S	FEATURES	ULCERATIVE COLITIS
normal	– goblet cells –	depleted
scanty	– crypt abscesses –	common
preserved	– glandular architecture –	distorted atrophic
patchy, heavy in places	– lymphocytic infiltrate –	uniformly heavy
present	– granulomas –	absent
normal	– muscularis mucosae –	thickened
disproportionately heavy	– submucosal inflammation –	little

Fig. 10.2 Histological features in the rectal biopsy that help to distinguish between ulcerative colitis and Crohn's disease. (Reproduced by permission of Blackwell Scientific Publications from Misiewicz J J, Pounder R E, Venables C W (eds) 1987 Diseases of the gut and pancreas.)

proctosigmoiditis. Involvement of other parts of the colon is termed colitis. The disease tends to progress proximally.

EPIDEMIOLOGY

Figures from north-western Europe, and the United States of America show similar prevalence rates of 79.9 and 87.0 per 100 000 population respectively.

Incidence rates based on hospitalized patients vary between 4.7 and 15.1 per 100 000 population for the United States of America and western Europe.

A twofold increase occurred during the 1950s and 1960s but it has remained steady over the last 20 years.

Contrary to the findings of early studies there is no variation between men and women, or between different socioeconomic groups. However, ulcerative colitis is more common in nonsmokers, quite the opposite to Crohn's disease.

All age groups are at risk. The peak age of onset is between 15 and 40 years.

AETIOLOGY

Genetic factors

Familial or genetic incidence of ulcerative colitis shows a wide variation from 1 to 16% amongst immediate family members with a possible tenfold increase in likelihood occurring when the parent has the disease.

Environmental factors

Infective agents, diet and psychosocial stress may be important but their present role remains ill-defined and unconfirmed. Like Crohn's sufferers, urban dwellers appear to be more at risk than rural dwellers. Similarly, evidence linking fibre, milk, and food intake to ulcerative colitis is lacking although countries whose fibre intake is high appear to have a low incidence.

PATHOPHYSIOLOGY

Although scientific and clinical evidence linking immunology with disease pathogenesis is lacking, some patients suffering from proctitis have a higher serum IgG concentration than controls. Serum antibodies against intestinal bacteria and colon epithelial component antigens have also been found but are considered secondary to a damaged mucosa.

Complement found in the basement membrane of colonic epithelium is evidence of deposition of immune complex in the mucosa. Monocyte stimulation by these complexes may explain increased prostaglandin synthesis that occurs in active disease.

Water and electrolyte balance is affected in extensive ulcerative colitis as a result of reduction in the absorption of sodium, chloride and water. Daily faecal weights of patients with ulcerative colitis are generally higher than in normal subjects. Proctitis sufferers sometimes demonstrate a slightly raised potassium to sodium ratio, probably due to a decreased sodium absorption.

Macroscopic examination of the rectum showing excoriated skin is often the first pathological evidence and, in acute active disease, blood, pus and mucus discharges from the colon to the rectum. Sigmoidoscopy will confirm the presence of granular haemorrhagic mucosa, and the extent of the disease. With inactive disease the rectal mucosa appears quite normal but close macroscopical examination reveals an abnormal vessel pattern, together with a fine granularity.

Microscopic examination allows subdivision of the disease into active colitis, resolving colitis, and colitis in remission. Active disease is characterized by dilatation of local blood capillaries and haemorrhages, reduction in goblet cell population and epithelial cell necrosis and the presence of crypt abscesses formed following polymorphonuclear cell infiltration of the lamina propria (see Fig. 10.2). Although generally confined to the mucosa if ulceration is present, inflammatory cells may infiltrate the submucosa. During treatment, microscopical examination reveals a reduction in cellular infiltration of the lamina propria and restoration of the goblet cell population. This phase is termed resolving colitis and remission is recognized by shortening of the crypts, with a defined gap between the crypt base and the muscularis mucosae.

CLINICAL MANIFESTATIONS

Depending on the severity and site of activity, patients can present with systemic and intestinal symptoms. A patient with proctitis may only show intestinal symptoms such as pain, diarrhoea and rectal bleeding, but if suffering from proctosigmoiditis there are likely to be more severe symptoms.

Abdominal pain is graded in degrees of severity relating to the extent of colonic involvement. Total colitis is usually accompanied by severe persistent pain whereas this rarely occurs in proctitis.

The majority of patients have diarrhoea with the severity related to the extent of the disease. Elderly patients, however, suffering from proctosigmoiditis may complain of constipation. Blood coating a formed stool usually suggests proctitis and patients may display systemic symptoms such as anorexia, weight loss, lethargy and fever.

Active disease is classified as mild, moderate or severe and of short- or long-term duration. Number of bowel motions, macroscopic appearance of blood in stools, anaemia and erythrocyte sedimentation rate are used quantitatively to determine disease severity.

INVESTIGATIONS

Endoscopy

Sigmoidoscopy is used to confirm a diagnosis of ulcerative colitis. Rectal biopsies support the diagnosis and are used to evaluate progress, assess the patient's response to treatment and to differentiate between ulcerative colitis and other causes of proctitis such as Crohn's disease. Disease assessment takes note of the appearance of the mucosa, changes in the vascular pattern, and severity of spontaneous bleeding.

Examination further along the colon from the rectum requires colonoscopy which allows assessment of the extent of disease, and the taking of multiple biopsies.

Radiology

Double contrast barium enemas will detect early mucosal changes and the extent of the disease. The typical radiograph of the chronic stage of ulcerative colitis shows a narrowing of the lumen, the walls becoming more rigid and the bowel shortened (Fig. 10.3).

Plain abdominal radiographs, not barium enemas, are used when initial diagnosis indicates the presence of acute disease or toxic dilatation.

Laboratory

Haematological and biochemical values pointing to ulcerative colitis include iron deficiency anaemia, elevated white cell count, raised erythrocyte sedimentation rate, and a low serum albumin. Microbiological examination of stool samples taken at initial diagnosis may provide evidence of infection as a cause of colonic inflammation.

CLINICAL ASSESSMENT

Treatment is aimed at resolving the disease and maintaining the patient in remission although a small number suffer continuous symptoms. Patient management revolves around the treatment of acute attacks, maintenance of remission and assessing the risk of colonic carcinoma.

Sudden deterioration in a patient's condition may occur as a consequence of toxic dilatation which if untreated can prove fatal following colonic perforation. Early diagnosis of inflammatory bowel disease is difficult and may delay treatment. This is particularly true in children and young adults.

TREATMENT OF INFLAMMATORY BOWEL DISEASE

A wide range of drugs and nutritional supplements are available to maintain the patient in long periods of remission in both Crohn's disease and ulcerative colitis. However, surgical intervention will eventually become necessary when the patient relapses and fails to respond to drug therapy.

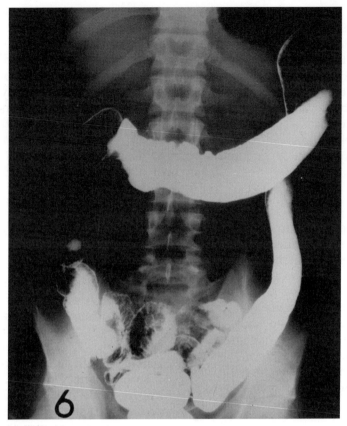

Fig. 10.3 Ulcerative colitis showing total involvement with loss of haustral pattern and fine ulceration (By courtesy of Professor John Rhodes.)

Nutritional needs

Although dietary control of the disease is usually inappropriate, some dietary refinements can be beneficial. For example, patients with small intestinal strictures should avoid indigestible foods that may cause obstruction by aggregation at strictures (see Table 10.2).

Carbohydrate intake is often higher than the population average but subsequent reduction is not associated with clinical improvement. Inadequate food intake is sometimes presented as a problem in Crohn's disease and patients with a poor appetite will often respond to supplemental enteral feeds.

Malnourished patients undergoing surgery should have their nutritional status improved which may even render surgery unnecessary.

Abnormal growth patterns in children with Crohn's disease can be corrected by concurrent enteral and medical therapy. Many nutritional deficiencies associated with inflammatory bowel

Table 10.2   Foods to avoid (reproduced by permission of Blackwell Scientific Publications from Misiewicz J J, Pounder R E, Venables C W (eds) 1987 Diseases of the gut and pancreas)
Foods that may cause bolus obstruction if there is an intestinal stricture
Segments of any citrus fruit Sweetcorn Coleslaw or uncooked vegetables Raw fruits, unless chewed thoroughly Nuts Popcorn Tough or gristly meat

disease are due to malabsorption following extensive small bowel resection. Iron depletion, hypoproteinaemia, deficiencies in water- and fat-soluble vitamins, trace elements and electrolytes can be corrected using a suitable replacement regimen. A total parenteral nutrition (TPN) regimen suitable for each patient can be established and maintained where appropriate. Often the most successful regimen is one based on using partial parenteral and enteral nutrition.

Drug treatment

Current drug treatment aims to ameliorate the disease's secondary effects rather than modify or reverse the underlying pathogenic mechanism. Corticosteroids, aminosalicylates, and immunosuppressive agents are routinely used. Other drugs such as metronidazole, cholestyramine, sodium cromoglycate and broad-spectrum antibiotics are helpful in some cases, whilst recent interest in cyclosporin, bismuth and arsenical salts, sucralfate, thalidomide, new steroid entities, cytoprotective agents and fish oils may well provide future alternative therapy.

Corticosteroids

The glucocorticoid properties of hydrocortisone and prednisolone are the mainstay of treatment. The preferred steroid is prednisolone, administered orally or rectally, and parenterally in emergency situations.

Moderately ill patients require prednisolone in doses of 30 to 40 mg/day orally, in divided doses for 2 to 3 weeks. Depending on the patient's response a gradual dose reduction can be introduced to 10 to 20 mg/day for 4 to 6 weeks. Milder cases can be controlled by morning administration only, mimicking the diurnal rhythm of the body's cortisol secretion. Severe extensive or fulminant disease will require hospitalization and the use of parenteral therapy using hydrocortisone sodium succinate, administered intramuscularly or intravenously in doses of 100 to 500 mg three to four times a day. Oral prednisolone therapy should be introduced as soon as possible.

Abrupt withdrawal of steroids must be avoided. Maintenance doses are normally in the range of 6 to 15 mg daily or on alternate days.

The incidence of adverse effects appears to increase when prednisolone doses are higher than 40 mg/day. An alternate-day regimen is helpful, causing less adrenal suppression. Azathioprine with its steroid-sparing property may be introduced together with a lower dose of steroid or as an alternative.

Formulation. Oral administration will control moderate inflammatory bowel disease but proctitis, left-sided disease and Crohn's disease of the anus and rectum are more appropriately treated using a topical preparation. The choice of locally applied formulations will depend on patient acceptability and preference (see Table 10.3).

Prednisolone sodium phosphate and metasulphobenzoate enemas, hydrocortisone acetate foam aerosol and prednisolone sodium phosphate suppositories are available. Pack presentation is important to the patient because the

---

Table 10.3 Comparison of available preparations for rectal administration in inflammatory bowel disease

Generic name	Formulation	Site of release
Sulphasalazine	Suppositories	Descending colon and rectum
	Retention enema	
Mesalazine	Retention enema	Descending colon and rectum
	Suppositories	
4-aminosalicylic acid	Retention enema	Descending colon and rectum
Prednisolone	Retention enema	Ascending transverse and descending colon
(Metasulphobenzoate or 21-phosphate)	Foam	Rectum and descending colon
Hydrocortisone	Foam	Rectum and descending colon
	Suppositories	

ease with which a patient can either open a suppository pack or insert an enema will influence compliance. Self-administration of a short tube enema may be difficult for rheumatic patients who may cope using the long tube version. The enema's volume and viscosity must allow easy application and retention. Foam formulations which adhere to the mucosa may be preferred.

Following rectal administration prednisolone metasulphobenzoate is poorly absorbed compared to prednisolone-21-phosphate, but gives comparative therapeutic results. These factors must be considered when recommending a suitable preparation. Rectal administration should be performed just before bedtime when the supine position allows much longer retention times.

Uncoated steroid tablets are suitable for most patients whilst enteric-coated preparations do not offer any proven advantage. Patients with short bowel or strictures should avoid enteric-coated preparations because of poor absorption and bolus formation at strictures respectively. Prednisolone steaglate appears to be more readily absorbed from the gut and is slowly metabolized to prednisolone.

Other steroids. New molecular configurations and formulations of steroids are being investigated. Methylprednisolone 40 mg enema appears as effective as hydrocortisone 100 mg in achieving remission and similarly betamethasone valerate enema, beclomethasone diproprionate and budesonide enema 2 mg/100 ml compare favourably with hydrocortisone, prednisone and prednisolone respectively. Budesonide also has fewer side effects.

Tixocortol pivolate, a new non-glucocorticoid and non-mineralocorticoid cortisol derivative, possesses anti-inflammatory activity equivalent to hydrocortisone. It appears as effective as other steroids, demonstrates a lower incidence of side effects and like betamethasone and budesonide undergoes extensive first-pass metabolism.

Aminosalicylates

Sulphasalazine is most effective in maintaining remission in ulcerative colitis. Its use in Crohn's disease is less well established.

Sulphasalazine consists of sulphapyridine diazotized to 5-aminosalicylic acid (5-ASA, mesalazine). When it reaches the colon the diazo bond is cleaved by bacterial azoreductase liberating mesalazine and sulphapyridine. Sulphapyridine is absorbed and metabolized by hepatic acetylation or hydroxylation followed by glucuronidation. Mesalazine is partly absorbed, metabolized by the liver and excreted via the kidneys as n-acetyl 5-aminosalicylic acid, although the majority is acetylated during passage through the intestinal mucosa. Sulphasalazine itself is poorly absorbed. That which is absorbed is recycled back into the gut via the bile either unchanged or as the n-acetyl metabolite.

Sulphasalazine metabolites are responsible for the yellow coloration of urine. Elimination of sulphapyridine depends on the patient's acetylator phenotype; those who inherit the 'slow' acetylator phenotype experience more side effects. Mesalazine is the active component of sulphasalazine exerting a local action independent of blood levels. Its effectiveness depends on the site of ulceration in relation to the drug's dissolution profile. This is very important when choosing aminosalicylate preparations as illustrated in Figure 10.4.

The optimal dose of sulphasalazine to achieve and maintain remission is usually in the range of 2 to 4 g per day in four divided doses. Acute attacks require 4 to 8 g per day in divided doses until remission occurs, but at these doses associated side effects begin to appear. Of the patients taking sulphasalazine, 30% experience adverse effects which are either dose-related reactions, dependent on acetylator phenotype or idiosyncratic non-dose-related reactions. The first group includes nausea, vomiting, headache, malaise, haemolytic anaemia, reticulocytosis, methaemoglobulinaemia, and the second includes skin rash, hepatic and pulmonary dysfunction, aplastic anaemia and reversible azoospermia. Adverse effects usually occur during the first 2 weeks of therapy, and are generally attributed to serum sulphapyridine levels.

Many of the adverse effects listed above can

PHYSIOLOGICAL PROBLEMS

FORMULATION PROBLEMS

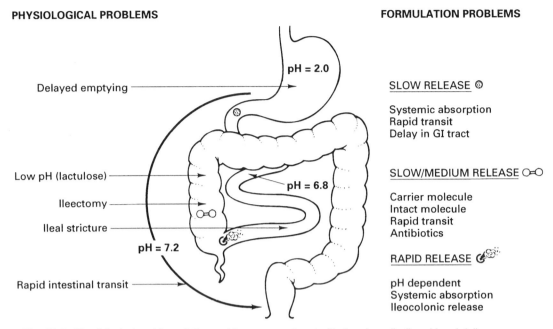

Fig. 10.4 Physiological and formulation problems encountered with 5-aminosalicylic acid oral delivery systems.

be avoided by using mesalazine or one of the other aminosalicylate preparations which are now available (Table 10.4).

As mesalazine is unstable in an acid medium and rapidly absorbed from the gastrointestinal tract the new preparations have been developed using three different approaches (see Fig. 10.4):

- a mesalazine tablet coated with a pH-dependent acrylic resin
- ethylcellulose-coated mesalazine granules
- diazotization of mesalazine to itself or to an inert carrier.

Asacol contains 400 mg of mesalazine coated with the acrylic resin Eudragit-S which dissolves at pH 7 and releases mesalazine in the terminal ileum and colon. Salofalk tablets are a similar formulation containing 250 mg mesalazine with sodium carbonate, glycine and a cellulose ether, coated with Eudragit-L which dissolves at pH 6 and above, releasing mesalazine in the jejunum and ileum.

Pentasa tablets 250 mg and 500 mg comprise ethylcellulosecoated granules of mesalazine which are released when the tablet disintegrates in the stomach. Mesalazine is leached slowly from the granules throughout the gastrointestinal tract at all physiological pHs.

Dipentum 250 mg tablets contain olsalazine sodium which is two diazotized mesalazine molecules. Like sulphasalazine it remains intact until it reaches the colon where it undergoes bacterial cleavage releasing two molecules of mesalazine.

Clinical studies have shown all three formulations to be as effective as sulphasalazine in maintaining remission in inflammatory bowel disease. Each preparation offers alternative therapy to sulphasalazine-intolerant patients if used as a new treatment. The dose range of mesalazine and olsalazine is 1 to 3 g daily in divided doses.

Mesalazine enemas (1 g in 100 ml) or suppositories (250 mg and 500 mg) are also effective alternatives for treating localized Crohn's disease or proctitis.

An interesting alternative to mesalazine is 4-aminosalicylic acid (para-aminosalicylic acid, PAS). Used as a 2 g enema it appears effective in the treatment of distal ulcerative colitis.

Table 10.4 Comparison of available oral aminosalicylate preparations for patients with inflammatory bowel disease

Generic and proprietary name	Formulation	Release profile	Site of release
Sulphasalazine (Salazopyrin)	Compressed tablet Plain and film-coated	Azo-linked, independent of pH	Terminal ileum and colon
Mesalazine (Asacol)	Compressed tablet Acrylic coating	Acrylic coating dissolving at pH 7	Terminal ileum and colon
Mesalazine (Salofalk)	Compressed tablet Acrylic coating	Acrylic coating dissolving at pH 6	Mid-jejunum, ileum and colon
Mesalazine (Pentasa)	Microgranules coated with ethyl cellulose and compressed into tablets	Disintegration not dependent on pH Slow dissolution rate	Stomach, duodenum, jejunum, ileum and colon
Olsalazine (Dipentum)	Hard gelatin capsules, uncoated	Azo-linked Disintegration independent of pH	Terminal ileum and colon
Balsalazide (Colazide)	Compressed tablet and/or capsule	Azo-linked Disintegration independent of pH	Terminal ileum and colon
Ipsalazide	Compressed tablet and/or capsule	Azo-linked Disintegration independent of pH	Terminal ileum and colon
Polyasa	Compressed tablet and/or capsule	Azo-linked Disintegration independent of pH	Terminal ileum and colon

An oral 500 mg acrylic-coated formulation is available in the USA.

Mesalazine inhibits components of the arachidonic acid cascade and interferes with the synthesis of prostaglandins in the inflamed rectal mucosa and it also acts as a scavenger of oxygen free radicals. The products of the arachidonic acid cascade are known to cause erythema, oedema and pain and stimulate adenyl cyclase in the small bowel leading to ion and water secretion and sodium absorption, thus contributing to diarrhoea. In addition to the inhibition of prostaglandin synthesis mesalazine also blocks the lipoxygenase pathway and inhibits leukotrienes which attract and recruit inflammatory cells.

Cyclo-oxygenase inhibitors such as flurbiprofen have failed to show a therapeutic benefit in inflammatory bowel disease.

Immunosuppressants

Azathioprine and 6-mercaptopurine are used in patients unresponsive to steroids and aminosalicylates. Azathioprine is metabolized to 6-mercaptopurine by the liver. Both possess steroid-sparing properties and are used either with prednisolone or alone in maintaining remission in Crohn's disease and occasionally in ulcerative colitis. Mercaptopurine is preferred although side effects occur more frequently.

Maintenance doses for azathioprine and 6-mercaptopurine are usually 2 and 1.5 mg/kg body weight respectively, with doses adjusted to the patient's response and tolerance and white cell and platelet counts.

Major concerns with immunosuppressive agents are their adverse effects. Skin rashes and nausea are common; raised liver enzymes and allergic hepatitis are less frequent and reversible. Thrombocytopenia and leucopenia have also been reported. Patients are monitored regularly for bone marrow depression, have routine blood counts and liver function tests including serum bilirubin and alkaline phosphatase.

The increased incidence of lymphomas in patients receiving immunosuppressants compared with other treatments is of concern and there is evidence of a greater incidence in patients taking azathioprine compared to 6-mercaptopurine.

Although the action of immunosuppressive agents in inflammatory bowel disease remains unclear it may be as a result of inhibition of DNA and purine synthesis which affect plasma cells and lymphocytes.

Metronidazole

Metronidazole has been used with some success in Crohn's patients using a dose of 10 to 20 mg/kg/day. Patients with severe perineal involvement have responded to metronidazole treatment experiencing less pain and tenderness and eventually decreased erythema and swelling, and wound healing.

An 800 mg dose of metronidazole has proved as effective as 3 g sulphasalazine in treating some cases of Crohn's disease but it is ineffective in ulcerative colitis. It is generally well tolerated with patients suffering only mild adverse effects such as metallic taste, glossitis, paraesthesia, darkening of urine and urticaria. Paraesthesia appears to be dose related, occurring frequently with prolonged treatment. Doses should be gradually reduced during treatment.

Oral and rectal doses of metronidazole are partly metabolized by gut bacterial flora and, following rapid absorption, by the liver. The metabolite's free nitro group is thought to be responsible for its local activity. It also inhibits phospholipase A, contributing to a reduction in damage induced by polymorphonuclear leucocytes.

Cyclosporin

The effectiveness of cyclosporin in treating inflammatory bowel disease has been studied in patients refractory to conventional drug therapy using doses ranging from 10 to 15 mg/kg/day. Patient response to this treatment has varied, adverse effects causing withdrawal of treatment in some cases. However, some patients have been able to discontinue concurrent steroid therapy and remained in remission for some time. Abdominal pain, diarrhoea and weight gain are common non-dose-related side effects whilst nephrotoxicity and hepatotoxicity are dose related, usually occurring when serum concentrations are greater than 400 ng/ml. Tremors and hirsutism occur at serum concentrations of 100 to 400 ng/ml.

Cyclosporin is a promising alternative treatment but careful monitoring of patients is needed.

Cyclosporin acts at an early stage on precursors of helper cells by interfering with the release of interleukin II, consequently inhibiting the formation of cytotoxic lymphocytes that cause tissue damage.

Sodium cromoglycate

Sodium cromoglycate has been shown to reduce the degranulation of mast cells in inflammatory bowel disease. It inhibits the passage of calcium ions across cell membranes, a process essential for the release of inflammatory mediators from mast cells. Intestinal lesions contain mast cells, macrophages and eosinophils and rectal biopsies show large numbers of IgE plasma cells in the lamina propria. This evidence points to a hypersensitivity response which is inhibited by sodium cromoglycate stabilizing the mast cell. Some patients suffering from proctitis respond when prescribed 100 mg sodium cromoglycate three times a day orally and 200 mg twice daily as enemas. However, many patients in remission or with active colitis have failed to show a therapeutic benefit. Its use in inflammatory bowel disease remains unproven but some patients may derive benefit. A recent re-evaluation of sodium cromoglycate as an enema revealed that it compared favourably to prednisolone.

Bismuth salts

Bismuth subsalicylate and bismuth chelate administered as enemas are effective treatments for ulcerative colitis. Bismuth salts inhibit sulphatase and sialidase enzymes which are secreted by colonic bacteria and contribute to the process of mucus degradation. Bismuth also demonstrates cytoprotective properties through a mechanism which increases tissue prostaglandin levels. A dose of 480 mg bismuth chelate suspension has been shown to be effective when administered nightly for 4 weeks. Similarly, 700 mg of bismuth subsalicylate suspension administered twice daily for 8 weeks has also been shown to give good results.

Arsenic salts

Arsenic salts, particularly acetarsol in the form of 250 mg suppositories have been used successfully to treat ulcerative proctitis, but toxicity limits its use. Acetarsol is bactericidal and chemically similar to bismuth which may account for its mode of action.

Thalidomide

The use of thalidomide has been restricted to monitored refractory cases. It probably antagonizes the chemical mediators of inflammation, stabilizes lysosomal membranes and at therapeutic doses inhibits the formation of superoxide and hydroxyl radicals, potent oxidants capable of causing tissue damage. Daily doses in the range of 50 to 400 mg have proved beneficial when used for periods of 1 week to several months.

Antibiotics

With the exception of metronidazole, antibacterials are not routinely used because causative bacterial agents have not been identified. However, systemic complications such as toxic colitis may respond to metronidazole or vancomycin. Active Crohn's disease accompanied by fever complications may be alleviated by the administration of cephazolin, tetracycline or ampicillin.

Antidiarrhoeals

Codeine, diphenoxylate, and loperamide should be used cautiously in inflammatory bowel disease as their use may mask inflammation and infection, delaying correct diagnosis.

Cholestyramine

Following ileal resection cholestyramine has been used in Crohn's patients to decrease diarrhoea associated with bile-acid malabsorption caused by the decrease in small bowel absorptive surface area and the cathartic effect of bile salts on the colon. At doses of up to 4 g three times a day it inhibits bile-acid stimulated secretion of water and electrolytes.

Fish oils

Fish liver oils which contain eicosapentaenoic acid and docosahexaenoic acid have recently been used with some initial success in the treatment of ulcerative colitis and Crohn's disease. It is postulated that fish oils might work by diverting fatty acid metabolism from leukotriene B_4 to the formation of the less inflammatory leukotriene B_5.

Other drugs

Alternative effective treatments for inflammatory bowel disease are still being sought. Current investigations involve sucralfate, nicotine, oxygen, oxygen-derived free radical scavengers, somatostatin analogues, lignocaine, chloroquine, methotrexate, d-penicillamine, and antituberculous agents. However, the strategy for future investigations may well focus on a drug's ability to block leukotriene synthesis by (a) interfering with phospholipase A_2, (b) modifying dietary intake of eicosanoids and (c) inhibition of 5-lipoxygenase.

The pharmacological profiles of drugs used in the management of adults with inflammatory bowel disease are shown in Table 10.5.

THE PATIENT

A consumer leaflet on inflammatory bowel disease has been prepared by the National

Table 10.5 Pharmacological profile of drugs used in adults with inflammatory bowel disease

Pharmacological group	Daily dose	$t_{1/2}$ (h)	Metabolism
Steroids			
Hydrocortisone	125–250 mg as foam 100–400 mg in 0.9% w/v sodium chloride i.v. 50 mg as suppositories	1.5	Hepatic metabolism 70% and 30% unchanged
Prednisolone	20–60 mg orally 20 mg as enema 5–10 mg as suppositories	3	Hepatic metabolism 70% and 30% unchanged
Aminosalicylates			
Mesalazine	150 mg–1.5 g as suppositories 1 g as enema 1.2–2.4 g orally	0.7–2.4	Local and systemic Hepatic acetylation glucuronidation
Olsalazine	1–3 g orally	1.0	Local and systemic Hepatic acetylation glucuronidation
Sulphasalazine	3 g as enema 1–2 g as suppositories 4–8 g orally	5–8	Colonic azoreduction Local and systemic acetylation Hepatic glucuronidation
4-aminosalicylic acid	1–2 g orally 1–2 g as enema	0.75–1.0	Rapid absorption and distribution Systemic acetylation
Immunosuppressants			
Azathioprine	2 mg/kg orally	3	Hepatic metabolism to 6-mercaptopurine
6-mercaptopurine	2.5 mg/kg orally	1.5	Hepatic metabolism to inactive metabolites
Cyclosporin	10–15 mg/kg	19–27	Mainly hepatic metabolism
Antibiotics			
Metronidazole	600 mg–1.2 g orally 2 g i.v.	6–14	Hepatic metabolism
Miscellaneous			
Arsenic salts	250 mg–1 g rectally	72	Tissue deposition excreted unchanged
Bismuth salts	200 mg–1.2 g rectally	Unknown	Tissue deposition excreted unchanged
Fish oils	3–4 g	Unknown	Used in arachidonic acid cycle
Sodium cromoglycate	200–800 mg orally 100–400 mg as enema	0.75–1.0	Poorly absorbed, excreted unchanged in urine and bile

Association for Colitis and Crohn's Disease (NACC).

Of particular importance is the 'Can't Wait' card which is a request for the use of a toilet in an emergency. The pharmacist should also be aware of the following points:

1. Patients taking steroids must be issued with a steroid card.

2. Relapse may be averted by ensuring that the patient retains a surplus of tablets and enemas. If, when in remission, symptoms recur, patients should have written instructions to increase the dose of their current oral therapy and commence rectal administration of a corticosteroid.

3. Effective home treatment of proctitis is important because tenesmus and occasional faecal incontinence, apart from being distressing, limit further treatment. Enemas or suppositories should be administered before retiring with clear instructions to warm the enema, insert it while lying in the left lateral position, and retain it as long as possible.

4. Infertility associated with sulphasalazine therapy should suggest the use of alternative aminosalicylate therapy.

5. Inflammatory bowel disease does not affect fertility or the course of pregnancy. There is no evidence that the frequency of congenital abnormalities, spontaneous abortions or stillbirths is increased, and neither sulphasalazine nor topical corticosteroids present a significant hazard to the fetus.

CASE STUDIES

CASE 10.1

Miss A. is a 26-year-old lady who presents with a prescription for sulphasalazine 500 mg four times a day. She has recently been referred to the gastroenterologist following a 3-month history of abdominal pain, diarrhoea and several episodes of rectal bleeding. Inpatient investigation found mild ulcerative colitis extending through most of the large bowel and most active proximally.

Q1 What monitoring should be carried out in patients starting sulphasalazine for ulcerative colitis?

Q2 What information about the drug should be provided to the patient?

Q3 Why is sulphasalazine often of limited usefulness in Crohn's disease?

CASE 10.2

Mr B. is 35 years old and has a 12-year history of Crohn's disease. He has been maintained in remission, apart from three or four acute exacerbations, for the last 3 years. His current therapy is:

- mesalazine 400 mg three times a day
- prednisolone 5 mg once a day (increased during acute exacerbations)
- ferrous sulphate 200 mg three times a day.

At his most recent clinic visit he was found to have glycosuria and mildly elevated blood pressure which, in association with a noticeable change in his facial features, were considered characteristic side effects of his long-term steroid therapy. It was decided to start him on azathioprine.

Q1 What is the rationale of this change in drug treatment?

Q2 What precautions should be taken?

Q3 If azathioprine fails to allow adequate reduction in the dose of steroid, what alternative could be tried?

CASE 10.3

Mrs C., 45 years old, was admitted to hospital for an ileostomy. Ulcerative colitis was diagnosed 15 years ago and since then she has had a number of hospital admissions with profuse diarrhoea, rectal bleeding and generalized symptoms such as reduced appetite, nausea and weight loss. She is no longer able to retain her prednisolone enemas for longer than a few minutes and is needing oral prednisolone 40 mg a day with codeine phosphate 15 mg tablets taken as required.

Q What prescription and over-the-counter drugs should be avoided in Mrs C. following her ileostomy?

CASE 10.4

Mr D. is 53 years of age and has suffered from ulcerative colitis for 25 years. Until recently he has been maintained in remission on a low dose oral prednisolone and sulphasalazine regimen but relapses are now occurring frequently. He has recently developed rheumatoid arthritis. Mr D. is found to be suffering from predominantly left-sided colitis and radiographic evidence reveals that a proximal stricture has formed.

Q1 What alternative therapy, in terms of (a) the formulation and (b) the drug should be considered for Mr D.?

Q2 Why should Mr D. be followed up at a hospital outpatient clinic?

ANSWERS TO CASE STUDIES

CASE 10.1

A1 Appropriate monitoring should be carried out for both efficacy and toxicity. Efficacy of sulphasalazine in ulcerative colitis can be assessed by a reduction in the degree of abdominal pain and in the frequency of diarrhoea and rectal bleeding. Miss A. should also show a reduction in acute phase proteins (e.g. C-reactive protein) and ESR and her biochemical tests and haemoglobin should return to normal.

A2 Patients should be warned about the potential dose-related side effects and also that the drug may colour the urine yellow and also cause discolouration of soft contact lenses.

A3 Sulphasalazine is less useful in Crohn's disease because of its pharmacodynamic properties. It is absorbed in the ileum and secreted unchanged in the bile, reaching the colon intact. Normal gut flora then split the drug into the active molecule which is absorbed in the colon, metabolized and then excreted in the urine. As a result the drug is most effective in disease of the colon and terminal ileum but Crohn's disease may affect the entire length of the gastrointestinal tract.

CASE 10.2

A1 The steroid-sparing effects of the azathioprine are being utilized.

A2 High doses of azathioprine produce bone marrow suppression and so a maximum of 2 mg/kg/day should be used. Liver function and blood counts should be monitored regularly.

A3 The immunosuppressant cyclosporin may be useful. It may be used in combination with steroids and azathioprine but gradual withdrawal of the azathioprine is preferred to reduce combined toxicity.

CASE 10.3

 Drugs altering fluid and electrolyte balance should be avoided. Laxatives and magnesium-containing antacids in particular can increase fluid loss through the stoma and lead to dehydration. Diuretics may aggravate dehydration. There may be reduced release of drug from sustained-release and enteric-coated preparations.

CASE 10.4

A1 a. The use of an enema foam, or suppository formulation should be considered for left-sided colitis. The stricture may prevent complete tablet disintegration, especially in the case of enteric-coated sulphasalazine formulations.

b. The choice of a mesalazine formulation which disintegrates proximally to the stricture may be helpful. An alternative drug worth considering would be bismuth citrate or subsalicylate enemas.

A2 Because the patient has rheumatoid arthritis it may be difficult, depending on how the disease progresses, for the patient to self-administer enema preparations. Compliance failure may then cause further relapses.

BIBLIOGRAPHY

Hawthorne A B, Hawkey C J. Immunosuppressive drugs in inflammatory bowel disease. Drugs 1989; 38: 267–288

Misiewicz J J, Pounder R E, Venables C W (eds). Diseases of the gut and pancreas. Oxford: Blackwell Scientific Publications 1987

Peppercorn M A. Advances in drug therapy for inflammatory bowel disease. Annals of Internal Medicine 1990; 112: 50–60

Rhodes J, Mayberry J F. Ulcerative colitis. Medicine International 1990; 79: 3269–3275

Sottile R F, Quandt C M, Present D H, Mehl B. Medical management of inflammatory bowel disease. DICP The Annals of Pharmacotherapy 1989; 23: 963–973

Chapter 11

Constipation and diarrhoea

D. K. Luscombe

Two of the most common disorders of the gastrointestinal tract are constipation and diarrhoea. Whilst simple constipation is relatively easy to treat, self-limiting and not life threatening, diarrhoea may be debilitating and occasionally fatal, particularly in the very young. Both disorders frequently occur as secondary features of more serious disorders such as strictures/ obstructions, diverticulosis (constipation) or ulcerative colitis, Crohn's disease and bowel carcinoma (diarrhoea). Many drugs may cause constipation or diarrhoea as side effects and should be suspected as possible causes whenever patients are receiving drug therapy.

CONSTIPATION

It is generally accepted that a patient is constipated if stools are passed less than three times a week and/or faecal weight is on average less than 30 g per day (normally 150 g daily for an adult). Another definition would be a reduced frequency of defaecation from the norm for an individual. The act of defaecation is often difficult or painful in constipation and the stools that are produced are dry and hard.

INCIDENCE

Constipation affects everyone at some time or other. It is commonly seen in the elderly, often secondary to other problems. Between 40 and 50% of acute admissions and approximately 80%

of long-stay elderly hospitalized patients suffer constipation. Children and patients who are bedridden are also susceptible as are pregnant females.

AETIOLOGY

It is probable that most cases of constipation arise from an inadequate intake of dietary fibre. Dehydration associated with low fluid intake or excessive sweating is also a major cause of constipation as the body attempts to conserve water by absorbing the maximum amount of fluid from the colon leading to dry, hard stools. Lack of exercise and poor mobility, especially in the elderly or the bedridden, lead to constipation. The young and elderly may fail to recognize or answer the normal call to stool resulting in constipation. Lack of toilet facilities or those of poor standards of hygiene may be the underlying cause of the reflex need to defaecate being overridden. Patients with haemorrhoids or anal fissures may elect to postpone the passing of stools to avoid causing pain, thus increasing the likelihood of constipation. The ageing process is accompanied by a loss of sensitivity of the sensory reflexes responsible for normal bowel function and a reduction in muscle tone in the small and large intestines. The result is decreased bowel motions and possibly faecal stasis.

Pregnant females are often inconvenienced by constipation. The reasons for this are various and include: exertion of pressure on the colon by the growing uterus; a possible reduction in dietary roughage and fluid intake; a reduction in physical activity; high levels of progesterone which inhibit gastrointestinal smooth muscle activity.

Many medical and surgical conditions may cause constipation as a secondary feature (Table 11.1). The fact that many drugs induce constipation is often overlooked. The list of drugs is extensive and includes opioid analgesics, anticholinergics, diuretics and some antidepressants (Table 11.2). Laxatives when used regularly over a long period may cause an atonic colon (loss of muscle tone in the colon) thus increasing constipation and exacerbating the underlying problem. The patient often increases the dose to

Table 11.1 Possible medical and surgical causes of constipation

Gastrointestinal disease	Irritable bowel syndrome Hernias Strictures/obstructions Diverticulosis Haemorrhoids Neoplasms (colon, rectal) Hirschsprung's disease
Neurological disorders	Parkinson's disease Multiple sclerosis Cerebral neoplasms
Psychological/psychiatric	Stress Depression
Metabolic disorders	Hypokalaemia Hypercalcaemia Diabetes Hypothyroidism
Surgical	Gastrointestinal or major abdominal surgery

Table 11.2 Classes of drugs that may cause constipation

Drug group	Examples
Opioid analgesics	Codeine, dihydrocodeine, morphine
Cough suppressants	Codeine, dextromethorphan, pholcodine
Anticholinergics	Orphenadrine, benzhexol
Antihistamines	H,-antagonists due to intrinsic anticholinergic activity
Tricyclic antidepressants	Imipramine, clomipramine
Monoamine oxidase inhibitors	Phenelzine, tranylcypromine
Diuretics	(If dehydration occurs)
Cations	Calcium, aluminium – in antacids
Antihypertensives	Clonidine, nifedipine, verapamil
Iron preparations	Ferrous sulphate
Laxative abuse	

achieve a laxative effect which leads to laxative abuse, a particular problem in the elderly.

PATHOPHYSIOLOGY OF CONSTIPATION AND DIARRHOEA

Constipation and diarrhoea both result from an upset in the balance of the absorption and secretion of water and electrolytes by the gastro-intestinal epithelium. Normally there is a net uptake of fluid in the intestine in response to osmotic gradients. These involve the absorption and secretion of ions and absorption of mainly sugars and amino acids. This process is under the influence of the autonomic nervous system (sympathetic and parasympathetic). If absorption is increased then this may lead to constipation whereas a net secretion of fluid will result in diarrhoea. Infectious organisms, chemicals and many drugs may interfere with the uptake and secretory processes. Furthermore, agents which alter intestinal motility, either directly or by acting on the autonomic nervous system, will affect the transit time of food material along the gastrointestinal tract. Since the extent of absorption and secretion of fluid from the gastrointestinal tract generally parallels the transit time, a slower transit time will lead to the formation of hard stools and constipation while rapid transit will result in diarrhoea. Motility is largely under parasympathetic (cholinergic) control, stimulation bringing about an increase in motility while antagonists such as the anticholinergic agents decrease motility and induce constipation.

Some 9 L of fluid normally enter the small intestine daily, 2 L from ingestion and the balance from intestinal secretions. Of the total volume, all but 1.0 to 1.5 L is absorbed in the ileum with the colon absorbing most of the remainder, leaving only 0.2 L of fluid to be expelled in the faeces. Since the colon is able to absorb only 4 to 5 L of fluid per day, any significant reduction in absorption within the small intestine, due for example to a reduced transit time, will result in an increased fluid content of the faeces. The aim of treating diarrhoea is to enhance intestinal absorption of fluid by reducing the content of intraluminal electrolytes by increasing the active absorption of sodium ions or decreasing the secretion of anions. Alternatively, absorption may be aided by decreasing intestinal motility. In contrast, in constipation the aim is to increase the water content of the faeces thus softening them, and encouraging intestinal motility by increasing the bulk of the intestinal contents and stimulating peristalsis.

SYMPTOMS OF CONSTIPATION

Most patients consider that a daily bowel movement is essential for a healthy life. In reality, normal bowel habits range from several stools daily to the passage of one stool every 2 to 3 days. For this reason, it is unwise to accept the patient's own diagnosis of constipation.

Symptoms associated with constipation include the inability to pass stools at regular intervals, the production of abnormally dry hard stools, straining at stool with or without abdominal pain or discomfort, having a sensation of incomplete evacuation of the bowel and the presence of mild abdominal distension, headache and slight anorexia.

When constipation is chronic or severe, or defaecation is accompanied by a loss of blood and mucus in the stool, or if there is fever and general malaise or anorexia, then constipation is symptomatic of some other underlying cause and further investigation is required.

INVESTIGATIONS

In cases where constipation is considered secondary to another gastrointestinal disorder then sigmoidoscopy, colonoscopy and barium enema should be performed to exclude inflammatory bowel disease and neoplasm of the large bowel. Determination of haemoglobin, white blood cell and platelet counts together with the erythrocyte sedimentation rate is also useful as well as electrolyte data.

Examination of the stool may provide useful information. Small hard pellets may indicate diverticular disease or the irritable bowel syndrome. Melaena is found in ulcerative colitis and haemorrhoids while ribbon-like stools may follow surgery or trauma and are common in patients with irritable bowel syndrome or haemorrhoids.

TREATMENT

Simple constipation is usually relieved by increasing the intake of dietary fibre. Other measures include increasing fluid intake and taking regular exercise. The use of laxatives should generally be avoided except where straining at stool will exacerbate a condition such as angina in the recovery phase following myocardial infarction or increase the risk of rectal bleeding as in haemorrhoids. The use of laxatives in children is undesirable and generally the introduction of fruit purée into the diet is sufficient to avoid constipation. Likewise in infants, an adjustment to the diet is often sufficient to remedy the problem. Laxatives are of value in treating drug-induced constipation and to expel material from the gastrointestinal tract prior to surgery or radiological procedures.

General measures

Most mild forms of constipation may be treated successfully by increasing the amount of high fibre foods in the diet. For example, the intake of fresh or dried fruit and vegetables should be encouraged and white bread should be replaced by wholemeal bread. Peas, beans and nuts are also high in fibre. The fibre acts to bind water and ions in the lumen of the colon, increasing stool bulk and fluid content. The increased volume results in stimulation of peristalsis and increased bowel movements. Since dehydration leads to the production of dry hard faeces, fluid intake should be encouraged to avoid this situation. Regular exercise, which does not need to be too vigorous, should be undertaken, particularly in the elderly and pregnant, since changes in lifestyle resulting in a lack of physical activity are a major cause of constipation.

Laxative drugs

Unfortunately, no perfect laxative is yet available and therefore when a preparation is being recommended the particular needs of the patient must be balanced against the relative risk of being dosed with the laxative agent. The passage of food through the intestine may be speeded up by:

- increasing the volume of non-absorbable solid residue with bulking agents

- using stimulant laxatives which stimulate the gastrointestinal mucosa to initiate peristalsis
- increasing the water content of the gastrointestinal contents with osmotic laxatives
- changing the consistency of the faeces with faecal softeners.

Examples of each class of laxative agent are presented in Table 11.3.

Bulking agents

Bulking agents are polysaccharide and cellulose derivatives which are not degraded by the normal processes of digestion in the upper gastrointestinal tract. They act in a similar manner to dietary roughage increasing the volume of the intestinal contents and prompting peristalsis. These agents are often the laxative of choice if a drug is required to treat simple constipation. They must always be taken with an adequate supply of fluid which causes them to swell substantially in the intestines to form a gel which increases stool bulk, distends the intestines and triggers peristalsis. Since the gel remains hydrated in the colon, soft moist stools are produced. Bulking agents require 12 to 72 hours to

Table 11.3 Some laxative agents	
Class of laxative	Active substance
Bulking agents	Methylcellulose Sterculia Ispaghula husk Bran
Stimulant laxatives	Senna Bisacodyl Sodium picosulphate Danthron Oxyphenisatin
Osmotic laxatives	Magnesium salts Lactulose Phosphates (rectal) Sodium citrate (rectal)
Faecal softeners and lubricants	Docusate sodium (dioctyl sodium sulphosuccinate) Liquid paraffin Arachis oil (enema)

exert their effect and are relatively safe and effective provided adequate fluid is taken. Failure to do so may result in faecal impaction or bowel obstruction, particularly in the elderly. They are a reasonable choice in relatively fit elderly patients, but in some, especially the frail elderly who may have atonic bowels, bulking agents may not be effective and may cause bowel obstruction. Bulking agents may be used in pregnancy and for breast-feeding women because they are not absorbed. They are also useful in patients unable to tolerate dietary roughage. Interestingly, bulking agents are also useful in the treatment of chronic diarrhoea associated with diverticular disease, irritable bowel syndrome and ulcerative colitis as well as being beneficial in the management of patients with ileostomy and colostomy. Examples of bulking agents include methylcellulose, sterculia, ispaghula husk and bran (Table 11.3).

Stimulant laxatives

Stimulant laxatives act directly to stimulate nerve endings in the intestinal wall probably by a local irritant effect. Impulses are then transmitted through the intestinal nerve plexuses resulting in increased smooth muscle activity in the small and large bowels. Onset of action is between 6 and 12 hours and so they may be conveniently administered at night. Since they may induce severe abdominal cramps, excessive fluid loss and electrolyte imbalance they are not the laxative of first choice although they may be considered when bulking agents are ineffective or unsuitable. Stimulant laxatives include senna, bisacodyl, danthron and sodium picosulphate. Other stimulants such as cascara, aloes and phenolphthalein, although no longer recommended, may be present in a number of proprietary laxatives. Senna and cascara contain anthracene derivatives combined with sugars to form glycosides. When taken orally the glycosides pass unchanged to the colon where they are hydrolysed by bacteria, releasing free anthracenes. The free anthracenes are absorbed and stimulate the intestinal nerve plexuses. Phenolphthalein is slightly absorbed and is an example of a drug which undergoes enterohepatic recycling, thus prolonging its action. It colours urine pink or red and has been associated with severe skin reactions, cardiovascular and respiratory collapse. Oxyphenisatin is a stimulant laxative administered rectally which is indicated only for diagnostic procedures or surgery because it causes hepatitis when used chronically.

Osmotic laxatives

Osmotic drugs consist of poorly absorbed solutes such as magnesium salts (saline purgatives) which retain fluid within the lumen of the bowel by an osmotic action. They should be taken on an empty stomach, generally before breakfast. Defaecation occurs in 2 to 4 hours. They act by accelerating the passage of the gastrointestinal contents through the small intestine with the result that an abnormally large volume of material enters the colon causing distension and triggering peristalsis. They should be taken with sufficient fluid to ensure that an isotonic or hypotonic solution is produced. Failure to do so may result in vomiting because hypertonic salt solutions when imbibed cause closure of the pylorus.

Lactulose is a non-absorbable semisynthetic disaccharide composed of fructose and galactose which passes unchanged into the colon where it is degraded by bacterial enzymes to form lactate and other compounds which are only poorly absorbed. Unchanged drug acts as an osmotic laxative while its breakdown products act as stimulants in the large bowel. Lactulose takes about 2 to 3 days to exert its laxative action and has enjoyed wide usage particularly in the elderly. It is safe and effective but offers no clinical advantage over other less expensive alternatives. In contrast, magnesium salts (i.e. hyroxide, sulphate) are inexpensive and useful where rapid bowel evacuation is required. However, in high doses they must be used with caution and their regular use should be avoided. They should not be used in patients with cardiac and renal problems, especially in the elderly since magnesium may be absorbed causing sedation and confusion. Hypertension may be induced if large doses of magnesium salts are taken. Glycerol (glycerin) acts to stimulate a reflex evacuation by a hyperosmotic action on the rectal mucosa. It also has lubricant properties to ease the passage of hardened faecal matter. In the form of suppositories, glycerol is particularly useful in children, the elderly and debilitated patients to promote rapid defaecation. Phosphate enemas are useful for bowel clearance before radiology, endoscopy, surgery, and the acute treatment of severe constipation.

Faecal softeners

Faecal softeners such as docusate sodium (dioctyl sodium sulphosuccinate) reduce the surface tension of hard stools thus acting as a wetting agent in a similar manner to a detergent. Docusate sodium probably also acts as a stimulant laxative. It acts in 2 to 3 days and possesses a mild action. Faecal softeners are useful when defaecation is painful such as in patients with haemorrhoids or anal fissures. They are also useful in the young and elderly, and are recommended for patients who have had a stroke or myocardial infarction and in whom straining at stool might be a hazard. Although once popular, liquid paraffin is no longer recommended because it may interfere with normal digestion and absorption. Liquid paraffin dissolves alpha and beta carotenes, the chief precursors of vitamin A, and prevents their absorption leading to vitamin A deficiency. The absorption of other fat-soluble vitamins (D, E, K) is also prevented. Liquid paraffin may be absorbed causing paraffinomas in mesenteric lymph nodes. It may also cause anal leakage and seepage into the lungs from the oesophagus.

Dosage forms

Whilst most laxatives are taken orally, some agents are administered rectally either as suppositories or enemas. Bisacodyl may be taken orally or administered as a suppository when rapid (15 to 30 minutes) defaecation is required. Bisacodyl suppositories should be avoided in patients with anal fissures or ulcerations since systemic absorption may occur. Other rectally administered laxatives include docusate sodium in an enema dosage form, magnesium sulphate as an enema and glycerol as suppositories. Bulk-forming laxatives may be formulated as tablets to be chewed before swallowing or as granules or powder to be taken in water.

Adverse reactions, contra-indications and warnings

Laxatives are generally safe and sensitivities are uncommon. Chronic use is contra-indicated particularly with the stimulants if laxative abuse is to be avoided. Laxatives are generally contra-indicated in patients with possible intestinal obstruction, appendicitis, intestinal perforation, faecal impaction, abdominal pain of unknown origin, nausea and vomiting. Sodium-containing laxatives should be avoided in patients with congestive cardiac failure, impaired renal function and those on a low sodium diet. Bisacodyl tablets must be swallowed whole to prevent stomach cramps and antacids and milk should be avoided. Preparations such as bulk-forming laxatives which swell when in contact with liquid should always be swallowed in a tumblerful of cold water and should not be taken immediately before retiring to bed. Stimulant laxatives often cause abdominal cramp. They are not generally recommended for use in children. Due to a potential risk of carcinogenicity, danthron is primarily indicated for the treatment of constipation in the elderly, and the prophylaxis and management of analgesic-induced constipation in terminally ill patients of all ages. Danthron must be avoided in pregnancy and breast-feeding mothers. Patients who receive this stimulant laxative should be warned that it may colour urine red.

Laxative abuse

Excessive laxative use may lead to symptoms such as abdominal pain, steatorrhoea, electrolyte loss (sodium and potassium), weakness, nausea, vomiting, diarrhoea and constipation. The elderly are particularly at risk since they often consider that for good health it is essential to pass one stool every day. Many elderly patients use laxatives in an attempt to keep themselves 'regular'. Following prolonged use in which the dose is generally increased, the patient complains of increasing constipation as degeneration of the myenteric plexus of the colon takes place. Treatment of constipation therefore becomes difficult. While replacement of stimulant laxatives with osmotic and then bulking agents may resolve the problem, many patients fail to respond. Electrolyte loss is not uncommon and there may be malabsorption due to the effect of laxatives on the small intestine.

PATIENT EDUCATION

Patients should be advised to focus on the fact that simple constipation is usually relieved by increasing the dietary intake of fibre. Examples of high fibre foods should be provided and the benefits of eating regular meals stated. The importance of an adequate fluid intake should also be stressed. Normally, adults should drink approximately six glasses of fluid per day. The association between constipation and physical activity should be emphasized and patients encouraged to take regular exercise such as walking. Delay of bowel action due to poor toilet facilities or fear of painful defaecation must be avoided. Counselling of the elderly poses a particular problem since atrophy of gastrointestinal smooth muscle and loss of nerve cells may have resulted from the ageing process, causing a delay in transit time and incomplete emptying of the bowels which may be contributing to constipation. The elderly may also find difficulties in coping with a high fibre diet and maintaining a reasonable level of physical activity.

DIARRHOEA

Diarrhoea is associated with an increased frequency of bowel movements with the production of soft or watery stools. This results in fluid and electrolyte loss. It is not a disease but a sign of an underlying problem such as an infection or gastrointestinal disorder.

INCIDENCE

Diarrhoea is a common problem particularly amongst people with poor standards of hygiene. As a direct consequence of dehydration resulting from diarrhoea, there are at least 5 million deaths per annum world-wide, particularly among young children under the age of 5 years. So-called traveller's diarrhoea frequently affects tourists visiting foreign countries with poor sanitation. The elderly and debilitated are also more susceptible to diarrhoea than other individuals.

AETIOLOGY

There are many causes of diarrhoea which may be classified as either simple and self-limiting (acute) or secondary to a more serious disease such as inflammatory bowel disease or diabetes mellitus (Table 11.4).

A number of drugs may also induce diarrhoea (Table 11.5). Infections are probably the commonest cause of diarrhoea, resulting from viral, bacterial or protozoan gastroenteritis. *Escherichia coli*, *Staphylococcus aureus* and *Clostridium* species produce toxins while others, such as *Salmonella* and *Shigella* species, invade the epithelial mucosa of the gastrointestinal tract leading to damage which restricts absorption. *Escherichia coli* is the most common cause of traveller's diarrhoea, the infection usually originating from contami-

Table 11.4 Some common causes of diarrhoea
Viral gastroenteritis
Bacterial gastroenteritis
Protozoan gastroenteritis
Irritable bowel syndrome
Crohn's disease
Ulcerative colitis
Surgery
Uraemia
Neoplasms
Drug withdrawal (opioids, barbiturates)
Endocrine/metabolic diseases (hyperthyroidism, diabetes)

Table 11.5 Drugs which may cause diarrhoea	
Drug group	Examples
Antibiotics	Most broad-spectrum agents
Antacids	Magnesium salts
NSAIDs	Indomethacin, mefenamic acid
Antihypertensives	Methyldopa, guanethidine
Chemotherapeutic agents	Methotrexate
Iron preparations	Ferrous salts
Asthma drugs	Theophylline
Diuretics	Frusemide
Laxative overuse or abuse	

nated food and drink resulting from a lack of adequate hygiene. Food poisoning may occur when frozen products such as turkey and chicken are cooked before being adequately defrosted. Many broad-spectrum antibiotics such as ampicillin, erythromycin and neomycin induce diarrhoea secondary to therapy. The primary cause is the overgrowth of antibiotic-resistant bacteria and fungi in the large bowel which takes place after several days of antibiotic treatment. Such acute episodes of diarrhoea are generally self-limiting. However, the overgrowth of *Clostridium difficile* and the accompanying production of a bacterial toxin may lead to the life-threatening condition, pseudomembranous colitis. Alcohol and caffeine also cause diarrhoea as do magnesium-containing antacids. Diarrhoea is frequently a symptom of drug withdrawal from alcohol, barbiturates, opioids and sedative hypnotics.

SYMPTOMS

Diarrhoea may be acute or chronic depending on the cause. Acute diarrhoea has a sudden onset of frequent, fluid stools usually accompanied by mild abdominal cramping pain, flatulence and general weakness. Nausea and vomiting may also be present. This form of diarrhoea which is usually of the infectious type is self-limiting and resolves within a few days. Chronic diarrhoea generally occurs secondary to some other disorder, for example, ulcerative colitis or thyrotoxicosis. Blood or mucus in the stool is indicative of a more serious medical problem.

INVESTIGATIONS

When diarrhoea is chronic or considered secondary to another disorder then a barium enema and sigmoidoscopy may be carried out to exclude conditions such as inflammatory bowel disease and neoplasm of the large bowel. When an infection is suspected then a stool culture may prove helpful.

TREATMENT

Since diarrhoea results in fluid and electrolyte loss it is important in its treatment to ensure an adequate fluid intake, either as water or in the form of a glucose–electrolyte mixture. This is particularly important when treating infants, children and the elderly. Antidiarrhoeal drugs are of secondary value due to their side effect profiles. However, they may offer benefit to some patients such as travellers.

General measures

Traditionally, food and drink is withheld for 4 to 6 hours followed by fluids only (ideally a glucose–electrolyte mixture) for a further 18 to 24 hours. However, current trends suggest that patients should be able to eat if they wish to without affecting recovery. In children, particularly infants, treatment is essentially the same. The frequent ingestion of small amounts of easily digested foods for 1 or 2 days is sensible advice. Food and drink containing milk are best avoided because in some patients a temporary disaccharidase deficiency in the inflamed bowel may result in lactose being neither digested nor absorbed leading to an osmotic diarrhoea, exacerbating the situation. Milk should not be withheld from infants (see Chapter 7). Fruits and green vegetables should also be avoided until symptoms subside. Since infection is the most likely cause of acute onset diarrhoea, normal hygienic measures should be employed to avoid the spread of infection to others.

Glucose–electrolyte mixtures

The oral rehydration solution recommended for

use in the treatment of diarrhoea by the World Health Organization is given in Table 11.6. It contains glucose, sodium, potassium, chloride and bicarbonate to give an almost isotonic solution. A number of similar mixtures are available commercially in the form of sachets which require reconstitution in clean water before use. Glucose concentrations between 80 and 120 mmol/L are needed to optimize sodium absorption in the small intestine. Glucose concentrations in excess of 160 mmol/L will cause an osmotic gradient leading to increased fluid and electrolyte loss. High sodium solutions in excess of 90 mmol/L may lead to hypernatraemia, especially in children, and should be avoided. While the WHO oral rehydration solution contains 90 mmol/L sodium, commercially available solutions in general contain no more than half this sodium concentration to reduce the risk of hypernatraemia. The presence of potassium prevents hypokalaemia occurring in the elderly especially in those taking diuretics. Replacement of potassium will also protect patients receiving digoxin from hypokalaemia-induced toxicity. For healthy adults, a satisfactory substitute for a rehydration sachet would be one level teaspoonful of table salt plus a tablespoon of sugar in a litre of drinking water or 4.5% glucose in half normal saline. The volume of oral solution to be taken in treating mild to moderate diarrhoea is dependent on age. Adults will require about 400 ml for every loose motion whereas children will require only 100 ml and infants 50 ml. The solution is best sipped every 5 to 10 minutes rather than drunk in large amounts less frequently. In severe diarrhoea where there are clinical signs of dehydration, patients should be admitted to hospital and administered electrolyte solution intravenously with both hydration status and electrolyte balance being closely monitored.

Drug treatment

For acute diarrhoea, the use of antidiarrhoeal drugs is unnecessary. Drug therapy is not generally recommended for children under the age of 12 years for whom rehydration sachets are the most satisfactory form of treatment. Antimotility drugs such as diphenoxylate and loperamide have a limited role in the treatment of diarrhoea. By slowing transit time, they help to reduce the amount of fluid passing into the colon. This results in increased water and electrolyte absorption throughout the gastrointestinal tract. However, these drugs may delay the clearance of infecting organisms and prolong the symptoms. For these reasons, they should be avoided unless required to decrease the inconvenience of frequent stool motions for social reasons and for travellers. They may be used with caution in patients suffering from chronic diarrhoea as a result of ulcerative colitis to prevent megacolon. Adsorbents such as kaolin which are considered to adsorb fluid and add bulk to the stool are no longer recommended for acute diarrhoea although they may provide some relief in mild chronic diarrhoea. Bulk-forming drugs used in the treatment of constipation, such as methylcellulose and sterculia, if taken with a relatively small volume of water are of use in controlling faecal consistency in ileostomy and colostomy, and in the control of chronic diarrhoea associated with diverticular disease. Antibiotics are generally unnecessary in simple gastroenteritis in which the symptoms are mild and self-limiting, the cause often being a viral infection. In contrast, systemic bacterial infections require antibiotic treatment. Bacterial infections caused by specific organisms such as *Campylobacter enteritis* may require erythromycin or ciprofloxacin while salmonella- and shigella-induced infectious diarrhoea are sometimes responsive to ciprofloxacin. The place of ampicillin and co-

Table 11.6 The World Health Organization's recommended oral rehydration solution for use in the treatment of diarrhoea (NB to be made up in clean water)		
Ingredient	Concentration	Ingredient in 1.0 L water
Glucose	111 mmol/L	20 g (glucose)
Sodium	90 mmol/L	3.5 g (NaCl)
Potassium	20 mmol/L	1.5 g (KCl)
Chloride	80 mmol/L	—
Bicarbonate	30 mmol/L	2.5 g (NaHCO$_3$)

trimoxazole in the clinical management of these disorders is largely unresolved (see Chapter 35).

Diphenoxylate

This is a synthetic opioid which is available in combination with a subclinical dose of atropine (Lomotil) to reduce the risk of abuse. It is readily absorbed after oral dosing and may produce systemic effects such as respiratory depression. Young children are particularly susceptible to overdosage (as few as 10 Lomotil tablets may be fatal) and symptoms may be delayed so that careful monitoring is required for at least 48 hours after dosing. Since diphenoxylate has no pharmacological effect on anal sphincter tone, some leakage may occur.

Loperamide

This is also a synthetic opioid which is slowly and incompletely absorbed after oral administration. It is slow to cross the blood–brain barrier and possesses little opioid activity at normal doses. In consequence, loperamide has little effect on the central nervous system. Anal sphincter tone is increased which may be useful in incontinent patients. Side effects include abdominal cramps and occasionally skin reactions including urticaria.

Codeine phosphate

The constipating side effect of the narcotic analgesic, codeine phosphate, may be used to treat diarrhoea. Although effective, tolerance and dependence may occur which limit its use in diarrhoea. Codeine phosphate is contained in some proprietary antidiarrhoeal preparations.

Morphine

Morphine possesses some gastrointestinal sedative activity. However, dependence and the associated problem of abuse with mixtures such as kaolin and morphine limit its usefulness. Hypokalaemia may also occur on prolonged use

due to an aldosterone-like constituent present in the liquorice extract used in the preparation of this mixture.

FOOD POISONING/ GASTROENTERITIS

Food poisoning generally occurs in small outbreaks and simultaneously in several patients. It presents with vomiting and/or diarrhoea and may be accompanied by fever. The causes of food poisoning are presented in Table 11.7. Non-infective causes and bacterial toxins which are preformed in the contaminated food produce symptoms rapidly after ingestion. Other infections may not result in the symptoms of food poisoning for up to 48 hours. The commonest bacterial cause of food poisoning in the United Kingdom is *Campylobacter jejuni*. Sources of infection include poultry, dogs, water and unpasteurized milk. Salmonellae are also common causes of food poisoning, the domestic fowl being the commonest source of infection. Food poisoning may result from eating inadequately defrosted and undercooked chicken or from raw or undercooked eggs. Acute staphylococcal food poisoning resulting from the toxin of *Staphylococcus aureus* frequently originates from a food

Table 11.7 Some causes of food poisoning
Infective
Non-toxin mediated
Viruses
Salmonella species
Bacillus cereus
Campylobacter jejuni
Listeria monocytogenes
Protozoa (*Giardia, Cryptosporidium*)
Toxin mediated
Staphylococcus aureus
Clostridium perfringens
Clostridium botulinum
Escherichia coli
Non-infective
Allergic
Shellfish
Strawberries
Non-allergic
Mushrooms
Scombrotoxin

handler with a septic lesion on the hand. If the contaminated food is allowed to stand at room temperature then growth of the organisms take place with the production of toxin. This may not be destroyed by cooking since it is relatively heat resistant. Likewise, many strains of clostridia which may contaminate meat are relatively heat stable. Precooking of stews and meat pies may fail to destroy all the spores which multiply on storage at room temperature causing gastro-enteritis. In general, the onset of symptoms is a guide to the cause of food poisoning. Onset of vomiting within 30 minutes of ingestion is likely to be due to a chemical poison. Vomiting within 2 to 6 hours usually with diarrhoea and abdominal pain later is probably due to staphylococcal or bacillus toxin. Salmonellae and campylobacter infections produce symptoms of vomiting, abdominal pain, fever and diarrhoea within 12 to 48 hours of ingesting contaminated food.

TRAVELLER'S DIARRHOEA

Tourists visiting countries with warm climates and poor sanitation frequently experience acute diarrhoea which is self-limiting and subsides within 24 to 48 hours. Action to avoid traveller's diarrhoea includes not drinking tap water or iced drinks, avoidance of salads and uncooked foods. Fruits and vegetables should be peeled or washed with boiled or bottled water. Persistence of symptoms on returning home may indicate the presence of dysentery, cholera, giardiasis or food poisoning.

PSEUDOMEMBRANOUS COLITIS

Following antibiotic therapy, the colon may become colonized with *Clostridium difficile* leading to severe diarrhoea as a result of the normal colonic flora being altered or suppressed. Characteristically, the rectum and colon show a membrane of fibrin and polymorphs which adheres to eroded mucosa. Whilst few antibiotics are free of this side effect, clindamycin, lincomycin and cephalosporins are a particular problem. Treatment consists of stopping the offending antibiotic and giving oral vancomycin or metronidazole.

CONCLUSIONS

Simple constipation and diarrhoea are usually self-limiting and may be controlled with minimal therapeutic intervention. However, it is important to confirm that the condition is not secondary to other more serious disorders such as constipation resulting from diverticular disease, Hirschsprung's disease, myxoedema, depression or hypercalcaemia. Treatment of simple constipation with laxatives is unnecessary and should generally be avoided except where straining at stool will exacerbate an underlying condition or increase the risk of rectal bleeding which may occur if haemorrhoids are present. Laxatives are useful in drug-induced constipation and in bowel evacuation before radiological procedures or surgery. The preferred method of resolving simple constipation is to educate the patient in the need to increase dietary fibre and fluid intake. This is usually sufficient and avoids the problem of possible laxative abuse which may lead to hypokalaemia and an atonic non-functioning large bowel.

Likewise, if diarrhoea is acute and not secondary to disorders such as carcinoma of the alimentary tract, ulcerative colitis, Crohn's disease, metabolic disorders (diabetes mellitus, thyrotoxicosis) or iatrogenic disease, then the first line of treatment is oral rehydration therapy to prevent or treat any fluid and electrolyte depletion. This is particularly important in children and the elderly. Antidiarrhoeal agents are of secondary importance although useful for travellers. In the case of systemic bacterial infections, clearly these require appropriate systemic treatment depending on the infecting organism.

CASE STUDIES

CASE 11.1

A 56-year-old lady complains of constipation. She normally has daily bowel movements but in the past 7 days she has passed only one stool. This was hard and difficult to pass but was free of blood or mucus. She does not complain of nausea, vomiting, abdominal pain or cramps. Since the death of her husband 4 months previously she has become introverted. A friendly neighbour runs errands and shops once a week on her behalf. She rarely cooks meals and survives on little more than snacks.

Q What factors may be contributing to the constipation?

CASE 11.2

A 76-year-old male requests a laxative. He comments that his stools appear normal but their passage has become irregular and infrequent. He has suffered from hypertension for a number of years and takes nifedipine retard 20 mg twice daily. 6 months ago he was prescribed Dytide (triamterene 50 mg; benzthiazide 25 mg), one to be taken on alternate days for oedema. He is a frequent taker of aluminium hydroxide gel for indigestion. He was recently troubled by moderately severe arthritic pain for which he was prescribed dihydrocodeine, one tablet every 4 to 6 hours.

Q What factors may be contributing to the constipation?

CASE 11.3

Mrs M. S. is suffering from severe chronic constipation. About 3 months ago she was found to have small-cell lung cancer and is undergoing palliative radiotherapy. For the past month she has been experiencing shortness of breath and severe pain in her chest. The pain is being controlled with 100 mg MST Continus taken orally every 12 hours.

Q What advice would you give on treating Mrs M. S.'s constipation?

CASE 11.4

Mrs A. T. is 8 months' pregnant and following a normal healthy pregnancy now complains of constipation. She also complains of external haemorrhoids which are painful. She has avoided taking any medicines apart from prescribed vitamins during her pregnancy but now considers that medication is necessary to relieve her constipation.

Q What advice would you give?

CASE 11.5

Mr D. M. is a 26-year-old comprehensive-school teacher who was admitted to hospital 2 days ago with an acute exacerbation of ulcerative colitis. His symptoms included rectal bleeding, pyrexia, weight loss and severe diarrhoea. He immediately received 200 mg hydrocortisone intravenously and is now being prescribed 40 mg prednisolone taken orally. Although showing some signs of improvement, the diarrhoea remains a problem.

Q What advice would you give concerning the treatment of Mr D. M.'s diarrhoea?

ANSWERS TO CASE STUDIES

CASE 11.1

A Psychological stress or alterations in daily routine are frequent causes of constipation and are doubtless contributing to the patient's problem following the death of her husband. The lack of exercise and a diet almost certainly low in fibre will contribute to constipation. Although not receiving treatment for depressive illness, both the disease and drugs such as tricyclic antidepressants used in its treatment, induce constipation. The patient does not appear to have constipation secondary to a more serious complaint, although investigations for thyroid function should be considered since hypothyroidism may cause symptoms such as tiredness, lethargy and constipation. In the absence of organic disease, it is probable that constipation can be resolved by patient counselling. The patient would benefit from advice on increasing the amount of fibre in her diet, and supplementing it with plenty of fruit and vegetables, preferably uncooked. She should also be encouraged to eat at regular times. Since a decreased fluid intake commonly contributes to constipation, the need to drink reasonable quantities of fluids should be emphasized. Likewise, the importance of regular exercise could be stressed. Since the use of a laxative is not contra-indicated in simple constipation, a short course of a stimulant laxative would be appropriate where a quick response is required.

CASE 11.2

A Drug therapy is frequently associated with constipation and should always be considered as the possible cause of this complaint. The patient is hypertensive and a number of antihypertensives are known to induce constipation as a side effect. These include clonidine, verapamil. diltiazem, and nifedipine. Diuretics likewise may cause constipation. However, the patient has been taking nifedipine retard and Dytide for at least 6 months and it is unlikely that either of these drugs has caused the present acute episode. Various inorganic ions such as iron, calcium and aluminium possess constipating properties while magnesium ions induce diarrhoea. For this reason, the patient would be better advised to replace aluminium hydroxide with a magnesium-containing antacid when requiring to treat his indigestion. The most likely cause of the constipation is dihydrocodeine. In common with other opioid analgesics, dihydrocodeine has a powerful constipating effect particularly on chronic use. This drug should be withdrawn and attempts made to control the pain with a non-opioid analgesic such as paracetamol (1.0 g) four times a day. While ibuprofen's anti-inflammatory action might be useful, the risk of treatment in an elderly patient already experiencing indigestion and hypertension may outweigh any potential benefits.

CASE 11.3

A Severe cancer pain may require treatment with an opioid analgesic. Morphine is particularly useful being given by mouth regularly every 4 hours. An alternative is dosing with a modified-release tablet of morphine such as MST Continus which has the advantage of requiring only twice-daily administration. The starting dose of these tablets is usually in the order of 20 mg every 12 hours with the dose being increased if breakthrough pain occurs. In patients with terminal illness the dose may be increased to 90 to 150 mg or higher if necessary. Unfortunately, a common side effect of morphine is constipation due to its pharmacological action of inhibiting gastrointestinal motility thus increasing transit time. The administration of a stimulant laxative such as co-danthrusate, 1 to 3 capsules usually at bedtime, should be beneficial. Danthron derivatives are particularly recommended in the prophylaxis and treatment of analgesic-induced constipation in terminally ill patients of all ages. They act within 6 to 12 hours and, due to rodent studies in which danthron was found to be potentially carcinogenic, the indications for its use are limited to use in the terminally ill, constipation in geriatric patients and constipation in cardiac failure and coronary thrombosis where bowel movements must be free of strain.

CASE 11.4

A Constipation frequently occurs during pregnancy. This is not unexpected since high circulating levels of progesterone decrease smooth muscle tone in the large bowel and the pressure of the uterus delays or inhibits bowel emptying. They may likewise inhibit contraction of abdominal muscles and the diaphragm. The patient has haemorrhoids which commonly occur in pregnancy. These may be painful and result in a voluntary suppression of the urge to defaecate. This overriding of the reflex involved in the process of defaecation is another cause of constipation. In the case of pregnant women, an agent which is not absorbed or possesses no stimulant activity would be useful. The regular use of lactulose, an osmotic laxative which acts to retain fluid in the lumen of the bowel, thus increasing faecal bulk, is both safe and effective in providing relief from constipation within 2 to 3 days of dosing. Bulking agents may also be safely used even during the early stages of pregnancy. However, the bulking effect is less likely to find favour in females who are heavily pregnant. Both lactulose and bulk laxatives may be continued postpartum. A number of other laxatives are secreted in breast milk and may cause diarrhoea in breast-fed offspring. This is particularly the case with anthraquinones.

CASE 11.5

A Whilst it is true that antidiarrhoeal drugs such as diphenoxylate and loperamide are effective in controlling diarrhoea associated with ulcerative colitis, there is a substantial risk that these drugs may precipitate paralytic ileus and megacolon. It is therefore unwise to administer diphenoxylate or loperamide in order to treat diarrhoea in patients with severe ulcerative colitis, although they may have a limited value in the mild disease. Antispasmodic agents should not be used to treat ulcerative colitis. The recommended treatment of severe ulcerative colitis is based on the so-called 5-day regimen. For this period, no food or fluid is permitted (nil by mouth); fluid, electrolytes and blood are administered parenterally as required. Drug therapy consists of intravenous hydrocortisone (200 to 400 mg) on the first day of treatment followed by 40 mg prednisolone orally reducing to nil over the next 3 to 4 weeks. Nurses should be advised that it is acceptable to give oral prednisolone despite the nil-by-mouth restriction. As soon as practical, prednisolone retention enemas or foam preparations should be administered rectally. Finally, sulphasalazine or the newer alternatives, mesalazine and olsalazine, are administered orally for long-term maintenance therapy.

BIBLIOGRAPHY

Brunton L L. Agents affecting gastrointestinal water flux and motility, digestants and bile acids. In: Gillman A G, Roll T W, Nies A S, Taylor P (eds) The pharmacological basis of therapeutics. New York: Pergamon 1990; 914–932

Edwards C. OTC treatment of constipation and diarrhoea. Pharmaceutical Journal 1988; 241: 46–49

Livingstone C, and Livingstone D. Diarrhoea in a diabetic patient. Pharmaceutical Journal 1991; 247: 628–629

Read N W. Constipation. Medicine International 1990; 79: 3259–3263

Shearman D J C, Crean G P. Diseases of the alimentary tract and pancreas. In: Edwards C R W, Bouchier I A D (eds) Davidson's Principles and practice of medicine. Edinburgh: Churchill Livingstone 1991; 417–486

Turnberg L A. Diarrhoea. Medicine International 1990; 79: 3256–3258

Wynne H, Edwards C. Which drug? Laxatives. Pharmaceutical Journal 1992; 248: 17–19

Chapter 12

Adverse effects of drugs on the liver

C. M. Way

The adverse effects of drugs on the liver may mimic almost any naturally occurring liver disease. Drug therapy should therefore always be considered as a cause of liver disease.

EPIDEMIOLOGY

The overall incidence of drug-induced liver disease varies from 2 to 5% of jaundiced hospital inpatients and up to 25% of fulminant hepatic failure cases in the USA. Abnormal liver function tests are seen commonly in patients commenced on certain drugs, but only in a minority of cases does significant hepatic injury follow.

The potential for adverse drug reactions in the liver is increased in patients with pre-existing liver disease, particularly cirrhosis, who are less able to metabolize drugs. The incidence of jaundice is higher in patients taking psychoactive or antituberculous drugs. In general the middle-aged and elderly are more likely to suffer from drug-induced hepatic injury than the young. Females are more susceptible than males. A middle-aged or elderly female presenting with symptoms of viral hepatitis, with no history of contact with viral infection, is particularly likely to be affected.

Some genetic differences in ability to synthesize enzymes may predispose certain individuals to drug-induced liver disease. In Japanese patients it was found that fast acetylators of isoniazid were more susceptible to isoniazid-induced liver damage than slow acetylators.

However, a higher incidence of isoniazid-induced liver damage was found in slow acetylators than in fast acetylators in a study of South Indian patients. Susceptibility to halothane-induced hepatitis may run in families. Such genetic defects may account for those hepatic reactions occurring only in a small number of people given a particular drug.

AETIOLOGY

Drug-induced liver disease may be acute or chronic. Hepatotoxicity can be classed as cytotoxic or cholestatic damage. Cytotoxic damage can be further subdivided into necrosis and steatosis (fatty liver). Some drugs cause a mixed cytotoxic and cholestatic injury.

Hepatic necrosis caused by paracetamol overdosage occurs because the normal metabolic pathway for paracetamol becomes saturated and the drug is metabolized via an abnormal pathway which results in the production of a toxic metabolite which covalently binds to liver cell proteins causing necrosis.

Tetracyclines are thought to cause steatosis by interfering with the synthesis of lipoproteins which normally remove triglycerides from the liver.

Cholestasis caused by anabolic and contraceptive steroids is due to inhibition of bilirubin excretion from the hepatocyte into bile. Rifampicin causes hyperbilirubinaemia by inhibiting uptake of bilirubin by the hepatocyte, as well as inhibiting bilirubin excretion into bile.

The mechanisms of drug-induced hepatic injury can be divided into two types, intrinsic and idiosyncratic hepatotoxicity.

In intrinsic hepatotoxicity the same injury always occurs, is dose dependent, occurs in everyone and can be reproduced in experimental animals.

Idiosyncratic hepatotoxicity produces variable injury, is not dose related, occurs rarely and is not reproducible in experimental animals. This type of hepatotoxicity may be due to either hypersensitivity or metabolic abnormality.

PATHOPHYSIOLOGY

In hepatic necrosis there is jaundice, modestly increased alkaline phosphatase values and markedly raised transaminases, up to 200 times the upper limit of normal. The prothrombin time also increases rapidly. Necrosis of hepatocytes can be seen on microscopy.

Steatosis caused by drugs such as tetracyclines is associated with moderately raised bilirubin and transaminase levels. Blood glucose may be low and blood ammonia levels high. Histologically, liver damage is similar to acute fatty liver of pregnancy. Small fat droplets are visible in liver cells.

In hepatic phospholipidosis such as that caused by amiodarone, raised serum transaminases may be the only biochemical abnormality. Histology is similar to that seen in acute alcoholic hepatitis, and cirrhosis can develop.

In fibrosis, serum transaminases may only be transiently raised and are not good predictors of hepatic damage. Microscopy shows deposition of fibrous tissue. Fibrosis may progress to cirrhosis. Such damage is seen with long-term methotrexate use.

Acute hepatitis occurs only in a small proportion of patients taking a particular drug. Such reactions are not dose dependent and are idiosyncratic. The reaction appears about a week after commencing drug therapy with agents such as isoniazid and is similar to viral hepatitis. Hepatocellular damage is indicated by raised transaminases.

Chronic active hepatitis may present as acute hepatocellular injury or progress to cirrhosis. Serum transaminases are usually raised and serum albumin low. Histology resembles that of autoimmune chronic active hepatitis. This type of damage can occur after many years of therapy with methyldopa, for example.

Hypersensitivity reactions occur 1 to 5 weeks after commencing drug therapy, are accompanied by eosinophilia and reappear in response to rechallenge with drugs. Examples of drugs causing such reactions are dantrolene and carbimazole.

Canalicular cholestasis is associated with a raised bilirubin and moderately raised alkaline phosphatase, usually no more than three times the upper limit of normal. Transaminases are rarely raised and no hepatocyte damage is seen.

Hepatocanalicular cholestasis is usually associated with alkaline phosphatase levels greater than three times the upper limit of normal. Serum bilirubin is raised and transaminases may be too. Microscopy shows a certain amount of liver damage as well as cholestasis.

CLINICAL MANIFESTATIONS

The signs and symptoms of drug-induced hepatotoxicity vary widely, depending on the type of liver damage caused.

In hepatocellular necrosis due to paracetamol overdosage, the patient initially suffers from malaise, nausea and vomiting, but remains conscious and within 48 hours appears to be recovering. Deterioration follows with jaundice and a tender, enlarged liver. Signs of other organ damage, including renal failure, may appear. Death may result from the complications of liver failure.

A patient presenting with steatosis shows fatigue, vomiting, jaundice, hypoglycaemia and disturbed consciousness.

In acute hepatitis the patient first experiences gastrointestinal symptoms followed by jaundice, pale stools, dark urine and an enlarged, tender liver. This type of reaction is normally severe. Death often occurs, particularly if the aetiology is unrecognized and the causative drug continued after liver damage has begun. Many drugs cause this type of reaction.

Drug-induced chronic active hepatitis presents in a similar manner to viral or autoimmune chronic active hepatitis. Jaundice usually occurs and symptoms of portal hypertension such as ascites and bleeding oesophageal varices appear as the disease progresses. Such injury has occurred after many years of drug treatment.

Many drugs can cause general hypersensitivity reactions of varying severity. Jaundice may occur with rash and fever.

Pure cholestasis due to interference with bile flow, without damage to liver cells, may be caused by anabolic and contraceptive steroids. Susceptible patients develop anorexia, malaise, nausea, pruritus and jaundice usually within the first month of treatment. The reaction is particularly prevalent in women with a history of cholestasis of pregnancy.

Drug-induced cholestatic hepatitis is similar in presentation to extrahepatic obstructive jaundice. Jaundice is often preceded by fever, pruritus, abdominal pain, anorexia and nausea.

INVESTIGATIONS

Various types of investigation are used in the diagnosis of drug-induced hepatotoxicity. Liver function tests (LFTs) are measured; these include serum bilirubin, transaminases, alkaline phosphatase, gamma-glutamyl transferase and albumin.

Bilirubin is transported to the liver in the unconjugated form, where it is conjugated with glucuronide and excreted in the bile. Drugs that damage liver cells reduce the organ's capacity to conjugate bilirubin leading to a raised serum level, which is visible as jaundice. In cholestasis there is obstruction to bile flow, which is usually intrahepatic in drug-induced injury. Conjugated bilirubin then appears in the blood in very high concentrations.

Aspartate transaminase (AST) and alanine transaminase (ALT) are normally present in liver cells and the highest levels are found in acute liver damage, such as that caused by hepatotoxic drugs.

The highest serum levels of alkaline phosphatase are seen in cholestasis.

Like alkaline phosphatase, gamma-glutamyl transpeptidase (gamma-GT) is most markedly raised in cholestasis. It may also be induced by therapy with anticonvulsants, rifampicin and other drugs. Such changes do not necessarily indicate hepatic damage. Levels return to normal on stopping treatment.

Prothrombin is a vitamin K dependent clotting factor. A prolonged prothrombin time may be caused by vitamin K deficiency as occurs in fat malabsorption due to cholestasis. Alternatively it may be due to severe liver cell damage, when the cells are unable to synthesize prothrombin.

A viral screen is normally performed on patients with symptoms of hepatitis to exclude an infective cause.

Radiological investigations such as ultrasound scans, percutaneous cholangiograms (PTCs) and endoscopic retrograde cholangiopancreatography (ERCP) are used to look for physical obstruction of bile ducts by gallstones, masses or strictures.

Liver biopsy and histological evaluation is useful in the diagnosis of acute hepatocellular dysfunction, which may be drug induced. Certain drugs cause characteristic lesions: microvesicular fat with tetracyclines; hepatic phospholipidosis with amiodarone for example.

TREATMENT

The goal in treating drug-induced hepatotoxicity is complete recovery. In order for this to be achieved the aetiology has to be recognized and the causative agent stopped. The importance of identifying the drug causing the adverse reaction cannot be stressed too highly. Adverse hepatic drug reactions will be made very much worse if the treatment is continued after symptoms appear or transaminases rise. Failure to recognize iatrogenic hepatotoxicity and discontinue treatment could give grounds for negligence claims. Although hepatic drug reactions are uncommon, the possibility of a drug-induced cause should be considered in any patient presenting with liver disease. As recovery normally follows discontinuation of a hepatotoxic drug, the single most important step in treating drug-induced hepatotoxicity is to stop the drug.

Supportive treatment is necessary in liver failure. Symptomatic treatment may be necessary after drug withdrawal, as recovery may be prolonged.

Treatment of the condition for which the offending drug was originally prescribed needs to be considered. In many cases this will still require drug therapy. For example a diabetic patient who develops hepatocanalicular cholestasis on chlorpropamide will still require treatment for diabetes and a safe alternative must be found. Care is necessary in choosing treatment to ensure any further adverse reaction is avoided.

Hepatocellular damage due to drugs will leave the patient's ability to handle other drugs impaired, as the liver is the body's main site of drug metabolism. This puts the patient at greater risk of developing further liver damage. The same care in choosing drug therapy for a patient with drug-induced hepatotoxicity will be required as in a patient with liver disease of any other aetiology. The type of liver damage needs

to be considered. Problems are most likely to occur in severe liver disease such as cirrhosis or in patients with jaundice, ascites or hepatic encephalopathy.

Withdrawal of drug

Once drug-induced hepatotoxicity is recognized and the offending drug withdrawn, recovery usually follows. Generally the causative drug should be avoided in future. In some cases caused by drug overdose specific therapies are available, but management is normally supportive. Symptomatic treatments are used for problems such as pruritus associated with jaundice. Ideally drug-induced hepatotoxicity should be avoided by careful drug use.

The first step in treating drug-induced liver disease is to recognize that the damage is indeed due to drug treatment. It is important to exclude other causes of liver disease by taking a clinical history and from the results of investigations. A comprehensive and accurate drug history is vital in patients with suspected iatrogenic hepatotoxicity. The history should include all drugs taken during the past 3 months, with details of dose, route and duration of treatment. The history should include specific questions about the use of over-the-counter (OTC) medication, herbal remedies, oral contraceptives and illicit drugs. Hepatic adverse drug reactions rarely occur more than 3 months after initiation of therapy.

The pharmacist should be familiar with drugs which are intrinsically hepatotoxic, the type of damage the drug produces, which patients are likely to be susceptible, and in what circumstances hepatotoxicity usually occurs. Paracetamol is an example of an intrinsic hepatotoxin (see Table 12.1). Toxicity from intrinsic hepatotoxins is dose related and may be avoided by ensuring that the doses listed in Table 12.1 are not exceeded.

Idiosyncratic drug reactions should also be considered and the literature consulted to match drug therapy with the type of hepatotoxicity seen. Table 12.2 lists some of the drugs commonly associated with the different types of liver damage.

If a drug is suspected of causing hepatic

Table 12.1   Intrinsic hepatotoxins

Drug	Toxic dosage
Anabolic steroids	High dose, > 1 month
Contraceptive steroids	High dose
Iron	Overdosage > 1 g
6-mercaptopurine	Dose > 2.5 mg/kg
Methotrexate	Cumulative dose > 2 g
Paracetamol	Overdosage > 10 g
Salicylates	Chronic use > 2 g/day
Tetracyclines	Dose > 1 g/day i.v.
	Dose > 2 g/day oral
Vitamin A	40 000 i.u./day for months

Table 12.2   Adverse drug reactions

Adverse reaction	Causative drugs
Hepatocellular necrosis	Paracetamol Salicylates Iron salts
Microvesicular fat	Sodium valproate Tetracyclines
Hepatic phospholipidosis	Amiodarone
Fibrosis	Methotrexate
Acute hepatitis	Isoniazid Methyldopa Halothane
Chronic active hepatitis	Methyldopa Nitrofurantoin Isoniazid
General hypersensitivity	Sulphonamides Phenytoin Dantrolene NSAIDs Carbimazole Diltiazem Carbamazepine Quinidine
Canalicular cholestasis	Contraceptive Anabolic steroids
Hepatocanalicular cholestasis	Chlorpromazine Erythromycin Nitrofurantoin Oral hypoglycaemics Imipramine Cimetidine Ranitidine

damage it should be stopped. If a patient is taking more than one potentially hepatotoxic drug, they all should be stopped. LFTs should be monitored following withdrawal. A return to normal levels lends support to a drug-induced cause. However, with some drugs such as the phenothiazines, LFTs may take many months to return to normal.

Rechallenge with a drug suspected of causing hepatotoxicity should normally be avoided. Although administering a challenge dose of a drug thought to be responsible for hepatic injury may help support the diagnosis, lack of response does not rule it out. Only half of patients show recurrence of the injury after a challenge dose and some drugs need to be given for up to 12 weeks to produce a recurrence. It is dangerous to give a challenge dose of a drug that causes hepatocellular injury as it may precipitate a severe reaction. It is safer to challenge if the drug induces cholestasis alone. In the majority of cases challenge is ethically difficult to justify. If there is no alternative, diagnostic challenge should be delayed until liver function tests have returned to normal following a reaction. The procedure should be carried out under inpatient supervision starting with subtherapeutic doses of the suspect drug. If a patient inadvertently receives treatment with a drug which has previously caused liver damage, particular attention should be paid to the outcome and to the effects of drug withdrawal.

Paracetamol overdosage is one of the few conditions where specific treatment is available. As little as 10 to 15 g may cause severe hepatocellular necrosis. If a patient presents within 4 hours of ingestion, the stomach should be emptied to prevent further absorption. A plasma paracetamol level is measured at least 4 hours after ingestion and this is plotted on a semilogarithmic graph of levels against time (see Fig. 12.1). If the level is greater than a reference line joining plots of 200 mg/L at 4 hours and 30 mg/L at 15 hours the patient is treated with intravenous acetylcysteine or oral methionine. These compounds are precursors of glutathione which conjugates paracetamol metabolites produced by normal metabolism. The aim of therapy is to replenish glutathione reserves in the liver thus preventing the formation of toxic paracetamol metabolites.

Iron overdosage is commonest in children and can lead to hepatic necrosis. The specific treatment is desferrioxamine, which chelates iron. After

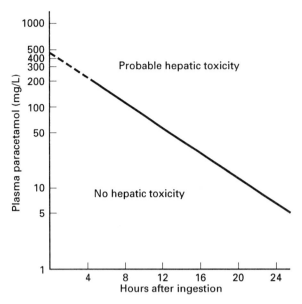

Fig. 12.1 Semilogarithmic plot of plasma paracetamol levels vs time. (Adapted from Rumack B H, Matthew H. Acetaminophen poisoning and toxicity. Pediatrics 1975; 871: 55.)

emptying the stomach by inducing vomiting, gastric lavage is performed and a solution of 10 g of desferrioxamine in 50 ml of water is left in the stomach. The serum iron concentration is then measured and parenteral desferrioxamine administered to chelate absorbed iron.

Pruritus occurs in jaundiced patients due to high systemic concentrations of bile acids which are deposited in tissues. Cholestyramine, an anionic exchange resin, is used in partial biliary obstruction to reduce bile acid concentrations by binding bile salts in the intestine and increasing faecal excretion. The starting dose should be one sachet daily, taken before breakfast so the arrival of the drug in the duodenum coincides with gall-bladder contraction and maximal duodenal bile acid concentration associated with food intake. An effect should be seen within 4 to 7 days. If necessary the dose can be increased to two sachets a day after 1 week, the second sachet being given before the midday or evening meal. The contents of a sachet are mixed with water or other drink immediately before taking. Cholestyramine is unpleasant to take, can cause nausea and constipation, and binds drugs as well as bile salts. Other drug therapy therefore

needs to be given at least 1 hour before or 4 to 6 hours after cholestyramine. Colestipol may be used as an alternative.

Anionic exchange resins are ineffective in complete biliary obstruction so alternative therapy needs to be considered. Antihistamines may be effective due to their sedative effect, for example chlorpheniramine 4 mg four times a day. Non-sedating antihistamines such as terfenadine 60 mg twice daily may also be effective. Rifampicin and anabolic steroids are normally reserved for the treatment of intractable pruritus. Topical measures such as aqueous cream, oilatum emollient or phenolated oily calamine lotion are also of use.

Patients with cholestasis or hepatocellular damage may have an increased prothrombin time. Vitamin K is given in an endeavour to correct this and reduce the risk of haemorrhage. Phytomenadione injection, 10 mg, is given daily intramuscularly or intravenously. When given by the intravenous route it must be given slowly over 10 minutes to avoid anaphylactoid reactions to the polyethoxylated castor oil included in the formulation as a surfactant. Parenteral vitamin K will correct prothrombin times in 5 days if the problem is due to deficiency, but will be unsuccessful if a prolonged prothrombin time is caused by hepatocellular damage. Oral phytomenadione is ineffective in cholestasis due to malabsorption of fat-soluble vitamins. Menadiol sodium phosphate, a water-soluble vitamin K analogue, may be effective in an oral dose of 10 mg daily.

Having identified drug-induced hepatotoxicity and stopped therapy, advice may be needed on alternative treatment. Drugs with similar chemical structures often cause similar hepatotoxicity.

Cholestatic hepatitis has been reported with chlorpromazine and other phenothiazines. As there is likely to be cross-sensitivity between them it is best to avoid any phenothiazine in a patient who develops jaundice with chlorpromazine.

Isoniazid, pyrazinamide and ethionamide are chemically related and all should be avoided if an adverse reaction to one occurs. Cross-hepato-toxicity has been reported between tricyclic antidepressants, and also between phenelzine and chemically related monoamine oxidase inhibitors.

Chlorpropamide and other sulphonylureas

cause cholestatic hepatitis. However, it has been reported that a patient who developed liver damage with both chlorpropamide and tolbutamide did not do so with glibenclamide.

Hepatotoxicity may vary with different derivatives of a drug. Erythromycin-induced cholestatic hepatitis has been most frequently associated with the estolate preparation, although jaundice has also been reported with erythromycin ethylsuccinate, propionate and lactobionate.

In general it is probably best to try a drug from a different chemical group which has a similar effect, for example insulin in a patient who has reacted to a sulphonylurea.

Isoniazid causes raised liver enzymes in up to 20% of recipients, but in the majority these return to normal despite continued therapy. A small minority go on to develop overt hepatitis. It is recommended that LFTs are checked monthly for the first 3 months of therapy, when toxicity is most likely to occur, especially in at-risk groups. Such patients include those with liver disease, on other hepatotoxic drugs, over 35 years of age or daily alcohol consumers. A combination of rifampicin and isoniazid is particularly likely to cause liver damage. Isoniazid and other antituberculous drugs should be temporarily discontinued if AST rises above three times the normal value. The drugs should be reintroduced one at a time at weekly intervals, with careful monitoring, to identify the drug responsible. This drug should then be discontinued.

Similar monitoring is recommended on initiating sodium valproate therapy in young children as deaths due to liver damage have been reported mainly during the first 2 months of treatment.

As well as 3- to 6-monthly LFTs, patients on long-term methotrexate therapy for psoriasis should have liver biopsies performed before treatment is started and after every 1.5 to 2 g cumulative dose of the drug to detect the development of fibrosis or cirrhosis. Weekly administration of larger doses causes less damage than smaller daily doses. Patients receiving methotrexate treatment for psoriasis appear to be at greater risk of hepatotoxicity than those being treated for rheumatoid arthritis. This may be due to psoriasis sufferers receiving higher cumulative doses.

THE PATIENT

Patients may be at risk of drug-induced hepatotoxicity from both prescribed and purchased drugs. Parents of young children should be reminded of the need to store medicines in child-resistant containers out of their reach, as deaths from liver damage have occurred due to overdosage with drugs such as iron tablets which are attractive to children.

Patients should be sufficiently well informed about their medication to minimize the risk of such serious adverse effects. Their attention should be drawn to minor side effects which could herald the start of hepatic damage. If a patient experiences drug-induced hepatotoxicity he should be informed of the causative agent and warned to avoid it in future. He should also be advised to inform any doctor or pharmacist supplying treatment about the occurrence of such an incident. Patients given treatment for drug-induced liver damage should be counselled to ensure that they understand how and when they should use the treatment.

Every year a small number of people die accidentally from paracetamol overdose because they take two or more paracetamol-containing preparations at the same time. Many OTC remedies contain paracetamol. Also the majority of compound analgesic preparations contain paracetamol and this may not be obvious from their names, e.g. co-proxamol. Although such preparations have to be labelled with a maximum dose, it is worth ensuring that patients who have been prescribed or have purchased preparations containing paracetamol understand the danger of overdosing that may occur if they take similar preparations simultaneously.

One group of patients at risk of developing hepatic damage are those undergoing treatment for tuberculosis, who will normally be receiving a number of potentially hepatotoxic drugs. Such patients require careful monitoring particularly during the first 3 months of treatment when hepatotoxicity is most likely to develop. As well as being counselled on timing of dosage and the importance of compliance, these patients should be alerted to report to their doctor any gastrointestinal symptoms such as anorexia, nausea, vomiting or abdominal discomfort which may be an indication of drug-induced hepatitis. Unfortunately deaths due to hepatotoxicity from antituberculous drugs continue to be reported. Patient education may avoid this in future.

Parents of children commenced on sodium valproate should be warned to report side effects such as vomiting or disturbed consciousness which may indicate the development of a reaction similar to Reye's syndrome, which can be fatal. Such a reaction usually occurs within the first 2 months of treatment. This is one of few hepatic drug reactions that affect children. It is more common in boys than girls and concomitant therapy with other anticonvulsant drugs greatly increases the risk.

Patients admitted for surgical procedures should be questioned about unexplained fever or jaundice following previous operations, and their previous admission notes inspected for reports of such occurrences. The anaesthetic agent halothane can rarely cause very severe liver damage. This reaction occurs on repeated exposure to the drug, especially when such exposures occur within a short time period. Many anaesthetists now avoid using halothane. There is some evidence that patients with a history of sensitivity to halothane may also develop hepatic damage when given enflurane. Isoflurane appears to be safe. A patient who is sensitive to halothane should be advised to inform medical staff of this.

Counselling is advised for patients commenced on cholestyramine or colestipol therapy for pruritus. They should be told to take any other medication 1 hour before or 4 to 6 hours after the anion exchange resin to avoid reduced absorption. The resins are most effective if taken before breakfast. If additional doses are needed they should be taken before meals. The contents of a sachet should be mixed with water, fruit juice, milk, soup, fizzy drinks or pulpy fruits immediately before taking.

Patients prescribed sedating antihistamines, e.g. chlorpheniramine, should be advised to avoid alcohol, warned about feeling drowsy and advised not to drive or operate machinery if affected.

Although hepatic adverse drug reactions are rare, when they do occur they can be very severe. Educating patients, as well as doctors and pharmacists, to recognize symptoms of such reactions may help to reduce the incidence of serious damage.

CASE STUDY

Mr H. C. is a retired dockworker who was admitted suffering from jaundice. He had been jaundiced once as a child but had never had an operation, transfusion or injection. He was born in Wales, had never been abroad and lived with his wife in a nursing home. He rarely drank alcohol. His drug history on admission was as follows:

- Tabs trimethoprim; 200 mg twice daily for 1 week, for a urinary tract infection
- Tabs co-amilofruse; 1 each morning for 1 month, for leg oedema
- Caps chlormethiazole; 2 at night for 1 month for agitation
- Tabs thioridazine; 25 mg twice daily for 1 week for agitation
- Tabs aspirin; 300 mg as required for pain, for years
- Beecham's pills (containing aloin 10 mg); p.r.n. for constipation, for years.

On examination he had yellow skin and sclerae, dark urine and pale stools. His liver function tests were as follows:

- albumin 36 g/L (35–55)
- bilirubin 132 μmol/L (< 17)
- alkaline phosphatase 159 units/L (25–100)
- aspartate transaminase 216 units/L (< 35)
- gamma-glutamyl transpeptidase 398 units/L (< 40).

Q1 What is the significance of the clinical history?

Q2 What type of liver disease do the signs, symptoms and liver function tests indicate?

Q3 Which drug is most likely to be responsible and why?

Q4 How should the patient's treatment be amended?

Q5 What other actions should be taken?

ANSWER TO CASE STUDY

A1 The patient had been a dockworker, an occupation unlikely to expose him to excessive risk of infection. A single episode of jaundice as a child is most likely to indicate hepatitis A infection, which has no long-term consequences. The fact that he had had no recent operations excludes postoperative jaundice. No history of transfusions or injections makes infections such as hepatitis B or C unlikely. Similarly Wales is not a high risk area for hepatitis B infection. As Mr H. C. has never been abroad he is unlikely to have contracted a tropical infection. He is married and living in a nursing home which makes homosexuality and associated disorders unlikely. He drinks little alcohol which excludes alcoholic liver disease. Overall his clinical history excludes many possible causes of liver disease.

A2 The dark urine and pale stools are characteristic of cholestasis. The yellow sclera and skin indicate jaundice. A serum albumin in the normal range excludes chronic liver disease. A raised bilirubin, with a raised alkaline phosphatase and gamma-glutamyl transferase indicate cholestasis. A raised aspartate transaminase suggests hepatocellular injury. The overall picture is of hepatocanalicular cholestasis.

A3 Phenothiazines including thioridazine are known to cause hepatocanalicular cholestasis. Such a reaction normally occurs soon after starting treatment and Mr H. C. commenced therapy a week previously. He has taken aspirin and Beecham's pills for many years, so it is unlikely that they would cause an acute reaction at this stage. Aspirin is an intrinsic hepatotoxin and needs to be taken regularly in doses of over 2 g a day to cause hepatocellular necrosis. Frusemide has been reported to cause jaundice, but hepatic damage is very rare, even when given in high dosage. Trimethoprim, amiloride and chlormethiazole are rarely associated with hepatic damage.

A4 The thioridazine should be stopped immediately. There is evidence of hepatocellular damage so chlormethiazole, which is hepatically metabolized, should be used with caution in a reduced dose. Aspirin should be discontinued because of the increased risk of gastric mucosal bleeding associated with liver damage. Co-amilofruse can be continued with electrolyte monitoring.

A5 Mr H. C.'s LFTs should be measured regularly to monitor recovery. He should be counselled on the need to avoid thioridazine and similar drugs in the future as they could provoke a severe reaction. It should be documented in his notes that he is allergic to thioridazine. Medical staff should be encouraged to complete a yellow card to notify the Committee on the Safety of Medicines of this reaction.

BIBLIOGRAPHY

Davis M. Drug-related liver disease. Medicine International 1990; 83 (Nov): 3444–3448

Sherlock S. Diseases of the liver and biliary system, 8th edn. Oxford: Blackwell Scientific Publications 1989

Davis M, Williams R. Hepatic disorders. In: Davies D M (ed) Textbook of adverse drug reactions, 4th edn. Oxford: Oxford University Press, 1991; 245–304

Zimmerman H J, Maddrey W C. Toxic and drug induced hepatitis. In: Schiff L, Schiff E R (eds) Diseases of the liver, 6th edn. Philadelphia: J B Lippincott, 1987; 591–667

Chapter 13

Hepatic disease

P. N. Bramley   R. D. Swallow

The liver is a key organ in regulating the homeostasis of the body. The function of the hepatocytes include protein synthesis, storage and metabolism of fats and carbohydrates, detoxification of drugs and toxins, and excretion of bilirubin, as well as playing a central role in hormone metabolism (Fig. 13.1). This diversity of physiological roles means that if liver function is impaired several homeostatic mechanisms will be affected.

Acute liver disease

Acute liver disease or acute hepatitis is usually a self-limiting episode of liver cell (hepatocyte) inflammation or damage which normally resolves completely. In rare cases the hepatocyte damage is so severe that it affects the whole liver causing hepatic coma and death (fulminant hepatic failure).

Chronic liver disease

Chronic liver disease occurs when permanent structural changes within the liver appear secondary to long-standing cell damage with loss of normal architecture. In most cases this progresses to cirrhosis, when fibrous scars divide the liver cells into areas of regenerative tissue called nodules. This process is irreversible and eventually leads to chronic liver failure and then death once the remaining liver tissue is unable to support the normal regulatory role of the liver.

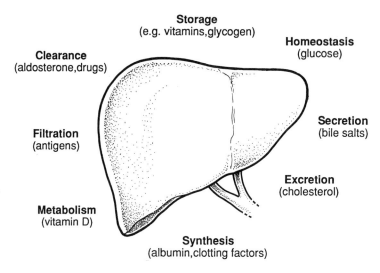

Fig. 13.1 The normal physiological functions of the liver, together with examples of each.

EPIDEMIOLOGY

Acute hepatitis

Acute hepatitis is a group of diseases which are found in all parts of the world. Hepatitis A is particularly prevalent wherever there is poor sanitation, or where human effluent is used for crop fertilization. As the virus is spread via the faecal–oral route, water- and food-borne epidemics occur. In western countries with high standards of hygiene, sporadic cases occur following person to person contact.

Hepatitis B is transmitted by contact with infected blood or intimate sexual contact. The prevalence of the disease varies around the world. Generally it is low in the USA and Britain with 0.1 to 0.2% of the population having markers which indicate that they are chronic carriers of hepatitis B. However, in Africa and the Far East, 15 to 20% of the population are chronic carriers whilst the majority of the population may have had a discrete acute hepatitis B infection at some time in their life. In these areas, vertical transmission of the infection is important, with infected mothers passing it on to their offspring at birth. Spread between family members is an important route in some communities and sharing toothbrushes, razors and towels all increase the risks of transmission. In western

countries, parenteral spread via tattooing, intravenous drug abuse, blood product infusions from infected donors and sexual contact are the commonest modes of transmission.

Hepatitis C and D have similar parenteral routes of transmission to hepatitis B, whilst hepatitis E appears to be water borne in underdeveloped countries.

Chronic liver disease

The commonest cause of cirrhosis of the liver in the western world is alcoholic liver disease, with a country's alcohol consumption per head of population correlating with the deaths from alcohol-related cirrhosis. The prevalence of alcoholic liver disease in a particular country depends on the cost of alcohol, and the social and religious customs surrounding drinking. France has the highest death rate from alcoholic cirrhosis of any European country (33 per 100 000 population per year), and the highest intake of alcohol (equivalent to 16 litres of pure alcohol per person per year). By comparison, England has 4 deaths per 100 000 population per year for a pure alcohol intake of 7 litres per person per year.

Chronic hepatitis B infection leading on to liver cirrhosis is the commonest cause of cirrhosis in the Far East. In these patients there is also a further risk of developing hepatocellular carcinoma, once a person has had a chronic hepatitis B infection for many years.

Other causes of chronic liver disease tend to vary in prevalence in different parts of the world. Immunological or autoimmune liver disease and metabolic liver diseases are found in all racial groups studied. Disease secondary to environmental factors such as iron overload due to cooking and fermenting in iron pots is peculiar to the Bantu people of Africa (Bantu siderosis). In the tropics infectious diseases such as schistosomiasis (bilharziasis) and liver flukes cause major morbidity and mortality from liver disease in the local populations.

AETIOLOGY

Acute liver disease

Most cases of acute hepatitis are virus related, many attacks being very mild and often passing unnoticed by the patient. Other causes of acute hepatitis are drugs (prescribed or taken as an overdose), toxins and chemicals. Sometimes it is not possible to be certain which agent is the cause of the hepatitis because the basic histological lesions in the liver and the biochemical markers of liver function in the blood are similar.

Chronic liver disease

This implies a previous or continuing insult to the liver. Chronic hepatitis is defined as persistent inflammation of the liver for over 6 months. It may follow an attack of acute viral hepatitis such as hepatitis B or C, or may be secondary to an autoimmune disease such as autoimmune chronic active hepatitis or a result of drug or toxin ingestion. Once the inflammation has progressed to fibrosis and nodule formation then a pathological diagnosis of cirrhosis can be made on liver biopsy. It is convenient to divide the causes into the following eight groups.

Causes of chronic liver disease

Viral hepatitis B and C. In a proportion of cases of acute viral hepatitis, instead of a gradual resolution of the inflammation, the virus is not cleared and chronic hepatitis ensues. This may take the form of chronic persistent hepatitis with a minimal degree of inflammation of the hepatocytes; this type of hepatitis tends to run a benign course, although the patient may still be considered infective to other people as virus is still being made (the carrier state). In some patients the inflammation is more marked and is described as chronic active hepatitis, which implies continuing destruction of the hepatocytes.

Alcohol. Excessive ingestion of ethanol over a prolonged period of time leads to progressive fibrosis around the hepatocytes. It appears that this process is reversible if the patient stops drinking. With continued insult the fibrosis becomes widespread with nodule formation.

Autoimmune. Autoimmune liver disease represents a state of altered immunity where the body's immune system develops autoantibodies against its own tissues. Primary biliary cirrhosis (PBC) and chronic active hepatitis (CAH) are examples of organ-specific immune-mediated disease. These occur predominantly in women, PBC in the 40 to 60 year age range, and CAH in younger women.

Biliary obstruction (cholestasis). Long-standing obstruction of the bile outflow from the liver can cause inflammation, scarring, and eventually cirrhosis. Examples of this occur following damage to the common bile duct during surgery, or associated with sclerosing cholangitis (a form of bile duct inflammation and scarring associated with inflammatory bowel disease). Biliary atresia (a developmental deficiency of the bile ducts which presents during infancy) is one cause of childhood liver disease.

Vascular. An obstruction to the veins draining the liver will cause eventual cell destruction and cirrhosis. The Budd–Chiari syndrome is caused by blood clots obstructing the hepatic veins and is associated with a state of abnormal clotting, or a malformation in the hepatic veins. Veno-occlusive disease occurs when the smaller veins become obliterated, this can be caused by toxins, irradiation or cytotoxic drugs. Prolonged right-sided heart failure or constrictive pericarditis can also be associated with so-called 'cardiac cirrhosis' secondary to increased venous backpressure on the liver parenchyma.

Metabolic. Inborn errors of metabolism (genetic) are called dominant if only one parent is required to carry the defective gene, and recessive if both parents have to carry the defective gene to pass it on to their offspring.

Haemochromatosis (iron overload). This is a recessive error of metabolism resulting in excess iron absorption and deposition throughout the body. A fibrosis tissue reaction is found wherever the iron is deposited leading eventually to fibrosis then cirrhosis, if iron accumulation continues.

Wilson's disease (copper overload). This is a recessive error which causes excess absorption of dietary copper and abnormal deposition in the liver, brain, kidneys and other tissues.

Alpha$_1$ antitrypsin deficiency. This is a dominant error which causes a reduction in a protein which protects tissues from attack by digestive enzymes (trypsin and others). Its reduction leads to either emphysematous lung disease or liver cirrhosis.

Glycogen storage disease. There are several forms of this disease, all are recessive with many presenting in childhood. All result in abnormal production and deranged homeostasis of glucose and glycogen causing metabolites to accumulate which then damage the hepatocytes.

Toxins and drugs. Several drugs have been identified as causing progressive liver damage, e.g. methotrexate, methyldopa, amiodarone and vitamin A.

Cryptogenic cirrhosis. After exhaustive investigations there are always patients in whom a definitive diagnosis can not be made. These patients are labelled as having cryptogenic cirrhosis. With advances in diagnostic tests, particularly with the diagnosis of new viruses, the label of cryptogenic cirrhosis will be used less often.

PATHOPHYSIOLOGY

In order to understand the changes that occur in the liver in acute hepatitis and in chronic liver disease, it is necessary to describe the normal liver architecture (Fig. 13.2).

There are two blood supplies to the liver, the arterial supply through the hepatic artery, and the portal venous system which collects venous blood draining from the abdominal viscera. The portal vein, hepatic artery, and the bile duct system which drains bile from the liver to the intestine, enter the liver through a structure called the porta hepatis. These three structures branch re-

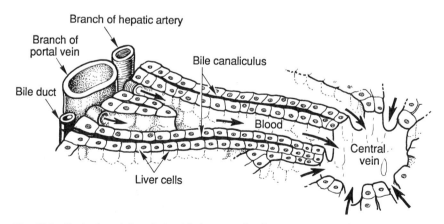

Fig. 13.2 Illustration of the relationship between the three structures which comprise the portal tract, with blood from both the hepatic artery and portal vein perfusing the hepatocytes before draining away towards the hepatic veins (central veins). Each hepatocyte is also able to secrete bile via the network of bile ducts. (Reproduced with permission from A Vander, Human physiology: mechanisms of body functions, third edition 1980, Figure 14.23, page 431, publishers McGraw-Hill Inc., New York.)

peatedly until they lie in the portal tracts which carry the finest branches of the vessels and ducts. From these portal tracts, columns of liver cells and blood-containing spaces extend towards a small hepatic vein (venule). This collects all the blood draining from the liver tissue into central veins which eventually form large hepatic veins which discharge into the inferior vena cava.

Acute liver disease

Hepatitis A serves as a good example of an acute liver disease which resolves completely.

Once the virus has entered the body, usually via contaminated water or food, there is a short incubation period of 2 to 7 weeks, during which the virus replicates and the liver function tests become progressively more abnormal. Jaundice then occurs due to a reduction in the capacity of the liver cells to excrete bilirubin, and enzymes which are normally found within the hepatocytes are released due to cell destruction. Microscopically, there is liver cell death and degeneration, and inflammatory white cells invade the liver tissue and remove the cellular debris. Eventually the surviving liver cells start to divide and replace the dead cells. Cell damage tends to occur mainly around the hepatic venules, as this part of the liver tissue receives blood which contains the least oxygen (see Fig. 13.2). In a severe attack, the cellular damage may be widespread, affecting all areas of the liver tissue including the portal tracts. In these rarer cases there may be enough cellular damage to cause acute hepatic failure as insufficient functioning liver tissue is left to maintain function. In paracetamol overdose, which provides an example of toxic cell damage following a well-defined insult, the maximum cell damage occurs at day 4 to 6 following the overdose. If the liver (and patient) survives the cell destruction, then the liver rapidly regenerates and returns to normal within a few months.

Chronic liver disease

Although the causes of cirrhosis are many, liver cell destruction, the development of diffuse fibrosis and nodule formation are common to all aetiologies and result in the same end point (see Fig. 13.3).

During the development of the cirrhosis, whilst active inflammation is occurring, the pattern of cell destruction may provide clues to the underlying aetiology. Once the inflammation disappears leaving inactive cirrhosis, it may be impossible to determine the original cause. Alcoholic liver cirrhosis provides a good example of the changes that occur in chronic liver disease.

With prolonged and excessive exposure to

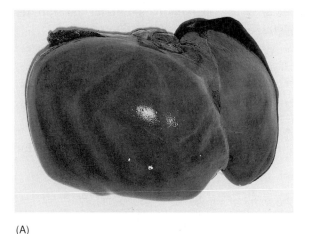

(A)

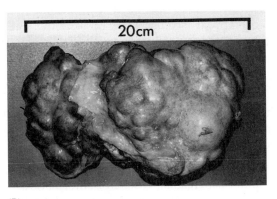

(B)

Fig. 13.3 The gross post-mortem appearances of a normal (A) and a cirrhotic (B) liver demonstrating scarring and nodule formation in B.

ethanol, inflammatory activity occurs within the liver tissue, hepatocytes accumulate large droplets of fat (fatty change) and inclusion bodies develop within swollen cells. A fine network of collagen fibres develops around the liver cells near the hepatic venule and gradually liver cells die and the amount of fibrosis increases. Eventually hepatic venules are obliterated and the areas of fibrosis around them link up to form bands of fibrous tissue. Areas of liver cells between the fibrous bands regenerate but with the destruction of the normal relationship between the portal tracts and the draining hepatic venules, the cells divide haphazardly and nodules or islands of liver tissue develop. The disordered anatomy means that blood from the portal system cannot flow as easily through the liver; this causes the pressure within the portal system to increase leading to a major complication of cirrhosis, the development of portal hypertension. The continuing reduction in the number of properly functioning liver cells leads to the other major complication of chronic liver disease, liver cell failure, where the number of hepatocytes becomes insufficient to maintain the essential synthetic, metabolic and excretory roles of the liver.

CLINICAL MANIFESTATIONS

Signs of liver disease

Generally it is necessary for liver impairment to be present for several weeks to months before many of the signs associated with chronic liver disease appear (see Fig. 13.4). Most of the signs can be related to a failure to synthesize, metabolize or excrete normally.

Cutaneous signs

There are a number of cutaneous signs which may indicate the presence of liver disease although none are specific. They include:

* Finger clubbing (swelling of the finger ends)
* Spider naevi (small vascular malformations in the skin)
* Palmar erythema (reddening of the palm of the hand).

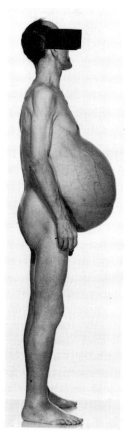

Fig. 13.4 Ascites, muscle wasting and distended abdominal collateral veins in chronic liver disease.

These are thought to be related to changes in the vascular system which cause the development of arterial–venous shunts in the skin and hands. They signify chronic liver disease.

* White nails – associated with low serum albumin states
* Dupuytren's contracture – abnormal fibrous tissue in palm of hand causing retraction of one or more fingers
* Easy bruising – secondary to deficiency of clotting factors and reduction in platelets due to portal hypertension.

Abdominal signs

Enlarged liver (hepatomegaly). This is a common finding in acute liver disease, indicating inflammation and regeneration. In cirrhosis the liver may be large or small depending on the stage of the chronic disease.

Enlarged spleen (splenomegaly). This is caused by the increased pressure in the portal venous system (portal hypertension) secondary to cirrhosis.

Distended abdominal wall veins. These are secondary to portal hypertension, as the portal blood joins other veins to drain around the liver.

General signs of liver cell failure

Jaundice. This signifies impaired liver cell function. This is a common finding in acute liver disease, but may be absent in chronic liver disease unless approaching the terminal stages of cirrhosis. See Figure 13.5 for other causes of jaundice.

Swollen abdomen (ascites). The accumulation of fluid within the abdominal cavity has many causes which include:

1. a reduction in the excretion of sodium by the kidney, due to enhanced activity of the renin–angiotensin–aldosterone system, secondary to central hypovolaemia (and also decreased aldosterone degradation) which causes increased retention of fluid in the body
2. reduction in the serum albumin which causes osmotic changes and allows fluid to leak out of blood vessels
3. portal hypertension which tends to drive fluid out of the capillaries into the abdominal cavity.

Swollen lower limbs (peripheral oedema). This condition is due to factors (1) and (2) mentioned above.

Hormonal changes. Those occurring in males are partly due to the inability of the cirrhotic liver to metabolize oestrogen which leads to the development of swollen breast tissue (gynaecomastia); in females of reproductive age, there is a reduction in fertility.

Mental changes or coma (hepatic encephalopathy). These occur in acute or chronic liver disease. In

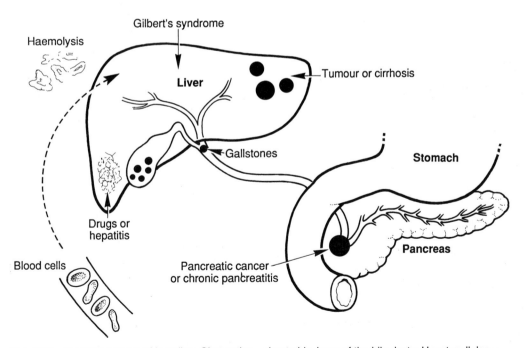

Fig. 13.5 Common causes of jaundice: Obstructive – due to blockage of the bile ducts; Hepatocellular – due to drugs, hepatitis, chronic liver disease or tumour formation; and Pre-hepatic – due to increased blood breakdown such as occurs in haemolysis.

acute liver disease, encephalopathy is associated with fulminant liver failure and signifies very severe liver damage. In this condition a common finding is the development of brain swelling (cerebral oedema) which poses a very significant threat to life. Encephalopathy in cirrhotic patients represents a decompensation in the function of the liver rather than a direct threat to life. Common causes are chest, urinary tract or ascitic infections, or excess faecal loading in the bowel, and it can be improved by treating the infection or constipation.

Symptoms of liver disease

Commonly, patients complain of being easily fatigued and generally run-down. They may have noted loss of appetite and weight loss, and in chronic liver disease loss of muscle from their arms and legs with swelling of their abdomen and lower body due to fluid retention. In individuals with enlarged livers the patient may complain of abdominal pain and tenderness particularly in acute hepatitis.

A distressing symptom for many patients is the intractable itching (pruritus) secondary to jaundice. This is probably due to the deposition of bile salts in the skin and can be very difficult to relieve. It appears to be related to the degree of jaundice, and is exacerbated by warming the skin, e.g. by taking a hot bath or lying in bed. Patients with chronic liver disease who have abnormal clotting or low platelet numbers often complain of increased bleeding from the gums and nose, and easy bruising.

INVESTIGATIONS

Most of the investigations to determine the cause and extent of liver disease are similar for both acute and chronic liver disease (Table 13.1).

Other investigations routinely performed

Visualization of the liver texture and the bile ducts is very important to exclude an obstructive cause for the impaired liver function. Ultrasound is the investigation of first choice, allowing investigation of areas of particular interest such as possible liver tumours, and extent of splenomegaly and portal hypertension. Computerized tomography (CT) scans are used to enable more detailed examination if necessary.

Table 13.1 Comparison of changes in standard liver function tests in acute and chronic liver disease

Test	Acute	Chronic	Remarks
Liver function tests			
Bilirubin	↑	↑	Marker of excretory function
Transaminases e.g. ALT, AST	↑	↔ or ↑	Indicate cell destruction
Alk. phos.	↔	↔ or ↑	Indicates biliary obstruction
Albumin	↔	↓	Indicates synthetic function
Prothrombin test	↔ or ↑	↑	Indicates synthetic function
Diagnostic tests			
Autoantibodies	–	+	Positive in: autoimmune primary biliary cirrhosis chronic active hepatitis diseases
Hepatitis B	+/–	+/–	Present if infected
Hepatitis C	+/–	+/–	Present if infected
Hepatitis A	+/–	–	Only in acute liver disease
Alpha-fetoprotein	–	+/–	Present if hepatoma (liver cancer)
Serum caeruloplasmin	↔ or ↓	↔ or ↓	Only reduced in Wilson's disease

Key: ↑ = increased; ↔ = normal or unchanged; ↓ = decreased; +/– = present/absent

Liver biopsy is routinely performed in order to determine the degree of tissue damage, and in many cases allows a definitive diagnosis to be made. It is performed percutaneously using a hollow needle between the lower ribs on the right chest wall.

TREATMENT

Preventive therapy

In liver disease, as in other diseases, prevention is better than cure. There are only now limited options to prevent certain types of acute hepatitis. As far as chronic liver disease is concerned, only alcoholic liver disease can be prevented by the simple expedient of stopping excessive alcohol intake. Providing liver damage is mild and has not progressed to cirrhosis, the liver will return to normal with continued abstinence.

With recent advances in vaccine technology, it is now possible to offer safe and effective vaccination against hepatitis B. As this disease is widespread throughout most of the Third World, and there is now strong evidence of an aetiological association between hepatitis B and hepatocellular (liver) carcinoma, the advent of effective vaccination will hopefully reduce the transmission of this serious disease.

Active immunization

This is achieved by stimulating the immune system to produce antibodies to the hepatitis B virus; vaccines are based on the hepatitis B surface (HBs) antigen (surface coat of the virus particle). Repeated exposure to this vaccine causes the immune system to produce antibodies against the surface antigen (anti-HBs), and these confer protection against future exposure to the active virus. At present, high risk groups such as health-care personnel and people at risk of being exposed to the virus such as partners of hepatitis B positive patients are offered the vaccine. The available vaccine is derived using recombinant DNA technology to express HB surface antigen in yeast cells. The vaccine requires three injections, at 0, 1 and 6 months, following which approximately 95% of people will have an adequate antibody response.

In non-responders, further booster injections may be required. Immunity is considered complete if a hepatitis B antibody response of over 100 IU/L is found following the course. It is suggested that booster injections will be required when the antibody level drops well below 100 IU/L.

Active immunization against hepatitis A virus (HAV) is also available using a vaccine prepared from a formaldehyde-inactivated strain of hepatitis A grown on human diploid cells. The immunization regimen involves two intramuscular injections of 720 ELISA units of hepatitis A viral protein in 1 ml, given two weeks to one month apart. This regimen provides antibodies for at least one year.

Passive immunization

This is used when a person who has not developed antibodies to the virus is suddenly exposed to hepatitis B, such as occurs when blood containing the virus is accidentally injected or inoculated, or when contamination of mucous membranes or eye occurs by splashes of blood.

Pooled serum from patients with high levels of anti-HBs immunoglobulin can be injected to give passive immunity. A dose of 500 IU has been used effectively in adults. Serum should be administered as early as possible following exposure, certainly within 48 hours. It is recommended that a second dose is given 30 days later. It is now standard practice to give passive immunization to babies of mothers who are hepatitis B positive to prevent transmission during the perinatal period. The immunoglobulin (200 IU) is given as soon after birth as is practical and certainly within 12 hours. The results of this prophylactic measure are very encouraging; recent studies combining passive with active immunization have been shown to confer successful protection in 90% of cases.

Passive immunization is also used to prevent hepatitis A infection in non-immune travellers to endemic areas. Approximately 50% of middle-aged people in England already have hepatitis A virus antibody (anti-HAV). The immunoglobulin contains at least 100 IU/ml of anti-HAV, and if given intramuscularly prior to or early in the incubation period will prevent or reduce the severity of an infection. The period of protection is only short, and boosters are recommended if still resident in an endemic area after 3 to 6 months.

Disease-modifying therapy

Treatment of viral hepatitis

In patients with hepatitis B, C and other (perhaps undefined) viral liver infections, various treatments have been attempted over the years to reduce the problems associated with chronic infection. Several antiviral agents have been used, mostly with disappointing results. Acyclovir can produce a transient and incomplete suppression in hepatitis B. In clinical trials, foscarnet has been used but has not been shown to produce any improvement in hepatitis B. Vidarabine in its water-soluble form (ara-AMP) produces an early and reproducible suppression of hepatitis B, but the improvement is only transient and long-term usage is associated with serious dose-dependent gastrointestinal and neuropathic complications. The most promising agents currently used in treating viral hepatitis are interferons (IFN), which are polypeptides (small proteins) produced naturally as a response to a viral infection. They exhibit direct viral inhibition and also enhance the body's immune responses to viruses. Following the development of recombinant DNA technology, large quantities of IFNs have been produced which have allowed clinicians to extensively study these agents. There are three classes of interferon, alpha produced from B-lymphocytes and monocytes, beta from fibroblasts and gamma from T-lymphocytes. Clinical trials have shown that alpha IFN appears to be more effective than the other classes.

Interferon treatment is associated with dose-dependent side effects, particularly with the first few doses. These tend to improve but may necessitate dose reduction. Careful monitoring is re-quired initially as reductions in white blood cells and platelets are common. The first few doses are associated with a 'flu-like' illness, with temperature, muscle pains and headaches developing within a few hours and lasting up to 24 hours. These symptoms are relieved by predosing with paracetamol, and injecting IFN late evening. Longer-term side effects include weight loss, anorexia, fatigue and depression. It should not be used in patients with a history of neurological or psychiatric illnesses.

In hepatitis B infection, the success of any therapy can be judged on the clearance of viral DNA from the blood, and the appearance of antibodies to the virus; in a small proportion of cases HBs antigen is replaced with anti-HBs antibody indicating complete clearance of the infection. It appears that certain patients have better response rates than others (See Table 13.2).

Treatment regimens are still being developed, but it appears that 5 million units of alpha IFN given subcutaneously three times per week for a minimum period of 4 months has been shown to enable approximately 40% of selected patients to lose HBe antigen and 10% to lose HBs antigen. A small proportion of these patients may relapse once the IFN is withdrawn. Recent and ongoing research suggests that pretreatment with steroids increases the response rate.

Trials of alpha IFN in patients with undefined

Table 13.2 Factors which are likely to determine the therapeutic response to interferon (IFN) therapy in chronic hepatitis B infection

	Good responders	Poor responders
Race	Caucasian	Oriental
Age at time of infection	Adult	Infant
Onset of infection	Recent	Long-standing
Sexual habit	Heterosexual	Homosexual
Degree of liver inflammation	Moderate/ severe	Mild
Elevation of serum ALT	High	Normal or mild
Other illnesses	None	HIV/cancer
Duration of IFN therapy	More than 4 months	Less than 3 months
Pretreatment with steroids	Yes	No

viral hepatitis (of whom the majority have antibodies to hepatitis C) have shown a rapid response to IFN in approximately 80% of patients at a lower dose than needed for hepatitis B, but the treatment needs to be continued for longer (9 to 12 months), and half of those responders will relapse once IFN is withdrawn. Maintenance IFN may be suitable for patients who demonstrate an initial response. It is not yet clear if IFN has a role to play in treating hepatitis D infections.

Treatment of other chronic liver diseases

There are only a few chronic liver diseases for which any disease-modifying treatment can be offered. Autoimmune chronic active hepatitis is one example where the inflammation present within the liver tissue can be suppressed by treatment with immunosuppressive drugs. The use of low to moderate doses of prednisolone (5 to 40 mg per day) reduces the inflammatory reaction around the hepatocytes and slows or prevents the progression to cirrhosis. The dose of prednisolone should be titrated against the serum alanine transaminase values. Occasionally azathioprine (50 to 100 mg per day) is added as a steroid-sparing drug. Frequent blood counts are essential to monitor the platelet and white cell count in patients on azathioprine. Steroid treatment also has distinct disadvantages, with exacerbation of the osteopenia (bone thinning) of chronic liver disease, and increased risk of infections.

Two of the genetically determined metabolic diseases can also be successfully treated. Haemochromatosis (presence of excessive iron overload) can be controlled by regular venesection (blood-letting). This causes excess body iron stores to be used in maintaining a normal blood haemoglobin. It is important to identify patients early in order to prevent the onset of tissue damage. Those diagnosed and treated in the pre-cirrhotic stage have normal life expectancy. All relatives should be screened to identify asymptomatic cases. Wilson's disease (presence of excessive copper) can be treated with penicillamine (dose 1.2 g increasing to 2 g per day in

four divided doses) which chelates copper and increases urinary copper excretion. Treatment is continued until there is evidence that the excessive copper has been removed, this may take many years. Maintenance penicillamine is then required together with regular liver biopsy to check liver copper levels. Monitoring of treatment is required specifically to watch for proteinuria, leucopenia and aplastic anaemia.

Symptomatic therapy

The main area of drug use in patients with liver disease is in the management of complications arising as a result of liver damage. These complications may be divided for the purpose of discussion into six areas which will be covered in this section.

Jaundice

A classification of the different types of jaundice is presented in Figure 13.5.

There are two main therapeutic lines of attack in patients with jaundice, the first of which is to attempt to improve bile flow in order to decrease the jaundice. If the biliary obstruction is clearly linked to a specific cause which may be removed (e.g. biliary stones) then this would usually facilitate drainage and consequently the alleviation of the jaundice. Where stones are causing the obstruction, these may be removed surgically, endoscopically or by medical dissolution using a supplementary bile acid such as ursodeoxycholic acid or chenodeoxycholic acid. Both these agents increase bile salt concentration and decrease cholesterol in bile. Medical treatment is only used if a surgical or endoscopic approach cannot be attempted. The use of methyl tertiary butyl ether to dissolve gallstones, instilled directly into the bile duct via a fine tube placed under endoscopic control, is currently being evaluated. If the obstruction is due to narrowing or inflammation of the biliary tree then drugs which modify bile flow may be used. Ursodeoxycholic acid has been used as a choleretic agent in patients with primary biliary cirrhosis at doses of approximately 10 mg/kg/day. Rifampicin is also throught to improve bile flow and is used at doses of 300 to 450 mg/day. It is thought that rifampicin may work by inducing liver enzymes and also possible by inhibiting bile salt uptake. Rifampicin is not without problems since it can increase biliary stone formation, decrease 25-hydroxy vitamin D levels and interact with many drugs. Rifampicin has also been noted to cause a mild hepatitis but this occurs usually in the context of a general hypersensitivity reaction.

Undoubtedly the most debilitating aspect of jaundice is the accompanying pruritus which can vary from mild inconvenience to intense itching. Prolonged scratching may even result in superficial skin ulceration (excoriation). Antihistamines form the mainstay of treatment and both non-sedating and sedating drugs are used. Until fairly recently it was assumed that an antihistamine should have sedating properties in order to work in pruritus of non-histamine-mediated origin. This view has, however, been challenged and in patients with jaundice the non-sedating antihistamines such as terfenadine (60 mg b.d.) and astemizole (10 mg daily) do seem to work in practice. The main reason for using non-sedating antihistamines as first line treatment is the reluctance to use agents which may precipitate encephalopathy. There are some situations where a sedative antihistamine is useful. Chlorpheniramine for example is often used at bedtime for its sedative effect and its ability to reduce the intensity of itching which increases as the skin is warmed whilst in bed. Hydroxyzine (25 mg 3 or 4 times a day) may also be used and in fact is frequently used for urticarial itching in dermatology patients.

Probably the most important therapy in patients with obstructive jaundice is the use of the ion-exchange resin cholestyramine (one sachet (4 g) two to four times daily). Cholestyramine works by binding bile salts within the intestinal lumen and preventing their absorption. There is evidence that the build up of bile salts in the skin is one cause of the itching. There may be other unknown substances involved with the pruritus of obstructive jaundice since cholestyramine is

also known to work in the pruritus of uraemia. Cholestyramine is often poorly tolerated because it can cause constipation and nausea whilst many patients complain of the texture of the product which is fairly 'gritty'. It is important to counsel the patient carefully and advice may by given on ways that the product may be incorporated into special recipes or mixed with drinks. These recipes and patient information leaflets may be readily obtained from the manufacturer. Careful explanation of the delay in therapeutic benefit is very important as relief may take up to 1 week to be apparent. The alternative ion-binding resin, colestipol, may be tried if patients remain intolerant to cholestyramine.

Cholestyramine has been reported to reduce the absorption of fat-soluble vitamins, calcium and a range of drugs including thiazide diuretics, cardiac glycosides, thyroxine and oral anticoagulants.

Steroids may be quite effective in treating patients with pruritus due to obstructive jaundice, but their side effects preclude long-term usage. In patients with chronic liver disease the risk of infections, and osteopenia are increased with their use. Methyltestosterone and stanozolol are extremely effective agents which will ameliorate pruritus but unfortunately may cause cholestasis in their own right.

In children who have a deficiency of a glucuronidase enzyme which allows excretion of bilirubin, ultraviolet (wave length 450 nm) phototherapy may be used (e.g. in the rare Crigler–Najjar syndrome); it is not clear whether phototherapy is of any practical benefit for obstructive jaundice of other aetiologies.

Although it is very much a palliative approach some success in patients with intractable pruritus has been achieved using a topically applied menthol cream (1 to 2% of menthol dissolved in a small amount of ethanol and diluted with aqueous cream). Some patients, however, get relief to excoriated areas with frequent application of calamine lotion.

Drugs commonly used in the treatment of jaundice are summarized in Table 13.3.

Ascending cholangitis is a serious complication of obstructive jaundice and the antibiotics used must be carefully chosen in terms of killing

Table 13.3 Drugs commonly used in the management of jaundice

Drug	Indication	Daily dose	Advantage	Disadvantage	Significant interactions
Ursodeoxycholic acid	Cholestatic jaundice	5–10 mg/kg	Choleretic-increased bile flow Initial reports suggest reduced itching, and possible beneficial effect on liver function in primary biliary cirrhosis	Results of larger clinical trials still awaited – role in liver disease uncertain	
Cholestyramine	Cholestatic jaundice Itching First line treatment	8–16 g	Reduces systemic bile salt levels	Poor patient compliance due to unpalatability Diarrhoea/constipation Increased flatulence Abdominal discomfort	Reduces bioavailability of most drugs Caution with digoxin, thiazides, thyroxine, fat-soluble vitamins
Terfenadine	Itching First line treatment	120 mg	Antihistamine with low incidence of sedation	Variable response in different patients	Avoid use with antiarrythmics, neuroleptics, tricyclic antidepressants, diuretics May interact with macrolide antibiotics and imadozole anti-fungals
Astemizole	Alternative to terfenadine	10 mg	Antihistamine with low incidence of sedation	Variable response in different patients	As for terfenadine
Chlorpheniramine	Itching	12–16 mg	Sedative effects may be helpful for night–time itching	May precipitate/ aggravate encephalopathy	Additive effects with alcohol and sedatives
Rifampicin	Cholestatic jaundice	300–450 mg	Improvement bile flow and possibly inhibits bile salt uptake	As for ursodeoxycholic acid	Many drug interactions due to enhancement of liver enzyme activity

organisms which are frequently encountered in biliary infections. Acute infections are treated with intravenous antibiotics, the choice of which will depend on whether the patient has had previous surgery to the biliary tree or has been taking prophylactic antibiotics. One approach is to use a cephalosporin (cefuroxime) plus metronidazole (after taking blood cultures) and modify treatment in the light of bacterial sensitivities.

In patients with recurrent cholangitis, prophylactic antibiotics are required; an oral cephalosporin or ciprofloxacin are frequently used long term. The important role of vitamin supplementation in patients with obstructive jaundice will be discussed later under nutrition.

Clotting abnormalities

The liver is the principal site of synthesis of all coagulating proteins except von Willebrand factor and fibrinolytic proteins. The liver also synthesizes protease inhibitors such as antithrombin III (See Fig. 13.6).

The most frequently used indicator of defective clotting factor synthesis is the prothrombin time. All patients with prolonged prothrombin time should receive intermittent vitamin K supplementation (20 mg i.m. twice daily for six doses), particularly those receiving long-term intravenous nutrition. Vitamin K will correct an abnormal prothrombin time which is secondary

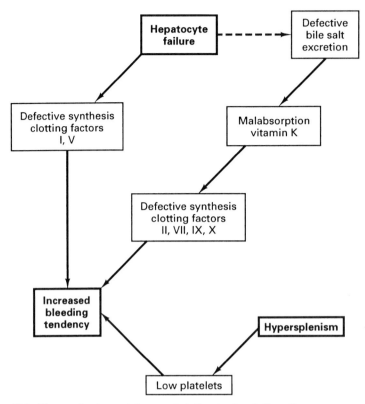

Fig. 13.6 The mechanisms of deranged clotting in chronic liver disease.

to fat malabsorption due to decreased bile salts excretion. However, if the prothrombin time is increased due to liver cell failure, vitamin K may only partially correct the abnormal prothrombin time. There are two forms of vitamin K which are currently available, namely phytomenadione and menadiol; fat-soluble and water-soluble forms respectively. Routinely phytomenadione is given intramuscularly (it may be given as a slow intravenous injection). It seems that the fat-soluble form of vitamin K is more efficient at correcting the prothrombin time in these patients than the water-soluble form. However, adverse reactions may be a problem, firstly due to anaphylaxis because of the presence of phenoxylated castor oil ('cremophor') which is used as a formulating agent in the injection and secondly an allergic type reaction which has been referred to as 'a belt and holster' rash which has been reported in some patients receiving

phytomenadione. Menadiol sodium phosphate can be administered orally but it is a provitamin which requires activation before it can exert vitamin-K-like effects.

If a liver biopsy is required in a patient with a raised prothrombin time even after vitamin K supplementation, there is a risk of life-threatening bleeding. The biopsy should be carried out using a plugged biopsy technique where a sterile absorbable sponge (e.g. 'gelfoam') is injected into the needle track after the tissue sample has been removed from the liver. If the prothrombin time is very prolonged, fresh frozen plasma may be given to the patient immediately prior to biopsy which will replenish the necessary clotting factors for a few hours. If the patient is thrombocytopenic secondary to hypersplenism platelets may be given.

A range of drugs are contra-indicated in patients with clotting abnormalities or can only be used with extreme caution, e.g. aspirin, non-steroidal anti-inflammatory agents, anticoagulants.

Portal hypertension

Portal hypertension occurs when there is increased pressure within the portal venous system secondary to increased resistance to flow through the damaged liver. Collateral veins develop and these can bleed due to the increased flow and pressure within them. Portal hypertension is one important contributory factor to the formation of ascites and the development of encephalopathy due to bypassing of blood from the liver to the systemic circulation. The major and potentially life-threatening complication of portal hypertension is the risk of torrential venous haemorrhage from the thin-walled veins which develop in the oesophagus and stomach. The management of bleeding oesophageal varices and gastric erosions in the cirrhotic patient constitutes a major medical management problem.

The treatment of bleeding varices resulting from portal hypertension may be broadly split into three stages:

Resuscitation. When the patient presents with bleeding varices, it is important that volume is repleted swiftly. Blood transfusions are frequently required but caution must be exercised in avoiding fluid overload, otherwise further bleeding may be provoked. Artificial plasma expanders may be used, such as modified gelatin solution, e.g. Haemaccel. It is important to avoid crystalloid fluids containing sodium chloride as this may aggravate fluid retention in the patient with liver disease. After the initial resuscitation the site of bleeding should be identified using endoscopy. A typical management strategy is outlined in Figure 13.7.

Acute drug treatment. Intravenous supplementation with phytomenadione is routinely carried out (20 mg twice a day up to four to six doses). If the varices do not stop bleeding spontaneously, attempts to stop the bleeding may be performed using balloon tamponade with a 'Linton' tube or Sengstaken–Blakemore tube or alternatively by using vasoconstrictor drugs.

Vasopressin has been used for many years to control bleeding from varices by lowering the pressure in the portal system as a result of vasoconstriction of splanchnic circulation. However, the drug has a very short half-life (10 to 20 minutes) and must be given by continuous infusion. Problems may arise with vasopressin due to general vasoconstriction which may result in cardiac ischaemia. To offset the latter effect, studies have been performed using nitrate therapy (administered sublingually as GTN, or topically) in addition to the vasopressin. Terlipressin is now available for use at a dose of 4 mg intravenous bolus, followed by 1 to 2 mg every 6 hours. Terlipressin is an inactive pro-drug which is slowly broken down in the body to lypressin, which has similar pharmacological actions to vasopressin. Other advantages of terlipressin are that it is reported to cause less cardiac ischaemia and less fluid retention. The mainstay of treatment in the acute phase after varices have bled is by sclerotherapy of the varices by endoscopic procedure. Commonly used agents for sclerosing the varices are STD (1% sodium tetradecylsulphate or 5% ethanolamine oleate). Sclerotherapy is useful in the acute emergency phase to stop variceal bleeds. Regular sclerotherapy sessions also prevent further variceal bleeds in the long term and will lead to the obliteration of the varices over a period of weeks to months.

Drugs commonly used to treat portal hypertension are summarized in Table 13.4.

Further treatment. Additional therapy may include antacids, which prevent gastric acid aggravating the condition and possibly causing varices to bleed, and drugs which aim to reduce portal blood pressure. Histamine H_2 antagonists are also frequently given to prevent further stress ulcers forming and prevent varices from rebleeding. Both cimetidine and ranitidine must be used with caution since there is an increased risk of confusion which may complicate a diagnosis of encephalopathy. Ranitidine is used in preference to cimetidine because it is less likely to be involved in interactions with concurrent therapy. There is increasing evidence to suggest that sucralfate (1 g four times a day) may be

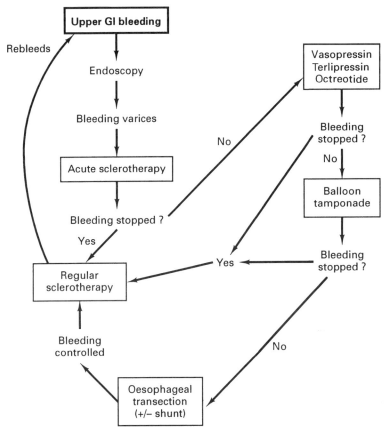

Fig. 13.7 Suggested flow chart for management of a variceal bleed. In practice, if a torrential bleed occurs, then the vasopressor drugs are used simultaneously with the insertion of a balloon tamponade. If a torrential bleed occurs in a patient known to have previously bled from varices, then the vasopressor drugs and balloon tamponade are used initially to prevent the patient exsanguinating, thus enabling endoscopy to be performed once the patient becomes stable.

useful in preventing stress ulcers. Omeprazole has recently been used with some success both orally and intravenously in the acute and further management of patients with bleeding varices who have extensive ulceration. In the past, somatostatin has been successfully given as an infusion to patients with bleeding varices. More recently a longer-acting analogue of somatostatin, octreotide, has been used. Octreotide appears to be at least as effective as other vasoactive agents in the management of bleeding varices and is less expensive. The optimal dose and duration of treatment is still unclear. However, treatment with 25 to 50 micrograms per hour for up to 5 days has been reported.

Early work was carried out in the 1980s on the use of beta-adrenoreceptor blockers to treat bleeding oesophageal varices by reducing portal pressure. Subsequent workers have had mixed success at further confirming the value of beta-adreno-receptor blockers in stopping bleeding varices or preventing them from rebleeding. Some clinicians are reluctant to use beta-adreno-receptor blockers as they reduce the cardiovascular response to blood loss and may mask the sympathetic signs of low blood pressure.

Fluid retention

Ascites is one of the most important conse-

Table 13.4   Drugs commonly used in the management of portal hypertension

Drug	Indication	Dose	Advantage	Disadvantage	Significant interactions
Vasopressin	Upper GI bleeding secondary to variceal haemorrhage	20 units over 15 min then 0.4 units/min until bleeding controlled, for up to 24 h	Reduces bleeding from varices by causing vasoconstriction action Effects can be stopped easily by stopping infusion	Short $t_{\frac{1}{2}}$; must be given by infusion Stomach cramps, belching, diarrhoea, nausea, increased sweating Caution in heart disease, asthma, epilepsy, migraine Can cause fluid retention due to ADH effects Profound hyponatraemia can occur	
Terlipressin	Upper GI bleeding secondary to variceal haemorrhage	4 mg i.v. bolus then 1–2 mg every 4–6 h until bleeding controlled, for up to 72 h	Longer duration of action and milder side effect than vasopressin Intermittent dosage	Longer duration of side effects than vasopressin More expensive than vasopressin	
Ranitidine	Prophylaxis and treatment of upper gastrointestinal erosions and ulceration	150–300 mg 12-hourly	No gynaecomastia or interference with hepatic drug metabolism compared to cimetidine	May increase confusion in liver cell failure	
Omeprazole	Treatment of severe ulceration, particularly post-sclerotherapy ulceration	40 mg/day oral or i.v.	Complete acid suppression	Long-term safety profile unclear	Effects of warfarin and phenytoin enhanced

quences of altered portal haemodynamics and liver cell failure in patients with chronic liver disease. Different studies vary in the figures reported but a 1-year survival probability for patients admitted for the treatment of ascites is approximately 50%. In patients with chronic liver disease and altered haemodynamics, the development of functional renal failure (hepato-renal syndrome) is an important factor which contributes towards fluid retention.

Since the 1960s the mainstay of treatment for fluid retention in patients with liver disease has been the use of diuretics with a low salt diet. A summary of the different diuretics that may be used for the treatment of ascites may be seen in Table 13.5.

There are problems with the use of diuretics in these patients with chronic liver disease. The incidence of side effects is high and approximately 20% of patients respond poorly to diuretic therapy. Some patients may only have slight ascites and fall into a category of 'easy responders'. These patients often respond to bed rest and a reduced salt diet.

Spironolactone has a central role in the diuretic management of patients with ascites. The starting dose is usually 100 or 200 mg spironolactone increased or decreased by increments of 100 mg every 4 days up to a maximum of 1.5 g per day. Frequently a loop diuretic, such as frusemide, is added and the doses titrated according to the weight loss and the effect on electrolyte levels. Patients can usually tolerate losing 1 kg of weight per day if peripheral oedema is present as well as ascites. However, if peripheral oedema is absent attempts are made

Table 13.5 Drugs commonly used in the management of fluid retention

Drug	Indication	Daily dose	Advantage	Disadvantage	Significant interactions
Spironolactone	Fluid retention	100 mg – 1 g	Aldosterone antagonist Slow diuresis	Painful gynaecomastia Variable bioavailability Hyperkalaemia	Potassium-containing preparations, ACE inhibitors and NSAIDs
Frusemide	Fluid retention	40–80 mg	Rapid diuresis, sodium excretion	Nephrotoxic Dehydration Hypokalaemia Hyponatraemia Caution in prerenal uraemia	Aminoglycosides
Bumetanide	Fluid retention	1–2 mg	Rapid diuresis, sodium excretion ?Better oral bioavailability than frusemide	Nephrotoxic Dehydration Hypokalaemia Hyponatraemia Caution in prerenal uraemia	Nephrotoxicity with NSAIDs Hyponatraemic effects with other diuretics
Amiloride	Mild fluid retention	5–10 mg	As K$^+$-sparing agent or weak diuretic if spironolactone contra-indicated	Not potent	As spironolactone
Metolazone	Unresponsive fluid retention	5 mg stat. day Repeated daily as required with caution	Useful in inducing diuresis in resistant cases	Severe electrolyte disturbances Hyponatraemia/ hypokalaemia	Profound synergy with loop diuretics

to limit the weight loss to approximately 0.5 kg per day. If further diuresis is required, a small intermittent dose of metolazone may be added to the spironolactone and the loop diuretic (thiazide diuretics such as bendrofluazide are not particularly effective in fluid retention with liver disease). Spironolactone has a greater natriuretic effect than frusemide in cirrhotic patients, whilst the reverse is true in non-cirrhotics. If loop diuretics are used alone in patients with ascites, only 50% of patients will respond adequately. The combined use of spironolactone and frusemide results in an increased natriuresis compared with either drug used alone. An important adjunct to the use of diuretics in patients with ascites is to give salt-poor albumin infusions which may increase the diuresis. Complications which may arise as a result of the use of diuretics include dehydration, hyponatraemia or hyperkalaemia. Electrolyte imbalance can also contribute to the development of encephalopathy.

The use of non-steroidal anti-inflammatory drugs (NSAIDs) in patients with fluid retention and chronic liver disease must be avoided. All NSAIDs (including sulindac) reduce renal blood flow by interfering with prostaglandins and this reduces the diuretic and natriuretic effect of loop diuretics and spironolactone in cirrhotic patients.

One of the problems of managing patients with gross ascites who are taking diuretics is that it may take several weeks of hospital treatment to gain adequate control. It has recently been shown that this time can be reduced if the ascites is removed by paracentesis (draining of the fluid) and at the same time giving exogenous intravenous albumin. Approximately 4 litres of ascites is removed on alternate days and 40 g of salt-poor albumin given over 1 hour at the same time.

Spontaneous bacterial peritonitis (i.e. infected ascites) is a major problem which is under-reported due to the difficulty in culturing ascitic fluid. The ascites may become infected as a result of being removed by paracentesis, or being seeded with bacteria ('translocation') from other parts of the body, such as the bowel, which may be more permeable to bacteria secondary to portal hypertension. A total white cell count of more than 0.3×10^9 cells per litre of ascitic fluid and an absolute neutrophil count of more than 0.25×10^9 cells per litre is an indication that the ascites is almost certainly infected. Standard anaerobic and aerobic cultures should be taken at the same time. Aminoglycosides must be avoided in patients with chronic liver disease. Such patients are extremely prone to the nephrotoxic effects of aminoglycosides even if blood levels are carefully monitored. First line treatment may include intravenous ciprofloxacin, ampicillin and metronidazole for the first few days followed by a change to oral treatment as sensitivity tests become available.

Encephalopathy

In the presence of poor liver cell function nitrogenous compounds absorbed from the gastrointestinal tract can accumulate. These nitrogenous compounds are known to play a central role in the pathogenesis of portal-systemic encephalopathy. For many years ammonia was thought to be the causative agent although recent evidence has suggested that there is a poor correlation between blood levels and the degree of encephalopathy. The role of methionine and its metabolites has also been discounted for similar reasons. The causative nitrogenous factor remains unknown although there has been speculation implicating the altered metabolism of neurotransmitters such as gamma-aminobutyric acid (GABA), and the false neurotransmitter octopamine. Factors which may precipitate encephalopathy in the patient with liver disease include infection, fluid depletion, electrolyte imbalance and also CNS depressant drugs, such as benzodiazepines and opiates. Treatment for encephalopathy may be broadly looked at under the following headings.

Diet. Dietary protein intake should be limited to approximately 40 g of protein per day whilst at the same time making sure that the intake of carbohydrate is not less than 1600 kcal/day given either orally or intravenously. It also seems that vegetable protein is better tolerated than meat protein and may in fact improve the degree of drowsiness and confusion, particularly in patients with chronic encephalopathy. However severe protein restriction is only suitable for short-term treatment.

Antibiotics. Nitrogenous material from the bowel is formed by the action of bacteria on protein. Consequently one approach to the treatment of encephalopathy is to use a non-absorbable antibiotic, such as neomycin, to kill the bacteria which would normally break down the protein. In severe acute encephalopathy the neomycin may be given orally in doses of not more than 4 g per day (usually doses of 2 g per day being used), with additional rectal washouts of neomycin, using 4 g per washout once or twice per day for the first 48 hours. The spectrum of neomycin is fairly narrow in that it covers mainly staphylococci and also Gram-negative bacteria such as *Esch. coli*, *Klebsiella*, *Haemophilus*, and *Proteus*. Although the majority of neomycin is not absorbed from the gastrointestinal tract, approximately 4 to 8% is absorbed and dose reduction is required if there is any evidence of renal impairment. Metronidazole may be used as an alternative antibiotic.

Laxatives. The aim of treatment with laxatives is to increase the throughput of bowel contents, and the most appropriate laxative which is used to treat encephalopathy is lactulose. Lactulose is a disaccharide which is broken down by colonic saccharophytic bacteria to form ultimately lactic and acetic acids. Lactulose works as an osmotic laxative and, in addition, the acidification of colonic contents by lactic and acetic acid leads to ionization of nitrogenous products with a consequent reduction in their absorption from the gastrointestinal tract. The usual dose of lactulose is that which causes the formation of approximately two soft stools per day. The use of lactulose is not without problems in that certain patients are unable to tolerate its sweet and sickly taste, and it also causes significant abdominal discomfort and flatulence.

Drugs commonly used to treat encephalopathy are summarized in Table 13.6.

Amino acids and neurotransmitters. The use

Table 13.6 Drugs commonly used in the management of encephalopathy

Drug	Indication	Daily dose	Advantage	Disadvantage
Neomycin	Kill bowel bacteria	Max. 4 g orally	Effective in acute encephalopathy Useful long term at low dosage in chronic encephalopathy	May accumulate in renal insufficieny → toxicity Use may lead to malabsorption
Metronidazole	Kill bowel bacteria	1.2 g orally	Useful alternative to neomycin	Nausea
Lactulose	Osmotic laxative	40–80 ml (sufficient to produce 2 soft stools/day)	Effective in acute encephalopathy Useful long term in chronic encephalopathy	Patient compliance poor due to unpalatability Causes flatulence and abdominal discomfort

of branched chain amino acids to treat encephalopathy will be considered in the section on nutrition.

It has been postulated that there is an imbalance in patients with encephalopathy between levels of 5-hydroxytryptamine and dopamine in the brain. The imbalance is thought to be in favour of the 5-hydroxytryptamine and consequently efforts have been made over the years to redress the balance by increasing dopamine receptor stimulation. This has been attempted by administering levodopa in large doses with or without dopa-decarboxylase inhibitors and also by using bromocriptine, in large doses. These agents tend to be used as a last resort in patients with unresponsive chronic encephalopathy. Flumazenil, a benzodiazepine antagonist which works by blocking GABA receptors, has been described in case reports as being of some use in alleviating acute and chronic encephalopathy. This adds weight to the theory that GABA may be an important factor in the formation of encephalopathy.

In addition to drugs such as benzodiazepines and opioids, which may precipitate a patient into encephalopathy, other important precipitating factors are constipation and bleeding, both of which increase the amount of nitrogenous matter which is produced by bacteria from protein in the bowel.

Nutrition

The nutritional requirements of patients with liver disease vary according to the stage of the disease and the underlying aetiology. Most patients in the later stages of decompensated liver disease have nutritional problems. Patients with compensated alcoholic liver disease also have nutritional problems which are managed according to whether a hepatitic or cirrhotic picture prevails.

Acute alcoholic hepatitis. In patients with acute alcoholic hepatitis, parenteral nutrition using amino acids and glucose is safe and may improve albumin levels although it is unclear if this latter effect is simply associated with an enforced period of abstinence from alcohol. Theoretically the aromatic amino acids given in parenteral feeds may lead to encephalopathy but this has not been shown in practice. Nasogastric feeds which give patients more than 80 g of protein each day have also been successfully used, again with no development of portal systemic encephalopathy.

Cirrhosis. Enteral and parenteral nutrition has been widely used in the management of malnourished patients with alcoholic liver disease and cirrhosis. Attention has focused on the possible contribution of feeds to the development of encephalopathy and the role of aromatic amino acids in particular. The supplement of patients' diets with branched chain amino acids whilst at the same time reducing aromatic amino acids has been tried without success.

Vitamin supplementation is important in alcoholic liver disease. There is a specific need for urgent thiamine supplementation in patients with suspected Wernicke–Korsakoff syndrome, particularly if receiving dextrose solutions. Thiamine is a cofactor in glucose metabolism and in deficiency states Wernicke's encephalopathy can be precipitated by a glucose load. Because of possible allergic reactions to multivitamin injections, routine supplementation is usually carried out with oral thiamine 100 to 300 mg per day after initial supplementation with parenteral vitamins. Folic acid is also often reduced in alcoholic liver disease patients and must be supplemented if required.

Patients with a cholestatic liver disease such as primary biliary cirrhosis may malabsorb fats due to the decreased secretion of bile salts into the bowel. It is therefore necessary for fat-soluble vitamin supplementation to be carried out in these patients: calciferol 100 000 units per month intramuscularly, and vitamin A 30 000 units per month intramuscularly can be used. Vitamin K is not routinely given unless the prothrombin time is raised and vitamin E is not necessarily given as a supplement although levels should routinely be checked.

THE PATIENT

The following section considers important aspects of patient monitoring and education. The four areas which patients or their relatives frequently complain of include itching, increased swelling of the abdomen and legs, pain and altered mental function.

Itching

Cause. Cholestatic liver disease.

Education. Cholestyramine is a mainstay of treatment; careful and repeated patient education is required. If prescribed granules, patients should be encouraged to incorporate them into various drinks or food as part of their normal diet (a useful handbook is available from the manufacturers). Health-care staff need reminding that cholestyramine dosage needs titrating and may take up to 7 days for any benefit to be appreciated. Although 'non-sedating' anti-histamines are usually prescribed as well, patients should be warned of possible sedative effects at first.

Increased swelling of abdomen and legs

Causes. Deteriorating liver cell function; infected ascites.

Education. Ensure diuretic tablets are taken regularly, check that patients are not drinking fluid excessively and check that they are complying with a low (40 mmol sodium) or 'no added' salt (70 to 100 mmol sodium) diet as appropriate. Review concurrent medication to exclude high-sodium-containing preparations (e.g. some antibiotic injections, antacids and effervescent preparations: NB some manufacturers replace sodium bicarbonate with potassium bicarbonate in effervescent formulations, but beware in patients on spironolactone). Daily or regular weighing is necessary to gauge progress. Regular blood tests are needed to avoid hyponatraemia and over-dehydration. If swelling is a result of alcoholic liver disease, ensure that the patient remains abstinent.

Infected ascitic fluid is usually a reflection of serious worsening of the underlying liver disease; long-term prognosis is extremely poor. Care must be taken with ototoxic and nephrotoxic antibiotics, e.g. vancomycin. Aminoglycosides must be avoided.

Pain

Causes. Abdominal distension; bone pain; muscle cramps; headaches; general aches and pains.

Education. Bone and muscle pain is common in these patients; vitamin D deficiency can occur due to malnutrition or malabsorption of fats. If appropriate give calcium (low-sodium-containing) supplementation. If patient complains of muscle cramps, try quinine sulphate (200 mg at bedtime) and correct any electrolyte imbalance. Headaches and other generalized aches and pains often require simple analgesia. Paracetamol may be used cautiously as required rather than as a regular prescription. Nefopam (30 to 60 mg three times daily) may be tried if the pain does not settle with paracetamol.

Aspirin and non-steroidal anti-inflammatory agents must not be used, due to fluid retention and gastric irritation. Opioids have prolonged and enhanced effects and should only be used if absolutely essential, e.g. crush fractures of vertebrae or after surgery. If the patient has terminal cancer, the usual palliation of pain and symptoms is indicated. Co-proxamol is used with caution as the dextropropoxyphene component can cause constipation and may precipitate/ aggravate encephalopathy.

Patients should be advised not to purchase any over-the-counter medication unless specifically instructed to do so by their doctor. Patients should be counselled to tolerate aches and pains rather than rely on medication.

Altered mental function

Confusion and drowsiness

Causes. Infection, bleeding into the gut and constipation commonly cause encephalopathy.

Education. Patients should be educated to see their physician as soon as they start to develop signs of urinary or chest infection or develop fever or rigors. If bleeding occurs, immediate attendance at hospital is advised. They should be counselled on how to regulate laxatives to produce one or two loose, formed stools per day. High fibre diets help and lactulose may be made more palatable by mixing with fruit juice, puddings or porridge.

Insomnia

Causes. Itching, cramps, early encephalopathy or depression.

Education. Depression is common, and may be severe: seek psychiatric advice. Major neuroleptic agents should be avoided. Dothiepin or amitriptyline may be used if slight sedation is desirable. Patients should be counselled to expect an altered sleep pattern; sedatives of any kind (including herbal sedatives) must be avoided.

Agitation

Causes. Electrolyte imbalance, acute or chronic encephalopathy and hypoglycaemia.

Education. Health professionals must be aware of the rapid deterioration that can occur in the patient's condition, and search for underlying causes. Benzodiazepines and major neuroleptic agents should not normally be used; however, chlormethiazole or haloperidol may be used cautiously to control a violent agitated patient.

Phenobarbitone may be useful as it is excreted unchanged renally.

LIVER TRANSPLANTATION AND IMMUNOSUPPRESSION

With the advent of effective immunosuppressive regimens, liver transplantation has now been accepted as the treatment of choice for many types of chronic liver disease. The survival rates for transplantation have improved substantially since cyclosporin became the first line immunosuppressive agent. The best survival results appear to be for patients with primary biliary cirrhosis in whom more than 80% survival at 1 year is claimed. It appears that once a patient's condition deteriorates with complications such as infected ascites, variceal bleeding and muscle wasting, the perioperative risks of transplantation increase so that the 1-year survival rate may only be 40 to 60%. Even in patients who have an uneventful clinical course following liver transplantion, side effects of immunosuppressive treatment are common and may be difficult to manage. New immunosuppressive agents are currently under investigation to replace cyclosporin.

Cyclosporin-related side effects

The major problem relates to the deterioration in renal function, with a relationship between increasing blood levels of cyclosporin and decreasing creatinine clearance. This appears to be partially reversible on stopping or reducing the drug. As the renal vasculature is affected by cyclosporin, systemic hypertension becomes a common finding, with over 80% of patients requiring antihypertensive therapy at 1 year. This is managed conventionally using diuretics, with the addition of beta-adrenoreceptor blockers required. Calcium channel antagonists are also effective, although their own side effects are enhanced and they may increase cyclosporin levels. A lower dose of calcium channel antagonist is recommended, and the dose of cyclosporin reduced depending on blood levels.

Hirsutism (overgrowth of body hair) is common in women taking cyclosporin and many women use depilatory creams for excessive facial hair. Less commonly a persistent coarse tremor can develop, and in the early stages when intravenous cyclosporin is given, neurological disturbances such as fits and confusion can occur. In some patients with severe renal impairment or resistant hypertension, cyclosporin may need to be withdrawn.

Steroid-related side effects

Depending on the immunosuppressive regimen, steroids are usually started at high dose (60 to 80 mg/day) and steadily reduced to an average of 10 to 20 mg over 6 months. Steroid-related side effects are therefore common within the first few months of transplantation. Elevation of blood glucose levels may require dietary restrictions, oral hypoglycaemic medication or even insulin. This tends to settle once the steroid dose is reduced. Excessive fat deposition on the body and face is common but this normally improves with reduction in dose. Cataracts are more frequent, especially if the patient has required a prolonged high dose secondary to rejection episodes. The additive effects of steroids, immobilization and pre-existing osteoporosis can lead to further bone loss and cause vertebral bone pain and even vertebral fractures. The skin becomes more fragile, with bruising and poor healing.

Azathioprine-related side effects

Azathioprine is often used as the third drug in an immunosuppressive regimen, so that the other drugs may be used in reduced dosage to try to prevent side effects. The major complications with azothioprine are thrombocytopenia (reduction in platelets) and leucopenia (reduction in white blood cells). Some patients are very sensitive to the drug, and are unable to tolerate even low doses without dropping their platelet and white cell counts. Hepatic toxicity is a well-recognized side effect of this drug.

Other drugs used in liver transplant recipients include methyl prednisolone, which is used as first line treatment for acute rejection episodes, usually in pulsed therapy, 500 mg daily for 3 days. If the rejection is not controlled with methyl prednisolone, then a 10-day course of OKT3 is used. This is a monoclonal antibody raised against CD3 white blood cells derived from mice. These cells regulate the rejection response. The side effects can be unpleasant for the patient with 'serum-sickness-like' reactions of fever and malaise; pulmonary oedema is a recognized complication if the patient is fluid overloaded at the start of therapy.

CASE STUDIES

CASE 13.1

A 30-year-old man with known alcoholic cirrhosis presents with a chest infection to casualty. He has been drinking one bottle of whisky a day for the last 6 months. The morning after admission he becomes confused and aggressive on the ward.

Q What treatment options are appropriate?

CASE 13.2

A 55-year-old woman with a 10-year history of autoimmune chronic active hepatitis with cirrhosis confirmed on liver biopsy, presents with a 7-day history of increasing central abdominal pain. She has required 400 mg/day spironolactone in order to adequately control her ascites over the last 2 years, but during the last 3 weeks the ascites has increased such that the abdominal wall has become tense. Her present drug treatment includes prednisolone 15 mg/day, and ibuprofen 200 mg b.d. for painful knees, in addition to spironolactone.

Q What therapeutic advice would you give on the management of this patient?

CASE 13.3

A 60-year-old woman with primary biliary cirrhosis has been complaining of increasing backache over the last 3 months. Her general condition has deteriorated over the past year during which she has suffered from ascites, and variceal bleeds and short spells of encephalopathy. Her main complaint is of continuous back pain which disturbs her sleep.

Q How would you manage her backache?

CASE 13.4

A 65-year-old man who is a long-standing patient on the liver unit is admitted from home with significantly increased encephalopathy. The patient has end-stage cryptogenic cirrhosis and has been suffering from chronic encephalopathy for the last 9 months. His admissions to hospital have been increasing due to his wife's inability to cope with his deteriorating mental function and confusion.

Q How would you advise the medical staff and family regarding the optimum treatment for the chronic encephalopathy?

ANSWERS TO CASE STUDIES

CASE 13.1

A a. Once other causes of the confusional state have been eliminated, treat for alcohol withdrawal state. Withdrawal reactions can occur within 6 hours of the last alcohol ingestion. Delirium tremens (DT) can occur within 24 to 36 hours. In patients with cirrhosis, there will need to be a judicious use of sedative agents. The initial management of acute aggression, when a patient is at risk of harming himself or others, requires prompt sedation with intravenous or intramuscular diazepam, the minimum dose (using boluses of 5 to 10 mg) being used to regain control of the patient.

Thereafter intravenous chlormethiazole (0.8% in 500 ml) should be commenced initially as a bolus of 10 to 50 ml then titrating the dose between 0.5 and 4 ml per minute (approximately 7 to 60 drops per minute) using the absolute minimum possible. The dose is reduced rapidly and stopped as soon as possible. If the patient is not aggressive or too confused to take oral therapy, chlormethiazole 2 to 3 capsules four times a day may be started, rapidly tailing off over 5 to 7 days. It is important to note that although the half-life of intravenous chlormethiazole is not impaired in cirrhosis, the bioavailability of oral chlormethiazole is significantly increased because of impaired first-pass metabolism and necessitates a reduction in the dose administered. Chlormethiazole is also an addictive agent and should not be used for longer than necessary. Chlordiazepoxide is a useful alternative agent for oral sedation used by some centres. It is less addictive.

If hallucinations are a major feature of the illness, then intramuscular haloperidol 2 to 4 mg, 4- to 8-hourly can be used to control the patient.

b. The chest infection should be treated with appropriate antibiotic therapy.

c. The patient should be given adequate vitamin replacement therapy. This involves immediate high dose intravenous vitamins given slowly over 10 minutes to prevent flushing and anaphylactoid reactions. It is important that the parenteral route is used in a patient such as this in order to achieve rapid thiamine supplementation, and prevent the onset of Wernicke's encephalopathy.

Oral supplementation should be commenced in all patients with multivitamin tablets and thiamine tablets at a dose 100 to 300 mg per day. An intravenous preparation of thiamine is commercially available from St James's University Hospital, Leeds.

CASE 13.2

[A] There are four distinct diagnostic possibilities to be excluded in the case of the patient described who develops abdominal pain with increasing ascites. The therapeutic advice given will depend on the underlying problem.

a. In any patient on steroids, an intra-abdominal infection or perforation can be masked by steroids which will reduce the inflammatory response. A careful history may provide clues that the patient has suffered from dyspeptic symptoms prior to the onset of the pain, and the pain may have had a sudden onset. The fact that this patient has been on non-steroidal anti-inflammatory agents together with steroids must raise the possibility of a 'silent perforation'.

b. Spontaneous bacterial peritonitis is a recognized complication of chronic liver disease in any patient with ascites. The onset tends to be insidious. A common finding is that the ascites becomes more difficult to control. There may be little systemic evidence of infection, with a normal peripheral blood white cell count. The only way to exclude the possibility of bacterial peritonitis is to remove 20 to 30 ml of ascites, and obtain an urgent white cell count on the sample, together with microscopy, culture and Gram staining for bacteria. It is usual to treat any ascites which contains more than 0.25×10^9 neutrophil white cells per litre.

The specific antibiotics used will depend on the centre concerned but may include ciprofloxacin, recent generation cephalosporins and vancomycin. Aminoglycosides are generally avoided. Treatment should be for at least 10 days.

c. Increasing ascites associated with abdominal pain may occur when there is a thrombosis of the portal venous system. Although this can occur during any stage of chronic liver disease it is more common when the flow of blood in the portal vein is reduced due to increased resistance to flow through the liver secondary to scarring in the liver substance.

d. If the patient has omitted to take her medication for any reason or the bioavailability of the diuretic is reduced, then ascites can rapidly accumulate. Accumulation of ascitic fluid itself may cause abdominal pain and discomfort due to stretching of the abdominal wall.

CASE 13.3

[A] a. Back pain secondary to osteopenia-related vertebral body fractures is common in cholestatic liver diseases especially primary biliary cirrhosis (PBC). This is perhaps due to the fact that most patients with PBC are postmenopausal females in their late fifties where bone thinning is likely, secondary to both menopausal and liver changes. Once the diagnosis has been confirmed and osteomalacia excluded, the patient should be counselled that the bone pain is chronic, tends to be intermittent, and takes several months to settle after each new fracture. Bed rest is useful in the initial acute situation, but prolonged bed rest can accelerate bone loss. The patient should be advised to take adequate calcium supplementation to provide approximately 1 to 1.5 g/day in addition to her normal diet. Various drug therapies have been tried for postmenopausal osteopenia but none have been validated in liver disease. Hormone replacement therapy is contra-indicated in liver cirrhosis. The patient should be encouraged to remain as mobile as possible, and given physiotherapy if appropriate.

b. Pain relief can be very difficult. Start with simple analgesics such as paracetamol and progress to co-proxamol. Dihydrocodeine may produce encephalopathy, as may other opioid analgesics. Nefopam has been used in chronic liver disease with good pain relief. Occasionally in the acute stages with very severe pain, morphine is used, at the minimum required dose for the shortest duration. If potent analgesics are used, increased laxatives are needed to prevent encephalopathy developing due to constipation.

Other treatments which occasionally work include transcutaneous electrical nerve stimulation (TENS). Injection of long-acting local anaesthetics under radiological guidance has helped in carefully selected cases.

c. Non-steroidal anti-inflammatory agents have to be used with extreme caution, particularly in patients with varices or renal impairment. There may be a role for mucosal protective agents such as misoprostol or sucralfate if non-steroidal anti-inflammatory agents have to be used. If the pain is a problem at night, then a long-acting non-steroidal taken only in the evening may help in addition to regular simple analgesia.

CASE 13.4

A a. Careful drug history must be obtained to ensure that drugs which increase mental confusion have not been inadvertently prescribed or bought over the counter, e.g. benzodiazepines, opiate-containing painkillers.

b. Obtain a dietary history to ensure low protein intake of less than 40 g per day. If the patient is confused despite low protein intake, consider changing to a diet of vegetable-derived protein to reduce nitrogenous load to bowels. This strategy will also increase roughage and hence faecal bulk which is beneficial if constipated. If there is no benefit from vegetarian protein, consider the use of branched chain amino acids. This latter approach is controversial with many studies showing no benefit and patients often find oral branched chain amino acid products very unpalatable.

c. If renal function is well preserved, try increasing oral neomycin up to 4 g per day in divided doses to reduce bacterial flora in the large bowel; metronidazole may be a useful alternative.

d. Close attention should be paid to effective colonic emptying in all patients with chronic encephalopathy. Use sufficient lactulose (up to 20 ml four times daily) to produce approximately two soft stools per day. If the patient remains constipated or remains encephalopathic despite loose stools, daily enemas, with or without 2 g neomycin added, can be performed at home by the district nurse, wife or carer.

e. If the patient still remains encephalopathic, bromocriptine or levodopa may be considered with a view to redressing a theoretical cerebral imbalance in the ratio of 5-hydroxytryptamine to dopamine.

In a few cases, it is not possible to produce any sustained improvement in mental function simply because the patient has reached an end stage of the disease process whereby there is insufficient functioning liver cell mass to prevent encephalopathy. These patients should be considered as terminally ill and treated symptomatically to keep them as comfortable as possible.

ACKNOWLEDGEMENT

The authors would like to thank Professor Losowsky and Dr J. Wyatt (St James's University Hospital, Leeds) for the loan of photographs used in this chapter.

BIBLIOGRAPHY

Bass N M, Williams R L. Guide to drug dosage in liver disease. Clinical Pharmacokinetics 1988; 15: 396–420

Fraser C L, Arieff A I. Hepatic encephalopathy. New England Journal of Medicine 1985; 313(14): 865–873

George C F, George R H. The liver and response to drugs. In: Wright R et al (eds) Liver and biliary disease, 2nd edn. London: Baillière Tindall 1985

Henderson J M. A perspective for the management of variceal bleeding. British Journal of Surgery 1989; 76: 323–324

McIntyre N et al (eds). Oxford textbook of clinical hepatology (Volumes I and II). Oxford: Oxford University Press 1991

Rocco V K, Ware A J. Cirrhotic ascites; pathophysiology, diagnosis and management. Annals of Internal Medicine 1986; 105: 573–585

Sherlock S. Landmarks in viral hepatitis. Journal of the American Medical Association 1984; 252(3): 402–406

Sherlock S, Dooley J. Diseases of the liver and biliary system, 9th edn. Oxford: Blackwell Scientific Publications 1993

Timbrell J A. Drug hepatotoxicity. British Journal of Clinical Pharmacology 1983; 15: 3–14

Chapter 14

Acute renal failure

A. Harper

Acute renal failure (ARF) is defined as a sudden decline in renal function leading to an increase in serum concentrations of urea, creatinine and other substances. This process occurs over a period of days, is often reversible or self-limiting, but may result in death. When such a decline in renal function occurs in patients with pre-existing renal impairment this condition is called acute on chronic renal failure.

CLASSIFICATION AND CAUSES

Renal function fails abruptly in a bewildering variety of clinical situations which lack any common clinical pattern. This renders it difficult to discuss causation generally. Nevertheless, it is diagnostically useful to classify the condition into prerenal, intrarenal and postrenal forms.

Prerenal ARF may be caused by any condition which reduces renal perfusion and thereby results in renal ischaemia. This in turn may lead to acute tubular necrosis. Contributing factors are as follows:

1. Decreased extracellular fluid volume caused by excessive sodium and water loss from the skin, urinary tract or gastrointestinal tract. Excessive loss through the skin by sweating occurs in hot climates and is rare in the UK, but can occur after extensive burns. Gastro-intestinal losses are associated with vomiting or diarrhoea whilst urinary tract losses often result from excessive diuretic therapy but may

also occur with the osmotic diuresis caused by hyperglycaemia and glycosuria in a diabetic patient.

2. Decreased effective plasma volume caused by a significant haemorrhage or by septicaemia in which the vascular bed is dilated thereby reducing the circulating volume.

3. Decreased cardiac output resulting from acute myocardial infarction or bilateral cardiac failure.

4. Renal hypoperfusion which may be produced by drugs. The three groups most commonly implicated are:

a. Excessive diuretic therapy which has already been mentioned.

b. Non-steroidal anti-inflammatory drugs (NSAIDs). These cause renal damage and ARF by inhibiting prostaglandin synthesis in the kidney, particularly prostaglandins E_2, D_2 and I_2 (prostacyclin). These prostaglandins are all potent vasodilators and consequently produce an increase in blood flow to the glomerulus and the medulla. In normal circumstances they do not play a large part in the maintenance of the renal circulation. However, increased amounts of vasoconstrictor substances such as angiotensin II or antidiuretic hormone in the blood occur in a variety of clinical conditions such as volume depletion, congestive cardiac failure or hepatic cirrhosis associated with ascites. These may render the patient reliant on the release of vasodilatory prostaglandins for the maintenance of renal blood flow. In these circumstances inhibition of prostaglandin synthesis may cause unopposed arteriolar vasoconstriction leading to renal hypoperfusion.

c. Angiotensin converting enzyme (ACE) inhibitors may also produce a reduction in renal function. This they do by preventing the angiotensin II mediated vasoconstriction of the efferent glomerular arteriole, which contributes to the high pressure gradient across the glomerulus. This problem is important only in patients with renal vascular disease, particularly those with bilateral stenoses, and is consequently rare.

Intrarenal ARF. Any form of damage to renal infrastructure may result in ARF. The condition may be subclassified according to which structure is primarily affected.

1. The commonest form of intrarenal damage, and indeed the classic form of ARF is acute tubular necrosis (ATN), which results from direct nephrotoxic damage to the tubule. The high metabolic activity of the proximal tubule renders it particularly vulnerable to ischaemia and toxins. The most frequent cause is renal hypoperfusion (see above and Fig. 14.1). ATN may also be caused by, or compounded by, a wide variety of potentially nephrotoxic drugs including aminoglycoside antibiotics, cyclosporin and radiographic contrast media.

2. Interstitial damage (interstitial nephritis) is also a hypersensitivity reaction to nephrotoxins with inflammation affecting those cells lying between the nephrons. There is usually secondary involvement of the tubules. Drugs which have been shown to be responsible antigens include penicillins (particularly methicillin), cephalosporins, allopurinol and azathioprine.

3. Glomerular lesions (glomerulonephritis)

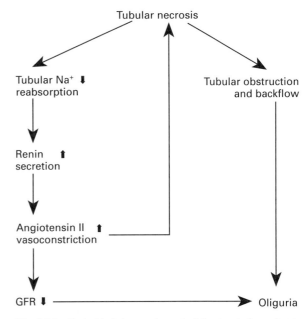

Fig. 14.1 Probable intrarenal events following ischaemic or nephrotoxic tubular damage.

are thought to be caused by the passive trapping of immune complexes in the glomerular tuft eliciting an inflammatory response. The antigens responsible for the immune complexes may be exogenous, precipitating a hypersensitivity reaction, or endogenous, resulting in an autoimmune condition. Specific aetiological factors can rarely be identified, although some drugs have been implicated including gold, penicillamine and phenytoin. Glomerulonephritis is a relatively rare cause of ARF. There are numerous other causes of ARF, including acute pyelonephritis with or without septicaemia, and vasculitis.

Postrenal ARF. Postrenal damage results from urinary tract obstruction. Causes include urinary stones, neoplasm, blood clots and even benign prostatic hypertrophy. Drug-induced causes of this condition are extremely rare.

DIAGNOSIS, INVESTIGATIONS AND MONITORING

In hospitalized patients, ARF is usually diagnosed incidentally, often by the detection of elevated serum creatinine or urea or by a decreased urine output including oliguria.

Creatinine is a by-product of normal muscle metabolism and is formed at a rate proportional to the mass of muscle. It is freely filtered by the glomerulus with little secretion or reabsorption by the tubule. When muscle mass is stable, any change in serum creatinine reflects a change in its clearance by filtration. Consequently, measurement of the creatinine clearance gives an estimate of the glomerular filtration rate (GFR). The ideal method of calculating creatinine clearance (CrCl) is by performing an accurate collection of urine over 24 hours and taking a serum sample midway through this period. The following equation may then be used:

$$CrCl = \frac{U \times V}{S}$$

where U = urine creatinine concentration (μmol/L); V = urine flow rate (ml/min); S = serum creatinine concentration (μmol/L).

A quicker method is to measure the serum creatinine concentration and collect those patient factors affecting the mass of muscle including age, sex and weight (preferably ideal body weight). This allows an estimation of creatinine clearance to be made from average population data. The equation of Cockroft & Gault is a useful way of making such an estimation:

$$CrCl = \frac{F \times (140 - Age\ (yr)) \times Weight\ (kg)}{Serum\ creatinine\ (\mu mol/L)}$$

where F = 1.04 (females) or 1.23 (males).

Assuming the normal creatinine clearance is 120 ml/minute, renal impairment can be classified as shown in Table 14.1.

Urea is commonly used to assess renal function. However, its production rate is considerably more variable than that of creatinine and fluctuates throughout the day in response to the protein content of the diet. It may also be elevated by dehydration or an increase in protein catabolism such as that which occurs in haemorrhage of the gastrointestinal tract or body tissues, severe infections, trauma (including surgery) and high dose steroid or tetracycline therapy. It is therefore an unreliable measure of renal function but it is often used as a crude test since it does give information on the patient's general condition and state of hydration. In the hospital situation, when the condition is detected incidentally, the cause(s) of the condition, e.g. fluid depletion, infection or the use of nephrotoxic drugs are often apparent on a close examination of the clinical history. In some patients, however, or in those

Table 14.1 Classification of renal impairment	
Degree of impairment	Glomerular filtration rate
Mild	50–20 ml/min
Moderate	20–10 ml/min
Severe	< 10 ml/min (patient is usually uraemic and will probably require dialysis)
End stage	< 5 ml/min (patient will die unless renal replacement therapy initiated)

occurring outside hospital practice, more extensive investigation is required to discover the cause. Although the majority of patients have acute tubular necrosis other rarer causes, e.g. rapidly progressive glomerulonephritis, acute nephritis or urinary tract obstruction, must be excluded, since, although the management of the ARF and its sequelae are common to all forms, longer-term treatment for the underlying cause may be required. Steps which should be taken include:

1. Full history including drug history.
2. Physical examination. Factors such as postural hypotension and diminished skin turgor would indicate a prerenal cause, while drug rashes or vasculitic lesions would render a renal cause more likely. Rectal and vaginal examination and the sizes of the bladder and kidneys would help permit the diagnosis of ARF due to a postrenal cause.
3. Examination of the urine. Anuria or crystalluria would indicate an obstructive uropathy. Patients with ATN usually have an abnormal urinary sediment with tubular epithelial cells and tubular casts. Glomerulonephritis or acute nephritis may produce both proteinuria and haematuria. Urine should also be sent for culture and sensitivity, and biochemical analyses such as urinary urea concentration, creatinine concentration and osmolarity are often useful.
4. Examination of the blood. Haematological tests such as white cell counts and erythrocyte sedimentation rate (ESR), biochemical tests such as serum creatinine, urea and albumin concentrations and serum osmolarity may be performed. Bacteriological and immunological tests are also of value.
5. Radiological studies including plain abdominal X-ray, renal arteriography and venography, ultrasonography and biopsy may be performed.

Various other parameters should be monitored through the course of ARF. Fluid balance charts are frequently used but they are often inaccurate and should not be relied upon exclusively. Records of daily weight are more reliable but are dependent on the mobility of the patient. Central venous pressure is of value in assessing circulating volume. The normal range is 10 to 15 cm of water. Serum electrolytes including potassium, bicarbonate, calcium, phosphate and the acid–base balance should similarly be monitored.

CLINICAL MANIFESTATIONS

The clinical signs and symptoms of ARF are often vague and nonspecific and the diagnosis is often made as a result of incidental findings. Some signs and symptoms of the precipitating condition may be present, for example patients in whom the ARF is due to volume depletion may exhibit tachycardia, postural hypotension, reduced skin turgor, and cold extremities. However, the commonest sign found in ARF is oliguria. Oliguria is the production of a urine volume of 200 to 400 ml in 24 hours, a volume in which the kidney is unable to concentrate the urine sufficiently to excrete the products of metabolism. This inevitably leads to elevation in serum urea and creatinine and diagnosis is often made on routine blood test results. Other substances which are normally renally excreted are similarly elevated in ARF including potassium ions and hydrogen ions (the latter causing acidosis). Other electrolyte disturbances which may occur include hypocalcaemia and hyperphosphataemia. Such an accumulation of substances, the classic example being urea, leads to uraemia, which implies not only the actual presence of excess urea and other metabolites in the blood but the variety of signs and symptoms associated with renal failure. These include nausea, vomiting, diarrhoea, gastrointestinal haemorrhage, muscle cramps, predisposition to infection, drowsiness and a declining level of consciousness. Pulmonary and/or systemic oedema is not an uncommon finding in ARF, caused by a normal or increased fluid intake, either orally or intravenously, in the presence of oliguria.

COURSE AND PROGNOSIS

The course of ARF may be divided into two phases. The first is the oliguric phase in which uraemia and hyperkalaemia inevitably occur unless adequate management is provided. The oliguric phase is usually no longer than 7 to 14 days but may last for 6 weeks. If the patient does not expire in this period, he or she will enter the second phase which is characterized by a urine volume which rises over a few days to several litres per day. This, the diuretic phase, lasts for up to 7 days and corresponds to the recommencement of tubular function. Patients who survive into this phase have a relatively good prognosis. Recovery of renal function takes place slowly over the following months although the GFR rarely returns completely to its initial level. The elderly recover renal function more slowly and less completely.

The mortality of ARF varies according to the cause but overall is about 50%. Death due to uraemia and hyperkalaemia is rare now; the major causes are septicaemia and to a lesser extent gastrointestinal haemorrhage. The high circulating levels of uraemic toxins which occur in ARF resulting in general debility, as well as the number of invasive procedures which may be necessary, such as bladder catheters and intravenous lines, render such patients prone to infection and septicaemia. Uraemic gastrointestinal haemorrhage is a recognized consequence of acute renal failure probably as a result of reduced mucosal cell turnover. Death is more common in patients aged over 60 years.

TREATMENT

The aim of medical treatment of ARF is to keep the patient alive long enough for the kidneys to recover their function. Treatment of ARF depends on a rapid diagnosis. If the underlying acute deterioration in renal function is detected early enough it is often possible to prevent the development of true ARF. If the condition is advanced, however, the therapy consists mainly of monitoring for the constellation of metabolic, fluid and electrolyte disturbances and treating appropriately. The following discussion will deal with the management of post-ischaemic ATN and the treatment of the sequelae which are common to all forms of ARF.

Early management

Initial treatment should consist of the rapid correction of fluid and electrolyte balance. A diagnosis of acute deterioration of renal function due to renal under-perfusion carries with it the implication that restoration of renal perfusion will reverse the renal impairment. Sodium chloride 0.9% is an appropriate choice of i.v. fluid since it replaces both water and sodium ions in a concentration approximately equal to serum. The effect of fluid replacement on urine flow and, whenever possible, central venous pressure should be carefully monitored. Although the measurement of central venous pressure carries the risks of any invasive procedure, it provides the best guide to the degree of fluid deficit and reduces the risk of pulmonary oedema by over-rapid transfusion. It should not be allowed to rise above the normal range of 10 to 15 cm of water. If the kidneys do not respond to replacement therapy other measures such as treatment with loop diuretics, mannitol and dopamine may be used.

Loop diuretics, as well as producing substantial diuresis, have been shown to increase renal blood flow, probably by stimulating the release of renal prostaglandins (this haemodynamic effect can be inhibited by NSAIDs). It is thought that the use of loop diuretics may thereby help salvage renal tissue although there is little evidence to support this hypothesis. However, any increase in urine volume produced will simplify the future management of patients, reducing the risk of fluid overload and hypokalaemia. Any diuretic therapy should of course only be used after the circulating volume has been restored. Doses up to 1 g of frusemide should be given intravenously at a rate of not more than 4 mg/minute since higher infusion rates may cause transient deafness. The addition of metolazone orally may also be considered. Metolazone, which by itself is a weak thiazide diuretic, has been shown to act synergistically with loop diuretics to produce a more effective diuresis.

The rationale for using mannitol arises from the theory that tubular debris may contribute to the oliguria of ARF by causing mechanical obstruction, and the use of an osmotic diuretic may wash out the debris. A dose of 0.5 to 1.0 g/kg as a 10 to 20% infusion has been recommended. However, intravenous mannitol will, before producing a diuresis, cause a considerable increase in the extracellular fluid volume by attracting water from the intracellular fluid. This expansion of the extracellular volume is potentially dangerous for patients with cardiac failure especially if a diuresis is not produced. For this reason mannitol is now less widely used.

Dopamine at low doses, e.g. 1 to 5 microgram/kg/minute, has a vasodilator effect in the kidney. At slightly higher doses, e.g. 5 to 20 microgram/kg/minute inotropic effects on the heart produce an increase in cardiac output. The dual effect increases renal perfusion. However, at higher doses still, e.g. 20 microgram/kg/minute and above, it also acts on alpha receptors causing peripheral and renal vasoconstriction resulting in impairment of renal perfusion. An initial dose of 2 microgram/kg/minute increasing to a maximum of 10 microgram/kg/minute with careful monitoring of central venous pressure is usually appropriate. Dobutamine does not produce renal vasodilation but may occasionally be added at an initial dose of 2.5 microgram/kg/minute for its inotropic effects.

Treatment of established acute renal failure

Uraemia

The symptoms of uraemia include nausea, vomiting and anorexia and are due mainly to the accumulation of substances, primarily urea, which occurs in renal failure. To reduce these symptoms it is consequently important to decrease protein intake but provide sufficient nutrition to prevent protein catabolism. The diet should provide all the essential amino acids in a total protein intake of about 40 g per day. A higher intake of protein, by exceeding the body's basic requirements, permits its use as an energy source resulting in increases in blood urea concentrations; further reduction in protein intake brings about endogenous protein catabolism and again causes blood urea to increase. Fat and carbohydrate should also be given to maintain a high energy intake of about 2000 to 3000 kcalories per day, or more in hypercatabolic patients, as this will help to prevent protein catabolism and will promote anabolism. Since uraemia causes anorexia, nausea and vomiting, many severely ill patients are unable to tolerate a diet of any kind and in these cases total parenteral nutrition should be considered at an early stage.

Hyperkalaemia

This is a particular problem in ARF, not only because of reduced urinary excretion, but also because of release of potassium from cells. Particularly rapid rises in extracellular potassium are to be expected when there is tissue damage as in burns, crush injuries and sepsis. Acidosis aggravates the situation by provoking potassium leakage from healthy cells. The condition may be life-threatening by causing cardiac arrhythmias and if untreated may result in asystolic cardiac arrest. Emergency treatment is necessary if the serum potassium is above 7.0 mmol/L (normal range 3.5 to 5.0 mmol/L) or if there are the progressive changes in the electrocardiogram (ECG) associated with hyperkalaemia including tall, peaked T waves, reduced P waves with increased QRS complexes or the 'sine wave' appearance which often presages cardiac arrest. The emergency treatment consists of:

1. 10 to 30 ml (2.25 to 6.75 mmol) of calcium gluconate 10% intravenously over 5 to 10 minutes; this has a stabilizing effect on the myocardium but no effect on the serum potassium concentration. The effect is short-lived, but the dose can be repeated.

2. 10 to 20 units of soluble insulin plus 50 ml of 50% glucose. This stimulates potassium uptake into cells removing it from the plasma, the effect lasting for 2 to 3 hours.

3. Calcium resonium 15 g three or four times a day orally or by enema. This ion exchange resin binds potassium in the gastrointestinal tract, releasing calcium in exchange and is used to lower serum potassium over a period of hours or days. It is required because the effect

of insulin/glucose is only temporary. Resins may cause constipation which may be treated with lactulose 10 to 20 ml three times a day.

Acidosis

The inability of the kidney to excrete hydrogen ions may result in a metabolic acidosis which in itself is not a serious problem although it may contribute to hyperkalaemia. It may be treated orally with sodium bicarbonate 1 to 6 g/day in divided doses, or 50 to 100 mmol of bicarbonate ion (50 to 100 ml sodium bicarbonate 8.4%) intravenously may be used. If calcium gluconate is being used to treat hyperkalaemia, care should be taken not to mix it with the sodium bicarbonate as the resulting calcium bicarbonate forms an insoluble precipitate. If elevations in plasma sodium preclude the use of sodium bicarbonate, extreme acidosis (plasma bicarbonate of less than 10 mmol/L) is best treated by dialysis.

Hypocalcaemia

Calcium malabsorption, probably secondary to disordered vitamin D metabolism, often occurs in ARF. It usually remains asymptomatic as tetany of skeletal muscles or convulsions do not normally occur until serum concentrations are as low as 1.6 to 1.7 mmol/L. Should it become necessary, oral calcium supplementation with calcium gluconate or lactate is usually adequate and although vitamin D may be used to treat the hypocalcaemia of ARF, it rarely has to be added. Effervescent calcium tablets should be avoided as they invariably contain a high sodium or potassium load.

Hyperphosphataemia

Phosphate is normally excreted by the kidney and phosphate retention and hyperphosphataemia may occur in ARF, but usually only slightly and the condition rarely requires treatment. Should it become necessary, phosphate-binding agents may be used to retain phosphate ion in the gut. The most common agents are calcium carbonate with glycine tablets (Titralac) or aluminium hydroxide in the form of mixture or capsules (Aludrox). The former is the drug of choice because of the slight risk that aluminium may be absorbed from the gut and deposited in bones to give a severe form of fracturing bone disease. Other problems which may be encountered when aluminium is used as a phosphate binder are described in Chapter 15.

Infection

Because of their general debility, patients in ARF are prone to infection and septicaemia, and these can be a cause of death in this condition. Bladder catheters and intravenous lines should be used with care to reduce the chance of bacterial invasion. Leucocytosis is sometimes seen in ARF and does not necessarily imply infection; but any unexplained pyrexia must be immediately treated with antibiotic therapy, especially if accompanied by toxic symptoms such as disorientation or hypotensive episodes. Samples from blood, urine and any other material such as catheter tips should be sent for culture before antibiotic therapy is started, and that therapy should cover as wide a spectrum as possible until a causative organism is identified.

Other problems

Uraemic gastrointestinal erosions are a recognized consequence of ARF probably as a result of reduced mucosal cell turnover due to high circulating levels of uraemic toxins. H_2 receptor antagonists are effective in this condition; it is unlikely that any one would be more advantageous than another. Sucralfate would be an effective alternative.

Muscle cramps are common in patients with renal failure probably as a result of electrolyte imbalances. Patients are generally prescribed quinine salts 200 to 300 mg at night. The efficacy of this form of treatment is dubious but its use is firmly entrenched in common medical practice. Fortunately, at the doses used for this purpose, toxicity is not a problem, although quinine poisoning may be fatal. The dose of quinine does not require alteration in renal failure. Other alternatives have been suggested for the treatment of cramps including benzodiazepines such as clonazepam (0.5 to 1 mg at night) or calcium antagonists such as verapamil (120 mg at night).

Nutrition

There are two major constraints concerning the nutrition of patients with ARF:

- such patients are frequently anorexic, vomiting and too ill to eat
- the oliguria of renal failure limits the volume of enteral or parenteral nutrition which can be given safely.

The introduction of haemofiltration and the ease with which fluid may be removed makes total parenteral nutrition (TPN) possible, and in anorexic patients, desirable. Large volumes of fluid may be administered without producing fluid overload. Factors which should be considered when formulating a TPN regimen include fluid balance, calorie and protein requirements, electrolyte balance and requirements and vitamin and mineral requirements.

The basic calorie requirements are similar to those in a non-dialysed patient, although protein requirements may occasionally be increased, in haemodialysis and haemofiltration because of amino acid losses and in peritoneal dialysis because of plasma protein loss. Protein is usually supplied as 12 to 20 g/day of an essential amino acid formulation although requirements may vary. Similarly, although lipid emulsions may theoretically reduce the efficiency of haemofiltration, in practice their use does not have any noticeable effect. It is useful, however, to infuse TPN solutions into the blood as it is being returned to the body after haemofiltration or haemodialysis, thereby ensuring that it is available to the patient before being presented to the filter.

Electrolyte-free amino acid solutions should be used as they allow the addition of electrolytes as appropriate. Potassium and sodium requirements can be calculated on an individual basis

depending on serum levels. There is usually no need to try to normalize serum calcium and phosphate as they will stabilize with the appropriate therapy or, if necessary, with haemofiltration or dialysis.

Water-soluble vitamins are removed by dialysis and haemofiltration but the standard daily doses normally included in TPN fluids more than compensate for this. Magnesium and zinc supplementation may be required not only because tissue repair often increases requirements, but because they may be lost during dialysis or haemofiltration.

It is necessary to monitor the serum urea, creatinine and electrolytes daily in order to make the appropriate alterations in the nutritional support. Glucose should also be checked at least every 6 hours as patients in renal failure sometimes develop insulin resistance. The pH should be checked initially to see whether the addition of amino acid solutions is causing or aggravating metabolic acidosis. It is also worth checking calcium phosphate and albumin levels regularly in case intervention becomes necessary, and, when practical, daily weighing gives a useful guide to fluid balance.

Dialysis and haemofiltration

Dialysis or haemofiltration should be commenced in a patient with ARF when there is hyperkalaemia of above 7 mmol/L, increasing acidosis (pH < 7.1 or serum bicarbonate < 10 mmol/L), severe uraemic symptoms such as impaired consciousness, fluid overload with pulmonary oedema or any combination of the above which may threaten life. It would appear that the current trend in ARF is to introduce dialysis therapy early as complications and mortality are reduced if the serum urea is kept below 35 mmol/L.

There are traditionally two types of dialysis: haemodialysis and peritoneal dialysis. In both, the patient's blood is on one side of a semipermeable membrane, and a dialysate solution on the other, across which exchange of metabolites occurs. In haemodialysis, blood is diverted out of the body and passed through an artificial kidney (dialyser) and returned to the patient, while in peritoneal dialysis the fluid is run in and out of the patient's abdominal cavity and the peritoneum itself acts as the semipermeable membrane.

In haemodialysis (Fig. 14.2), blood is taken from an arterial line and heparinized. Alternatively, in patients at high risk of haemorrhage when heparinized, e.g. post-surgical patients, epoprostenol, a prostaglandin with a short plasma half-life of 2 to 3 minutes which inhibits platelet aggregation, may be used. The blood is then actively pumped through a dialyser and returned to the patient. The dialyser contains synthetic semipermeable membranes which allow the blood to come into close proximity with the dialysate in a countercurrent flow. Metabolites and excess electrolytes, particularly H^+ and K^+, pass from the blood to the dialysate, while sufficient Ca^{2+} is present in the dialysate to permit diffusion into the blood. By increasing the hydrostatic pressure of the blood, water can also be removed from the patient. Haemodialysis is usually performed two or three times a week and the duration of a single dialysis is usually about 4 hours. The disadvantages of haemodialysis include its dependence on expensive technology and the production of rapid fluid and electrolyte shifts which may be dangerous.

The principle of peritoneal dialysis, (Fig. 14.3) is identical to haemodialysis but the technique is simpler. A semi-rigid catheter is inserted into the abdominal cavity. 1 or 2 litres of warmed dialysate are run into the abdomen, left for a period usually of about 30 minutes and then run into a collecting bag. This may be done manually or by semi-automatic equipment. The procedure may be repeated up to 20 times a day, depending on the condition of the patient.

The capital cost of haemodialysis is considerable and it requires specially trained staff, so it is seldom undertaken outside a renal unit. It does, however, treat renal failure much more rapidly and is therefore essential in hypercatabolic renal failure where urea is produced faster than peritoneal dialysis can remove it; it can also be used in patients who have recently undergone abdominal surgery in whom peritoneal dialysis is ill-advised. Peritoneal dialysis, however, is relatively cheap and simple, does not require specially trained staff nor the facilities of a renal unit and is consequently more widespread. It does, however, have the disadvantages of being uncomfortable and tiring for the patient, producing a fairly high incidence of peritonitis and permitting protein loss, as albumin crosses the peritoneal membrane.

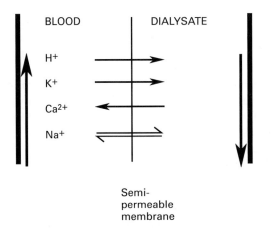

Fig. 14.2 Schematic diagram of blood and dialsate flow through dialyser. Long arrows show relative directions of flow of blood and dialysate. Short arrows represent electrolyte movements.

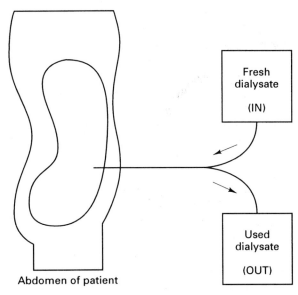

Fig. 14.3 Schematic diagram of peritoneal dialysis.

Haemofiltration has advantages over dialysis because of its simplicity of use, the fine control of fluid balance it offers, and its low cost. Haemofiltration is a relatively recent technique, the simplicity of which is ensuring its increasing use in the treatment of ARF. Usually arterial blood is obtained from the femoral artery, heparinized, passed over a semipermeable filter similar to the membrane used in haemodialysis, and returned to the femoral vein. The hydrostatic pressure of the blood drives a filtrate similar to interstitial fluid across the filter which can, if necessary, then be replaced with an appropriate fluid added to the blood on its return to the venous system. Various replacement fluids are marketed commercially for this purpose and contain electrolytes, including sodium, potassium, calcium, magnesium and chloride in differing quantities, thereby enabling an appropriate solution to be selected for the patient's needs. In addition to avoiding the expense and complexity of haemodialysis, this system enables continuous but gradual removal of fluid, thereby allowing very fine control of fluid balance in addition to electrolyte control and removal of metabolites. Very often this control of fluid balance facilitates the use of TPN. The advantages of haemofiltration over peritoneal dialysis make it likely that continuous haemofiltration, which is becoming increasingly available, will replace peritoneal dialysis as the most appropriate form of dialysis in the majority of patients with ARF.

Whether a drug is significantly removed by dialysis or haemofiltration is an important clinical problem. Drugs which are not removed will require dose reductions in order to avoid accumulation and possible toxic effects. Alternatively, drug removal may be significant enough to require a dosage supplement to ensure adequate efficacy. In general, since haemodialysis, peritoneal dialysis and haemofiltration depend on filtration, the process can be considered analogous to glomerular filtration; drug characteristics which favour clearance by the glomerulus are similar to those which favour clearance by dialysis or haemofiltration. These include:

- low molecular weight

- high water solubility
- low protein binding
- small volume of distribution
- low metabolic clearance.

Unfortunately a number of other factors inherent in the dialysis process itself affect clearance by dialysis. For dialysis, these include:

- duration of dialysis procedure
- rate of blood flow to dialyser
- surface area and porosity of dialyser
- composition and flow rate of dialysate

and for peritoneal dialysis they include:

- rate of peritoneal exchange
- concentration gradient between plasma and dialysate.

In view of the above, it is usually possible to predict whether a drug will be removed by dialysis, but it is very difficult to quantify the process except by direct measurement and this is rarely practical. It is not surprising, therefore, that a single, comprehensive guide to drug dosage in dialysis is non-existent. However, limited data for specific drugs are available in the literature while many drug manufacturers have information on the dialysability of their products and some now even include dosage recommendations on their data sheets. The most practical method, therefore, for treating patients undergoing dialysis, is to accumulate appropriate dosage guidelines for a number of drugs which are likely to be used in patients with renal impairment and use those drugs only.

Although drug clearance by haemofiltration is relatively more predictable than in dialysis, the fact that it is still a relatively new technique means that sufficient information to produce general guidelines is again not readily available. Therefore a similar set of individual drug dosage guidelines would be useful in practice.

Factors affecting use of drugs

How the drug to be used is absorbed, distributed, metabolized and excreted and whether it is intrinsically nephrotoxic are all factors which must be considered. The pharmacokinetic behaviour of many drugs may be altered in renal failure.

Absorption

Oral absorption in ARF may be reduced due to vomiting or diarrhoea, although this is of limited clinical significance.

Metabolism

The main hepatic pathways of drug metabolism appear to be unaffected in renal impairment. The kidney is also a site of metabolism in the body but the effect of renal impairment is clinically important in only two cases. The conversion of 25-hydroxycholecalciferol to 1,25-dihydroxycholecalciferol (the active form of vitamin D) occurs in the kidney and the process is impaired in renal failure. Patients in ARF occasionally require vitamin D replacement therapy and this should be in the form of 1α-hydroxycholecalciferol (alfacalcidol) or 1,25-dihydroxycholecalciferol (calcitriol). The latter is the drug of choice in the presence of concomitant hepatic impairment. Also the kidney is the major site of insulin metabolism and the insulin requirements of diabetic patients in ARF are often reduced.

Distribution

Changes in distribution may be altered by fluctuations in the degree of hydration or by alterations in tissue or serum protein binding. The presence of oedema or ascites would increase the volume of distribution while dehydration would reduce it. In practice these changes would only be significant if the volume of distribution were small, less than 50 litres. Serum protein binding may be reduced due either to protein loss or to alterations in binding due to uraemia. For certain highly bound drugs the net result of reduced protein binding is an increase in free drug so that care must be taken when interpreting serum concentrations of such drugs. Most analyses measure total serum concentration, i.e. free plus bound drug. A drug level may therefore fall within the accepted concentration range but still result in toxicity due to the increased proportion of free drug. However, this is usually only a temporary effect. Since the unbound drug is now available for elimination, its concentration will eventually return to its original value, albeit with a lower total bound and unbound level. The total drug concentration may therefore fall below the therapeutic range while therapeutic effectiveness is maintained. It must be noted that the time required for the new equilibrium to be established is about four or five elimination half-lives of the drug and this may be altered itself in renal failure. Some drugs which show reduced serum protein binding include diazepam, morphine, phenytoin, thyroxine, theophylline and warfarin. Tissue binding may also be affected, for example the displacement of digoxin from skeletal muscle binding sites by metabolic waste products results in a significant reduction of its volume of distribution in renal failure.

Excretion

Alteration in renal clearance of drugs in renal impairment is by far the most important parameter to consider when making dosage considerations. Generally, a fall in renal drug clearance indicates a decline in the number of functioning nephrons. The glomerular filtration rate (GFR) of which creatinine clearance is an approximation, can be used as an estimate of the number of functioning nephrons. Thus a 50% reduction in GFR will suggest a 50% decline in renal clearance.

Renal impairment therefore often necessitates drug dosage adjustments. Loading doses of renally excreted drugs are often necessary in renal failure because of the prolonged elimination half-life leading to a prolonged time to reach steady state. The equation for a loading dose is the same in renal disease as in normal patients, thus:

Loading dose (mg) =
Target concentration (mg/L) × Volume of distribution (L)

The volume of distribution may be altered but generally remains unchanged. It is possible to derive other formulae for dosage adjustment in renal impairment. One of the most useful is:

$$DRrf = DRn \times \{(1 - Feu) + (Feu \times RF)\}$$

Where:

DRrf = dosing rate in renal failure
DRn = normal dosing rate
RF = extent of renal impairment

$$= \frac{\text{Patient's creatinine clearance (ml/min)}}{\text{Ideal creatinine clearance (120 ml/min)}}$$

Feu = fraction of drug normally excreted unchanged in the urine

e.g. when RF = 0.2 and Feu = 0.5, 60% of normal dosing rate should be given.

An alteration in dosing rate can be achieved by either altering the dose itself, or the dosage interval, or a combination of both as appropriate. Unfortunately for this method, it is not always possible readily to obtain the fraction of drug excreted unchanged in the urine. In practice, it is simpler to use the guidelines to prescribing in renal impairment found in the British National Formulary, and these are adequate for most cases, although the specialist may need to refer to other texts.

Nephrotoxicity

Some drugs are known to damage the kidney by a variety of mechanisms. The commonest forms of damage are interstitial nephritis and glomerulonephritis. The list of potentially nephrotoxic drugs is a long one but the majority cause damage by producing hypersensitivity reactions and are quite safe in the majority of patients. Some drugs, however, are directly nephrotoxic and their effects on the kidney are consequently more predictable. Such drugs include the aminoglycosides, amphotericin, colistin, the polymixins and cyclosporin. The use of any drug with recognized nephrotoxic potential should be avoided in all patients if at all possible. This is particularly true in patients with preexisting renal impairment or renal failure. Inevitably occasions will arise when the use of potentially nephrotoxic drugs becomes necessary, and

Table 14.2 Characteristics of the ideal drug to use in a patient with renal failure
Less than 25% excreted unchanged in the urine
No active metabolites
Disposition unaffected by fluid balance changes
Disposition unaffected by protein binding changes
Response unaffected by altered tissue sensitivity
Wide therapeutic margin
Not nephrotoxic

on these occasions constant monitoring of renal function is essential.

In conclusion, when selecting a drug for treating a patient in renal failure, an agent should be chosen which approaches the ideal characteristics listed in Table 14.2.

CASE STUDIES

CASE 14.1

Mr N., a 66-year-old clergyman, was admitted to hospital for recanulation of sclerosed varicose veins. He suffered a myocardial infarction 2 years previously and has had congestive cardiac failure since. His regular drug therapy comprises:

- Frusemide 80 mg each morning
- Spironolactone 100 mg twice daily
- Isosorbide mononitrate 20 mg twice daily

In addition to the above, his postoperative therapy included:

- Gentamicin 80 mg every 8 hours
- Dextrose 4%/saline 0.18% 1 litre every 8 hours.

His perioperative serum biochemistry was as follows:

Day		1	2	4	6	8
Na	(135–145 mmol/L)	124.0	123.0	122.0	116.0	114.0
K	(3.5–5.0 mmol/L)	4.0	4.4	4.4	5.8	6.0
Urea	(3.0–6.5 mmol/L)	6.6	13.6	23.9	23.6	25.2
Creat.	(50–120 μmol/L)	113.0	186.0	221.0	196.0	201.0

When examined on day 8, he was noted to be cyanosed with decreased skin turgor. His pulse was 96/minute and regular, his BP was 80/50 mmHg (standing) and 100/60 mmHg (lying) and his JVP was –2 cm; oliguria was not present.

Q What was the diagnosis and treatment?

CASE 14.2

Mrs K. is a patient on the Intensive Care Unit with ARF. A routine electrolyte screen shows the following:

Sodium	137	mmol/L	(135–145)
Potassium	7.1	mmol/L	(3.5–5.0)
Bicarbonate	19	mmol/L	(22–31)
Urea	31.7	mmol/L	(3.0–6.5)
Creatinine	567	μmol/L	(50–120)
pH	7.28		(7.36–7.44)

The patient was connected to an ECG monitor and it was observed that P waves were absent and the QRS complex was broadened.

Q What is the explanation of the ECG abnormalities and what steps should be taken?

CASE 14.3

Mrs R. is a patient on the Intensive Care Unit with ARF. She has recently had diarrhoea which was described by the nursing staff as black and tarry in appearance. A full blood count revealed a normochromic and normocytic anaemia with a haemoglobin of 8.1 g/dl.

Q What is the cause of this condition and how should it be treated?

CASE 14.4

Mr F. is a patient on the Intensive Care Unit with ARF being treated by haemofiltration. Since he was suffering from anorexia the dietitian found it difficult to give him adequate nutrition and it was felt that he would be a good candidate for total parenteral nutrition. A Hickmann catheter was inserted.

Q What factors should be taken into account when formulating a TPN regimen for Mr F.?

CASE 14.5

Mr B. is a patient on the Intensive Care Unit with ARF whose arms are observed to flex in intermittent involuntary tonic contractions. Urea and electrolyte results revealed the following:

Sodium	142	mmol/L	(135–145)
Potassium	5.1	mmol/L	(3.5–5.0)
Calcium	1.72	mmol/L	(2.20–2.55)
Phosphate	1.8	mmol/L	(0.9–1.5)
Urea	34.9	mmol/L	(3.0–6.5)
Creatinine	485	μmol/L	(50–120)

Q What is the cause of this condition and how should it be treated?

ANSWERS TO CASE STUDIES

CASE 14.1

A The cyanosis, diminished skin turgor, tachycardia, postural hypotension and low JVP suggest dehydration; this will lead to reduced perfusion of the kidney and prerenal failure. The volume depletion, hyponatraemia and hyperkalaemia give the diagnosis of diuretic abuse. The fluid replacement was not sufficient in the face of the diuretic therapy, especially since the fluid was sodium deficient. Gentamicin may have contributed to the renal impairment; plasma levels should have been requested.

Treatment consists primarily of stopping diuretic therapy and giving appropriate fluid replacement (sodium chloride 0.9% 1 L q.d.s.), with electrolyte monitoring. If oliguria had been present and fluid replacement had not produced a diuresis, the use of loop diuretics would be appropriate, provided, of course, the fluid had been adequately replaced.

CASE 14.2

A Hyperkalaemia is a particular problem in ARF, not only because of reduced urinary excretion but also because of potassium release from cells. Acidosis, which also occurs in ARF, aggravates the situation by provoking potassium leakage from healthy cells. Without treatment the ECG changes observed would be followed with life-threatening ventricular arryhthmias and possibly asystolic cardiac arrest. Emergency treatment is necessary if the serum potassium is above 7.0 mmol/L or if there are ECG changes. The emergency treatment consists of:

1. 10 to 30 ml of calcium gluconate 10% intravenously over 5 to 10 minutes; this has a stabilizing effect on the myocardium but no effect on serum potassium concentration.

2. 10 to 20 units of soluble insulin plus 50 ml of 50% glucose. This stimulates potassium uptake into cells removing it from the plasma.

3. Calcium resonium 15 g three or four times a day orally or by enema. This ion exchange resin binds potassium in the gastrointestinal tract, releasing calcium in exchange and is used to lower serum potassium over a period of hours or days. It is required because the effect of insulin/glucose is only temporary. Lactulose may be used to prevent constipation.

4. 50 to 100 ml sodium bicarbonate 8.4% intravenously may be used as well as insulin/glucose. This helps to correct the acidosis of acute renal failure thereby stimulating potassium re-uptake by cells. However, it is rarely used because of its fluid and electrolyte load.

CASE 14.3

A Mrs R's low haemoglobin may be a result of reduced erythropoietin secretion, although this is unlikely, or of gastrointestinal bleeding. Erythropoietin, the hormone which stimulates production of red blood cells, is produced virtually exclusively by the kidney, and a normochromic, normocytic anaemia due to reduced erythropoietin secretion is a very common symptom in chronic renal failure. However, the normal time course of acute renal failure is often too short for this type of anaemia to become a problem. Uraemic gastrointestinal haemorrhage is a recognized consequence of acute renal failure probably as a result of reduced mucosal cell turnover due to high circulating levels of uraemic toxins. The presence of melaena stool was diagnostic of a gastrointestinal bleed and this was the most likely cause of the anaemia. H_2 receptor antagonists are effective in this condition; it is unlikely that any one would be more advantageous than another. Sucralfate would be an effective alternative.

CASE 14.4

A The aim of dietary supplementation whether enteral or parenteral is to provide sufficient nutrition to prevent breakdown of body tissue, especially protein. Orally the essential amino acids should be provided in a total protein intake of about 40 g/day, while parenterally 12 to 20 g/day of an essential amino acid formulation are usually given. Protein requirements may occasionally be increased in haemofiltration because of amino acid losses. Fat and carbohydrate should also be given to maintain a high energy intake of about 2000 to 3000 kcalories/day. Lipid emulsions do not interfere with dialysis and may be used; similarly, although lipid emulsions may theoretically reduce the efficiency of haemofiltration, in practice their use does not have any noticeable effect. It is useful, however, to infuse TPN solutions into the blood as it is being returned to the body after haemofiltration or haemodialysis, thereby ensuring that it is available to the patient before being presented to the filter. Electrolyte-free amino acid solutions should be used as they allow the addition of the precise quantities of sodium and potassium required depending on serum levels. Water-soluble vitamins are removed by haemofiltration but the standard daily doses normally included in TPN fluids more than compensate for this. Magnesium and zinc supplementation may be required because tissue repair often increases requirements.

CASE 14.5

A Mr B's calcium and phosphate levels are abnormal, and the condition, tetany, is probably due to hypocalcaemia. Calcium malabsorption, probably secondary to disordered vitamin D metabolism, often occurs in acute renal failure. It is usually asymptomatic as tetany of skeletal muscles or convulsions do not normally occur until plasma concentrations are as low as 1.6 to 1.7 mmol/L. Oral calcium supplementation with calcium gluconate or lactate is usually adequate and although vitamin D may be used, it rarely has to be added. Effervescent calcium tablets should be avoided as they invariably contain a high sodium and potassium load. Phosphate is normally excreted by the kidney and phosphate retention and hyperphosphataemia may also occur in ARF, but usually only slightly and the condition rarely requires treatment. Should it become necessary, phosphate-binding agents may be used to retain phosphate ion in the gut. The most common agents are calcium carbonate with glycine tablets (Titralac) or aluminium hydroxide in the form of mixture or capsules. The former is the drug of choice because of the slight risk that aluminium may be absorbed from the gut and deposited in bones to give a severe form of fracturing bone disease.

BIBLIOGRAPHY

American hospital formulary service drug information. American Society of Hospital Pharmacists 1991
Bennett W M. Drugs and renal disease, 2nd edn. Churchill Livingstone 1986
Bennett W M et al. Drug prescribing in renal failure – dosing guidelines for adults. Philadelphia: American College of Physicians 1987
Cattell W R, Baker L R I, Greenwood R N. Renal disease. In: Kumar P J, Clark M L (eds) Clinical Medicine, 2nd edn. Baillière Tindall 1990; 425–489
Davies D M. Textbook of adverse drug reactions, 4th edn. Oxford University Press 1991; 305–343
Dische F E. Concise renal pathology. Castle House Publications 1987
Dollery C et al. Therapeutic drugs. Churchill Livingstone 1991
Fillastre J P, Singlas E. Pharmacokinetics of newer drugs in patients with renal impairment – Part 1. Clinical Pharmacokinetics 1991; 20: 293
Fillastre J P, Singlas E. Pharmacokinetics of newer drugs in patients with renal impairment – Part 2. Clinical Pharmacokinetics 1991; 20: 389
Mammenem G J (ed). Clinical pharmacokinetics drug data handbook. New Zealand: Adis Press 1990

Chapter 15

Chronic renal failure

A. Harper

Chronic renal failure (CRF) may be defined as a condition characterized by anaemia, acidosis, osteodystrophy, neuropathy and general debility frequently accompanied by hypotension, oedema and susceptibility to infection resulting from a significant reduction in the excretory, homeostatic, metabolic and endocrine functions of the kidney.

INCIDENCE AND AETIOLOGY

Accurate information on the incidence of CRF is not readily available but it has been estimated that in the adult population approximately 45 patients per million of the population aged between 15 and 55 years in the UK will present with renal failure for the first time each year. In older patients the incidence rises markedly to approximately 280 per million in the 60 to 70 year age group and approximately 590 per million in the 80 to 90 year age group. This increase with age is attributable to non-immunological causes including vascular disease and undiagnosed prostatic disease in men.

The altered function of the kidney described above is the result of any process which damages the infrastructure of the nephrons. It is generally thought that the diseased kidney loses nephrons as complete units so that all functions are lost simultaneously. The remaining nephrons cope initially with the increased demand upon them. The patient remains well until so many nephrons are lost that the glomerular filtration rate (GFR) can no longer be maintained, and the GFR progressively declines. The patient may well remain symptomless until the GFR falls as low as 15 to 20 ml/min. Any discussion of the relative incidence of the various causes of CRF is of limited value since many patients present with renal impairment so advanced that even detailed examination cannot elicit the cause.

Causes include:

Chronic glomerulonephritis

This is the most common cause of CRF in both adults and children. It should not be regarded as a single disease as it may result from many conditions, both idiopathic and as part of systemic disease. The precise aetiology is unknown but it is thought to result from the passive trapping of immune complexes in the glomerular tuft and the subsequent inflammatory response. Responsible antigens include certain strains of streptococci, other infections such as malaria, endogenous antigens (for example from neoplastic lesions), DNA (in systemic lupus erythematosis) and drugs. Patients with glomerulonephritis present with a variety of clinical syndromes which are characterized to various extents by proteinuria, haematuria, oliguria and hypertension. When proteinuria is profound the condition is referred to as the nephrotic syndrome which is characterized by:

- pitting oedema
- proteinuria 3 to 5 g/day
- hypoalbuminaemia 25 to 30 g/L.

Hypertension

Hypertension is both a common result and a frequent cause of CRF. It may be prevented by adequate treatment thereby preventing further decline in renal function.

Chronic pyelonephritis

Chronic pyelonephritis refers to the chronic inflammation of the renal parenchyma with scarring of the kidney. It is generally caused by recurrent urine infection which may be secondary to outflow obstruction.

Urinary obstruction

Urinary obstruction may develop insidiously when it does not cause symptoms such as oliguria or pain. Causes include:

- prostatic hypertrophy
- renal calculi
- congenital abnormalities
- vesicoureteric reflux
- indwelling urinary catheters.

Interstitial nephritis

Inflammation of the interstitium of the kidney, with secondary involvement of the tubules is almost invariably caused by toxins including drugs.

Congenital abnormalities

The principal congenital abnormality encountered is polycystic kidney disease.

Metabolic diseases

Diabetes mellitus and amyloidosis are probably the most common metabolic diseases which may lead to chronic glomerulonephritis.

DIAGNOSIS, INVESTIGATIONS AND MONITORING

Diagnosis is usually straightforward. The history almost always includes a long period of nocturia, sometimes for years. Patients may appear normal or fatigued, breathless, anaemic, cachectic, pigmented and with hypertension. In some patients 'knobbly' kidneys may be palpable.

Functional assessment of the kidney may be performed by testing serum and urine. Serum creatinine is a more reliable indicator of renal function than serum urea though both are normally measured. Hyperkalaemia, acidosis with correspondingly low serum bicarbonate, hypercalcaemia and hyperphosphataemia may also be present.

Urine should be cultured and a 24-hour collection made. Some proteinuria occurs in any form of CRF but the presence of more than 2 g in a 24-hour collection is usually taken to indicate a chronic glomerulonephritic aetiology. Urinary creatinine excretion and serum creatinine concentration may be used to calculate creatinine clearance, although this may also be calculated approximately from the serum creatinine concentration and other patient parameters (see Ch. 14, 'Acute renal failure').

Structural assessments of the kidney may be performed by carrying out radiological procedures. An intravenous urogram (IVU) will show the following:

- the presence, length and position of the kidneys; in CRF the kidneys shrink in proportion to nephron loss
- the presence or absence of renal scarring and the shape of the calyces and renal pelvis; renal cortical scarring and calyceal distortion indicate chronic pyelonephritis
- any obstruction to the ureters, e.g. by a stone, a tumour or retroperitoneal fibrosis; these require surgical intervention
- the shape of the bladder and the presence of residual urine; enlargement and a post-micturition residue suggest urethral obstruction such as prostatic hypertrophy.

With advanced renal failure, ultrasound may be more useful in visualizing the renal tract than an IVU, and as experience grows with this procedure, it may gradually replace the use of the contrast technique.

If an IVU or ultrasound fails to give a cause for the reduction in renal function, a renal biopsy may be performed, although in advanced disease, scarring of the renal tissue may render diagnosis difficult.

All patients with CRF should be monitored regularly to detect any of the sequelae of the disease, e.g. serum biochemistry and haematology. Renal function itself may be monitored by plotting creatinine clearance against time. The decline in renal function is usually linear in most patients. If an abrupt decline in the slope is noted, its cause must be detected and remedied.

CLINICAL MANIFESTATIONS

Nocturia

Nocturia is almost invariable. As the nephrons diminish in number, plasma urea increases. The osmotic effect of this produces a diuresis throughout the day and night. When plasma urea is constantly above 40 mmol/L the patient will be wakened two or three times a night with a full bladder.

Oedema

As the GFR falls further the kidneys become unable to excrete water adequately resulting in peripheral and central oedema.

Uraemia

Many substances besides urea, creatinine and water are normally excreted by the kidney and tend to accumulate as renal function decreases. It is thought that some of the substances responsible for the toxicity of uraemia are intermediate in size between small molecules which are readily dialysed and large non-dialysable proteins, and hence are described as 'middle molecules'; examples include phosphate, guanidines, phenols and organic acids. These and other molecules are generally described as uraemic toxins, indicating that urea is not the only such toxin, although its accumulation is often used as a guide for their accumulation. The symptoms of uraemia are many and various including anorexia, nausea, vomiting, constipation, foul taste and skin discolouration presumed to be due to pigment deposition compounded by the pallor of anaemia. The characteristic complexion is often described as muddy, and is associated with severe pruritus.

Anaemia

Several factors are thought to contribute to the

pathogenesis of anaemia in uraemia including shortened red cell survival and marrow suppression by uraemic toxins. However, the main cause is inadequate secretion of erythropoietin. This hormone, which is produced mainly, though not exclusively, in the kidney, is the main regulator of red cell production. Renal impairment results not only in a reduction in excretory function but also in a reduction in erythropoietin production. The resulting anaemia is the major cause of fatigue and dyspnoea on exertion observed in virtually all patients with renal failure. Nevertheless it should be noted that the development of the anaemia is slow and insidious permitting some adaptation; many patients cope relatively well with profoundly low haemoglobin concentrations.

Electrolyte disturbances

Serum sodium levels are frequently normal, despite very low creatinine clearance. Potassium levels are generally elevated, and levels of over 7.0 mmol/L are life threatening and should be treated as an emergency. Hydrogen ions (H^+) are a common end product of very many metabolic processes and are normally excreted via the kidney. In renal failure (H^+) is retained causing acidosis; the combination of (H^+) with bicar-bonate (HCO_3^-) results in the removal of some hydrogen as water, the elimination of CO_2 via the lungs and a low plasma bicarbonate. Serum phosphate is usually elevated due to the failure to excrete dietary phosphate. Serum calcium levels are usually low because of insufficient 1,25-dihydroxycholecalciferol (calcitriol), the physiologically active form of vitamin D.

Hypertension

The vast majority of patients with CRF will have hypertension. The probable mechanism is that renal ischaemia activates the renin–angiotensin system with subsequent hyperaldosteronism and sodium retention (Fig. 15.1). This, in combination with the diminished ability to excrete dietary sodium, causes an increase in both extracellular fluid volume and blood pressure. Since hypertension may exacerbate renal damage and precipitate CRF, blood pressure in such patients should be carefully monitored and controlled.

Bone disease (renal osteodystrophy)

Several types of bone disease are associated with CRF. Cholecalciferol, the percursor of active vitamin D, is both absorbed from the gastrointestinal tract and produced in the skin by the action of sunlight. Production of 1,25-dihydroxychole-

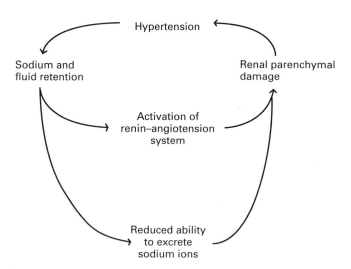

Fig. 15.1 Cycle of events leading to hypertension in chronic renal failure.

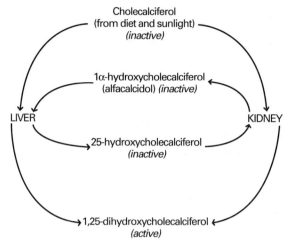

Fig. 15.2 Renal and hepatic involvement in vitamin D metabolism.

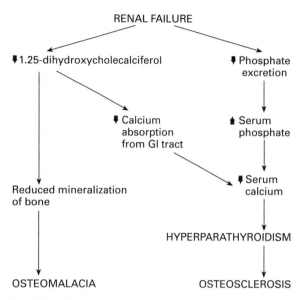

Fig. 15.3 Disturbance of calcium and phosphate balance in chronic renal failure.

calciferol (calcitriol) requires the hydroxylation of the cholecalciferol molecule at both the 1-α and the 25 position (Fig. 15.2). Hydroxylation at the 25 position occurs in the liver, while hydroxylation of the 1-α position occurs in the kidney; this latter process is impaired in renal failure. The resulting deficiency in vitamin D leads to defective mineralization of bone and osteomalacia.

The deficiency in vitamin D with the consequent reduced calcium absorption from the gut in combination with the reduced renal tubular reabsorption, results in hypocalcaemia (Fig. 15.3). This is compounded by hyperphosphataemia due to reduced phosphate excretion, which in turn reduces the concentration of ionized serum calcium by sequestering calcium phosphate in bone or, eventually, in soft tissue. Hypocalcaemia and a reduction in the direct suppressive action of 1,25-dihydroxycholecalciferol on the parathyroid gland results in an increased secretion of parathyroid hormone (PTH).

Since the failed kidney is unable to respond to PTH by increasing renal calcium reabsorption, the serum PTH levels remain persistently elevated and hyperplasia of the parathyroid glands occur. The resulting secondary hyperparathyroidism produces a disturbance in the normal architecture of bone termed osteosclerosis (literally, hardening of the bone). Bone pain is

the main symptom and distinctive appearances on X-ray may be observed (e.g. the 'rugger-jersey' spine where there are alternate bands of excessive and defective mineralization in the vertebrae).

A further possible, though by no means inevitable, consequence of the secondary hyperparathyroidism produced in response to hypocalcaemia is that sufficient bone resorption may be caused to maintain adequate calcium levels. This, in combination with the hyperphosphataemia, may result in calcium phosphate deposition and soft tissue calcification.

Neurological changes

The most common neurological changes are nonspecific and include an inability to concentrate, memory impairment, irritability and stupor probably due to uraemic toxins. Fits due to cerebral oedema or hypertension may occur. Most patients have evidence of peripheral neuropathy although this is usually asymptomatic.

Muscle function

Muscle cramps and restless legs are common and may be a major symptom causing distress to patients. These are probably caused by a general nutritional deficiency and changes in electrolytes, notably divalent cations and especially by hypocalcaemia. A proximal myopathy of shoulder and pelvic girdle muscles may rarely develop.

PROGNOSIS

When the GFR has declined to about 20 ml/ minute a continuing deterioration in renal function to end-stage renal failure appears inevitable in most patients even when the initial cause of the kidney damage has been removed. The mechanism for this is obscure but hypertension, deposition of calcium phosphate or urate crystals in the kidney and damage due to increased blood flow through the remaining intact nephrons have been suggested and are probably all relevant. Serum creatinine and creatinine clearance should be monitored to ensure the detection of the most appropriate point at which to commence renal replacement therapy.

TREATMENT

Although CRF is a comparatively rare disorder, the treatment modalities available which include dialysis, transplantation and the use of human recombinant erythropoietin are effective at reducing mortality and morbidity as well as improving the quality of life in patients. Management of these patients has therefore assumed economic and political aspects as well as medical.

The aims of treatment may be summarized thus:

- to reverse or arrest the process causing the renal damage; this is rarely possible
- to relieve symptoms of the condition
- to implement regular dialysis treatment and/ or transplantation in a patient at the most appropriate point in the patient's disease progress.

Reversal or arrest of primary disease factors

As has already been mentioned, reversal or arrest of the primary cause of renal failure is rarely possible. However, early detection of some causes may enable remedial action to be taken. A postrenal obstructive lesion, e.g. a ureter obstructed by a stone or a ureteric tumour, may be successfully treated surgically. Glomerulonephritis may respond to immunosuppressants and/or steroids. Clearly when drug-induced renal disease is suspected the drug in question should be stopped.

Relief of symptoms

Hypertension

Adequate control of blood pressure is one of the most important therapeutic measures since there is a vicious cycle of events whereby hypertension causes damage to the intrarenal vasculature resulting in thickening and hyalinization of the walls of arterioles and small vessels. By effectively reducing renal perfusion, this stimulates the renin–angiotensin–aldosterone system leading to sodium conservation and vasoconstriction which in turn increases the degree of hypertension.

The drugs used to treat hypertension in renal disease are generally the same as those used in other forms of hypertension although allowances must be made for the effects of renal failure on drug disposition.

Diuretics. High dose loop diuretics are of value in the treatment of fluid overload and are effective even in severe failure although under these circumstances large doses may be necessary, e.g. 500 to 1000 mg of frusemide or higher. Patients who do not respond to oral therapy may benefit from concomitant administration of metolazone which acts synergistically to produce a profound diuresis, or the loop diuretic may be given intravenously. Care must be taken to avoid hypovolaemia (monitor body weight) and electrolyte disturbances such as hypokalaemia and hyponatraemia. Concomitant treatment with potassium supplements or potassium-sparing diuretics for hypokalaemia is potentially dangerous in renal failure because of the risk of hyperkalaemia.

Thiazide diuretics with the apparent exception of metolazone are ineffective at low GFR and may accumulate causing an increased incidence of side effects.

Beta-adrenoreceptor blockers. Beta-adrenoreceptor blockers are commonly used in the treatment of hypertension in CRF. As in most patients it is advisable to use the more cardioselective beta-adrenoreceptor blockers, atenolol or metoprolol. Atenolol is excreted renally and therefore should require dosage adjustment in renal failure. In practice, however, it is effective and tolerated well by renal patients at standard doses. Nevertheless metoprolol would theoretically be a better choice since it is cleared hepatically and needs no dosage adjustment, although small initial doses are advised in renal failure since there may be increased sensitivity to its hypotensive effects.

Calcium antagonists. Calcium channel blocking agents are a useful adjunct to beta-adrenoreceptor blockers. Nifedipine is probably the agent of choice as it rarely precipitates heart failure, its negative inotropic effect being offset by the reduction in cardiac workload. As well as headache, facial flushing and oedema, nocturia can occur, but in practice significant problems are rarely encountered.

Angiotensin converting enzyme (ACE) inhibitors. ACE inhibitors reduce the amount of circulating angiotensin II which results in vasodilatation and reduced sodium retention. There is little to choose clinically between those currently on the market. ACE inhibitors can cause profound hypotension in patients with renal failure and it is important to give a test dose before initiating routine therapy. Captopril, with its shorter half-life and rapid onset of action is probably the agent of choice for the test dose. A dose of 6.25 mg is given and the blood pressure closely monitored for about 4 hours. For long-term management, it is usually preferable to use an agent with a longer duration of action such as enalapril or lisinopril which permit once-daily dosing. It has been reported that ACE inhibitors may reduce thirst, which may be useful in those patients who have a tendency to fluid overload as a result of excessive drinking. ACE inhibitors

are potassium sparing and therefore plasma potassium should be monitored carefully. A low potassium diet may be necessary.

The role of ACE inhibitors in hypertensive patients with renal insufficiency is unclear. They can produce a reduction in renal function by preventing the angiotensin II mediated vasoconstriction of the efferent glomerular arteriole, which contributes to the high pressure gradient across the glomerulus. This problem is important only in patients with renal vascular disease, particularly those with bilateral stenoses, and is consequently rare. However ACE inhibitors have been shown to reduce proteinuria and increase GFR in hypertensive patients with renal insufficiency indicating beneficial intrarenal haemodynamic effects in addition to their effects on arterial blood pressure.

Vasodilators. The vasodilators hydralazine, prazosin and minoxidil have been used with varying degrees of success but they rarely add significantly to the control of hypertension. They are usually only used when other measures have failed. Sensitivity of patients to all these drugs is increased in renal failure so, if used, therapy should be initiated with small doses. Minoxidil particularly is very potent and is usually only added when other measures have failed; a beta-adrenoreceptor blocker may need to be co-prescribed, as minoxidil can cause a reflex tachycardia.

Other drugs. Methyldopa is not commonly used as an antihypertensive because of its many side effects. If used in renal failure, initial doses should be small, because of an increased sensitivity to its effects.

Uraemia

The symptoms of uraemia described above are due to the accumulation of uraemic toxins which occurs in renal failure. Although urea is only one of these toxins, many patients experience a symptomatic improvement when dietary protein intake is reduced. The aim of protein restriction is to provide all the essential amino acids in a total protein intake of 40 g/day. A higher intake of protein stimulates its use as an energy source resulting in increases in blood urea concentrations; further reduction in protein intake brings about endogenous protein catabolism and again causes blood urea to increase. There is some evidence that, as well as reducing the symptoms of uraemia, protein restriction slows the progression of CRF but this remains controversial. Fat and carbohydrate should also be given to maintain a high energy intake of about 2000 to 3000 kcalories/day, or more in hypercatabolic patients, as this will help to prevent protein catabolism and promote anabolism. Other dietary precautions which may be taken include sodium restriction to reduce the risk of fluid overload, and potassium restriction to reduce the risk of hyperkalaemia. Sodium intake may often be reduced to a satisfactory level of 80 mmol/day by not adding salt to food at the table, and avoiding convenience foods and snacks. This is usually tolerable to patients. Low potassium diets are sometimes used (see hyperkalaemia).

Vitamin supplements are sometimes necessary as water-soluble vitamins may be lost during dialysis. This is becoming less of a problem as dialysis techniques and dietary control improve.

Nausea and vomiting may persist after starting a low protein diet. In this situation metoclopramide is useful but sometimes accumulation of the drug and its metabolites may occur leading to a higher incidence of extrapyramidal side effects. Patients should be started on a low dose which should then be increased slowly. Prochlorperazine or cyclizine may also be useful. The anaemic patient often becomes less nauseated when treated with erythropoietin.

Constipation is a common problem in patients with renal disease, partly as a result of fluid restriction and anorexia and partly as a consequence of drug therapy, such as aluminium supplements as phosphate binders. It is particularly important that patients controlled by peritoneal dialysis do not become constipated as this can reduce the efficacy of dialysis and predispose to peritonitis. Standard therapy may be used such as bulk-forming laxatives or increased dietary fibre for less severe constipation, or a stimulant such as senna with enemas or glycerin suppositories for severe constipation. Higher doses of stimulant laxatives such as 2 to 4 tablets of senna at night may be required. It should be noted that ispaghula husk preparations contain up to 7 mmol of potassium in each sachet, and should be avoided in renal failure because of the risk of hyperkalaemia. Sterculia preparations are an effective alternative.

Pruritus in renal failure can be severe. It is sometimes produced by high serum phosphate levels and improves after treatment with aluminium hydroxide or calcium carbonate. Generally however no cause is found. Conventionally, chlorpheniramine is used to treat pruritus. However, it is seldom very effective and is often very sedating. Terfenadine is sometimes useful as an alternative, but is generally less effective than the sedating antihistamines. Trimeprazine may be useful as may topical crotamiton lotion. Treatment is usually given at night when itching is most troublesome and sedation less of concern.

Anaemia

The normochromic normocytic anaemia of CRF does not respond to iron or folic acid unless there is a coexisting deficiency. Traditionally the only treatment was to give red blood cell transfusions but this is time consuming, may lead to fluid and iron overload and promotes antibody formation which may give problems in later transplantation. Recently, recombinant human erythropoietin (rhuEPO), a genetically engineered form of the hormone, has become available; it is immunologically and biologically indistinguishable from physiological erythropoietin. It may be given by the intravenous or subcutaneous route; the latter route is preferred as it provides equally effective clinical results while using similar or smaller doses. It is usually given three times a week. Most patients report a dramatically improved quality of life.

Patients on rhuEPO generally require iron supplements because of the greatly increased marrow requirements. A slow rise in haemoglobin should be the aim of therapy to avoid haemodynamically induced side effects, such as hypertension, seizures and clotting of vascular accesses. Blood pressure should be closely monitored. An initial subcutaneous or intravenous dose of 50 units/kg body weight three times weekly increased as necessary in steps of 25 units/kg every 4 weeks should be given to produce the advised rise of no more than 1 g/dl per month. The target haemoglobin is commonly 9 to 11 g/dl, and, once this has been reached, a maintenance dose in the region of 50 to 100 units/kg/week subcutaneously or 90 to 300 units/kg/week intravenously in three divided doses should maintain the level.

Correcting the anaemia usually helps control the symptoms of lethargy and myopathy, and often greatly reduces nausea. Improved appetite on rhuEPO therapy can, however, increase potassium intake, and will necessitate dietary control.

Fluid retention

Oedema may occur as a result of sodium retention and the associated water retention. Renal patients also often have hypoalbuminaemia following renal loss and this can result in extravasation of fluid and retention. Pulmonary and peripheral oedema are best controlled with dialysis but diuretics can be useful (see hypertension above).

In patients with fluid overload, moderate salt restriction is sensible. It is important to be aware of the sodium-containing medications including some antibiotics, soluble or effervescent preparations, magnesium trisilicate mixture, Gaviscon, sodium bicarbonate and the plasma expanders hetastarch and gelatin.

Hyperkalaemia

Hyperkalaemia often occurs in CRF and may cause life-threatening cardiac arrhythmias. If untreated, asystolic cardiac arrest and death may result. Patients are often put on a potassium-restricted diet by avoiding potassium-rich foods, such as fruit and fruit drinks, vegetables, chocolate, beer, instant coffee and ice cream. Many drugs have a high potassium content such as potassium citrate mixture, Sandocal tablets, some antibiotics and ispaghula husk sachets.

The use of these drugs is less of a problem in dialysed patients.

Emergency treatment is necessary if the serum potassium is above 7.0 mmol/L or if there are ECG changes. The most effective treatment is dialysis but if this is not available, other measures may be tried as discussed in Chapter 14.

Acidosis

Since the kidney is the main route for excreting H^+ ions, CRF may result in a metabolic acidosis which is seen as a reduction in serum bicarbonate. It may be readily treated with sodium bicarbonate 1 to 6 g/day orally. As the dose is not critical, it is easy to experiment with different dosage forms and strengths to suit individual patients.

Neurological problems

Neurological changes are generally due to uraemic toxins and improve on the treatment of uraemia by dialysis or diet. Muscle cramps and restless legs are common and often treated with quinine sulphate (see Ch. 14).

Osteodystrophy

The osteodystrophy of renal failure is due to three factors; hyperphosphataemia, vitamin D deficiency and hyperparathyroidism.

Hyperphosphataemia. The management of hyperphosphataemia depends upon the binding of orally ingested phosphate in the gut, using a phosphate-binding agent to prevent its systemic absorption. Such agents are invariably salts of a di- or trivalent metallic ion, usually either aluminium or calcium.

Aluminium hydroxide has been widely used as a phosphate binder. Unfortunately the slight degree of systemic absorption of aluminium which occurs has toxic effects in CRF including encephalopathy, osteomalacia, proximal myopathy and anaemia. Dialysis dementia is a disease endemic among haemodialysis patients which is believed to be due to aluminium deposition in the brain. Desferrioxamine (4 to 6 g in 500 ml saline 0.9% per week) has been used to treat this condition by removing aluminium from tissues by chelation. Aluminium can no longer be recommended as a phosphate binder.

Calcium carbonate has been used as a phosphate binder in the form of Titralac or Calcichew. Unfortunately, it is less effective as a phosphate binder than aluminium and sometimes requires the use of doses up to 10 g daily. One advantage of calcium carbonate, however, is its contribution to the treatment of the hypocalcaemia of CRF due to limited systemic calcium absorption.

Vitamin D deficiency. Vitamin D deficiency may be treated with the synthetic vitamin D analogues 1α-hydroxycholecalciferol (alfacalcidol) at 0.25 to 1 microgram/day or 1,25-dihydroxycholecalciferol (calcitriol) at 1 to 2 microgram/day. The serum calcium should be monitored, and the dose of alfacalcidol or calcitriol adjusted accordingly. Hyperphosphataemia should be controlled before starting vitamin D therapy since the resulting increase in serum calcium may result in soft tissue calcification.

Hyperparathyroidism. The rise in plasma 1,25-dihydroxycholecalciferol and calcium which results from starting vitamin D therapy suppresses the production of PTH by the parathyroids; parathyroidectomy, once commonly performed on CRF patients, is now very rare.

Implementation of regular dialysis treatment and/or transplantation

End-stage renal failure is the point at which, despite the conservative measures discussed above, the patient will die without the institution of renal replacement by dialysis or transplantation (see Fig. 15.4). This may occur very rapidly after presentation or after a period of several years.

The principle of dialysis is simple. The patient's blood is on one side, and a dialysate solution on the other side, of a semipermeable membrane across which exchange of metabolites occurs. There are traditionally two types of dialysis: haemodialysis and peritoneal dialysis both of which are discussed in detail in Chapter 14.

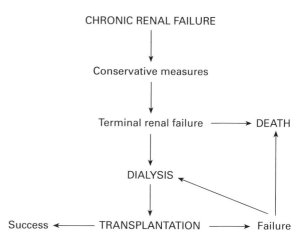

Fig. 15.4 Possible events for patients with chronic renal failure. Occasionally a patient may receive a transplant kidney before dialysis.

Because patients with CRF may require dialysis treatment for many years, adaptations to the process of peritoneal dialysis have been made which enable the patient to follow a lifestyle as near normal as possible. A flexible non-irritant silicone rubber catheter (a 'Tenckhoff' catheter) is surgically inserted into the abdominal cavity. Dacron cuffs on the body of the catheter become infiltrated with scar tissue during the healing process causing the catheter to be firmly anchored in place. Such catheters may remain viable for many years. During the dialysis process thereafter, a bag containing a volume of warmed dialysate, usually 2 litres, is connected to the catheter and the fluid run into the abdomen under gravity. The empty bag and tube are rolled up and tucked into a belt or pocket and the patient continues his or her normal life for the next few hours. Then the bag is unrolled and the fluid drains out of the abdomen, again under gravity, the bag is disconnected, a new bag connected and the process repeated. The procedure is repeated continuously so that dialysate is kept in the abdomen 24 hours a day usually by repeating the process four times a day with an average dwell time of 6 to 8 hours. During this time the patient is able to walk about freely which gives the process its name of continuous ambulatory peritoneal dialysis (CAPD).

Since CAPD is by definition continuous and

corrects fluid and electrolyte levels constantly, dietary and fluid restrictions are less stringent. Blood loss is avoided making the technique safer in anaemic patients. Unfortunately peritoneal dialysis is not an efficient process; it only just manages to excrete the substances required and, as albumin crosses the peritoneal membrane, up to 10 g of protein may be lost in the dialysate daily. It is also uncomfortable and tiring for the patient, and is contra-indicated in patients who have recently undergone abdominal surgery.

Peritonitis is the most frequently encountered complication of peritoneal dialysis. Its diagnosis usually depends on the presence of two of the three main signs, i.e. abdominal pain, cloudy dialysate and positive culture. Empirical antibiotic therapy should therefore be commenced as soon as peritonitis is clinically diagnosed. Gram-positive cocci (particularly *Staphylococcus epidermidis*) and Enterobacteriaceae are the causative organisms in the majority of cases. Ceftazidime is a broad-spectrum cephalosporin with good Gram-negative activity while vancomycin has excellent activity against Gram-positive species, and these agents are usually administered in combination via the intraperitoneal route of administration. The antibiotic regimen should be adjusted appropriately after the results of microbiological culture and sensitivity.

Oral ciprofloxacin in a dose of 500 mg four times a day for 14 days has recently been shown to be effective in the treatment of CAPD peritonitis (it should be noted that this dose is above the manufacturer's recommended dose). When this regimen is used it is important that any oral aluminium preparations are discontinued, as they reduce the absorption of ciprofloxacin by chelation.

Haemodialysis is suitable for patients producing a lot of metabolites such as those with high nutritional demands or a large muscle mass where these substances are produced faster than peritoneal dialysis can remove them. It also provides a backup for those patients in whom peritoneal dialysis has failed.

Haemofiltration is a technique related to haemodialysis and is discussed in detail in Chapter 14.

Transplantation

Renal transplantation remains the treatment of choice for end-stage renal disease as it enables patients to resume a normal lifestyle. The most important therapeutic aspect of transplantation is immunosuppression to prevent rejection. The major disadvantage of all immunosuppressive agents is their nonspecificity in that they cause a general depression of the immune system, exposing the patient to an increased risk of infection which remains an important cause of morbidity and mortality.

Immunosuppressants

The major pharmacological immunosuppressive agents are steroids, azathioprine and cyclosporin. Biological agents which suppress T-cell activity are also starting to become more widely used.

Steroids. Prednisolone is the oral agent commonly used for immunosuppression after transplantation, while methylprednisolone is used intravenously in regimens to reverse acute rejection. The maintenance dose of prednisolone is about 10 to 20 mg/day given as a single dose in the morning to minimize adrenal suppression. The use of steroid therapy often leads to complications, particularly if high doses are given for long periods. In addition to a cushingoid state there may be gastrointestinal bleeding, hypertension, diabetes, osteoporosis and mental disturbances. Patients who are temporarily unable to take oral prednisolone should be given an equivalent dose of hydrocortisone or methylprednisolone intravenously.

Azathioprine. Azathioprine should be given in a dose of 2.5 mg/kg/day either orally or intravenously; the two routes have the same bioavailability. There is no advantage in giving it in divided doses. Since azathioprine interferes with nucleic acid synthesis, it may be mutagenic, and pharmacy and nursing staff should avoid handling the tablets; this is readily achieved by using the blister-packed product.

Cyclosporin. Cyclosporin is now the mainstay of post-transplant immunosuppression. Its action is partially selective in that it suppresses T-cytotoxic cell production but to some extent spares B-lymphocyte activity permitting a greater response to infection than can normally be mounted by patients using other forms of immunosuppression. There is thus a relatively low incidence of severe infection. The use of cyclosporin in immunosuppression regimens has greatly increased transplant survival rates. It is available in both liquid and capsule presentations for oral use; these forms are equally bioavailable. The capsules are useful for visually handicapped patients or a glass U100 insulin syringe of the type which can be preset may be of value in drawing up the prescribed dose of liquid. It is common to mix the liquid with milk or fruit juice to mask the unpleasant taste. An intravenous preparation is also available. An equivalent dose is one-third of the oral dose.

Cyclosporin carries a high risk of side effects including nephrotoxicity, hypertension, fine muscle tremor, gingival hyperplasia, nausea and hirsutism. Nephrotoxicity occasionally necessitates the withdrawal of cyclosporin. There is tremendous inter- and intrapatient variation in absorption of cyclosporin. Blood level monitoring is essential to achieve the maximum protection against rejection with the minimum risk of side effects. The range regarded as acceptable varies between centres but is commonly taken as 100 to 200 ng/ml.

Cyclosporin is known to interact with a number of drugs (Table 15.1). It has been suggested that a reduction in the dose of cyclosporin would be achievable by co-administration of ketoconazole, making clinical use of the interaction.

Cyclosporin and azathioprine are used in various combinations and regimens for long-term immunosuppression but are ineffective in treating acute rejection episodes. Methylprednisolone or one of the novel anti-T-cell antisera are required to try to reverse acute rejection.

Anti-T-cell sera

Antithymocyte globulin (ATG) is an antilymphocyte globulin produced from rabbit serum immunized with human T-cells. It contains anti-

Table 15.1 Examples of drug interactions involving cyclosporin

Reduce serum levels of cyclosporin (induction of hepatic metabolism):
     Phenytoin
     Phenobarbitone
     Rifampicin
     Isoniazid
     Co-trimoxazole (mechanism unknown)

Increase serum levels of cyclosporin (inhibition of, or competition for, the same route of hepatic metabolism):
     Diltiazem
     Erythromycin
     Corticosteroids
     Ketoconazole
     Synthetic hormones

Enhance nephrotoxicity of cyclosporin:
     Aminoglycosides
     Amphotericin B
     Co-trimoxazole
     Melphalan

bodies to human T-lymphocytes which on injection will attach to, neutralize and eliminate most T-lymphocytes thereby weakening the immune response. Antilymphocyte globulin (ALG) is similar but is of equine origin, and not specific to T-lymphocytes, acting on lymphocytes generally.

The main drawback to the use of anti-T-cell sera is the relatively high incidence of side effects, notably anaphylactic reactions including hypotension, fever and urticaria. These reactions are more frequently observed with the first dose and may require supportive therapy with steroids and antihistamines. Severe reactions may necessitate stopping the treatment. Steroids and antihistamines may be given prophylactically to minimize reactions. Pyrexia often occurs on the first day of treatment but usually subsides without requiring treatment. Tolerance testing by administration of a test dose is advisable, particularly in patients who commonly experience allergic reactions, e.g. asthmatics. ALG and ATG can be substituted for each other should adverse reactions occur.

OKT3 is a monoclonal antibody directed against the T3 antigen on human T-cells. It blocks the function and generation of the T-cytotoxic cells responsible for kidney transplant rejection. As with other anti-T-cell sera the main drawbacks to the use of OKT3 are its side effects which include nausea, vomiting and diarrhoea, marked pyrexia (often over 40°C), chills, dyspnoea and chest pain (treatment should be withheld from patients with pulmonary oedema) and rigors. It is common practice to prescribe agents against these side effects prophylactically, especially with the early doses of the course.

Anti-T-cell sera are reserved for the treatment of acute transplant rejection. It is likely that research will continue into biological immuno-suppression, producing agents as effective or more so than the agents described here, but with fewer or less severe side effects.

CASE STUDIES

CASE 15.1

Mr F., an unemployed man (date of birth 5/7/55) weighing 65 kg, was admitted to hospital in March 1992 for investigation of rapid deterioration of renal function. His medical history included the following:

- Angina (diagnosed 1985)
- Wolff–Parkinson–White syndrome (1988)
- Hypertension (1988)
- IgA nephrosis and chronic renal failure (1989)
- Atypical chest pain (non-cardiac, probably musculoskeletal) (1991).

His medication included:

- Amiodarone 200 mg once daily
- Atenolol 100 mg once daily
- Co-proxamol as required
- GTN transdermal patch 5 mg once daily
- GTN sublingual as required
- Indomethacin 50 mg twice daily
- Isosorbide mononitrate 40 mg twice daily
- Nifedipine SR 20 mg three times daily
- Nortriptyline 25 mg three times daily
- Temazepam 20 mg at night.

His serum creatinine concentrations were taken from his case notes retrospectively:

Date	Serum creatinine (μmol/L)
18.01.88	162
19.08.88	167
15.01.89	186
29.10.89	192
23.03.90	211
13.04.91	237
07.10.91	343
11.01.92	559
24.02.92	904

Q Could his drug therapy have contributed to the acute deterioration in his chronic renal condition?

CASE 15.2

Mr D., a 71-year-old retired sub-postmaster with a stable weight of around 65 kg, was admitted to hospital feeling 'generally dreadful'. He has a history of chronic renal failure secondary to chronic glomerulonephritis. On admission he complained of severe itching, nausea and loss of appetite.

Laboratory results on admission included a serum urea of 41.1 mmol/L and a serum creatinine of 692 μmol/L.

Q Explain Mr. D's signs and symptoms and suggest appropriate therapy.

CASE 15.3

Mr A. is a patient with chronic renal failure secondary to chronic interstitial nephritis. He complains of chronic fatigue and breathlessness on exertion; his haemoglobin concentration is found to be 5.6 g/dl.

Q How should he be treated?

CASE 15.4

Mr T. is a patient with chronic renal failure secondary to polycystic kidney disease. On routine examination he is found to have a serum phosphate concentration of 2.1 mmol/L (normal range 0.9 to 1.5 mmol/L) and a serum calcium concentration of 2.01 mmol/L (normal range 2.20 to 2.55 mmol/L). On investigation he admits to aches in his thighs on walking, and radiographic examination suggests slight reduction in bone density.

Q What is the cause of the condition and what is its treatment?

CASE 15.5

Mrs K. is a 43-year-old patient with CRF who has had a cadaveric renal transplant 4 days previously. Postoperative immunosuppression consisted of methylprednisolone 20 mg daily, azathioprine 75 mg daily and cyclosporin 150 mg twice daily, all administered intravenously.

Q What drug and dose regimen should be instituted for long-term immunosuppression now the patient may take oral medication, and what counselling points should be made?

ANSWERS TO CASE STUDIES

CASE 15.1

A The plasma creatinine concentrations may be used to calculate creatinine clearances by means of the equation of Cockroft & Gault (note that age is not constant throughout). If these are plotted against time, it may be observed that the slow decline in renal function accelerates from about mid-1991. This coincides with the diagnosis of atypical chest pain which was probably musculoskeletal in origin. It would be reasonable to suppose that the chest pain was being treated with the indomethacin, and this was indeed the case.

This case illustrates two main points. Firstly NSAIDs may be nephrotoxic especially in the presence of pre-existing renal impairment. Secondly plots of creatinine clearance may be used to detect changes in the rate of renal deterioration; in fact they are also useful in predicting the optimum time when replacement therapy should be started. Mr F. was started on haemodialysis shortly after the last creatinine measurement – probably some years earlier than would otherwise have been felt necessary.

CASE 15.2

A The signs and symptoms described in Mr D. are due to uraemia, i.e. the accumulation of uraemic toxins which occurs in renal failure. Most renal units avail themselves of the services of a dietitian who can institute a low protein diet designed to provide all the essential amino acids in a total protein intake of about 40 g/day. Fat and carbohydrate should also be given to maintain a high energy intake of about 2000 to 3000 kcalories/day or more to help prevent protein catabolism.

Nausea and vomiting may persist after starting a low protein diet. In this situation metoclopramide, prochlorperazine or cyclizine may be useful.

Pruritus in renal failure can be severe. It is sometimes produced by high serum phosphate levels and improves after treatment with aluminium hydroxide or calcium carbonate. Terfenadine is less sedating than chlorpheniramine, but it is also generally less effective than the sedating antihistamines. Trimeprazine or topical crotamiton lotion may be useful. Treatment is usually given at night when itching is most troublesome and sedation less of concern.

CASE 15.3

A The normochromic normocytic anaemia of CRF does not respond to iron or folic acid unless there is a coexisting deficiency. Red blood cell transfusions may be given but this procedure carries substantial problems and risks. However, the recent introduction of recombinant human erythropoietin (rhuEPO) renders it the agent of choice. As the haemoglobin concentration increases, lethargy, dyspnoea and other symptoms such as nausea and anorexia improve and most patients report a dramatically improved quality of life. Ideally rhuEPO should be administered by the subcutaneous route as this enables smaller doses to be used to give the same clinical result. An initial subcutaneous or intravenous dose of 50 units/kg body weight three times weekly increased as necessary in steps of 25 units/kg every 4 weeks is adequate to produce the advised rise of no more than 1 g/dl/month. The target haemoglobin is commonly 9 to 11 g/dl, and once this has been reached, a maintenance dose in the region of 50 to 100 units/kg/week subcutaneously or 90 to 300 units/kg/week intravenously in three divided doses should maintain the level. Patients on rhuEPO generally require iron supplements because of the greatly increased marrow requirements. A slow rise in haemoglobin should be the aim of therapy to avoid haemodynamically induced side effects, such as hypertension, seizures and clotting of vascular accesses. Blood pressure should be closely monitored.

CASE 15.4

A The apparent reduction in bone density and the bone aches suggest a diagnosis of osteomalacia. The generalized aches which occur in this condition are more marked in the legs and pelvis making walking painful. Bone tenderness is common. Loss of bone density is the earliest sign but it is often difficult to detect. The symptoms of osteomalacia are due to the reduction in 1,25-dihydroxycholecalciferol which occurs in renal failure. Renal bone disease can almost always be alleviated by correcting plasma calcium and phosphate imbalances and instituting vitamin D therapy

Hyperphosphataemia is managed with oral phosphate-binding agents which prevent its systemic absorption. Aluminium hydroxide is now less widely used for this purpose because of its numerous disadvantages. Calcium carbonate is probably the drug of choice although it is a less effective phosphate binder than aluminium. It does have the advantage however of contributing to the treatment of the hypocalcaemia of CRF.

Vitamin D deficiency may be treated with the systemic vitamin D analogues 1α-hydroxycholecalciferol (alfacalcidol) at 0.25 to 1 microgram/day or 1,25-dihydroxycholecalciferol (calcitriol) at 1 to 2 microgram/day. This rapidly brings about an increase in serum calcium.

CASE 15.5

A Prednisolone should be substituted for methylprednisolone when converting to oral therapy. Since prednisolone has a potency ratio 5:4 compared to methylprednisolone, an equivalent dose would be 25 mg. Patients should be issued with a steroid card, advised to take their medication with food and it should be emphasized that they should not stop taking the tablets unless advised by a doctor.

Although azathioprine absorption is variable in the majority of patients, patients are usually prescribed the same dose as intravenously, i.e. 75 mg. Patients should be advised to take their dose with food. There is considerable inter- and intrapatient variation in oral absorption of cyclosporin. An initial oral dose should be three times the intravenous dose but the dose should be individualized by measuring plasma levels after 3 days and adjusted accordingly. Patients should be advised that they can mix the liquid with milk or fruit juice before taking to mask the taste, and that they should check with their doctor or pharmacist before taking any other drugs or medicines.

BIBLIOGRAPHY

American hospital formulary service drug information. American Society of Hospital Pharmacists 1991

Bennett W M. Drugs and renal disease, 2nd edn. Churchill Livingstone 1986

Bennett W M et al. Drug prescribing in renal failure – dosing guidelines for adults. Philadelphia: American College of Physicians 1987

Cattell W R, Baker L R I, Greenwood R N. Renal disease. In: Kumar P J, Clark M L (eds) Clinical medicine, 2nd edn. Baillière Tindall 1990; 425–489

Davies D M. Textbook of adverse drug reactions, 4th edn. Oxford University Press 1991; 305–343

Dische F E. Concise renal pathology. Castle House Publications 1987

Dollery C et al. Therapeutic drugs. Churchill Livingstone 1991

Fillastre J P, Singlas E. Pharmacokinetics of newer drugs in patients with renal impairment – Part 1. Clinical Pharmacokinetics 1991; 20: 293

Fillastre J P, Singlas E. Pharmacokinetics of newer drugs in patients with renal impairment – Part 2. Clinical Pharmacokinetics 1991; 20: 389

Mammenem G J (ed). Clinical pharmacokinetics drug data handbook. New Zealand: Adis Press 1990

Cardiovascular disorders

Chapter 16

Hypertension

E. M. Graham-Clarke   B. S. Hebron

Primary hypertension is not a disease, it has no symptoms and patients do not die directly from it. Its importance lies in that it is the major risk factor for cerebrovascular accidents and cardiovascular events. The degree of hypertension is based on blood pressure, a continuous variable, which fluctuates from minute to minute depending on the patient's mental and physical state and environmental factors.

Hypertension is defined by an arbitrarily selected blood pressure reading, above which the benefits of treating the patient outweigh the risks of treating.

The World Health Organization defines hypertension as a diastolic blood pressure reading greater than 95 mmHg, on more than one occasion. Diastolic blood pressure readings between 90 and 95 mmHg are described as mild or borderline. Raised systolic blood pressures can exist in the absence of raised diastolic blood pressures and, therefore, systolic blood pressures greater than 160 mmHg are also classed as hypertensive.

EPIDEMIOLOGY

Hypertension occurs in 10 to 20% of middle-aged adults in developed countries and becomes more common with increasing age.

Primary or essential hypertension accounts for approximately 95% of the hypertensive population, the remainder consisting of patients with secondary hypertension.

AETIOLOGY

Primary hypertension

Primary or essential hypertension has no single identifiable cause but may be affected by a number of factors.

Age

Blood pressure tends to increase with increasing age. This is probably due to decreased compliance of the blood vessels which leads to an alteration in peripheral resistance and hence an increase in blood pressure. Diastolic blood pressure may start to fall again in those over 80 years old although the systolic blood pressure can remain elevated.

Hypertension in the elderly should be treated as vigorously as that in the younger population. The European Working Party on Hypertension in the Elderly (EWPHE) and the Primary Care Study both demonstrated the benefits of treating the elderly patient with hypertension. Three further studies have confirmed that there are significant benefits in treating isolated systolic hypertension in elderly patients; they are the Medical Research Council (MRC) Hypertension in Older Adults Study, the Systolic Hypertension in the Elderly Program (SHEP) and the Swedish Trial in Old Patients with Hypertension (STOP). Each of these studies showed a reduction in cerebrovascular accidents and cardiovascular events.

Genetics

There is a tendency for hypertension to run in families, although such a genetic link is often disputed. There is closer correlation for hypertension between siblings than parents and children. It is possible that environmental factors, learned or acquired from the family, are instrumental in providing the apparent genetic link.

Environment

Stress. Mental and physical stress cause transient increases in blood pressure. This effect is not generally sustained and taking the hypertensive individual out of the stressful environment does not always result in a decreased blood pressure.

Sodium intake. Severe dietary sodium restriction in patients who usually have a high salt intake does lead to a beneficial drop in blood pressure. However, reducing salt intake in patients whose consumption is not high does not have the same effect.

Some studies suggest that restricting sodium intake to 100 mmol/day has no effect, whereas reducing sodium intake to 60 to 80 mmol/day may reduce blood pressure. However, patients have difficulty in complying with severely sodium-restricted diets and find food so prepared unpalatable.

Alcohol. Patients who drink large amounts of alcohol have a raised blood pressure which will fall if alcohol consumption is reduced. Patients who drink no alcohol at all tend to have slightly higher blood pressures than those who drink in moderation.

Weight

Obese patients have higher blood pressures than non-obese patients, and weight reduction can lead to a decrease in blood pressure.

Obese patients may have their blood pressure overestimated by the use of an incorrectly sized blood pressure cuff. It is important that the bladder in the cuff encircles at least two-thirds of the arm, and if necessary, a larger cuff should be used in obese patients to ensure accurate readings.

Race

In developed countries Caucasians tend to have lower blood pressures than black people. However, black populations living in rural Africa have lower blood pressures than their counterparts living in the cities.

It may be that black people are more responsive to stress than Caucasians, hence the increase in blood pressure when black people move to the city and a more stressful way of living. This increase may also be associated with changes in diet. Black people may be genetically geared to salt preservation as a result of their hot climate, and may become easily overwhelmed by the salt content of the western diet, again leading to hypertension.

Secondary hypertension

Secondary hypertension has an identifiable underlying cause. However, removing the cause will not necessarily result in a fall in blood pressure. This is because the raised blood pressure can damage organs such as the kidneys, which creates a vicious circle by causing a further rise in blood pressure and leads to more damage.

Some of the more common causes of secondary hypertension are presented in Table 16.1.

Malignant or accelerated phase hypertension

Malignant or accelerated phase hypertension can occur in patients with primary or secondary hypertension and is often associated with renovascular disease. It is characterized by a rapid rise in blood pressure with associated damage to small blood vessels which is seen most markedly in the retina of the eye and appears as retinal exudates. The kidney is also damaged leading to haematuria and proteinuria.

The condition is usually seen in younger patients and is closely associated with smoking.

Table 16.1 Common causes of secondary hypertension

Renal disease	Polycystic kidneys
	Renal artery stenosis
	Pyelonephritis
	Renin-secreting tumour
Drug induced	Oral contraceptives
	Carbenoxolone and liquorice derivatives
	Corticosteroids
Pregnancy	Pre-eclampsia
Hormonal	Cushing's syndrome
	Phaeochromocytoma
	Hyper- and hypothyroidism
	Acromegaly
Other	Coarctation of the aorta

If left untreated 90% of patients will die within 1 year. The long-term prognosis depends on the success of treatment in limiting end-organ damage, particularly in the kidney.

PATHOPHYSIOLOGY

Blood pressure is the product of cardiac output and peripheral resistance. If the output from the heart rises, but the resistance from the small blood vessels remains the same then the blood pressure will rise. However, in most patients with essential hypertension the peripheral resistance increases whilst cardiac output remains the same. Peripheral resistance comprises several components that include the viscosity of the blood and the diameter and compliance of the blood vessels. High viscosity blood will require a higher blood pressure in order to force it through the vascular bed. A high pressure is also needed to push blood through constricted and non-compliant blood vessels.

A variety of mechanisms exist to maintain normal blood pressure control, two of which are susceptible to drug therapy. Blood pressure mainly falls under the control of the sympathetic nervous system. Peripheral baroreceptors detect changes in the blood pressure and send appropriate messages to the cardiovascular centre in the medulla of the brain. This, in turn, triggers nerves, leading to a change in circulating blood pressure. Stimulation of $beta_1$-adrenoreceptors increases the heart rate. In the blood vessels stimulation of $beta_2$-adrenoreceptors will cause dilatation, whilst stimulation of alpha-adrenoreceptors causes vasoconstriction.

The kidney also plays a major role in blood pressure regulation, through the renin–angiotensin system. Renin is released from the juxtaglomerular apparatus in the kidney when a reduction in serum sodium concentration or blood volume is detected. Renin acts on angiotensinogen to release angiotensin I, which is converted by angiotension converting enzyme, to angiotensin II. Angiotensin II produces a potent rise in blood pressure through several routes including vasoconstriction, stimulation of the noradrenergic sympathetic nervous system and stimulation of the adrenals to release aldosterone. A similar renin–angiotensin system has been detected in the blood vessel walls where it is probably mainly responsible for local vaso-constriction.

CLINICAL MANIFESTATIONS

Hypertension has no symptoms and until patients are diagnosed as hypertensive, most patients feel perfectly well. The exceptions to this are patients with malignant hypertension in whom the rapid rise in blood pressure may lead to headaches.

The symptoms usually associated with hypertension by the layman, such as headaches and nosebleeds, are probably no more frequent than found in the general population.

INVESTIGATIONS

The diagnosis of hypertension relies solely on blood pressure readings. It is important that the correct technique is used, with suitable equipment. Sphygmomanometers should be well maintained. In the case of mercury (the most popular) this means ensuring that the glass is kept clean and that the mercury zeroes correctly. The reading should be taken to the nearest 2 mmHg as rounding up or down to the nearest 10 mmHg could lead to misdiagnosis. As the scale is marked in 2 mmHg intervals it also makes no sense to round to 5 mmHg. The cuff should be placed around the arm at a height which is level with the heart. It should then be inflated until the pulse cannot be felt and then deflated slowly until the first sounds are heard in the brachial artery, the reading at this point being the systolic blood pressure. The cuff is then deflated until the sounds disappear (5th Korotkoff phase, K5), the reading at this stage being the diastolic blood pressure. Many people still record diastolic blood pressure at the point at which the sounds become muffled (4th Korotkoff phase, K4), but this is less reliable and K5 is now recommended in the UK.

Some patients tend to have higher blood pressure readings when measured at the clinic or surgery than they have normally. This is referred to as 'white coat hypertension' and may result in the patient being classed as hypertensive when in fact they are not. Ambulatory blood pressure monitoring eliminates this bias and can prove more reliable than single one-off readings at the surgery.

Several further investigations are usually carried out, in order to detect any potential causes for the hypertension.

Raised serum urea and creatinine levels may indicate some form of renal damage.

Serum potassium must be measured before treatment is started. Low levels of potassium will not only be aggravated by some drug treatments, but also suggest the presence of hyperaldosteronism.

High serum uric acid levels are common in patients with renal hypertension, and less common in untreated primary hypertensive patients. Diuretic treatment may elevate uric acid levels further but need not be treated unless gout is precipitated.

An electrocardiogram (ECG) will indicate whether left ventricular hypertrophy has occurred. Long-standing untreated, or poorly treated hypertension leads to a strain on the heart as it tries to pump blood around the body against the increased peripheral resistance. This results in an enlargement of the left ventricular muscle. The presence of hypertrophy is an important indicator of poor long-term survival.

Dipstick testing of the urine is important, to reveal the presence or absence of glucose, protein and blood. The latter two indicate renal disease, and the former suggests diabetes mellitus.

TREATMENT

The aim of treatment is to reduce the blood pressure to what is considered a normal level and thereby reduce the risk of suffering a cerebrovascular accident or a cardiovascular event, and to prevent organ damage. In addition, treatment should aim to reduce other risk factors which may be present.

Over-treatment might prove to be as hazardous as under-treatment, although this has not been conclusively proven. It is probably prudent to lower diastolic blood pressure to within the range 85 to 90 mmHg.

Patients with borderline hypertension probably require only non-drug therapy, associated with regular blood pressure checks. Non-drug therapy may involve changes to a patient's lifestyle such as weight reduction, decreased alcohol and salt intake and relaxation therapy. In addition, patients should be advised to stop smoking. Although smoking has no impact on hypertension itself, combined with hypertension it becomes a potent risk factor for both cardiovascular and cerebrovascular accidents. If patients continue to smoke whilst receiving antihypertensive therapy, the benefits of therapy are greatly reduced.

In patients with hypertension a significant change in lifestyle is often called for and may be difficult to achieve, especially if an individual felt perfectly well prior to diagnosis. When drug therapy has been initiated the patient may feel worse because of drug-induced side effects. Considerable time needs to be taken to explain the benefits of therapy and the need for changes in lifestyle. Drug therapy should aim for a single drug regimen which has minimal side effects.

Drug treatment

The British Hypertensive Society currently recommends a stepwise approach to treatment of essential hypertension starting with a diuretic, then a beta-adrenoreceptor blocker, then a combination of the two, with the addition of a vasodilator if the combination is not effective. Although this remains a commonly prescribed sequence it is not appropriate for all patients. Indeed, recent trials have focused on the unexpectedly high incidence of treatment withdrawal among patients. This has led to the consensus that diuretics and beta-adrenoreceptor blockers, especially propranolol, are probably less universally well tolerated than previously thought. There are also many patients in whom a stepped approach is undesirable.

It is probably more appropriate to approach drug therapy from the point of view of the patient and his or her concomitant disease state. However, some knowledge of the mode of action of the various classes of drugs is essential.

Diuretics

Thiazides are the commonest group of diuretics used in the treatment of hypertension. Loop diuretics are occasionally used but appear to have a smaller antihypertensive effect than thiazides but are useful in patients with renal impairment and when the patient requires a more potent diuresis as in heart failure. The potassium-sparing diuretics may be used in combination with either a thiazide or loop diuretic to prevent the occurrence of hypokalaemia in susceptible individuals. Thiazides are more effective than loop diuretics in lowering blood pressure and have been used for many years. They have the advantage that they are cheap and can be given once daily to aid compliance. Diuretics have been shown to significantly reduce the incidence of stroke but their use has been associated with a large number of treatment withdrawals because of side effects. It is now thought that the high incidence of side effects is dose related and drugs such as bendrofluazide need not be prescribed in doses exceeding 2.5 mg with some suggestions that 1.25 mg may be more than sufficient. The main adverse effects of thiazides are listed in Table 16.2.

The initial mode of action of diuretics is probably connected with a reduction in circulating fluid volume and sodium as a result of diuresis. However, their long-term mode of action appears to be a reduction in peripheral resistance as a result of vasodilatation of the small blood vessels.

Beta-adrenoreceptor blockers

Along with thiazide diuretics, beta-adrenoreceptor blockers have been the mainstay of hypertensive therapy for many years. Their mode of action is more complicated than originally thought, and is still not fully understood. They act by blocking the beta-adrenoreceptors of the

Table 16.2 Common adverse effects of drugs used to treat hypertension

Drug class	Adverse effects	Drug class	Adverse effects
Thiazide diuretics	Hypokalaemia Hyperuricaemia Decreased glucose tolerance Impotence Lethargy Hyperlipidaemia	Alpha-adrenoreceptor blockers	Profound first dose hypotension Dizziness Headache Lethargy Oedema
Beta-adrenoreceptor blockers	Bronchoconstriction Hyperlipidaemia Impotence Increased insulin resistance Decreased peripheral blood flow Masking of hypoglycaemic symptoms in diabetic patients	Methyldopa	Sedation Headache Impaired mental agility Nightmares Bradycardia Orthostatic hypotension Oedema Haemolytic anaemia Impotence

Lipophilic beta-adrenoreceptor blockers	Central side effects:
	    nightmares
	    sleep disturbance
	    hallucinations
		Clonidine	Rebound hypertension on sudden withdrawal
			Drowsiness
			Sleep disturbance
			Headache
			Euphoria

ACE inhibitors	Profound first dose hypotension if administered with diuretics Dry cough Hyperkalaemia Taste disorders Worsening of pre-existing renal dysfunction Angioneurotic oedema	Hydralazine	Lupus-like syndrome Tachycardia Headache Dizziness Flushing Liver damage
Calcium channel blockers	Headache Dizziness Flushing Postural hypotension Ankle oedema	Minoxidil	Hirsutism Oedema Tachycardia

adrenergic nervous system. However, there is more than one type of beta-adrenoreceptor and the beta-adrenoreceptor blockers vary in their selectivity. Beta$_1$-adrenoreceptors are found in the heart where stimulation causes an increased rate and cardiac output. They are also found in the juxtaglomerular apparatus where stimulation leads to an increase in renin production. Beta$_2$-adrenoreceptors are widespread throughout the body and stimulation leads to a variety of effects, including dilatation of the bronchioles, arterioles and veins, and increased secretion of glucagon and insulin. Non-selective beta-blockade will, therefore, have a variety of unwanted effects on the lungs and small blood vessels. For this reason beta$_1$-selective blockers (cardioselective) are now preferred in the treatment of hypertension (e.g. atenolol). As with the

thiazide diuretics, the initial doses of atenolol that were recommended are now considered excessive, and therapeutic responses can be achieved with 50 mg daily (possibly even as low as 25 mg) and no advantage is found in using doses greater than 100 mg daily.

Angiotensin converting enzyme (ACE) inhibitors

These drugs act by blocking the conversion of angiotensin I to angiotensin II and so prevent the vasoconstrictive effect of angiotensin II and the sodium retention caused by aldosterone. ACE is now thought to be one of the prostaglandin family, and as such the ACE inhibitors may have other mechanisms of bringing blood pressure down that are currently unknown. Captopril was the first commercially available

ACE inhibitor and was found to have a wide range of side effects including renal impairment. In patients taking a diuretic it is preferable to stop the diuretic and try a small test dose of the ACE inhibitor. Providing there is no great hypotensive effect it is then safe to proceed with regular therapy, increasing the dose gradually until the desired result is achieved.

Calcium channel blockers

These act by blocking the calcium channels in smooth muscle, hence reducing or preventing muscle contraction. There are thought to be at least three different receptor sites where they act and the different groups of calcium channel blockers do show different effects, for example on heart rate and peripheral vasodilatation. The dihydropyridines (e.g. nifedipine and amlodipine) have relatively little direct action on the heart compared to the phenylalkylamines (e.g. verapamil) and benzothiazepines (e.g. diltiazem) but an increased effect on peripheral vasodilatation, making them in theory more suitable for the treatment of simple hypertension.

Alpha-adrenoreceptor blockers

Alpha-adrenoreceptor antagonists block the action of alpha-adrenergic receptors in the small blood vessels which, when stimulated, would normally cause vasoconstriction. Prazosin is associated with a profound first dose hypotension in some patients and requires to be given three times daily. Doxazosin and terazosin, on the other hand can be given once daily, and may prove to have a reduced first dose hypotensive effect. The advantage of all these drugs is that they appear to have a beneficial influence on the blood lipid profile by lowering LDL cholesterol.

Centrally acting agents

The two drugs in this class that are still in use are methyldopa and clonidine, although the use of both agents is declining. Reserpine and the rauwolfia alkaloids have been used in the past, but are now seldom seen as their side effect profile has caused them to be superseded by safer and newer drugs. The exact mechanism of antihypertensive action for methyldopa is unclear but it is thought to involve stimulation of central alpha-adrenoreceptors by a metabolite, alpha-methyl-noradrenaline, which inhibits sympathetic outflow to the heart, kidneys and peripheral vasculature. Clonidine similarly stimulates central alpha-adrenoreceptors and reduces sympathetic outflow.

Vasodilators

As their name suggests, these act by causing peripheral vasodilatation. As a result of their side effect profile they are confined to second or third line treatment of hypertension when other drugs have failed. The two orally active agents that are currently used are minoxidil and hydralazine. Both drugs cause a direct vasodilatation of arterioles and reduce peripheral resistance with little effect on veins. Nitroprusside causes vasodilatation by a direct effect on arterial and venous smooth muscle and can be used by intravenous infusion in a hypertensive emergency.

The comparative pharmacokinetics of the antihypertensive agents are summarized in Table 16.3 and common drug interactions listed in Table 16.4.

Treatment of malignant hypertension

Blood pressure in malignant hypertensive patients needs to be brought down and under control quickly, but rarely requires the use of intravenous drugs. An extremely rapid rise in blood pressure, for example during surgery, does require immediate correction, usually with nitroprusside. If the blood pressure has been rising (at an accelerated rate) over a number of days, then the body will to some extent compensate, and a very rapid fall in blood pressure will lead to decreased perfusion of vital organs including the brain and, therefore, to organ damage. In these circumstances, treatment with oral antihypertensive agents such as the calcium channel blockers is suitable, with dose titration

Table 16.3 Comparative pharmacokinetics of antihypertensive agents

Drug	Elimination half-life (h)	Frequency of administration	Clearance routes	Active metabolites
Thiazide diuretics				
Bendrofluazide	3.9	Once a day	Hepatic, 30% renal	Yes
Hydrochlorothiazide	10	Once a day	Renal	
Indapamide	17	Once a day	Hepatic	Yes
Beta-adrenoreceptor blockers				
Atenolol	6–9	Once a day	Renal	No
Labetolol	3–4	Twice a day	Hepatic	No
Metoprolol	3–4	Once to twice a day	Hepatic	No
Oxprenolol	2–3	Twice a day	Hepatic	No
Timolol	4–5	Once to twice a day	Hepatic, 20% renal	No
Propranolol	3–4	Twice a day	Hepatic	Yes
ACE inhibitors*				
Captopril	4	Twice a day	50–70% renal	No
Enalapril	11 (enalaprilat)	Once a day	60% renal/bile	Yes
Lisinopril	12.5	Once a day	Renal	No
Quinapril	1 (pro-drug) 2 (quinaprilat)	Once a day	Renal, bile	Yes
Calcium channel blockers				
Verapamil	3–7	Two to three times a day	Hepatic	Yes
Amlodipine	35–50	Once a day	Hepatic	
Nifedipine	5.4	Twice a day (modified release)	Hepatic	Yes
Alpha-adrenoreceptor blockers				
Prazosin	3	Two to three times a day	Hepatic	
Doxazosin	22	Once a day	Hepatic, bile	
Terazosin	10–18	Once a day	Hepatic, bile	
Others				
Clonidine	6–13	Three times a day	45% renal	Yes
Methyldopa	1.3	Two to three times a day	Hepatic, 20–60% renal	Yes
Hydralazine	2.5	Twice a day	Hepatic, 25% renal	Yes
Minoxidil	3.5	Once a day	Hepatic, 15–20% renal	

* Excretion of ACE inhibitors unclear.

and additional drugs as necessary in order to bring the blood pressure down over 2 or 3 days.

Patients and their disease states

Many patient-related factors and clinical conditions influence the choice of antihypertensive agent. Some of the clinical conditions which influence the selection of antihypertensive agents are summarized in Table 16.5.

Afro-Caribbeans

In the mid 1980s it was noticed that a subgroup of Afro-Caribbeans responded better to hydrochlorothiazide than to acebutolol. This lack of response to beta-adrenoreceptor blockers has subsequently been supported in other trials, although labetalol, which also blocks alpha-adrenoreceptors does seem to be as effective as it is in the white population. Trials comparing calcium channel blockers to beta-adrenoreceptor blockers in the two races have confirmed the resistance of hypertension in the black population to beta-blockade. In general diuretics and calcium channel blockers are more effective than beta-adrenoreceptor blockers as monotherapy in Afro-Caribbeans.

Table 16.4   Common drug interactions with antihypertensive agents

Drug class	Interacting drug	Interaction
Thiazide diuretics	NSAIDs	Decreased hypotensive effect
	Digoxin	Digoxin toxicity if hypokalaemia occurs
	Antiarrhythmics	Increased toxicity of amiodarone, disopyramide, flecainide and quinidine if hypokalaemia occurs
		Action of lignocaine, mexiletine and tocainide antagonized by hypokalaemia
	Lithium	Increased lithium levels
	Corticosteroids	Increased risk of hypokalaemia
Beta-adrenoreceptor blockers	Anaesthetics	Increased hypotensive effect
	Antiarrhythmics	Bradycardia
		Increased risk of lignocaine toxicity with propranolol
	Alpha-adrenoreceptor blockers	Increased risk of first dose hypotension
	Verapamil	Asystole
	Sympathomimetics	Severe hypertension
	NSAIDs	Decreased hypotensive effect
ACE Inhibitors	NSAIDs	Hyperkalaemia
	Lithium	Increased lithium levels
	Anaesthetics	Increased hypotensive effect
	Potassium supplements	Hyperkalaemia
	Potassium-sparing diuretics	Hyperkalaemia
Alpha-adrenoreceptor blockers	Diuretics and beta-adrenoreceptor blockers	Increased risk of first dose hypotension
	Corticosteroids	Decreased hypotensive effect
Prazosin	Indomethacin	Decreased hypotensive effect
Calcium channel blockers	Digoxin	Digoxin levels increased by diltiazem, nicardipine and verapamil
	Antiepileptics	Effect of carbamazepine enhanced by diltiazem and verapamil
		Effect of isradipine, nicardipine and nifedipine reduced by primidone, carbamazepine, phenytoin and phenobarbitone
Methyldopa	Antidepressant monoamine oxidase inhibitors	Decreased hypotensive effect which can lead to a hypertensive crisis
	Levodopa	Potential hypotension
	Lithium	Increased lithium levels
	Nitrates	Increased hypotensive effect

The elderly

Selection of appropriate antihypertensive medication in the elderly is difficult because of the age-related deterioration in glomerular filtration rate, hepatic mass and blood flow and the co-existence of other diseases. Most studies of the treatment of hypertension in the elderly have shown that there is no reduction in overall death rate although there is a reduction in cardiovascular death rate. If drug treatment is necessary it should be with low doses of a thiazide diuretic, with the addition of a potassium-sparing agent, e.g. triamterene or amiloride, if hypokalaemia is a problem. However, as renal function deteriorates with age, it should be noted that thiazides are less effective in the presence of compromised renal function.

Numerous studies have demonstrated that beta-adrenoreceptor blockers are less potent in the elderly despite a reduction in drug clearance. Low doses of beta-adrenoreceptor blockers should be used but probably not as first line agents unless there are associated cardiovascular conditions, such as angina or arrhythmias, which would benefit from beta-blockade.

Table 16.5 Clinical conditions that influence the choice of antihypertensive agent

Disorder	Advantageous effect	Disadvantageous effect	Dangerous effect
Cardiovascular disease			
Angina	Beta-adrenoreceptor blockers Calcium channel blockers		
Heart failure	Diuretics ACE inhibitors	Calcium channel blockers	Beta-adrenoreceptor blockers
Heart block			Beta-adrenoreceptor blockers Verapamil
Tachycardia	Beta-adrenoreceptor blockers Verapamil	Calcium channel blockers, e.g. dihydropyridines Prazosin	
Previous heart attack	Beta-adrenoreceptor blockers without ISA	Beta-adrenoreceptor blockers with ISA	
Raynaud's phenomenon	Calcium channel blockers	Non-selective beta- adrenoreceptor blockers Clonidine	
Respiratory disease			
Asthma			Beta-adrenoreceptor blockers
Chronic obstructive airways disease		Beta-adrenoreceptor blockers	
Metabolic diseases			
IDDM			Non-selective beta- adrenoreceptor blockers
NIDDM		Thiazides	
Gout		Thiazides	
Thyrotoxicosis	Non-selective beta- adrenoreceptor blockers		
Hyperlipidaemia	Alpha-adrenoreceptor blockers	Thiazides Beta-adrenoreceptor blockers	
Porphyria			Calcium channel blockers ACE inhibitors Hydralazine Clonidine Methyldopa
Hepatic impairment		Hydralazine Calcium channel blockers	Methyldopa
Genitourinary disease			
Prostatism	Alpha-adrenoreceptor blockers	Diuretics	
Renal impairment		ACE inhibitors Methyldopa	
Central nervous system			
Migraine	Non-selective beta- adrenoreceptor blockers		
Depression		Propranolol Clonidine	Methyldopa

Methyldopa, a centrally acting agent, was one of the earlier antihypertensive drugs and many of the elderly were started on this drug in the past. It has numerous side effects including sedation, which is of particular importance in the elderly, and stopping this drug can often lead to a noticeable improvement in mental agility.

Vasodilators such as the calcium channel blockers can prove extremely useful in the eld-erly in reducing blood pressure with the minimum of side effects without putting too much strain on the heart. Peripheral resistance is increased with the decreasing compliance of blood vessels in the elderly, thus vasodilatation of the arterioles by a calcium channel blocker can produce a significant reduction in blood pressure.

ACE inhibitors can be effective, even though low renin levels are common in the elderly and a reduced effect might be expected. Careful monitoring is necessary because of the decrease in renal function with increasing age, which could potentiate the ability of ACE inhibitors to cause potassium retention and lead to hyperkalaemia. ACE inhibitors are contra-indicated in renal stenosis, a condition which is difficult to diagnose in the elderly.

Diabetic patients

Hypertension and diabetes mellitus commonly coincide. In non-insulin-dependent diabetes (NIDDM) thiazides can further impair glucose tolerance and, whenever possible, should be avoided. In insulin-dependent diabetes (IDDM), hypoglycaemic side effects have been reported with non-selective beta-adrenoreceptor blockers. This is a result of impairment of the beta$_2$-mediated breakdown of glycogen to glucose and release of glucose from the liver. In insulin treated patients beta$_1$-selective blockers (e.g. atenolol, bisoprolol, metoprolol) may be used, unless the patient is particularly vulnerable to hypoglycaemia. Beta-adrenoreceptor blockers also mask the tachycardia associated with hypoglycaemia such that patients may be unaware that their blood glucose levels are decreasing. In addition, beta-adrenoreceptor blockers can aggravate pre-existing peripheral vascular disease which may be present in the diabetic patient.

Myocardial infarction

Ten different beta-adrenoreceptor blockers have been evaluated at various dosages with the aim of reducing post-infarct mortality. Those trials comparing beta-adrenoreceptor blockers with intrinsic sympathomimetic activity (ISA) (e.g. oxprenolol, pindolol) with placebo have shown either an unfavourable mortality trend or no statistically significant differences between the drug and placebo. In contrast, most of the trails of beta-adrenoreceptor blockers without ISA (e.g. propranolol, timolol) have shown a reduction in mortality. Thus, in hypertensive patients surviving a heart attack, a beta-adrenoreceptor blocker without ISA would be beneficial not only in reducing blood pressure but also in reducing the risk of death and rate of non-fatal reinfarctions.

Asthmatic patients

Stimulation of bronchial beta$_2$-adrenoreceptors is the principal mechanism by which bronchodilatation can be effectively produced to treat an asthma attack. Blockade of beta$_2$-adrenoreceptors with a beta-adrenoreceptor blocker will impair the efficacy of such treatment. Indeed, non-selective beta-adrenoreceptor blockers such as propranolol can cause bronchoconstriction in certain patients who have no history of asthma. All beta-adrenoreceptor blockers, including those with beta$_1$ selectivity and ISA, can cause bronchoconstriction in asthmatic patients. Although patients who develop asthma while taking a beta$_1$-selective blocker respond more readily to beta$_2$-stimulants such as salbutamol, the risk of severe bronchoconstriction should preclude the use of all beta-adrenoreceptor blockers in asthmatics.

Renal disease

Propranolol diminishes renal blood flow and reduces the glomerular rate by 10 to 20%. The more selective beta-adrenoreceptor blockers, or those with ISA or an alpha-adrenoreceptor blocking action, produce smaller reductions in renal blood flow. However, nadolol, which is non-selective, can maintain renal blood flow, presumably by stimulating dopamine receptors in the renal vasculature. The dosage of water-soluble beta-adrenoreceptor blockers, which are excreted in the urine, may need to be reduced in patients with impaired renal function.

ACE inhibitors may cause a reduction in renal blood flow and must be used with caution in patients with renal disease. In renal artery stenosis ACE inhibitors are contra-indicated because the reduction in blood flow can be such that the affected kidney receives no blood at all.

Pregnancy

Patients with pre-existing primary hypertension

may become pregnant or pregnancy itself may induce gestational hypertension. In either case it is desirable to control blood pressure, as the hypertension is associated with complications for both the mother and the fetus.

Methyldopa remains the drug of choice for treating hypertension presenting in pregnancy. Atenolol is used but has been associated with the birth of smaller babies and it is excreted in breast milk. ACE inhibitors are potentially damaging to the fetus and inhibition of the renin–angiotensin system may cause problems in the neonate.

If the hypertension leads to eclampsia parenteral hydralazine is usually effective, continuing until the mother recovers sufficiently to take oral medication. The disadvantage of using parenteral hydralazine is the reflex tachycardia which invariably occurs.

CASE STUDIES

CASE 16.1

A 55-year-old West Indian man with NIDDM is found on three consecutive visits to the clinic to have a blood pressure of 172/100 mmHg. It is decided to initiate drug therapy to control his hypertension.

Q What antihypertensive drugs should be avoided?

CASE 16.2

Mr A. D. is a fit healthy 35-year-old obese male who is found to have a blood pressure of 178/114 mmHg. He smokes heavily and drinks 10 or more units of alcohol each evening.

Q What advice do you give him?

CASE 16.3

Mr D. C. is a 30-year-old patient who was found to have hypertension and was started on atenolol 50 mg daily. 3 weeks after starting therapy he complained of being tired and having cold hands. His wife mentioned that he now seemed to be having problems with lovemaking.

Q How could his drug treatment be changed to help him?

CASE 16.4

Mrs S. V. is 45 years old and was recently diagnosed as having hypertension, for which she was prescribed atenolol 100 mg daily. A few days later she was rushed to hospital with a severe asthma attack.

Q What has precipitated the attack, and what changes should be made to her drug therapy?

CASE 16.5

A 58-year-old hypertensive female has suffered side effects from a variety of antihypertensive drugs. She is now well controlled on enalapril, 20 mg daily, but complains of a dry cough. Her serum potassium has also risen.

Q Should her treatment be changed?

ANSWERS TO CASE STUDIES

CASE 16.1

A Although thiazide diuretics are effective antihypertensive agents in Afro-Caribbeans, they should be avoided in diabetic patients because they reduce glucose tolerance. This is particularly important in patients with NIDDM because it may make the difference between control by diet or medication. Beta-adrenoreceptor blockers should also be avoided in diabetics because of their effects on hypoglycaemia, and because they will aggravate any pre-existing peripheral neuropathy. There is also evidence that some calcium channel blockers may impair glucose tolerance, but the clinical significance of this is thought to be minor.

CASE 16.2

A Mr A. D. will need to change his lifestyle quite dramatically. In order to acquire the appropriate motivation, he needs to understand why the treatment of hypertension is so important. Weight reduction down to his ideal body mass will help to reduce his blood pressure. Regular exercise will help protect his cardiovascular system, and also aid weight reduction. He should stop smoking which would then reduce his chances of having a cardiovascular accident. He should also reduce his alcohol intake to within the recommended limit of 21 units each week (14 units each week for women).

CASE 16.3

A The feeling of tiredness and the cold extremities described by the patient are both adverse effects of beta-adrenoreceptor blockers. Impotence is also another recognized, but probably under-reported, side effect. The treatment is actually making Mr D. C. feel worse and, in order to gain his confidence and ensure his compliance with treatment, a different class of drug needs to be tried. Although thiazide diuretics are effective, their side effect profile, in particular lethargy, impotence and effects on the lipid profile, makes them unsuitable in the young. The flushing and headaches seen with calcium channel blockers are not necessarily a class effect and changing to an alternative within the class can improve matters. However, Mr D. C. has already experienced side effects to one class of drugs, and a trial of another with noticeable side effects may decrease his confidence even further. An ACE inhibitor may possibly be a better choice for this patient.

CASE 16.4

A The atenolol has blocked the beta-adrenoreceptors in the lung preventing bronchial dilatation and precipitating the attack. Mrs S. V. needs to be changed to a more suitable drug therapy which will not affect her bronchioles. A thiazide diuretic, calcium channel blocker or ACE inhibitor would be suitable. It would also be worthwhile taking a little time to reassure the patient that the new drug would not have the same effect on the lungs as atenolol.

CASE 16.5

A The dry cough is a side effect of all ACE inhibitors (up to 20% of patients, particularly middle-aged women, suffer this) but does not necessarily require that the treatment should be stopped. It appears to be an adverse effect of all ACE inhibitors, so changing to another will not resolve the problem. The decision depends on the patient and the severity and disturbance associated with it: she may feel that the dry cough is a small price to pay for a better quality of life. The rise in the serum potassium level is potentially more serious and a possible explanation, such as concurrent therapy with a potassium-sparing agent, must be explored.

BIBLIOGRAPHY

Amery A, Burkenhager W, Brixko P, Bulpitt C, Clement D, Deruyttere M et al. Mortality and morbidity results from the European working party on high blood pressure in the elderly trial. Lancet 1985; 1: 1349–1354

Coope J, Warrender T S. Randomised trial of treatment of hypertension in elderly patients in primary care. British Medical Journal 1986; 293: 2562–2571

Dahlof B, Lindholm L H, Hansson L, Schersten B, Ekbom T, Wester P-O. Morbidity and mortality in the Swedish Trial in Old Patients with hypertension (STOP-Hypertension). Lancet 1991; 338: 1281–1285

Lewis R V, Maclean D. Treatment of mild–moderate hypertension. Hospital Update April 1990; 331–345

Medical Research Council Working Party. MRC trial of mild hypertension: principal results. British Medical Journal 1985; 291: 97–104

SHEP Cooperative Research Group. Prevention of stroke by antihypertensive drug treatment in older persons with isolated systolic hypertension. Final results of the Systolic Hypertension in the Elderly Programme (SHEP). JAMA 1991; 265: 3255–3264

The British Hypertension Society Working Party. Treating mild hypertension – agreement from the large trials. British Medical Journal 1989; 298: 694–698

Chapter 17

Ischaemic heart disease

D. K. Scott

Ischaemic heart disease (IHD) is a condition with many underlying causes which all have in common the ability to impair the supply of oxygenated blood to cardiac tissue. The most common situation in which oxygen demand exceeds supply occurs when the vascular supply to the heart is impeded by atheroma, thrombosis or spasm of coronary arteries. Myocardial ischaemia can also arise if oxygen demand is abnormally increased as may occur in severe ventricular hypertrophy due to hypertension or where the oxygen carrying capacity of blood is impaired as in iron-deficiency anaemia. Two or more causes usually coexist and progress to precipitate myocardial ischaemia.

EPIDEMIOLOGY

The epidemiology of IHD has been studied extensively and has led to much debate concerning the associated risk factors. Absence of established risk factors does not guarantee freedom from IHD for any individual and some individuals with several major risk factors seem perversely healthy. None the less, it is generally believed that in developed countries education and publicity about the major risk factors has led to changes in social habits, particularly with respect to a reduction in smoking and fat consumption, and this has contributed to a decrease in the incidence of IHD. Better treatment has also contributed to a decrease in cardiac mortality although IHD still remains the most common cause of death in adults and accounts for some 200 000 deaths per year in the UK including 70% of sudden natural deaths. Around one-third of 50- to 59-year-old men have evidence of IHD and this proportion increases with age.

The increase in mortality with age is probably not due to a particular age-related factor but the cumulative effect of risk factors which lead to atheroma and thrombosis and hence to coronary artery disease. The main risk factors are family history, hypertension, cigarette smoking and raised serum cholesterol. Of these, the determining factor appears to be serum cholesterol because hypertension and smoking have little effect on the incidence of IHD in populations with low average cholesterol concentrations but a major effect in populations such as the UK with high cholesterol levels.

Other cholesterol-related risk factors include elevated serum triglyceride concentrations, high saturated fat intake and a high saturated:polyunsaturated dietary fat ratio. These and other dietary factors, including energy intake and obesity, are difficult to separate out since they are all interrelated. However, it is clear that obese persons have a higher risk of IHD, whatever the prime cause, and all dietary factors should be addressed simultaneously in an attempt to decrease risk.

Females appear to be less susceptible to IHD than men although they seem to lose this protection after the menopause, presumably because of hormonal changes. The effect of combined hormone replacement therapy is unclear although there is increasing evidence that postmenopausal oestrogen therapy substantially reduces the risk of death from cardiovascular disease. Race has not proved to be a clear risk factor since the prevalence of IHD seems to depend much more strongly on location and lifestyle than on ethnic origin or place of birth. Diabetes mellitus is a positive risk factor in developed countries with high levels of IHD but not in countries with little IHD. Whilst frequent aggressive physical exercise is probably harmful to some, an active lifestyle which includes moderate exercise is beneficial, although the optimum level has not been determined and its beneficial effect appears to be readily overwhelmed by the presence of other risk factors. A family history of IHD is a positive risk factor, independent of diet and other risk factors.

AETIOLOGY

The vast majority of IHD occurs in patients with atherosclerosis of the coronary arteries which starts before adulthood. The cause of spontaneous atherosclerosis is unclear although it is thought that in the presence of hypercholesterolaemia a non-denuding form of injury occurs to the endothelial lining of coronary arteries and other vessels. This injury is followed by subendothelial migration of monocytes and the accumulation of lipid in fatty streaks. Thereafter, there is migration and proliferation of smooth muscle cells into the intima with further lipid deposition. The smooth muscle cells, together with fibroblasts, synthesize and secrete collagen, proteoglycans, elastin and glycoproteins that make up fibrous tissue and contribute to the progression of atherosclerosis. The presence of atherosclerosis results in narrowing of vessels and a reduction in blood flow. Associated with the atherosclerotic lesion is a loss of endothelium which can serve as a stimulus for the formation of a thrombus and result in more acute manifestations of IHD, including unstable angina and myocardial infarction.

CLINICAL MANIFESTATIONS

IHD may present with the death of cardiac tissue (an infarction) or as a painful but reversible ischaemia (angina). There are three main branches of the coronary artery which supply blood to the heart. A major thrombus in one of these arteries can lead to a regional infarction which may be transmural and affect the full thickness of the myocardium, or non-transmural in which only the subendocardial layer is affected. A more diffuse subendocardial infarction may be produced by a general reduction in perfusion, perhaps as a result of widespread atherosclerosis, or perhaps as a result of myocardial hypertrophy or increased ventricular diastolic pressures. Perfusion of the subendocardium occurs only during diastole and any increase in ventricular wall tension, as could arise in congestive cardiac failure, or a reduction in the length of diastole during a tachyarrhythmia, will reduce the oxygen supply. Ventricles are affected more than atria because of their higher workload. Infarcted areas begin to heal rapidly and collateral vessels develop to supply the tissue but the process may take several months and will not permit regeneration of a fully functioning myocardium.

Unstable angina, sometimes called crescendo angina if progression is rapid, with its variable intensity and generally progressive nature, is thought to be caused by thrombosed plaques which may occlude vessels intermittently. Alternatively, platelets or small particles may break from the thrombus and occlude other small vessels.

Stable or exercise-induced angina is caused by a narrowing of the vessels which becomes critical at a certain level of demand.

Variant or Prinzmetal's angina is caused by spasm of the coronary arteries and may occur even at rest.

PROGNOSIS

Many patients with IHD experience no clinical symptoms and up to one-third of patients who have had angina-type chest pains deny it at a later examination when it appears to have resolved spontaneously. IHD is not necessarily fatal despite the large number of deaths it causes but proven coronary artery disease has an annual mortality rate of 3% (single vessel disease) to 10% (triple vessel disease).

The prognosis of an individual who has suffered a myocardial infarction is improving as thrombolytic therapy becomes more widely used and its use refined. Figure 17.1 shows the outcome of 'heart attacks' in a London suburb and indicates that some 25% of individuals will die before any medical intervention occurs. The most dangerous time after a myocardial infarction is the first few hours when ventricular fibrillation is most likely to occur. Higher death rates occur in patients who are older, have had a

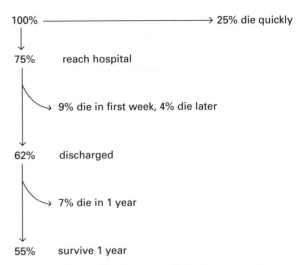

Fig. 17.1 Prognosis of heart attacks in the community (based on a London suburb; similar data are reported from the USA). (Adapted from Hampton J. Prognosis in ischaemic heart disease. Medicine International 1989; 68: 2820.)

previous infarction, suffer an anterior infarction, develop hypertension, heart failure or tachycardia, or who fail to stop smoking. Mortality is proportional to the size of the infarction which may be estimated by measuring the extent of release of cardiac enzymes into blood from damaged myocardial cells. The varying prognosis in patients treated with thrombolytic agents, in relation to the time of treatment after the infarction, is described later.

SIGNS, SYMPTOMS AND INVESTIGATIONS

IHD is very variable in presentation and there are three main diagnostic factors in the evaluation of suspected IHD: the patient's symptoms and history, the electrocardiograph (ECG) and blood enzyme assays.

The patient with a classical presentation of IHD complains of pain of a gripping or tight nature which occurs in the retrosternal region of the chest and may radiate to the neck, back or left shoulder with possible involvement of the jaw, teeth or epigastrium. The pain is typically brought on by exertion, a heavy meal or a change in temperature and is relieved by stopping the exertion. Sweating, pallor and anxiety are common but nonspecific signs after an infarction. Fever may follow within 12 hours and last for several days whilst pericarditis or heart failure may also occur. IHD is very variable in presentation and whilst classically associated with the symptoms described above, chest pain in particular is not always present. It has been reported that 25% of all infarcts are 'silent' and pain free. Such patients may just feel nonspecifically 'unwell' for a while and not seek medical attention or they may not remember the incident at all. Patients with or without angina may also get episodes of silent ischaemia without infarction.

The history of the pain is important because of the differing prognoses and the implications for treatment. Stable (exercise-induced) angina does not normally occur at rest, is generally predictable in relation to activities that induce pain, resolves on cessation of the causative activity and worsens only slowly. Unstable angina occurs unpredictably, including at rest, worsens rapidly over hours or days (crescendo angina) and has a 10% 1-year mortality rate.

The ECG is of considerable value in identifying ischaemia or infarction. It is, however, not unambiguous and may be difficult to interpret, especially after a previous infarction. In general, ECG changes are seen in three-quarters of patients with significant coronary artery disease but a resting ECG is normal in 50 to 75% of patients presenting for the first time with unequivocal angina. An ECG recorded during an episode of pain is more likely to be diagnostic and an ECG during an exercise tolerance test may be useful.

A standard 12-lead ECG which records the electrical activity of the heart from different aspects can identify the region of the heart affected. In leads facing an infarcted area there will usually be S–T segment elevation early on, followed within days by inversion of the T wave and then within weeks or months by a return to normal. S–T segment depression may occur in the opposite leads and in subendocardial infarctions. The only definitive ECG change, however, is the development of a Q wave within a few days of the infarction. Q waves generally persist and their presence gives no real clue as to the time of an infarction without a clinical history or enzyme studies. In ischaemia without infarction there are no QRS changes but there are many possible changes in the S–T segment and T wave.

The most conclusive retrospective evidence that an individual has suffered an infarction is an increase in cardiac enzymes in the blood. Several cardiac enzymes are assayed routinely including aspartate transaminase (AST), lactate dehydrogenase (LDH) and creatine kinase (CK). Serial estimations of these enzymes are of greatest diagnostic value since their rate and extent of release varies, as does their serum half-life (Fig. 17.2). All three enzymes can originate from sites other than the heart and therefore it may be necessary to type the enzyme (isoenzyme) by electrophoresis to identify its site of origin. For example, creatine kinase of cardiac origin (CK-MB) may be distinguished from the isoenzymes found in the brain (CK-BB) and skeletal muscle (CK-MM).

More elaborate and invasive tests may be used to determine cardiac function in appropriate patients. A catheter may be introduced into a peripheral vein and passed through to the heart and lungs where pressures and flow rate can be measured in different chambers and vessels of the heart. A radiopaque dye may be used to outline the coronary circulation and identify blockages (angiography). Radioisotopes such as technetium[99] are used to label blood cells and plasma for studying blood flow whilst thallium[201] is used for studying perfusion in myocardial tissue to identify infarcted or non-functioning areas of muscle. Echocardiography by ultrasound is noninvasive and is used to examine the gross structure and function of the myocardium and valves.

TREATMENT

As in most diseases, the aim of treatment is to decrease mortality and morbidity. However, whilst mortality is easy to measure, morbidity is not. Several measures of quality of life have been used to assess the outcome of IHD treatment,

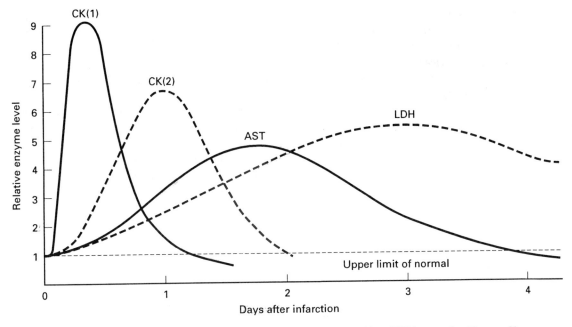

Fig. 17.2 Typical enzyme activity in serum following myocardial infarction. Key: CK(1) = creatine kinase with thrombolytic therapy; CK(2) = creatine kinase without thrombolytic therapy; AST = aspartate transaminase; LDH = lactate dehydrogenase.

combining indicators of pain, breathlessness, exercise tolerance and ability to perform normal daily activities with duration of survival. A minimum aim for treatment would therefore be to prevent myocardial infarction and associated mortality and to increase the length of pain-free survival with a lifestyle acceptable to the patient.

Modification of risk factors

Common to all stages of treatment of IHD is the need to reduce risk factors (Table 17.1). The patient needs to appreciate the value of the proposed strategy in terms of their lifestyle and to agree a plan for changing habits, which may

Table 17.1   Effect of interventions on risk of myocardial infarction (adapted from Manson J E et al. The primary prevention of myocardial infarction. New England Journal of Medicine 1992; 326: 1406–1416)

Intervention	Control	Benefit of intervention
Stopping smoking for ≥ 5 years	Current smokers	50–70% lower risk
Reducing plasma cholesterol		2% lower risk for each 1% reduction in plasma cholesterol
Treatment of hypertension		2–3% lower risk for each 1 mmHg decrease in diastolic pressure
Active lifestyle	Sedentary lifestyle	45% lower risk
Mild to moderate alcohol consumption (approx. 1 unit/day)	Total abstainers	25–45% lower risk
Low dose aspirin	Non-users	33% lower risk in men
Postmenopausal oestrogen replacement	Non-users	44% lower risk

Note: The quality of data leading to these summaries varies greatly and figures may not apply to all patient groups.

not be easy after years of smoking or eating a particular diet. The professional carer must appreciate that preventing IHD is important but neither instant nor spectacular. It involves repeated sessions of counselling over many years to initiate and maintain healthy habits. It may also involve persuasion of patients to continue taking medication for disorders such as hypertension or hyperlipidaemia to prevent an outcome that 'won't happen to me'. The general public, with government as its agent, needs to agree that a reduction in the incidence of IHD is worth some general changes in lifestyle or liberty. There is considerable evidence that passive smoking is harmful, but the only way to control it effectively is to reduce the number of public places in which smoking is permitted. National campaigns to encourage healthy eating or exercise are expensive, as is the long-term medical treatment of hypertension or hyperlipidaemia and such strategies must have the backing of governments to succeed.

For every individual there is a need to act against the causative factors of IHD. Thus, attempts should be made to control or remedy hypertension, heart failure, arrhythmias, hyperlipidaemia, obesity, diabetes mellitus, thyroid disease, anaemia and cardiac valve disorders. Apart from medication, these will require careful attention to diet and exercise and will necessitate stopping smoking. Antithrombotic therapy, most commonly with aspirin, is of proven benefit in unstable angina and myocardial infarction but trials of its use in primary prevention in asymptomatic populations have not provided conclusive evidence of benefit, partly because the subject groups were not representative of the general population. As might be expected, gastrointestinal haemorrhage, stroke and poor compliance tended to offset any reduction in IHD although the benefits were still considerable in one trial amongst male US physicians.

Whilst it is essential to deal with the above risk factors in order to reduce the impact of IHD in an individual or a community, it should be realized that several of the factors relate to the formation of atheroma and cannot easily be undone. Decisions on lifestyle and treatment have to be taken in the light of each individual's circumstances and aspirations.

Treatment of angina

Treatment is similar for both main varieties but whereas stable angina can be managed by a GP or in an outpatient clinic, unstable angina should be treated in hospital to facilitate the rapid changes in treatment that may be required. Aspirin, as a prophylaxis of infarction at 150 to 300 mg/day, is of proven benefit in unstable angina (and following myocardial infarction) but is often also used in stable angina despite a lack of evidence that it decreases the severity or frequency of anginal attacks. Changing lifestyle to reduce the demand on the heart is of value in stable angina but complete short-term bed rest is required in unstable angina in which more invasive investigations such as coronary angiography may be performed once the acute episode has settled.

Drug treatment is directed towards decreasing the workload of the heart and, to a lesser extent, improving the coronary blood supply. The main agents are organic nitrates, calcium channel blockers and beta-adrenoreceptor blockers. Unless contra-indicated, beta-adrenoreceptor blockers are first-line agents for stable and unstable angina although they are contra-indicated in the rare Prinzmetal's angina. Patients may dislike the side effects of beta-adrenoreceptor blockers but should be urged to continue wherever reasonable. Nitrates, calcium channel blockers, or both, may be added. Verapamil should be avoided (or used with extreme care) with beta-adrenoreceptor blockers but may be indicated instead of a beta-adrenoreceptor blocker. Treatment of acute attacks is by small doses of sublingual nitrates which may also be used prior to an activity (e.g. walking) which would be expected to cause an attack. Treatment of unstable angina is much more vigorous, often with several agents given simultaneously rather than by stepwise addition, generally includes parenteral nitrates and may include a sedative, such as diazepam.

Beta-adrenoreceptor blockers

Beta-adrenoreceptor blockers are useful for preventing angina in exercise because they decrease the rise in blood pressure as well as reducing the resting heart rate and decreasing the force of ejection in systole. The decreased heart rate not only reduces the energy demand but also permits better perfusion of the subendocardium by the coronary circulation. A beta-adrenoreceptor blocker may also reduce energy-demanding supraventricular or atrial arrhythmias and counteract the cardiac effects of hyperthyroidism or phaeochromocytoma.

Whilst beta-adrenoreceptor blockers are widely used, their tendency to cause bronchospasm and peripheral vascular spasm means that they are contra-indicated in patients with asthma, chronic obstructive airways diseases and peripheral vascular disease as well as in heart failure and bradycardia. They are used with caution in insulin-dependent diabetics, in whom the signs of a hypoglycaemic attack may be masked, and in patients with a history of heart block. Cardioselective agents (e.g. atenolol, metoprolol) are preferred because of their reduced tendency to cause bronchoconstriction but that does not override the above contra-indications because no

agent is completely specific for the heart. Agents with low lipophilicity (e.g. atenolol) penetrate the CNS to a lesser extent than others (e.g. propranolol) and do not so readily cause the nightmares, hallucinations and depression that are sometimes found with lipophilic agents which should not be used in patients with psychiatric disorders. CNS-mediated fatigue or lethargy are found with all beta-adrenoreceptor blockers although it must be distinguished from that of myocardial suppression. Beta-adrenoreceptor blockers should not be stopped abruptly for fear of precipitating angina through rebound receptor hypersensitivity. All beta-adrenoreceptor blockers tend to reduce renal blood flow but this is only important in renal impairment. Drugs eliminated by the kidney (Table 17.2) may require to be given at lower doses in renal impairment or in the elderly who are particularly susceptible to the CNS-mediated lassitude. Drugs eliminated by the liver have a number of theoretical interactions with other agents that affect liver blood flow or metabolic rate but these are rarely of clinical significance since the dose should be titrated to the effect. Likewise, although there is theoretical support for the use of agents with high intrinsic sympathomimetic activity (ISA) to reduce the incidence or severity of drug-induced

Table 17.2 Beta-adrenoreceptor blockers: properties and pharmacokinetics

	Blockade	Lipophilicity	ISA	Oral absorption	Elimination
Atenolol	β_1	−	−	50%	Renal $t_{1/2}$ 5–7 h
Betaxolol	β_1	+	−	100%	Hepatic+renal $t_{1/2}$ 15 h
Esmolol	β_1	−	−	i.v.	Blood enzymes $t_{1/2}$ 9 min
Labetalol	β_1 β_2 α_1	−	−	100%*	Hepatic $t_{1/2}$ 6–8 h
Metoprolol	β_1	+	−	95%*	Hepatic $t_{1/2}$ 3–4 h
Nadolol	β_1 β_2	−	−	30%	Renal $t_{1/2}$ 16–18 h
Oxprenolol	β_1 β_2	+	++	90%*	Hepatic $t_{1/2}$ 1–2 h
Propranolol	β_1 β_2	+	−	90%*	Hepatic $t_{1/2}$ 3–6 h
Sotalol	β_1 β_2	−	−	70%	Renal $t_{1/2}$ 15–17 h
Timolol	β_1 β_2	+	−	90%*	Hepatic + renal $t_{1/2}$ 3–4 h
Carteolol	β_1 β_2	−	++	80%	Hepatic + renal $t_{1/2}$ 3–7 h
Bisoprolol	β_1	+	−	90%	Hepatic + renal $t_{1/2}$ 10–12 h
Pindolol	β_1 β_2	+	+++	90%	Hepatic + renal $t_{1/2}$ 3–4 h
Carvedilol	β_1 β_2 α_1	+	−	80%*	Hepatic $t_{1/2}$ 4–8 h

Notes: All figures are approximate and subject to interpatient variability. Therapeutic ranges are not well defined.
Key: ISA = intrinsic sympathomimetic activity; $t_{1/2}$ = elimination half-life.
* Extensive first-pass metabolism may result in a significant decrease in bioavailability.

heart failure, there is no beta-adrenoreceptor blocker which is free from that problem and clinical trials of drugs with ISA have generally failed to show any benefit.

Nitrates

Organic nitrates are valuable in angina because they dilate veins (decreasing preload), dilate arteries to a much lesser extent (decreasing afterload) and promote flow in collateral coronary vessels, diverting blood from the epicardium to the endocardium. They are available in many forms but all relax vascular smooth muscle by releasing nitric oxide (also known as endothelium-derived relaxing factor) which acts via cyclic GMP. The production of nitric oxide from nitrates is probably mediated by intracellular thiols and it has been observed that when tolerance occurs to the action of nitrates, a thiol donor (such as N-acetyl cysteine) may partially restore the effectiveness of the nitrate. Tolerance is one of the main limitations to the use of nitrates, which remain the most useful class of agents in all forms of angina. Whilst it was formerly thought that it was important to have high blood levels of nitrate at all times, it is now recognized that tolerance develops rapidly and a 'nitrate-free' period of a few hours in each 24-hour period is beneficial in maintaining the effectiveness of treatment. The 'nitrate-free' period should coincide with the period of lowest risk and this is usually night-time, but not early morning which is a high risk period for infarction. Many patients receiving nitrates three times a day would do well to have their doses between 7 a.m. and 6 p.m. but this is generally not practised in unstable angina where there is no low risk period and where continuous dosing is used, with increasing doses if tolerance develops. There are many nitrate preparations available including intravenous infusions, conventional or slow-release tablets and capsules, transdermal patches and ointments, sublingual tablets and sprays and adhesive buccal tablets. The majority of stable angina patients should be controlled by conventional tablets or capsules which are cheap, can usually be administered 2 or 3 times daily and

which permit a 'nitrate-free' period at night. There is no advantage in using more than one preparation. Slow-release preparations and transdermal patches are expensive, do not generally offer such flexible dosing rates and may not permit a 'nitrate-free' period. Ointments are messy and buccal tablets are expensive and offer no real therapeutic advantage in regular therapy. Like sublingual sprays and tablets, however, they have a rapid onset of action and the drug bypasses the liver which has an extensive first-pass metabolic effect on oral nitrates. The sublingual preparations (sprays, suckable or chewable tablets) are used for the prevention or relief of acute attacks of pain but may elicit the two principal side effects of nitrates, hypotension (with dizziness and fainting) and a throbbing headache. To minimise these effects, patients should be advised to sit down, and to spit out (or swallow) the tablet once the angina is relieved. Sublingual glyceryl trinitrate tablets have a very short shelf life on exposure to air and should be stored carefully and replaced frequently. All nitrates may also induce tachycardia.

Three main nitrates are used: glyceryl trinitrate (mainly for sublingual, buccal, transdermal and intravenous routes), isosorbide dinitrate and isosorbide mononitrate. All are effective if given in appropriate doses at suitable dose intervals (Table 17.3). Since isosorbide dinitrate is metabolized to the mononitrate, there is a preference in some quarters for using the more predictable mononitrate, but this is not a significant clinical factor. A more relevant feature may be that whereas the dinitrate is usually given three to four times a day, the mononitrate is given two to three times a day. More expensive slow-release preparations exist for both drugs.

Calcium channel blockers

Calcium channel blockers act on a variety of smooth muscle and cardiac tissues and there are a large number of agents which have differing specificities for different body tissues. Those of importance in angina are arterial vasodilators (Table 17.4) but some also possess antiarrhythmic activity and most are myodep-

Table 17.3 Properties of commonly used nitrates

Drug	Speed of onset	Duration of action	Notes
Glyceryl trinitrate (GTN)			
i.v.	Immediate	Duration of infusion	
transdermal	30 minutes	Designed to release drug steadily for 24 h	Tolerance develops if applied continuously
SR tablets and capsules	Slow	8–12 h	
sublingual tablets	Rapid (1–4 min)	Less than 30 min	Inactivated if swallowed Less effective if dry mouth
spray	Rapid (1–4 min)	Less than 30 min	
buccal tablets	Rapid (1–4 min)	4–8 h	Nearly as rapid in onset as sublingual tablets
Isosorbide dinitrate			
SR tablets	} Similar to GTN		
i.v.			
sublingual	Slightly slower than GTN	As for GTN	
chewable tablets	2–5 min	2–4 h	Less prone to cause headaches than sublingual tablets
oral tablets	30–40 min	4–8 h	
Isosorbide mononitrate			
oral tablets	30–40 min	6–12 h	
SR tablets or capsules	Slow	12–24 h	Some brands claim a nitrate-free period if given once daily

Table 17.4 Properties of calcium antagonists used in angina

Drug	Absorption	Protein binding	Elimination route and half-life ($t_{1/2}$)	Effective serum concentrations
Nifedipine	60–70% available after first pass Rapid*	>90%	Hepatic $t_{1/2}$ = 3–5 h (capsules)*	—
Nicardipine	Rapid, well absorbed Extensive first-pass effect	>90%	Hepatic $t_{1/2}$ = 4–5 h	—
Diltiazem	45% available after first pass Very rapid	80–85%	Hepatic (active metabolite) + gut $t_{1/2}$ = 4–7 h	50–300 ng/ml
Verapamil	10–20% available after first pass Slow	90%	75% renal, 25% hepatic $t_{1/2}$ = 3–7 h	80–400 ng/ml

*Apparent $t_{1/2}$ and time to onset of action are greater after tablets because of slow absorption.

ressants. Nifedipine and nicardipine (and other dihydropyridines) have no effect on the conducting tissues and are very effective arterial dilators, decreasing afterload and improving coronary perfusion but also causing flushing, headaches and reflex tachycardia. The tachycardia is overcome by use of a beta-adrenoreceptor blocker. They have a particular role in the management of Prinzmetal's (variant) angina which is thought to be due to coronary artery spasm. Nicardipine has a smaller effect on myocardial contractility but neither drug has the myodep-

ressant effect of diltiazem or verapamil, both of which also have significant effects on conducting fibres and are not suitable for use in ventricular failure. Great caution should be exercised in considering their use with beta-adrenoreceptor blockers because of the additive effects on bradycardia and myodepression. Verapamil is suitable for patients in whom beta-adrenoreceptor blockers are contra-indicated on grounds of respiratory or peripheral vascular disease. Chapter 16 describes the side effects of calcium antagonists, the most important non-cardiovascular effect being marked constipation associated with verapamil.

Treatment of myocardial infarction

Treatment of infarction may be divided into three categories:

- immediate care which is designed to remove pain, prevent deterioration and improve cardiac function
- management of complications notably heart failure and arrhythmias
- prevention of a further infarction (secondary prophylaxis).

The management of heart failure and arrhythmias is covered in Chapters 18 and 19 and general measures for the prevention of infarctions are described above. The remaining therapeutic aims are pain relief, thrombolysis, minimization of infarct size and prophylaxis of arrhythmias.

The timing of treatment is vital, since myocardial damage after onset of an acute ischaemic episode is progressive and there are pathological data to suggest that it is irreversible at 6 hours. Clinical data from large studies of thrombolysis (see below) have shown that the sooner treatment is started after the onset of pain, the better. 60% of post-infarction deaths occur within 1 hour, but whilst treatment within an hour has been found to be particularly advantageous it is extremely difficult to achieve for logistic reasons.

Pain relief should be administered rapidly with intravenous diamorphine or morphine together with an antiemetic such as prochlorperazine or cyclizine. There is no benefit in leaving a patient in pain while the diagnosis is considered. The rhythm and blood pressure should be stabilized and diagnostic tests performed. Several large

Table 17.5 Vascular deaths at 35 days in ISIS-2 study	
Placebo	13.2%
Aspirin	10.7%
Streptokinase	10.4%
Aspirin + streptokinase	8.0%

studies have shown the benefit of an aspirin tablet (usually 162 mg) chewed as soon after the infarct as possible and followed by a daily enteric-coated dose for at least 1 month (but probably for life). Benefit, measured as reduced mortality, is found in addition to any thrombolytic therapy (Table 17.5).

Studies such as ISIS-3 and GISSI-2 have demonstrated the great benefit of thrombolytics given soon after the onset of pain, and the lack of a discernible difference between streptokinase and the more expensive tissue plasminogen activator (r-TPA, duteplase, alteplase) and anistreplase (anisoylated plasminogen streptokinase activated complex, APSAC) in reducing mortality. There is, however, some controversy over the optimum method of administration, over adjunct therapy, and over other measures of benefit. Since mortality studies require a large number of patients and a long term, other studies have used coronary artery patency (as measured by angiography) or left ventricular function as outcome measures. The patency studies suggest that tissue plasminogen activator produces earlier and more frequent recanalization of the arteries, especially if intravenous heparin is administered. Heparin also seems to reduce the incidence of reocclusion after tissue plasminogen activator but has no effect on streptokinase or anistreplase. Those findings are consistent with data on the relative clot-specificity of the three agents but whether they lead to measurable differences in mortality is controversial. All three agents cause haemorrhage, which may present as a stroke or a GI bleed, and some studies show an increased risk with regimens that use high dose subcutaneous or intravenous heparin. The increased mortality from heparin-associated bleeding is of similar magnitude to the decrease in cardiac mortality in the same studies and at present there seems to be no advantage in the routine use of heparin in addition to aspirin, with the possible exception of their use in rapid r-TPA regimens. Recent strokes, bleeds, pregnancy and surgery are contra-indications to thrombolysis. Anistreplase has the advantage that it can be administered by bolus rather than infusion and studies are awaited on its use by paramedics and primary care physicians prior to hospital admission. Anistreplase and streptokinase induce cross-reacting antibodies which reduce their potency and may cause an anaphylactoid response. Patients with exposure to either agent within the past 3 days to 12 months, or with a history of rheumatic fever or recent streptococcal infection, should not receive either drug. The use of hydrocortisone with the drug, to reduce allergic responses, has fallen out of favour but patients should be carefully observed for hypotension during the administration of streptokinase and anistreplase. Old age is no longer considered to be a contra-indication to thrombolysis.

Studies on nitrates in myocardial infarction were mostly completed before thrombolysis was widely used. Nevertheless, meta-analysis of those controlled studies carried out shows a reduction in mortality if nitrates are given, with some evidence that they confer additional benefit on a thrombolytic regimen. Nitrates improve collateral blood flow and aid reperfusion, thus limiting infarct size and preserving functional tissue. Sublingual nitrates may be given as a first-aid measure and the use of intravenous or buccal nitrates considered in patients whose pain does not resolve rapidly or who develop ventricular failure.

Beta-adrenoreceptor blockers have been the subject of many studies because of their anti-arrhythmic potential and because they permit increased subendocardial perfusion. In pre-thrombolysis studies, the early administration of an intravenous beta-adrenoreceptor blocker was shown to limit infarct size and to reduce mortality from early cardiac events. Long-term therapy has been shown in several studies to decrease mortality but most of the trials were too small to exclude the possibility of the difference arising by chance. When the results are combined, however, beta-blockade appears to be useful and should be used in patients in whom there is no contra-indication. Beta-blockade should be avoided in heart block, heart failure, bradycardia, asthma, obstructive airways disease and peripheral vascular disease. The most convincing trial evidence concerns timolol at 5 to 10 mg

twice a day, but other agents have been used successfully. If a beta-adrenoreceptor blocker is contra-indicated because of respiratory or vascular disorders, verapamil may be used, since it has been shown to reduce late mortality and reinfarction in patients without heart failure, although it showed no benefit when given immediately after an infarct. This is clearly not a class effect, however, since other calcium channel blockers have produced different results and nifedipine may even increase mortality in patients with heart failure following a myocardial infarction (MI). Diltiazem has been shown to reduce late mortality in non-Q-wave infarctions but further studies are required to define the role of calcium channel blockers after myocardial infarction. Other antiarrhythmics have not been found to be beneficial as prophylactic agents.

Formal anticoagulation with warfarin is not generally recommended, despite promising results in some trials. This is partly because of the poor design of those trials but also because of the success of aspirin therapy which does not have the same need for expensive and time-consuming follow-up and has fewer drug interactions. Studies on dipyridamole and sulphinpyrazone have suffered methodological flaws and their use is not recommended.

Studies on ACE inhibition have yielded promising results, especially in reduction of the left ventricular dilatation that often follows an infarction and which has a poor prognosis. Further studies are under way to investigate whether this benefit translates to increased survival and whether early administration leads to a reduction in infarct size.

PATIENT EDUCATION

Patients should be encouraged to adopt a lifestyle which makes the most of their abilities without undue hazard to their health. Most of the guidelines on prevention of IHD (see above) apply to all stages of the disease although the degree of exercise taken must be tailored according to the patient's threshold for angina. In general, although some patients are too cavalier, most patients are likely to err on the cautious side and may need to be encouraged to do more, lest their fears turn them into functional 'cripples'.

Many patients find that beta-adrenoreceptor blockers cause fatigue, dizziness, depression or nightmares and may not take their medication because it makes them feel worse not better. Such patients should be encouraged to continue with medication and discuss the problems with their doctor.

Patients requiring GTN should be counselled on the best way to administer sublingual doses, i.e. whilst sitting, not standing or lying. Tablets should be placed under the tongue only until relief is obtained (to avoid headaches), and a fresh supply should be kept in a convenient place (pocket, handbag, etc.) at all times. Oral nitrates and transdermal patches should be taken or applied at the appropriate times to ensure a low nitrate period at night and a high nitrate period soon after rising.

A diary of anginal attacks is very useful as a record of progress and may be used to adjust treatment. The use of sublingual GTN should be recorded as well as details of the activities or circumstances which provoked angina. In view of the success of early thrombolysis in MI, patients should be encouraged if they experience chest pain that is similar to a previous infarction, or worse than their usual angina, to call for an ambulance without summoning a general practitioner first. Until anistreplase is generally available to general medical practitioners, there is little they can do that the ambulance and casualty service cannot and any delay may worsen the patient's prognosis.

Patients should avoid over-the-counter preparations containing sympathomimetic drugs (e.g. 'cold-cures') but occasional aspirin for analgesia does not affect the antiplatelet action of low-dose aspirin.

CASE STUDIES

CASE 17.1

The following patients present with a history of stable angina that requires prophylactic drug therapy. Which drugs would be suitable as first line agents?

 a. A 60-year-old man with mixed COAD and asthma.

b. A 45-year-old woman with first degree heart block.

c. An 80-year-old man with non-insulin-dependent diabetes mellitus (NIDDM) and poor renal function.

CASE 17.2

Which of the following are suitable candidates for streptokinase thrombolytic therapy in the event of a suspected myocardial infarction?

 a. A 30-year-old woman with an irregular menstrual cycle.

b. A 55-year-old man with hypertension.

c. An 80-year-old man with no history of angina prior to the infarction.

d. A 65-year-old man who had an infarction 3 months ago.

ANSWERS TO CASE STUDIES

CASE 17.1

The main agents available for treating patients with stable angina are beta-adrenoreceptor blockers (e.g. atenolol, metoprolol), calcium channel blockers (e.g. verapamil, nifedipine) and nitrates. Although not strictly mandated by clinical trials, aspirin (150 mg daily) is frequently used in patients with stable angina as prophylaxis against infarction. Aspirin should only be used with caution in patients with a history of asthma because of the risk of provoking bronchoconstriction (patient a). A careful enquiry should always be made as to each patient's previous experience of taking aspirin. Patients with COAD should be treated similarly because of the difficulty of excluding reversible obstruction.

Beta-adrenoreceptor blockers should not be used in patients with asthma because of their potential for bronchoconstriction (patient a). Even cardioselective agents are not without bronchial effects and should not be used as first choice. Nitrates and calcium channel blockers are not contra-indicated.

Beta-adrenoreceptor blockers are contra-indicated in heart block (patient b) because of the risk of intensifying the block and producing symptomatic disease. Verapamil and diltiazem are similarly contra-indicated but not nifedipine and analogues which do not significantly affect the heart's conduction system and may be considered appropriate agents. Nitrates are also suitable agents to use in patients with heart block.

Beta-adrenoreceptor blockers are not contra-indicated in NIDDM (patient c) unless they reduce perfusion of peripheral organs, including the kidneys. Calcium channel blockers may increase peripheral perfusion and do not impair glucose tolerance, and are thus the preferred agents in an elderly diabetic with presumed peripheral vascular disease. Nitrates are also suitable agents. Renal impairment leads to accumulation of atenolol but this is not usually clinically significant at doses of 25 to 50 mg daily.

CASE 17.2

A Thrombolytic therapy with any agent is contra-indicated in pregnancy or if there is a high risk of bleeding. An irregular menstrual cycle may indicate either of these problems and further enquiry should be made (patient a). A history of hypertension may indicate a risk of bleeding, e.g. haemorrhagic stroke or retinal bleeding, and enquiries should be carried out to ensure this has not been a problem with the patient in question (patient b). Uncomplicated moderate hypertension is not a contra-indication; neither is old age nor the presence or absence of a history of ischaemic heart disease (patient c). Streptokinase, however, is contra-indicated within 12 months of a previous dose (patient d) or in any patient where streptococcal antibodies may be present. There are at least theoretical risks of a serious allergic reaction to a second dose of streptokinase and of a reduction in efficiency because of circulating antibodies. The precise time period is subject to debate but cross-sensitivity with anistreplase (APSAC) also occurs. Alteplase may be given without regard to previous thrombolytic therapy and would be suitable if the treatment used in a previous infarction was uncertain.

BIBLIOGRAPHY

Fuster V, Badimon L, Badimon J J, Chesebro J H. The pathogenesis of coronary artery disease and the acute coronary syndromes. New England Journal of Medicine 1992; 326: 242–250, 310–318

GISSI-2. A factorial randomised trial of alteplase versus streptokinase and heparin versus no heparin among 12,490 patients with acute myocardial infarction. Lancet 1990; 336: 65–71

ISIS-2 Collaborative Group. Randomised trial of intravenous streptokinase, oral aspirin, both or neither among 17,187 cases of suspected acute myocardial infarction. Lancet 1988; 332: 349–360

ISIS-3 Collaborative Group. ISIS-3: a randomised comparison of streptokinase vs tissue plasminogen activator vs anistreplase and of aspirin plus heparin vs aspirin alone among 41,229 cases of suspected acute myocardial infarction. Lancet 1992; 339: 753–770

Opie L H (ed). Drugs for the heart (3rd edn). Philadelphia: W B Saunders 1991

Chapter 18

Congestive cardiac failure

S. Hudson

Cardiac failure occurs when the heart fails to deliver adequate blood, and therefore oxygen and nutrients, to the tissues. Venous congestion gives rise to symptoms in the lungs and tissues. By convention, congestive cardiac failure describes the involvement of both the left and right ventricles.

EPIDEMIOLOGY

Cardiac failure is a common condition which occurs in 3 to 5% of the population over 65 years old and accounts for 5% of adult medical admissions to hospital. There is loss of cardiac reserve with age which increases the risk of cardiac failure complicating other conditions in the elderly. A common identifiable cause of cardiac failure is coronary artery disease with consequent myocardial infarction and irreplaceable loss of cardiac muscle. Cardiac failure is also commonly associated with chronic obstructive airways disease. Myocardial ischaemia and dysrhythmia contribute to the risk of sudden death in patients with heart failure.

For patients with cardiac failure, the outlook is progressive deterioration with an overall median survival after diagnosis of around 5 years. Survival varies according to aetiology and severity. For patients with severe cardiac failure the annual mortality may be as high as 50%. Effective drug therapy can improve survival although the differences between treatments are ill defined.

261

In young patients with end-stage disease, cardiac transplantation may be an option.

AETIOLOGY

Cardiac failure may be acute or chronic. Gradual onset over a number of years may occur without an identified underlying cause. Commonly, cardiac failure is a complication of other conditions such as chronic hypertension; ischaemic heart disease; mechanical defect, such as heart valve disease; and chronic sustained arrhythmias, of which the most common is atrial fibrillation. Cardiac failure can contribute to deterioration in lung function in chronic chest disease.

Conditions which place increased demands on the heart can create a shortfall in cardiac output. In hyperthyroidism the tissues place a greater metabolic demand and in severe anaemia there is an increased circulatory demand on the heart.

PATHOPHYSIOLOGY

The left ventricle is most vulnerable to failure and symptoms arise from diminished blood supply to tissues and organs, particularly the liver, kidney and gut. There is congestion of blood in the lungs leading to breathlessness and fatigue. Pulmonary congestion increases vascular resistance in the lungs and leads to failure of the right ventricle. Right-sided failure is associated with peripheral venous congestion and oedema.

The ventricle may fail if the muscle itself is diseased, as with ischaemia, or if there is structural damage affecting the mechanical flow of blood through the heart.

The ventricle may also fail if there is a sustained arrhythmia causing a bradycardia or a tachycardia that is sufficient to compromise cardiac output. In atrial fibrillation, which often accompanies hyperthyroidism and mitral valve disease, a rapid and irregular ventricular response compromises cardiac efficiency.

In health, cardiac output at rest is approximately 5 L/minute with a mean heart rate of 70 beats per minute and a stroke volume of 70 ml. Since the filled ventricle normally has a volume of 130 ml, the fraction ejected is over 50% of the ventricular contents, while 60 ml remains as residual volume. In cardiac failure the ejection fraction is reduced to below 40% and the residual volume is increased accordingly. In severe cardiac failure, the ejection fraction falls below 25% and mitral regurgitation contributes to the ventricular dysfunction.

Ventricular performance is affected by the tension on the ventricular wall. The tension during systole, the afterload, is determined by the degree of resistance to outflow at the exit valve and within the arterial tree, the systemic vascular resistance. Conditions in which the afterload is raised include arterial hypertension, narrowing of the aorta and disorders of the aortic valve.

Effective filling requires active diastolic expansion of the ventricular volume, which may be impaired in cardiac failure. The filling process normally contributes to the contractile strength by stretching and increasing the elasticity of cardiac muscle fibres. However, this elasticity becomes limited as the degree of stretch increases.

The volume of blood in the ventricle prior to each ventricular contraction is the cardiac preload. The tension on the ventricular wall at the end of diastole stretches the muscle fibres. The increased end-diastolic volume causes the failing ventricle to overfill and overstretch, which contributes to the loss of cardiac efficiency. The increased stress on the ventricular wall raises myocardial oxygen requirements, with the risk of ischaemia leading to angina pectoris or myocardial infarction.

The performance of the ventricle can be improved by reducing the tension on the ventricular wall by venodilatation to lower the preload, and by arteriodilatation to reduce the afterload.

Chest X-ray shows cardiomegaly, cardiac enlargement due to dilatation, which can be reversed by successful treatment. With gradual progression of cardiac failure, particularly in patients with long-standing hypertension, there is an increase in cardiac muscle mass, which is termed cardiac hypertrophy.

A reflex sympathetic discharge caused by the

diminished tissue perfusion in cardiac failure helps to sustain cardiac output by exposing the heart to the positive inotropic and chronotropic effects of catecholamines. Tachycardia is accompanied by arterial constriction to divert blood from the skin to the organs. However, the vasoconstriction adds to the resistance in the arteries and therefore increases the afterload on the heart.

Renin is released from the kidney, in response to reduced renal artery perfusion. Circulating renin leads to the formation of the vasoconstrictor angiotensin II which in turn prompts adrenal aldosterone secretion. Aldosterone retains salt and water at the distal renal tubule and so expands the blood volume. Arginine vasopressin release from the anterior pituitary adds to the vasoconstriction and has an antidiuretic effect by retaining water at the renal collecting duct.

In cardiac failure, compensating mechanisms for maintaining the circulation become inadequate and lead to clinical manifestations. If untreated these mechanisms become counterproductive by adding to the burden on the heart. The long-term consequences are for the failing heart to suffer biochemical and histological changes. Myocardial cell dysfunction and injury contribute to the risk of myocardial ischaemia.

CLINICAL MANIFESTATIONS

The reduced cardiac output, impaired oxygenation and diminished blood supply to muscles causes fatigue. Shortness of breath, dyspnoea, occurs on exertion whilst if it occurs when lying down it is called orthopnoea. When the patient lies down, abdominal pressure on the diaphragm contributes to the breathlessness caused by redistribution of oedema to the lungs. At night, the pulmonary symptoms also cause cough, and an increase in urine production, nocturia, also disturbs sleep by prompting micturition.

Gradual accumulation of fluid in the lungs at night may awaken the patient with gasping attacks, referred to as paroxysmal nocturnal dyspnoea (PND). PND causes the patient to seek fresh air but is relieved by sitting or standing up, so that patients may have to sleep propped up

by three or more pillows to prevent sleep disturbance.

The patient in cardiac failure may appear pale and the hands may be cold and sweaty. Reduced blood supply to the brain and kidney leads to confusion and renal failure. Congestion of the gastrointestinal tract causes hepatomegaly. The enlargement of the liver may be accompanied by abdominal bloating, anorexia, nausea, abdominal pain and distension.

Oedema affects the lungs, ankles and abdomen, arising from increased pressure in the capillary beds associated with sodium and water retention. Signs in the lungs include crepitations at the lung bases. In acute cardiac failure, symptoms of pulmonary oedema are prominent and may be life threatening. The sputum may be frothy and tinged red from the leakage of fluid and blood from the capillaries. Severe dyspnoea may be complicated by bronchospasm and accompanied by cyanosis and shock. The clinical manifestations of cardiac failure are presented in Figure 18.1.

A patient's cardiac status may be categorized according to symptoms, where:

- category 1 = no symptoms with ordinary physical activity such as walking or climbing stairs
- category 2 = slight limitation with symptoms on climbing stairs rapidly or walking uphill
- category 3 = moderate limitation of activity, restricting walking distance and limiting climbing to one flight of stairs
- category 4 = severe disability, unable to carry on physical activity without discomfort.

INVESTIGATIONS

Patients with chronic congestive cardiac failure are diagnosed and monitored on the basis of signs and symptoms from physical examination and history. A lateral and downward displacement of the apex beat of the heart is evidence of cardiac enlargement. Additional third and/or fourth heart sounds are typical of cardiac failure and arise from valvular dysfunction. Venous congestion can be demonstrated in the

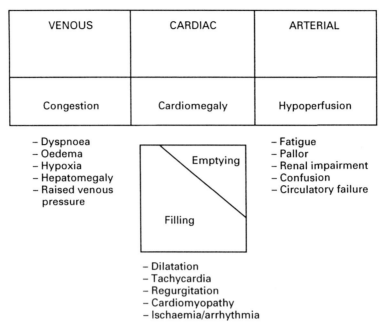

Fig. 18.1 Clinical manifestations of cardiac failure.

jugular vein by the jugular venous pressure (JVP), measured by the elevation of the visible distension in cm above the sternum, while the patient is reclining.

Investigations of the patient with cardiac failure include chest X-ray to look for enlarged cardiac shadow and consolidation in the lungs; measurement of plasma creatinine and urea to assess the renal function; measurement of plasma alanine/aspartate aminotransferase and other enzymes to test liver function. Full blood counts and thyroid function tests are used to investigate possible associated anaemia or thyrotoxicosis.

Cardiac catheterization is an invasive pressure monitoring technique for investigating cardiac function. The procedure is used on coronary and intensive care units. A Swan–Ganz balloon-tipped catheter is directed via a suitable vein into the right atrium and out of the right ventricle to wedge into the pulmonary artery. From this position on the right side of the heart, inflation of the balloon enables the distal catheter tip to monitor the filling pressure in the left ventricle by briefly blocking pulmonary arterial flow. In acute heart failure, haemodynamic

monitoring from the Swan–Ganz catheter and a simultaneous arterial line allows the degrees of pulmonary congestion and systemic vascular resistance to be measured.

Continued assessment of patients during chronic treatment is guided by improvement in symptoms with particular emphasis on exercise tolerance.

TREATMENT

The goal of treatment is to relieve symptoms, and effective therapy can considerably improve quality of life as well as improve survival. The pharmacological aims are to control oedema and to improve cardiac output.

Attention is given to treatment of any underlying disorder contributing to cardiac failure, such as hyperthyroidism, anaemia and dysrhythmia. Atrial fibrillation is commonly associated with hyperthyroidism and with valvular heart disease. Those patients with atrial fibrillation or other supraventricular arrhythmias are distinct from those in sinus rhythm. Atrial fibrillation requires control of tachycardia by suppression of AV node conduction, usually with digoxin and/or a calcium slow channel blocking drug, such as verapamil. For patients in sinus rhythm, consideration of coexisting ischaemic heart disease or chest disease may have a bearing on the choice of drug therapy for cardiac failure.

The oedema of cardiac failure results from complex circulatory and neurohumoral reflex mechanisms affecting the general circulation and the kidney. The disorder can be controlled by pharmacological improvement in cardiac output and intervention in the reflex mechanisms illustrated in Figure 18.2.

Drug treatment

The objectives are to relieve pulmonary congestion, increase the patient's tolerance to exercise and mobilize peripheral oedema.

Improved cardiac output can be achieved by lowering the pressures on the ventricular muscle during filling and emptying, which has the beneficial effect of improving the efficiency of the heart. Cardiac output can also be improved by strengthening cardiac contractility using inotropic agents.

The treatment of congestive cardiac failure relies on the use of diuretics, vasodilators and inotropic agents.

Diuretic therapy

In chronic cardiac failure, diuretics increase sodium and chloride excretion by blockade of sodium reabsorption in the renal tubule. Normally about 70% of sodium is reabsorbed, along with water, in the proximal tubule. Although thiazides have a minor action at this site they fail to produce a very marked diuresis since a compensatory increase in sodium reabsorption can occur in the loop of Henle. The ascending limb of the loop of Henle removes about 25% of filtered sodium. Loop diuretics, such as frusemide and bumetanide act at this site and are known as 'high-ceiling' agents because their blockade of sodium reabsorption continues as the dose is increased.

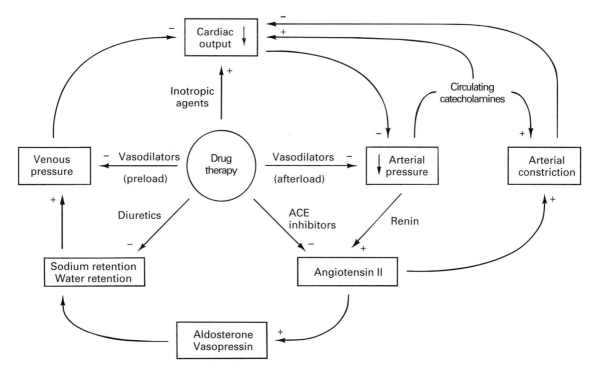

Fig. 18.2 Reflex mechanisms and interventions in cardiac failure.

Thiazides are low-ceiling agents because maximum diuresis occurs at low doses. These diuretics act mainly on the cortical diluting segment. At this site, where the ascending limb merges into the distal tubule, a further 5 to 10% of sodium is normally removed.

Less than 5% of sodium is removed in the distal convoluted tubule where sodium is exchanged for potassium and hydrogen. Potassium-retaining diuretics such as amiloride and triamterene affect this mechanism directly; whereas spironolactone affects the exchange mechanism by antagonizing aldosterone. Table 18.1 summarizes the diuretics in common clinical use for cardiac failure.

Diuretics are used in lower doses than formerly, although doses used in cardiac failure are often higher than those used to treat hypertension. A thiazide diuretic is often selected initially for the treatment of mild cardiac failure and avoids an intense diuresis. Thiazides act within 1 to 2 hours and maintain their action over 6 to 24 hours. The duration of action varies but with little clinical significance except where diuresis at night produces inconvenience. In doses above the equivalent of bendrofluazide

5 to 10 mg, thiazides present greater risk of unwanted effects with little or no additional benefit.

A thiazide can usefully be combined with a potassium-retaining agent to achieve an additive diuresis and to safeguard against hypokalaemia. When this combination fails to control symptoms, a loop diuretic offers the potential to increase the diuresis. Metolazone acts similarly to thiazides but works even at low glomerular filtration rates for 12 to 24 hours. It has a pronounced action on the proximal tubule. Sodium reabsorption in the loop of Henle normally compensates for its proximal tubular action and for this reason it is usually administered with a loop diuretic.

Loop diuretics are often required in the management of cardiac failure for the control of oedema. These diuretics produce less hypokalaemia than thiazides but in high doses their intensity of action may produce hypovolaemia with the risk of postural hypotension, worsening of symptoms and renal failure.

In general, a combination of thiazide and loop diuretic offers no advantages and increases the risk of untoward effects. However, a loop diuretic

Class & agent	Agent remarks	Class comments
Thiazide & related		
Hydrochlorthiazide	Duration 6–12 h	Oral only. Onset 1–2 h lasting 6–24 h.
Bendrofluazide	Duration 12–18 h	Loss of action in renal failure (GFR < 25 ml/min)
Cyclopenthiazide		
Chlorthalidone	Duration 24–72 h	
	Ca^{2+} retaining	
Metolazone	Duration 12–24 h	
	Intense action when added to 'loop' agent	
	Effective at low GFR	
Loop diuretics		
Frusemide	Slow i.v.	Parenteral/oral
Bumetanide		Onset <1 h lasting 4–8 h
Ethacrynic acid	GI disturbances	Increase Ca^{2+} excretion
		Effective at low GFR
Potassium retaining		
Amiloride	Renally excreted	Weak. Duration 12–24 h
Triamterene	Renal calculi	Avoid in renal failure
Spironolactone (oral)	Metabolized to canrenoate	Antagonists of aldosterone. Onset about 12 h.
Canrenoate (i.v. form)	Menstrual problems and gynaecomastia	Full action after 1–3 days.
	Useful in liver failure	

Table 18.1   Diuretics: classes and agents used in cardiac failure

greatly enhances the effectiveness of metolazone by blocking the compensatory sodium reabsorption in the loop of Henle. This combination is useful in severe or resistant oedema. However, because of profound diuresis careful attention must be paid to the metolazone dose.

Diuretics have a mild vasodilator action in left ventricular failure. The mild arterial vasodilator effect of thiazides helps improve cardiac function by reducing afterload. Acutely, the intravenous administration of a loop diuretic reduces the preload and locally relieves pulmonary congestion prior to producing a diuresis.

Vasodilator therapy

Cardiac output can be improved by unloading the heart by venodilatation, arteriodilatation or a combination of both. The combined approach is most effective and can be achieved by the use of one or more vasodilators. These agents are usually used with diuretic therapy and may also be combined with inotropic agents. Since certain vasodilators also have cardioprotective effects, the choice of vasodilator may be governed by the need to treat accompanying ischaemic heart disease or hypertension. Arterial vasodilatation may provoke a reflex tachycardia. However, in patients with cardiac failure the reflex is offset by the increased cardiac output, especially where vasodilator therapy has a combined effect on both arterioles and venules.

ACE inhibitors

Angiotensin converting enzyme (ACE) inhibitors act as ligands for the zinc ion at the active centre of ACE. The zinc ligand is a sulphydryl group for captopril, whereas for enalapril and most others it is a carboxyl group.

Captopril and enalapril have been used widely and successfully. By inhibiting the activation of angiotensin II, ACE inhibitors block arterial and venous constriction, reducing preload and afterload, and they also decrease aldosterone formation. By increasing cardiac output renal function is increased, which further helps to relieve oedema. Inhibition of ACE may also

potentiate the vasodilator bradykinin and intervene locally on ACE in cardiac and renal tissues. The pharmacological effects of these drugs may be the result of a combination of interventions on the circulatory dysfunction in cardiac failure.

ACE inhibitors have been shown to be well tolerated by most patients and to improve quality of life and survival. Nevertheless, their use does require careful attention to dosage and patient monitoring. The introduction of an ACE inhibitor may produce hypotension. This effect is most pronounced after the first dose and may be severe, especially in patients with prior activation of the renin–angiotensin system. Patients at risk include those on high doses of loop diuretics, those with a low plasma sodium and those with liver disease. Ideally diuretics should be discontinued for a few days beforehand. In moderate–severe cardiac failure diuretic treatment often cannot be interrupted. Treatment must then be started with a low dose administered at bedtime and usually under medical supervision. It is preferable to start treatment in patients at particular risk of hypotension with the short-acting agent, captopril. Transfer to an equivalent dose of a longer-acting agent can be made once treatment has been safely initiated.

Blockade of the renin–angiotensin system may also lead to reversible deterioration in renal function in 5% of patients. ACE inhibitors are therefore hazardous in pre-existing renal disease and particularly in bilateral renal artery stenosis in which renal perfusion is maintained by an activated renin–angiotensin system. Since most ACE inhibitors or their active metabolites depend on the kidney for elimination, the risks of toxicity are further increased in renal disease.

Patients receiving ACE inhibitors are at risk of hyperkalaemia if renal function deteriorates and if a potassium supplement or a potassium-sparing diuretic is co-prescribed. A dry cough may occur in about 10% of patients receiving an ACE inhibitor. The cough is more common in women and may be accompanied by a voice change. Patients may also complain of taste disturbances and mouth ulcers. Rashes, loss of taste and proteinuria can occur, particularly with captopril, perhaps because of its sulphydryl group. These unwanted effects are more common in patients with connective tissue disorders.

With the exception of captopril and lisinopril, many of the ACE inhibitors are administered as esters to improve their absorption. Differences in absorption are not clinically significant to long-term treatment. Captopril absorption may be slowed by food or antacids, perhaps decreasing its intensity of action advantageously. Most ACE inhibitors are dependent on the kidney for elimination and require careful dosage in renal failure. The differences in the pharmacokinetic characteristics of ACE inhibitors do not fully explain their differences in duration of action, which are related to ACE binding affinity.

Nitrates

The nitrates are less effective vasodilators than ACE inhibitors but are particularly useful in patients whose cardiac failure is associated with ischaemic heart disease. In general they need to be used in higher doses than those used to treat angina and often in combination with other vasodilators. The prominent nitrate venodilator action is useful where symptoms of pulmonary congestion predominate over loss of exercise tolerance. To achieve a balanced effect on afterload, nitrates must be used in combination with an arterial vasodilator such as hydralazine.

In tissues nitrate vasodilators work by interaction with sulphydryl groups, releasing nitric oxide which causes vasodilatation by activating guanylate cyclase in vascular smooth muscle. Plasma concentrations are not clearly related to pharmacological effects because of their indirect action on the vasculature. Depletion of sulphydryl groupings can occur during continued treatment and explains the tolerance to sustained exposure to high nitrate doses. Restoration of sulphydryl groupings occurs within hours of treatment being interrupted. Nitrate tolerance can be prevented by suitable timing of doses to ensure a dose interval which provides a daily nitrate-free period of more than 8 hours.

Nitrates undergo first-pass metabolism, which is extensive with glyceryl trinitrate. The short duration of action of glyceryl trinitrate is a dis-

advantage to its oral use but allows dosage titration during intravenous use.

Isosorbide dinitrate (ISDN) is completely absorbed orally but only 25% appears as ISDN in plasma. There is rapid conversion, with a half-life of 1 hour, of 70% of the dose to mononitrate metabolites during the absorption process. Conversion to isosorbide-5-mononitrate (5-ISMN), which has a half-life of 5 hours, eventually accounts for over 60% of the dose. The effects of ISDN and 5-ISMN are due to their nitrate content but since the latter is longer acting, most of the effects of ISDN are attributable to the 5-ISMN metabolite. Equivalent doses of ISMN are approximately twice those of ISDN.

Other vasodilators

Direct acting vasodilators include sodium nitroprusside, which is used in acute conditions by continuous infusion. Nitric oxide also mediates the action of nitroprusside but its formation is independent of sulphydryl compounds. In impaired renal function thiocyanate accumulates over several days causing nausea, anorexia, fatigue and psychosis.

Agents such as hydralazine and the alpha-adrenoreceptor antagonist prazosin are less well tolerated and have been superseded as first-line vasodilators. Hydralazine has a predominantly arterial vasodilator action and the sympathetic reflex may exaggerate the tachycardia in patients with cardiac failure. While this reflex is less apparent than in patients treated for hypertension, it is potentially hazardous in patients with ischaemic heart disease. Hydralazine must be prescribed in high doses for cardiac failure and its use is associated with a risk of drug-induced systemic lupus erythematosus (SLE). SLE is an uncommon multisystem connective tissue disorder, which is more likely to occur in slow acetylators of hydralazine. Hydralazine with a nitrate, to produce a balanced effect on arteries and venules, is an effective combination. Prazosin has an effect on preload and afterload but tolerance develops on long-term administration.

Patients with coronary artery disease may be candidates for calcium blocking antianginal vasodilators. However, some of these agents can exacerbate coexisting cardiac failure, since their negative inotropic effects offset the potentially beneficial arterial vasodilatation. Amlodipine, nicardipine and nifedipine have a less pronounced effect on cardiac contractility than other calcium antagonists.

The vasodilators are summarized in Table 18.2.

Inotropic agents

Digoxin. Digoxin acts by increasing the availability of calcium within the myocardial cell through an inhibition of sodium extrusion, thereby increasing sodium–calcium exchange. Digoxin increases cardiac output in atrial fibrillation by suppressing atrioventricular conduction and controlling the ventricular rate. In some patients in sinus rhythm the benefit of digoxin may not be sustained, so that the drug may be discontinued without worsening of symptoms. Digoxin

treatment is potentially hazardous and patients on digoxin should therefore be regularly reviewed.

Digoxin may cause potentially fatal cardiac arrhythmias. Other toxic symptoms include nausea, vomiting, confusion and visual disturbances. Digoxin toxicity is more pronounced in the presence of metabolic or electrolyte disturbances and in patients with cardiac ischaemia. Patients with hypokalaemia, hypomagnesaemia, hypercalcaemia, alkalosis, hypothyroidism and hypoxia are at particular risk of toxicity. Treatment may be required to restore plasma potassium. Intravenous digoxin antibody fragments can be used for rapid reversal of life-threatening toxicity.

The pharmacokinetics of digoxin affect the choice of dose. Urinary excretion of digoxin is 70% and the digoxin half-life of 36 hours is extended further in renal failure. In the elderly the digoxin half-life averages approximately 48 hours. The use of loading doses is therefore

Table 18.2 Vasodilators: classes and agents used in cardiac failure

Class & agent	Agent remarks	Class comments
ACE inhibitors		
Captopril	Duration 8–12 h	First dose hypotension
	Greater risk of allergy	May worsen renal failure
		Adjust dose in renal failure
Enalapril	Duration 12–24 h	Hyperkalaemia, cough, taste disturbance &
Quinapril		allergies may occur
Lisinopril	Duration 24 h	Shown to improve survival
Perindopril		
Nitrates		
Isosorbide dinitrate	Oral/sublingual/i.v.	High doses needed
(ISDN)	ISDN $t_{1/2}$ 1–2 h metabolism	Tolerance can be prevented by overnight dose
	to ISMN	interval > 8 h
Isosorbide	Oral $t_{1/2}$ 4–6 h	
5-mononitrate (ISMN)	i.v. & topical for sustained effect	Protective effect against cardiac ischaemia
Glyceryl trinitrate	in acute/severe cardiac failure but	
	limited by tolerance	
Others		
Nitroprusside	i.v. only. Light sensitive	
	Acts on veins & arteries	
	Cyanide accumulation and	
	acidosis limit treatment duration	
Hydralazine	Direct action on arteries	
	Tolerance occurs	
	May cause drug-induced lupus &	
	sodium retention	
Prazosin	Alpha-adrenoreceptor antagonist	
	First dose hypotension	
	Tolerance occurs	

necessary to digitalize the patient. Digoxin is 99% bound to tissues, particularly skeletal muscle, with a high apparent volume of distribution of approximately 600 L per 70 kg. The digitalizing dose therefore depends on the patient's lean body weight.

Digoxin plasma concentrations associated with therapeutic effects show wide interpatient variation. Therapeutically effective steady state plasma concentrations are usually within 1 to 2 microgram/L. Most patients with digoxin cardiac toxicity usually have concentrations > 2 microgram/L; although toxicity occurs at lower concentrations in patients with hypokalaemia. Equally, some patients may require to be maintained on higher plasma concentrations, particularly those with atrial fibrillation. Plasma digoxin concentrations > 3 microgram/L are associated with increased cardiotoxicity.

Digitalizing doses are therefore difficult to predict and vary according to the patient's clinical condition and lean body weight. With a single loading dose, digitalization occurs within 4 to 6 hours, the time for equilibration of plasma and tissue digoxin concentrations. This delay in equilibration means that plasma samples should be drawn at least 6 hours after a dose, see Figure 18.3.

In the absence of loading doses, digitalization occurs over 4 to 5 half-lives. In practice, the opti-

mum digitalizing dose is obtained by the use of small repeated doses to achieve symptomatic improvement and to minimize the risk of toxicity. This approach is shown in Figure 18.4.

The difficulty in defining the target digoxin plasma concentration undermines the value of routine digoxin plasma concentration monitoring, but does not detract from its value for confirming suspected digoxin toxicity. Digoxin is absorbed in the upper small intestine. Oral bioavailability of digoxin is 65 to 75% and is affected by dissolution. Appropriate dosage adjustment must be made when changing between oral and intravenous routes of administration.

Sympathomimetic agents. In hospital practice, acute cardiac failure may require intravenous combination therapy including the continuous infusion of one or more inotropic agents, particularly the sympathomimetic agents isoprenaline, dobutamine and dopamine. These agents have inotrope–vasodilator effects which differ according to their profile of action on alpha, $beta_1$, $beta_2$ and dopamine receptors. $Beta_1$ agonists increase cardiac contractility, $beta_2$ agonists produce arterial vasodilatation and dopamine agonists enhance renal perfusion. Noradrenaline is an alpha-adrenoreceptor agonist whose vasoconstrictor action limits its usefulness to severely

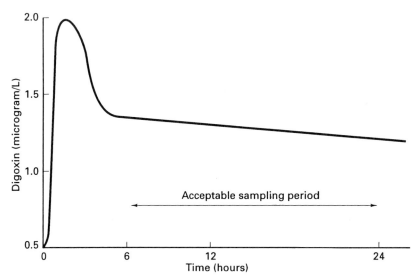

Fig. 18.3 Plasma digoxin profile at steady state on oral daily dosing, showing the biphasic distribution and elimination with equilibration after 4 to 6 hours.

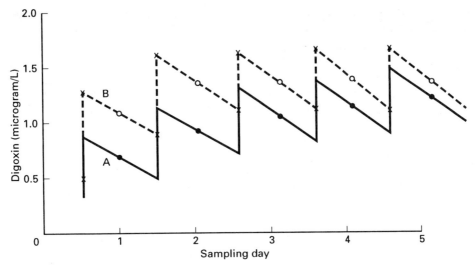

Fig. 18.4 Comparison of plasma digoxin profiles from samples taken daily after the start of treatment: (A) 250 micrograms orally once daily – steady state after day 5; (B) 375 micrograms orally once daily on days 1, 2 and 3, 250 micrograms once daily thereafter – steady state after day 2.

hypotensive states. With dopamine, high doses have a predominant action on alpha-adreno-receptors. Dobutamine has a predominantly ino-tropic and vasodilator action due to the action of the (+) isomer selectively for beta adrenoreceptors. Tolerance to sympathomimetic inotropic agents may develop on prolonged administration. Toler-ance and cardiotoxicity have limited the useful-ness of oral beta-agonists.

Phosphodiesterase inhibitors. The phospho-diesterase inhibitors are newer inotropes which activate intracellular cAMP and facilitate the slow calcium channels. The effects of these drugs are both inotropic and vasodilator. Enoximone is administered intravenously and has a direct va-sodilator effect which can produce hypotension. Enoximone and dobutamine are synergistic. The use of enoximone to interrupt dobutamine treat-ment may help to avoid tolerance to the sympa-thetic agonist. Clinical trials have yet to establish the place of these agents but they are potential adjuncts where other treatments have failed. The properties of inotropic drugs are summarized in Table 18.3.

Adverse effects of therapy

Elderly patients are at particular risk from un-

wanted effects of diuretics. In the elderly the in-crease in urine volume can also worsen inconti-nence or precipitate urinary retention. Rapid diuresis with loop diuretics leading to more than 1 kg loss in body weight daily, may exacerbate cardiac failure by causing an acute reduction in the blood volume, hypotension and diminished renal perfusion with increased renin release.

The biochemical effects of excessive diuresis are uraemia, hypokalaemia and alkalosis. Thi-azide and loop diuretics may worsen glucose tolerance or precipitate the diabetic state in pre-disposed individuals. These diuretics increase plasma urate and the incidence of gout is about 2%. Hyponatraemia may occur with diuretics and is usually due to water retention rather than sodium loss. Severe hyponatraemia, with plasma sodium < 115 mmol/L, causes confusion and drowsiness and most commonly arises when potassium-sparing agents are used in diuretic combinations.

Diuretics cause potassium loss as a result of the urinary sodium increasing the rate of K^+/Na^+ exchange in the distal tubule. Plasma potas-sium concentrations below 3.0 mmol/L occur in less than 5% of patients receiving diuretics. Hy-pokalaemia is hazardous for those receiving dig-oxin and for those with ischaemic heart disease.

Table 18.3   Inotropic agents: classes and agents used in cardiac failure

Class & agent	Agent remarks	Class comments
Digitalis		
Digoxin	$t_{1/2}$ 36 h, prolonged in renal failure, plasma levels help to monitor for toxicity i.m. absorption poor, avoid	Beneficial in atrial fibrillation Exact benefits long term need to be defined
Ouabain	i.v. onset < 1–2 h $t_{1/2}$ 21 h	Risk of arrhythmias
Digitoxin	Oral, $t_{1/2}$ 4–6 days Dose unaffected by renal failure	CNS, visual & GI symptoms of digitalis toxicity
Phosphodiesterase inhibitors		
Enoximone	Oral use under trial Alkaline i.v. loss of solubility on dilution or admixture Avoid contact with glass	Severe heart failure only
Milrinone	i.v. only for short-term use	Adjunctive therapy Arrhythmias & increased long-term mortality
Sympathetic agonists		
Noradrenaline	β_1 and α	Continuous i.v. only
Isoprenaline	β_1, β_2	Require close monitoring in critical care setting
Dopamine	β_1, (β_2), α, dopamine	
Dobutamine	β_1, (β_2) and (α)	
Dopexamine	β_2, dopamine	

In these patients a plasma potassium < 3.5 mmol/ L requires treatment. However, hypokalaemia is more common with thiazide than with loop diuretics and more likely when diuretics are used for cardiac failure than for hypertension, because of the activated renin–angiotensin system.

Potassium-retaining diuretics are more effective at preventing hypokalaemia than potassium supplements. Prevention of hypokalaemia requires at least 25 mmol and treatment requires 60 to 120 mmol potassium daily. Since proprietary diuretic–potassium combination products usually contain less than 12 mmol in each dose, their use is often inappropriate. Potassium supplements are poorly tolerated at the high doses often needed to treat hypokalaemia. Local high concentrations of potassium salts can damage the gastrointestinal tract in patients with swallowing difficulties or delayed gastrointestinal transit. Potassium supplementation and potassium-sparing diuretics can cause hyperkalaemia in patients with renal failure.

Volume depletion due to prior diuretic treatment increases the risk of a large drop in blood pressure following the first dose of ACE inhibitor. ACE inhibitors predispose to hyperkalaemia by reducing circulating aldosterone. An ACE inhibitor usefully controls any potassium loss from a diuretic regimen. Potassium supplements or potassium-retaining agents should not be used with ACE inhibitors unless careful monitoring of plasma potassium is to be undertaken. Heparin therapy can also increase the risk of hyperkalaemia with ACE inhibitors.

Digoxin treatment is particularly hazardous, toxicity is difficult to recognize and may cause fatal arrhythmias. Digoxin slows AV conduction and produces bradycardia but may also cause various ventricular and supraventricular arrhythmias. Digoxin toxicity typically causes conduction disturbances with enhanced automaticity leading to premature ventricular contractions. Patients at particular risk are those with myocardial ischaemia, hypoxia, acidosis, or renal failure. Digoxin dosage should be guided by assessment of the patient's renal function from plasma creatinine or creatinine clearance determinations. Digoxin toxicity causes arrhythmias, nausea, anorexia, tiredness, weakness, diarrhoea, confusion and visual disturbances.

The major unwanted effects of drugs used in cardiac failure are summarized in Table 18.4. The major clinically important drug interactions and contra-indications are shown in Table 18.5. Interactions involve drugs causing negative inotropic effects, salt and fluid retention, alterations of potassium and digoxin plasma concentrations, excessive blood pressure reduction and impairment of renal function.

THE PATIENT

Patients with cardiac failure are often elderly with other complications, particularly cardiovascular disorders and polypharmacy. Renal function is often compromised and attention is required to dosages of drugs excreted largely unchanged in the urine. Patients with cardiac failure are at particular risk of fluid or electrolyte imbalance, contra-indications, adverse effects and drug interactions. Consequently careful monitoring is indicated to help detect problems associated with poor patient compliance, unwanted drug effects and the need for dosage adjustments.

Patient monitoring

Patients receiving treatment for congestive cardiac failure should be carefully monitored in order to:

- assure effective control of symptoms and appropriateness of dose and dose interval
- identify and attribute signs and symptoms of toxicity
- assure patient cooperation with the treatment.

Effective control

Therapeutic control is monitored by improvements in exercise tolerance and shortness of breath. Oedema is often visible and remarked upon by patients. Increased oedema may be reflected by an increase in the patient's body weight. Questions about tolerance to exercise are useful in identifying patients who may be experiencing difficulties and are possibly in need of review of their medication. However, the identification of loss of control is complicated by other factors in the elderly that affect mobility, such as arthritis

Table 18.4   Monitoring therapy in cardiac failure: unwanted effects

Complication	Drugs implicated					
	Digitalis	Vasodilators	ACE inhib.	Thiazides	Loop	K⁺ retaining
Hyponatraemia				+	+	+
Hypokalaemia				+	+	
Hyperkalaemia			+			+
Hypercalcaemia				+		
Hypomagnesaemia				+	+	
Postural hypotension		+	+	+	+	+
Alkalosis				+	+	
Hyperglycaemia				+	+	
Hyperlipidaemia				+		
Gout				+	+	
Uraemia			+	+	+	+
Dehydration				+	+	+
Proteinuria			+			
Arrhythmias	+					
Diarrhoea	+		+		+	
Mental changes	+					
Nausea/anorexia	+		+		+	
Impotence			+	+		
Pancreatitis				+	+	
Tinnitus/deafness					+	

Table 18.5 Monitoring therapy in cardiac failure: drug–disease and drug–drug interactions

Clinical effect	Interaction/contra-indication
Reduced cardiac output (-ve inotropic effect)	Quinidine, procainamide, beta-adrenoreceptor blockers, calcium slow channel blockers, disopyramide, anthracycline antineoplastic agents
Exacerbation of oedema	Salt/fluid retention with corticosteroids, liquorice & carbenoxolone Sodium-containing antacids & i.v. antibiotics Non-steroidal anti-inflammatory drugs (NSAIDs) Oestrogens Water retention with carbamazepine, chlorpropamide, vinca alkaloids
Digoxin Toxicity	Quinidine, quinine, verapamil diltiazem, amiodarone (all increase plasma levels) i.v. calcium salts
Loss of effect	Cholesterol binding resins, some antibiotics
Potassium Hypokalaemia	Corticosteroids, liquorice, carbenoxolone, salbutamol
Hyperkalaemia	Potassium-retaining diuretics, NSAIDs especially indomethacin, ACE inhibitors (increased risk with heparin)
Glucose intolerance	Corticosteroids, thiazide and loop diuretics, beta-adrenoreceptor blockers
Renal failure	NSAIDs with ACE inhibitors, thiazides, loop diuretics or triamterene

and parkinsonism. Onset or deterioration of symptoms is often slow and patients are inclined to gradually adapt their lifestyle by reducing their mobility to compensate. In patients with chest disease, cardiac failure may be a complicating factor that adds to the shortness of breath.

Loss of control may arise from overuse of diuretics and is also a feature of digoxin toxicity. Failure to restrict sodium intake may undermine treatment. Simple dietary advice to avoid processed foods and added salt at the table should be reinforced. Cardiac failure is often incipient in nature and may be precipitated or exacerbated by drug therapy for other conditions.

Signs and symptoms of toxicity

Chronic excessive doses of diuretics can worsen cardiac failure and contribute to symptoms of fatigue through electrolyte disturbances and dehydration. Diuretic-induced glucose intolerance may affect diabetic control in non-insulin-dependent diabetes. More commonly diuretics reveal glucose intolerance in patients not known to be diabetic. Hyperuricaemia may not require a change in therapy in the absence of symptoms of gout.

Symptoms of fainting or dizziness on standing may indicate a need to review diuretic or vasodilator therapy. Patients should be reassured about mild postural effects and given advice to avoid standing from the chair too quickly. Impaired renal function may also be due to drug therapy or to loss of control of the condition.

Excessive digoxin dose should be considered a possibility in any patient whose health deteriorates or who shows signs of social withdrawal. Important indicators of toxicity are abdominal pain, nausea, anorexia, tiredness, weakness, diarrhoea, confusion and any change in vision, mobility or temperament.

Patient cooperation

To secure cooperation patients must be helped to understand the potential benefits from their medication. Education of patients should enable them to recognize the importance of each item of medication and the relevance of the labelled instructions. Specific advice should direct patients on the timing of doses and forewarn them of symptoms of anticipated potentially troublesome unwanted but self-limiting effects.

In general, diuretic therapy should be timed for the morning to avoid inconvenient micturition. Twice daily regimens of vasodilators are best timed with the second dose taken at bed time to minimize postural effects. However, timing the last dose of a nitrate regimen at tea time provides an overnight dose interval long enough to avoid nitrate tolerance. Patients with prominent nocturnal symptoms require separate consideration. Table 18.6 provides a general patient education and monitoring checklist.

The pharmaceutical care of the patient with congestive cardiac failure includes a wide range of skills. Cardiac failure is commonly a contributing cause of hospital admission, frequently complicating other serious illness. Acutely, the patient's treatment is monitored by routine objective measurements including fluid and electrolyte balance, renal and hepatic dysfunction, radiography, electrocardiography and, in critical care settings, by haemodynamic mea-

surements. The pharmacist must be familiar with these objective measures in order to contribute advice on dosage and drug combinations. Pharmaceutical advice helps to ensure safe intravenous administration, preparation and dilution in order to avoid problems of dose-related toxicity, stability and physical incompatibility.

In community practice, many elderly patients are maintained long term in the community and may see their pharmacist more frequently than their general practitioner. Patients may have other complications; their multiple drug therapy makes patient counselling and the provision of practical advice to improve compliance especially important. Careful attention to the patient's well-being, discussion and recording of symptoms and advice given are important to maintaining a long-term profile of treatment. Pharmacy patient medication records are important and can enable the pharmacist to contribute fully to the care of these patients.

Table 18.6 Patient education and monitoring checklist		
	Advise on	Monitor for symptoms of
Diuretics	Appropriate timing Avoidance of added salt, e.g. in processed foods and tomato juice	Incontinence Muscle weakness Confusion Dizziness Gout
ACE inhibitors	Avoiding standing rapidly	Hypotension Dizziness Cough Taste disturbance Sore throat Rashes Tingling in hands, joint pains
Nitrates	Timing of doses Avoiding standing rapidly (especially when combined with other vasodilators)	Headache Hypotension Dizziness Flushing of face/ neck GI upset
Digitalis	Report any symptoms to doctor or pharmacist	Anorexia, nausea Visual disturbances Diarrhoea Confusion Deterioration or social withdrawal
Potassium salts	Swallow whole immediately after food Soluble forms in at least ¼ tumbler of water/fruit juice & allow fizzing to stop	Gastrointestinal disturbances Swallowing difficulty Diarrhoea Tiredness Limb weakness

CASE STUDIES

CASE 18.1

Mrs E. L., a 53-year-old, 60 kg woman, has recently been discharged from hospital on the following medication:

- **Digoxin 0.375 mg**
- **Carbimazole 10 mg t.d.s.**
- **Frusemide 40 mg daily**
- **Propranolol 40 mg three times daily.**

Q Is this a rational combination of drug therapy? How would you respond to this prescription? What information would you seek to maintain your patient records? What matters would you discuss with the patient or prescriber?

CASE 18.2

Mrs E. L., from Case 18.1, complains of tiredness, increased breathlessness and malaise. She is readmitted to hospital after an outpatient consultation.

Q Is digoxin toxicity likely and what are the acute symptoms of digoxin overdosage? What investigations are required to confirm digoxin toxicity and how is it treated?

CASE 18.3

Mrs A. B., a 69-year-old woman, has been receiving digoxin 0.25 mg and frusemide 80 mg daily for her heart failure for the past 6 months according to your patient records. She now presents the following prescription to your pharmacy:

- Enalapril 10 mg twice daily
- Frusemide 80 mg in the morning
- Potassium chloride (slow release) 2 three times daily.

Q Describe your response. Would you dispense the prescription, offer advice, contact the prescriber? Explain the implications for the pharmaceutical care of this patient.

CASE 18.4

Mrs F. M., a 70-year-old woman with chronic asthma and mild heart failure, has been receiving:

- Bendrofluazide 10 mg each morning
- Prednisolone 5 mg daily
- Salbutamol inhaler 2 puffs four times daily
- Beclomethasone inhaler 2 puffs four times daily
- Magnesium trisilicate 10 ml when required.

The patient is breathless at night and kept awake with a painful knee. Her general practitioner has prescribed naproxen 250 mg three times daily.

Q Would you dispense the prescription? What advice would you give the patient or the prescriber? Explain your actions.

ANSWERS TO CASE STUDIES

CASE 18.1

A Mrs E. L. is receiving the antithyroid agent carbimazole. She is receiving the diuretic presumably for cardiac failure with a high likelihood that the digoxin is being used for atrial fibrillation (AF), since AF is associated with thyrotoxicosis.

The dose of digoxin is relatively high but is consistent with the higher dosage requirements in thyrotoxicosis. These higher dosage requirements are in part due to the higher plasma concentrations needed to suppress atrioventricular conduction.

Propranolol, as with all beta-adrenoreceptor blockers, has a negative inotropic effect which makes it contra-indicated in cardiac failure. However, in the case of Mrs E. L, propranolol is necessary to improve the tremor and anxiety of thyrotoxicosis. Propranolol may also be beneficial to her AF since it helps to control tachycardia. The positive inotropic action of digoxin affords some protection against the negative inotropic action of the beta-adrenoreceptor blocker.

Patients with thyrotoxicosis also show a relative resistance to the pharmacological effects of digoxin. After a diagnosis of thyrotoxicosis, antithyroid treatment will lead to gradual attainment of the euthyroid state over about 6 weeks. During this period, although cardiac function might be expected to improve, sensitivity to digoxin may increase.

Mrs E. L. is receiving a loop diuretic, frusemide, and is at risk of hypokalaemia which is particularly hazardous while she is receiving digoxin.

The pharmacist should establish as much background information from the patient as possible in order to confirm the purpose and duration of her drug therapy and the reason for her recent hospital admission. Information about her current symptoms, past medical and drug history, renal function, thyroid status, her body weight, plasma electrolyte and digoxin determinations would help complete the picture.

Signs of digoxin toxicity may include a loss of appetite, nausea, a change in bowel habit or general malaise. Visual disturbances such as haloes or yellow/green colour blindness are characteristic of digoxin toxicity but are infrequently volunteered by patients. The need to prevent hypokalaemia should be raised with the prescriber.

CASE 18.2

A The acute symptoms of digoxin toxicity are nausea and vomiting due to an action on the chemoreceptor trigger zone. The emetic effect can occur independently of cardiotoxicity. Other gastrointestinal disturbances include anorexia, diarrhoea or constipation. There may be breathlessness due to loss of control of cardiac failure, bradycardia or any of a variety of arrhythmias, in particular heart block and ventricular extrasystoles. Bigeminy, the coupling of QRS complexes, is a characteristic ECG feature of digoxin toxicity. Propranolol may contribute to bradycardia and cardiac failure. Hospital tests include ECG and plasma digoxin as well as serum potassium, urea and creatinine to identify hypokalaemia or dehydration and to assess the renal function.

If toxicity is suspected, digoxin and propranolol must be discontinued and potassium administered. Potassium may be given orally or intravenously in profound hypokalaemia and life-threatening toxicity. Intravenous potassium should be administered at no more than 30 mmol per hour diluted with dextrose 5% or sodium chloride 0.9%. It is necessary to monitor plasma potassium at least every 4 hours. Digoxin elimination can be increased by administration of oral anionic exchange resins. Cholesterol binding agents such as colestipol and cholestyramine will adsorb digoxin in the gut and increase its faecal elimination. The effect is to shorten the digoxin half-life. Life-threatening arrhythmias or the presence of high plasma digoxin (> 5 microgram/ litre) with renal impairment requires immediate treatment with intravenous digoxin antibody fragments in a single or repeated dose as an antidote.

CASE 18.3

A The combination of ACE inhibitor and potassium supplement carries a serious risk of hyperkalaemia. The prescriber needs to be contacted and meanwhile the potassium supplement should be withheld.

The enalapril should only be introduced under supervision especially in this elderly patient. The patient's past history of large doses of frusemide places her at particular risk of first dose hypotension. Is the patient still taking the digoxin? The history of digoxin treatment raises the question of whether the prescription of ACE inhibitor is because digoxin was poorly tolerated or because of worsening of symptoms. The patient should be asked if she has been advised that the enalapril is intended to replace her digoxin.

Has the patient already been started on an ACE inhibitor? If not, has the patient received any advice from the prescriber? The prescription for enalapril for the first time requires the pharmacist to alert the precriber to the risk of hypotension and the need for the supervised administration of a low initial dose of 2.5 mg at bed time. The use of the shorter-acting captopril in a dose of 6.25 mg is safer for those, like this lady, who are at particular risk of the first dose effect. Enalapril can then be exchanged for captopril in equivalent daily dosage (enalapril 5 to 10 mg to replace captopril 25 to 50 mg). Contact with the prescriber will also enable the pharmacist to confirm that the ACE inhibitor is intended to replace the digoxin treatment. If the patient is known to have poor renal function, the dosage of captopril will need to be low and adds further caution against the use of potassium supplements or potassium-sparing diuretics.

CASE 18.4

 Is the patient's breathlessness an exacerbation of her asthma or a worsening of her cardiac failure? The non-steroidal anti-inflammatory agent, naproxen, can further exacerbate the asthma and the cardiac failure by inducing bronchospasm and by causing retention of salt and water. The naproxen also risks exacerbating upper gastrointestinal problems, particularly in combination with the oral steroid. The naproxen may not be necessary if the painful knee is responsive to a simple analgesic such as paracetamol. Alternatively a weaker NSAID, such as ibuprofen in low dosage, is likely to have less effect on respiratory and renal function.

The patient is receiving four drugs with the potential to reduce serum potassium; the thiazide, the oral and the inhaled steroids and the salbutamol. Thiazides and steroids increase renal losses of potassium, while salbutamol increase the movement of potassium into cells. However, with low inhaled doses of the steroid and the salbutamol there is little systemic absorption and they are unlikely to contribute to hypokalaemia. The age of the patient, the dose of thiazide and the oral steroid make the patient a candidate for a potassium-sparing diuretic, such as amiloride.

How much magnesium trisilicate is the patient taking? Each 10 ml of magnesium trisilicate contains 6 mmol sodium. 30 ml daily therefore contains sodium equivalent to about 1 g of table salt. An alternative aluminium and magnesium hydroxide antacid with low sodium, such as Maalox, is preferable.

The dose of the beclomethasone is not stated and, since there are several different doses of inhaler available, the dose needs to be confirmed with the prescriber. Contact with the prescriber provides the opportunity to consider the following additional points.

Is the patient receiving maximum benefit from the steroid inhaler? If not the inhaler technique must be checked and improved if necessary. If possible, the dose of beclomethasone should be maximized to allow the need for oral steroid to be reviewed. Reduction of the oral steroid dose may benefit the cardiac failure but must be undertaken gradually to avoid exacerbation of the asthma. Removal of the oral steroid may also benefit any dyspepsia and perhaps remove the need for antacid. A regular regimen of salbutamol is not advisable since it may impair control of asthma by masking the onset of exacerbations.

Assuming continuation of the oral steroid is necessary, is there evidence of exacerbation of the cardiac failure? Lack of response to the addition of a potassium-sparing diuretic would indicate the need to change from a thiazide to a loop diuretic such as frusemide.

BIBLIOGRAPHY

Burnier M, Biollaz J. Pharmacokinetic optimisation of angiotensin-converting enzyme (ACE) inhibitor therapy. Clinical Pharmacokinetics 1992; 22: 375–384

Cohn J N. Inotropic therapy for heart failure. New England Journal of Medicine 1989; 320: 729–731

Dobbs R J, O'Neill C J A, Deshmukh A, Nicholson P W, Dobbs S M. Serum concentration monitoring of cardiac glycosides. How helpful is it for adjusting dosage regimens? Clinical Pharmacokinetics 1991; 20: 175–193

Katz R J. Mechanisms of nitrate tolerance: a review. Cardiovascular Drugs and Therapy 1990; 4: 247–252

Leading Article. Failure to treat heart failure. Lancet 1992; 339: 278–279

Packer M. Pathophysiology of chronic heart failure and treatment of chronic heart failure. Lancet 1992; 340: 88–92, 92–95

Schrier R W. Pathogenesis of sodium and water retention in high-output and low-output cardiac failure, nephrotic syndrome, cirrhosis and pregnancy. New England Journal of Medicine 1988; 319: 1058–1064

Smith T W. Digitalis: mechanisms of action and clinical use. New England Journal of Medicine 1988; 318: 358–365

SOLVD Investigators. Effect of captopril on survival in patients with reduced left ventricular ejection fractions and congestive heart failure. New England Journal of Medicine 1991; 325: 303–310

Sutton G C. Epidemiologic aspects of heart failure. American Heart Journal 1990; 120: 1538–1540

Warner Stevenson L, Fonarow G. Vasodilators: a re-evaluation of their role in heart failure. Drugs 1992; 43: 15–36

Chapter 19

Cardiac arrhythmias

D. K. Scott

An arrhythmia is an abnormal cardiac rhythm, usually involving a change in rate or regularity, and is monitored by an electrocardiograph (ECG). The term dysrhythmia is probably a better term since arrhythmia implies 'without rhythm' but is not in general use in the UK.

PHYSIOLOGY

The heart contains many different types of cell, including muscle cells and some specialized cells that generate or conduct electrical stimuli and cause the muscles to contract. Several types of cardiac cell are capable of generating impulses (automaticity) and the overall heart rhythm is determined by the cells which do so most rapidly. When a cell is stimulated it passes on the impulse to adjacent cells and then enters a latent phase (refractory period) during which it cannot be restimulated. Cells which possess automaticity depolarize steadily until they reach a threshold potential at which they depolarize rapidly and generate an impulse (Fig. 19.1). In the normal heart (Fig. 19.2), SA node cells depolarize quickest and thus control the heart rhythm. The impulses are conducted from the SA node across the atria to the atrioventricular (AV) node and then down the bundle of His to the Purkinje fibres and the ventricles. This is termed sinus rhythm.

The activity of the heart is controlled by the sympathetic nervous system which stimulates the SA node and penetrates most cardiac tissue,

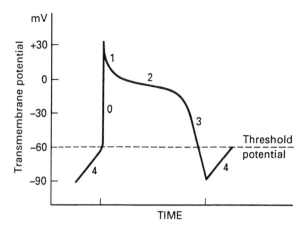

Fig. 19.1 Cardiac cell potential (see Table 19.3 for dominant ion movement in each phase 0–4).

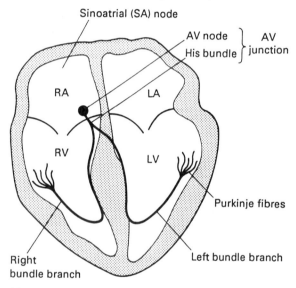

Fig. 19.2 Heart conduction system.

and the parasympathetic vagus nerve which reduces conduction through the AV node and slows the SA node. When functioning normally, the AV node prevents the conduction of excess atrial beats (e.g. in atrial fibrillation) to the ventricles but permits the passage of beats from a normal sinus rhythm. Excessive vagal stimulation results in bradycardia. This may occur in abdominal surgery, following oesophageal intubation or even in some very fit athletes when they stop exercise. Anticholinergic drugs such as tricyclic antidepressants or atropine may remove vagal control and cause tachycardia.

If the SA node is prevented from operating normally the AV node will usually take over as pacemaker or, if both are disabled, the ventricular conducting tissues will serve as pacemaker. Whenever the SA node is not the controlling pacemaker, the heart beat is less well coordinated and this may result in inefficient pumping with an increase in energy expenditure to maintain an adequate circulation or ineffective pumping with an inadequate circulation.

AETIOLOGY

Arrhythmias result from abnormal impulse formation or abnormal impulse conduction and these changes may be brought about in several ways:

1. An infarction may cause the death of pacemaker cells or of conducting tissue.

2. A cardiac tissue disorder, e.g. fibrosis or rheumatic fever, or a multisystem connective tissue disorder, e.g. sarcoidosis, disrupts the conduction network.

3. Sympathetic or parasympathetic control changes, e.g. stress, anxiety, exercise or smoking.

4. Circulating drugs, e.g. antiarrhythmics or inotropes, or other substances, e.g. caffeine, alcohol or bile salts, affect the heart directly or via the nervous system.

5. Hypothyroidism, hyperthyroidism, hypoadrenalism, hyperkalaemia and hypokalaemia or other electrolyte disturbances may predispose to arrhythmias.

Patients who have pre-existing cardiac disorders or who have had a recent infarction are at greater risk of arrhythmias because of their damaged tissue. Some patients have occasional arrhythmias which may be attributed to temporary ischaemia (angina), or some physical activity or stress but others have paroxysmal arrhythmias for no discernible reason. Most apparently normal adults have occasional ectopic beats whilst in some studies up to 20% have brief periods of atrial fibrillation and nearly half have both ventricular and supraventricular arrhythmias. Most such arrhythmias are asymptomatic and treatment is not recommended. Many young adults have resting sinus rhythms of as little as 40 beats per minute which would be defined as bradycardia in an older or active patient.

Description of arrhythmias

Whilst the terminology of arrhythmias seems confusing at first sight, all cardiac rhythms can be described by a phrase which includes terms that relate to rate, origin and pattern.

Table 19.1 lists terms that may be combined into a single phrase. For example, 'atrial flutter' denotes a fast, regular rhythm originating in the atria. The term flutter includes both rate and pattern. Even complex phrases can be broken down into the same three elements, for example 'paroxysmal atrial tachycardia with block' denotes a fast rhythm which originates from a single atrial focus and which occurs in bursts with some other rhythm in between. There is also a delay in conducting the beat from the atria to the ventricles.

Traditional names are still used for a few arrhythmias, e.g. torsades de pointes which is a fast ventricular rhythm with polymorphic QRS complexes and a characteristic ECG pattern. Some terms, e.g. supraventricular, have a general meaning 'originating above the ventricles' but can commonly denote something more specific, 'from the AV node'. This terminology arises partly because all descriptions depend on an indirect measure of the heart's function, namely the ECG recording. The ECG records patterns of electrical activity in the heart, it does not refer to how well the heart is functioning as a pump nor to the physical state of heart tissues. The heart's pumping ability may be measured by pulse and blood pressure and it is important that patients are treated on the basis of their heart function and not just on the basis of an electrical recording.

The ECG is useful, however, in providing clues to the nature and cause of an arrhythmia (see Fig. 19.3). The P wave represents atrial depolarization and the QRS complex represents ventricular depolarization. The interval between the two (PR interval) is the time taken to conduct the beat through the AV node and is lengthened in AV block. The QRS complex is generally narrow when the ventricles are controlled from above and wide when not. The T wave denotes ventricular repolarization, and the QT interval (i.e. the time between depolarization and polarization of the ventricles) may be altered by some drugs including tricyclic antidepressants and

Table 19.1 Nomenclature for describing arrhythmias	
Term	Notes
Rate	
Tachycardia	Both terms imply an SA node
Bradycardia	rhythm unless otherwise stated
	Often a regular rhythm
	Normal limits for rate vary according to the age and activity of the patient
	Bradycardia is slow, tachycardia is fast
Origin	
Sinus	Sinoatrial (SA) node
Atrial	From the atria but not the SA node
Nodal	Atrioventricular node
Supraventricular	Usually, but not necessarily, from AV node
Re-entrant	A circuit involving retrograde (backward) conduction and an accessory pathway whereby impulses travel in a loop, e.g. Wolf–Parkinson–White syndrome
Ventricular	From the ventricular tissue
Pattern	
Ectopic	From a focus other than SA node
Premature contraction	May be isolated or repeated
Paroxysmal	Occurs in bursts
Flutter	A fast, regular rhythm from a single ectopic focus
Fibrillation	A fast, chaotic rhythm from multiple foci
Block	A delay in, or absence of, conduction through the AV node
Mobitz, Wenkebach	Terms used to describe particular varieties of second degree block
Torsades de pointes	A form of ventricular tachycardia with complexes of varying amplitude
Electromechanical dissociation	Electrical impulses (as recorded by ECG) do not lead to mechanical activity (as detected by pulse)

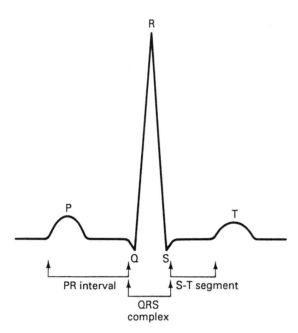

Fig. 19.3 ECG.

antiarrhythmics. The QT interval varies with heart rate and a corrected figure (QTc) is used. A prolonged QTc predisposes to torsades de pointes.

Signs of arrhythmias and criteria for treatment

Signs and symptoms of arrhythmias may include dizziness or collapse because of a poor blood supply to the brain; shortness of breath because of poor oxygenation; angina associated with a poor coronary circulation and/or increased cardiac workload arising from a tachycardia, and weakness and palpitations. It is estimated that 80% of an individual's cardiac output comes from ventricular action, even when that is not coordinated with the atria. Thus many patients with an abnormal but regular ventricular rhythm experience little difficulty in normal daily living. Atrial fibrillation (AF) is sometimes described as 'slow' or 'fast' depending on the ventricular rate. A patient with slow AF in which an effective AV node block permits only a small proportion of impulses to pass from the atria to the ventricles may not need treatment. In contrast, fast AF which occurs in patients with an ineffective AV node block features rapid and irregular ventricular beats and consequent inefficient filling of the ventricles and inefficient circulation.

Since arrhythmias can occur without apparent ill effect, it follows that their mere presence does not mandate treatment, indeed the use of an antiarrhythmic agent may generate a worse arrhythmia. In the case of post-infarction ventricular ectopics, 10% of patients may deteriorate if treated. The Cardiac Arrhythmia Suppression Trial (CAST) in the USA showed that the use of flecainide or encainide in such patients increased the risk of sudden death.

Suitable criteria for treatment of an arrhythmia would include the following:

1. The arrhythmia causes haemodynamic failure (poor circulation).
2. Haemodynamic failure has not occurred but the present arrhythmia is known to be a predictor of a more serious arrhythmia. For example, patients who experience an episode of ventricular tachycardia following myocardial infarction have a 30% risk of dying within 1 year, probably from ventricular fibrillation.
3. The patient is distressed by an awareness of extra or missed beats (palpitations).

The aim of treatment is to restore a satisfactory circulation and to prevent further episodes of poor circulation or distress.

TREATMENT
Bradyarrhythmias

Bradyarrhythmias are generally caused by tissue damage, a decrease in sympathetic autonomic tone or an increase in parasympathetic tone mediated by the vagus nerve. Such changes in autonomic function may be caused or mimicked by drugs such as hyoscine, beta-adrenoreceptor blockers, digoxin and verapamil or by deficiencies in thyroid or corticosteroid hormones. Increased vagal tone causes AV block of varying degree which reduces the rate of impulses reaching the ventricles. A ventricular escape rhythm involving ectopics, an idioventricular rhythm or even a tachycardia may then result which should be recognized as secondary to the fault at the AV node and not treated as a primary disorder.

AV block may be classified into three types. First degree block describes instances where all beats are conducted through the AV node, but with some delay. This does not require treatment but may be a warning to avoid drugs which would worsen the block, such as beta-adrenoreceptor blockers and class IV agents.

Second degree block implies that some, but not all, beats are conducted through the AV node and there are further subdivisions of this class, e.g. Mobitz and Wenkebach. The need for treatment depends upon whether a satisfactory ventricular rate and output can be maintained.

Third degree block implies that there is no conduction of sinus or atrial beats through the AV node and treatment is usually required.

The treatment of bradycardia should include identification and treatment of the cause, such as treatment of jaundice or hypothyroidism, and removal of causative drugs. Immediate treatment is normally to decrease vagal tone with intravenous atropine which will decrease AV block and increase SA rate. It is important to note that it will take a minute or longer to see initial signs of benefit and at least 5 minutes to observe maximum effect. Doses of 300 to 600 micrograms of atropine may be given up to six times at 1 minute intervals until benefit is observed. If atropine is ineffective, intravenous adrenaline or isoprenaline may be used. The only oral treatment available for bradycardia is slow-release isoprenaline which is not generally satisfactory.

Ultimately a pacemaker may be required to pace the heart from the right ventricle or from both right atrium and ventricle. This approach may also be used where the patient has bouts of tachycardia and bradycardia (e.g. in sick sinus syndrome). In such cases the tachycardia may be controlled by beta-adrenoreceptor blockers, amiodarone or class IV drugs but an undesirable consequence may be the worsening of the bradycardia for which the only suitable treatment is a pacemaker.

Tachyarrhythmias

The primary treatment of any tachyarrhythmia is to remove the cause. Removal of arrhythmogenic drugs or stimulants such as caffeine, alcohol and smoking may solve the problem and investigation of other medical causes, including abnormal thyroid function, is essential. Behavioural modifications to avoid stress and anxiety may help and physical procedures such as the Valsalva manoeuvre have been useful in terminating re-entrant tachycardias.

Tachyarrhythmias that compromise cardiac output will require DC cardioversion or, more often, antiarrhythmic drug treatment. The first choice to be made is that of the class of drug to be used according to the Vaughan-Williams system (see below). That choice is based upon the origin of the arrhythmia, regardless of its pattern. Table 19.2 lists the classes of drug considered useful for arrhythmias of various origins. For any origin, the preference of one class to another may vary, depending on personal clinical experience with particular drugs, on the presentation of the arrythmia and on patient characteristics. Such factors also govern the choice of drug within a class. The drug chosen should have the dosing schedule and adverse-effect profile that best suit the patient (or inconvenience him least). Thus, for example, a patient with glaucoma or prostatism should not be given disopyramide which possesses marked anticholinergic properties, and a patient with obstructive airways disease should preferably not have a beta-adrenoreceptor blocker (class II), though if considered essential they could have a cardioselective agent.

Table 19.2 Choice of antiarrhythmics by class, based on the origin of the tachyarrhythmia

SA node	Atria	AV node	Accessory pathways (re-entrant)	Ventricles
II	IA	II	IA	IB
IV	II	IV	III	IA
Digitalis	IV	Digitalis		III
	Digitalis	IC		IC
	III			
	IC			

It should be noted that it is not necessary to cure all arrhythmias to satisfy the criteria for treatment. Atrial arrhythmias may be well tolerated provided the ventricular rate is controlled and the patient is not distressed. Thus, digoxin or other digitalis derivatives may provide satisfactory therapy by controlling the number of impulses that pass through the AV node to the ventricles but without converting the patient to a sinus rhythm.

Emergency treatment of arrhythmias in adults

Acute life-threatening arrhythmias may result in haemodynamic failure, the so-called cardiac arrest. Fast, but careful, management is required to prevent permanent damage or death and the following scheme is simplified from guidelines issued by the European Resuscitation Council.

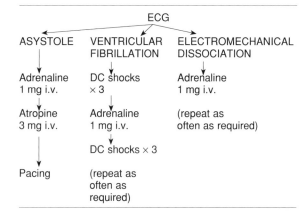

In all cases, cardiopulmonary resuscitation should be continued throughout and any specific cause removed or countered.

Adrenaline, atropine and lignocaine can be administered by endotracheal tube at double the i.v. dose in 10 ml isotonic saline. The use of lignocaine or bretylium as an adjunct to electrical defibrillation is controversial but common.

Acidosis may cause widespread problems, including serious arrhythmias, and sodium bicarbonate (50 mmol) may be given to counteract acidosis after prolonged resuscitation. Overdose is hazardous, however, and arterial blood gas measurements should be made where possible.

Table 19.3 Effect of different drug classes on phases of action potential in His–Purkinje fibres

Phase	Dominant ion movement	Drug class	Effect
0	Sodium inward	IA	Marked block
		IB	Block
		IC	Very marked block
2	Calcium inward	IV	Block
3	Potassium outward	III	Marked slowing
4	Sodium inward Potassium outward	I,II,IV	Slows

Severe bradycardia should be managed with atropine first and adrenaline second.

CLASSIFICATION OF ANTIARRHYTHMIC DRUGS

The most widely accepted classification is the Vaughan-Williams system based on electrophysiological data illustrated in Tables 19.3 and 19.4 and Figure 19.1. It is not only physiologically acceptable but it provides a good basis for clinical choices since drugs in the same class

Table 19.4 Electrophysiological effects of some antiarrhythmics

Class	Antiarrhythmic agents	Effects on duration of		Sinus rate
		QRS	QT	
IA	Quinidine, procainamide, disopyramide	+	+	+
IB	Lignocaine, mexiletine, tocainide, phenytoin, aprindine	0/–	0	0
IC	Flecainide, encainide, lorcainide, propafenone	++	+	0
II	Atenolol, metoprolol, sotalol, esmolol	0	++	– –
III	Amiodarone, bretylium sotalol	0	+++	–
IV	Verapamil, diltiazem, adenosine	0	0	– –

Key: + = increased; – = decreased; 0 = no change

have similar therapeutic effects. Table 19.3 and Figure 19.1 relate to His–Purkinje fibres ('fast fibres') which have a sodium-dependent phase 0. Other fibres have different characteristics notably in the SA node and upper AV node where phase 0 is calcium dependent and overlaps phase 1 and 2 ('slow fibres'). The clinical consequences are that class I drugs (especially IB) have less effect on SA or AV nodal arrhythmias than those which originate from ventricular cells, whilst class IV drugs have major effects on the SA and AV nodes.

Most drugs have several modes of action and their effectiveness as antiarrhythmic agents depends upon the summation of these effects. For example, class IB agents shorten the duration of the action potential thereby decreasing the refractory period and increasing the risk of sustaining a tachyarrhythmia. In contrast, they also slow phase 4 which increases the overall refractory period. The net result is a decrease in the risk of sustaining a tachyarrhythmia.

The action of drugs also varies according to the activity of the tissue concerned. Class IB are more active in ischaemic tissue than in well-perfused tissue and thus are of particular value in arrhythmias following a myocardial infarction. It is important to note that all antiarrythmics are also pro-arrythmics.

Class I

All class I agents slow down sodium currents in phases 0 and 4 of the action potential but vary in their effects on phases 2 and 3. All are useful in ventricular tachyarrhythmias but class IB are of no value in atrial disorders and are more effective in ischaemic tissue than in normal tissue. Lignocaine is the most commonly used agent in the UK for prophylaxis of ventricular tachycardia (VT) or ventricular fibrillation (VF) and for management of ventricular ectopics and VT. Whilst it is also indicated in the management of VF, it is only an adjunct to DC electric shock. Lignocaine is not available orally and is usually administered by an i.v. infusion regimen in which the dose is decreased with time, e.g.:

- 4 mg/minute for 30 minutes then
- 2 mg/minute for 2 hours then
- 1 mg/minute to continue.

It is unusual to continue for longer than 24 to 48 hours, after which an oral agent should be used if required. Mexiletine is commonly chosen for oral administration because tocainide may cause thrombocytopenia. Phenytoin is difficult to control because of its non-linear elimination and is now rarely used except in digitalis-induced arrhythmias.

Class IA agents are all potentially toxic but have an important role in patients who have no contra-indication to their use (Table 19.5). They may be used on their own or combined cautiously with digoxin for atrial arrhythmias. Quinidine and disopyramide are particularly prone to cause torsades de pointes but disopyramide is valuable in treating Wolf–Parkinson–White syndrome in which it inhibits both anterograde and retrograde conduction. All three class IA agents may be used in VT but individual variation in response to these agents is probably greater than in any other class. It may be useful, therefore, to try a second class IA agent if the first is not successful.

Class IC agents are effective in atrial and ventricular tachyarrhythmias but they also cause arrhythmias in a significant number of patients. The CAST study demonstrated that flecainide and encainide increased mortality when used in the management of ventricular ectopics after myocardial infarction. These agents are usually restricted to the management of ventricular arrhythmias resistant to other drugs although intravenous flecainide may be used to terminate atrial or supraventricular tachycardias.

Class II

Beta-adrenoreceptor blockers are useful for treating arrhythmias that are provoked or exacerbated by sympathetic autonomic nervous stimulation or by circulating catecholamines. They are valuable in arrhythmias originating from the SA or AV nodes which are provoked by anxiety, stress or exercise. They are also useful,

Table 19.5 Adverse effects of antiarrhythmic drugs (class I)

Drug	Cardiac	Non-cardiac	Caution or avoid in
Disopyramide	Torsades de pointes Myodepressant	Anticholinergic (urinary retention, constipation, dry mouth, blurred vision)	Glaucoma, prostatism, hypotension
Procainamide		Lupus, nausea, diarrhoea	Myasthenia gravis, slow acetylators (increased risk of lupus)
Quinidine	Torsades de pointes Vasodilatation (i.v.)	Diarrhoea, nausea, tinnitus, headache, deafness, confusion, visual disturbances, blood dyscrasias	Myasthenia gravis
Lignocaine		Convulsions in overdose, paraesthesiae	Liver failure (reduce dose)
Mexiletine		Nausea, paraesthesiae	2nd or 3rd degree heart block
Tocainide		Thrombocytopenia, nausea, pulmonary fibrosis, paraesthesiae	Use only if other agents have failed
Flecainide	Pro-arrhythmic Myodepressant	Paraesthesiae, tremor	Use only if other agents have failed
Propafenone	Pro-arrhythmic Myodepressant	GI disturbances	Use only if other agents have failed

along with alpha-adrenoreceptor blockers, in the arrhythmias of phaeochromocytoma. Beta-adrenoreceptor blockers are contra-indicated in heart failure and in patients with extensive infarcts because of their myodepressant actions but have a cardioprotective effect in uncomplicated acute myocardial infarction (see Ch. 17) which is probably due, at least in part, to their antiarrhythmic activity.

Beta-adrenoreceptor blockers are contra-indicated in patients with asthma or obstructive airways disease unless other agents have failed and a cardioselective beta-adrenoreceptor blocker is used at low doses. It should be noted that cardioselectivity is a relative term and no agent is free from respiratory effects. Membrane stabilizing activity and intrinsic sympathomimetic activity have no impact upon the choice of drug (see Table 17.2, Ch. 17) for arrhythmias. The risk of bradycardia is a threat with all beta-adrenoreceptor blockers and especially in patients with myocardial disease, heart block or a mixed tachycardia–bradycardia (sick sinus syndrome). Beta-adrenoreceptor blockers with partial agonist activity have not proved useful in such cases despite theoretical promise. In general, beta-adrenoreceptor blockers may also exacerbate peripheral vascular disease and cause nightmares or depression. There is little value

in changing to a second beta-adrenoreceptor blocker if the first agent has not been successful.

Atenolol, metoprolol and esmolol are available for intravenous use and esmolol, with its short duration of action, is the most appropriate beta-adrenoreceptor blocker for urgent use in SA, atrial or atrioventricular arrhythmias. Verapamil and adenosine (class IV) are also suitable, however, and have even shorter durations of action. Care must be taken if both class II and IV agents are to be used since they have additive effects in suppressing the AV node and in depressing contractility. The combination is most dangerous if i.v. verapamil follows i.v. or oral beta-adrenoreceptor blockers which have a prolonged action.

Sotalol has some class III activity as well as class II effects and bretylium is considered to have class II activity in addition to class III.

Class III

Class III drugs (amiodarone, bretylium, sotalol) prolong the action potential and bring greater uniformity amongst different cell types, thus reducing the means for generation of arrhythmias. Although they are all powerful anti-arrhythmics, there the similarities end. Each drug has different side effect profiles and other electrophysiological properties. Amiodarone can

Table 19.6   Adverse effects of antiarrhythmic drugs (classes II–IV)

Drug	Cardiac	Non-cardiac	Caution or avoid in
Beta-adrenoreceptor blockers (general)	Myodepressant Heart block	Bronchoconstriction (β_2) Vasoconstriction Hallucinations/vivid dreams (lipophilic compounds) Decreased renal blood flow Changes in serum lipid profile Drowsiness, fatigue	Asthma, COAD, Raynaud's disease, gangrene, diabetes mellitus, depression
Sotalol	Torsades de pointes		Combination with disopyramide or amiodarone
Amiodarone	Torsades de pointes	Hyper-/hypothyroidism Pneumonitis, myopathy, neuropathy, hepatitis, corneal deposits, photosensitivity	Thyroid disease
Bretylium	Hypotension	Initial sympathomimetic response Nausea	
Verapamil & diltiazem	Heart block	Constipation, headaches, flushing, ankle oedema, lightheadedness	

cause sodium channel blockade, bretylium is an adrenergic neurone blocking agent whilst sotalol is a beta-adrenoreceptor blocker. Amiodarone has an extensive range of side effects, both trivial and fatal, that prevent its wider use. It is commonly restricted to serious ventricular arrhythmias that have proved resistant to other therapy, although it is increasingly being used in atrial arrhythmias and has a role in re-entrant rhythms such as the Wolf–Parkinson–White syndrome. A significant disadvantage to its use is its long half-life (about 1 month) which necessitates intensive oral loading, e.g. 200 mg three times daily for a week, then 200 mg twice daily for a week, reducing to 200 mg daily in many cases. The long half-life results in a slow onset of action and very prolonged effects after discontinuing therapy. Intravenous doses are effective immediately but there are hazards associated with rapid i.v. doses and incompatibility problems with common infusion fluids.

In contrast to amiodarone, bretylium has a rapid onset of action and short half-life, is only available parenterally and is not effective in atrial arrhythmias. It has been used mostly in emergency resuscitation for ventricular tachycardia or fibrillation, either to aid electric defibrillation or to cardiovert patients on its own. The major problem has been severe hypotension although, paradoxically, there may be an initial

sympathetic stimulation that precedes the sympathetic block and causes hypertension and arrhythmias. Whereas amiodarone and bretylium have minimal myodepressant activity, sotalol is a significant myodepressant and also has the standard side effect profile of a beta-adrenoreceptor blocker. It is less effective than amiodarone but, despite its problems, is a lot safer, it is available orally, and it may be of particular benefit in treating arrhythmias in hypertensive patients, in angina and after acute myocardial infarcts. It is rarely used for non-antiarrhythmic purposes.

All three agents, by virtue of their class III activity, prolong the QT interval and increase the risk of torsades de pointes, especially in hypokalaemic patients or when combined with a bradycardic drug such as a class IA agent.

Class IV

Verapamil and diltiazem inhibit slow channel conduction through the AV node and are referred to by a number of terms, including the general name 'calcium antagonists'. Other calcium antagonists such as nifedipine and other 4, 5-dihydropyridines have no antiarrhythmic effect. The potassium channel openers adenosine and its pro-drug ATP act as indirect calcium antagonists and resemble verapamil in their antiarrhythmic scope. Intravenous adenosine's ultra-short duration of action makes it very suitable as a diagnostic aid and for interrupting supraventricular arrhythmias without the myosuppressant effects of verapamil. Adenosine is, however, a bronchoconstrictor and causes dyspnoea, flushing, chest pain and further transient arrhythmias in a high proportion of patients. All class IV agents should be avoided in second or third degree heart block and sick sinus syndrome, unless the patient has a pacemaker to overcome bradycardia. Likewise, combined therapy with a beta-adrenoreceptor blocker is hazardous because of the risk of excessive AV block, although in some cases it may be useful to treat chronic atrial fibrillation or flutter with digoxin and a calcium antagonist where either agent alone has failed. Calcium antagonists may cause conversion to sinus rhythm but are used chiefly to control ventricular rate. Verapamil has a greater dilatory effect on systemic arteries than diltiazem and may be especially useful in patients with hypertension or angina. Both agents cause myocardial suppression and are thus contra-indicated in heart failure although their depressant actions on the SA node are usually offset by the reflex response to arterial vasodilatation. Side effects are mostly predictable and include ankle oedema, flushing, dizziness, lightheadedness and headache. Constipation is relatively more common in patients receiving verapamil.

Digoxin

Digoxin is one of a group of cardiac (digitalis) glycosides and has a well-defined role in the management of atrial tachyarrhythmias, in the presence of congestive heart failure. Digoxin inhibits conduction through the AV node and thus protects the ventricles from rapid atrial rhythms. In addition, some patients with established atrial fibrillation may convert to sinus rhythm although this is unusual in atrial flutter and in atrial fibrillation of recent origin (less than 1 week). It is less effective in the presence of high sympathetic nervous activity and its use is diminishing as that of amiodarone, sotalol and

Table 19.7   Adverse effects of digoxin

Cardiac
  Ventricular ectopics including bigeminy
  Ventricular tachycardia
  AV junctional beats or tachycardia
  2nd or 3rd degree heart block
  Atrial tachycardia (often paroxysmal) with block
  SA node arrest

Non-cardiac
  Anorexia, nausea, vomiting
  Diarrhoea (less common)
  Fatigue, confusion
  Abnormal colour vision (excess yellow/green)

class II drugs increases. Digoxin also causes both atrial and ventricular ectopic beats and is a potent cause of arrhythmias (Table 19.7). Both beneficial and toxic effects are enhanced by hypokalaemia and hypercalcaemia and the AV block is enhanced by beta-adrenoreceptor blockers and calcium antagonists. There are numerous other drug interactions (Table 19.8), some of which are pharmacokinetic and some of which are pharmacological. Digoxin is the only antiarrhythmic for which therapeutic drug monitoring is widely used. It has a narrow therapeutic range of 1 to 2 ng/ml. This range is, however,

Table 19.8   Interactions involving digoxin

Serum levels increased by:	Amiodarone, verapamil, diltiazem, quinidine, propafenone, broad-spectrum antibiotics (erythromycin, tetracyclines), decreased renal blood flow (beta-adrenoreceptor blockers), renal failure, heart failure
Serum levels decreased by:	Cholestyramine, sulphasalazine, neomycin, rifampicin, antacids improved renal blood flow (vasodilators)
Effects of digoxin increased by:	Hypokalaemia, hypercalcaemia, hypomagnesaemia Antiarrhythmic classes IA, II, IV Diuretics that cause hypokalaemia, corticosteroids Myxoedema, hypoxia (acute or chronic), acute myocardial ischaemia or myocarditis
Effects of digoxin decreased by:	Hyperkalaemia, hypocalcaemia, thyrotoxicosis

Table 19.9 Pharmacokinetics of antiarrhythmics

	Oral absorption	% protein-binding	Approx. therapeutic range	Elimination, metabolism, half-life
Amiodarone	Slow, variable	> 95	0.5–2.5 mg/L	Extensive metabolism, very variable rate, $t_{1/2}$ = 2 days initially increasing to 40–60 days
Bretylium	i.v./i.m. only	Unbound	Not determined	Renal, $t_{1/2}$ = 5–10 h
Digoxin	Variable, 70%	25	0.8–2 ng/ml	70% renal, variable, $t_{1/2}$ = 36 h
Diltiazem	40% absorbed	80	0.05–0.3 mg/L	Hepatic, $t_{1/2}$ = 3 h
Disopyramide	Rapid, > 80%	30–90	2–4 mg/L (depends on extent of binding)	50% renal, 15% bile, active metabolite, $t_{1/2}$ 4–10 h
Flecainide	Complete, slow	40	0.2–1 mg/L	30% renal, $t_{1/2}$ = 20 h
Lignocaine	i.v./i.m. only	60–80	1.5–5 mg/L	10% renal, rapid hepatic metabolism to CNS-toxic products, $t_{1/2}$ = 8–100 min increases with duration of dosing
Mexiletine	> 90%	60–70	0.5–2 mg/L	10% renal, $t_{1/2}$ = 10–12 h, hepatic metabolites mostly inactive
Phenytoin	Variable rate and extent	> 90	10–12 mg/L	Capacity-limited hepatic metabolism, $t_{1/2}$ = 10–60 h but variable because of non-first-order elimination
Procainamide	Rapid, > 75%	15–20	3–10 mg/L	50% renal, 25–40% converted to N-acetylprocainamide (active, $t_{1/2}$ = 6 h), procainamide $t_{1/2}$ = 2.5–4.5 h
Propafenone	Complete, rapid	> 95	0.06–1 mg/L	Extensive first-pass metabolism, capacity-limited $t_{1/2}$ 2–12 h
Quinidine	Rapid, > 80%	80–90	2–6 mg/L	Mixed renal & hepatic, $t_{1/2}$ = 6 h
Tocainide	Complete, rapid	> 10	4–10 mg/L	40% renal, 60% hepatic, $t_{1/2}$ = 15 h
Verapamil	Rapid, > 90%	90	0.1–0.4 mg/L	Hepatic, $t_{1/2}$ = 4–12 h, marked first-pass effect

Notes:
All values quoted are subject to marked interindividual variability. Most therapeutic ranges are poorly defined.
Oral absorption does not account for drug lost by first-pass hepatic metabolism.
Rapid absorption indicates a peak plasma concentration in less than 2 hours.
$t_{1/2}$ = elimination half-life at normal renal function.
For the pharmacokinetics of beta-adrenoreceptor blockers and other calcium channel blockers see Chapter 17.

modified by serum electrolyte concentrations and by the concurrent use of other drugs, but the extent of the modification is not defined. Since digoxin is excreted by the liver and the kidney (70% renal elimination in normal renal function) reduced renal function increases digoxin levels and necessitates reduced doses, notably in the elderly.

Table 19.10 Interactions involving antiarrhythmic agents (excluding digoxin)

Antiarrhythmic	Other drug	Effect
Disopyramide	Anticholinergics	Increased anticholinergic effects
	Pyridostigmine	Decreased anticholinergic effects of disopyramide
		Decreased cholinergic effects of pyridostigmine
	Class II, IV	Increased hypotension
	Class III	Torsades de pointes
Procainamide	Class III	Torsades de pointes
	Cimetidine	Decreased renal clearance
Quinidine	Class II, IV	Increased hypotension
	Class III	Torsades de pointes
	Warfarin	Increased anticoagulation
	Enzyme inducers	Decreased serum levels
	Enzyme inhibitors	Increased serum levels
Lignocaine	Beta-adrenoreceptor blockers, cimetidine	Decreased elimination of lignocaine
	Enzyme inducers	Increased elimination of lignocaine
Mexiletine	Theophylline	Increased theophylline levels
Propafenone	Warfarin	Enhanced anticoagulation
Amiodarone	Warfarin	Enhanced anticoagulation

Notes:
Additive antiarrhythmic or myosuppressant effects are not included.
Interactions between antiarrhythmics are listed under the first named drug only.
Enzyme inducers include barbiturates, rifampicin, smoking.
Enzyme inhibitors include cimetidine.

CASE STUDIES

CASE 19.1

A 68-year-old man with a history of atrial fibrillation controlled until recently by digoxin (250 micrograms daily) complains at an outpatient clinic of recurrent palpitations. He is diagnosed as suffering from uncontrolled atrial fibrillation, confirmed on ECG.

Q1 What course of action should be pursued now?

The patient is given quinidine (250 mg SR twice daily) and returns a week later with better control of fibrillation but suffering from a disabling pneumonia. He is admitted to hospital where an ECG shows controlled AF and a digoxin level is 1.8 ng/ml, 8 hours after his last dose. He is given erythromycin for the infection and although the chest sounds and sputum improve over the next 4 days, he becomes more unwell, complaining of tiredness, nausea and confusion.

Q2 What is the differential diagnosis and what tests should be performed?

CASE 19.2

A teenage patient in casualty complains of nausea 2 hours after ingesting about 15 of her grandmother's heart tablets and a quantity of alcohol. She now regrets her attempt at suicide and has come with her boyfriend to seek help. A rapid digoxin assay indicates a serum digoxin of 2.6 ng/ml (normal range 1 to 2 ng/ml) and serum potassium is 3.4 mmol (normal range 3.5 to 5.0).

Q1 What tests and treatment would be appropriate?

After a few hours she becomes more unwell, complaining of bursts of palpitations, wooziness and shortness of breath. An ECG shows a slow sinus rate with ventricular escape beats and some bigeminy. There is also evidence of electromechanical dissociation, i.e. the pulse does not match the ECG trace but suggests fewer beats.

Q2 What tests and treatment should be pursued?

ANSWERS TO CASE STUDIES

CASE 19.1

A1 A serum digoxin concentration should be measured 6 to 8 hours after a dose and electrolytes and creatinine checked. A check should be made on compliance if there is any reason to suspect a change and on any potential interactions (e.g. changes in diet, use of antacids or other drugs). A recent change in causative factors for AF should be considered, e.g. coffee, tea, smoking and alcohol.

If serum potassium is low, a supplement should be provided. If the digoxin level is low, despite apparently good compliance, the dose may be increased. Renal function should be calculated from serum creatinine and reconciled with the digoxin dose, level and claimed compliance.

If none of the above approaches suggests a solution to the problem, the use of another drug should be considered because the patient is symptomatic and requesting treatment. The choice of drug is to add a beta-adrenoreceptor blocker, add class IA, add class IV, or use a class IA, IC or III drug alone.

Amiodarone (III) and flecainide (IC) are too toxic to contemplate as first choices and verapamil (IV) causes marked constipation.

There is no evidence of sympathetic overactivity associated with stress or exercise which would favour a beta-adrenoreceptor blocker so it is decided to use a class IA drug. Disopyramide is excluded because of the possibility of sub-clinical prostatism; quinidine has a good success rate in such cases and is selected in addition to digoxin.

A2 If there is no other obvious cause, digoxin toxicity is likely (high serum level or normal level with low potassium) and a cause should be sought. (ECG changes may or may not be apparent.) Four main possibilities exist:

- Illness may lead to decreased renal function and increased digoxin levels.
- Quinidine increases digoxin levels markedly.
- Previous non-compliance now results in toxicity because dose administration is supervised and given as prescribed.
- Erythromycin, a broad-spectrum antibiotic, kills gut organisms that metabolize digoxin to inactive products. More digoxin is therefore available for absorption and toxicity ensues. This may be remedied by stopping the antibiotic.

CASE 19.2

A1 Blood pressure, pulse and ECG should be recorded and repeated frequently, including upon any sign of clinical deterioration. A digoxin level may be repeated 2 hours later, since absorption may not yet be complete, and serum potassium rechecked. It may be worth checking for other drugs by a urine screen. It is desirable to reduce further absorption of digoxin but emesis is undesirable and gastric lavage, or any process involving pharyngeal stimulation, may lead to increased AV block. Activated charcoal (50 g) should be given immediately and may be repeated at 1 to 2 hour intervals in an attempt to remove digoxin from the circulation and decrease further absorption.

Potassium chloride may be given orally (since it is not adsorbed by charcoal) or by infusion in dextrose or sodium chloride to prevent hypokalaemia but should not be given if the ECG shows AV block.

No specific treatment should be given unless symptoms occur. Calcium supplements must be avoided.

A2 These are signs of digoxin toxicity. Digoxin and potassium levels should be measured but should not delay treatment. Calcium should be avoided. Nausea and vomiting are treated as usual. Digoxin-binding antibody fragments ('Digibind') may be given intravenously to inactivate digoxin and enhance its elimination. The effect is very rapid and should be titrated to circulatory function indicated by pulse and blood pressure and not to the ECG. It is expensive to administer enough Digibind to bind all the digoxin taken (40 mg Digibind to 1 mg digoxin) but symptomatic treatment with small doses (20 to 40 mg) should suffice until the digoxin is eliminated by the kidneys to a sufficient extent to represent no further problem.

Immune-complex assay methods such as radioimmune assays continue to detect bound digoxin and are unhelpful in monitoring treatment once Digibind has been given. Other antiarrhythmics should not be necessary but phenytoin may be useful since it reverses AV block and reduces ventricular escape rhythms.

BIBLIOGRAPHY

Antonaccio M J. Cardiovascular pharmacology, 3rd edn. New York: Raven Press 1990

Arrythmia Octet. London: Lancet 1993

CAST Investigators. Preliminary report: Effect of encainide and flecainide on mortality in a randomised trial of arrhythmia suppression after myocardial infarction. New England Journal of Medicine 1989; 321: 406–412

Opie L H (ed). Drugs for the heart, 3rd edn. Philadelphia: W B Saunders 1991

Chapter 20

Thrombosis

P. A. Routledge

Thrombosis is the development of a 'thrombus' consisting of platelets, fibrin, red cells and white cells in the arterial or venous circulation. If part of this thrombus in the venous circulation breaks off and enters the right heart, it may be lodged in the pulmonary arterial circulation causing pulmonary embolism. In the arterial circulation, an embolus may result in peripheral arterial occlusion, either in the lower limbs or in the cerebral circulation (where it may result in stroke). Since the pathophysiology of each of these conditions differs, they will be discussed separately under venous thromboembolism and arterial thromboembolism.

VENOUS THROMBOEMBOLISM

EPIDEMIOLOGY

Venous thromboembolism is common, with an incidence of 2 to 5%. Pulmonary embolism is now the commonest cause of maternal death and deep vein thrombosis may result not only in pulmonary embolism but in subsequent morbidity as a result of the post-phlebitic limb. Thromboembolism appears to increase in prevalence over the age of 50 years and the diagnosis is more often missed in this age group.

AETIOLOGY

Venous thromboembolism occurs primarily due to a combination of stagnation of blood flow and hypercoagulability. Vascular injury is also a recognized causative factor but is not necessary for the development of venous thrombosis. Sluggishness of blood flow may be related to bed rest, surgery or reduced cardiac output (e.g. heart failure). Factors increasing the risk of hypercoagulability include surgery, pregnancy, oestrogen administration, malignancy, myocardial infarction and several acquired or inherited disorders of coagulation (e.g. antithrombin III deficiency, protein C deficiency or circulating lupus anticoagulant). In venous thromboembolism, the thrombus is different in structure from that in arterial thromboembolism. In the former, platelets seem to be uniformly distributed through a mesh of fibrin and other blood cell components, whereas in arterial thromboembolism the white platelet 'head' is more prominent and it appears to play a much more important initiatory role in thrombus formation.

Oestrogens increase the circulating concentrations of clotting factors I, II, VII, VIII, IX and X and reduce fibrinolytic activity. They also depress the concentrations of antithrombin III which is protective against thrombosis. This effect is dose related and venous thrombosis was more often seen with the high (50 micrograms) oestrogen-containing contraceptive pill than with the present lower dose preparations. Venous thromboembolism is also commoner in malignancy (the risk may be up to fivefold greater). Although first described in association with carcinoma of the pancreas, all solid tumours seem to be associated with this problem. The reason for the association is unknown although migrating thrombophlebitis is also sometimes associated with underlying carcinoma.

The increased risk of venous thromboembolism in surgery is related in part to stagnation of venous blood in the calves during the operation, but also to tissue trauma, since it appears to be more common in operations which involve marked tissue damage (e.g. orthopaedic surgery). This may in turn be related to release of tissue thromboplastin and to reduced fibrinolytic activity. The most important risk factors associated with clinical thromboembolism after surgery are age and obesity.

Antithrombin III deficiency is a rare autosomal dominantly inherited abnormality associated with a reduced plasma concentration of this protein. The defect may not result in clinical problems until either pregnancy occurs or patients enter their fourth decade when venous (and to a lesser extent) arterial thrombosis become more common.

Protein C deficiency is also inherited by an autosomal dominant transmission. Not only are such patients at increased risk of venous thromboembolism but also of warfarin skin necrosis. This occurs because protein C (and its closely related co-factor protein S) are vitamin K dependent antithrombotic factors which can be further suppressed by the administration of warfarin. Thrombosis in the small vessels of the skin may occur if large loading doses of warfarin are given to such patients when the suppression of the antithrombotic effects of these factors occurs before the antithrombotic effects of blockade of vitamin K dependent clotting factor (II, VII, IX and X) production has occurred.

Lupus anticoagulant is so named because it increases the clotting time in blood when measured by some standard clotting tests. Patients affected are more prone to thromboembolism as well as (in females) to recurrent spontaneous abortion. This factor is found in 10% of patients with systemic lupus erythematosus (SLE) but may occur in patients without any skin, nervous system or renal manifestations of SLE.

CLINICAL MANIFESTATIONS

In 90% of patients, deep vein thrombosis occurs in the veins of the lower limbs and pelvis. In up to half the cases, this may not result in local symptoms or signs and the onset of pulmonary embolism may be the first evidence of the presence of venous thromboembolism. In other cases, patients classically present with pain involving the calf or thigh associated with swelling, redness of the overlying skin and increased warmth. In a large deep venous thrombosis which prevents venous return, the leg may become discoloured and oedematous. Massive venous thrombus can occasionally result in gangrene although this occurs very rarely now that effective drug therapies are available.

Pulmonary embolism may occur in the absence of clinical signs of venous thrombosis. It may be very difficult to diagnose because of the non-specificity of symptoms and signs. Clinical diagnosis is often made because of the presence of associated risk factors. Obstruction with a large embolus of a major pulmonary artery may result in acute massive pulmonary embolism, presenting with sudden shortness of breath and dull central chest pain together with marked haemodynamic disturbance (e.g. severe hypotension and right ventricular failure). It may increase the risk of unconsciousness and the patients may die of acute circulatory failure unless rapidly treated.

Acute sub-massive pulmonary embolus occurs when less than 50% of the pulmonary circulation is occluded by embolus and the embolus normally lodges in a more distal branch of the pulmonary artery. It may result in some shortness of breath but if the lung normally supplied by that branch of the pulmonary artery becomes necrotic, pulmonary infarction results with pleuritic pain, haemoptysis (coughing up blood) and there may be a pleural 'rub' (a sound like 'Velcro' being torn apart when the patient breathes in) as a result of inflammation of the lung. Patients may rarely develop recurrent thromboembolism. This may not result in immediate symptoms or signs but the patient may present with increasing breathlessness and signs of pulmonary hypertension (right ventricular hypertrophy) and (if untreated) progressive respiratory failure.

INVESTIGATIONS

The clinical diagnosis of venous thrombosis is relatively unreliable and venography is the most specific diagnostic test. This involves injection of radiopaque contrast medium, normally into a vein on the top of the foot and subsequent X-ray of the venous system. Doppler ultrasound has been used but this is less reliable and is normally only used as a screening test. Although several conditions may mimic deep vein thrombus (e.g. a rupture of the posterior aspect of the synovial capsule of the knee, or 'Baker's' cyst), deep vein thrombosis is the commonest cause of pain, swelling and tenderness of the leg. Venography may be contra-indicated in patients with allergy to contrast media and in pregnancy (to avoid exposure of the fetus to radiation).

The diagnosis of pulmonary embolism is most often made using one of two techniques (pulmonary arteriography or ventilation–perfusion scanning). Pulmonary arteriography is the most specific test. This requires catheterization of the right side of the heart and an injection of contrast medium into the pulmonary artery. Adequate facilities and experienced personnel are therefore required.

Ventilation–perfusion scanning involves the injection of a radiolabelled substance into the vein and measurement using a scintillation counter of the perfusion via the pulmonary circulation. This is often combined with a ventilation scan in which radiolabelled gas (normally xenon) is inhaled by the patient. Pulmonary embolism classically results in an area of under- or non-perfusion of a part of the lung which nevertheless (because the airways are patent) ventilates normally. This pattern is called 'ventilation–perfusion mismatch' and is a specific sign of pulmonary embolism.

Other findings do occur in pulmonary embolism such as changes in the chest X-ray, the commonest of which is a raised right hemidiaphragm as a result of loss of lung volume (pulmonary embolism more commonly affects the right than the left lung). Hypoxia is also seen and this is worse, the larger the pulmonary embolus. The electrocardiogram may show signs of right ventricular strain. However, all these changes are nonspecific and do not obviate the need for the specific tests mentioned earlier.

DRUG TREATMENT

The aim of treatment of venous thrombosis is to allow normal circulation in the limbs and wherever possible to prevent damage to the valves of the veins thus reducing the risk of the swollen 'post-phlebitic limb'. Secondly, it is important to try to prevent associated pulmonary embolism and also recurrence of either venous thrombosis or pulmonary embolism in the risk period after the initial episode.

In acute massive pulmonary embolism the initial priority is to correct the circulatory defect which has caused haemodynamic upset and, in these circumstances rapid removal of the obstruction using thrombolytic drugs or surgical removal of the embolus may be necessary. In acute sub-massive pulmonary embolism, the goal of treatment is to prevent further episodes, particularly of the more serious acute massive pulmonary embolism. In both deep vein thrombosis and pulmonary embolism, a search must be made for underlying risk factors, such as carcinoma which may occur in up to 10% of patients and particularly in those with repeated episodes of venous thromboembolism.

The treatment of venous thromboembolism consists of the use of anticoagulants and in severe cases, thrombolytic drugs. Anticoagulant therapy involves the use of immediate acting agents (particularly heparin), and oral anticoagulants, the commonest of which is warfarin. Not only do these treat the acute event, but they prevent recurrence and may be necessary for some time after the initial event, depending on the persistence of risk factors for recurrent thromboembolism.

Heparin

Heparin is a mixture of large mucopolysaccharide molecules with immediate anticoagulant properties. It acts via antithrombin III by increasing the rate of the interaction of thrombin with antithrombin III by a factor of 1000-fold. It thus prevents the production of fibrin (factor I) from fibrinogen. Heparin also has effects on the inhibition of production of activated clotting factors IX, X, XI and XII (and these effects occur at concentrations lower than its effects on thrombin).

Because heparin consists of high molecular weight molecules which are highly ionized (it is the strongest organic acid found naturally in the body), it is not absorbed via the gastrointestinal tract and must be given by intravenous infusion or deep subcutaneous (never intramuscular) injection. Heparin is highly protein bound and it appears to be restricted to the intravascular space with a consequently low volume of distribution. It does not cross the placenta and does not appear in breast milk. Its pharmacokinetics are complex but it appears to have a dose-dependent increase in half-life. The half-life is normally around 60 minutes but is shorter in patients with pulmonary embolism. It is removed from the body by metabolism (possibly in the reticuloendothelial cells of the liver) and by renal excretion. The latter seems to be more important after high doses of the compound.

The major adverse effect of heparin is haemorrhage which is commoner in patients with severe heart or liver disease, renal disease, general debility and in women aged over 60 years. The risk of haemorrhage is increased in those with prolonged clotting times and in those given heparin by intermittent intravenous bolus rather than by continuous intravenous administration. Heparin is monitored by derivatives of the activated partial thromboplastin time (e.g. kaolin cephalin clotting time or KCCT) and in those patients with KCCT three times greater than control there is an eightfold increase in the risk of haemorrhage. The therapeutic range for KCCT during heparin therapy therefore appears to be between 1.5 and 2.5 times the control values. Rapid reversal of heparin's effect can be achieved using protamine sulphate but this is rarely necessary because of the short duration of action of heparin.

Heparin may also cause thrombocytopenia (low platelet count). This may occur in two forms, the first occurring 3 to 5 days after treatment and not normally resulting in complications. The second type of thrombocytopenia occurs after about 6 days of treatment and often results in much more profound decreases in platelet count and an increased risk of thromboembolism.

Heparin-induced osteoporosis is rare but may occur when the drug is used during pregnancy and may be dose related. The exact mechanism is unknown. Other adverse effects of heparin are urticaria and anaphylaxis but these are rare.

It has been shown that there is a non-linear relationship between the dose of heparin infused

Table 20.1   Guidelines to control heparin treatment

Loading dose: 5000 u. over 5 minutes.
Infusion: Start at 1400 u./h (e.g. 8400 u. in 100 ml over 6 hours). Check kaolin cephalin clotting time after 6 hours. Adjust dose according to ratio of kaolin cephalin clotting time to control value using table below.

KCCT ratio	Change in heparin (infusion rate)
> 7.0	Discontinue temporarily and reduce by > 500 u./h
5.1–7.0	Reduce by 500 u./h
4.1–5.0	Reduce by 300 u./h
3.1–4.0	Reduce by 100 u./h
2.6–3.0	Reduce by 50 u./h
1.5–2.5	No change
1.2–1.4	Increase by 200 u./h
< 1.2	Increase by 400 u./h

Wait 10 hours before next estimation of kaolin cephalin clotting time unless ratio is greater than 5.0, in which case more frequent estimation is advisable.
NB developed using Diogen (Bell and Alton), local validation may be necessary.

and the KCCT. This means that disproportionate adjustments in dose are required depending on the KCCT if underdosing or overdosing is to be avoided (Table 20.1). Since the half-life of heparin is 1 hour it would take 5 hours (5 half-lives of the drug) to reach a steady state. A loading dose is therefore administered to reduce the time to achieve adequate anticoagulation.

Heparin in full dose can also be given by repeated subcutaneous injection and in these circumstances the calcium salt appears to be less painful than the sodium salt. Opinions differ as to whether the subcutaneous or intravenous route is preferable. The subcutaneous route may take longer to reach effective plasma heparin concentrations.

Heparin is normally used in the immediate stages of venous thrombosis and pulmonary embolism until the effects of warfarin become apparent. In the past it has been continued for 7 to 10 days but recent evidence indicates that 3 to 5 days of therapy may be sufficient in many instances. This shorter treatment may also reduce the risk of the rare but potentially very serious complication of severe heparin-induced thrombocytopenia which normally occurs after the sixth day.

Recently, low molecular weight heparins and heparinoids have been developed. It is claimed that they are more specific on clotting factors X and XI than on factor II (prothrombin) and are said to be associated with a lower risk of haemorrhage. They are also claimed to be less likely to produce hypersensitivity and heparin-induced thrombocytopaenia. Most have a longer half-life than heparin and the half-life is not dose dependent. Their relative benefits, however, other than the convenience of once daily administration remain unclear.

Warfarin

Although not the only coumarin anticoagulant available, warfarin is by far the most widely used drug in this group because of its potency and its more reliable bioavailability. When given by mouth it is completely and rapidly absorbed, although food decreases the rate (but not the extent) of absorption. It is highly plasma protein bound (99%) and therefore has a small volume of distribution (7 to 14 litres). It consists of an equal mixture of two enantiomers, R and S warfarin. They have different anticoagulant potencies and routes of metabolism. Both enantiomers act by inducing a functional deficiency of vitamin K and thereby prevent the normal carboxylation of the glutamic acid residues of the amino-terminal ends of clotting factors II, VII, IX and X. This renders the clotting factors unable to cross-link with calcium and thereby to bind to phospholipid-containing membranes. Warfarin prevents the reduction of vitamin K epoxide to vitamin K by epoxide reductase. S-warfarin appears to be at least five times more potent in this regard than R-warfarin. Since warfarin does not have any effect on already carboxylated clotting factors, the delay in onset of the anticoagulant effect of warfarin is dependent on the rate of clearance of the fully carboxylated factors already synthesized. In this regard the half-life of removal of factor VII is approximately 6 hours; factor IX, 24 hours; factor X, 36 hours; and factor II, 50 hours.

The effect of warfarin is monitored using the one-stage prothrombin time (the international

Table 20.2 Recommended range of international normalized ratio for different indications (British Society for Haematology 1990)

	INR range
Prophylaxis of postoperative deep vein thrombosis (general surgery)	2.0–2.5
Prophylaxis of postoperative deep vein thrombosis in hip surgery and fractures	2.0–3.0
Post-myocardial infarction: prevention of venous thromboembolism	2.0–3.0
Treatment of venous thrombosis	2.0–3.0
Treatment of pulmonary embolism	2.0–3.0
Transient ischaemic attacks	2.0–3.0
Tissue heart valves	2.0–3.0
Atrial fibrillation	2.0–3.0
Valvular heart disease	2.0–3.0
Recurrent deep vein thrombosis and pulmonary embolism	3.0–4.5
Arterial disease including myocardial infarction	3.0–4.5
Mechanical prosthetic valves	3.0–4.5
Recurrent systemic embolism	3.0–4.5

normalized ratio or INR). This test is sensitive chiefly to factors II, VII, IX and X (and to a lesser extent factor V which is not a vitamin K dependent clotting factor). However, factor VII, to which the INR is sensitive, is the most important factor in the extrinsic pathway of clotting. The optimum therapeutic range for INR differs for different clinical indications since the lowest international normalized ratio consistent with therapeutic efficacy is the best in reducing the risk of haemorrhage. Examples of therapeutic ranges recommended for certain indications are given in Table 20.2.

Warfarin is metabolized by the liver via the cytochrome, P450 system. Only very small amounts of the drug appear unchanged in the urine. The average clearance is 4.5 L/day and the half-life ranges from 20 to 60 hours (mean 40 hours). It thus takes approximately 1 week (around five half-lives) for steady state to be reached after warfarin has been administered. The enantiomers of warfarin are metabolized stereospecifically, R-warfarin being mainly reduced at the acetyl side chain into secondary warfarin alcohols while S-warfarin is predominantly metabolized at the coumarin ring to hydroxywarfarin. The clearance of warfarin may

be reduced in liver disease as well as during administration of a variety of drugs known to inhibit either the S or R, or both enantiomers. These are shown in Table 20.3. Renal function is thought to have little effect on the pharmacokinetics of, or anticoagulant response to, warfarin.

The major adverse effect of warfarin is haemorrhage which often occurs at a predisposing abnormality such as an ulcer or tumour. The risk of bleeding is increased by excessive anticoagulation, although this may not need to be present for severe haemorrhage to occur. Close monitoring of the degree of anticoagulation of warfarin is therefore important and guidelines for reversal of excessive anticoagulation are shown in Table 20.4. It is also important to reduce the duration of therapy of the drug to the minimum effective period in order to reduce the period of risk.

Skin reactions to warfarin may also occur but are rare. The most serious skin reaction is warfarin-induced skin necrosis which may occur over areas of adipose tissue (the breasts, buttocks or thighs) especially in females and which is related to relative deficiency of protein S. This is important because these deficiencies result in an increased risk of thrombosis and therefore warfarin may more often be used in such subjects. The severity of the reaction may be reduced by preventing excessive anticoagulation in the initial stages of induction of therapy. A scheme which helps to achieve this aim is shown in Table 20.5.

Warfarin may also be teratogenic, producing in some instances a condition called chondrodysplasia punctata. This is associated with 'punched out lesions at sites of ossification' particularly of the long bones but also of the facial bones and may be associated with absence of the spleen. Although it has been associated predominantly with warfarin use during the first trimester of pregnancy, other abnormalities including cranial nerve palsies, hydrocephalus and microcephaly have been reported at later stages of pregnancy, if the child is exposed to warfarin in utero. The pharmacology of heparin and warfarin are compared in Table 20.6.

Since patients vary markedly in their maintenance requirements for warfarin, a fixed-

Table 20.3   Some clinically important interactions with warfarin

Interacting drug	Effect of interaction on warfarin's effects	Mechanism(s)
Cholestyramine Colestipol	Reduced anticoagulant effect	Impaired absorption and increased elimination of warfarin NB long-term treatment may cause impaired vitamin K absorption and enhance anticoagulant effect
Barbiturates Carbamazepine Primidone Rifampicin	Reduced anticoagulant effect	Induction of warfarin metabolism
Cimetidine Sulphonamides Erythromycin Metronidazole Mefenamic acid Azapropazone Phenylbutazone Amiodarone Ketoconazole Fluconazole Sulphinpyrazone Chloramphenicol Ciprofloxacin	Increased anticoagulant effect	Inhibition of warfarin metabolism
Salicylates Clofibrate Bezafibrate Gemfibrozil D-thyroxine L-thyroxine Stanozolol Danazol	Increased anticoagulant effect	Pharmacodynamic potentiation of anticoagulant effect
Oral contraceptives Vitamin K	Reduced anticoagulant effect	Pharmacodynamic antagonism of anticoagulant effect

induction dose scheme is likely to be satisfactory for only one-third or less of patients. Flexible induction schemes have therefore been devised to reduce excessive anticoagulation in those patients with increased sensitivity to the drug and to help in dose prediction. An example of this approach is shown in Table 20.5.

Although other oral anticoagulants are available (nicoumalone, phenprocoumon, dicoumarol and phenindione) these have not been shown to have any clear benefits over warfarin in the vast majority of cases. They may be used occasionally where a patient does not tolerate warfarin.

The necessary duration of anticoagulation in venous thrombosis and pulmonary embolus is still uncertain. On the basis of the available evidence, therapy may be required for approximately 3 months after the first deep vein thrombosis or pulmonary embolus. It may be possible to reduce the duration of therapy in patients who have had a postoperative episode since it is likely that the risk factor has been reversed (unless immobility continues). In patients with a second episode, therapy may be required for even longer and in patients with more than two episodes lifelong treatment may be necessary in order to reduce the risk of recurrence.

Fibrinolytic drugs

Thrombolytic therapy is used in life-threatening acute massive pulmonary embolus. It has been used in deep vein thrombosis, particularly in those patients where a large amount of clot exists and venous valvular damage is likely. However, fibrinolytic drugs are potentially more

Table 20.4 Reversal of oral anticoagulant therapy (recommendations of the British Society for Haematology)

Cause	Treatment
Life-threatening haemorrhage	Immediately give phytomenadione (Vitamin K_1) 5 mg by slow intravenous injection and a concentrate of factors II, IX, X (with factor VII concentrate if available). If no concentrate is available, fresh frozen plasma should be infused (approximately 1 litre for an adult) but this may not be as effective
Less severe haemorrhage (e.g. haematuria and epistaxis)	Withhold warfarin for one or more days and consider giving phytomenadione (vitamin K_1) 0.5–2 mg by slow intravenous injection
INR 4.5–7 without haemorrhage	Withhold warfarin for 1 or 2 days then review
INR > 7 without haemorrhage	Withhold warfarin and consider giving phytomenadione (vitamin K_1) 500 micrograms by slow intravenous injection
Unexpected bleeding at therapeutic levels	Investigate possibility of underlying cause, e.g. unexpected renal or alimentary tract pathology

Table 20.5 Suggested warfarin induction schedule (see Shetty et al 1989)

Warfarin day	International normalized ratio preferable (measured 9–10 a.m.)	Warfarin dose preferably given at 5–6 p.m. (milligrams)
1	< 1.4	10.0
2	< 1.8	10.0
	1.8	1.0
	> 1.8	0.5
3	< 2.0	10.0
	2–2.1	5.0
	2.2–2.3	4.5
	2.4–2.5	4.0
	2.6–2.7	3.5
	2.8–2.9	3.0
	3.0–3.1	2.5
	3.2–3.3	2.0
	3.4	1.5
	3.5	1.0
	3.6–4.0	0.5
	> 4.0	0
		Predicted maintenance dose (milligrams)
4	< 1.4	> 8.0
	1.4	8.0
	1.5	7.5
	1.6–1.7	7.0
	1.8	6.5
	1.9	6.0
	2–2.1	5.5
	2.2–2.3	5.0
	2.4–2.6	4.5
	2.7–3.0	4.0
	3.1–3.5	3.5
	3.6–4.0	3.0
	4.1–4.5	Miss out next day's then give 2 milligrams
	> 4.5	Miss out 2 days' doses then give 1 milligram

Notes:
Caution in patients with heart failure, liver disease, or immediately postoperative since their sensitivity to warfarin may vary with time.
If international normalized ratio on day 4 is less than 2.0, heparin can be used until the international normalized ratio is within the desired range.
If the international normalized ratio on day 1 is 1.4 or greater, the initial dose of warfarin should be reduced and the schedule is no longer relevant.

dangerous than anticoagulant drugs and evidence is not available in situations other than acute massive embolism to show a sustained benefit from their use.

Streptokinase was the first agent available in this class. It was produced from streptococci, and is a large protein which binds to and activates plasminogen thus encouraging the breakdown of formed fibrin to fibrinogen degradation products. It also acts on the circulating fibrinogen to produce a degree of systemic anticoagulation. Since it is a large protein molecule, it cannot be administered orally and has to be given by intravenous infusion. The half-life of removal from the body is 30 minutes. It is cleared chiefly by the reticuloendothelial system in the liver.

Its major adverse effect is to increase the risk of haemorrhage but it may also be antigenic and produce an anaphylactic reaction. It may also cause hypotension during infusion and in

some patients, particularly those who have been administered the drug within the previous 12

Table 20.6 Comparison of the pharmacology of heparin and warfarin

	Heparin	Warfarin
Mode of action	Immediate Acts via antithrombin III to inactivate prothrombin (II), and activate factors IX, X, XI and XII	Delayed Inhibits carboxylation of vitamin K dependent clotting factors II, VII, IX and X
Absorption	Not orally absorbed Must be given parenterally	Completely absorbed from gut 100% bioavailability
Distribution	Very low Vd Does not cross placenta or enter breast milk	Very low Vd Highly protein bound Does not enter breast milk in significant amounts
Metabolism	Dose dependent, by reticuloendothelial system $T_{\frac{1}{2}}$ 60 mins	Dose independent Completely metabolized via cytochrome P450 mediated metabolism in liver $T_{\frac{1}{2}}$ 36 hours
Excretion	Renal excretion significant after larger doses	Excreted as metabolites only No excretion of unchanged warfarin
Adverse effects	Haemorrhage Thrombocytopenia Osteoporosis Alopecia	Haemorrhage Teratogenicity
Drug interactions	Very few	Many (see Table 20.3)
Monitoring	Activated partial thromboplastin time (e.g. KCCT) Keep 1½–2½ times control	One-stage prothrombin time (e.g. INR) Degree depends on indication (see Table 20.2)
Antidote	Protamine	Vitamin K

months, a relative resistance to the drug may occur. Thrombolytic therapy is contra-indicated in patients who have had major surgery or with active bleeding sites in the gastrointestinal or genitourinary tract; in patients who have a history of stroke; in patients with a history of renal or liver disease; and in patients with hypertension. It should also be avoided in patients during pregnancy or during the postpartum period.

Tissue plasminogen activator (tPA) is a human tissue type plasma plasminogen activator which was developed using recombinant DNA technology. Although this agent is much more expensive it can be used in those situations where streptokinase may be less effective because of development of antibodies (e.g. within 1 year of previous streptokinase use) or where allergy to streptokinase has previously occurred. Because it produces a lesser degree of systemic anticoagulation (it is more active against plasminogen associated with the clot), immediate use of heparin subsequently is necessary to prevent recurrence of thrombosis.

Anistreplase (APSAC) is a precursor of streptokinase which can be administered more rapidly by intravenous injection over 4 to 5 minutes. It may cause a higher frequency of allergic reactions than streptokinase, however, and is much more expensive.

THE PATIENT

The patient on oral anticoagulants should be given full information on what to do in case of problems and what circumstances and drugs to avoid. An anticoagulant card with previous INR values and doses should also be provided. The patient should be told of the colour code for the different strengths of warfarin tablet and should be told to carry his or her treatment card at all times. The likely duration of anticoagulant therapy should be made clear to the patient to avoid unnecessary and potentially dangerous prolongation of treatment. Patients who have received a fibrinolytic agent should also carry a card identifying the drug given and the date of administration.

ARTERIAL THROMBOEMBOLISM

EPIDEMIOLOGY

Acute myocardial infarction is the commonest cause of acute arterial thrombosis. Stroke is commonly caused by atherothromboembolism from the great vessels or embolism arising from the heart (approximately 80% of strokes). The annual incidence of stroke in the developed world is approximately 1 per 2000 population, and incidence is likely to increase as the population ages. Peripheral arterial occlusive thrombosis is normally associated with atherothromboembolism but is rare, even in patients with increased risk of thromboembolism (e.g. atrial fibrillation).

AETIOLOGY

Arterial thromboembolism is normally associated with vascular injury and hypercoagulability. Vascular injury is most often due to atheroma. Although the exact mechanism is not clear, it is thought that platelet aggregation may be induced by the sheer stresses caused by stenosis of an atherosclerotic vessel. This thrombotic material may embolize to cause occlusion further downstream. Hypercoagulability is also a risk factor. It may be associated with increased plasma fibrinogen levels, and an increase in circulating cellular components (e.g. polycythaemia or thrombocythaemia). As mentioned earlier, the thrombus formed in the artery contains a much larger proportion of platelets, possibly reflecting the fact that other blood components which are not as readily adherent may be dissipated by the higher flow rates in the arterial circulation.

Oestrogens, by the mechanisms described earlier, are likely to increase the risk of arterial as well as venous thrombosis. Hyperlipidaemia may also increase the risk of hypercoagulability as well as enhancing thrombotic risk through its role in the progression of atheroma and vascular injury.

CLINICAL MANIFESTATIONS

Arterial thromboembolism affecting the cerebral circulation results in either transient ischaemic attacks (TIAs) or in severe cases cerebral infarction (one form of 'stroke'). A transient ischaemic attack is defined as symptoms of acute ischaemia of the brain lasting for less than 24 hours with complete recovery. The distinction between transient ischaemic attack and a stroke is therefore one of degree. It may involve weakness of the limbs or cause disturbance of vision. If the vertebrobasilar territory is affected, nausea, vomiting and dizziness may be the most prominent features. In stroke, features are similar but persist for longer than 24 hours. Clinical findings, however, vary markedly and it may be difficult on clinical grounds to separate cerebral infarction from the even more serious cause of 'stroke', cerebral haemorrhage, although patients with haemorrhage more often have severe headache and coma, and less often have a preceding history of transient ischaemic attacks.

Arterial thromboembolism affecting the limb (normally a lower limb) most often presents as sudden onset of pain in the limb associated with loss of peripheral pulses and coldness of the affected limb.

INVESTIGATIONS

The diagnosis of a transient ischaemic attack is a clinical one since by definition, no permanent damage to the brain substance is caused by these episodes. The investigations therefore help to identify risk factors for transient ischaemia and will include investigations of factors known to increase blood viscosity or hypercoagulability, investigation of the carotid vessels (normally by ultrasound) and a search for any cardiac sources of emboli (echocardiography). Evidence of arterial disease elsewhere increases the suspicion of transient ischaemic episodes.

The diagnosis of cerebral infarction includes the investigations previously mentioned for transient ischaemic attacks but computerized tomography (CT scanning) is the investigation of choice. In cerebral infarction, areas of low density occur within a day or two of the episode. In cerebral haemorrhage, an area of high density occurs, often immediately after the episode.

The diagnosis of arterial thromboembolism is usually made clinically but angiography may help to delineate the site and extent of the blockage.

DRUG TREATMENT

Treatment of transient ischaemic attacks is normally unnecessary and a major aspect of management is prophylaxis (see 'Aspirin'). In cerebral infarction the treatment is initially supportive. Anticoagulant therapy may increase the risk of conversion of infarction of brain substance to haemorrhage. Anticoagulant therapy if required for prophylaxis is not normally instituted until some time after the event. Although heparin has been recommended for the treatment of thrombotic stroke in 'evolution', there is no clear evidence of benefit. Other risk factors for recurrent cerebral infarction are hypertension which should be controlled. It is possible in the future that calcium antagonists may have a role in protecting critical ischaemic areas of the brain but this indication remains experimental. If the source of embolism is from the heart, subsequent prophylaxis against transient ischaemia or cerebral infarction may be considered using warfarin. This is particularly useful in patients with atrial fibrillation when the risk of subsequent stroke can be reduced by up to 80%. If the source of emboli is from the great vessels, then treatment with aspirin is more likely to be of benefit. There is no evidence that fibrinolytic drugs are effective in the acute management of cerebral infarction and their use may predispose to cerebral haemorrhage.

Aspirin (acetylsalicylic acid)

Aspirin is a potent inhibitor of the enzyme cyclo-oxygenase which catalyses the production of prostaglandins. It reduces the production of thromboxane A2 in the platelet, an effect which lasts for the life of the platelet. It also prevents the production of the antiaggregatary prostaglandin epoprostenol (prostacyclin) in the endothelium of the blood vessel but there is still debate as to what is the optimal dose for aspirin to achieve the maximum ratio of inhibition of thromboxane versus epoprostenol production.

Aspirin is well absorbed after oral administration. It is rapidly metabolized by esterases in blood and liver to salicylic acid and other metabolites which are excreted in the urine. In the doses used in prophylaxis against thromboembolism, aspirin is largely metabolized by the liver but in overdose, urinary excretion of salicylate becomes a limiting factor in drug elimination.

The major adverse effect of aspirin is gastrointestinal irritation and bleeding. This problem is much more common with higher doses of aspirin (600 mg or more) which were once used in the prevention of arterial thromboembolism but are less common with the doses (150 to 300 mg) now recommended. There is evidence that concomitant use of ulcer-healing drugs (e.g. misoprostol, H_2 receptor antagonists or omeprazole) can reduce the risk of NSAID-induced peptic ulceration in patients susceptible to the problem. However, the vast majority of patients tolerate low dose aspirin well and it is normally given as a single oral dose of soluble aspirin.

Aspirin may also rarely induce asthma, particularly in patients with coexisting reversible airways-obstruction but this effect is rare. Other patients have a form of aspirin hypersensitivity which may result in urticaria and/or angio-edema. In this situation, there may be cross-reactivity with other NSAIDs.

THE PATIENT

Aspirin is normally well tolerated at the doses used for stroke prevention (150 to 300 mg). However, it should not be given to patients with gastrointestinal ulceration. Since it may induce bronchospasm in susceptible individuals, it should be used cautiously in such circumstances. It is best tolerated if taken once daily as soluble aspirin after food.

CASE STUDIES

CASE 20.1

A patient receiving warfarin to prevent deep vein thrombosis and previously well controlled comes to the clinic with an INR of 12, despite having the same dose of drug. There is no evidence of bleeding.

Q What should be done?

CASE 20.2

A patient receiving heparin for 10 days for extensive venous thromboembolism develops arterial thrombosis.

Q What would you suspect in this situation and what should be done?

CASE 20.3

A patient who is admitted with suspected myocardial infarction says that he had a myocardial infarction 6 months earlier and was treated with a drug to 'dissolve the clot in the coronary artery'.

Q What relevance may this have to his management on this occasion?

CASE 20.4

Q What should a 64-year-old male patient be asked before starting aspirin therapy following an acute myocardial infarction?

ANSWERS TO CASE STUDIES

CASE 20.1

A The patient should be given phytomenadione (vitamin K) 500 micrograms by *slow* intravenous injection. This should return the INR to the therapeutic range by 24 h without causing warfarin resistance subsequently. A search for clinical conditions or drugs which might cause warfarin sensitivity should also be made. Measurement of plasma warfarin concentration may help in difficult cases.

CASE 20.2

A The rare but serious heparin-induced thrombocytopenia may be responsible. The platelet count should be measured urgently and heparin discontinued immediately. Fibrinolytic therapy has been used successfully in cases of occlusive thrombosis, and surgery has also been necessary. The CSM recommends monitoring the platelet count regularly in patients given heparin for more than 5 days.

CASE 20.3

A The patient has received a thrombolytic, possibly streptokinase, within the last year. He should be asked if he was given a card with the identity of the therapy to carry with him. If the prior treatment was with streptokinase, consideration should be given to the use of tPA as an alternative agent because of the relative resistance to streptokinase which may last up to 12 months after prior treatment.

CASE 20.4

A The patient should be asked if he has had aspirin before and, if so, whether he tolerated it. Aspirin is contra-indicated in patients with gastrointestinal ulceration. It may induce bronchospasm or angioedema in susceptible individuals and caution should be exercised in these circumstances. Gastric irritation is minimized by taking the dose after food.

CASE 20.5

A 56-year-old woman on warfarin therapy for atrial fibrillation with mitral stenosis appears to become resistant to warfarin after previously good control on 5 mg daily and her INR does not rise above 1.4 even when her warfarin dose is increased to 20 mg daily.

Q What can be done to find the cause of the resistance?

CASE 20.5

A The patient should be asked about any new medications which might have been introduced recently. Some proprietary medicines may contain vitamin K which could cause resistance. One cause of apparent resistance to warfarin is poor compliance and this should therefore be considered. Supervised administration of the dose and/or measurement of plasma warfarin concentration may be of value if the latter is suspected.

BIBLIOGRAPHY

British Society for Haematology. Guidelines on oral anticoagulation, 2nd edn. Journal of Clinical Pathology 1990; 43: 177–183

Fennerty A G, Renowden S, Scolding N, Bentley D P, Campbell A, Routledge P A. Guidelines for the control of heparin treatment. British Medical Journal 1986; 292: 579–580

Fuster V, Verstraete M (eds). Thrombosis in cardiovascular disorders. Philadelphia: W B Saunders 1991

Shetty H G M, Routledge P A. Adverse effects of anticoagulants. Adverse Drug Reactions Bulletin 1989; 137: 512–515

Shetty H G M, Fennerty A G, Routledge P A. Clinical pharmacokinetic considerations in the control of oral anticoagulant therapy. Clinical Pharmacokinetics 1989; 16: 238–253

Shetty H G M, Backhouse G, Bentley D P, Routledge P A. Effective reversal of warfarin induced excessive anticoagulation with low dose vitamin K. Thrombosis and Haemostasis 1992; 67: 13–15

Hyperlipidaemia

R. Walker

Hyperlipidaemia is considered to arise when serum cholesterol or triglycerides, or both, reach levels associated with an increased risk of ischaemic heart disease (IHD).

Hyperlipidaemia also embraces the terms hypercholesterolaemia and hyperlipoproteinaemia. If the cholesterol level is raised this is referred to as hypercholesterolaemia. Hyperlipoproteinaemia denotes an elevated level of lipoproteins (a combination of lipids and proteins), the form in which virtually all of the lipids in serum are present.

In contrast to hyperlipoproteinaemia, hypolipoproteinaemia represents a depressed concentration of circulating lipoproteins. The term dyslipoproteinaemia is used to encompass both hyper- and hypolipoproteinaemia.

EPIDEMIOLOGY

Lipid and lipoprotein concentrations vary amongst different populations with countries consuming a 'western diet' generally having higher values than those where the regular consumption of fat and cholesterol is low.

The mean total serum cholesterol concentration in the United Kingdom is considered to be too high. A reduction in the population cholesterol mean would reduce the development of coronary atherosclerosis and the incidence of ischaemic heart disease (IHD) which accounts for more than 200 000 deaths of adults in the UK each year, more than from cancer and road accidents combined. The identification of hyper-cholesterolaemia as a risk factor for IHD has attracted much attention, particularly as to whether widespread screening should be undertaken. A relationship between serum cholesterol concentrations and the incidence of IHD is well established in western populations at concentrations above 5.2 mmol/L. It is unclear whether below this level of cholesterol further reductions continue to lower the incidence of IHD. However, studies in populations with a low mean serum cholesterol concentration have revealed that even between 3.8 to 4.7 mmol/L there is no evidence of a level below which a further reduction of cholesterol concentration is not associated with a lower risk of ischaemic heart disease.

Population studies have shown that the total serum cholesterol level increases with age in males and females over the age of 20 years. The rate of rise slows in men after the age of 45 to 50 years and appears to decline after 70 years, presumably because the men with hypercholesterolaemia have died from cardiovascular disease. In women, the cholesterol level continues to rise up to the age of 70 years. Between the ages of 50 and 70 years the mean total cholesterol in women exceeds that of men of a similar age.

The British Hyperlipidaemia Association have formulated guidelines for identifying the risk associated with particular cholesterol concentrations (Table 21.1). Approximately 27% of the UK population have a serum cholesterol level equal to or above 6.5 mmol/L.

LIPID TRANSPORT AND LIPOPROTEIN METABOLISM

The major lipids in serum (cholesterol, tri-glycerides and phospholipids) are transported in the form of lipoproteins. There are six main classes of lipoproteins: chylomicrons, chylomicron remnants, very low density lipoproteins (VLDL), intermediate density lipoproteins (IDL), low density lipoproteins (LDL) and high density lipoproteins (HDL).

The protein components of lipoproteins are known as apoproteins, of which apoprotein A-I, E, C and B are perhaps the most important. Apoprotein B exists in two forms: B-48 which is present in chylomicrons and associated with the transport of ingested lipids; and B-100 which is found in endogenously secreted VLDL and associated with the transport of lipids from the liver (see Fig. 21.1).

When dietary cholesterol and triglycerides are absorbed from the intestine they are transported in the intestinal lymphatics as chylomicrons which pass through blood capillaries in adipose tissue and skeletal muscle where the enzyme lipoprotein lipase is located bound to the endothelium. Lipoprotein lipase is activated by apoprotein C-II (a component of apoprotein C) on the surface of the chylomicron. The lipase catalyses the breakdown of the triglyceride in the chylomicron to free fatty acid and glycerol which then enter adipose tissue and muscle. The cholesterol-rich chylomicron remnant is taken up by receptors on hepatocyte membranes and in this way dietary cholesterol is delivered to the liver and cleared from the circulation.

VLDL is formed in the liver and transports triglycerides and contains some cholesterol. The triglyceride content of VLDL is removed by lipoprotein lipase in a manner analogous to that described for chylomicrons above, and forms IDL particles. IDL particles acquire cholesterol esters from HDL under the influence of the enzyme lecithin-cholesterol acyltransferase (LCAT). The IDL may be transported to the liver or be further hydrolysed and modified to lose triglyceride and apoprotein E_1 and become an LDL particle. LDL is the major cholesterol-carrying particle in plasma.

LDL provides cholesterol, an essential component of cell membranes and a precursor of steroid hormones, to those cells which require

Table 21.1 Incidence and risk associated with different cholesterol concentrations		
Risk	Incidence/1000	Cholesterol level
Desirable	330	< 5.2 mmol/L
Borderline	400	5.2 to 6.4 mmol/L
Intermediate risk	220	6.5 to 7.8 mmol/L
High risk	50	> 7.8 mmol/L

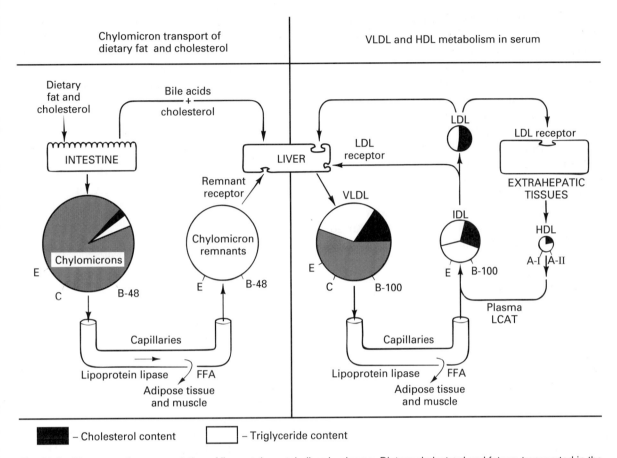

Fig. 21.1 Diagrammatic representation of lipoprotein metabolism in plasma. Dietary cholesterol and fat are transported in the chylomicron pathway. Cholesterol produced in the liver is transported in the VLDL/LDL pathway. Relative sizes of lipoproteins are shown together with their respective triglyceride and cholesterol ester content. (Modified from Goldstein J L, Kita T, Brown M S. Defective lipoprotein receptors and atherosclerosis. New England Journal of Medicine 1983; 309: 288.)

it. LDL is also probably the main lipoprotein involved in atherogenesis. For reasons which are not totally clear, but probably related to minor trauma, anoxaemia or hypertension, the arterial endothelium becomes permeable to lipoproteins. Monocytes migrate through the permeable endothelium and engulf the lipoproteins. This results in the formation of lipid-laden macrophages which have a principal role in the development of atherosclerosis. The aim of treatment in hyperlipidaemia is often to reduce serum concentrations of LDL cholesterol (and consequently atherogenesis) and thus normally reduce total cholesterol.

Whilst VLDL and LDL are considered the 'bad' lipoproteins, HDL is often considered to

be the 'good' antiatherogenic lipoprotein. HDL transports cholesterol from peripheral tissues to the liver and plays a major role in maintaining cholesterol homeostasis in the body. It is therefore considered desirable to maintain levels of the protective HDL. Drugs which reduce HDL levels are considered to have an undesirable effect on lipid metabolism. It is now clear that there are at least two subfractions of HDL (HDL_2 and HDL_3) of which probably only HDL_2 protects against atheroma formation.

AETIOLOGY

In 1967 the Fredrickson classification of hyperlipoproteinaemia was established which described five phenotypic patterns of hyperlipoprotein-aemia. This classification has subsequently been revised by the World Health Organization (Table 21.2). The WHO classification of lipoprotein phenotypes is not a diagnostic classification but provide a useful means of describing the profile of the commonly occurring hyperlipidaemias. Unfortunately it does not permit differentiation between those hyperlipidaemias of primary (genetic) origin and those caused by underlying disorders or environmental factors. The classification also takes no account of variations in high-density lipoprotein (HDL) cholesterol.

Once treatment with diet or drugs has started, the WHO phenotype of an individual may change. For example, a type IIa hyperlipoproteinaemia often changes to type IIb when cholestyramine is given because of a rise in VLDL associated with the use (side effect) of the drug while some elevation of LDL may remain despite an overall reduction. It is therefore a pointless exercise to attempt to repeat the phenotyping of a patient once treatment has started.

Primary hyperlipidaemia

Up to 60% of the variability in serum fasting lipids may be genetically determined although expression is often influenced by interaction with environmental factors. The familial disorders can be classified as follows:

- the primary hypercholesterolaemias such as familial hypercholesterolaemia in which cholesterol is raised
- the primary mixed (combined)

hyperlipidaemias in which both cholesterol and triglycerides are raised
- the primary hypertriglyceridaemias such as type III hyperlipoproteinaemia, familial lipoprotein lipase deficiency and familial Apo C-II deficiency.

Familial hypercholesterolaemia

Heterozygous familial hypercholesterolaemia affects approximately 1 in 500 of the population and is associated with a deficiency of LDL receptors which play a major role in the catabolism of LDL. In contrast homozygous familial hypercholesterolaemia is extremely rare (1 per million) and associated with an absence of LDL receptors.

In heterozygous familial hypercholesterolaemia the deficiency of LDL receptors results in the accumulation of LDL in serum and hypercholesterolaemia from birth. Total serum cholesterol levels correlate with the LDL receptor deficit and are approximately twice normal in adult heterozygotes. In patients with heterozygous familial hypercholesterolaemia it has been estimated that IHD occurs about 20 years earlier than in the general population and is accompanied by an equivalent decrease in life expectancy. In addition to hypercholesterolaemia, the adult heterozygote usually develops the signs of cholesterol deposition such as corneal arcus (crescentic deposition of lipids in the cornea), tendon xanthomata (yellow papules or nodules of lipid deposited in tendons) and xanthelasma (yellow plaques or nodules of lipids deposited on eyelids) in their third decade.

Table 21.2	World Health Organization classification of hyperlipoproteinaemia			
Type	Plasma cholesterol	LDL cholesterol	Plasma triglyceride	Lipoprotein abnormality
I	Raised	Low or normal	Raised	Excess chylomicrons
IIa	Raised or normal	Raised	Normal	Excess LDL
IIb	Raised	Raised	Raised	Excess LDL & VLDL
III	Raised	Low or normal	Raised	Excess chylomicron remnants & IDL
IV	Raised or normal	Normal	Raised	Excess VLDL
V	Raised	Normal	Raised	Excess chylomicrons & VLDL

In some adults with familial hypercholesterolaemia there are elevated levels of triglycerides associated with a type IIb (familial combined hyperlipidaemia) phenotype.

In the patient with homozygous familial hypercholesterolaemia, atheromatous involvement of the aorta is evident by puberty and is usually accompanied by cutaneous and tendon xanthomata. Myocardial infarction has been reported in homozygous children as early as 1.5 to 3 years of age. Until the 1980s sudden death from acute coronary insufficiency before the age of 20 was normal.

Familial combined hyperlipidaemia

Familial combined hyperlipidaemia has an incidence of 1 in 200 and is associated with excessive synthesis of VLDL. The condition is associated with an increased risk of atherosclerosis and it is estimated that it occurs in 15% of patients with IHD below the age of 60 years.

Familial type III hyperlipoproteinaemia

Familial type III hyperlipoproteinaemia is relatively uncommon with an incidence of 1 in 5000. It is characterized by the accumulation in plasma of chylomicron and VLDL remnants which fail to get cleared at a normal rate by hepatic receptors due to the presence of less active polymorphic forms of apoprotein E. Serum cholesterol and triglyceride levels are both elevated and accompanied by corneal arcus, xanthelasma, tuberoeruptive xanthomata (groups of flat or yellowish raised nodules on the skin over joints, especially the elbows and knees) and palmar striae (yellow raised streaks across the palms of the hand). The disorder predisposes to premature atherosclerosis.

Familial lipoprotein lipase deficiency

Familial lipoprotein lipase deficiency is characterized by marked hypertriglyceridaemia and chylomicronaemia and usually presents in childhood. It has an incidence of 1 per million and is due to a deficiency of the extrahepatic enzyme lipoprotein lipase which results in a failure of lipolysis and the accumulation of chylomicrons in plasma. The affected patient presents with recurrent episodes of abdominal pain, eruptive xanthomata, lipaemia retinalis (retinal deposition of lipid) and enlarged spleen. This disorder is not associated with an increased susceptibility to atherosclerosis, the major complication being acute pancreatitis.

Familial ApoC-II deficiency

In the heterozygous state familial ApoC-II deficiency is associated with reduced levels of apolipoprotein C-II, the activator of lipoprotein lipase, which are 50 to 80% of normal. This level of activity can maintain normal serum lipid levels. In the rare homozygous state there is an absence of ApoC-II and despite normal levels of lipoprotein lipase it cannot be activated. Consequently, homozygotes (type V phenotypes) have triglyceride levels in the range 15 to > 100 mmol/L (normal range < 2.3 mmol/L) and may develop acute pancreatitis. Premature atherosclerosis is unusual but has been described.

There are many other familial disorders of lipid metabolism which are rare. Raised levels of lipoprotein a (Lp(a)) are emerging as a major genetically inherited determinant of IHD.

Lipoprotein a

Lp(a) was first described more than 30 years ago and is best considered as a modified LDL particle. Lp(a) is found in the serum of virtually everybody in a wide concentration range (0.01 g/L to 2 g/L) with up to 70% of the variation in serum concentration being genetically determined. The concentration of Lp(a) is not normally distributed. The contribution of inheritance of circulating Lp(a) levels is more pronounced than for any other lipoprotein or apoprotein. Parental history of early onset coronary heart disease is associated with raised concentrations which appear to play a role in both atherogenesis and thrombosis. Concentrations of Lp(a) above 0.3 g/L occur in about 20%

of caucasians and increase the risk of coronary atherosclerosis twofold which may increase further to fivefold if LDL concentrations are also raised.

Secondary hyperlipidaemia

Hyperlipidaemias which occur secondary to a number of disorders, dietary indiscretion or as a side effect of drug therapy, account for up to 40% of all hyperlipidaemias. Fortunately, the lipid abnormalities in secondary hyperlipidaemias can often be corrected if the underlying disorder is treated, effective dietary advice implemented or the offending drug withdrawn.

On occasions a disorder may be associated with hyperlipidaemia, but not the cause of it. For example, hyperuricaemia (gout) and hypertriglyceridaemia coexist in approximately 50% of men. In this particular example neither is the cause of the other and treatment of one does not resolve the other. There are, however, two exceptions to the rule with this example: nicotinic acid and fenofibrate. Both drugs reduce triglyceride levels but nicotinic acid increases urate whilst fenofibrate reduces it by an independent uricosuric effect.

Disease states

Many of the disease states associated with secondary hyperlipidaemias are listed in Table 21.3. The impact and severity of the lipid disorder will depend on the individual's genetic or nutritional

---

Table 21.3 Examples of disorders which cause secondary hyperlipidaemia

Non-insulin-dependent diabetes
Insulin-dependent diabetes
Hypothyroidism
Pregnancy
Inappropriate diet
Alcohol abuse
Chronic renal failure
Nephrotic syndrome
Renal transplantation
Cardiac transplantation
Hepatocellular disease
Cholestasis
Myeloma

---

predisposition to hyperlipidaemia. Some of the more common disorders which cause secondary hyperlipidaemia will be discussed below.

Diabetes mellitus. Diabetes is a disorder of carbohydrate, lipid and protein metabolism. Disorders of lipid metabolism such as atherosclerosis and ketoacidosis are, in fact, two of the major complications of diabetes.

Patients with poorly controlled diabetes mellitus may present with severe hypertriglyceridaemia. Insulin administration lowers the serum triglyceride levels probably by reducing hepatic synthesis of VLDL and by inducing lipoprotein lipase activity.

Hypertriglyceridaemia is less likely to arise in patients with insulin-dependent diabetes mellitus (IDDM) than those with non-insulin-dependent diabetes mellitus (NIDDM). This may occur because insulin therapy is the norm in IDDM whilst patients with NIDDM often have other factors present which predispose to hypertriglyceridaemia such as being obese or receiving beta-adrenoreceptor blocker or diuretic therapy.

Hypothyroidism. Abnormalities of plasma lipid and lipoprotein levels are common in patients with untreated hypothyroidism. It is an important cause of secondary hypercholesterolaemia which can also lead to combined hyperlipidaemia, or less commonly, severe hypertriglyceridaemia in susceptible individuals. However, once adequate thyroid replacement has been instituted, hypercholesterolaemia, hypertriglyceridaemia and any accumulation of remnant lipoproteins should resolve.

Chronic renal failure. Hyperlipidaemia is frequently seen in patients with renal failure in the predialysis phase, during haemodialysis or when undergoing chronic ambulatory peritoneal dialysis. The hypertriglyceridaemia which most commonly occurs is associated with reduced lipoprotein lipase activity and often persists despite starting chronic maintenance renal dialysis.

Nephrotic syndrome. In patients with the nephrotic syndrome, the hypercholesterolaemia appears to be caused by an increased production of apolipoprotein B-100 and associated LDL. The increased production, in turn, is related to the extent of proteinuria (which depletes plasma of apolipoproteins) and the plasma albumin level. The necessary use of glucocorticoids in patients with the nephrotic syndrome may exacerbate underlying lipoprotein abnormality.

Obesity. Chronic, excessive intake of calories leads to increased plasma concentrations of triglycerides and reduced HDL cholesterol. Obesity, per se, can exacerbate any underlying primary hyperlipoproteinaemia.

Alcohol. In the heavy drinker the high calorie content of beer and wine may be a cause of obesity with its associated adverse effect on the lipid profile. In addition, alcohol increases hepatic triglyceride synthesis which, in turn, produces hypertriglyceridaemia. Overall plasma LDL cholesterol levels tend to be low in chronic alcoholics whilst HDL cholesterol is often raised.

Drugs

A large number of drugs can affect serum lipid and lipoprotein concentrations (Table 21.4). In particular, much attention has been given to the adverse effects of diuretic and beta-adrenoreceptor blocker antihypertensive drugs on lipoprotein metabolism but the clinical significance of these effects is unclear.

Antihypertensive agents. Hypertension is a major risk factor for atherosclerosis and the beneficial effects of lowering blood pressure are well recognized. It is, however, a concern that treatment of patients with hypertension has reduced the incidence of cerebrovascular accidents and renal failure but had no major impact in reducing the incidence of IHD. It has been suggested

that many of the antihypertensive agents used have an adverse effect on lipids and lipoproteins which override any beneficial reduction of blood pressure.

Diuretics. Thiazide and loop diuretics increase VLDL and LDL by mechanisms which are not completely understood. Whether these adverse effects are dose-dependent is also unclear. Triamterene and amiloride are potassium-sparing diuretics that are frequently taken in combination with diuretics. If these agents have any adverse effect on the lipid profile it would appear to be minor.

Beta-adrenoreceptor blockers. The effects of beta-adrenoreceptor blockers on lipoprotein metabolism are reflected in an increase in serum triglyceride concentrations, a decrease in HDL cholesterol and with no discernible effect on LDL. Beta-adrenoreceptor blockers with intrinsic sympathomimetic activity (ISA) appear to have little or no effect on VLDL or HDL. Pindolol has the most ISA but is rarely used as an antihypertensive agent since it may exacerbate angina. Acebutolol and oxprenolol have half of pindolol's ISA and may be useful if a beta-adrenoreceptor blocker has to be used in a patient particularly susceptible to altered lipoprotein metabolism. Alternatively, the combined alpha- and beta-adrenoreceptor blocking effect of labetalol may be of use since it would appear to have a negligible effect on serum lipoproteins.

Overall, the need to use a diuretic or a beta-adrenoreceptor blocker must be balanced against patient considerations. A patient in heart failure should receive a diuretic if indicated regardless of the lipid profile. Similarly, in patients who have had a myocardial infarction and have no signs of cardiac failure, the beneficial protective effect of a beta-adrenoreceptor blocker will usually outweigh any benefit of drug withdrawal.

If an antihypertensive agent is required which is without adverse effects on lipoproteins many studies would suggest that ACE-inhibitors (e.g. captopril), alpha-adrenoreceptor blockers (e.g. prazosin), calcium channel blockers (e.g. nifedipine) or direct acting vasodilators (e.g. hydralazine) could be used.

Oral contraceptives. Oral contraceptives

Table 21.4   Drugs known to adversely affect the lipoprotein profile

Amiodarone
Androgens
Beta-adrenoreceptor blockers
Cyclosporin
Diuretics
  thiazide
  loop
Glucocorticoids
Oral contraceptives
Progestogens
Vitamin A derivatives

containing an oestrogen and a progestogen provide the most effective contraceptive preparations for general use and have been well studied with respect to their harmful effects.

Oestrogens and progestogens both posses mineralocorticoid and glucocorticoid properties which predispose to hypertension and diabetes mellitus, respectively. However, the effects of the two hormones on lipoproteins are different. Oestrogens cause a slight increase in hepatic production of VLDL and HDL, and reduce serum LDL levels in postmenopausal women. In contrast, progestogens increase LDL and reduce serum HDL and VLDL.

The specific effect of the oestrogen or progestogen varies with the actual dose and chemical entity used. Ethinyl oestradiol at a dose of 30 to 35 micrograms or less would appear to create few problems with lipid metabolism, whilst norethisterone would appear to be one of the more favourable progestogens even though it may cause a pronounced decrease in HDL concentrations.

Corticosteroids. The effect of glucocorticosteroid administration on lipid levels has been studied in patients treated with steroids for asthma, rheumatoid arthritis and connective tissue disorders. Administration of glucocorticosteroids (e.g. prednisolone) has been shown to increase serum cholesterol and triglycerides by elevating LDL and, less consistently, VLDL. The changes are generally more pronounced in women. Alternate-day therapy with glucocorticosteroids has been suggested to reduce the adverse effect on lipoprotein levels in some patients.

Cyclosporin. Cyclosporin is primarily used to prevent tissue rejection in recipients of renal, hepatic and cardiac transplants. Its use has been associated with increased LDL levels, hypertension and glucose intolerance. These adverse effects are often exacerbated by the concurrent administration of glucocorticosteroids. Without doubt the combined use of cyclosporin and glucocorticosteroid contributes to the adverse lipid profile seen in transplant patients. Moreover, the administration of the lipid-lowering drug lovastatin to patients treated with cyclosporin has been shown to increase the incidence of

myositis and even cause rhabdomyolysis (dissolution of muscle associated with excretion of myoglobin in the urine) and therefore its use is contra-indicated in such patients.

Hepatic microsomal enzyme inducers. Drugs such as carbamazepine, phenytoin, phenobarbitone, rifampicin and griseofulvin which can increase hepatic microsomal enzyme activity can also increase serum HDL concentrations. The administration of these drugs may also give rise to a slight increase in LDL and VLDL. The overall effect is one of favourable increase in the HDL to serum LDL ratio. It is interesting to note that patients treated for epilepsy have been reported to have a decreased incidence of IHD.

TREATMENT

The aim of treating a patient with hyperlipidaemia is to reduce the serum concentration of elevated atherogenic lipoproteins and triglycerides and increase the concentration of the antiatherogenic HDL. The serum concentration of cholesterol, HDL and triglycerides should initially be measured to determine the lipid profile of a patient.

Serum concentrations of triglycerides increase after the ingestion of a meal and therefore patients must fast for 12 to 15 hours and be seated for at least 5 minutes prior to taking a blood sample. Cholesterol levels are little affected by food intake and this is therefore not a consideration if only cholesterol is to be measured. It is important, however, that whatever is being measured reflects a steady state value. For example, during periods of weight loss, lipid concentrations decline as they do following a myocardial infarction. In the case of the latter, samples drawn within 24 hours of infarct onset will reflect the pre-infarction state. In general, measurement should be deferred for 2 weeks after a minor illness and for 2 months after a myocardial infarction, serious illness or pregnancy.

Once the total cholesterol, HDL and triglyceride values are known it is possible to calculate the value for LDL cholesterol using the Friedewald equation:

$$LDL = \frac{Total}{cholesterol} - HDL - \frac{Triglycerides}{2.19} \ mmol/L$$

The Friedewald formula is not valid in the presence of chylomicrons, intermediate density lipoproteins or a serum triglyceride concentration > 4.6 mmol/L.

Once the lipid profile of a patient has been determined and compared to the optimal serum lipid profile (Tables 21.1 & 21.5), the individual risk factors for IHD should be considered (Table 21.6), and the appropriate management strategy implemented following recommended guidelines (Table 21.7).

Dietary therapy

The obese patient generally has elevated serum triglycerides, possibly a raised serum LDL and a tendency to have a low HDL level. Weight reduction in such an individual will improve their hyperlipidaemic profile.

Some form of classification of obesity is required. The body mass index (BMI) in all but the most muscular individual gives a clinical measure of adiposity:

$$BMI \ (kg/m^2) = \frac{Weight \ (kg)}{Height^2 \ (m)}$$

and where

BMI ≤ 19.1	= underweight
BMI = 20 to 24.9	= acceptable
BMI = 25 to 29.9	= low health risk
BMI = 30 to 40	= moderate health risk
BMI > 40	= high health risk

Diet modification alone may be successful in controlling hyperlipidaemia associated with an inappropriate diet or obesity. Dietary management may even be beneficial in familial forms of hyperlipidaemia and drugs, when used, should be given in addition to a lipid-lowering diet.

The recommended diet (Table 21.8) should contain less total fat, saturated fat and cholesterol, and more polyunsaturated and monounsaturated fat. Protein intake should be kept constant and more of the total energy administered in the form of carbohydrates, particularly complex carbohydrates. The energy provided should be sufficient to achieve and maintain the desirable body weight.

Exercise

Moderate amounts of aerobic exercise (walking, jogging, swimming, cycling) on a regular basis have a desirable effect on serum lipids. These beneficial effects have been demonstrated within 2 months in middle-aged men exercising for 30 minutes three times a week. A decrease in LDL has been shown to be proportional to the distance run, although it appears necessary to run over 10 miles per week before significant increases in HDL occur.

Overall, comprehensive lifestyle changes (low fat vegetarian diet, stopping smoking, stress management training and moderate exercise) have been shown to bring about regression of even severe coronary atherosclerosis after 1 year without use of lipid-lowering drugs.

Drugs

Over recent years there have been many major

Table 21.5   Optimal serum lipid profile

Total serum cholesterol	< 5.2 mmol/L
LDL cholesterol	< 3.5 mmol/L
Total serum triglycerides	< 2.3 mmol/L
HDL cholesterol	> 0.9 mmol/L

Table 21.6   Risk factors which influence the management of lipid disorders

History of:
   ischaemic heart disease
   stroke
   peripheral vascular disease
Positive family history exemplified by:
   ischaemic heart disease in first-degree relative under
   55 years
Cigarette smoking
Diabetes mellitus
Hypertension
Low HDL (< 0.9 mmol/L)
Male
Body mass index > 25 kg/m²

Table 21.7 Summary of guidelines for management of hyperlipidaemias

	Assessment	Management
Hypercholesterolaemia Cholesterol level (mmol/L)		
5.2 to 6.5	Assess overall risk of IHD including risk factors and age	Correct overweight and other modifiable risk factors Dietary improvement
6.5 to 7.8	Assess overall risk of IHD including risk factors and age	Correct overweight and other modifiable risk factors Lipid-lowering diet Drugs required if response inadequate and other risk factors present
> 7.8	Assess overall risk of IHD including risk factors and age	Correct overweight and other modifiable risk factors Lipid-lowering diet Drug treatment
Hypertriglyceridaemia Triglyceride level (mmol/L)		
2.3 to 5.6	Assess overall risk of IHD, take account of age Find cause of raised triglycerides	Correct overweight, modifiable risk factors and underlying cause Lipid-lowering diet Monitor lipid levels
> 5.6	Assess overall risk of IHD, take account of age Find cause of raised triglycerides	Drug treatment Correct overweight, modifiable risk factors and underlying cause
Hypercholesterolaemia with hypertriglyceridaemia Cholesterol 5.2 to 7.8		
Triglycerides 2.3 to 5.6	Assess overall risk of IHD, take account of age Find cause of raised lipids	Correct overweight, modifiable risk factors and underlying cause Lipid-lowering diet Drug treatment if inadequate response or other risk factors present
Cholesterol > 7.8	Assess overall risk of IHD, take account of age	Drug treatment
Triglycerides > 5.6	Find cause of raised lipids	Correct overweight, modifiable risk factors and underlying cause Lipid-lowering diet

Table 21.8 General guidelines for a lipid-lowering diet

1. Attain ideal body weight; reduce energy intake or increase energy output by exercise
2. Reduce total fat to ≤ 30% of total dietary energy intake
3. Reduce saturated (mainly animal) fat to < 10% of total energy; partially replace saturated fat by monounsaturated and polyunsaturated fats (vegetable, olive and fish oils)
4. Reduce dietary cholesterol to < 300 mg/day
5. Increase intake of complex carbohydrates and soluble fibres (fruit, cereals, vegetables)

studies (Table 21.9) which have assessed the effect of treatment with either diet alone, a combination of diet with drug therapy or treatment of lipid abnormalities together with modification of other risk factors. Clinical end points of IHD have been assessed after intervention in individuals without (primary prevention) or with (secondary prevention) evidence of coronary disease. The majority of trials have involved males of between 30 and 65 years of age. The general findings of these major studies reveal that:

Table 21.9 Examples of lipid modification trials which have shown a significant reduction in IHD

	Number in study	Duration (years)	Treatment
Primary prevention trials			
WHO Cooperative Trial	15 745	5	Clofibrate
Lipid Research Clinics Coronary			
Primary Prevention Trial	3806	7.4	Cholestyramine
Helsinki Heart Study	4081	5	Gemfibrozil
Secondary prevention trials			
Coronary Drug Project	3908	5	Niacin
Stockholm Ischaemic Heart			
Disease Secondary Prevention Study	555	5	Clofibrate + nicotinic acid

- a 1% reduction in serum cholesterol is associated with a 2% reduction in IHD risk
- the lowering of triglycerides is associated with a variable reduction in IHD risk
- lowering the lipid level of an individual can slow the rate of progression of atherosclerosis and achieve a regression within 2 years
- there has been no demonstrable impact on mortality.

Before starting drug therapy, patients should receive 3 to 6 months of dietary therapy. If dietary management does not have a beneficial effect on the lipid profile then drug therapy may be added. Once a decision to initiate drug therapy has been made this implies a long-term commitment to the treatment.

There are four main classes of lipid-lowering agents available:

- anion-exchange resins
- fibrates
- HMG-CoA reductase inhibitors
- nicotinic acid and derivatives.

The choice of agent will depend upon the underlying hyperlipidaemia, the response obtained and patient acceptability.

Anion-exchange resins

Anion-exchange resins are also known as ion-exchange resins or bile acid sequestrants. The two members of this group in current use are cholestyramine and colestipol. Both have been considered first line agents in the management of patients with primary hypercholesterolaemia (type IIa hyperlipidaemia) at risk of IHD. They reduce serum cholesterol concentrations but cause no change or a slight increase in triglyceride concentrations and are therefore unsuitable in patients with elevated triglycerides.

Following oral administration neither cholestyramine nor colestipol are absorbed from the gut. They bind bile acids in the intestine, prevent their reabsorption and produce an insoluble complex which is excreted in the faeces. The depletion of bile acids results in an increase in hepatic synthesis of bile acids from cholesterol. The depletion of hepatic cholesterol increases LDL receptor activity on the liver which removes LDL from the blood. Both cholestyramine and colestipol can also increase hepatic VLDL synthesis and increase serum triglycerides.

Cholestyramine and colestipol can reduce serum cholesterol concentrations within 24 to 48 hours and thereafter continue to gradually reduce the levels for up to 1 year. The starting dose of cholestyramine is one 4 g sachet twice a day. Over a 3- to 4-week period the dose should normally be built up to 12 to 24 g daily taken in water as a single dose, or up to 4 divided doses each day. Occasionally 36 g a day may be required although the benefits of increasing the dose above 16 g a day may be offset by gastrointestinal disturbances and poor patient compliance. Colestipol is also administered in granular form at a dose of 5 g once or twice daily. This is increased every 1 to 2 months to a maximum of 30 g in a single or twice daily regimen.

Adverse effects. Side effects with the resins are more likely to occur with high doses and in patients aged over 60 years. Bloating, flatulence, heartburn and constipation are common complaints. Constipation is the major subjective side effect and although usually mild and transient it may be severe.

Cholestyramine and colestipol are known to interact with many drugs primarily by interfering with absorption (Table 21.10). Consequently, medication should be taken 1 to 2 hours before or 4 to 6 hours after the anion-exchange resin. For patients on multiple drug therapy resins may not be the best choice.

Fibrates

This group comprises bezafibrate, ciprofibrate, clofibrate, fenofibrate and gemfibrozil. They all increase HDL and are effective in reducing triglyceride levels and, to a lesser extent, LDL levels.

The mechanism of action for the fibrates is not completely understood. They are thought to reduce triglyceride levels by increasing lipoprotein lipase activity which, in turn, enhances VLDL catabolism; decrease release of free fatty acids from adipose tissue causing reduced production of VLDL in the liver; and increase output of hepatic cholesterol into the bile. The fibrates take 2 to 5 days to have a measurable effect on VLDL, with their optimum effect present after 4 weeks.

Adverse effects. The use of clofibrate is now limited due to concern over long-term serious side effects, notably a suspicion of causing malignant neoplasms, cholelithiasis and pancreatitis. Overall, the side effects of fibrates are mild and vary between members of the group. Their apparent propensity to increase the cholesterol saturation index of bile renders them unsuitable for use in patients with gallbladder disease. Gastrointestinal symptoms such as nausea, diarrhoea and abdominal pain are common but transient, and often resolve after a few days of treatment. Myositis has been described and is associated with muscle pain, unusual tiredness or weakness.

Table 21.10   Drug interactions involving hypolipidaemic agents

Drug	Interacting drug	Comment
Anion-exchange resin	Warfarin	Increased anticoagulant effect due to depletion of vitamin K or reduced anticoagulant effect due to binding of warfarin in gut
	Digoxin	Absorption of all agents reduced due to binding in gut: clinical significance unclear
	Thiazide diuretics	All medication is probably best taken 1 to 2 hours before or 4 to 6 hours after a resin
	Propranolol	
	Tetracycline	
	Vancomycin	
	Vitamins (fat soluble)	
	Sulphasalazine	
Fibrates	Warfarin	Increased anticoagulant effect
	Chenodeoxycholic acid/ ursodeoxycholic acid	Reduced effect of the bile acids because fibrates increase cholesterol saturation of bile
	Sulphonylureas	Enhanced hypoglycaemic response
	Pravastatin/simvastatin	Increased risk of rhabdomyolysis
HMG-CoA reductase inhibitors	Warfarin	Increased anticoagulant effect
	Cyclosporin/other immunosuppresants	Increased risk of rhabdomyolysis
	Erythromycin	
	Fibrates	
	Nicotinic acid	
Simvastatin	Digoxin	Increased digoxin levels
Nicotinic acid and derivatives	Antihypertensive agents	Additive hypotensive effect
	Chenodeoxycholic acid/ ursodeoxycholic acid	Reduced effect of the bile acids because of increased cholesterol saturation of bile
	HMG-CoA reductase inhibitors	Increased risk of rhabdomyolysis

With respect to drug interactions fibrates have been implicated in two potentially serious drug interactions. They are known to significantly increase the effect of anticoagulants, whilst concurrent use with pravastatin and simvastatin is associated with an increased risk of myositis and rarely rhabdomyolysis.

Overall there appears to be little to differentiate between members of the group with regard to their effect on the lipid profile. In addition to their effect on lipids, they have all been reported to produce an improvement in glucose tolerance, although bezafibrate probably has the most marked effect. In the patient with elevated triglycerides and gout only fenofibrate has been reported to have a sustained uricosuric effect on chronic administration.

HMG-CoA reductase inhibitors

The discovery of a class of drugs that selectively inhibits 3-hydroxy, 3-methylglutaryl-CoA reductase (HMG-CoA reductase), the rate-limiting enzyme in cholesterol biosynthesis, has heralded a significant advance in the treatment of severe hypercholesterolaemia. Once the intracellular levels of cholesterol are reduced, more LDL receptors are expressed and LDL uptake from the circulation is increased. The reductase inhibitors reduce LDL, VLDL and triglyceride concentrations and slightly increase HDL. Their primary site of action is the liver.

Simvastatin was the first member of this group of drugs to be marketed in the UK and was closely followed by pravastatin. Both drugs inhibit HMG-CoA reductase and consequently reduce LDL concentrations in a dose-dependent manner over a dose range of 10 to 40 mg. Triglycerides are reduced in a dose-independent manner.

Pravastatin and simvastatin require the presence of LDL receptors for their optimum clinical effect and consequently they are not as effective in patients with homozygous familial hypercholesterolaemia who have no such receptors. However, even in the homozygous patient they can reduce serum cholesterol although the mechanism is unclear. Their use with anion-ex-change resins can be very effective in reducing LDL cholesterol.

Adverse effects. Although relatively new, side effects appear mild and transient and include rashes and gastrointestinal symptoms. Rises in serum transminases and creatinine phosphokinase are common. Reversible, threefold increases in transaminases have been noted and may necessitate discontinuation of the drug. The rise in creatinine phosphokinase may be the result of myositis and very occasionally rhabdomyolysis, both of which have been reported with concurrent cyclosporin, gemfibrozil and nicotinic acid.

Nicotinic acid and derivatives

Nicotinic acid in pharmacological doses (0.3 to 6 g) lowers both serum LDL and VLDL, and increases HDL.

Acipimox is structurally related to nicotinic acid, has similar beneficial effects on the lipid profile, has a better side effect profile but appears to be much less potent. Nicofuranose is another analogue of nicotinic acid but its side effects limit its use.

Adverse effects. Despite the established long-term safety of nicotinic acid it is of limited use in practice because of its side effects. These are very common and unpleasant and range from troublesome flushing of the skin, headache, postural hypotension, diarrhoea, exacerbation of peptic ulcers, hepatic dysfunction, gout and increase in blood glucose. Whilst acipimox shares many of these side effects, but to a lesser extent, it does not have an adverse effect on blood glucose levels nor share the propensity to exacerbate peptic ulcers.

Probucol

Probucol has been shown to reduce both LDL and HDL and cause significant regression of xanthomata. The underlying mechanism of action is unclear but because of its ability to reduce the beneficial HDL it is now little used.

Fish oils

A fish oil preparation rich in omega-3-fatty acids has been shown to markedly reduce triglyceride levels by decreasing VLDL synthesis. Although LDL may be lowered and HDL increased, these effects are inconsistent. A rise in LDL often accompanies its use. On current evidence there is little support for advocating the use of pharmacological doses of fish oils in the treatment of hyperlipoproteinaemias.

Combination therapy

The various groups of drugs available to control abnormal lipid and lipoprotein synthesis work at different sites and have a different effect on the lipid profile of an individual (Table 21.11).

THE PATIENT
Diet

In primary prevention of IHD the benefits of screening and detecting hypercholesterolaemia are probably greatest in young, male patients. However, such patients will require considerable long-term support from health-care staff. Initial management should be targeted at lifestyle changes once underlying causes have been eliminated. Dietary advice (Table 21.12) is the cornerstone of management and should be supported by advice to stop smoking, undertake regular exercise and moderate alcohol intake. Patients

Table 21.11 Reported change in lipids and lipoproteins at optimal dose of single drug

Drug group	Cholesterol (%)	Triglycerides (%)	LDL (%)	HDL (%)
Anion-exchange resin	↓ 15 to 30%	↑ 5 to 30%	↓ 15 to 30%	↑ 3 to 8%
Fibrate	↓ 10 to 20%	↓ 30 to 50%	↓ 20 to 25%	↑ 10 to 25%
HMG-CoA reductase inhibitor	↓ 20 to 35%	↓ 10 to 30%	↓ 25 to 45%	↑ 2 to 15%
Nicotinic acid and derivatives	↓ 15 to 30%	↓ 20 to 60%	↓ 15 to 40%	↑ 10 to 20%
Probucol	↓ to 5 to 15%	↓ 0 to 5%	↓ 10 to 15%	↓ 10 to 25%
Fish oils	↑ or ↓	↓ 10 to 60%	Variable	↑ 5 to 10%

Table 21.12 Examples of dietary modifications to lower cholesterol intake

Avoid/decrease	Preferred alternative
Meat Fatty cuts of meat, ham, pork, bacon, duck Liver kidney Sausages Scotch eggs Meat pies, pasties	Chicken and turkey without skin Lean cuts of meat Fish
Dairy produce Whole milk, cream Full fat yoghurt Hard cheese, cream cheese or processed cheese Egg yolks	Skimmed or semi-skimmed milk Low fat yoghurt Low fat cheeses Cottage cheese Egg white
Fats Butter, dripping, lard, suet, margarine, ghee, coconut oil	All fats should be limited Unsaturated vegetable oils and margarines such as corn, sunflower, safflower, soya, olive and rapeseed oils
Nuts Coconut, peanut	Nuts should be limited Walnuts, almonds, hazelnuts
Fish Fish roe, caviar, potted fish, fried fish Shellfish in excess	Fresh, frozen or smoked fish

should be encouraged to increase their intake of complex carbohydrates, fruit and vegetables and use protein sources low in saturated fats. Soluble fibre found in lentils, beans, peas and oats are considered by many to be particularly effective in reducing cholesterol. The evidence to support this is, however, by no means conclusive.

Alongside the soluble fibre debate is the issue of whether coffee or caffeine consumption increases the risk of coronary heart disease or stroke. Coffee is thought by many to raise the serum cholesterol concentration, although its effect is probably influenced by the method of brewing and the actual volume consumed. A study involving 45 000 men revealed no increased risk of IHD with increasing coffee and caffeine intake.

Drugs

Anion-exchange resins

Anion-exchange resins are frequently prescribed as first line therapy. However, since palatability is often a major problem, patients need to be well motivated and prepared for the problems they may encounter.

Cholestyramine is available in an orange flavour and as a low sugar powder. Colestipol is without taste and is odourless. Each sachet of cholestyramine or colestipol should be added to at least 120 ml of liquid and stirred vigorously to avoid the powder clumping. The powder does not dissolve but disperses in the chosen liquid which may be water, fruit juice, skimmed milk usually in hot or regular breakfast cereals, thin soups or puréed food with a high fluid content.

A recipe book is available from the manufacturers of cholestyramine which outlines how it can be incorporated in the sauces of meals. Many patients find the 'gritty' texture of the resin in a drink unacceptable. In this situation palatability can be improved by mixing the day's supply of resin with the desired liquid and storing overnight in a fridge.

All patients receiving colestipol or cholestyramine must be aware that any concurrent medication must be taken 1 to 2 hours before or 4 to 6 hours after the anion-exchange resin. Gemfibrozil can be administered with colestipol if the two drugs are administered 2 hours apart.

Other lipid-lowering agents

To achieve optimum effect, patients taking a fibrate should be advised to take their medication 30 minutes before a meal. In patients receiving pravastatin or simvastatin a once-daily regimen involving an evening dose is preferred. The HMG-CoA reductase inhibitors are more effective when given as a single dose in the evening compared to a similar dose administered in the morning. This has been attributed to the fact that cholesterol biosynthesis increases at night.

The adverse effect profile of nicotinic acid has already been discussed. For those patients who find the flushing particularly troublesome a single dose of aspirin 300 mg, taken some 30 minutes before the nicotinic acid, has been shown to give relief. This advice is based on the rationale that the flushing is prostaglandin mediated. Extended-release dosage forms of nicotinic acid have also been shown to reduce the incidence of flushing and pruritus. Finally, patients should be advised to take their nicotinic acid with skimmed milk or meals to avoid the possibility of stomach upset.

CASE STUDIES

CASE 21.1

Mr S. C. is 36 years old and regularly participates in long distance 'fun runs'. At a routine health check he was found to have type IIa hyperlipidaemia for which he was prescribed simvastatin 20 mg once a day and cholestyramine 12 g twice daily. 4 weeks after starting therapy he complained of widespread muscle pain, generalized weakness and was having difficulty walking. On examination he was found to have sluggish tendon reflexes. His urine was red-brown in colour and revealed high concentrations of haem and myoglobin, and the presence of erythrocytes. Renal function was normal but serum muscle enzyme concentrations were raised.

Q What is the likely cause of Mr S. C.'s problem and how should it be managed?

CASE 21.2

Mrs C. W. is 52 years old and known to have familial hypercholesterolaemia. Her current blood lipid profile reveals a total cholesterol level of 7.1 mmol/L (ideal < 5.2 mmol/L), triglycerides of 1.9 mmol/L (ideal < 2.3 mmol/L) and HDL of 0.9 mmol/L (ideal > 0.9 mmol/L). She is taking simvastatin 20 mg once a day. Her physician is contemplating starting hormone replacement therapy (HRT).

Q What effect is HRT likely to have on Mrs C. W.'s lipid profile and how will it influence her subsequent risk of suffering from ischaemic heart disease (IHD)?

CASE 21.3

Mr W. G. is 45 years old and was found on a routine health check to have the following serum lipid profile: total cholesterol 7.1 mmol/L (ideal < 5.2 mmol/L); triglycerides 1.4 mmol/L (ideal < 2.3 mmol/L); and HDL 0.9 mmol/L (ideal > 0.9 mmol/L). There was no evidence of vascular disease, no physical signs of hyperlipidaemia and no family history of coronary heart disease. He has a body mass index of 35 kg/m², He smokes more than 20 cigarettes each day and drinks an average of 40 units of alcohol per week.

Q1 What type of hyperlipidaemia does Mr W. G. have?

Q2 Identify the risk factors for IHD in Mr W. G. and determine the important aspects of his future lipid management.

CASE 21.4

Mr T. B. is 45 years old and has a past medical history of cholecystitis and appendicectomy. On a routine health screen he was found to have the following lipid profile: total cholesterol 7.8 mmol/L (ideal < 5.2 mmol/L), triglycerides 4.8 mmol/L (ideal < 2.3 mmol/L) and HDL 0.9 mmol/L (ideal > 0.9 mmol/L). He takes no other medication and was prescribed gemfibrozil 600 mg twice a day.

Q Is it appropriate to use gemfibrozil in Mr T. B.?

ANSWERS TO CASE STUDIES

CASE 21.1

A Simvastatin-induced rhabdomyolysis was probably the cause of Mr S. C.'s problem. There is little evidence to implicate cholestyramine in this type of adverse reaction. The HMG-CoA reductase inhibitors have rarely been reported to cause rhabdomyolysis when used alone although it is a recognized problem when they are used in combination with fibrates or cyclosporin.

The reductase inhibitors probably interfere with muscle metabolism. Vigorous exercise itself, such as long-distance running, can cause myoglobinuria. Patients who receive an HMG-CoA reductase inhibitor alone or with other drugs should probably avoid strenuous muscular work.

Mr S. C.'s drug treatment was immediately stopped and he was confined to bed and treated with intravenous fluids. The myoglobinuria resolved within 24 hours. The muscle pain and weakness resolved over the following 2 weeks and the serum enzyme concentrations returned to normal.

CASE 21.2

A Much of the available data which has looked at the influence of HRT on lipid metabolism has focused on the use of oestrogens alone. The available data suggest that oestrogens lower total cholesterol and LDL whilst increasing HDL levels. They may, of course, also have unfavourable effects on blood pressure, glucose tolerance and blood clotting. The balance of opinion is that cardiovascular risk is reduced in postmenopausal women receiving oestrogens.

The use of oestrogen-only HRT has declined with the recognized increased incidence of uterine cancer. In order to overcome this risk but obtain the benefits of oestrogen therapy, particularly in women who have not had a hysterectomy, progestogens are usually prescribed during the last 10 or 12 days of each cycle. Progestogens such as norethisterone (but not medroxyprogesterone acetate) have an adverse effect on the lipid profile and decrease HDL levels although they may have a beneficial effect of reducing Lp(a) levels. The clinical relevance of this latter observation is unclear.

Oestrogens when used alone confer some degree of protection against IHD and stroke. The role of progestogens again is less clear, although it has been suggested that adding an adequate dose of synthetic progestogen to oestrogen replacement therapy is likely to significantly reduce the beneficial effects of oestrogens on IHD risk.

Mrs C. W. probably has significant risk of underlying coronary disease. In this situation the risk of thromboembolism probably outweighs any advantage of receiving HRT.

CASE 21.3

A1 Mr W. G.'s triglyceride and HDL levels are within the 'normal range' and only his total cholesterol would appear elevated. This is the typical picture of a patient who presents with common hypercholesterolaemia (type IIa).

A2 Mr W. G. has a number of risk factors for IHD including being male, smoking cigarettes, having a body mass index > 25 kg/m² and having a borderline low HDL. The alcohol intake of Mr W. G. is above the recommended maximum intake per week (> 21 units per week) and must be considered as a contributory factor.

The reality of Mr W. G.'s case is that he will probably die prematurely of IHD if he does not make a concerted effort to stop smoking, reduce his alcohol intake and reduce his body mass index.

The benefits of stopping smoking need not be dwelt on here.

Obesity is a common cause of hypertriglyceridaemia and reduced HDL levels. The reduction of serum HDL in obesity is independent of other variables know to affect serum HDL. There is no evidence of any increase in HDL during weight loss associated with low energy diets although it has been reported in individuals who have reduced their weight and maintained the loss. The key to a successful weight loss programme is to set realistic goals for the patient which can be achieved.

Alcohol is also a common cause of hyperlipidaemia and is usually associated with hypertriglyceridaemia. The high alcohol intake of Mr W. G. may in itself be a significant part of his dietary energy intake and thus have contributed to his obesity.

If Mr W. G. can be encouraged to stop smoking, reduce his overall calorie intake and his saturated fat intake this should improve his lipid profile and drug therapy may not be necessary.

CASE 21.4

A Mr T. B. has a raised total cholesterol and a raised triglyceride concentration. The picture is typical of a combined hyperlipidaemia (type IIb).

Fibric acid derivatives such as gemfibrozil are effective in lowering elevated serum triglycerides, increasing HDL and lowering LDL concentrations. There is also increasing evidence that fibrates can protect against IHD not only through their effects on lipid levels, but also by altering LDL structure and various haemostatic factors. It would therefore appear rational to use gemfibrozil in a patient with type IIb hyperlipidaemia.

However, fibric acid derivatives are known to increase the cholesterol saturation index of bile although it has been suggested that this effect may not be sustained beyond the initial few months of therapy. They are contra-indicated in patients with pre-existing gallstones. Since Mr T. B. has a history of acute cholecystitis (an acute inflammation of the gallbladder wall usually as a response to cystic duct obstruction by a gallstone) it would appear wise to initially try an alternative agent such as a statin or nicotinic acid.

BIBLIOGRAPHY

Bilheimer D W. Clinical considerations regarding treatment of hypercholesterolaemia in the elderly. Atherosclerosis 1991; 91: S35–S57

Carlson L A, Rosenhamer G. Reduction in mortality in the Stockholm Ischaemic Heart Disease Secondary Prevention Study by combined treatment with clofibrate and nicotinic acid. Acta Medica Scandinavica 1988; 223: 405–418

Committee of Principal Investigators. WHO cooperative trial on primary prevention of ischemic heart disease with clofibrate to lower serum cholesterol: mortality follow-up. Lancet 1984; ii: 600–604

Durrington P N. Hyperlipidaemia: diagnosis and management. London: Butterworth 1989

Frick M H, Elo O, Haapa K, Heinonen O P, Heinsalmi P, Helo P et al. Helsinki Heart Study: primary prevention trial with gemfibrozil in middle-aged men with dyslipidaemia. Safety of treatment, changes in risk factors and incidence of coronary heart disease. New England Journal of Medicine 1987; 317: 1237–1245

Henkin Y, Como J A, Oberman A. Secondary dyslipidemia: inadvertent effects of drugs in clinical practice. JAMA 1992; 267: 961–968

The Coronary Drug Project Research Group. Clofibrate and niacin in coronary heart disease. JAMA 1975; 231: 360–381

The Lipid Research Clinics Coronary Primary Prevention Trial. I. Reduction in incidence of coronary heart disease. JAMA 1984; 251: 351–364

Thompson G R. A handbook of hyperlipidaemia. London: Current Science 1989

Rossouw J E, Rifkind B M. Does lowering serum cholesterol levels lower coronary heart disease risk? Endocrinology and Metabolism Clinics of North America 1990; 19: 279–296

Chapter 22

Asthma

K.P. Gibbs   J. C. Portlock

'Asthma' literally means 'panting'. It is a broad term used to refer to a disorder of the respiratory system which leads to episodic difficulty in breathing. A lack of knowledge of the exact defect which causes the airways to be hyper-reactive to various stimuli has led to an imprecise definition. In fact the definition is actually a description of the clinical symptoms. Asthma has been defined as a chronic inflammatory disorder of the airways in which many cells play a role, including mast cells and eosinophils. In susceptible individuals this inflammation causes symptoms which are usually associated with widespread but variable airflow obstruction that is often reversible either spontaneously or with treatment, and causes an associated increase in airway responsiveness to a variety of stimuli.

EPIDEMIOLOGY

The exact prevalence of asthma remains uncertain because of the difficulty in defining the disease. Until the 1950s the definition included a necessity to diagnose allergy. Consequently, there are few long-term population based statistics which have used uniform criteria for diagnosis. It has been estimated that about 5% of the American and the British population have asthma. Mortality from asthma is estimated at approximately 0.4 per 100 000 and is currently estimated at 2000 per annum in the UK. However, it has been stated that more than 80% of deaths from asthma may be preventable. Most deaths occur outside hospital and the most common reason for death is thought to be inadequate assessment of the severity of airway obstruction by the patient and/or clinician and inadequate therapy of an acute attack.

The probability of children having asthma-like symptoms is estimated to be 5 to 12%, with a higher occurrence in boys than girls and in children whose parents have an allergic disorder. Between 30 and 70% of children will become symptom free by adulthood. However, individuals who develop asthma at an early age do have a poorer prognosis.

The prevalence of asthma actually appears to be rising despite advances in therapy. However, there is some doubt about this due to the differing criteria for the diagnosis of asthma used in different studies. Asthma is considered to be one of the consequences of western civilization and appears to be related to a number of environmental factors. Air pollution resulting from industrial sources and transport may be interacting with smoking, dietary and other factors to increase the incidence of this debilitating problem.

AETIOLOGY

The specific abnormality underlying asthma is hyperreactivity of the lungs to one or more stimuli. This can also occur in certain patients with chronic bronchitis and allergic rhinitis but usually to a lesser extent. There are a number of possible trigger factors, see Table 22.1.

One of the most common trigger factors is the allergen found in the faeces of the house dust mite which is almost universally present in bedding, carpets and soft furnishing. Pollen from grass (prevalent in June and July) can lead to seasonal asthma. The role of occupation in the development of asthma has become apparent with increased industrialization. There are many causes of occupational asthma, and bronchial reactivity may persist for years after exposure to the trigger factor. Food allergy usually results in gastrointestinal disturbances and eczema rather than asthma. Drug-induced asthma can be severe and the most common causes are beta-adrenoreceptor blocking drugs and prostaglan-

Table 22.1   Examples of trigger factors which may cause asthma

Allergens (e.g. pollens, moulds, house dust mite, animals' dander, saliva and urine, bacteria)
Cold, dry air
Exercise
Viral respiratory tract infections
Psychological stimuli (e.g. stress, anxiety)
Drugs (e.g. aspirin, ibuprofen and other prostaglandin synthetase inhibitors, beta-adrenoreceptor blockers)
Industrial chemicals (e.g. isocyanates, epoxy resins, aluminium, hair sprays, penicillins, cimetidine)
Other industrial triggers (e.g. wood or grain dust, colophony in solder, cotton dust, grain weevils, mites)

din synthetase inhibitors. The administration of beta-adrenoreceptor blockers to a patient even in the form of eye drops can cause $beta_2$-receptor blockade and consequently bronchoconstriction. Selective beta-adrenoreceptor blockers are thought to pose slightly less risk but as these lose their selectivity at higher doses it is generally recommended that this group of drugs is avoided altogether in asthma patients. Aspirin and related non-steroidal anti-inflammatory drugs (e.g. ibuprofen) can cause severe bronchoconstriction in susceptible individuals. Aspirin inhibits the enzyme prostaglandin synthetase which normally converts arachidonic acid to prostaglandins. When this pathway is blocked an alternative reaction predominates leading to an increase in production of bronchoconstrictor leukotrienes. More than 15% of the adult asthma population are sensitive to aspirin.

It is generally thought that emotional disturbances cannot cause asthma but it is well known that they can provoke or worsen bronchoconstriction and may affect the effectiveness of bronchodilators used to treat asthma.

PATHOPHYSIOLOGY

The discovery of the antibody 'IgE' led to the description of 'extrinsic' or allergic asthma and non-IgE-mediated 'intrinsic' asthma (also known as asthma of unknown origin). However, these definitions are considered to be of secondary importance to the classification of asthma according to the frequency and severity of symptoms.

Extrinsic asthma is common in children and is precipitated by known allergens (see 'Aetiology') whereas intrinsic asthma tends to develop in adulthood, symptoms being triggered by non-allergenic factors such as a viral infection, or irritants (due to epithelial damage and mucosal inflammation), emotional upsets (thought to be mediated by excess parasympathetic input) and exercise (thought to be due to water and heat loss from the airways triggering mediator release from mast cells).

The main features of asthma are marked hypertrophy and hyperplasia of bronchial smooth muscle, mucous gland hypertrophy leading to excessive mucus production and inflammatory cell migration which leads to damaged epithelium, mucosal oedema and impaired mucociliary clearance. A specific cellular defect has not yet been discovered but there are a number of pathophysiological features which are prevalent in asthma. For example, there may be a defect in cholinergic activity in the airways. This is supported by the apparently lower threshold for irritant stimuli in asthmatics. Smooth muscle in the lungs is innervated by parasympathetic nerves and the normal resting tone is maintained by the vagus. Vagally mediated bronchoconstriction is most apparent in the small bronchi. The afferent system detects irritant stimuli (chemical, mechanical or pharmacological) due to the presence of irritant receptors immediately beneath the epithelial layer. Asthma may also result from abnormal beta-receptor–adenylate cyclase function which leads to a decrease in adrenergic responsiveness. There is some evidence that alpha-receptors trigger bronchoconstriction in some patients.

It is thought that the final common pathway in asthma is altered regulation of intracellular calcium. Most of the signs and symptoms in asthma are calcium-dependent processes and include release of mediators from mast cells, smooth muscle contraction, mucus secretion, vagus nerve impulse conduction and inflammatory cell infiltration. Mast cells play a significant role in allergen-induced asthma. It has been proposed that the release of mast cell components is the key mechanism in asthma. However, this does not explain the asthma induced by ozone, viral infection, sulphur dioxide, cold air or emotional disturbances.

Mast cell components are released as a result of an IgE-antibody-mediated reaction on the surface of the cell. Histamine and other mediators of inflammation are released from mast cells, e.g. leukotrienes, prostaglandins, bradykinin, adenosine, prostaglandin generating factor of anaphylaxis, as well as various chemotactic agents which attract eosinophils and neutrophils. These mediators have a number of activities. For example histamine triggers rapid bronchoconstriction whereas leukotrienes (LT) such as LTC_4, LTD_4 and LTE_4 constrict at a slower rate. The chemotactic agents cause a slower reaction which is characterized by the infiltration of macrophages into the lumen of the airways. Macrophages release prostaglandins, thromboxane and platelet activating factor (PAF). PAF appears to sustain bronchial hyperreactivity and causes respiratory capillaries to leak plasma which increases mucosal oedema. It also facilitates the accumulation of eosinophils within the airways which is a characteristic pathological feature of asthma. Eosinophils release various inflammatory mediators such as LTC_4 and PAF. Epithelial damage results and a thick viscous mucus is produced which causes further deterioration in lung function.

Mucus production is normally a defence mechanism but in asthma patients there is an increase in size of bronchial glands and goblet cells which produce mucus. Mucus transport is dependent on its viscosity. If it is very thick it plugs the airways which also become blocked with epithelial and inflammatory cell debris. Mucociliary clearance is also decreased due to inflammation of epithelial cells. The epithelial cell damage can be severe which in turn can increase access of various irritants to the cholinergic receptors. This can result in further bronchoconstriction mediated by the parasympathetic nervous system.

CLINICAL MANIFESTATIONS

Asthma can present in a number of ways. It

may manifest as a persistent cough. Most commonly it is described as recurrent episodes of difficulty in breathing (dyspnoea) associated with wheezing (a high-pitched noise due to turbulent airflow through a narrowed airway). Diagnosis is usually made by a combination of a full history from the patient or patient's representative together with lung function tests before and after administration of bronchodilators. The history of an asthma patient often includes the presence of atopy and allergic rhinitis in the patient or within the close family. Symptoms of asthma are often intermittent and the frequency and severity of an episode can vary from individual to individual. Between periods of wheezing and breathlessness patients may feel quite well. Tightness of the chest, shortness of breath and abnormal lung function tests which improve by 15% with administration of suitable treatment confirm the diagnosis of asthma. However, no improvement in ventilation cannot rule out asthma, and in younger children it is sometimes very difficult to perform lung function tests.

Acute severe asthma is a dangerous condition which requires hospitalization and immediate emergency treatment. It occurs when bronchospasm has progressed to a state where the patient is breathless at rest and has a degree of cardiac stress. This is usually progressive and can build up over a number of hours or even days. The breathlessness (peak flow rate < 100 litres per minute) is so severe that the patient cannot talk or lie down. Expiration is particularly difficult and prolonged as air is trapped beneath mucosal inflammation. The pulse rate can give an indication of severity. Severe acute asthma can increase the pulse rate to more than 110 beats per minute. Pulsus paradoxus of over 10 mmHg may also be apparent (this is a term used to describe a drop in systolic blood pressure upon inspiration). It is common to see hyperexpansion of the thoracic cavity and lowering of the diaphragm which means that accessory respiratory muscles are required to try to inflate the chest. Breathing can become rapid (> 30 breaths/minute) and shallow leading to low arterial oxygen tension (PO_2) with the patient

becoming fatigued, cyanosed, confused and lethargic. The arterial carbon dioxide tension (PCO_2) is usually low in acute asthma. If it is high it should respond quickly to emergency therapy. Hypercapnia (high PCO_2 level) which does not diminish is a more severe problem and indicates progression towards respiratory failure.

INVESTIGATIONS

The function of the lungs can be measured in order to help diagnose and monitor various respiratory diseases. A series of routine tests has been developed to assess asthma as well as other respiratory disease such as chronic obstructive airways diseases (COAD). The most useful test for abnormalities in airways function is the forced expiratory volume (FEV). This is measured by means of lung function assessment apparatus such as a spirometer. The patient inhales as deeply as possible and then exhales as forcefully and completely as possible into a mouthpiece connected to the spirometer. The FEV_1 is a measure of the forced expiratory volume in the first second of exhalation. Another volume which is commonly measured is the forced vital capacity (FVC). This is an assessment of the maximum volume of air exhaled with maximum effort after maximum inspiration. The FEV_1 is usually expressed as a percentage of the total volume of air exhaled and is reported as the FEV_1/FVC ratio. This ratio is a useful and highly reproducible measure of the capabilities of the lungs. Normal individuals can exhale at least 75% of their total capacity in 1 second. Any reduction indicates a deterioration in lung performance (see Fig. 22.1).

The peak flow meter is a useful means of self-assessment for the patient. It gives slightly less reproducible results than the spirometer but has the advantage that the patient can do regular tests at home with the hand-held meter. The peak flow meter measures peak expiratory flow rate (PEFR). This is the maximum flow rate which can be forced during expiration. The PEFR can be used to assess the improvement or deterioration in the disease as well as the effectiveness of treatment. For all three measurements (FEV_1,

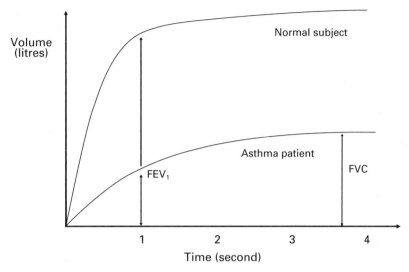

Fig. 22.1 Typical lung spirometry in normal subjects and asthma patients. FEV_1/FVC is an index of airways obstruction. A decrease in FEV_1/FVC indicates obstruction. Key: FFV_1 = forced expiratory volume in 1 second; FVC = forced vital capacity.

FVC and PEFR) there are 'normal' values with which the patient's results can be compared. However, these 'normal' values do vary with age, race, gender, height and weight. The measurement of FEV_1, FVC or PEFR do not detect early deterioration of lung function such as bronchospasm and mucus-plugging in the smaller airways. Other investigations include assessment of the partial pressures of oxygen PO_2 (reference range = 12 to 16 kPa) and carbon dioxide PCO_2 (reference range = 4.6 to 6.0 kPa) in arterial blood. These values together with pH (reference range = 7.35 to 7.45) are routinely monitored in hospital inpatients. There is a homeostatic mechanism for maintaining these values within very narrow limits. In patients with severe asthma the PCO_2 values tend to increase as a result of poor lung ventilation causing a reduction in gas exchange. Respiratory acidosis can occur because of accumulation of carbonic acid produced from the excess CO_2. Compensatory mechanisms such as those found in the kidneys counteract this by excreting hydrogen ions and generating bicarbonate ions to neutralize the pH. Arterial bicarbonate levels can be measured (HCO_3^- reference range = 22 to 28 mmol/L). Arterial oxygen levels (PO_2) can fall as a result of poor lung ventilation

due to bronchospasm, and poor diffusion into the respiratory capillaries due to inflammation, oedema and mucus-plugging.

TREATMENT

Since asthma involves inflammation and bronchoconstriction treatment should be directed towards reducing inflammation and increasing bronchodilatation. Restoration of normal airways function and prevention of severe acute attacks are the main goals of treatment. It has become apparent that anti-inflammatory drugs should be given to most patients. Bronchodilators probably do little to influence inflammation and, in briefly relieving the symptoms, may mask deterioration in the condition. Other measures, such as avoidance of recognized trigger factors, may also contribute to the control of this disease. The lowest, effective doses of drugs should be given to minimize short-term and long-term side effects. However, it should always be remembered that asthma is a potentially life-threatening illness and is often undertreated.

Chronic asthma

The pharmacological management of asthma

depends upon the frequency and severity of a patient's symptoms. Infrequent attacks can be managed by treating each attack when it occurs, but with more frequent attacks preventive therapy needs to be used.

The preferred route of administration of the agents used in the management of asthma is by inhalation. This allows the drugs to be delivered directly to the airways in smaller doses and with fewer side effects than if systemic or parenteral routes were used. Inhaled bronchodilators also have a faster onset of action than when administered systemically and give better protection from bronchoconstriction.

Treatment of chronic asthma can be given in a stepwise progression, as outlined in Figure 22.2, according to the severity of the patient's asthma symptoms. At each stage the patient's inhaler technique should be assessed. If necessary the type of inhalation device used should be changed to improve patient compliance.

Beta-adrenoreceptor agonist bronchodilators

Beta-adrenoreceptor agonists are the mainstay of the management of asthma. Selective beta$_2$-agonists such as salbutamol and terbutaline have now replaced the older, non-selective agents such as adrenaline, isoprenaline and orciprenaline. The selective agents have fewer beta$_1$-mediated side effects, particularly cardiotoxicity. However, beta$_2$-receptors are also present in myocardial tissue. Therefore, cardiovascular stimulation resulting in tachycardia and palpitations is still the main dose-limiting toxicity with these agents. The degree of selectivity varies with the agent, dose, route and duration of therapy.

An inhaled beta$_2$-agonist is the first line agent in the management of asthma. These are used as required by the patient for the symptomatic relief of breathlessness and wheezing, for example salbutamol 200 micrograms when required. This may be the only treatment necessary for those with infrequent symptoms.

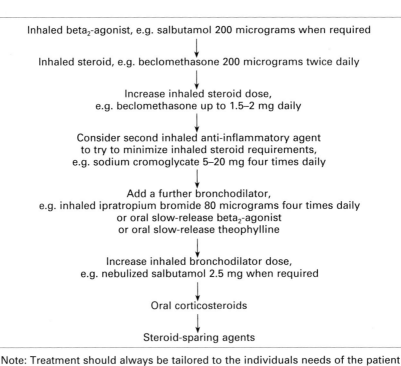

Inhaled beta$_2$-agonist, e.g. salbutamol 200 micrograms when required

↓

Inhaled steroid, e.g. beclomethasone 200 micrograms twice daily

↓

Increase inhaled steroid dose,
e.g. beclomethasone up to 1.5–2 mg daily

↓

Consider second inhaled anti-inflammatory agent
to try to minimize inhaled steroid requirements,
e.g. sodium cromoglycate 5–20 mg four times daily

↓

Add a further bronchodilator,
e.g. inhaled ipratropium bromide 80 micrograms four times daily
or oral slow-release beta$_2$-agonist
or oral slow-release theophylline

↓

Increase inhaled bronchodilator dose,
e.g. nebulized salbutamol 2.5 mg when required

↓

Oral corticosteroids

↓

Steroid-sparing agents

Note: Treatment should always be tailored to the individuals needs of the patient

Fig. 22.2 Guidelines for the management of chronic asthma in adults.

A report of increased numbers of asthma deaths resulting from the use of regular fenoterol has led to a debate over the use of beta$_2$-agonists in a regular dosage regimen compared to their 'when required' use in symptomatic relief. Until it is clearly established whether this finding is limited to fenoterol or is a general property of the beta$_2$-agonists, these drugs should only be used for symptomatic relief.

Inhaled anti-inflammatory agents

Regular anti-inflammatory treatment must be given to patients who require an inhaled bronchodilator more than once a day or who have nocturnal symptoms. The agents used include corticosteroids, sodium cromoglycate and nedocromil sodium (see Table 22.2).

At present, inhaled corticosteroids are the drugs of choice in adults. Beclomethasone or budesonide are used at doses of 100 to 400 micrograms twice daily. Higher doses are used if symptoms persist. The dose of inhaled corticosteroid should be reduced, if possible, once symptoms and peak expiratory flow rates have improved.

If a patient's asthma cannot be controlled by the above dose of inhaled corticosteroid and the inhaler technique and compliance are adequate, the dose can be increased to a maximum of 1.5 to 2 mg a day. Adrenal suppression may occur at these maximum doses so a steroid warning card should be carried by the patient. Oropharyngeal side effects such as candidiasis are also more common at the higher doses of steroids (see Table 22.3) but can be minimized if patients use a large volume spacer device and rinse their mouths with water after inhalation.

Inhaled sodium cromoglycate and nedocromil sodium could be used instead of corticosteroids and are effective at controlling symptoms in mild to moderate asthma and exercise-induced asthma but less effective in severe asthma. They can be used as an adjunct to inhaled corticosteroid therapy in those who are not fully controlled on steroid treatment, in an attempt to reduce the amount of steroid required, or in children, especially those with exercise-induced or allergic asthma.

Table 22.2 Drugs used for the prophylaxis of asthma

Drug/route		Total daily dosage range
Beclomethasone diproprionate		
Inhaled	Adult	Standard dose: 300 to 800 micrograms in 2 to 4 divided doses High dose: 1000 to 2000 micrograms in 2 to 4 divided doses
	Child	100 to 400 micrograms in 2 to 4 divided doses
Nebulized	Child	100 to 400 micrograms in 2 to 4 divided doses
Budesonide		
Inhaled	Adult	Standard dose: 400 to 800 micrograms daily in 2 to 4 divided doses High dose: 800 to 1600 micrograms daily in 2 to 4 divided doses
	Child	100 to 800 micrograms daily in 2 to 4 divided doses
Nebulized	Adult	1 to 4 mg in 2 divided doses
	3 to 12 years	0.5 to 2 mg in 3 divided doses
Sodium cromoglycate		
Inhaled	Adult & child	Maintenance dose: 20 mg in 4 divided doses increased to 120 to 160 mg in severe cases or periods of risk
Nedocromil sodium		
Inhaled	Adult	8 to 16 mg in 2 to 4 divided doses

Additional bronchodilators

Additional bronchodilators may be required if the above therapy does not adequately control symptoms (see Tables 22.4 and 22.5).

Inhaled anticholinergic agents. These block muscarinic receptors in bronchial smooth muscle and can be added to the treatment regimen. Ipratropium bromide 80 micrograms four times daily or oxitropium 200 micrograms twice daily are available. They have slower onsets of action than beta$_2$-agonists but last longer. The anticholinergics may be especially helpful in the elderly where asthma may be complicated by a degree of obstructive airways disease.

Oral bronchodilators. Either beta$_2$-agonists or theophylline (including aminophylline which is

Table 22.3 Adverse reactions associated with drugs used in the management of asthma

Beta$_2$-agonists

- By inhalation: Adverse drug reactions are uncommon.
- More commonly (mainly by nebulization, orally or parenterally): Fine tremor (usually the hands), nervous tension, headache, peripheral vasodilatation, tachycardia. The adverse reactions often diminish as tolerance develops with continued administration.
- With high doses: hypokalaemia, aggravation of angina.

Inhaled corticosteroids

- Hoarseness, oral or pharyngeal candidiasis.
- Adrenal suppression may occur with high doses, for example beclomethasone diproprionate above 1500 micrograms daily.

Oral corticosteroids

- Prolonged use of these results in exaggeration of some of the normal physiological effects of steroids.
- Mineralocorticoid effects include: hypertension, potassium loss, muscle weakness, and sodium and water retention. These effects are most notable with fludrocortisone, are significant with hydrocortisone, occur only slightly with prednisolone and methylprednisolone and are negligible with dexamethasone and betamethasone.
- Glucocorticoid effects include: precipitation of diabetes, osteoporosis, development of a paranoic state, depression, euphoria, peptic ulceration, immunosuppression, Cushing's syndrome (moon face, striae & acne), growth suppression in children, worsening of infection, skin thinning, striae atrophicae, increased hair growth, perioral dermatitis and acne.
- Adrenal suppression occurs with high doses and/or prolonged treatment. Steroid therapy must be gradually withdrawn in these patients to avoid precipitating an adrenal crisis of hypotension, weight loss, arthralgia and sometimes, death.

Ipratropium bromide

- Occasionally: dry mouth.
- Rarely: systemic anticholinergic effects such as urinary retention & constipation.

Methotrexate

- Myelosuppression, mucositis and rarely, pneumonitis.

Nedocromil sodium

- Mild and transient nausea, coughing, transient bronchospasm, throat irritation, headache and a bitter taste.

Oxitropium

- Dry mouth, local irritation of the throat and nose may occur.
- Occasionally: nausea.
- Rarely: systemic anticholinergic effects, e.g. blurring of vision, hesitancy of micturition. These are more likely in the elderly.

Sodium cromoglycate

- Coughing, transient bronchospasm and throat irritation due to inhalation of the powder.

Theophylline

- Although around 5% of the population experience minor adverse effects; nausea, diarrhoea, nervousness and headache, increasing the serum concentration results in more serious effects. The following is a guide to the serum levels at which the adverse reactions usually occur:
  — Above 20 mg/L: persistent vomiting, insomnia, gastrointestinal bleeding, cardiac arrhythmias.
  — Above 35 mg/L: hyperglycaemia, hypotension, more serious cardiac arrhythmias, convulsions, permanent brain damage and death.
- Individual patients may suffer these effects at serum levels other than those quoted, for example convulsions have occurred in patients at 25 mg/L.

Table 22.4 Comparison of inhaled bronchodilators

Drug	Onset of action (min)	Peak action (min)	Duration of action (h)
Fenoterol	3–5	1–2	4–8
Ipratropium	3–10	60–120	4–6
Oxitropium	5–10	60–120	7.5–12
Reproterol	1–10	30–60	4*
Rimiterol	1–5	90–120	1–3
Salbutamol	5–15	60*	4–6
Salmeterol	14*	150*	12*
Terbutaline	5–30	60–120	3–6

* Approximate or median value.

theophylline combined with ethylenediamine) can also be added for additional symptom control. Slow-release forms should be used; these are especially useful in a single night-time dose if nocturnal symptoms are particularly troublesome although twice-daily dosing is more usual. Oral bronchodilators may also become necessary in patients who are unable to use inhaler therapy effectively.

Theophylline should be started at a dose of 3 mg/kg/day in adults and increased after 7 days to 6 mg/kg/day (children 13 mg/kg/day).

Table 22.5   Daily dosage range for bronchodilators

Drug/route	Age	Total daily dosage range
Aminophylline		
Intravenous injection		5 mg/kg as a single dose
Intravenous infusion	Adult	500 microgram/kg/hour
	6 months to 9 years	1 mg/kg/hour
	10 to 16 years	800 microgram/kg/hour
Oral	Adult	225 to 900 mg (modified release) in 1 to 2 divided doses
	Child	12 to 24 mg/kg (modified release) in 2 divided doses
Fenoterol		
Inhaled	Adult & child	100 to 800 micrograms daily in divided doses
Nebulized	Adult	Up to 5 mg daily in divided doses
	Child	Up to 3 mg daily in divided doses
Ipratropium bromide		
Inhaled	Adult	60 to 3200 micrograms in 3 to 4 divided doses
	Child	20 to 120 micrograms in 3 to 4 divided doses
Nebulized	Adult	100 to 2000 micrograms in up to 4 divided doses
	3 to 14 years	100 to 1500 micrograms in up to 3 divided doses
Oxitropium		
Inhaled		400 to 600 micrograms in 2 to 3 divided doses
Pirbuterol		
Inhaled		1200 to 2400 micrograms in 3 to 4 divided doses
Oral		30 to 60 mg in 3 to 4 divided doses
Reproterol		
Inhaled	Adult	0.5 to 8 mg in 3 to 8 divided doses
	Child	1.5 mg in 3 divided doses
Oral	Adult	30 to 90 mg in 3 divided doses
	Child	30 mg in 3 divided doses
Rimiterol		
Inhaled		200 to 600 micrograms as a single dose, up to a maximum of 4800 micrograms daily
Salbutamol		
Inhaled		100 to 800 micrograms in 3 to 4 divided doses
Nebulized	Adult	2.5 to 10 mg as a single dose, with a maximum of 40 mg daily in up to 4 divided doses
	Child	2.5 to 5 mg as a single dose
Intravenous injection		250 micrograms, repeated if necessary
Intravenous infusion		3 to 20 micrograms per minute
Subcutaneous or intramuscular injection		500 micrograms repeated every 4 hours if necessary
Oral	Adult	6 to 16 mg in 3 to 4 divided doses
	Up to 2 years	400 microgram/kg in 4 divided doses
	2 to 6 years	3 to 8 mg in 3 to 4 divided doses
	6 to 12 years	6 to 8 mg in 3 to 4 divided doses
Salmeterol		
Inhaled		100 to 200 micrograms in 1 to 2 divided doses
Terbutaline		
Inhaled		250 to 4000 micrograms in 4 divided doses
Nebulized	Adult	10 to 40 mg in 2 to 4 divided doses
	Up to 3 years	4 to 8 mg in 2 to 4 divided doses
	3 to 6 years	6 to 12 mg in 2 to 4 divided doses
	6 to 8 years	8 to 16 mg in 2 to 4 divided doses
	Over 8 years	10 to 20 mg in 2 to 4 divided doses
Intravenous, subcutaneous or intramuscular injection	Adult	250 to 2000 micrograms in up to 4 divided doses
	Child	10 microgram/kg up to a maximum of 300 micrograms
Intravenous infusion	Adult	1.5 to 5 microgram/min for up to 8 to 10 hours

Table 22.5 *(cont'd)*

Drug/route	Age	Total daily dosage range
Theophylline		
Oral	Adult	250 to 1000 mg (modified release) in 1 to 2 divided doses
	2 to 6 years	60 to 240 mg (modified release) in 1 to 2 divided doses
	7 to 12 years	125 to 500 mg (modified release) in 1 to 2 divided doses
Tulobuterol		
Oral	Adult	4 to 6 mg in 2 to 3 divided doses
	Over 10 years	2 to 4 mg in 2 divided doses

Theophylline has a narrow therapeutic index and its hepatic metabolism varies greatly between individuals. Theophylline clearance is affected by a variety of factors including disease states and concurrent drug therapy. The dose used should, therefore, take into account these factors, which are outlined in Table 22.6. Serum levels may be taken after 3 to 4 days at the higher dose and it has been normal practice to adjust the dose to keep the serum level within a therapeutic window of 10 to 20 mg/L. Some patients, however, show a good clinical response with levels which are less than 10 mg/L while others tolerate levels in excess of 20 mg/L. The patient should be monitored for the emergence of serious toxic effects, such as tachycardia and persistent vomiting. Only modified-release preparations should be used and once stabilized on a particular product the patient should not be changed to another theophylline preparation as there are large differences in serum profiles with the different preparations. Normal-release theophylline preparations should not be used because of their rapid absorption and highly variable clearance, giving short and unpredictable durations of action.

High dose beta$_2$-agonists. These are only considered if conventional doses do not achieve adequate symptom control. Nebulized drugs such as salbutamol 2.5 to 5 mg per dose are given. Multiple actuations of a metered-dose inhaler into a large volume spacer can be used instead of a nebulizer.

Terbutaline has been given by subcutaneous infusion in the treatment of 'brittle' asthma, where there is an unpredictable and rapid onset of airway narrowing.

Oral corticosteroids

Oral corticosteroids should only be used if symptom control cannot be achieved with maximum doses of inhaled bronchodilators and steroids. The dose should be given as a single morning dose to minimize adrenal suppression. Alternate-day dosing produces less side effects but is less effective in controlling asthma.

Short courses of high-dose oral steroids, 40 to 60 mg can be safely used during exacerbations of asthma.

Steroid-sparing agents

Some agents are being investigated in patients

Table 22.6 **Factors affecting theophylline clearance**

Decreased clearance	Increased clearance
Congestive cardiac failure	
Cor pulmonale	
Chronic obstructive airways disease	
Viral pneumonia	
Acute pulmonary oedema	
Cirrhosis	
Premature and term babies	Children 1 to 12 years
Elderly	
Obesity	
	Cigarette smoking
High carbohydrate, low protein diet	High protein, low carbohydrate diet
	Barbecued meat
Cimetidine	Carbamazepine
Erythromycin	Phenobarbitone
Oral contraceptives	Phenytoin
Ciprofloxacin	Sulphinpyrazone
Propranolol	

who are dependent on systemic steroids in an attempt to reduce the steroid dose. Low-dose methotrexate, 15 mg once weekly has been shown to be effective. Other agents being investigated include gold, hydroxychloroquine and azathioprine and cyclosporin.

Long-acting beta-adrenoreceptor agonist bronchodilators

Long-acting inhaled beta$_2$-agonists such as salmeterol are available. Salmeterol should be used in conjunction with conventional beta$_2$-agonists as the latter have a faster onset of action. The current place of salmeterol in therapy is unclear but probably should be as an addition to maximal high-dose inhaled steroids to help manage nocturnal and early morning symptoms, or instead of oral theophyllines or beta$_2$-agonists.

Acute severe asthma

The management of acute asthma depends on the severity of the attack and its response to treatment as well as an appreciation of the patient's past history and present treatment. If an acute attack becomes persistent and difficult to treat it is known as acute severe asthma.

The aims of treatment are to prevent any deterioration in the patient's condition and hasten recovery.

Prevention of an acute attack

The ideal way of treating an acute attack is to educate the patient to recognize that his/her condition is deteriorating so that treatment can be initiated by the patient to prevent the attack becoming severe.

This can be achieved with an individualized self-management plan which will be discussed later.

The doses of inhaled beta$_2$-agonist and inhaled corticosteroid should be increased and a short course of oral steroids commenced at a dose of 40 to 60 mg every morning for 1 week.

If the condition deteriorates further, hospital admission may become necessary. Ideally this should be a self-referral from the patient, responding to criteria drawn up by the doctor, such as a peak expiratory flow rate falling to 100 to 150 litres per minute. The education of patients and their relatives in the management of acute attacks should always stress the prompt initiation of further treatment and early referral.

Immediate management of acute severe asthma

The immediate treatment of acute severe asthma should take place in the patient's home, during the ambulance journey or immediately on admission to hospital. One suggested treatment protocol is outlined in Figure 22.3.

Oxygen is administered in a high concentration, at high flow rates, whenever possible. A nebulized beta$_2$-agonist is administered, which should give prompt bronchodilatation lasting for 4 to 6 hours.

Nebulizers are used in preference to conventional inhalers because they permit a high dose (10 to 20 times the dose of a metered dose inhaler) and they require no coordination on the part of the patient between inspiration and actuation which is helpful in those distressed or for those who panic. Patients undergoing an acute attack often have an inspiratory rate which is too low to use a metered-dose inhaler effectively. If a nebulizer is not immediately available, multiple actuations of a metered-dose inhaler into a large volume spacing device is an acceptable alternative. Salbutamol at doses of 2 to 5 mg (20 to 50 puffs, given five puffs at a time in the spacer) is used.

Corticosteroids are also given in the acute attack. Intravenous hydrocortisone 3 to 4 mg/kg (commonly 200 mg), oral prednisolone 0.6 mg/kg (commonly 40 to 60 mg) or both are given. These reduce and prevent the inflammation that causes oedema and hypersecretion of mucus and hence help to relieve the resultant smooth muscle spasm. The clinical response to both oral and parenteral steroids has an onset at 1 to 2 hours with a peak effect at 6 to 8 hours.

If life-threatening features are present, such as cyanosis, bradycardia, confusion, exhaustion or unconsciousness, intravenous bronchodilators

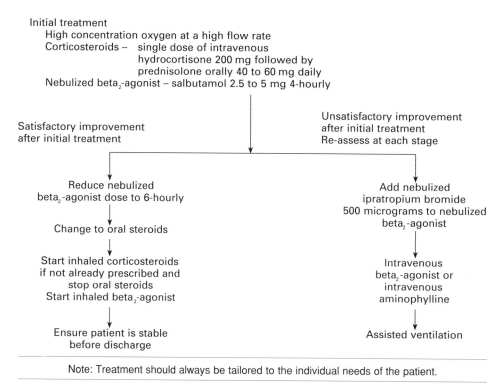

Initial treatment
    High concentration oxygen at a high flow rate
    Corticosteroids –   single dose of intravenous
                             hydrocortisone 200 mg followed by
                             prednisolone orally 40 to 60 mg daily
    Nebulized beta$_2$-agonist – salbutamol 2.5 to 5 mg 4-hourly

Satisfactory improvement
after initial treatment

Unsatisfactory improvement
after initial treatment
Re-assess at each stage

Reduce nebulized
beta$_2$-agonist dose to 6-hourly

Change to oral steroids

Start inhaled corticosteroids
if not already prescribed and
stop oral steroids
Start inhaled beta$_2$-agonist

Ensure patient is stable
before discharge

Add nebulized
ipratropium bromide
500 micrograms to nebulized
beta$_2$-agonist

Intravenous
beta$_2$-agonist or
intravenous
aminophylline

Assisted ventilation

Note: Treatment should always be tailored to the individual needs of the patient.

Fig. 22.3 Guidelines for the management of acute severe asthma in adults.

can be used. Intravenous aminophylline can be given with a bolus dose of 250 mg over 30 minutes. A beta$_2$-agonist such as salbutamol 200 micrograms over 10 minutes is often preferred if the patient is already taking an oral theophylline. Potential adverse effects of intravenous beta$_2$-agonists include cardiovascular effects such as tremor and tachycardia and metabolic effects such as hypokalaemia.

Antibiotics are only indicated where there is evidence of a bacterial infection.

Subsequent management of acute severe asthma

The subsequent management depends on the patient's clinical response. All patients should be monitored throughout their treatment with objective measures of their peak expiratory flow rates before and after bronchodilator treatment and with continual monitoring of their arterial blood gas concentrations to ensure adequate

oxygen is being given. Initially, beta$_2$-agonists are given every 4 hours, and the corticosteroids given orally every morning or every 6 hours if intravenous treatment is required, for example in very severe asthma or if the patient is vomiting.

If the response to the initial treatment is good, treatment is tailed off gradually. Intravenous steroids are discontinued, oral and inhaled steroids started if indicated, and the nebulized beta$_2$-agonist is reduce in frequency to 6-hourly. As improvement continues, an inhaled beta$_2$-agonist is substituted for the nebulized form and the oral corticosteroids stopped or reduced to a maintenance dose if clinically necessary.

If the patient's condition has not responded to the initial treatment within 15 to 30 minutes, nebulized ipratropium bromide 500 micrograms may be given together with each beta$_2$-agonist dose. The addition of the anticholinergic often gives a response that is greater than that of the two agents used alone. Intravenous aminophylline or intravenous beta$_2$-agonist is then added

Table 22.7 Intravenous aminophylline dosing in acute severe asthma

	Aminophylline dose	Patient characteristics
Loading dose	6 mg/kg over 10–15 minutes	Adults and children
	3 mg/kg over 10–15 minutes	Previous theophylline therapy
Maintenance dose	0.5 mg/kg/hour	Non-smoking adults
	0.7 mg/kg/hour	Children under 12 and smokers
	0.2 mg/kg/hour	Cardiac failure, liver impairment, pneumonia

if progress is still unsatisfactory. Both drugs may be used earlier if life-threatening signs such as cyanosis, bradycardia or exhaustion are seen. The choice between intravenous aminophylline and beta$_2$-agonist depends on concurrent therapy and side effect profiles.

The dose of intravenous aminophylline used must also take into account recent theophylline therapy in addition to other factors (see Table 22.7). Serious toxicity can occur with parenteral aminophylline and patients must be carefully monitored for nausea and vomiting, the most common early signs of toxicity. If the aminophylline infusion is continued for more than 24 hours, the serum theophylline level may be measured to maintain the serum theophylline level in the optimum range of 10 to 20 mg/L.

Further deterioration in the condition may require assisted mechanical ventilation on an intensive care unit. Regular monitoring of arterial blood gases and oxygen saturation are performed to help detect any deterioration in condition.

As the patient responds to treatment infusions can be stopped and other treatment changed or tailed off as described above. Throughout the treatment programme potential drug interactions should be anticipated and managed appropriately (see Table 22.8).

All patients should have their inhaler technique checked and any observed deficiencies corrected before discharge. A self-management plan should be drawn up and discussed with each patient.

THE PATIENT

The correct use of drugs and the education of patients is the cornerstone of the management of asthma. There are three main steps in the education of the asthmatic patient:

1. The patient should have an understanding of the action of each of the medicines they use.
2. The appropriate choice of inhalation device(s) should be made and the patient educated to use them correctly.
3. An individualized self-management plan should be developed for each patient.

Several groups of health-care professionals should contribute to the education process including pharmacists, clinicians, nurses and physiotherapists, each imparting their own specialist knowledge to the patient.

Patient knowledge of asthma treatment

Increasing the knowledge of patients about their asthma therapy is a necessary component of asthma management. However, education alone has not been shown to have a beneficial effect on morbidity. Education programmes must, therefore, also look at modifying a patient's behaviour and attitude to asthma. Counselling should lead to increased patient confidence in the ability to self-manage asthma, decrease hospital admission rates and emergency visits by general practitioners, increase compliance and improve quality of life.

Specific counselling on drug therapy should concentrate on three areas; drugs used to relieve symptoms, drugs used to prevent asthma attacks and those drugs which are given only as reserve treatment for severe attacks.

Choice of inhalation device

The choice of a suitable inhalation device is vital in the management of a patient's asthma. The incorrect use of inhalers will lead to suboptimal treatment. This has been demonstrated to occur in up to 75% of patients using metered dose inhalers. Several factors need to be considered

Table 22.8 Common interactions with drugs used in the management of asthma

Drug	Interacting drug	Probable mechanism and clinical result
Beta$_2$-agonists	Corticosteroids	Increased risk of hypokalaemia with high dose corticosteroids
	Theophylline	Increased risk of hypokalaemia with high dose beta$_2$-agonists
	Beta-adrenoreceptor antagonists	Antagonism of bronchodilator effect. More marked with non-selective antagonists
Corticosteroids	Antidiabetic agents	Corticosteroids have hyperglycaemic activity
	Antihypertensives	Antagonism of hypotensive effect
	Beta$_2$-agonists	Increased risk of hypokalaemia with high doses
	Carbamazepine Phenobarbitone Phenytoin Primidone Rifampicin	Reduced steroid effect due to increased metabolism
	Carbenoxolone	Increased risk of hypokalaemia
	Diuretics	Excessive potassium loss possible
	Oestrogens and oral contraceptives	Enhanced steroid effects, possibly due to reduced steroid metabolism
	Salicylates	Enhanced salicylate elimination
Theophylline	Beta-adrenoreceptor antagonists Cimetidine Ciprofloxacin Enoxacin Erythromycin Oral contraceptives Verapamil Vidarabine	Inhibition of theophylline metabolism resulting in increased plasma levels
	Barbiturates Carbamazepine Phenytoin Smoking Rifampicin	Induction of theophylline metabolism resulting in decreased plasma levels
	High dose beta$_2$-agonists	Increased risk of hypokalaemia
	Lithium carbonate	Theophylline enhances the renal clearance of lithium thus reducing serum lithium concentrations
	Thyroxine (starting thyroxine while on theophylline)	Increased theophylline elimination
Methotrexate	Non-steroidal anti-inflammatory drugs & aspirin	Increased risk of methotrexate toxicity
	Cholestyramine	Binding of methotrexate reducing the serum levels
	Probenecid	Inhibits renal secretion of methotrexate, increasing serum levels
	Live vaccines	Immunosuppression by methotrexate increases risk of infections from live vaccines

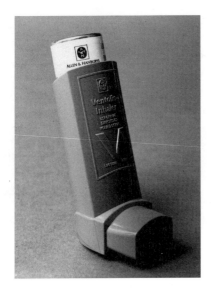

Fig. 22.4 Pressurized, metered-dose inhaler.

when choosing the appropriate device including the patient's age, severity of disease, manual dexterity and coordination.

Metered-dose aerosol inhalers

The pressurized, metered-dose inhaler (MDI), illustrated in Figure 22.4, is the most widely prescribed inhalation device. It contains a suspension of active drug, with a particle size of 2 to 5 microns, in a liquefied freon propellant. Operation of the device releases a metered dose of the drug with a droplet size of 35 to 45 microns. The increased droplet size is due to the propellant which evaporates when expelled from the inhaler.

MDIs have the advantage of being multidose, small and widely available for most of the drugs used for asthma management. Their main disadvantage is that correct use requires a good technique, mainly coordinating the beginning of inspiration with the actuation of the inhaler. Even when this is done correctly MDIs only deliver around 10% of drug to the airways with 80% deposited in the oropharynx. Other disadvantages include irritation in the pharynx and

bronchi which inhibits further inspiration and is caused by the cold propellant. Corticosteroids administered by MDI can cause dysphonia and oral candidiasis. The candidiasis can be minimized either by counselling patients to gargle with water after using the inhaler and to expel the water from the mouth afterwards, or by using a spacer device.

Technique for using metered-dose inhalers:

1. MDIs have a mouthpiece dust-cap which has to be removed before use. Often this is not performed by patients.
2. The MDI must be vigorously shaken. This distributes the drug particles uniformly throughout the propellant. The MDI must be held upright.
3. The patient should breathe out gently, but not fully.
4. The tongue should be placed on the floor of the mouth and the inhaler placed between the lips which are then closed round the mouthpiece.

Holding the inhaler 3 to 4 cm away from the mouth has been advocated to give the propellant time to evaporate, thus slowing down the aerosol, reducing the oropharyngeal deposition and increasing the deposition in the lungs. This 'advanced technique' also requires careful instruction, to avoid spraying the aerosol on to the tongue or face.

5. The patient should now start to breathe in slowly and deeply through the mouth.
6. The canister is pressed to release the dose whilst the patient continues to breathe in. This synchronization of inspiration and actuation, so that there is a supporting stream of air to carry the drug to the lungs, is probably the most common failure in those with bad inhalation technique. Asthmatics very short of breath, for example during a severe attack, find this particularly difficult.
7. The breath is held for at least 10 seconds. This allows the drug particles reaching the periphery of the lung to settle under gravity. Using this technique around 15% of a dose may reach the lungs. Exhalation should be through the nose.

8. If a second dose is called for, at least 1 minute should elapse before repeating the inhalation procedure. During actuation, the temperature of the MDI actuator stem and valve drops and should theoretically be allowed to warm up. In practice, however, this may not be very important.

Studies indicate that personal tuition does improve inhaler technique. Other methods of instruction include videos, package inserts and information leaflets or booklets provided by the pharmaceutical industry and the National Asthma Campaign.

The scoring of inhalation technique has been advocated using checklists (see Table 22.9) which can be kept as a permanent record by any of the health-care professionals.

Metered-dose inhaler with a spacer extension

Extension devices allow greater evaporation of the propellant, so reducing particle size and velocity. This also reduces oropharyngeal deposition and potentially increases lung deposition. Oral candidiasis and dysphonia (impaired voice) from inhaled corticosteroids may be reduced by using these devices. Spacers are useful for people who have poor coordination between inspiration and actuation. Several types are available.

A 10 cm long, 80 ml tube spacer is available as an integral part of the design of some MDIs, as illustrated in Figure 22.5. This tube is collaps-

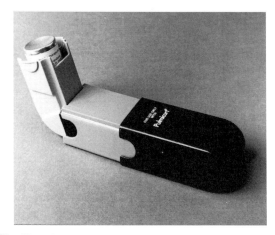

Fig. 22.5 Spacer extension as integral part of metered-dose inhaler.

ible and hence easily portable. Some coordination between inspiration and inhalation is required. The tube spacer has been shown to be superior to conventional MDIs in increasing the forced expiratory volume in one second (FEV_1) in children and has been used to try to compensate for poor inhalation technique in adults.

Large volume (750 ml) spacers are available. The Volumatic (see Fig. 22.6) and the Nebuhaler are two such devices. These have one-way inhalation valves which allow several inhalations of one dose from the spacer's chamber. No coordination is required between actuation of the MDI and inhalation. This type of spacer has been shown to produce greater bronchodilatation than either a conventional MDI or a nebulizer. A large volume spacer has been used instead of a nebulizer to deliver high doses of

---

Table 22.9 MDI technique score chart

1. Shake vigorously
2. Remove cap
3. Hold upright
4. Breathe out gently, not fully
5. Start breathing in slowly & deeply
6. Actuate during inspiration
7. Continue slow inhalation
8. No aerosol loss is visible
9. Hold breath 10 seconds
10. Next dose after 1 minute

Score 1 for each correct step undertaken

This gives a score out of 10 which can be used to monitor a patient's performance and highlight any problem areas.

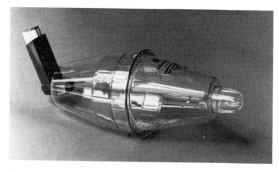

Fig. 22.6 Large volume spacer (Volumatic).

a beta$_2$-agonist in acute severe asthma attacks. The disadvantage of these devices is their large size which renders them less portable.

Breath-actuated metered-dose inhalers

This is a MDI which is fired by a spring mechanism, triggered by inspiratory flow rates of 22 to 36 L/minute. It eliminates the need for coordination of inspiration–actuation.

Dry powder inhalers

Several types of breath-operated dry powder inhalers are available. These are freon propellant free and are designed to be easier to use than conventional MDIs. They are useful for those with difficulties in coordinating MDIs and can be used by children as young as 2 years old.

In dry powder inhalers, such as the one illustrated in Figure 22.7, the drug is supplied in a gelatin capsule which is pierced or broken by the device and inhaled by fast inspiration of more than 60 L/minute. It is important to regularly clean these inhalers to avoid the powder clogging the device. Multiple-dose dry powder

devices are also available, one of these is illustrated in Figure 22.8.

Nebulizers

A nebulizer produces an aerosol by blowing air or oxygen through a solution to produce droplets of 5 microns or less in size. Nebulizers require little coordination from the patient as any drug is inhaled through a face mask or mouthpiece using normal tidal breathing. Only around 13% of the dose used is deposited in the lungs but because the doses used are higher than those used in other aerosol devices, patients will receive 10 to 20 times the dose received from a MDI.

Nebulizers are, therefore, useful in patients who are unable to use conventional inhalers, for example children under 2 years old, patients with severe attacks of asthma unable to produce sufficient inspiratory effort and those lacking the coordination to use other inhalers. Nebulized bronchodilators can be used in acute severe asthma attacks, often avoiding the need for intravenous drugs, and in conjunction with prophylactic agents in the treatment of chronic

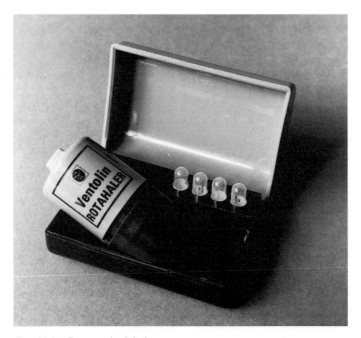

Fig. 22.7 Dry powder inhaler.

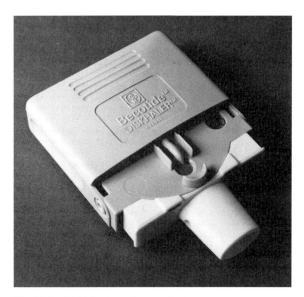

Fig. 22.8 Multiple dose dry powder inhaler.

asthma unresponsive to or poorly controlled by conventional treatment.

Most of the beta$_2$-agonists as well as ipratropium bromide, beclomethasone, budesonide and sodium cromoglycate are available for nebulization. The majority of these preparations are made up in isotonic 0.9% sodium chloride and are available in preservative-free, unit dose presentations. The use of solutions which are either hypertonic or hypotonic (particularly after dilution with water) or contain a preservative such as benzalkonium chloride or EDTA have been associated with bronchoconstriction.

The safe and correct use of nebulizers requires careful counselling, especially if they are to be used in the home environment. The following points are critical for the correct use of a nebulizer:

1. Nebulizers should only be driven by compressed air or by oxygen at flow rates of at least 5 to 6 L/minute to ensure that droplets of the correct size are produced.

2. For all drugs a minimum volume of 3 to 4 ml should be nebulized, using 0.9% sodium chloride as a diluent if necessary. This volume is required to reduce the amount of drug which is unavoidably left in a 'dead-space' fluid volume of around 1 ml at the end of nebulization. The side of the nebulizer should be repeatedly tapped

during use to ensure that no fluid builds up on the sides of the nebulizer chamber.

3. Most nebulizer chambers are disposable but will last 3 to 4 months when used by a patient at home. The chamber must be emptied after use and each day the chamber should be rinsed in hot water and dried by blowing air through the device. Several centres advocate that once a week the chamber should be sterilized using 0.02% hypochlorite to prevent bacterial contamination. The chamber is then thoroughly rinsed to remove all traces of hypochlorite and then dried.

4. The nebulizer should be serviced at least once a year.

5. Each patient should be given a self-management plan for the correct use of his/her nebulizer. If the nebulizer is only for use in severe attacks, the patient should be advised to use it only when the peak flow reading falls below a specified amount and not to exceed a maximum dose, e.g. 5 mg salbutamol. Patients must be informed to contact their doctor if the nebulizer fails to give the expected relief or the relief lasts for less than 4 hours.

There are disadvantages with the use of nebulizers. There may be overreliance on the nebulizer by the patient which can result in a delay in seeking medical advice, whilst the high doses of bronchodilators used increase the incidence of side effects.

Self-management plans

Every asthmatic should have an individualized self-management plan. These plans are a means of giving the patient more confidence by involving them in the management of their own asthma. The patient should then be able to deal with any fluctuation in his/her condition and know when to seek medical advice.

Key elements of a self-management plan include being able to monitor their symptoms, peak flow measurements, drug usage and knowing how to deal with fluctuations in severity of their asthma according to written guidance. Symptom diaries, treatment/management guidance cards and peak flow reading diary cards are available from the National Asthma

Campaign and from some of the pharmaceutical companies who manufacture asthma products.

A self-management plan would also include details of when to increase the dose of an inhaled steroid, when to take a short course of oral corticosteroids and when to use a nebulizer, how to monitor the effects of the nebulized dose and when to self-refer to a general practitioner or local hospital.

CASE STUDIES

CASE 22.1

L. J. is a 7-year-old schoolgirl. She suffers from mild childhood asthma, mainly induced by exercise. She currently uses a metered-dose inhaler containing 500 micrograms terbutaline per actuation at a dose of one inhalation when required.

However, L. J.'s symptoms have gradually become more frequent over the last few months. She has episodes of wheezing every 3 to 4 weeks, occurring during exercise and at rest. She is also having more time off school because of her asthma.

Q1 What treatment should L. J. now be given?

Q2 If, after 3 months, the symptoms have not reduced in frequency and wheezing is particularly troublesome in the mornings, what other treatment should be given?

CASE 22.2

J. R., a 16-year-old girl, was admitted via the accident and emergency department severely short of breath and unable to speak. She had a respiratory rate of 36 breaths per minute using accessory respiratory muscles, a pulse rate of 160 beats per minute and a pulsus paradoxus of 22 mmHg.

She is a non-smoker and normally uses a salbutamol inhaler 200 micrograms 6-hourly, ipratropium bromide inhaler 40 micrograms 6-hourly, beclomethasone inhaler 500 micrograms 6-hourly, sustained-release theophylline 250 mg twice daily and is currently taking pivampicillin 500 mg twice daily for a suspected pulmonary infection.

She was diagnosed as having acute severe asthma. Her immediate treatment was:

- 35% Oxygen
- Salbutamol 5 mg via a nebulizer
- Hydrocortisone 200 mg i.v.
- Ampicillin 500 mg i.v.

Q How should J. R.'s initial management be continued?

CASE 22.3

Mrs C. N. (age 24 years) was admitted to hospital with an acute exacerbation of asthma. She was first diagnosed as being asthmatic at the age of 6 years. Recently the disease has become progressively worse and required numerous hospital admissions. On this admission her drug therapy was as follows:

- **Salbutamol MDI 200 micrograms four times a day**
- **Ipratropium bromide MDI 40 micrograms four times a day**
- **Beclomethasone MDI 200 micrograms four times a day**
- **Prednisolone tablets 10 mg every morning**
- **Ranitidine tablets 150 mg twice a day.**

On examination she was found to be very anxious, tachypnoeic, cyanosed and unable to speak. She was pyrexial (temperature 40°C) and had coughed up a small amount of cloudy sputum. Her PEFR was unrecordable. Her blood pressure was normal (120/70 mmHg) with 20 mm of paradox. Chest X-ray showed no evidence of pneumonia. Her blood gases were PCO_2 = 7.49 kPa (high), PO_2 = 14.50 kPa (normal), pH = 7.3 (low), HCO_3^- = 23 mmol/L (low end of normal range).

Q1 What is the most appropriate first course of action in this patient?

Q2 Explain how respiratory acidosis has occurred.

CASE 22.4

A. F. is 27-year-old man who suffers from chronic, severe asthma with acute exacerbations. He has no known allergies and his asthma is considered to be intrinsic rather than extrinsic. His previous treatment has included various bronchodilators and inhaled steroid preparations. Over the last 2 years his asthma has deteriorated further and regular oral steroids have been used. Increasing doses have been required and there is concern about short-term and long-term side effects. His current therapy is:

- Salbutamol nebules 5 mg four times a day
- Beclomethasone inhaler 1 mg twice daily
- Aminophylline modified-release tablets 450 mg twice daily
- Methotrexate tablets 15 mg once a week
- Prednisolone tablets 10 mg once daily
- Amiloride tablets 5 mg once a day.

Q1 What is the role of methotrexate and other steroid-sparing agents in the treatment of severe, chronic asthma?

Q2 Why is amiloride used in this case?

ANSWERS TO CASE STUDIES

CASE 22.1

A1 Inhaled beta$_2$-agonists are the initial treatment of choice in children with infrequent asthma or mild exercise-induced asthma when they are given prior to exercise. If symptoms occur with greater frequency than every 4 to 6 weeks, prophylactic treatment, as well as bronchodilator treatment, is necessary. Inhaled sodium cromoglycate is the usual first treatment of choice for prophylaxis and is effective in up to 70% of children. Dry powder (20 mg 6-to 8-hourly) or breath-actuated (5 to 10 mg 6-to 8-hourly) inhalers could be tried for L. J.

A2 A 6- to 8-week trial is sufficient to see if sodium cromoglycate will be effective. If this proves not to be the case it should be stopped and inhaled corticosteroids should be used in preference to oral therapy due to the high incidence of side effects with oral dosing. With inhaled corticosteroid therapy, clinically significant side effects are rare at doses of less than 1 mg per day. Concern has been expressed about inhaled steroids having a detrimental effect on growth but this has not been causally established (asthma itself can stunt growth).

Nocturnal and early morning symptoms which persist despite maximal steroid and bronchodilator treatment will often respond to slow-release beta$_2$-agonists or slow-release theophylline, given as a single night-time dose. Oral therapy will result in a greater incidence of side effects which will need monitoring. Children metabolize theophylline relatively quickly compared with adults and serum levels may be required for nocturnal doses and when using theophylline more frequently.

CASE 22.2

A High-dose bronchodilators should be used in acute severe asthma. In the hospital situation these are normally given by nebulization. In J. R.'s case she should be given salbutamol 2.5 mg 4-hourly and ipratropium bromide 500 micrograms 4-hourly. This combination gives synergistic bronchodilator activity. In practice both solutions are usually mixed immediately prior to administration, this is not recommended by the manufacturers but is widely performed. The solution is nebulized 'to dryness', when no mist is being produced. This results in around 1 ml of solution left in the chamber (the dead space).

J. R. could also be given a salbutamol infusion at an initial rate of 5 micrograms per minute. Salbutamol is preferred as she is already taking oral theophylline therapy. Intravenous salbutamol has been shown to be more effective than nebulized salbutamol in acute severe asthma but has higher incidence of side effects, notably tachycardia. Hypokalaemia is also a complication of both nebulized and intravenous salbutamol and some clinicians routinely give an infusion of potassium chloride to counteract this.

Oral prednisolone, 40 mg daily should also be given. If the patient can swallow oral medication no benefit is gained by using intravenous corticosteroids. When the acute exacerbation is resolved, J. R.'s steroid dose should be stopped. Other treatment used could include amoxycillin 500 mg 8-hourly for the pulmonary infection together with her usual sustained-release theophylline 250 mg twice daily.

Inhaled beclomethasone (twice daily, not four times daily as on admission) salbutamol and ipratropium bromide could be recommended on day 4. Salmeterol could also be started at 100 micrograms twice daily.

CASE 22.3

A1 A management plan should be drawn up. The patient's arterial blood gases should be regularly monitored. Oxygen should be administered via a face mask (e.g. 28% oxygen) and blood gases should be checked after 30 minutes. Mechanical ventilation should be considered if the blood gases deteriorate further. Drug therapy should be administered either intravenously or by nebulizer, e.g. salbutamol 5 mg nebulizer 4-hourly, ipratropium bromide 500 micrograms nebulized 6-hourly, hydrocortisone 200 mg intravenously 6-hourly and aminophylline 6 mg/kg intravenously over 20 minutes followed by 500 microgram/kg/hour by continuous intravenous infusion (she has not previously been treated with theophylline). Intravenous fluid replacement may be necessary as patients with acute severe asthma can become dehydrated due to increased respiratory fluid loss and sweating.

A2 Respiratory acidosis occurs when CO_2 is not effectively removed from the body. Normally the CO_2, which is produced from dietary protein and tissue metabolism, is removed via the lungs during ventilation. If there is a deficit in ventilation (such as occurs due to bronchoconstriction) CO_2 will be retained resulting in an elevated PCO_2 in arterial blood. CO_2 combines with water to form carbonic acid which dissociates to form hydrogen ions ($CO_2 + H_2O \rightleftharpoons H_2CO_3 \rightleftharpoons H + HCO_3^-$). Therefore excess CO_2 leads to a fall in pH until compensatory mechanisms occur. Compensation includes excretion of hydrogen ions and generation of bicarbonate ions by the kidneys in an attempt to neutralize the pH. Renal compensation had not yet occurred in Mrs C. N. as her plasma bicarbonate was not elevated. Acidosis should be corrected to prevent neurological symptoms (ranging from anxiety and confusion to seizures and coma). Mechanical ventilation may be required to correct the acidosis.

CASE 22.4

A1 Methotrexate is thought to have an anti-inflammatory as well as an immunosuppressant effect. Studies have shown that low oral doses such as 15 mg per week may allow a reduction of the prednisolone dose by one-third. The mechanism of action is not certain, though its anti-inflammatory effect seems to be important for this particular indication. Long-term use has not yet been established due to the many side effects of this drug. These include gastrointestinal disturbance, skin rashes, renal and liver impairment and myelosuppression. Regular assessment of the patient is required. Full blood count, urea, creatinine and electrolyte levels as well as liver function tests need to be measured.

Hydroxychloroquine is an immunosuppressant and also an anti-inflammatory agent. It is thought to inhibit enzymes which normally lead to the production of arachidonic acid and the bronchoconstricting leukotrienes. However, its use is limited by side effects including gastrointestinal disturbances and skin reactions and, in long-term use, retinopathy. Regular ophthalmic examination is required during treatment. Response to hydroxychloroquine, when used for its licensed indications, often takes 4 to 6 weeks. Therefore it is likely that some time will elapse before respiratory function is seen to improve. Doses of 300 to 400 mg daily for several months have been used. Studies have shown that oral prednisolone doses could be decreased by up to a half. Further studies are required to establish a role for this drug in asthma therapy.

A third drug, auranofin, has also been examined for its steroid-sparing activity. It has been shown to inhibit antibody production as well as reducing the release of lysosomal enzymes and inflammatory mediators from macrophages and mast cells. These properties may explain the potential steroid-sparing activity of auranofin. Serious side effects again limit its use. They include diarrhoea, abdominal pain, blood dyscrasias, proteinuria, dermatitis and pruritus. Therefore, regular monitoring of full blood count and urinalysis are required when auranofin is used. Immediate improvement in respiratory function tests is not seen although some improvement can be expected after 12 weeks' treatment. Studies have shown some benefit in steroid-dependent asthma. However, as with methotrexate and hydroxychloroquine, the value of auranofin has yet to be established in longer-term studies.

A2 Beta$_2$-agonists such as salbutamol can activate the sodium–potassium pump, increasing potassium transport into the cells. Long-term hypokalaemia should be prevented (which can lead to hypotension and arrhythmias as well as flaccid paralysis). Amiloride has only mild diuretic activity but inhibits potassium excretion in the distal tubules of the kidneys.

BIBLIOGRAPHY

Barnes P J. A new approach to the treatment of asthma. New England Journal of Medicine 1989; 321: 1517–1527

British Thoracic Society, British Paediatric Association, Research Unit of the Royal College of Physicians of London, King's Fund Centre, National Asthma Campaign, Royal College of General Practitioners, General Practitioners in Asthma Group, British Association of Accident and Emergency Medicine and British Paediatric Respiratory Group. Guidelines on the management of asthma. Thorax 1993; 48 (suppl): S1–S24

Clark T J H (ed). Steroids in asthma: a reappraisal in the light of inhalation therapy. Auckland, NZ: ADIS Press Limited 1983

Clark T J H, Cochrane G M (eds). Bronchodilator therapy: the basis of asthma and chronic obstructive airways disease management. Auckland, NZ: ADIS Press Limited 1984

Crompton G K, McHardy G J R. Diseases of the respiratory system. In: MacLeod J, Edwards C, Bouchier I (eds) Davidson's principles and practice of medicine. London: Churchill Livingstone 1987; 197–268

Kelly H W, Hill M R. Asthma. In: DiPiro J T, Talbert R L, Hayes P E, Yee G C, Matzke G R, Posey L M (eds) Pharmacotherapy – a pathophysiological approach. New York: Elsevier 1992; 408–449

National Heart, Lung, and Blood Institute, National Institutes of Health. International consensus report on diagnosis and treatment of asthma. European Respiratory Journal 1992; 5: 601–641

Phelan P D. Asthma in children. Medicine International 1991; (89): 3703–3707

Tattersfield A. Asthma in adults. Medicine International 1991; (89): 3708–3712

Chapter 23

Chronic obstructive airways disease

K. P. Gibbs   J. C. Portlock

Chronic obstructive airways disease (COAD) is an umbrella term which includes a number of respiratory diseases. Alternative terms include chronic obstructive pulmonary disease (COPD) and chronic obstructive lung disease (COLD). Bronchitis and emphysema are the two main conditions which are considered in this category. The two conditions often occur together although it is easier to describe them separately when discussing pathophysiology, aetiology and clinical manifestations. In fact, pure chronic bronchitis or pure emphysema, are less common and it is likely that a patient will exhibit signs and symptoms of both conditions with one condition predominating.

Chronic bronchitis is diagnosed after determination of the symptoms. The accepted definition is 'a chronic or recurrent cough with expectoration on most days for at least 3 months of the year during at least 2 consecutive years'. Emphysema is defined as a permanent change in the anatomy of the lungs with enlargement and destruction of the alveoli and respiratory bronchioles which results in deterioration in gas exchange and impaired ventilation.

EPIDEMIOLOGY

Chronic bronchitis has been a major cause of mortality in Europe for at least two centuries. It affects all industrialized countries and is the largest single cause of lost working days in Great Britain.

Respiratory diseases including chronic bronchitis are more common in areas of high atmospheric pollution and in dusty occupations, e.g. foundry workers and coal miners. Areas of Northern England and Scotland which are highly industrialized show the highest incidence of chronic obstructive airways disease. Smoking is one of the most important risk factors and is now considered to be more important than air pollution. In fact, the highest incidence of COAD occurs where a combination of air pollution and a high incidence of smoking occur together. It has been calculated that COAD results in 14% of all non-violent deaths in Great Britain.

AETIOLOGY
Chronic bronchitis

Chronic bronchitis is associated with cigarette smoking and air pollution. Normally cilia and mucus in the bronchi protect against inhaled irritants which are trapped and expectorated. Persistent irritation such as that caused by cigarette smoke causes an exaggeration in the response of these protective mechanisms. Hypersecretion of mucus results from hypertrophy and proliferation of mucus-producing glands. Cigarette smoke also inhibits mucociliary clearance which causes a further build-up of mucus in the lungs. Irritation from smoke leads to inflammation of the small bronchioles (bronchiolitis) and alveoli (alveolitis). As a result macrophages and neutrophils infiltrate the epithelium and trigger a degree of epithelial destruction. This, together with a proliferation of mucus-producing cells, leads to plugging of smaller bronchioles and alveoli with mucus and particulate matter.

There are a number of other risk factors for the development of bronchitis. It is known that not all smokers with a similar smoking history develop the same degree of pulmonary impairment.

An additional risk factor is the natural ageing process of the lungs. Males are currently more at risk of developing chronic bronchitis but as the number of females who smoke increases the incidence of chronic bronchitis in females will also rise. Occupational exposure to chemical fumes

and dust are established risk factors for chronic airflow obstruction and increased mortality from COAD. Other risk factors are shown in Table 23.1.

Emphysema

Emphysema has a different aetiology to chronic bronchitis but is often found to coexist with it. Emphysema results from a gradually progressive loss of elastic tissue within the lungs due to an imbalance between proteolytic enzymes and protective factors. Macrophages and neutrophils release lysosomal enzymes such as elastase which are capable of destroying connective tissue in the lungs. Under normal circumstances a protective factor called α_1-antitrypsin (or α_1-protease inhibitor) inhibits proteolytic enzymes and so prevents damage. A deficiency of α_1-antitrypsin is known to predispose to emphysema. Measurement of α_1-antitrypsin is sometimes useful in younger patients since it may indicate those who are predisposed to emphysema caused by smoking. Cigarette smoke has been shown to inactivate this protein. Its production is determined by the protease inhibitor gene (M). One in 2500 individuals are homozygous for the recessive (Z) gene which causes low blood levels of α_1-antitrypsin (10 to 15% of normal levels) and can result in early emphysema. Heterozygous individuals with the MZ gene also have an established risk of emphysema which is increased by smoking. It is thought that females may have

---

Table 23.1   Risk factors for the development of chronic obstructive airways disease

Smoking
Age
Male gender
Existing impaired lung function
Occupation
α_1-antitrypsin deficiency
Air pollution
Alcohol consumption
Race
Nutritional status
Family history
Socioeconomic status
Recurrent respiratory tract infection

protection conferred by oestrogen which stimulates the synthesis of protease inhibitors such as α_1-antitrypsin.

PATHOPHYSIOLOGY

Bronchitis

There are two pathological processes underlying the development of chronic bronchitis. The first is a hypersecretory disorder characterized by expectoration with increasing susceptibility to respiratory infections. The second is an obstructive disorder which results from smooth muscle constriction and may or may not be associated with emphysema. Bronchoconstriction is not apparent in all patients but where it does occur it adds further to deterioration in ventilation.

Hypersecretion of thick and viscous mucus results from proliferation of the mucus-secreting glands and goblet cells in the bronchial epithelium. Excessive mucus production is not thought to contribute significantly to airways obstruction although it does cause distension of the alveoli and loss of their gas exchange function. Pus and infected mucus accumulate leading to recurrent or chronic viral and bacterial infections. The primary pathogen is usually viral but bacterial infection often follows. Common bacterial pathogens include *Streptococcus pneumoniae* and *Haemophilus influenzae*. Ulceration occurs where there is a focal point for infection and/or inflammation. Normal columnar epithelium may be replaced by squamous epithelium.

In addition, thickening of the bronchiole and alveolar walls results from chronic inflammation and oedema. This leads to blockage and obstruction of the airways. Alveolar distension and destruction results in distortion of the blood vessels which are closely associated with the alveoli. This causes a rise in the blood pressure in the pulmonary circulation. Reduction in gas diffusion across the alveolar epithelium leads to a low partial pressure of oxygen in the blood vessels (hypoxaemia) due to an imbalance between ventilation and perfusion. By a mechanism which is not clearly established, chronic vasoconstriction results and causes a further increase in blood

pressure and further compromises gas diffusion from air spaces into the blood stream. The chronic low oxygen levels lead to polycythaemia (increase in number of erythrocytes) which makes the blood more viscous. The result of increased pulmonary blood pressure and increased blood viscosity is an increase in right ventricular pressure within the heart. The consequence of continued high right ventricular pressure is eventual myocardial hypertrophy and progressive right ventricular failure (cor pulmonale).

Bronchiectasis is a pathological change in the lungs where the bronchi become permanently dilated. It is common after early attacks of acute bronchitis during which mucus both plugs and stretches the bronchial walls. In severe infections the bronchioles and alveoli can become permanently damaged and do not return to their normal size and shape. The loss of muscle tone and loss of cilia can contribute to COAD because mucus has a tendency to accumulate in the dilated bronchi.

Emphysema

Emphysema is a term used to describe progressive destruction of the respiratory bronchioles, the alveolar duct and alveolar sac. Adjacent alveoli can become indistinguishable from each other with two main consequences. The first is loss of available gas exchange surfaces which leads to an increase in dead space and impaired gas exchange. The second consequence is the loss of elastic recoil in the small airways (vital for maintaining the force of expiration) which leads to a tendency for them to collapse particularly during expiration. Increased thoracic gas volume and hyperinflation of the lungs results.

There are two main types of emphysema. Centrilobular emphysema involves the destruction of respiratory bronchioles, due to lack of α_1-antitrypsin, although alveoli are not generally destroyed. This type of emphysema is especially common in the upper lobes of the lungs of cigarette smokers and coal miners. Panlobular (panacinar) emphysema is also associated with α_1-antitrypsin deficiency but in this case the alveoli are also affected. As described above, macrophages and neutrophils release the proteo-lytic enzyme elastase which is normally inhib-ited by α_1-antitrypsin. Evidence suggests that macrophages and neutrophils release a greater amount of elastase in response to smoke in smokers than in non-smokers. Elastase breaks down elastin which is an integral protein of the alveoli. In addition to destruction, matrix repair may be inhibited particularly amongst those who smoke cigarettes. In emphysema destruc-tion of the alveoli also results in the loss of the capillary network essential for adequate perfu-sion. The decrease in lung perfusion along with loss of ventilation capacity due to loss of elastic recoil means that, unlike bronchitis, the ventila-tion/perfusion ratio is normally maintained. Therefore the patient with emphysema experi-ences greater dyspnoea than a bronchitic, but is better able to preserve gas exchange as the res-piratory centres are more responsive to lack of oxygen in the tissues (hypoxia). As a result, pure emphysema does not tend to lead to cor pulmo-nale or polycythaemia at such an early stage as bronchitis.

CLINICAL MANIFESTATIONS

The signs and symptoms of COAD depend on whether bronchitis or emphysema predominate. Chronic bronchitic patients exhibit excess mucus production and a degree of bronchospasm re-sulting in wheeze and dyspnoea. Hypoxia and hypercapnia (high levels of carbon dioxide in the tissues) are common. This type of patient has a productive cough, is often overweight and finds physical exertion difficult due to dyspnoea. The bronchitic patient is sometimes referred to as a 'blue bloater'. This term is used because of the tendency of the patient to retain carbon di-oxide caused by a decreased responsiveness of the respiratory centre to prolonged hypoxaemia (leading to cyanosis) and also the tendency for peripheral oedema to occur. Bronchitic patients lose the ability to increase the rate and depth of ventilation in response to persistent hypoxaemia. The reason for this is not clear but decreased ventilatory drive may result from abnormal pe-ripheral or central respiratory receptors. In se-

vere disease the chest diameter is often increased giving the classical barrel chest. As obstruction worsens, hypoxaemia increases, leading to pul-monary hypertension. Right ventricular strain leads to right ventricular failure which is char-acterized by jugular venous distension, hepato-megaly and peripheral oedema all of which are consequences of an increase in systemic venous blood pressure. Recurrent lower respiratory tract infections can be severe and debilitating. Signs of infection include an increase in the volume of thick and viscous sputum which is yellow or green in colour and may contain bacterial pathogens, squamous epithelial cells, alveolar macrophages and saliva, but pyrexia may not be present.

The clinical features of emphysema are dif-ferent from those of bronchitis. A patient with emphysema will experience increasing dyspnoea even at rest but often there is minimal cough and the sputum produced is scanty and mucoid. Cough is usually more of a problem after dysp-noea is apparent. The patient will breathe rap-idly (tachypnoea) because the respiratory centres are responsive to mild hypoxaemia and he or she will have a flushed appearance. Typically a patient with emphysema will be thin and have pursed lips in an effort to compensate for a lack of elastic recoil and exhale a larger volume of air. Such a patient will tend to use the accessory muscles of the chest and neck to assist in the work of breathing. Hypoxaemia is not a problem until the disease has progressed. Pulmonary hypertension is usually mild and cor pulmonale is uncommon until the terminal stages of the disease.

Generally bronchial infections tend to be less common in emphysema. The patient with em-physema is sometimes referred to as a 'pink puffer' because he hyperventilates to compen-sate for hypoxia by breathing in short puffs. As a result he appears pink with little carbon dioxide retention and little evidence of oedema. Even-tually the patient reaches a stage where he cannot obtain enough oxygen in spite of rapid breathing.

The 'blue bloater' and 'pink puffer' represent two ends of the spectrum. In reality the underlying pathophysiology may well be a mixture and the resulting signs and symptoms will be somewhere between the two extremes described.

Two specific problems are common in patients with COAD:

- sleep apnoea syndrome
- acute respiratory failure.

Sleep apnoea syndrome is a respiratory disorder characterized by frequent or prolonged pauses in breathing during sleep. It leads to a deterioration in arterial blood gases and a decrease in the saturation of haemoglobin with oxygen. Hypoxaemia is often accompanied by pulmonary hypertension and cardiac arrhythmias which may lead to premature cardiac failure.

Acute respiratory failure is said to have occurred if the PO_2 suddenly drops and there is an increase in PCO_2 which decreases the pH to 7.30 or less. The most common cause is an acute exacerbation of chronic bronchitis with an increase in volume and viscosity of sputum. This further impairs ventilation and causes more severe hypoxaemia and hypercapnia. The clinical signs and symptoms of acute respiratory failure include restlessness, confusion, tachycardia, cyanosis, sweating, hypotension and eventual unconsciousness.

INVESTIGATIONS

Lung function tests are used to determine the severity of the respiratory disease and can also indicate response to treatment. A spirometer is used to measure lung volumes and flow rates. Various values are obtained such as:

- Tidal volume (volume of air inhaled and exhaled during normal breathing)
- Functional residual capacity (FRC – the volume of air left in the lungs after normal exhalation)
- Vital capacity (VC – the volume of air inhaled and exhaled during maximal ventilation)
- Residual volume (RV – the volume of air left in the lungs after maximal exhalation)
- Total lung capacity (TLC – the vital capacity (VC) plus the residual volume (RV)).

Normal values depend on a number of factors such as age and sex and the values obtained from the patient are usually compared to tabulated normal readings.

Vital capacity decreases in bronchitis and emphysema. Residual volume increases in both cases but tends to be higher in patients with emphysema due to air being trapped distal to the terminal bronchioles. Total lung capacity is often normal in patients with bronchitis, but is usually increased in emphysema again due to air being trapped. Other respiratory function tests which are carried out are the same as those for asthma. In patients with chronic bronchitis and/or emphysema there are reductions in FEV1 (forced expiratory volume in first second of exhalation), FVC (forced vital capacity) and FEV1/FVC ratio. The mean rate of decline in FEV1 provides a very useful measure of the progression of COAD. The major criticism of measuring FEV1 and FVC is that they detect changes only in airways greater than 2 mm in diameter. As the airways which are less than 2 mm in diameter contribute only 10 to 20% of normal resistance to airflow, there is usually severe obstruction and extensive damage to the lungs by the time the lung function tests (FEV1 and FVC) detect abnormalities. Whole body plethysmography can be used to measure airways resistance and the functional residual capacity (FRC). The patient sits in an airtight box and breathes normally. Gas flows through the mouthpiece and box pressure changes are recorded. The pressure changes within the box reflect the compression and decompression of gas in the alveoli (as the expansion of the lungs during inspiration displaces the thorax which exerts pressure on the surrounding air). Emphysema patients may have bullae within their lungs (large areas of destroyed tissue) which will contract as the patient exhales. This will result in less displacement of the thorax and abnormal values for FRC.

Arterial blood gases can be measured at rest and after exercise and are useful to determine the severity of disease and response to treatment. However, they are not considered to be useful in assessing disease progression. In a chronic bronchitic there is usually a low partial pressure of oxygen (PO_2: reference range = 12 to 16 kPa) and an elevated partial pressure of carbon dioxide (PCO_2: reference range = 4.6 to 6.0 kPa). Haemoglobin level (reference range 13.5 to 18 g/dl for an adult male) and haematocrit (reference range 40 to 80%) can increase due to polycythaemia secondary to chronic hypoxaemia. Emphysema usually leads to a higher PO_2 than is seen in patients with bronchitis and normal values for PCO_2 until later stages of the disease.

In both bronchitis and emphysema the oxygen and carbon dioxide partial pressure changes progress slowly over a period of years. The pH of blood stays near normal (pH = 7.35 to 7.45) in chronic disease because the kidneys compensate for the acidity caused by retention of carbon dioxide by retaining bicarbonate ions (reference range = 22 to 28 mmol/L). In acute respiratory failure (e.g. due to pneumonia) where PCO_2 rises rapidly there may be a temporary acidosis until the kidneys can compensate which may take more than 24 hours Acid/base defects can be corrected by mechanical ventilation to reverse carbon dioxide accumulation.

Chest X-rays reveal differences between the two disease states. A patient with emphysema will have a flattened diaphragm with a loss of peripheral vascular markings and the appearance of bullae. These are indicative of extensive trapping of air. A bronchitic patient will have increased bronchovascular markings and may also have cardiomegaly (increased cardiac size due to right ventricular failure) with prominent pulmonary arteries.

TREATMENT

The clinical progress of COAD depends on whether bronchitis or emphysema predominates. Bronchitic patients will experience an increasing frequency of exacerbations of acute dyspnoea triggered by excess mucus production and obstruction. There is a progressive decline in lung function with complications such as cor pulmonale, hypercapnia and polycythaemia. Eventually cardiorespiratory failure with hypercapnia will occur which may be severe, unresponsive to treatment and result in death.

Emphysema patients will become progressively dyspnoeic without exacerbations triggered by increased sputum production. Eventually cor pulmonale will develop very rapidly, usually in the late stages of the disease and lead to intractable hypercapnia and respiratory arrest.

Drug treatment together with other measures such as physiotherapy and artificial ventilation have been shown to lengthen survival although they do not offer a cure. However, quality of life and symptoms improve with suitable treatment and it is likely that the correct management of the patient will lead to a reduction in hospital admissions and may prevent premature death.

The aims of treatment for patients with COAD are shown in Table 23.2. Drug treatment itself can only relieve symptoms, it does not modify the underlying pathology. Most patients with COAD are considered to have irreversible obstruction compared with asthmatics, but a significant number do seem to respond to bronchodilators.

Smoking

Smoking is the most important factor in the development of obstructive airways disease. Every smoker with chronic airflow obstruction must be advised to stop smoking.

Individually targeted advice may prove to be more successful in persuading individuals to give up, especially in those motivated to do so.

There are three types of therapeutic agent designed to help people stop smoking: nicotine substitutes, nicotine replacement and aversion products, each having varying success rates.

Table 23.2   Treatment aims for patients with COAD

1. Stop cigarette smoking
2. Limit exposure to environmental or industrial pollutants
3. Correct reversible obstruction, if present (bronchodilators such as sympathomimetics, anticholinergics and corticosteroids)
4. Prevent acute exacerbations due to infection (prophylactic antibiotics are not considered suitable in most cases)
5. Maintain nutritional intake (especially in emphysema which can be associated with considerable weight loss)

Smokers who have a strong physical type of dependence will benefit from agents such as nicotine chewing gum. When the gum is chewed nicotine is released by the action of alkaline saliva. The nicotine absorbed reduces the effects associated with cigarette smoking such as irritability, sleep disturbances, fatigue, headache and increased appetite.

Antibiotics and vaccines

Prophylactic antibiotics have no place in the management of COAD. Antibiotic therapy is, however, vital if a patient develops purulent sputum. If patients frequently develop acute infective exacerbations of bronchitis they should be given a supply of antibiotics to keep at home and start on the first sign of an exacerbation.

Initial routine sputum cultures are unhelpful in these patients as they are unreliable in identifying the pathogenic organisms.

The normal pathogens involved are *Streptococcus pneumoniae, Haemophilus influenzae* or *Haemophilus catarrhalis*. The usual antibiotics of choice are ampicillin, amoxycillin, erythromycin or trimethoprim. If the infection follows influenza, *Staphylococcus aureus* may be present and an anti-staphylococcal agent such as flucloxacillin should be added to the regimen. If the infection is considered atypical in presentation or if the purulent sputum is still present after 1 week of treatment then sputum cultures should be taken to try to identify the pathogenic organisms.

The benefit of immunization in preventing acute infective exacerbations has not yet been demonstrated in all patient groups. A single dose of pneumococcal vaccine has been shown to prevent infection in the elderly and should be offered to those with chronic airflow obstruction. Influenza vaccine should also be given annually to patients with COAD and this has been shown to reduce clinical infection rates in the elderly. The prevalent strains of influenza change so the vaccine composition is, correspondingly, altered annually.

Bronchodilators

Bronchodilators in COAD are used to reverse airflow limitation. As the degree of limitation varies widely their effectiveness should be assessed in each patient using respiratory function tests and assessing any subjective improvement reported by the patient. Patients may report an improvement in exercise tolerance or relief of symptoms such as wheeze and cough. The use of diary cards to document daily symptoms may help.

Inhaled beta$_2$-adrenoreceptor agonists

Selective beta$_2$-agonists should be tried initially since they provide rapid relief and have a low incidence of side effects. The low doses of beta$_2$-agonists used in asthma such as 200 micrograms salbutamol may not be high enough for COAD; higher doses (400 to 800 micrograms) may be required. Poor patient response to bronchodilators may be due to poor inhalation technique and this should always be assessed and the inhaler device changed if necessary. If nocturnal symptoms are troublesome, oral sustained release beta$_2$-agonists could be added to the treatment regimen.

In acute exacerbations these agents may need to be administered in higher doses via a nebulizer.

Anticholinergic drugs

In COAD patients, parasympathetic (vagal) airway muscle tone is the major reversible component. Inhaled anticholinergic drugs reverse this vagal tone and have a significant bronchodilator effect, especially in the elderly. The drugs of choice are the quaternary atropine derivatives, ipratropium bromide and oxitropium, which when inhaled, give local effects with little systemic absorption. The inhaled anticholinergics have a slower onset of bronchodilatation than the beta$_2$-agonists. Higher doses of anticholinergics may be required than are used in patients with asthma, e.g. 80 to 120 micrograms ipratropium bromide.

Patients vary in their response to beta$_2$-agonists and anticholinergics. Combination therapy may produce additive bronchodilatation but responses must always be properly assessed.

Theophyllines

Theophylline and aminophylline are weak bronchodilators and may only offer limited benefit in COAD. Whenever theophylline is tried in the management of COAD, an initial therapeutic trial of several weeks should be carried out. If subjective and objective measures of lung function show an improvement, then theophylline can be continued as maintenance therapy.

Care must be taken when prescribing theophylline. The clearance of theophylline is affected by many factors, including cigarette smoking, viral pneumonia, heart failure and concurrent drug treatment (see Ch. 22).

Theophylline can be tried in individual patients who either cannot use inhaled therapy or who are troubled by their symptoms despite maximal doses of bronchodilators and a trial of steroids.

Theophylline may also be of value in the control of persistent nocturnal symptoms, such as cough and wheeze. In this situation a single night-time dose of a sustained-release theophylline product may be of benefit.

In an acute exacerbation of obstructive airways disease, intravenous aminophylline may be required.

Corticosteroids

A therapeutic trial of corticosteroids should be tried in patients with COAD whose condition is clinically stable and who are already on maximal bronchodilator therapy. It is difficult to predict which patients will benefit from steroid therapy. Patients should be given oral steroids (for example, 40 mg prednisolone every morning) for 2 weeks. Lung function tests should be performed together with patient records of peak flow measurements, exercise tolerance and a diary of symptom frequency and severity. Maintenance steroids should, then, only be given if both subjective and objective measurements are improved, for example a 20 to 25% increase in lung function tests.

If a patient benefits from the trial of steroids, inhaled steroids should ideally be used as maintenance treatment. Long-term side effects are minimized using inhaled therapy although local effects such as oral candidiasis and speech impairment are possible. For the transition from oral to inhaled therapy, the oral steroids should be gradually tailed off and inhaled treatment started (for example beclomethasone 200 to 500 micrograms twice daily initially, increased to 1500 micrograms when sole therapy). At high inhaled doses (above 1500 to 2000 micrograms beclomethasone) side effects such as adrenal suppression are possible.

Only if maximal inhaled doses fail to control symptoms should oral steroids be used. These should be used in the smallest dose possible to minimize long-term adverse effects and should be used in conjunction with inhaled steroids.

Treatment for dyspnoea

Some patients with COAD, particularly with emphysema, have severe breathlessness which does not respond to the conventional treatment. Such patients may benefit from low-dose opioids. Methadone and diamorphine have been used but any opioid can be tried. These reduce the respiratory drive and perception of dyspnoea and will reduce oxygen consumption at rest and on exercise. This therapy requires close monitoring of arterial blood gases and should not be used if hypercapnia exists.

Acute exacerbations of COAD

Acute exacerbations of airflow limitation can occur in any patient with COAD. These exacerbations can be spontaneous but are often precipitated by infection and lead to respiratory failure with hypoxaemia and retention of carbon dioxide.

Bronchodilatation is required using a beta$_2$-agonist given by nebulization (e.g. salbutamol 2.5 mg 4- to 6-hourly) and if necessary, intravenously. The addition of a nebulized anticholinergic agent may be beneficial, depending on the clinical condition of the patient. Antibiotics and high-dose steroids may also be required if the patient does not respond to bronchodilator therapy.

If intravenous aminophylline is considered, the loading dose and maintenance dose required should be carefully chosen as these depend on various factors (see Ch. 22).

Oxygen therapy is necessary to improve hypoxia. In patients with a hypoxic drive, the administration of high concentration oxygen will cause a fall in ventilation, carbon dioxide retention and respiratory acidosis. A maximum concentration of 24% oxygen is therefore used.

During an acute attack, pyrexia, hyperventilation and the excessive work of breathing can result in an inability to eat or drink and lead to dehydration. Intravenous hydration is usually given and any inspired gases administered are humidified. Care must be taken to avoid fluid retention, especially if pulmonary oedema is present.

Chest physiotherapy is employed to mobilize secretions, promote expectoration and expand collapsed lung segments.

A respiratory stimulant (analeptic) can be tried in patients with acute respiratory failure, carbon dioxide retention and depressed ventilation. These are nonspecific central nervous system stimulants. The drug of choice is doxapram which stimulates the respiratory and vasomotor centres in the medulla. Doxapram increases the depth of breathing and may slightly increase the rate of breathing. Arterial oxygenation is usually not improved because of the increased work of breathing induced by doxapram. These agents have a narrow therapeutic index and the alternative drug, nikethamide is no longer used because of a high incidence of side effects such as arrhythmias, vasoconstriction, dizziness and convulsions. Doxapram is used as a continuous infusion at a rate of 1 to 4 mg per minute. The patient's arterial blood gases and blood pH must be monitored during treatment to allow correct dosage adjustment. Doxapram may be harmful if used when the PCO_2 is normal or low and should be used with care in patients with epilepsy, hypertension, coronary artery disease or those taking monoamine oxidase inhibitors.

If the patient's condition still does not improve, assisted ventilation may be considered.

Treatment of cor pulmonale

Treatment of cor pulmonale is symptomatic and involves managing the underlying airways obstruction (COAD is responsible for over 90% of cases of cor pulmonale), hypoxaemia and any pulmonary oedema which develops. Peripheral oedema is managed by using thiazide or loop diuretics. Plasma aldosterone concentrations are often raised in chronic hypoxaemia and hypercapnia and the patient with resistant oedema may benefit from spironolactone. Alternatively an angiotensin converting enzyme inhibitor may be tried. Oxygen is used to treat hypoxaemia and this should also promote a diuresis.

Domiciliary oxygen therapy

The use of oxygen should be regarded as a drug therapy. The aim of therapy is to improve oxygen delivery to the cells, increase alveolar oxygen tension and decrease the work of breathing to maintain a given PO_2. Domiciliary oxygen therapy can be given in two ways.

Intermittent administration. Intermittent administration is used to increase mobility and capacity for exercise and to ease discomfort. Intermittent administration is of most benefit in patients with emphysema.

Continuous long-term oxygen therapy (LTOT). LTOT for at least 15 hours per day has been shown to improve survival in patients with severe, irreversible airflow obstruction, hypoxaemia and peripheral oedema. The Department of Health has issued guidelines for the prescribing of LTOT (Table 23.3). One of the aims of treatment is to achieve a PO_2 of at least 8 kPa without causing a rise in PCO_2 of more than 1 kPa, achieved by adjusting the oxygen flow rate. Before selecting patients for LTOT, each individual must also be assessed with respect to age, quality of life and smoking habits. Patients who smoke are a fire risk if they use LTOT. Moreover, the carbon monoxide present in tobacco smoke binds to haemoglobin and forms

Table 23.3 Department of Health guidelines for prescribing long-term oxygen

1. Absolute indication – chronic obstructive airways disease with $PO_2 < 7.3$ kPa, $PCO_2 > 6.0$ kPa, $FEV_1 < 1.5$ L, FVC <2.0 L and oedema
   Measurements should be made with stable disease on at least two occasions, 3 weeks apart, with all reversible factors (e.g. reversible airways disease) fully treated
2. Relative indication – as in (1) with hypoxaemia but without hypercapnia or oedema
3. Palliative use – in other severe hypoxaemic lung disease
4. Palliation of chronic respiratory failure

carboxyhaemoglobin which decreases the amount of oxygen that can be transported by the blood which will partially or completely negate the beneficial effects of LTOT.

Oxygen can be prescribed as oxygen cylinders but 15 hours per day at 2 L/minute requires 10 'F' size (1340 L) cylinders a week. A more convenient system is to use a concentrator which converts ambient air to 90% oxygen using a molecular sieve. The concentrator is sited in a well-ventilated area in the home with plastic tubing to terminals in rooms such as the living room and bedroom. Tubing from the terminals delivers oxygen to the patient who wears a mask or uses the more convenient nasal prongs. This tubing should be long enough to allow some mobility.

THE PATIENT

Stopping smoking

Government advertising has alerted smokers to the health hazards involved with smoking. To give up smoking, which has been described as a form of drug addiction, requires self-motivation. Members of the health-care team can educate smokers of the dangers and actively encourage and motivate those that want to give up.

The use of inhaled therapy

For those patients with obstructive airways disease which has a degree of reversibility, the correct use of inhaled therapy is a vital part of overall management.

In common with asthmatic patients (see Ch. 22), these patients are often receiving an inhaled beta^2-agonist and an anticholinergic. In addition, the patient may also be receiving an inhaled or oral steroid.

Counselling needs to highlight the modes of action of the bronchodilators, particularly the more rapid onset of action of the $beta_2$-agonists to relieve breathlessness rather than the slower-acting anticholinergics. If inhaled steroids are prescribed, the importance of regular administration must be stressed.

The incorrect use of any inhaler will lead to subtherapeutic dosing. The correct use of inhalers is, therefore, as vital in the management of obstructive airways disease patients as outlined for patients with asthma (see Ch. 22). The advantages and disadvantages of each type of inhaler device are summarized in Table 23.4.

Domiciliary oxygen therapy

Studies have shown that only about 50% of patients on LTOT comply with the requirement for 15 hours of treatment a day. Counselling will be required to persuade the patient to comply with this minimum figure. Emphasis must be given to the improvement in quality of life gained from treatment rather than the idea of being continually 'tied' to the oxygen supply.

The long term, chronic nature of COAD may leave a patient with a fear of exercise as this will cause dyspnoea (breathlessness). Thus the patient with COAD may decide not to undertake any exercise. Mobility should be encouraged but is limited by the need to use domiciliary bottled oxygen or oxygen concentrators. Portable oxygen cylinders can be used to increase exercise tolerance during walking. These must be purchased privately. If an oxygen concentrator is used, limited mobility can be gained by installing at least two terminals for the unit (usually in the living room and bedroom) with long tubing between the terminal and nasal prongs.

Portable cryogenic liquid oxygen units are available which are refilled from a larger reservoir system kept in the patient's home. These must also be privately purchased.

Inhaler type	Compact	Hand–lung coordination required	Easy to use	CFC free	Reduces oropharynx deposition
MDI	+	+	−	−	−
MDI + small spacer	+	±	±	−	+
MDI + large spacer	−	−	±	−	+
Breath-actuated MDI	+	−	+	−	−
Dry powder	+	−	±	+	−
Breath-actuated dry powder	+	−	+	+	−
Nebulizer	−	−	±	+	−

Table 23.4 Comparison of inhaler devices

Note: CFC = chlorofluorocarbon propellant
Key: + = feature present; ± = feature present for some patients; − = feature absent

CASE STUDIES

CASE 23.1

Mr M. R. is a 52-year-old man with chronic bronchitis. He asks if it would be worthwhile to purchase some nicotine gum to help him stop smoking. Questioning reveals that he has already tried to give up but has only managed to cut down from 30 cigarettes a day to around 20 or 25.

Q1 Why is it important for a patient with COAD to give up smoking and what general counselling should be given to Mr M. R.?

Q2 Nicotine replacement gum is available over the counter as Nicorette. What specific counselling should be given with this product?

Q3 Would Nicorette be suitable for Mr M. R.?

CASE 23.2

Mr E. B. has a history of chronic obstructive airways disease (COAD) and congestive cardiac failure.

He was admitted to a medical ward with increasing breathlessness, wheeze, productive sputum and cyanosis. He was diagnosed as having an infective exacerbation of his airways disease and started on intravenous cefuroxime 750 mg 8-hourly together with the nebulizers he normally takes (salbutamol 2.5 mg 8-hourly and ipratropium bromide 500 micrograms 8-hourly) which were increased to a 4-hourly regimen.

1 hour after admission his arterial blood gases were:

		(Reference range)
pH	7.37	(7.35–7.45)
PCO_2	7.5 kPa	(4.6–6.0)
PO_2	4.5 kPa	(12–16)
Standard bicarbonate	32.3 mmol/L	(22–28)
Base excess	+6.5	(−2 to +2)
Oxygen saturation	63.7%	

He is diagnosed as being in respiratory failure.

Q1 What type of respiratory failure does the patient have?

Q2 Is there any value in using a respiratory stimulant in Mr E. B.?

Q3 What is the role of artificial ventilation in COAD?

CASE 23.3

Mr H. A. is 62 years of age and has a long history of obstructive airways disease. He has bronchiectasis and had a right upper lung lobe removed 29 years ago. For the last 6 months he has been unable to do the shopping but could get out of doors when he was feeling at his best. He smoked 20 cigarettes a day until 3 years ago and now only smokes occasionally.

For the past 3 days he has been increasingly out of breath and has a productive green/yellow coloured sputum. His present medication includes:

- Home oxygen therapy
- Salbutamol 2.5 mg nebulized four times daily
- Ipratropium bromide 500 micrograms nebulized four times daily
- Aminophylline slow-release tablets 225 mg twice daily
- Prednisolone tablets 5 mg every morning until 3 days ago when it was increased to 30 mg daily by his doctor.

He was admitted to hospital with dyspnoea, cyanosed and breathing using accessory muscles. He had a pulse rate of 100 beats per minute and a PEFR of 190 L/minute but was apyrexial.

He was diagnosed as having an infective exacerbation of his COAD.

Q1 What would be the initial choice of antibiotic for Mr H. A.?

Q2 Should a sputum sample for microbiology culture and sensitivity testing be taken before initiation of treatment or only if the patient fails to improve on the initial antibiotic choice?

Q3 What is the role of long-term antibiotics?

CASE 23.4

Mr M. A. is 72 years old with a long-standing history of mild COAD who has been suffering from increased shortness of breath over the last 6 months. He has an outpatient appointment in the chest clinic of the local hospital because of increased dyspnoea at rest. On physical examination he was found to be tachypnoeic with a pink, flushed appearance. There was minimal production of clear, mucoid sputum. His arterial blood gases were as follows:

		(Reference range)
pH	7.39	(7.35–7.45)
PCO_2	5.4 kPa	(4.6–6.0)
PO_2	9.5 kPa	(12–16)
Standard bicarbonate	23 mmol/L	(22–28)

His respiratory function tests indicated decreased FEV1, decreased FVC and greatly increased residual volume.

His current therapy included: salbutamol metered-dose inhaler 200 micrograms 3 to 4 times daily, and a sustained-release theophylline tablet 250 mg twice a day.

Q1 Identify the features in Mr M. A. which indicate the presence of emphysema.

Q2 Discuss the stepwise treatment for COAD with particular reference to emphysema.

ANSWERS TO CASE STUDIES

CASE 23.1

A1 Smoking is the major avoidable risk factor for chronic obstructive airways disease. Smoking is responsible for one-third of all deaths in the age group 40 to 69 years and one tenth of deaths in the over 70s. One-fifth of all deaths from coronary heart disease are smoking related, as are nine out of ten deaths from chronic bronchitis, emphysema and lung cancer.

Mr M. R. should be told that stopping smoking will not prevent the onset of heart disease but that it will 'reduce the odds' for him personally. Stopping smoking now will not have an immediate effect, a reduction in COAD mortality is not seen until around 10 years or more after cessation of smoking. Giving up at his age will slow down the gradual decline in FEV_1 which is seen in smokers and the onset of disability from COAD may be postponed by 10 to 15 years.

Giving up smoking should be done at a time which is free from stress as far as possible. Motivation is the key to giving up.

A2 When Nicorette gum is chewed it releases nicotine which is absorbed through the buccal mucosa, this does not produce the pleasure that cigarettes do, so the patient must be counselled to continue.

The technique of chewing the gum is important. One piece is chewed whenever a cigarette is desired, chewing slowly a few times. The gum has to be 'parked' (not chewed) between the gum and cheek when the taste becomes strong. When the taste has faded, the gum is chewed again. This procedure should be continued for about 30 minutes. Most people should only need around 10 pieces a day, with 15 a day the maximum number.

Nicorette is used in this manner for 3 months. After this the patient should reduce the number of pieces chewed per day by one every week until none is chewed at all.

Nicorette should not be given to pregnant women, breast-feeding mothers, children under 18 years old, people with persistent indigestion or chest pain or those with heart disease.

If palpitations, chest pain, leg pain or severe indigestion are experienced by the patient he should be counselled to stop the gum, not to smoke and to consult his general practitioner. Minor side-effects, which do not warrant cessation of therapy, include a bitter taste, hiccups, sore throat, headaches, dizziness, sickness and mild indigestion.

A3 No. Mr M. R. smokes 20 to 25 cigarettes a day. He will have to be referred to his general practitioner who can prescribe Nicorette Plus which contains 4 mg nicotine per piece and is required by most heavy smokers.

CASE 23.2

A1 Respiratory failure occurs when pulmonary gas exchange is sufficiently impaired to cause hypoxaemia with or without hypercapnia. There are two types of respiratory failure: type I (acute hypoxaemic) failure occurs when hypoxaemia follows interference with gas exchange resulting from damage to lung tissue; type II (ventilatory) failure occurs when alveolar ventilation is insufficient to excrete the amount of carbon dioxide being produced by metabolism.

Both types of failure commonly occur together in patients with COAD ('mixed respiratory failure'). The initial pulmonary disease causes hypoxaemic respiratory failure but the patient becomes exhausted and is no longer able to overcome the impaired lung function and increased dead space and therefore retains carbon dioxide (hypercapnia). This is the case with Mr E. B.

A2 Respiratory stimulants could be tried. These stimulate the respiratory centre and increase the depth of breathing and to a lesser extent the rate of breathing. They are sometimes used in patients with acute respiratory failure to try to avoid the necessity for artificial ventilation but their efficacy is doubtful. Oxygenation is often not improved as they increase the work of breathing. Doxapram is the treatment of choice, given by continuous intravenous infusion at 1 to 4 mg per minute. Doxapram has a narrow therapeutic index with side effects such as hypertension, tachycardia, tremor, agitation, anxiety and convulsions.

If a severe metabolic alkalosis exists a carbonic anhydrase inhibitor such as acetazolamide or dichlorphenamide could be given. These agents decrease the rate of carbonic anhydrase formation thus promoting the renal excretion of bicarbonate. The plasma bicarbonate then falls and a metabolic acidosis results thereby stimulating respiration.

A3 Artificial ventilation may become necessary if a patient's condition deteriorates despite the usual treatment of oxygen, bronchodilators, physiotherapy, respiratory stimulants, etc. If the patient had reasonable respiratory function before the acute deterioration he may benefit from aggressive treatment and ventilation. If, however, the patient has advanced and incapacitating disease then he may not recover fully after ventilation or enjoy a reasonable quality of life. Weaning this kind of patient off a ventilator can be difficult.

CASE 23.3

A1 The most common pathogens associated with COAD infections are *Streptococcus pneumoniae*, *Haemophilus influenzae*, and *Bramhamella catarrhalis*. Suitable first line antibiotics include, amoxycillin, ampicillin, trimethoprim, co-trimoxazole or erythromycin. It must be remembered that around 10% of isolates of *Haemophilus influenzae* are resistant to amoxycillin/ampicillin, and co-amoxiclav may be a suitable alternative. Mr H. A. received one intravenous dose of 500 mg ampicillin and was then given amoxycillin 500 mg 8-hourly.

One factor which may need to be taken into account in COAD pneumonia is the extent to which the chosen antibiotic penetrates the sputum. This property appears to be more important in COAD than in other respiratory infections, possibly because subtherapeutic antibiotic concentrations in mucus may lead to relapse. Penetration into sputum also becomes worse as tissue damage progresses. The beta-lactam antibiotics only reach sputum concentrations around 5 to 20% of those in serum. Trimethoprim passes readily into sputum. Erythromycin and the tetracyclines may reach concentrations which are sufficient to treat streptococci but concentrations needed to treat *Haemophilus influenzae* tend to be higher. Intravenous therapy may be required in some patients, although good results have been seen with some antibiotics given by inhalation, such as amoxycillin and gentamicin. High-dose oral amoxycillin 3 g twice a day, has been successfully used in bronchiectasis with daily purulent sputum, where the severity of tissue damage forms an increased barrier to sputum penetration.

A2 Initial sputum culture is often unhelpful in identifying the pathogen involved in infective exacerbations of obstructive airways disease. One reason for this is that the pathogen is frequently overgrown on culture with upper respiratory tract organisms such as Gram-negative bacilli.

In Mr H. A.'s case the initial culture showed purulent normal flora only. After 5 days of amoxycillin his condition had not improved. A second sputum culture was taken which showed a moderate growth of *Haemophilus parainfluenzae*, which was sensitive to amoxycillin, co-trimoxazole and cefaclor. His antibiotic was changed to co-trimoxazole 480 mg twice a day and he was discharged 7 days later.

A3 Antibiotic treatment in infective exacerbations of chronic bronchitis is usually successful with a 7- to 10-day course. In bronchiectasis this may not be an adequate length and relapse will occur if the course is too short. If persistent or repeated infections are seen in patients with bronchiectasis they may be given antibiotics for 4 to 6 months. Several antibiotics could be used in rotation. Ciprofloxacin may be included in the rotation as infections with pseudomonas are common.

CASE 23.4

A1 Patients with emphysema are breathless but usually have no appreciable cough or sputum production. Weight loss is often a problem, partly due to the energy consumed in ventilatory effort and partly due to reduced food intake as a result of constant dyspnoea. The degree of weight loss affects the time of survival; almost 50% of patients die within 5 years of the onset of substantial weight loss. Acute respiratory failure has been associated with malnutrition in COAD patients as weight loss can lead to decreased respiratory muscle function and a depressed immune system. Arterial blood gas values can be normal but there may be some values characteristic of emphysema. PO_2 may be slightly low, PCO_2 may be slightly high and pH may indicate mild respiratory acidosis. Mr M. A.'s values are typical in mild emphysema with mild hypoxaemia, normal PCO_2, normal pH and normal bicarbonate. Cor pulmonale is uncommon until later on in the disease. The most characteristic pulmonary function test is a marked increase in residual volume due to air trapping.

A2 Drug therapy for emphysema is similar to that for chronic bronchitis; however, all treatment depends on the response of the individual patient. The treatment options available include beta2-agonists, anticholinergics, corticosteroids and theophylline.

BIBLIOGRAPHY

Burrows B. Airways obstructive diseases: pathogenetic mechanisms and natural histories of the disorders. Medical Clinics of North America 1990; 74(3): 547–559

Clausen J L. The diagnosis of emphysema, chronic bronchitis and asthma. Clinics in Chest Medicine 1990; 11(3): 405–416

Gross N J. Chronic obstructive pulmonary disease – current concepts and therapeutic approaches. Chest 1990; 97(2): 195–235

Gotz V P. Chronic obstructive airways disease. In: Young L Y, Koda-Kimble M A, (eds) Applied therapeutics: the clinical use of drugs. Vancouver: Applied Therapeutics 1988; 393–413

Holland W W. Chronic obstructive airways disease prevention. British Journal of Diseases of the Chest 1988; 82: 32–44

Howard P, Stewart A G. Cor pulmonale and long-term domiciliary oxygen therapy. Medicine International 1991; (89): 3727–3731

Lewis L D, Cochrane M. Management strategies and therapeutics of chronic airflow obstruction. Medicine International 1991; (89): 3722–3726

MacFarlane J T. Pneumonia. Medicine International 1991; (89): 3732–3739

Stratton M A. Chronic obstructive lung disease. In: DiPiro J T, Talbert R L, Hayes P E, Yee G C, Matzke G R, Posey L M (eds) Pharmacotherapy – a pathophysiologic approach. New York: Elsevier 1992; 450–465

Chapter 24

Drug-induced lung disease

N. P. Keaney

An adverse drug reaction (ADR) can involve the lung in a variety of ways and the clinical presentation is mainly determined by the site of the damage. Thus the airways may be principally affected as in an allergic reaction to penicillin; or the parenchyma of the lung may be the sole site of involvement in various chronic fibrotic reactions. The symptoms and signs of an ADR may not, therefore, be easily distinguished from those of a naturally occurring illness. Likewise, the changes in pulmonary function, as measured by spirometry or by the carbon monoxide transfer factor, and the radiological abnormalities seen on a chest X-ray are usually nonspecific. A high index of suspicion is therefore required if an ADR is to be diagnosed and it can be very difficult to establish a cause and effect relationship without re-exposing the patient to one or more suspected drugs. Because of many uncertainties this is not a technique that is regularly used to confirm a suspected pulmonary ADR, e.g. a chronic reaction may have so disabled a patient that the risk:benefit ratio is unfavourable or provocation of an asthma attack may cause a life-threatening situation. Other dilemmas of drug rechallenge relate to the size and duration of dosage which must be chosen to ensure on one hand that an ADR is identifiable and on the other that only a safe reaction occurs.

In some circumstances rechallenge may not be necessary, either because the ADR is merely an aspect of the therapeutic effect of a suspected drug or because of previous reports of ADRs to the drug. ADRs are typically classified into those which are predictable on the basis of the known pharmacological action of the drug (Type A) and those which are of an idiosyncratic nature (Type B). Allergic (anaphylactic) reactions are defined as Type B, although in the airways, some apparently allergic reactions, i.e. asthmatic reactions, may be due to a recognized non-allergic mechanism (see Table 24.1). For most ADRs, however, the underlying mechanism is ill understood and the classification into Type A and B reactions cannot be easily applied. For example, some pulmonary reactions to cytotoxic drugs, although unpredictable in any particular patient, in essence may be a direct consequence of some, as yet unidentified, action of the drug.

It is convenient, therefore, to discuss induced lung disease on the basis of the respiratory structure principally affected and giving rise to the clinical syndrome characteristic for that site. Thus the bronchi and small airways, the parenchyma of the lung, the pulmonary circulation and the pleural space will be treated separately as much as is possible.

All the ADRs described below are infrequent or rare phenomena and the descriptions of incidence, whether explicit or implied, should be read with that in mind.

BRONCHI AND SMALL AIRWAYS

Airflow obstruction

Local anaphylaxis causing asthma is due to release of preformed and newly synthesized mediators and involves IgE, mast cells, polymorphs, neutrophils, eosinophils and platelets. It is helpful to consider the various ways in which drugs may interact with the above processes as they modify the physiological control of the calibre of the airways (Table 24.1).

Drugs as antigens

Antibiotics are the drugs most often responsible for allergic reactions. These vary in severity, and acute asthma can accompany such local or systemic anaphylaxis. With penicillins, the group most commonly involved, there is almost always a history of uneventful exposure to a previous course of treatment. Fatal reactions seem to occur in patients with a recognized allergic predisposition such as asthma or a previous ADR to a penicillin. Sensitivity to penicillin is sometimes due to persisting impurities such as a polyvalent penicilloyl antigen and is sometimes due to the beta-lactam itself. Identification of penicillin sensitivity by patch or prick skin testing is not reliable and intradermal testing has been associated with fatality. From the above discussion it can be appreciated that cross-reactivity with another group of beta-lactam antibiotics, the cephalosporins, is not an inevitable consequence of allergy to penicillin.

Direct release of mediators

Histamine can be released from mast cells by a number of drugs and this phenomenon is readily demonstrated by intradermal injection of mor-

Table 24.1 Various mechanisms whereby bronchospasm may occur as an ADR		
Site of reaction	Mechanism	Drug
Interaction with IgE	Drug as antigen	Penicillin, dextrans
Direct release of mediators	Displacement of histamine	Iodinated contrast media, quaternary amines
Altered mediator synthesis	Cyclo-oxygenase inhibition	Aspirin, NSAIDs
Reflex bronchoconstriction	Nonspecific irritation	Dry powder propellant, metabisulphite
Direct effect on smooth muscle	Agonist	Pilocarpine
Inhibit hydrolysis of mediator	Inhibition of enzyme	Neostigmine, captopril
Antagonism at beta-adrenoreceptors	Antagonist	Timolol, propafenone
Agonists at beta-adrenoreceptors	Agonist	Isoprenaline, fenoterol, salmeterol (?)

phine or quaternary ammonium compounds such as tubocurarine; also in the clinical context marked bronchoconstriction has been reported after intravenous injection of muscle relaxants. This latter group of drugs is used in conjunction with intravenous anaesthetic agents which themselves can cause anaphylaxis. The combination of thiopentone and suxamethonium is commonly used and most often implicated in anaesthetic ADRs affecting the airways. Individual patients often cross-react with other induction agents and relaxants which means that an allergic process is unlikely. Direct release of mediators is probable with this combination of drugs and is clearly the mechanism for the high incidence of anaphylactoid reactions with the former anaesthetic agent Althesin. Althesin was a combination of two steroids solubilized with polyoxyethylated castor oil (Cremophor EL), in which disruption of the membrane of mast cells was thought to be affected by the surface-active agent Cremophor EL with release of granules and mediators ensuing.

Iodinated intravenous radiological contrast media have been systematically studied and in one study an incidence of anaphylaxis of 1 in 14 000 has been identified accompanied in 12% of cases by severe bronchospasm. Individuals who are thought to be sensitive to contrast media can be tested with small intravenous doses and/or pretreated with an H_1 antagonist such as chlorpheniramine. However, this therapy may only be effective for two-thirds of susceptible patients.

Other drugs in which a mechanism of direct mediator release has been invoked include hydrocortisone, methylprednisolone and acetylcysteine. Benzalkonium, used as a preservative in a number of formulations, probably acts in the same way and has been removed from solutions which are intended to be administered by nebulization (e.g. ipratropium).

Altered mediator synthesis

Aspirin and other non-steroidal anti-inflammatory drugs (NSAIDs) can precipitate asthma in sensitive individuals. These attacks develop about half an hour after ingestion and are frequently accompanied by flushing and rhinorrhoea. Cross-sensitivity between aspirin and the many differently structured NSAID molecules argues against an allergic mechanism. One theory suggests that their common action as inhibitors of cyclo-oxygenase and prostaglandin synthesis creates an imbalance between bronchodilator and bronchoconstrictor prostanoids and leukotrienes respectively with both series deriving from the same precursor, arachidonic acid.

Some individuals with this type of sensitivity to aspirin cross-react to the food colourant tartrazine (E102). About 10% of asthmatics have been estimated to be affected. A syndrome of late-onset asthma, nasal polyposis and intermittent attacks of rhinorrhoea, angioedema or urticaria has been reported. Extrinsic asthmatics are also susceptible. The severity of an attack is variable but even mild asthmatics have been known to suffer a fatal reaction. A genetic predisposition may be relevant to familial clustering of cases but the expression of the abnormality is variable with positive challenge results in those unaware of any history and negative in a significant proportion of those reporting previous aspirin-sensitivity. Analgesia in this group of patients can be safely provided by the use of codeine or dihydrocodeine and paracetamol for all but a few.

Reflex bronchoconstriction

The modern management of bronchial asthma utilizes the inhaled route of administration. In view of the hyperreactivity of the airways in asthmatics it should not be surprising that with a number of inhaled drugs bronchoconstriction may be brought about by a vagal reflex due to a nonspecific stimulation of bronchial mucosal irritant receptors. This is especially problematic with dry powders. As an example of the need to overcome this side effect the dry powder sodium cromoglycate administered via a Spinhaler (Fisons) was formerly available as a combination formulation with isoprenaline, a bronchodilator with a rapid onset of action.

Wheeze following inhalation of beclomethasone dipropionate is well recognized and may be of some concern if an allergic reaction is responsible. In one study the abnormal reaction could be prevented by prior inhalation of cromoglycate suggesting that an allergic basis was possible. However, the patients had a similar response to a placebo inhaler containing propellant alone. This suggested that a nonspecific irritant action was the cause. A dry powder formulation of beclomethasone using a Diskhaler (Allen & Hanbury) could be regarded as a safe alternative in this situation.

Similarly, use of the multi-dose Turbohaler (Astra), which has no filler (lactose) should be without ill effect. The prior use of a bronchodilator would, of course, prevent this particular ADR.

Paradoxical bronchoconstrictor reactions to inhaled ipratropium have been reported with the nebulizer solution and, as mentioned above, the preservative benzalkonium was implicated. However, the major factor in this adverse response was undoubtedly the hypotonicity of the solution. Unit-dose vials with an isotonic preservative-free sterile formulation have more or less eliminated this ADR. Sporadic reports are now likely to be due to nonspecific irritation and to involve metered-dose inhalers.

Direct effect on smooth muscle

Cholinoceptor agonists such as carbachol, pilocarpine (eye drops) and methacholine (bronchial challenge testing) have all been identified as causative agents which can aggravate asthma or produce unexpectedly severe bronchoconstriction.

Inhibition of mediator hydrolysis

Anticholinesterases such as neostigmine are used after general anaesthesia to reverse the effects of competitive muscle antagonists. Because of the risks of bradycardia and bronchospasm the muscarinic antagonist atropine is given simultaneously. The novel antimuscarinic drug, glycopyrronium, has failed to prevent such bronchospasm.

Angiotensin converting enzyme (ACE) inhibitors such as captopril and lisinopril also inhibit other proteases such as those which inactivate bradykinin and other vasoactive peptides. The incidence of cough with this group of drugs has been reported to vary from 0.2 to 3%. This adverse effect has been ascribed to sensitization of non-myelinated (C) nerve fibres by excess kinins. Modulation of the response can be effected by prostaglandins. The NSAID sulindac has been shown to prevent the induction of cough caused by ACE inhibitors. There is conflicting evidence as to whether ACE inhibitors affect bronchial hyperreactivity. It is clear, however, that asthma is a much less likely side effect than cough to these agents.

Antagonism at beta-adrenoreceptors

Non-selective beta-adrenoreceptor antagonists given orally block the beta-adrenoreceptors in the heart, peripheral vasculature, bronchi, pancreas and liver. There may be some argument for using a selective $beta_1$-agonist such as atenolol, metoprolol or bisoprolol in a patient with reversible airflow obstruction due to chronic bronchitis and not asthma. In, this situation an inhaled $beta_2$-agonist would have to be administered in a large dose to overcome the $beta_2$-blockade which occurs to some extent even with 'selective' $beta_1$-blockers. Whilst it would appear logical to use the anticholinergic agent ipratropium as the bronchodilator in this situation, the solution is really to avoid the use of beta-adrenoreceptor blockers. This latter recommendation is consistent with advice from the Committee on the Safety of Medicines.

Nowadays there are many alternatives to beta-adrenoreceptor blockers which can be used in the treatment of disorders such as hypertension and angina. It is eminently more rational to withdraw the beta-adrenoreceptor blocker and permit a bronchodilator effect to a beta-agonist to go unhindered. In asthmatic subjects there is an added risk to the use of a beta-adrenoreceptor blocker, namely that acute severe bronchospasm may be precipitated. This can occur even with the low systemic concentrations achieved following topical application of timolol eye drops. The mechanism of this ADR is uncertain. It is unlikely to be due to simple antagonism of circulating adrenaline or neurally released noradrenaline. It may possibly relate to an effect on mast cells which are stabilized by beta-agonists at therapeutic concentrations, since pretreatment of asthmatic subjects with cromoglycate protects from bronchoconstriction induced by propranolol. Interestingly, ipratropium has also been shown to be protective.

One must be aware that some drugs may have beta-adrenoreceptor blocking properties and can exacerbate asthma even though this may not be obvious at first sight. Examples of such agents include xamoterol, a drug which was formerly indicated for use in mild cardiac failure and propafenone, a class I_C antiarrhythmic drug.

Agonists at beta-adrenoreceptors

Overuse of inhaled isoprenaline has been found to be associated with findings that suggest tolerance may develop in a proportion of patients who overuse the drug. The evidence for this is very indirect and is based on an increase in the duration of action seen in those who revert to using the drug appropriately. The suggestion has been made in the past, and resurrected recently, that regular use of bronchodilators may result in a deterioration in the control of asthma. Experiments designed to test tolerance by establishing successive dose–response curves before, during and after chronic dosing with oral or inhaled beta-agonist have failed to demonstrate tolerance. However, the role of pressurized aerosols of isoprenaline as a factor in the epidemic of sudden death from asthma which was recorded in a number of countries in the 1960s is relevant to this discussion. Mortality from asthma is an area of much concern and recent epidemiological findings from New Zealand attributed an increase in asthmatic deaths to self-treatment with nebulized high-dose beta-agonists. With isoprenaline it seemed likely that inadequate education of patients about prophylactic and emergency steroid therapy was combined with an over-reliance on high doses of a nonselective beta-

agonist bronchodilator. Similar arguments have been presented for the data from New Zealand, where nebulized fenoterol, which may be less $beta_2$-selective than salbutamol or terbutaline, is more widely used in severe asthmatics than salbutamol and terbutaline.

The discussion about the safety of beta-adrenoreceptor agonists has been further developed by evidence that regular bronchodilator therapy might itself result in a deterioration of asthma control even when prophylactic inhaled steroid therapy is constant. This concern has given rise to much argument especially relating to the novel drugs salmeterol and formoterol which have a duration of bronchodilator action of up to 12 hours, i.e. they provide virtually constant stimulation of beta-adrenoreceptors when taken twice daily.

Another concern relates to the rate of onset of bronchoconstriction during an acute asthmatic attack especially in the presence of a bronchodilator. In this circumstance the functional antagonism between the bronchodilator and endogenous spasmogens means that dilated airways require a higher concentration of mediators to achieve a given degree of bronchoconstriction. It has been shown for the bronchoconstrictors histamine and methacholine that, following pretreatment with salbutamol, the rate of decline of FEV_1, once it begins, is more rapid with the higher concentrations required to overcome the pre-existing salbutamol-induced bronchodilatation. This evidence could be extrapolated to justify the guidelines for the management of asthma issued by the British Thoracic Society (1990). The guidelines recommend that in an informed, motivated, self-monitoring patient bronchodilators should be used on an intermittent basis, as required for symptomatic relief, provided that there is an additional therapeutic background of anti-inflammatory prophylaxis.

LUNG PARENCHYMA

A broad systemic classification into two main groupings is possible with acute and chronic reactions reflecting hypersensitivity and fibrosis as the predominant mechanisms of toxic response respectively. Subacute reactions, intermediate between acute and chronic in their onset, also occur. Although there is little understanding of the processes underlying the aetiology and pathogenesis of these ADRs certain clinical patterns are identifiable.

Hypersensitivity pneumonitis

In general, these acute reactions are of an allergic nature, have a dramatic clinical presentation, and demand urgent diagnosis and withdrawal of the offending agent. If he or she receives early treatment the affected individual will respond quickly and have an excellent chance of a complete recovery.

When a patient develops a cough with breathlessness and wheezing many probable causes are considered before this symptom complex is attributed to an ADR. If eosinophilia on a blood count is a feature of the clinical picture, allergy is certain and a patchy bilateral infiltrate distributed peripherally on the chest radiograph should lead to review of recent drug therapy. Such a presentation in an individual whose lungs have previously been normal and in whom infection has been excluded will be confidently identified as an ADR if the history reveals ingestion of a candidate drug. A diagnosis will usually be made on the grounds of high clinical suspicion but further investigations will include pulmonary function testing with spirometry and measurement of the transfer factor for carbon monoxide. However, these results will merely show the type of defect and will not be diagnostic for an ADR. In recent years the technique of bronchoscopic bronchoalveolar lavage has been applied to these cases. It has proved possible to identify an increase in the cellular yield (pleocytosis) in hypersensitivity pneumonitis and eosinophilia and/or lymphocytosis in the fluid obtained at bronchoalveolar lavage. With more sophisticated facilities the pattern of various lymphocytic subtypes can be seen or an in vitro analysis of the transformation of lavaged lymphocytes can be performed and the effects of challenge with the suspected drug studied.

Pleural effusions sometimes are a feature and eosinophilia may be found in the pleural fluid or on pleural biopsy.

The rapid onset of the symptoms will usually ensure the speedy withdrawal of the offending drug (usually by the patient) and it seems likely that many minor reactions are never reported. The probability of complete recovery is excellent and the rate of improvement may be accelerated by systemic corticosteroid therapy. Drug-induced hypersensitivity pneumonitis is not a sufficiently frequent occurrence for trials of treatment to be compared. It seems logical to use a corticosteroid with a view to suppressing the inflammatory reaction and so prevent a subacute illness or chronic inflammation which could progress to pulmonary fibrosis and a permanent defect.

Non-steroidal anti-inflammatory agents

Among the drugs which are recognized causes of hypersensitivity pneumonitis, NSAIDs are prominent. In a survey which documented information gathered by the yellow-card reporting system of the Committee on the Safety of Medicines many NSAIDs were identified in a series of 29 episodes of alleged hypersensitivity pneumonitis. The drugs involved included indomethacin, azapropazone, diclofenac, piroxicam and ibuprofen. While a detailed analysis of the indications for prescribing these drugs was not feasible, it is of interest that only 12 of these patients had rheumatoid arthritis, whereas 11 had osteoarthritis for whom an alternative analgesic might have been more appropriate.

The NSAIDs are a dangerous group of drugs making it very important that they are prescribed for positive indications and that their continued use is kept under review.

Gold

Parenteral gold (aurothiomalate) when used in the treatment of rheumatoid arthritis has also been found to cause acute breathlessness with bilateral 'alveolar' infiltrates on the chest X-ray. The symptoms can follow the second to the fifth or sixth injection. There is approximately a 50% chance of complete resolution if the gold treatment is discontinued. A genetic predisposition to this ADR is probable.

Salazopyrin

Salazopyrin is now widely used in the management of patients with rheumatoid arthritis. It too has been implicated as a cause of pulmonary eosinophilia although the majority of reports have related to its use in inflammatory bowel disease. The reaction is mostly related to the sulphonamide rather than the 5-aminosalicylate moiety (mesalazine).

Other drugs

Many other drugs have featured in sporadic reports of drug-induced pulmonary eosinophilia especially antibiotics. Nitrofurantoin causes both acute pneumonitis (90% of cases) and rarely, chronic pulmonary fibrosis. Nitrofurantoin is of particular interest as it resembles paraquat in its capacity to undergo cyclical reduction and oxidation. The reoxidation liberates a free electron and generates toxic $O_2^{\bullet-}$ radicals. The acute reaction usually occurs after 4 weeks or so of continuous treatment although even more rapid reactions have been observed.

With cytotoxic drugs acute reactions are uncommon. Methotrexate is implicated most often but this reflects its higher usage compared with procarbazine, mitomycin, bleomycin or azathioprine all of which have been associated with the development of eosinophilic pneumonitis. Corticosteroid therapy will hasten clinical improvement of these ADRs and re-exposure to the offending drug is not recommended.

Pulmonary fibrosis

Drug-induced pulmonary fibrosis is an ADR which is somewhat more reliably diagnosed than other parenchymal reactions, particularly with cytotoxic drugs. For such drugs the cumulative dose, the patient's age, renal dysfunction, previous radiotherapy, oxygen administration and concurrent cytotoxic therapy have been implicated as predisposing factors. The anti-

arrhythmic agent amiodarone has also been frequently implicated as a cause of pulmonary fibrosis.

Bleomycin

Bleomycin was found to cause pulmonary damage during early animal experiments but nevertheless it was introduced into clinical practice. The predictability of this reaction to bleomycin led to its experimental use and research into mechanisms of toxicity. The high ambient oxygen tension in the lung facilitates the generation of superoxide radicals by bleomycin and this effect also accounts for the risks of oxygen therapy mentioned above. A relationship between the dose of bleomycin and its toxicity becomes evident when more than 450 mg has been administered – below this dose toxicity occurs in 3 to 5% of patients, whereas at 450 to 550 mg and over 550 mg incidences of 13% and 17% respectively have been observed.

The clinical onset of the chronic pneumonitis/pulmonary fibrosis syndrome is insidious with symptoms of malaise, dry cough, fever and breathlessness developing and progressing over a period of several weeks or months. The chest X-ray is usually abnormal with basal infiltrates initially and widespread infiltrates in more severely affected patients. CT scanning is a more sensitive method of detecting pulmonary abnormalities. (Nodules resembling metastatic deposits from the primary tumour have also been seen on CT scanning.) Pulmonary function testing has shown abnormalities in asymptomatic individuals with no radiological changes, yielding presumed prevalences of toxicity of 33% and 71% in two surveys. However, some of the effects attributed to bleomycin were minor and unlikely to be clinically deleterious, e.g. a 10% reduction in gas transfer occurred after the first dose of bleomycin in one study but did not decrease further.

The course of the pulmonary damage caused by bleomycin is variable. With mild disease the radiological changes may resolve over a period of 6 to 12 months if the drug is withdrawn – and symptoms may disappear. High-dose corticosteroid therapy in more severely affected patients has led to improvement. Mortality from bleomycin-induced pulmonary fibrosis ranges from 1 to 2% in large series to 10% in patients receiving 550 mg. Despite this profile of toxicity bleomycin is widely used in a variety of malignant tumours as it is often curative.

Busulphan

Pulmonary parenchymal damage caused by other cytotoxic drugs is regularly observed and reported in the literature. The alkylating agent busulphan has a low risk estimated at 4% but autopsy studies have found a much higher incidence of abnormalities (46%) which had not been clinically evident during life. Chlorambucil, cyclophosphamide and melphalan are the subjects of sporadic reports of fibrotic ADRs involving the lung. In one bizarre incident, a pharmacist treated himself with melphalan because myelomatosis had been mentioned in a differential diagnosis. He died from progressive pulmonary fibrosis and did not have any disorder requiring cytotoxic therapy.

Carmustine

The nitrosoureas, especially carmustine, seem to be capable of causing a syndrome of delayed pulmonary fibrosis. Carmustine is usually used alone in primary cerebral malignant tumours which rarely affect the lung either directly or via radiotherapy. The attribution of a pulmonary ADR to this drug can be made much more clearly and confidently in this circumstance than, for example, when multiple cytotoxic drugs are used for an intrathoracic tumour which is subsequently irradiated. For carmustine the total dose is related to the early development of pulmonary fibrosis but the incidence of this ADR increases as survivors are followed up. In one series of 31 children treated with carmustine only 17 were cured of their tumour. Of these survivors, six died from pulmonary fibrosis (two within 3 years of treatment) and six of the remaining eight patients, who could be traced, were found to have evidence of severe fibrotic damage to the lungs with an active fibrotic process recognized up to 17 years after treatment.

Amiodarone

The antiarrhythmic drug amiodarone has an unusual pharmacokinetic profile due to its high lipid solubility. The parent drug and its principal desethyl metabolite have exceptionally low rates of elimination ($t_{1/2}$ 45 to 60 days) from huge volumes of distribution (5000 litres) resulting in concentrations in the lung 1000 times greater than in serum. This accumulation favours a direct toxic effect and daily doses in excess of 400 mg for more than 2 months result in pulmonary toxicity in 6% of patients. A mortality rate of 10 to 20% is expected. Chronic pneumonitis with fibrosis is the usual toxic manifestation and this can be readily diagnosed on transbronchial biopsy. Foamy alveolar macrophages with dense lamellar cytoplasmic inclusions containing phospholipid (with amiodarone and desethylamiodarone) are a consequence of pulmonary accumulation and are seen even in the absence of clinical evidence of pneumonitis or fibrosis.

Up to 25% of patients with amiodarone-induced pulmonary damage may have 'organizing pneumonia' a steroid responsive condition with characteristic histological features. This type of reaction is thought to have an immunological basis and treatment with prednisolone is recommended for all patients in case some areas of pneumonitis are of this nature. This treatment should be continued for some months after withdrawal of amiodarone, because of its prolonged elimination half-life.

Amiodarone is heavily iodinated and increases the density of tissues, e.g. pulmonary opacities seen on CT scans can be ascribed to this drug's toxicity from the radiological appearances. Oxygen therapy, e.g. during general anaesthesia, may aggravate pulmonary toxicity and in some instances precipitate respiratory failure in patients with subclinical amiodarone toxicity.

Bromocriptine, like methysergide, is an ergot derivative and has also been found to cause pulmonary fibrosis. An unusual feature of this ADR has been the presence of pleural effusions and/

or pleural thickening. It is tempting to relate the reaction to an effect involving 5HT receptors but which cell-type is involved is unclear. Other drugs associated with pleural effusion are listed in Table 24.2.

PULMONARY VASCULATURE

Eosinophilia/myalgia with L-tryptophan

In 1989 a new syndrome occurred typified by pain in muscles and a rash with cough and breathlessness being common. There was marked eosinophilia of peripheral blood but even in the most breathless patients the chest X-ray looked surprisingly normal. Pulmonary hypertension was often found and was the cause of the respiratory distress. Treatment with an anti-inflammatory high-dose corticosteroid was rapidly beneficial. The majority of patients were taking L-tryptophan as a 'health food' supplement but subsequently cases were described from psychiatric clinics where L-tryptophan was prescribed for a depressive illness. The causative factor of this eosinophilia/myalgia syndrome is obscure. It is intriguing that such an adverse reaction should be due to a naturally occurring amino acid. An individual producer of L-tryptophan was linked epidemiologically to many cases in the USA but it remains unclear whether an impurity arising from the manufacturing process was the cause.

Pulmonary vasculitis

Drug-induced pulmonary vasculitis is caused by

Table 24.2 Examples of drugs associated with pleural effusion and/or thickening

L-tryptophan
Amiodarone
Bromocriptine
Cytotoxics
Dantrolene
Interleukin-2
Mesulergine
Methysergide
Nitrofurantoin
Oesophageal sclerosants
Drugs causing systemic lupus erythematosus

an immune mechanism, e.g. due to the formation of immune complexes formed when excess antigen (drug or metabolite) and antibody combine and are deposited on the vascular endothelium. The complement system is activated and the sequential changes set up an inflammatory reaction. The result is a vasculitis which produces different clinical manifestations, the pattern of which depends on the size and site of the blood vessels targeted by the immune complexes and on the persistence of the cellular response. Our understanding of these and other parenchymal reactions is limited by the absence of suitable animal models and the paucity of adequate histological evidence in most patients, so that many cases of pulmonary vasculitis will be overlooked.

Pulmonary vasculitis is almost always a capillaritis and the conventional diagnostic appearances associated with an arteritis will be absent. The involvement of capillaries weakens them and as they are largely unsupported by connective tissue, bleeding into the alveolar walls and alveoli occurs. If this diffuse intrapulmonary haemorrhage is associated with glomerulonephritis it is called Goodpasture's syndrome. The diagnostic marker is a circulating antibody against the glomerular basement membrane (anti-GBM). This anti-GBM is not detected in cases of drug-induced diffuse intrapulmonary haemorrhage (with or without glomerulonephritis) due to penicillamine, aminoglutethimide, nitrofurantoin, amphotericin or cocaine smoking.

Pulmonary embolism

In the early 1960s there were many reports of venous thrombosis in association with the use of oral contraceptive agents. The sporadic reports were followed by many systematic surveys both retrospective and prospective which established a causative relationship with a risk of venous thrombosis five to six times greater in women on the contraceptive pill. Further studies related the risk to the dose of oestrogen and despite a general dose reduction a small risk persists. In a prospective study of 17 000 married women aged 25 to 39 years, 105 episodes of venous thromboembolism occurred, the incidence (events per thousand woman-years) being 0.43 in users and 0.06 in non-users of oral contraceptives. 71 of the certain or probable diagnoses were in postoperative patients and confined to current users of oral contraceptives. Further evidence suggests that the risk of pregnancy (and associated incidence of thromboembolic disease) is such that a combined oral contraceptive should not be discontinued preoperatively. The use of a progestogen-only pill would undoubtedly carry less risk.

Pulmonary hypertension

A small epidemic of pulmonary hypertension occurred in the late 1960s particularly in Switzerland. The problem seemed to be confined to countries where the appetite-suppressant aminorex fumarate was marketed. The evidence for this ADR was circumstantial as no animal model was found that reproduced the syndrome. Withdrawal of the drug brought the epidemic to an end. Now sporadic cases associated with other anorectic drugs such as amphetamines, fenfluramine and most recently dexfenfluramine have been reported.

Pulmonary hypertension progresses to a clinical syndrome characterized by increasing breathlessness, right-sided cardiac failure and sudden death. It usually follows severe or recurrent pulmonary thromboembolism and is therefore linked with oestrogen therapy and the oral contraceptive. Intravenous drug abusers inject particulate matter, e.g. from crushed tablets, and impaction in pulmonary arterioles may give rise to a clinical presentation typical of pulmonary embolism. Progression to severe pulmonary hypertension does occur and corn starch, talc and microcrystalline cellulose have each been found in the lung on histological examination.

Pulmonary oedema

Noncardiogenic pulmonary oedema or adult respiratory distress syndrome (ARDS) occurs as a consequence of increased pulmonary alveolar

Table 24.3 Drugs causing noncardiogenic pulmonary oedema

Adrenaline
Amitriptyline*
Antilymphocytic globulin
Aspirin
Codeine*
Dextropropoxyphene*
Diamorphine (heroin)
Hydrochlorothiazide
Indomethacin
Interleukin-2
Methadone
Mono-octanoin
Ritodrine
Salbutamol
Terbutaline

* ADR occurs with overdose.

capillary permeability. Classically the air spaces in the lung become filled with a proteinaceous fluid. Breathlessness and hypoxaemia may progress to respiratory failure. In 1880 Osler described pulmonary oedema as a complication of heroin abuse and it still seems to be common in that group of addicts who end up admitted to hospital as an urgency. This particular ADR occurs with both intravenously and orally administered opiates. It has been reported after overdose of dextropropoxyphene and codeine and even with naloxone (although this drug is only likely to be given to patients who have already taken an opiate). Other drugs known to cause noncardiogenic pulmonary oedema are listed in Table 24.3.

BIBLIOGRAPHY

Allen J, Cooper D Jun (eds). Clinics in Chest Medicine 1990; 11(1)
Gibson G J. Adverse pulmonary effects of drugs and radiation. In: Brewis R A L, Gibson G J, Geddes D M (eds) Respiratory medicine. London: Baillière Tindall 1990; 1149–1165
Keaney N P. Respiratory disorders. In: Davies D M (ed) Textbook of adverse drug reactions. Oxford: Oxford University Press 1991
White D A, Matthy R. Drug induced pulmonary disease. American Review of Respiratory Diseases 1986; 133: 321–340, 488–505

Chapter 25

Insomnia and anxiety

C. H. Ashton

DEFINITIONS AND EPIDEMIOLOGY

Insomnia and anxiety are among the commonest symptoms seen in general practice. Each can arise from a number of causes and often, though not always, they occur together. Insomnia refers to difficulty in falling asleep or staying asleep, or to lack of refreshment from sleep. Complaints of poor sleep increase with increasing age and are twice as common in women as in men. Thus by the age of 50 years a quarter of the population are dissatisfied with their sleep, the proportion rising to 30 to 40% (two-thirds of them women) among individuals over 65 years.

Anxiety, a feeling of apprehension or fear, combined with symptoms of increased sympathetic activity, is a normal response to stress. A clinical problem may arise if the anxiety becomes severe or persistent, and interferes with everyday performance. Clinical subtypes of anxiety include panic disorder, agoraphobia, other phobias, and generalized anxiety. The prevalence of such syndromes in the general population is about 10%, rising to over 20% if other symptoms of high psychic distress (excluding major depression) are added. The overall female to male ratio is nearly 2:1. The age of onset of most anxiety disorders is in young adulthood (20s and 30s), although the maximum prevalence of generalized anxiety and agoraphobia-panic in the general population is in the 50- to 64-year age group.

PATHOPHYSIOLOGY

Anxiety and insomnia reflect disturbances of arousal and/or sleep systems in the brain. These systems are functionally interrelated and their activity determines the degree and type of alertness during wakefulness and the depth and quality of sleep.

Arousal systems

Arousal is maintained by at least three interconnected systems: a general arousal system, an 'emotional' arousal system and an endocrine/autonomic arousal system (Fig. 25.1). The general arousal system, mediated by the brain stem reticular formation, serves to link the cerebral cortex with incoming sensory stimuli and provides a tonic influence on cortical reactivity or alertness. Excessive activity in this system, due to internal or external stresses, can lead to a state of hyperarousal as seen in anxiety and insomnia. Emotional aspects of arousal, such as fear and anxiety are contributed by the limbic system which serves to focus attention on selected aspects of the environment. There is evidence that

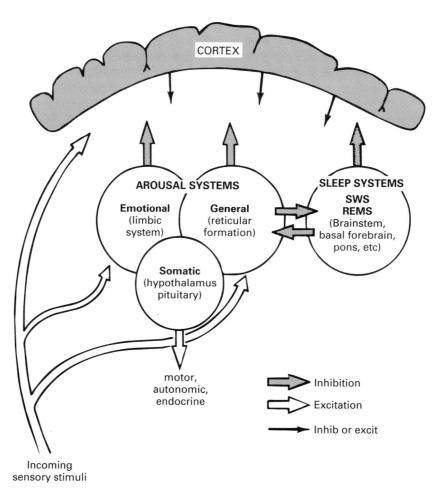

Fig. 25.1 Diagram of arousal and sleep systems. Arousal systems receive environmental and internal stimuli, cause cortical activation, and mediate motor, autonomic and endocrine responses to arousal. Reciprocally connected sleep systems generate slow wave sleep (SWS) and rapid eye movement sleep (REMS). Either system can be excited or inhibited by cognitive activity generated in the cortex.

increased activity in certain limbic pathways is associated with anxiety and panic attacks.

These arousal systems activate somatic responses to arousal, such as increased muscle tone, increased sympathetic activity, and increased output of anterior and posterior pituitary hormones. Inappropriate increases in autonomic activity are often associated with anxiety states; the resulting symptoms (palpitations, sweating, tremor, etc.) may initiate a vicious circle which increases the anxiety.

Several neurotransmitters have been particularly implicated in arousal systems. There is evidence that heightened arousal is associated with increased noradrenergic and serotonergic activity, and drugs which antagonize such activity have anxiolytic effects. In addition, the inhibitory neurotransmitter GABA (γ-aminobutyric acid) exerts an inhibitory control on other transmitter pathways, and increased GABA activity may have a protective effect against excessive stress reactions. Drugs which increase GABA activity (including alcohol and benzodiazepines) are potent anxiolytics.

Sleep systems

At the other end of the arousal spectrum, the phenomenon of sleep is actively induced and maintained by neural mechanisms in several brain areas including the lower brain stem, pons and parts of the limbic system. These mechanisms have reciprocal inhibitory connections with arousal systems, so that activation of sleep systems at the same time inhibits waking, and vice versa (Fig. 25.1). Normal sleep includes two distinct levels of consciousness, orthodox sleep and paradoxical sleep, which are promoted from separate neural centres.

Orthodox sleep normally takes up about 75% of sleeping time. It is somewhat arbitrarily divided into four stages (1 to 4) which merge into each other, forming a continuum of decreasing cortical and behavioural arousal. Stages 3 and 4 are associated with increasing amounts of high voltage slow delta waves (1 to 3 Hz) shown on the electroencephalograph (EEG). These latter stages represent the deepest level of sleep and are also termed slow wave sleep (SWS).

Paradoxical sleep (rapid eye movement sleep, REMS) normally takes up about 25% of sleeping time and has quite different characteristics. The EEG shows unsynchronized fast activity similar to that found in the alert conscious state and the eyes show rapid jerky movements. Peripheral autonomic activity is increased during REMS and there is an increased output of catecholamines and free fatty acids. Vivid dreams and nightmares most often occur in REMS, although brief frightening dreams (hypnagogic hallucinations) can occur in orthodox sleep, especially at the transition between sleeping and waking. Both SWS and REMS show a rebound after a period of deprivation, usually at the expense of lighter (stage 1 and 2) sleep which appears to be expendable.

AETIOLOGY AND CLINICAL MANIFESTATIONS

Insomnia

Insomnia may be caused by any factor which increases activity in arousal systems or decreases activity in sleep systems. Many causes act on both systems. Increased sensory stimulation activates arousal systems, resulting in difficulty in falling asleep. Common causes include pain or discomfort and external stimuli such as noise, bright lights and extremes of temperature. Anxiety may also delay sleep onset as a result of increased emotional arousal.

Drugs are an important cause of insomnia. Difficulty in falling asleep may result directly from the action of stimulants including caffeine, theophylline, sympathomimetic amines and some antidepressants, especially monoamine oxidase inhibitors. Drug withdrawal after chronic use of central nervous system depressants, including hypnotics, anxiolytics, and alcohol commonly cause rebound insomnia with delayed or interrupted sleep, increased REMS and nightmares. With rapidly metabolized depressants, such as alcohol or short-acting benzodiazepines, this rebound may occur in the latter part of the night, resulting in early waking. Certain drugs, including neuroleptics, tricyclic antidepressants, triazolam and propranolol, may occasionally cause nightmares.

Difficulty in staying asleep is characteristic of depression. Patients typically complain of early waking but sleep records show frequent awakenings, early onset of REMS, and reduced SWS. Alteration of sleep stages, increased dreaming and nightmares may also occur in schizophrenia while recurring nightmares are a feature of post-traumatic stress disorder. Interference with circadian rhythms, as in shift work or rapid travel across time zones, can cause difficulty in falling asleep or early waking.

Frequent arousals from sleep are associated with myoclonus, 'restless legs syndrome', muscle cramps, bruxism (tooth-grinding), head banging and sleep apnoea syndromes. Reversal of the sleep pattern, with a tendency to poor nocturnal sleep but a need for daytime naps is common in the elderly in whom it may be associated with cerebrovascular disease or dementia.

Anxiety

Anxiety is commonly precipitated by stress, but vulnerability to stress appears to be linked to genetic factors such as trait anxiety, and many patients presenting for the first time with anxiety symptoms have a long history of high anxiety levels going back to childhood. Anxiety may also be induced by central stimulant drugs (caffeine, amphetamines), withdrawal from chronic use of central nervous system depressant drugs (alcohol, hypnotics, anxiolytics) and metabolic disturbances (hyperventilation, hypoglycaemia, thyrotoxicosis). It may form part of a depressive disorder and may occur in temporal lobe lesions and in rare hormone-secreting tumours such as phaeochromocytoma or carcinoid.

Apart from the psychological symptoms of apprehension and fear, somatic symptoms may be prominent in anxiety and include palpitations, chest pain, shortness of breath, dizziness, dysphagia, gastrointestinal disturbances, loss of libido, headaches and tremor. Panic attacks are experienced as storms of increased autonomic activity combined with a fear of imminent death or loss of control. If panics become associated with a particular environment, commonly a crowded place with no easy escape route, the patient may actively avoid similar situations and eventually become agoraphobic.

INVESTIGATIONS, DIFFERENTIAL DIAGNOSIS

Many patients complaining of insomnia overestimate their sleep requirements. Although most people sleep for 7 to 8 hours daily, some healthy subjects require as little as 3 hours of sleep and sleep requirements decline with age. Such 'physiological insomnia' does not usually cause daytime fatigue, although the elderly may take daytime naps. If insomnia is causing distress, primary causes such as pain, drugs which disturb sleep, psychiatric disturbance including anxiety and depression, and organic causes such as sleep apnoea should be identified and treated before hypnotic therapy is prescribed.

In patients presenting with symptoms and clinical signs of anxiety, it is important to exclude organic causes such as thyrotoxicosis, excessive use of stimulant drugs such as caffeine, and the possibility of alcoholism or withdrawal effects from benzodiazepines. More rarely attacks of anxiety or panic may be associated with temporal lobe epilepsy or phaeochromocytoma. However, unnecessary investigations should be avoided if possible. Extensive gastroenterological, cardiological and neurological tests may increase anxiety by reinforcing the patient's fear of serious underlying physical disease.

TREATMENT
Hypnotic drugs

Hypnotic drugs provide only symptomatic treatment for insomnia. Although often efficacious in the short term, they do little to alter the underlying cause which should be sought and treated where possible. Simple explanation of sleep requirements, attention to sleep hygiene, reduction in caffeine or alcohol intake, and the use of analgesics where indicated may obviate the need for hypnotics. Nevertheless, about 15 million pre-scriptions for hypnotics are issued each year in the UK, and these drugs can improve the quality of life if used rationally.

The ideal hypnotic would gently suppress all arousal systems while simultaneously stimulat-ing the systems for deep and satisfying sleep. It would allow a natural return of normal sleep patterns and would be suitable for long-term use. Unfortunately, no such hypnotic exists; all presently available hypnotics are general central nervous system depressants which inhibit both arousal and sleep mechanisms. Thus they do not induce normal sleep and often have adverse effects including daytime sedation ('hangover') and rebound insomnia on withdrawal. They are unsuitable for long-term use because of the development of tolerance and dependence.

Benzodiazepines

By far the most commonly prescribed hypnotics are the benzodiazepines. A number of different benzodiazepines are available (Table 25.1). These drugs differ considerably in potency (equivalent dosage) and in rate of elimination but only slightly in clinical effects. All benzodiazepines have sedative/hypnotic, anxiolytic, amnesic, muscular relaxant and anticonvulsant actions with minor differences in the relative potency of these effects.

Pharmacokinetics. Most benzodiazepines mar-keted as hypnotics are well absorbed and rapidly penetrate the brain, producing hypnotic effects within half an hour after oral administration. Rates of elimination, however, vary with elimi-nation half-lives of from 2 to 100 hours (Table 25.1). The drugs undergo hepatic metabolism via oxidation or conjugation, and some form pharmacologically active metabolites with even longer elimination half-lives. Oxidation of benzodiazepines is decreased in the elderly, in patients with hepatic impairment and in the presence of some drugs including alcohol.

Pharmacokinetic characteristics are important in selecting a hypnotic drug. A rapid onset of action combined with a medium duration of action (elimination half-life about 8 hours) is usually desirable. Too short a duration of action

Table 25.1 Profile of some hypnotic drugs			
Drug	Site of action	Elimination half-life (h)	Recommended hypnotic dose*
Benzodiazepines	GABA/BZ receptor		
Diazepam†		20–100 (36–200)‡	5–10 mg
Loprazolam		6–12	1 mg
Lorazepam		10–18	1 mg
Lormetazepam		10–12	1 mg
Nitrazepam		15–38	5–10 mg
Temazepam		8–15	10–30 mg
Triazolam§		2–5	0.25 mg
Non-Benzodiazepines	GABA/BZ receptor		
Zopiclone		5–6	7.5–15 mg
Chloral hydrate		(8)‡	0.5–1 g
Chlormethiazole		4	192–384 mg
Barbiturates	GABA/BZ receptor		
Amylobarbitone		17–34	100–200 mg
Antihistamines	Histamine (H₁) receptor		
Promethazine		12	50 mg

* Doses are suggested adult doses. Dosage should be reduced in the elderly. The recommended doses are approximately equivalent hypnotic potency.
† Diazepam, though classed as an anxiolytic drug, has useful hypnotic properties when administered as a single dose.
‡ ( ) half-life of pharmacologically active metabolite.
§ Triazolam was withdrawn in the United Kingdom in 1991.
BZ = benzodiazepine.

(triazolam) may lead to, or fail to control, early morning waking, while a long duration of action (nitrazepam) may produce residual effects the next day and may lead to cumulation if the drug is used regularly. However, frequency of use and dosage are important. For example, diazepam (5 to 10 mg) produces few residual effects when used occasionally, despite its slow elimination, although chronic use impairs daytime performance. Large doses of short-acting drugs may produce 'hangover' effects, while small doses of longer-acting drugs may cause little or no 'hangover'.

Effects on sleep. A major site of the hypnotic action of benzodiazepines is the brain stem reticular formation which, as mentioned above, is of central importance in arousal. The reticular formation is extremely sensitive to depression by benzodiazepines which decrease both spontaneous activity and responses to afferent stimuli. Similar depression of limbic arousal systems adds to hypnotic efficacy in patients with insomnia due to anxiety. However, active sleep mechanisms are also suppressed, and this effect leads to disruption of the normal sleep pattern.

Benzodiazepines are effective hypnotics: they hasten sleep onset; decrease nocturnal awakenings; increase total sleeping time; and often impart a sense of deep, refreshing sleep. However, they produce changes in the relative proportion of different sleep stages. Stage 2 (light sleep) is prolonged and mainly accounts for the increased sleeping time. By contrast, the duration of SWS may be considerably reduced. REMS is also decreased; the latency to the first REMS episode is prolonged and dreaming is diminished. This abnormal sleep profile probably arises because of the unselective depression of both arousal and sleep mechanisms. The suppression of REMS may be an important factor in determining rebound effects on drug withdrawal (see below).

Mechanism of action. Most of the effects of benzodiazepines result from their interaction with specific binding sites associated with post-synaptic GABA$_A$ receptors in the brain. All benzodiazepines bind to these sites although with varying degrees of affinity.

The GABA$_A$ receptor consists of a multimolecular complex which controls a chloride ion channel and contains specific binding sites for benzodiazepines and barbiturates (Fig. 25.2). The

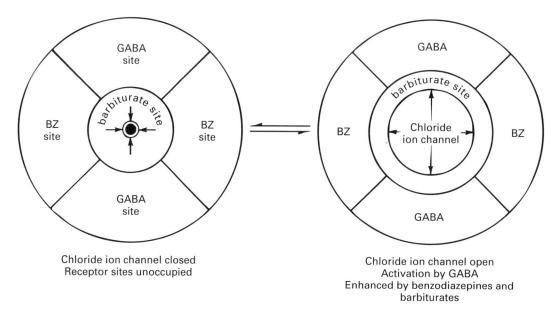

Fig. 25.2 Cross-sectional diagram of the GABA/benzodiazepine (BZ) receptor complex. On the left, the diagram shows the inactive state of the receptor, with chloride ion channel closed and receptor sites unoccupied. Activation of the receptor by GABA, benzodiazepines or barbiturates (diagram on right) opens the chloride channel causing hyperpolarization (inhibition) of the neurone.

various effects of benzodiazepines (hypnotic, anxiolytic, anticonvulsant) probably result from GABA potentiation in specific brain sites, and some actions may result from secondary effects on other neurotransmitter systems. For example, a reduction in serotonergic activity may underlie the anxiolytic effects.

Adverse effects of hypnotic use

Tolerance. Tolerance to the hypnotic effects of benzodiazepines develops rapidly. Sleep latency, stage 2 sleep, SWS, REMS, dreaming and intrasleep awakenings all tend to return to pretreatment levels after a few weeks of regular use. Nevertheless poor sleepers may report continued efficacy and the drugs are often used long term because of difficulties in withdrawal.

Rebound insomnia. Rebound insomnia, in which sleep is poorer than before drug treatment, is common on withdrawal of benzodiazepines. Sleep latency is prolonged; intrasleep wakenings become more frequent; REMS duration and intensity is increased, with vivid dreams or nightmares which may add to frequent awakenings. These symptoms are most marked when the drugs have been taken in high doses or for long periods but can occur after only a week of low-dose administration. They are conspicuous with moderately rapidly eliminated benzodiazepines (temazepam, lorazepam) and may last for many weeks. With rapidly eliminated benzodiazepines (triazolam) rebound effects may occur in the later part of the night and cause early morning waking and daytime anxiety. With slowly eliminated benzodiazepines (diazepam), SWS and REMS may remain depressed for some weeks and then slowly return to baseline, sometimes without a rebound effect. Tolerance and rebound effects are probably a reflection of down-regulation of GABA/benzodiazepine receptors, a homeostatic response to regular drug use. They encourage continued hypnotic usage and contribute to the development of drug dependence (see later section on benzodiazepines).

Oversedation, 'hangover' effects. Many benzodiazepines used as hypnotics can give rise to a subjective 'hangover', and after most of them,

even those with short elimination half-lives, psychomotor performance and memory may be impaired on the following day. Oversedation is most likely with slowly eliminated benzodiazepines, especially if used chronically, and is most marked in the elderly in whom drowsiness, incoordination and ataxia, leading to falls and fractures, and acute confusional states may result even from small doses. Paradoxical excitement may occur occasionally.

Some benzodiazepines in hypnotic doses may decrease alveolar ventilation and depress the respiratory response to hypercapnia increasing the risk of cerebral hypoxia, especially in the elderly and in patients with chronic respiratory disease.

Drug interactions. Benzodiazepines have additive effects with other central nervous system depressants. Combinations of benzodiazepines with alcohol, other hypnotics, sedative tricyclic antidepressants, antihistamines, or opiates can cause marked sedation and may lead to accidents or severe respiratory depression.

Pregnancy and lactation. The regular use of benzodiazepines is contra-indicated in pregnancy since the drugs are concentrated in fetal tissues where hepatic metabolism is minimal. They can cause neonatal depression, hypotonia and feeding difficulties if given in late pregnancy, and infants exposed in utero to regular hypnotic maternal doses may develop withdrawal symptoms 2 to 3 weeks after birth (irritability, crying, muscle twitches). They also enter breast milk, and long-acting benzodiazepines are contra-indicated during lactation, although short- to medium-acting benzodiazepines appear to be safe.

Barbiturates

Although barbiturates are now obsolete as hypnotics or anxiolytics, several thousand elderly people continue to take them nightly as a legacy of pre-benzodiazepine prescribing. The actions of barbiturates are very similar to those of benzodiazepines: they have hypnotic, anxiolytic muscle relaxant and anticonvulsant properties. These effects, like those of benzodiazepines, are mediated through an interaction at the GABA$_A$ receptor which also has a specific barbiturate binding site (Fig. 25.2).

The effects of barbiturates on sleep are similar to those of benzodiazepines. They are effective hypnotics but depress both SWS and REMS. Tolerance develops on continued use and rebound insomnia occurs on drug withdrawal. Most barbiturates used as hypnotics are only slowly eliminated and 'hangover' effects with oversedation and residual psychomotor impairment are common. Other adverse effects include a low therapeutic index (fatal respiratory and vasomotor depression can occur in doses about 10 times the hypnotic dose), a high risk of drug dependence, and a propensity to drug interactions due to hepatic enzyme induction as well as additive effects with other central nervous system depressants.

Chloral derivatives (chloral hydrate, triclofos, dichloralphenazone)

Chloral derivatives still have considerable use as hypnotics in general practice. They are all metabolized to trichlorethanol which has an elimination half-life of 8 hours (Table 25.1). These drugs are moderately effective as hypnotics and their effects on sleep are similar to those of benzodiazepines and barbiturates. They can produce 'hangover' effects, drug dependence and an abstinence syndrome on withdrawal and may cause gastrointestinal disturbance. The mechanism of action is similar to that of barbiturates, and respiratory and cardiovascular depression occurs on overdose.

Chlormethiazole

Chlormethiazole has hypnotic and anticonvulsant properties and a mode of action similar to that of barbiturates. It is fairly rapidly eliminated (half-life 4 hours; Table 25.1) and produces little respiratory depression at therapeutic doses. For these reasons it has been advocated for use in the elderly and is sometimes used in alcohol and narcotic detoxification. However, it has a low therapeutic index, produces a profound respi-

ratory depression in overdose, and carries an appreciable risk of dependence, especially in combination with alcohol.

Zopiclone

Zopiclone, a cyclopyrrolone, is a non-benzodiazepine which nevertheless binds to a site on benzodiazepine receptors. It has hypnotic and other therapeutic effects similar to benzodiazepines but carries the same potential for adverse effects including dependence and abstinence effects on withdrawal. Psychiatric reactions including hallucinations, and behavioural disturbances have been reported to occur shortly after the first dose. This drug appears to have no particular advantages over benzodiazepines, although it may cause less alteration of sleep stages.

Promethazine

Promethazine is one of the few drugs with useful hypnotic properties which does not act on GABA/benzodiazepine receptors. It is a sedative antihistamine with antagonistic effects on H$_1$ receptors in the brain. Promethazine is related to the phenothiazines and has additional slight neuroleptic and anticholinergic effects. In suitable dosage (Table 25.1), promethazine has mild to moderate hypnotic efficacy, but the onset of action is slow (1.5 to 3 hours) and it is only slowly eliminated (elimination half-life 12 hours). 'Hangover' effects are common and it occasionally produces excitement rather than sedation. Nevertheless, promethazine is sometimes of value in paediatric practice and in cases where other hypnotics are contra-indicated. Other sedative antihistamines with similar effects include diphenhydramine and chlorpheniramine.

Other drugs used as hypnotics

Prescribing data suggests that tricyclic antidepressants with sedative effects and neuroleptic drugs in low dosage are being increasingly used as hypnotic alternatives to benzodiazepines. Such drugs may be indicated when insomnia is due to depression or severe anxiety, but are not recommended for general hypnotic use since they have potentially serious adverse effects. Alcohol is used as a 'nightcap' by many individuals, often with the tacit approval of their doctors. Alcohol (which also acts on $GABA_A$ receptors) may indeed help to induce sleep but may lead to late-night restlessness, and excessive use of alcohol is a common cause of insomnia.

Rational drug treatment of insomnia

A hypnotic drug may be indicated for insomnia when it is severe, disabling, unresponsive to other measures, or likely to be temporary. In choosing an appropriate agent, individual variables relating to the patient and to the drug need to be considered (see Table 25.2).

THE PATIENT

Type of insomnia

The duration of insomnia is important in deciding on a hypnotic regimen. Transient insomnia may be caused by changes of routine such as overnight travel, change in time zone, alteration of shift work or temporary admission to hospital. In these circumstances a hypnotic with a rapid onset and medium duration of action and few residual effects could be used on one or two occasions.

Short-term insomnia may result from temporary environmental stress. In this case a hypnotic may occasionally be indicated, but should be prescribed in low dosage for 1 or 2 weeks only, preferably intermittently on alternate nights or 1 night in 3.

Chronic insomnia presents a much greater therapeutic problem. It is usually secondary to other conditions (organic or psychiatric) at which treatment should initially be aimed. In selected cases a hypnotic may be helpful but it is recommended that such drugs should be prescribed at the minimal effective dosage and administered intermittently (1 night in 3) or temporarily (not more than 2 or 3 weeks). Occasionally it is necessary to repeat short, intermittent courses at intervals of a few months.

The elderly

The elderly are especially vulnerable both to insomnia and to adverse effects from hypnotic drugs. They may have reduced metabolism of some drugs and may be at risk of cumulative effects. They are also more susceptible than younger subjects to central nervous system depression including cognitive impairment and ataxia (which may lead to falls and fractures). They are sensitive to respiratory depression, prone to sleep apnoea and other sleep disorders, and are more likely to have 'sociological', psychiatric and somatic illnesses which both disturb sleep and may be aggravated by hypnotics. For some of these elderly patients, hypnotics can improve the quality of life but the dosage should be adjusted (usually half the recommended adult dose) and hypnotics with long elimination half-lives should be avoided. A considerable number

Table 25.2 Drug treatment in insomnia		
Type of insomnia	Choice of drugs	Administration
Transient insomnia	Benzodiazepine (temazepam, diazepam)	Once or twice only
Short-term insomnia	Benzodiazepine (long or medium duration of action)	1–2 weeks only, or intermittent
Chronic insomnia	1. Treat primary cause (education, sleep hygiene, pain relief, psychiatric treatment) 2. Benzodiazepine (medium duration of action) 3. Chlormethiazole 4. Sedative antihistamine	2–3 weeks maximum; preferably intermittent; lowest effective dose

of elderly patients give a history of regular hypnotic use going back for 20 or 30 years. In some of these, gradual reduction of hypnotic dosage or even withdrawal may be indicated.

The young

Hypnotics are generally contra-indicated for children. Where sedation is required, sedative antihistamines are usually recommended. However, a single dose of a benzodiazepine (with appropriate dosage reduction) may be more effective.

Pregnancy and lactation

Regular use of slowly eliminated hypnotics are contra-indicated. If hypnotics are required, intermittent doses of relatively rapidly eliminated hypnotics may be used and have been shown to be safe during breast feeding.

Disease states

In patients with chronic pain or terminal conditions suitable analgesics including non-steroidal anti-inflammatory agents or opiates, sometimes combined with neuroleptics, usually provide satisfactory sedation. In such patients the possibility of drug dependence becomes a less important issue and regular use of hypnotics with a medium duration of action should not be denied if they provide symptomatic relief of insomnia.

Choice of drug

There is little difference in hypnotic efficacy between most of the available agents. The main factors to consider in the rational choice of a hypnotic regimen are duration of action and the risk of adverse effects, especially oversedation and the development of tolerance and dependence. Cost may be a factor with new drugs.

Rate of elimination

In general, very short-acting drugs such as triazolam should be avoided as they tend to cause late-night insomnia and daytime anxiety. Regular use of slowly eliminated drugs should also be avoided because of the increased risk of oversedation and 'hangover' effects. Drugs with a medium elimination half-life (8 to 12 hours) appear to have the most suitable profile for hypnotic use. These include temazepam, lormetazepam and loprazolam which are the drugs of first choice in most situations where hypnotics are indicated. Chlormethiazole is sometimes suitable as a second choice provided that its relatively short duration of action and toxicity in overdose are taken into account. A sedative antihistamine such as promethazine is a safe third choice and it is useful in children although it may produce daytime drowsiness.

Dosage

The minimum effective dosage should always be used as there is considerable individual variation in response and susceptibility to oversedation. It is best to start with a small dose which may be increased if necessary. Dosage should, in general, be halved in the elderly and caution exercised in the presence of respiratory or hepatic disease.

Duration and timing of administration

In order to prevent the development of tolerance and dependence, the maximum duration of treatment should be limited to 2 or 3 weeks and treatment should where possible be intermittent (1 night in 2 or 3). Doses should be taken 20 minutes before retiring in order to allow dissolution in the stomach and absorption to commence before the patient lies down in bed.

Anxiolytic drugs

As with insomnia, drugs provide only symptomatic treatment for anxiety. They may temporarily help a patient to cope with an otherwise overwhelming stress and can provide a short-term cover which allows time for more specific treatments to take effect, but they do not cure the underlying disorder. Most anxiety states are more effectively treated in the long term by non-pharmacological interventions including counselling, psychotherapy, behavioural and cognitive methods, relaxation, and anxiety management training. Essentially, all these methods involve a learning process which enables the patient to develop improved stress-coping techniques. However, these methods are time consuming, labour intensive and costly.

The ideal anxiolytic drug would selectively damp down excess activity in limbic (emotional) and somatic arousal systems, without inhibiting learning processes or producing undue sedation. The onset of action would be rapid and the drugs would be suitable for long-term use. No available drug meets all these requirements. The 'classical' anxiolytics, such as the benzodiazepines, have a rapid onset of action but impair cognitive processes and have undesirable long-term effects. Antidepressants are effective in some types of anxiety but have a delayed onset of action, are potentially toxic, and may be difficult to withdraw. Some of the somatic manifestations of anxiety can be alleviated by beta-adrenorecep-tor antagonists, but these drugs have little effect on subjective symptoms. Some anxiolytic drugs are shown in Table 25.3.

Benzodiazepines

Benzodiazepines are still the most commonly prescribed drugs for anxiety. About 10 million prescriptions for benzodiazepines classed as anxiolytics are issued each year in the UK, and may anxious patients are also prescribed hypnotics.

Benzodiazepines have potent anxiolytic effects which are exerted at low doses that produce minimal sedation. A major advantage in acute situations is the rapid onset of action which occurs within an hour of the first effective dose. Many clinical trials have shown efficacy in patients with anxiety disorders. Anxiolytic effects have also been reported in normal volunteers with high trait anxiety and in patients with anticipatory anxiety before surgery. However, in subjects with low trait anxiety and in non-stressful conditions benzodiazepines may para-

Table 25.3 Profile of some anxiolytic drugs

Drug	Elimination half-life (h)	Recommended anxiolytic dosage*
Benzodiazepines		
Alprazolam	6–12	0.25–0.5 mg three times daily
Chlordiazepoxide	5–30 (36–200)[†]	10 mg twice daily
Diazepam	20–100 (36–200)[†]	2–5 mg twice daily
Lorazepam	10–18	1 mg three times daily
Oxazepam	4–15	15–30 mg three times daily
Buspirone	2–11	5 mg three times daily
Beta-adrenoreceptor blockers		
Propranolol	2–4	20 mg three times daily
Tricyclic antidepressants[2]		
Amitriptyline	10–25 (13–93)[†]	50–100 mg daily
Dothiepin	14–40	75–125 mg daily
Doxepin	8–25	75–125 mg daily
Mianserin	8–19	30–40 mg daily
Trazodone	4	150–300 mg daily
Trimipramine	7–9	75–125 mg daily
Monoamine oxidase inhibitors		
Phenelzine	‡	15 mg three times daily

* Dosage should be reduced in the elderly. Recommended doses are approximately equivalent in anxiolytic potency, except for lorazepam for which 0.5 mg tablets (equivalent to 5 mg diazepam) are not available in the UK.
[†] ( ) half-life of pharmacologically active metabolite.
‡ Causes irreversible enzyme inhibition; antidepressant effects last up to 2 weeks after cessation of treatment.
[2] Specific serotonin reuptake inhibitors (SSRIs) fluoxetine, fluvoxamine, paroxetine, sertraline, are also effective in anxiety disorders and are safer in overdose.

doxically increase anxiety and impair psychomotor performance.

The major site of anxiolytic action is the limbic system (see above). This effect is mediated by a primary action at GABA receptors resulting in enhancement of inhibitory GABA activity (Fig. 25.2). Secondary suppression of noradrenergic and/or serotonergic pathways appears to be of particular importance in relation to anxiolytic effects.

Adverse effects of anxiolytic use

Tolerance. Tolerance to the anxiolytic effects of benzodiazepines seems to develop more slowly than to the hypnotic effects. In clinical use, most patients reporting initial drowsiness find that it wears off in a few days while the anxiolytic effect remains for some weeks. However, benzodiazepines are usually no longer effective in the treatment of anxiety after 1 to 4 months of regular use.

Psychomotor impairment. Although oversedation is not usually a problem in anxious patients, there is evidence that long-term use of benzodiazepines results in psychomotor impairment and may have adverse effects on memory. Many patients on long-term benzodiazepines complain of poor memory (which improves after withdrawal), and incidents of shoplifting have been attributed to memory lapses caused by benzodiazepine use. There is some evidence that benzodiazepines also inhibit the learning of alternative stress-coping strategies, such as behavioural treatments for agoraphobia. Additive effects with other central nervous system depressants including alcohol occur, as with hypnotic use of benzodiazepines, and may contribute to traffic and other accidents.

Disinhibition, paradoxical effects. Occasionally, benzodiazepines produce paradoxical stimulant effects. These effects are most marked in anxious subjects and include excitement, increased anxiety, irritability and outbursts of rage. Violent behaviour, including baby battering, have sometimes been attributed to disinhibition by benzodiazepines of behaviour normally suppressed by social restraints, fear or anxiety.

Increased daytime anxiety and psychiatric symptoms can occur with rapidly eliminated benzodiazepines, such as triazolam, and are probably withdrawal effects.

Affective reactions. Chronic use of benzodiazepines can aggravate depression and provoke suicide in depressed patients, and can cause depression in patients with no previous history of depressive disorder. Aggravation of depression is a particular risk in anxious patients who often have mixed anxiety/depression. Some patients on long-term benzodiazepines complain of 'emotional anaesthesia' with inability to experience either pleasure or distress. However, in some patients benzodiazepines induce euphoria and they are increasingly used as drugs of abuse when taken in high doses or self-administered intravenously.

Dependence. The greatest drawback of chronic benzodiazepine use is the development of drug dependence. It is now generally agreed that the regular use of therapeutic doses of benzodiazepines as hypnotics or anxiolytics for more than a few weeks can give rise to dependence, with withdrawal symptoms on cessation of drug use in over 30% of patients. It is estimated that there are about 1.2 million long-term benzodiazepine users in the UK at present and many of these are likely to be dependent. People with anxious or 'passive-dependent' personalities seem to be most vulnerable to dependence and withdrawal symptoms. Such individuals make up a large proportion of anxious patients in psychiatric practice, are often described as suffering from 'chronic anxiety', and are the type of patient for whom benzodiazepines are most likely to be prescribed. Such patients often continue to take benzodiazepines for many years because attempts at dosage reduction or drug withdrawal result in abstinence symptoms which they are unable to tolerate. Nevertheless, these patients continue to suffer from anxiety symptoms despite continued benzodiazepine use, possibly because they have become tolerant to the anxiolytic effects and may also suffer from other adverse effects of long-term benzodiazepines use such as depression or psychomotor impairment.

Benzodiazepine withdrawal. Many patients on long-term benzodiazepines are now seeking help with drug withdrawal. Increasing clinical experience shows that withdrawal is feasible in most patients if carried out with care. Abrupt withdrawal in dependent subjects is dangerous and can induce acute anxiety, psychosis or convulsions. However, gradual withdrawal, coupled where necessary with counselling or psychological treatments, can be successful in the majority of patients. The duration of withdrawal should be tailored to individual needs and may last many months. Dosage decrements may be of the order of 1 to 2 mg diazepam per month. Even with slow dosage reduction, a large variety of withdrawal symptoms may be experienced, including increased anxiety, insomnia, hypersensitivity to sensory stimuli, perceptual distortions, paraesthesiae, muscle twitching, depression and many others. The temporary use of other drugs, particularly sedative tricyclic antidepressants may be indicated during the withdrawal period. Withdrawal symptoms appear to be most pronounced in patients with personality disorders, and are related to duration of benzodiazepine use. However, the eventual outcome does not appear to be influenced by dosage, type of benzodiazepine, duration of use, personality disorder, psychiatric history, age, severity of withdrawal symptoms or rate of withdrawal. Hence benzodiazepine withdrawal is worth attempting in patients who are motivated to stop, and most patients report that they feel better after withdrawal than when they were taking the benzodiazepine.

Choice of benzodiazepine in anxiety

Despite the drawbacks of chronic use, benzodiazepines can be valuable in the short-term management of anxiety because of their anxiolytic efficacy and rapid onset of action. The choice of an appropriate benzodiazepine, as with hypnotics, depends largely on pharmacokinetic characteristics. Potent benzodiazepines such as lorazepam and alprazolam (Table 25.3) have been widely used for anxiety but are probably inappropriate. These drugs are moderately rap-idly eliminated and need to be taken several times daily. Blood concentrations fluctuate and lead to craving between doses probably because patients start to undergo withdrawal symptoms as the anxiolytic effect of each tablet wears off. The high potency of lorazepam (approximately 10 times that of diazepam), and the fact that it is available only in 1 mg and 2.5 mg tablet strengths has often led to excessive dosage. It is not unusual to see patients taking 7.5 mg lorazepam daily (approximately equivalent to 75 mg diazepam). Such doses lead to adverse effects, a high probability of dependence and difficulties in withdrawal. A slowly eliminated benzodiazepine such as diazepam is more appropriate in most cases. Diazepam has a rapid onset of action and its slow elimination ensures a steady blood concentration. It should be prescribed in the minimal effective dosage to avoid cumulative effects, and it can also be used as a hypnotic, thus avoiding the need for a separate hypnotic drug. However, as with hypnotics, the anxiolytic use of benzodiazepines should generally be limited to short-term (maximum 2 weeks) or intermittent use.

Buspirone

Buspirone is a relatively recently introduced anxiolytic drug with a structure and mode of action completely different from that of the benzodiazepines. It has mixed agonist/antagonist actions at serotonergic receptors which are thought to be involved in anxiety. In clinical trials it appears to have anxiolytic effects comparable with those of benzodiazepines, but it is without sedative/hypnotic, anticonvulsant or muscle relaxant effects. A major disadvantage is that anxiolytic effects are delayed for up to 3 weeks and in some patients buspirone produces dysphoria and may actually increase anxiety. Furthermore, it does not alleviate anxiety associated with benzodiazepine withdrawal. Buspirone does not appear to produce dependence or a withdrawal syndrome, although most clinical studies have been of limited duration, and the drug is recommended for short-term use only. The place of buspirone in the treatment of anxiety is doubtful at present, but serotonin receptor antagonists which are possibly more efficacious are under development.

Antidepressant drugs

A number of tricyclic and other antidepressants have additional sedative or anxiolytic effects (Table 25.3). They appear to be as effective as benzodiazepines in generalized anxiety and superior in panic disorder and agoraphobia. They are also of value in depressive states associated with anxiety and in anxiety/depression associated with benzodiazepine withdrawal. Monoamine oxidase inhibitors are also effective in phobic states and panic disorders. A disadvantage of these drugs is their slow onset of action which may be delayed for 2 or 3 weeks (tricyclic antidepressants) or up to 6 weeks (monoamine oxidase inhibitors), and they may initially exacerbate anxiety symptoms. The mode of action of these drugs is thought to be an initial increase in central serotonergic and noradrenergic activity, which may cause further anxiety, followed by a down-regulation of adrenergic and serotonergic receptors, accounting for the delayed anxiolytic effect. Nevertheless, the sedative effect of some tricyclic antidepressants may be a separate action and is often manifested early in the treatment; monoamine oxidase inhibitors, on the other hand, often cause insomnia. A second disadvantage of this group of drugs is that they are toxic in overdose and have many adverse effects including anticholinergic actions, which are common, cardiovascular actions, especially in the elderly, drug interactions, and interactions with certain foods. They are, however, more suitable for long-term use than benzodiazepines and can be continued for several months. They are often effective in low to moderate doses and do not cause cognitive impairment. Some anxious patients may have difficulty in stopping these drugs because of withdrawal symptoms which include rebound excessive cholinergic activity and increased anxiety or depression. Withdrawal should therefore be carried out gradually.

Beta-adrenoreceptor blockers

Some somatic symptoms of anxiety such as palpitations and tremor are due to excessive sympathetic activity acting on peripheral beta-adrenoreceptors. These symptoms can be effectively controlled by beta-adrenoreceptor blockers such as propranolol. These drugs, when used in small doses which do not induce hypotension, can be of value in acutely stressful situations or panic attacks where physical symptoms dominate the picture, although they have little effect on subjective anxiety symptoms. If used regularly in anxious patients, withdrawal should be gradual to prevent rebound tachycardia and return of palpitations.

Antipsychotic drugs

Some antipsychotic drugs such as chlorpromazine and haloperidol have sedative and anxiolytic effects and may, on occasion, be of short-term use in severe anxiety disorders associated with panic. They have a rapid onset of action (within an hour) but should be used in minimal dosage and only for a few weeks since they carry a risk of inducing dyskinesias. Anxious patients may have withdrawal problems after regular use. The growing tendency to prescribe these drugs as alternatives to benzodiazepines is to be deprecated.

Rational use of drugs in anxiety

It is clear that drugs do not provide a long-term solution for anxiety. In acute anxiety states, often precipitated by stress, short-term benzodiazepines may help to cope with the immediate situation as they have high efficacy and a rapid onset of action (Table 25.4). Diazepam, prescribed in hypnotic or anxiolytic doses, depending on the circumstances, is probably the drug of choice. A single dose may be sufficient, and it should not be continued regularly for more than 1 or 2 weeks. It can be given intermittently and intermittent courses can be repeated if necessary. Potent, short-acting benzodiazepines such as alprazolam, lorazepam and triazolam should be

Table 25.4 Drug treatment in anxiety

Drug	Efficacy	Onset of therapeutic effect	Risk of dependence	Administration
Benzodiazepines	++	Immediate	++	Single dose, intermittent, short term (2 weeks)
Buspirone	+	Delayed (2–3 weeks)	–	Short term (4 weeks)
Beta-adrenoreceptor blockers	+ (some patients)	Immediate	±	Medium term (weeks–months)
Tricyclic antidepressants	++	Delayed (2–3 weeks)	±	Medium to long term (3–12 months)
Monoamine oxidase inhibitors	++ (selected cases)	Delayed (3–6 weeks)	+	Medium to long term (3–12 months)

NB: Wherever possible, psychological treatments are preferred (counselling, anxiety management training, cognitive and behaviour therapy, psychotherapy).

avoided. Benzodiazepines are not recommended in bereavement because their amnesic actions may interfere with subsequent readjustment. The aims and limitations of benzodiazepine treatment for anxiety, and the risk of drug dependence should be explained to patients.

If longer-term treatment is required in generalized anxiety, anxiety/depression or phobic states, sedative tricyclic antidepressants are preferred. These drugs are efficacious, can be used for several months, and do not interfere with non-pharmacological treatments. However, their therapeutic effects may be delayed for 2 or 3 weeks and they can initially exacerbate anxiety. Monoamine oxidase inhibitors are effective in phobic disorders but have a delayed onset of action, commonly cause adverse effects, and carry a risk of dependence.

Beta-adrenoreceptor blockers are effective in controlling somatic symptoms such as palpitations and tremor and have a role for patients in whom such symptoms are prominent. Newer anxiolytics such as buspirone and serotonin receptor antagonists are appearing on the market but their clinical efficacy and dependence-producing potential have yet to be evaluated.

The most effective long-term treatment of anxiety is by psychological methods which can include self-help groups, counselling, behavioural and cognitive techniques, anxiety management training and psychotherapy. These measures all take time to be effective: the main role of drugs is to alleviate symptoms during the learning process involved.

CASE STUDIES

CASE 25.1

A female patient aged 60 years has been taking nitrazepam (10 mg nocte) for 15 years. The drug was originally prescribed for insomnia following a domestic crisis which has since passed. However, the patient has continued taking the drug and is afraid that she would now be unable to sleep without it. She is physically fit.

Q Outline a suitable approach to this problem.

CASE 25.2

A male patient aged 30 years was prescribed lorazepam (1 mg three times daily) 5 years ago for anxiety precipitated by business worries and still takes the drug daily in the same dosage. He now finds that he becomes increasingly anxious as the usual time for each dose approaches. He carries the tablets with him and becomes extremely anxious and distressed if, for any reason, he is prevented from taking his tablets or if his supply runs low. He feels that his life has begun to revolve around the tablets and would like to stop but is worried that he could not cope without them.

Q Outline a suitable approach to this problem.

ANSWERS TO CASE STUDIES

CASE 25.1

A Slow withdrawal of the nitrazepam is advisable after explanation of normal sleep requirements and long-term effects of benzodiazepines. It would be convenient to substitute nitrazepam with diazepam in equivalent dosage and to reduce dosage of diazepam in decrements of 1 mg (half a 2 mg tablet) every 2 to 4 weeks. With this slow reduction, withdrawal symptoms, if they occur at all, are likely to be mild and temporary; a normal drug-free sleep pattern will be restored; and adverse effects of long-term benzodiazepine usage (which become more pronounced as age advances) will be avoided.

CASE 25.2

A The patient's anxiety is probably largely due to withdrawal symptoms as the anxiolytic effect of each dose of lorazepam wears off. He should be given a full explanation about benzodiazepine tolerance and withdrawal symptoms and offered appropriate anxiety management counselling. He should be advised to withdraw the lorazepam slowly while receiving psychological support. Slow reduction could be achieved either by using a lorazepam suspension which allows dosage reduction in 0.1 mg decrements, or by converting his dosage gradually to an equivalent dose of diazepam (Table 25.1) and reducing this at the rate of 1 to 2 mg every 2 to 4 weeks. The temporary use of adjuvant drugs, such as propranolol for palpitations or tremor, or a sedative tricyclic antidepressant drug for depression may be helpful during the withdrawal period. The chances of a successful outcome with eventual improvement in anxiety and everyday performance are high.

BIBLIOGRAPHY

Ashton H. Benzodiazepine withdrawal: outcome in 50 patients. British Journal of Addiction 1987; 82: 665–671

Feely M, Pullar T. Pharmacokinetic differences between benzodiazepines. In: Hindmarch I, Beaumont G, Brandon S, Leonard B E (eds) Benzodiazepines: current concepts. Chichester: John Wiley & Sons 1990; 61–72

Haefely W. Benzodiazepine receptor and ligands: structural and functional differences. In: Hindmarch I, Beaumont G, Brandon S, Leonard B E (eds) Benzodiazepines: current concepts. Chichester: John Wiley & Sons 1990: 1–18

Horne J. Why we sleep. Oxford: Oxford University Press 1988

Kales A, Soldatos C R, Bixler E O, Kales J A, Vela-Bueno A. Diazepam: effects on sleep and withdrawal phenomena. Journal of Clinical Psychopharmacology 1988; 8: 340–346

Lader M H, Petursson H. Benzodiazepine derivatives – side effects and dangers. Biological Psychiatry 1981; 16: 1195–1212

Marks J, Nicholson A N. Drugs and insomnia. British Medical Journal 1984; 288: 261

Owen R T, Tyrer P. Benzodiazepine dependence: a review of the evidence. Drugs 1983; 25: 385–398

Tyrer P. Benefits and risks of benzodiazepines. In: Freeman H, Rue Y (eds) The benzodiazepines in current clinical practice. London, New York: Royal Society of Medicine Services 1987

Tyrer P. Choice of treatment in anxiety. In: Tyrer P (ed). The psychopharmacology of anxiety. Oxford: Oxford University Press 1989; 255–282

Neurological and psychological disorders

Chapter 26

Affective disorders

J. P. Pratt

The central feature of an affective disorder is the alteration in mood. The most common presentation is that of a low mood or depression. Less commonly the mood may become high or elated as in mania.

Depression

The term depression can in itself be misleading. Everyone in the normal course of daily life will experience alterations in mood. Depressed mood in this context does not represent a disorder or illness, in fact lowered mood as a normal response to the ups and down of living can be considered normal and is more correctly termed sadness or unhappiness. Sometimes clinical depression may present in a mild form, so it is important to differentiate this from normal unhappiness.

Mania

If the mood becomes elated or irritable this may be a symptom of mania. The term mania has been used to describe severe cases, with hypomania used to describe a less severe form of the disorder. This distinction is arbitrary and in everyday practice the two terms can be considered synonymous.

Bipolar and unipolar disorders

If a patient develops one or more manic episodes this may be termed a bipolar disorder; although this may be accompanied by depressive episodes, the existence of repeated manic episodes alone is sufficient to be termed bipolar disorder. The term manic depressive is a somewhat outdated way of describing a bipolar disorder.

The term unipolar is now confined to single episodes of depression.

EPIDEMIOLOGY

Differences in diagnosis, particularly of depression make it difficult to estimate the true incidence of affective disorders.

The lifetime risk of developing a bipolar disorder is said to be about 0.6 to 0.9% with an annual incidence of between 9 and 15 per 100 000 for men and up to 30 per 100 000 population for women. In the United States the incidence is said to be the same for both men and women, other studies suggest the disorder may be slightly more common in women.

By comparison, the overall incidence of depression is much higher and there does appear to be a significant difference between the sexes. In the United States the prevalence of major depressive disorder is between 3 and 6%, with a lifetime risk of between 8 and 12% for men and between 20 and 26% for women. The annual incidence is said to be between 80 and 200 per 100 000 for men and between 250 and 7800 per 100 000 for women. These differences between the sexes have been explained by the fact that women are more likely to express their feelings of depression to a doctor whereas men may present as alcoholics.

Although depression can occur at any age, including infancy, it is estimated that the average age of onset of depression is in the late 20s. Some earlier studies found the incidence and prevalence of depression in women peaking at the age of 35 to 45 years. In bipolar disorder an earlier age of onset is suggested, perhaps in late adolescence, but with the incidence increasing with age. Generally speaking the episodes tend to become more frequent as people grow older.

AETIOLOGY

Like most psychiatric disorders the cause, or causes of affective disorders are unknown. Despite this uncertainty several factors can be identified which may have a role in the development of an affective disorder and there appears to be more data about depression than bipolar disorders.

Genetic causes

The incidence of major depression in first-degree relatives of someone with severe depression may be 10 to 15%, which is much higher than the risk for the general population. Comparisons of the risk of affective disorder in the children of both parents with an affective disorder show a four times greater risk, and the risk is doubled in children with one parent with an affective disorder.

Social, environmental and genetic factors could all account for the findings of higher familial rates of affective disorders. Studies looking at twins have found fairly strong evidence for a genetic factor.

Evidence of a genetic link has been found in studies of children from parents with affective disorder who were adopted by healthy parents. A higher incidence of affective disorder was found in the biological parents of adopted children with affective disorder than in the adoptive parents.

Environmental factors

Although environmental stresses can often be identified prior to an episode of mania or depression, a causal relationship between a major event in someone's life and the development of an affective disorder has not been firmly established.

The lack of prospective studies makes it difficult to interpret data linking early life events, such as loss of a parent, to the development of an affective disorder.

The fact that specific environmental stresses have not been identified should not lead to the conclusion that the environment or lifestyle is irrelevant to the course or development of affective disorders. Indeed employment and close and confiding relationships have been noted to offer some protection.

Biochemical factors

In its simplistic form the biochemical theory of depression postulates a deficiency of neurotransmitter amines in certain parts of the brain. This theory has been developed to suggest receptor sensitivity changes may be important.

The hypothesis focuses on an involvement of the neurotransmitters noradrenaline and 5-hydroxytryptamine. This arose out of the findings that both the monoamine oxidase inhibitors (MAOIs) and the tricyclic antidepressants appeared to increase neurotransmitter amines (particularly noradrenaline) at important sites in the brain. When it was found that reserpine, previously used as an antihypertensive, caused both a depletion of neurotransmitter and induced depression, this was also taken as an apparent confirmation of the theory.

By looking at the metabolites of noradrenaline and 5-hydroxytryptamine some investigators have suggested different types of depression may exist. It has been found that some depressed patients appear to have reduced cerebral concentrations of 5-hydroxyindolacetic acid (5HIAA) (the metabolite of 5-hydroxytryptamine) whereas others appear to have reduced levels of methoxyhydroxyphenylglycerol (MHPG), a metabolite of noradrenaline.

This idea of noradrenergic and serotonergic forms of depression has not gained widespread support and there is little justification in measuring noradrenaline or serotonin metabolites in routine practice.

Overall the data suggest that biochemical abnormalities and receptor changes are associated with affective disorders, particularly depression, but the evidence to date does not confirm a biochemical cause.

Endocrine factors

Although some endocrine disorders such as hypothyroidism and Cushing's syndrome have been associated with changes in mood, there is no direct evidence linking thyroid hormones or adrenal glucocorticoids with affective disorder.

Some investigators have found a proportion of depressed people have increased cortisol levels. This finding has been used as the basis for the dexamethasone suppression test in depression.

Physical illness and side effects of medication

Disorders of mood, particularly depression, have been associated with several types of medication and a number of physical illnesses (Table 26.1).

CLINICAL MANIFESTATIONS
Depression

A low mood is the central feature of depression. This is often accompanied by a loss of interest or pleasure in normally enjoyable activities. Thinking is pessimistic and in some cases suicidal. A depressed person may complain that he or she has little or no energy.

Anxiety or agitation may accompany the disorder and the so-called biological features of sleep disturbances, weight loss and loss of appetite are often present. Depressed people typically complain of somatic symptoms, particularly gastric problems and nonspecific aches are common.

Normal sexual drive is reduced and some people may lose interest in sex altogether. In some cases the biological features are reversed

Table 26.1 Drugs and physical illnesses associated with disorders of mood	
Drugs	
Analgesics	Antidepressants
Antihypertensives	Anticonvulsants
Antipsychotics	Benzodiazepines
Antiparkinson agents	Steroids
Opiate withdrawal	
Amphetamine withdrawal	
Benzodiazepine withdrawal	
Physical illness	
Viral illness	Carcinoma
Neurological disorders	Diabetes
Thyroid disease	Addison's disease
Systemic lupus erythematosus	Pernicious anaemia

and excessive eating and sleeping may occur. In contrast to agitation, psychomotor retardation may be a presenting feature.

Bipolar disorder

At least one episode of mania must have occurred for a diagnosis of bipolar disorder to be made; depression may also occur, but it is not essential for this diagnosis to be made.

In mania the mood is elated or irritable and the accompanying overactivity is usually unproductive. Disinhibition may result in excessive spending sprees or inappropriate sexual activity. Manic people may describe their thoughts as racing, with ideas rapidly changing from one topic to another. Speech may be very rapid with frequent punning and rhyming.

An individual's ideas may become grandiose, they may develop fantastic projects which lead nowhere and inevitably are left incomplete and disjointed.

Clothing is usually flamboyant and if make-up is worn it is usually excessive and involves bright colours.

Severity

The severity of the disorder may vary from mild through moderate to severe. In most circumstances mild forms of the disorders are unlikely to come to the attention of specialist services, but many cases of mild depression will be seen by the primary health-care team.

In severe cases hallucinations and delusions may be present, making a differential diagnosis difficult. If left untreated it is important to remember that affective disorders carry a risk of mortality. As well as suicidal attempts by someone who is depressed, the lack of self-care and physical exhaustion resulting from mania may be life-threatening.

INVESTIGATIONS

There are no universally accepted tests which will confirm the presence of an affective disorder.

Various rating scales have been developed which may help demonstrate the severity of depressive disorder or distinguish a predominantly anxious patient from a depressed patient.

As discussed before, biochemical tests have not been particularly helpful in the treatment or management of affective disorders. The dexamethasone suppression test is still used by some clinicians as an aid to diagnosis, but it must be considered as having limited value in practice.

The American Psychiatric Association have developed a precise system of diagnosis, based on the description of symptoms in the *Diagnostic and statistical manual of mental disorders*, now in its third edition, revised form (DSM III R). This systematic approach to the diagnosis of affective disorders is particularly helpful when considering the effectiveness of medication, as most new clinical trials will require a DSM III R diagnosis as an entry criterion.

Rating scales

Various rating scales have been developed which may help the psychiatrist assess the severity of the disorder. Two of the more common ones in practice are the Beck depression inventory and the Hamilton depression rating scale.

Beck depression inventory

This is a self-reporting scale looking at 21 depressive symptoms. The subject is asked to read a series of statements and mark on a scale of one to four how severe the symptoms are. Obviously the higher the score the more severely depressed a person may be.

Hamilton rating scale for depression

This rating scale is used by the psychiatrist at the end of an interview to rate the severity of the depression.

Dexamethasone suppression test

This test involves the administration of 1 mg of

dexamethasone at 11 p.m., which is said to coincide with the low point of cortisol secretion. It would be expected that normally dexamethasone would suppress the secretion of cortisol for around 24 hours. Blood samples are taken the following day at 8 a.m., 4 p.m. and 11 p.m. If it is found that plasma cortisol levels are elevated between 9 and 24 hours after the administration of dexamethasone then this is taken as a positive result (i.e. dexamethasone has failed to suppress normal cortisol secretion).

It is important to note that this test is not specific to depression and other disorders may account for an apparent positive result. Similarly, there may be a high proportion of depressed people who show a negative result with the test.

Diagnostic and statistical manual of mental disorders

The majority of modern drug trials demonstrating the benefit of antidepressant treatment will use the DSM III R criterion for the diagnosis of affective disorder.

DSM III R diagnostic criteria for a major depressive episode

A. At least five of the following symptoms have been present during the same 2-week period and represent a change from previous functioning; at least one of the symptoms is either (1) depressed mood or (2) loss of interest or pleasure.

1. Depressed mood most of the day, nearly every day, as indicated by subjective account or observation by others.
2. Markedly diminished pleasure or interest in all or almost all activities, most of the day, nearly every day.
3. Significant weight loss or weight gain when not eating or increase or decrease in appetite nearly every day.
4. Insomnia or hypersomnia nearly every day.
5. Psychomotor retardation or agitation nearly every day.
6. Fatigue or loss of energy nearly every day.
7. Feelings of worthlessness or excessive or inappropriate guilt (which may be delusional) nearly every day.
8. Diminished ability to think or concentrate or indecisiveness, nearly every day.
9. Recurrent thoughts of death (not just fear of dying), recurrent suicidal ideation without a specific plan, or a suicide attempt or a specific plan for committing suicide.

B. It cannot be established that an organic factor initiated and maintained the disturbance.

The disturbance is not part of a normal reaction to the death of a loved one.

C. At no time during the disturbance have there been delusions for as long as 2 weeks, in the absence of prominent mood symptoms.

D. Not superimposed on schizophrenia, schizophreniform disorder, delusional disorder or psychotic disorder.

DSM III R diagnostic criteria for a manic episode

A. A distinct period of abnormality and persistently elevated, expansive, or irritable mood.

B. During the period of mood disturbances, at least three of the following symptoms have persisted (four if only the mood is irritable) and have been present to a significant degree:

1. Inflated self-esteem or grandiosity
2. Decreased need for sleep
3. More talkative than usual or pressure to keep talking
4. Flight of ideas or subjective experience that thoughts are racing
5. Distractibility
6. Increase in goal-directed activity or psychomotor agitation
7. Excessive involvement in pleasurable activities which have a high potential for painful consequences.

C. Mood disturbance sufficiently severe to cause marked impairment in occupational functioning or in usual social activities or relationships with others, or to necessitate hospitalization to prevent harm to others or self.

D. At no time during the disturbance have there been hallucinations or delusions for as long as 2 weeks in the absence of prominent mood symptoms (i.e. before the mood symptoms developed or after they have remitted).

E. Not superimposed on schizophrenia or schizophreniform disorder, delusional disorder or psychotic disorder.

F. It cannot be established that an organic factor initiated and maintained the disturbance. Note: somatic antidepressant treatments (e.g. drugs or electroconvulsive therapy (ECT)) that apparently precipitate a mood disturbance should not be considered an aetiological organic factor.

Although DSM III R does distinguish mania from hypomania as being more severe, in normal practice in the UK the two terms are frequently considered synonymous.

TREATMENT

The primary aim of treatment is to prevent harm and to relieve distress. Treatment will not change a person's normal personality; therefore it is important to differentiate symptoms of the disorder from the premorbid personality.

Many drugs which are used to control the symptoms of mania are not specifically anti-manic. They are also used in schizophrenia and other disorders; therefore the diagnosis will primarily influence the way in which these drugs are used rather than the choice of drug per se.

In the treatment of depression all the anti-depressants are equally effective. There is no con-vincing evidence that any one drug is any faster acting, or any better or any worse than any other in relieving the symptoms of depression. The major difference between agents is in their side-effect profile and toxicity in overdose. There can also be significant variations in the costs of different agents.

In addition to treating the disorders of mania or depression, treatment may also be considered prophylactic to prevent or reduce the intensity or frequency of an episode.

Treatment of depression

In moderate and severe depression, antidepressant medication should be considered the mainstay of treatment. In depressive states of mild severity some non-drug therapies are as effective as drug treatment.

Unfortunately there is a view that non-drug treatments and antidepressant medication are mutually exclusive. Quite clearly this is wrong, just as antidepressants should never be seen as the sole answer to a depression, the use of non-drug strategies should not be used as the reason for withholding treatment with antidepressant drugs.

Drug treatment

Despite the many new antidepressants available today, the therapeutic effectiveness of these agents has changed little since the discovery of the antidepressant properties of imipramine over 30 years ago.

Given an accurate diagnosis, any antidepressant currently available can be considered to be effective in 70 to 80% of patients. They will take some 2 to 4 weeks (up to 8 weeks in some patients) to produce a full response.

As discussed earlier there is no strong evidence for a particular biochemical sub-type of depression. However, for some unknown reason certain patients do respond to one antidepressant and not another. This has led to the widely held view that previous response to treatment is a strong indication to use that particular drug in the treatment of a future episode.

As well as previous response, the other important considerations to take into account are side effects, contra-indications and toxicity in overdose.

Generally speaking the older drugs have a poorer side effect and toxicity profile than the more recently introduced agents.

Traditionally the antidepressant drugs are categorized by their chemical structure (e.g. tricyclic) or their predominant pharmacological action (e.g. monoamine oxidase inhibitor or selective 5HT reuptake inhibitor).

Tricyclic antidepressants. A greater understanding of the pharmacology of antidepressants has led much support to the biochemical theory of depression.

Although substantial data on the pharmacological effects of the tricyclic antidepressants exist, it is still not clear how the drugs relieve the symptoms of depression.

Originally it was thought that the primary effect of the drugs was related to their ability to block the reuptake of noradrenaline and/or 5-hydroxytryptamine following their release and action as neurotransmitters. As this effect occurs some weeks before the antidepressant response, clearly this is not the whole story.

Following on from reuptake blockade, further changes take place particularly with pre- and postsynaptic receptor sensitivity. Reduction of presynaptic alpha$_2$ sensitivity takes place and this increases the production of noradrenaline. Other effects which may be relevant include an increase in alpha$_1$- and beta$_1$-receptor sensitivity. It is now felt that these receptor changes may be more related to the antidepressant response than simple reuptake inhibition.

There are at least 12 different antidepressants in clinical use today. Although the basic chemical structure of all these compounds is similar there are differences between them. All the tricyclic antidepressants block the reuptake of noradrenaline and 5-hydroxytriptamine to a greater or lesser degree.

Imipramine. This is probably the most well-established antidepressant. Its antidepressant effect was demonstrated over 30 years ago and it is still widely prescribed today. Although less sedating than some other tricyclic drugs, some patients may still experience problems. As well as cardiovascular problems, significant anti-muscarinic effects such as dry mouth, blurred vision and constipation occur.

For an effective antidepressant response it is important that the drug is given in full therapeutic doses, at least 150 mg daily and higher in some cases (up to 300 mg). Even though the dose needed by the elderly is likely to be lower, some patients, particularly the elderly, will be unable to tolerate adequate doses.

Tolerance may develop to some of the unpleasant side effects and this may be facilitated by starting with a lower dose of the drug and gradually increasing the dose over 1 week.

In addition to the unpleasant side effect profile

imipramine is toxic following overdose. Bearing in mind that the drug is used to treat a disorder which involves suicide this relative lack of safety is an important disadvantage.

Imipramine is metabolized by demethylation to an active metabolite desipramine. Both the parent drug and its metabolite have a long half-life which permits single daily dosing. Unfortunately the drug is only available in 10 mg or 25 mg tablets and some patients do not like taking large numbers of tablets at once.

Amitriptyline. Another well-established and widely prescribed antidepressant, it has a similar poor side effect and toxicity profile to imipramine, but is more sedative. Additional sedative properties are sometimes considered an advantage in selected patients.

The half-life and dose range is similar to imipramine but the existence of 50 mg tablets facilitates single daily dosing. Higher dose slow release versions of amitriptyline exist, but apart from the convenience of swallowing fewer tablets they offer little advantage over conventional tablets.

Amoxapine. Although recently introduced into the UK this potent noradrenaline reuptake inhibitor has been available in the USA for some time. Unlike many of the other recently introduced antidepressants amoxapine does not appear to have a significantly improved side effect or toxicity profile in overdose.

Like other drugs in this class it is an effective antidepressant. There is conflicting evidence over the speed of onset of action. Some data suggest the drug may have a particularly rapid onset of action, but this remains to be confirmed.

In standard doses amoxapine may be less cardiotoxic than some other tricyclics but its effects following overdose are particularly severe, with renal failure and a high rate of seizures making management more difficult.

Another difference between amoxapine and the rest of the group is its dopamine-blocking effect. At first sight having an antidepressant with inherent antipsychotic effects would appear to be useful, but in practice this is unlikely and the potential for anti-dopaminergic side effects is a significant disadvantage.

Butriptyline. Butriptyline is a tricyclic antidepressant similar to amitriptyline or imipramine.

Clomipramine. This was one of the first antidepressants found to be a potent 5HT reuptake inhibitor. Some clinicians believe this drug to be more effective than other antidepressants, but there is little data to support this view.

In addition to its antidepressant effect the drug has also been found to be of value in obsessional states.

Data from a fatal toxicity index (see Cassidy and Henry 1987) show clomipramine to have a lower than expected toxicity per million prescriptions. This may be accounted for by the high rate of prescribing in non-depressive states, rather than any specific effect of the drug.

Desipramine. An active metabolite of imipramine. Although the drug is rather more specific for noradrenergic reuptake inhibition there is little difference in clinical effect between the parent drug and its major metabolite.

Dothiepin. Although produced over 20 years ago this is now the most widely prescribed antidepressant in the UK. Originally the drug could be considered an improvement over amitriptyline and imipramine, due to its improved side effect profile.

Since the introduction of many of the newer antidepressants, further improvements in the side effect profile of antidepressants have been made. As dothiepin has a particularly poor toxicity profile there would now appear to be little reason for using this drug, over the newer agents.

Doxepin. Doxepin has similar effects and side effects to the traditional tricyclics. There is some evidence to suggest that doxepin may have less effect on patients with cardiac disease than traditional tricyclics. Although there have been no direct comparisons, one of the newer agents should be considered as an alternative to doxepin in patients with cardiac disease.

Lofepramine. Although desipramine is a metabolite of lofepramine, the latter should not be considered purely as a pro-drug. Important differences exist between lofepramine and the other traditional tricyclics.

Although antimuscarinic effects do occur with lofepramine, these are less than with other tricyclics. Similarly the hypotensive effect of lofepramine has been found to be less pronounced than the other agents in this class.

The fact that lofepramine is not just a prodrug for desipramine has been highlighted by the significant safety of lofepramine following overdose, compared with desipramine.

Lofepramine does not have a significant sedative effect, which may be an advantage in some patients but in others, lack of sedation may be seen as a disadvantage. Some patients may complain of an alerting effect from lofepramine particularly if the majority of the dose is given at bedtime.

Despite a few reports of hepatic problems, given the favourable side effect profile and low toxicity in overdose, lofepramine may be considered as an important therapeutic advance in the treatment of depression.

Nortriptyline. Nortriptyline is the major metabolite of amitriptyline. Nortriptyline appears to have little effect on blood pressure. Plasma levels seem to show an inverted 'U' relationship with antidepressant effect. Patients respond best to intermediate levels of the drug but higher or lower levels may be associated with a poorer response. Apart from these differences, nortriptyline shares many of the properties of the traditional tricyclic antidepressants.

Protriptyline. In contrast to the other tricyclics, protriptyline appears to have a stimulant effect in addition to its antidepressant properties. Moreover the normal daily dose of protriptyline (30 mg) is considerably less than the usual dose of 150 mg for the traditional tricyclics.

Trimipramine. This is a particularly sedative tricyclic antidepressant with little difference from the rest of the traditional tricyclics.

Monoamine oxidase inhibitors (MAOIs). In practice the MAOIs are used much less than the tricyclic antidepressants. Some clinicians believe that the MAOIs are less effective than other antidepressants in moderate to severe depression. This is probably based on some of the original work which showed the MAOIs to be little different from a placebo. Certainly the drugs do have anxiolytic properties and if used in adequate doses are antidepressant. Some workers have suggested that MAOIs may be more effective in atypical depression or mild depression with a significant anxiety component. Other psychiatrists believe that when given in adequate dose the MAOIs are effective treatments, but due to the potential for drug and food interactions they reserve MAOIs for use when first line antidepressant treatments have failed.

The potential for MAOIs to interact has been well known since the 1960s. It is important that patients are aware of the advice printed on the MAOI warning card and follow the dietary restrictions. Unfortunately other foods occasionally creep on to the list of banned foods. For the majority of patients, it is most unhelpful to needlessly extend this list and include other foods or drinks.

Like the tricyclics, an understanding of the effects of the MAOIs added weight to the biochemical hypothesis of depression. Although the effect of these drugs on monoamines is well understood, it is still not established how the MAOIs exert their antidepressant effect.

MAOIs inhibit the enzymes responsible for the oxidation of noradrenaline, 5HT and other biogenic amines. Two forms of monoamine oxidase have been found to exist, MAO-A and MAO-B. Although the antidepressant MAOIs currently available are all nonselective, it is thought that the antidepressant effects are related to inhibition of MAO-A, the enzyme which is also responsible for metabolizing tyramine and producing the cheese interaction. Selegeline, a selective MAO-B inhibitor, does not seem to produce this interaction with foods, but neither does it appear to have a significant antidepressant effect.

Generally speaking the MAOIs have little anticholinergic effect but, even so, some patients do experience dry mouth, constipation and urinary retention. In contrast to the hypertension which follows an interaction of tyramine-rich foods and the MAOIs, the drugs are liable to cause postural hypotension as a side effect. This side effect may be particularly noticeable with phenelzine and may prevent adequate dosages being achieved.

Tranylcypromine. Tranylcypromine has a structure which closely resembles amphetamine. It has a significant stimulant effect and is more likely to give rise to dependence because of this. Unlike the other MAOIs it does not irreversibly inhibit monoamine oxidase, which is said to recover some 5 days after withdrawal of the drug. Even so the precautions associated with the MAOIs must still be continued for 2 weeks after discontinuing the drug.

Due to the amphetamine-like alerting effect of tranylcypromine the last dose should not be given after about 3 p.m. Some clinicians believe that the onset of action of this drug may be somewhat faster than the other MAOIs. However, the risk of interaction is also said to be greater with tranylcypromine than with other MAOIs.

Phenelzine. Unlike tranylcypromine, phenelzine belongs to the hydrazine group of MAOIs. The distinction is important as the hydrazines have been associated with hepatocellular jaundice. Although hydrazine MAOIs like phenelzine should be avoided in patients with hepatic impairment, jaundice is rarely seen with their use in practice.

In most patients, phenelzine is neither sedative nor stimulant and may be considered as an alternative to tranylcypromine, when its amphetamine-like effects are undesirable. As with other antidepressants it is important that phenelzine is prescribed in an adequate dosage (at least 1 mg per kg body weight).

Isocarboxazid. This is the least potent of the MAOIs and may be considered if side effects from the other agents are particularly troublesome. Unfortunately the drug may also be less effective than the other MAOIs.

Specific serotonin reuptake inhibitors (SSRIs). In an attempt to reduce some of the problems associated with the tricyclic antidepressants, a series of agents which are specific to 5-hydroxytriptamine have been developed, the so-called specific serotonin reuptake inhibitors (SSRIs).

As a group these drugs are no more, but no less, effective than the tricyclics. Generally speaking they have less troublesome side effects and are significantly less toxic following overdose than the traditional agents.

All the SSRIs currently available have a different chemical structure, but they all have a specific effect which inhibits serotonin reuptake. The SSRIs have a similar side effect profile, but there may be slight differences in the intensity of different side effects. However, lack of direct comparisons between the drugs make it difficult to comment on the relative incidence of side effects for each of the drugs in this class. Although all the SSRIs appear to have a similar effect on serotonin, there are differences which may be important in some circumstances.

Data on fluoxetine indicate that a maximum response is achieved at 20 mg with little benefit to be gained by increasing the dose further. Limited data on the drop-out rates from clinical trials suggest that fluoxetine and paroxetine may be better tolerated than tricyclic comparators, whereas fluvoxamine and sertraline had similar drop-out rates to tricyclic comparators.

Fluvoxamine. This was the first SSRI available in the UK. Although patients experience few antimuscarinic side effects, other problems related to serotonergic enhancement such as nausea, headache and nervousness have been reported.

Fluoxetine. The main difference between fluoxetine and the other SSRIs is the long half-life of both the parent drug and its primary active metabolite desmethylfluoxetine. In the initial stages of treatment some patients may experience a greater feeling of nervousness with fluoxetine than with the other SSRIs, but in most cases tolerance to this develops.

In practice the long half-life of fluoxetine is a problem if severe side effects develop or the prescriber wishes to change to an MAOI. It will take 5 weeks to clear fluoxetine and in some patients this delay makes management difficult.

Paroxetine. In the UK paroxetine is licensed for the treatment of depression associated with anxiety. With continued treatment all the SSRIs are likely to be anxiolytic so it is not yet clear whether or not this is an important difference between paroxetine and the rest of the SSRIs.

Sertraline. Like the other SSRIs, sertraline is an effective antidepressant. It has been shown to be prophylactic when given for extended periods. Unfortunately there are less data available on the use of sertraline in specific situations such as renal and hepatic impairment. Although doses of up to 200 mg have been used, doses of 150 mg and above should not be given for longer than 8 weeks.

Lithium. Lithium does have antidepressant properties, but will be discussed in more detail under the antimanic section.

Other drugs. As well as the drugs mentioned below, viloxazine, low-dose flupenthixol and iprindole are antidepressants which do not fall into any of the categories mentioned so far.

Maprotiline. Although maprotiline does have slightly less antimuscarinic side effects than the tricyclics it does appear to have many of the cardiovascular problems associated with these drugs. It also appears to induce seizures to a greater extent particularly at higher doses.

Trazodone. Pharmacologically trazodone is an interesting drug. In vitro the drug appears to operate as a mixed serotonin agonist/antagonist, but clinically it is thought to operate as a serotonin agonist. Trazodone is much safer than the tricyclics following overdose but it does have pronounced sedative and hypotensive effects in some patients. Priapism has also been noted as a rare but distressing side effect. This is probably due to its potent alpha-receptor blocking properties.

Mianserin. Mianserin was one of the first antidepressants to have a significantly improved toxicity profile following overdose. Like many of the newer drugs, mianserin has less antimuscarinic side effects than the traditional tricyclics. One drawback in using mianserin is the need for monthly blood counts during the first 3 months of treatment, due to a high reported incidence of blood dyscrasias, particularly in the elderly.

Other treatments.

Electroconvulsive therapy. Electroconvulsive therapy (ECT) would only be considered after referral to a psychiatrist. Although it is said to have a faster onset of action, its effects are fairly short-lived and antidepressants are normally required to prevent relapse. Although the treatment itself is considered safe, there are risks from the anaesthetic agent and some patients suffer short-term memory loss following treatment.

Non-drug treatments. In addition to drug treatment, most patients will need help and support to cope with depression. As well as this type of 'therapy' other forms of psychotherapy are available from specialist services.

Choice of antidepressants. As there is no antidepressant that is any more effective than any other, the choice will depend primarily on side effects and toxicity. In general, the newer drugs have a better side effect profile and less toxicity following overdose. Recent experiences with some new antidepressants, now withdrawn due to severe and unexpected side effects, quite rightly serve as a caution against significant changes in traditional prescribing habits, based on limited data.

There is now substantial experience of using some of the newer drugs like lofepramine, trazodone and fluoxetine. Overall, the advantages of these agents clearly outweigh the disadvantages of the older, but well-established drugs.

In some circumstances the higher costs of the newer drugs have been used as a rationale for reserving them for use as second line agents, if a patient is unable to tolerate a cheaper traditional tricylic. Considering the fact that an overdose attempt with a traditional tricylic is likely to be fatal, the avoidance of the use of newer drugs on the grounds of cost alone cannot be justified.

So long as there are no contra-indications, then previous response to a particular drug is a strong indication for use. In the absence of previous treatment (and obvious contra-indications) where sedation is not required then lofepramine or one of the well-established SSRIs should be considered as first line treatment. If the patient requires additional sedative effects then trazodone may be more appropriate.

Treatment of mania

There are no drugs currently available which are specifically antimanic agents. The neuroleptics, lithium and sedatives all have a place in the management of mania. In most cases the neuroleptics are to be preferred to control the acute stages and lithium is undoubtably the drug of choice for long-term use to prevent recurrence or relapse.

Neuroleptics. All these drugs share a common effect of blocking dopamine D_2 postsynaptic receptors. There is little evidence supporting the use of any one neuroleptic over any others, but in practice haloperidol or chlorpromazine tend to be used most frequently.

In most circumstances haloperidol is probably the drug of choice as it is free from many of the cardiovascular problems of chlorpromazine. As haloperidol is less sedating than chlorpromazine it may occasionally be necessary to control severe behaviour disturbances with additional sedatives like lorazepam injection.

Zuclopenthixol (Acuphase) is formulated as a long-acting injection (up to 3 days) and may be appropriate as an alternative to repeated attempts to control disturbed behaviour with other injections.

Dosage and duration of treatment are important when treating acute mania. The dose of neuroleptic should be reduced as the patient improves and in most cases the neuroleptic can be stopped as the patient becomes euthymic.

Lithium. There is no universally accepted indication for lithium treatment. Generally speaking, lithium prophylaxis should be considered in bipolar patients who have had two or more episodes within 2 to 4 years. It may also be reasonable to consider lithium therapy as prophylaxis in any patient following a severe manic episode.

As lithium treatment is long term, the cooperation of the patient is essential and so a thorough explanation of the risks and benefits of this treatment is vital.

Before lithium treatment is initiated an assessment of the patient's physical state is essential. Thyroid, renal and cardiac function should all be within normal limits, but it is still possible to use lithium, with caution, in patients with mild to moderate renal failure or cardiovascular impairment. Thyroid deficiency should be corrected before lithium treatment is commenced.

Plasma levels. There is a narrow therapeutic window for lithium plasma levels. Levels above 1.5 mmol per litre are considered to be toxic and levels below 0.4 mmol per litre are not considered to be effective. If lithium levels are kept in the range 0.5 mmol to 0.8 mmol per litre, then lithium is usually well tolerated with minimal side effects.

Although the range of 0.5 to 0.8 mmol per litre is appropriate for prophylaxis, in the acute phase of mania, levels may need to be around 1.0 mmol per litre. Although lithium is effective in the acute phase, it may take up to 2 weeks to take effect and therefore neuroleptics are more commonly used.

In order to interpret lithium levels correctly it is important that the correct schedule is followed. In order to establish accurate and consistent results the 12-hour standard serum lithium protocol has been devised. This means that lithium levels should be taken in the morning as near as possible to 12 hours after the last dose of lithium.

As the absorption and bioavailability may vary from brand to brand of lithium, it is important that patients do not change brands or dosage forms without levels being checked.

Even though lithium has a narrow therapeutic range and is particularly toxic in overdose, it is still well tolerated by most people if the blood levels are kept in the lower end of the therapeutic range.

The most common side effects reported by patients are tremor, thirst, polyuria, weight gain and lethargy. As well as complaints of side effects some patients may not like taking lithium as they like the slight 'highs' in their illness. Another problem is that patients taking lithium may occasionaly stop taking their medication as they feel they no longer need it, or they want to see if they can overcome the disorder without the need for drugs. Most people have several trials on lithium before they accept the fact that they will need it long term and that they do relapse when they stop taking it.

Carbamazepine. Although carbamazepine has been shown to be both antidepressant and antimanic, its main use is as an alternative to lithium in the prophylaxis of bipolar disorders. It may be more effective than lithium in the treatment of rapid-cycling patients. In most patients a dose of 400 to 600 mg daily in divided doses is adequate for prophylaxis.

THE PATIENT

In the acute phase of an affective disorder a patient will have little insight into his or her condition and this often makes it difficult to prescribe medication following an informed discussion on the risks and benefits of treatment.

Depressed patients may say they are not worth treating; most manic patients will insist they do not need medication and consistently refuse treatment. Thus, in the initial stages of treatment, some patients are treated against their will. As people respond to treatment it is important to continue to explain the risks of treatment, but also emphasize the benefits. This is particularly important with long-term treatment like lithium where a patient may feel well for many months (apart from the side effects of medication!).

Patients with an affective disorder may have a low attention span and will often forget what they have been told about medication. This is important as patients may continue to seek information and reassurance even after someone has already fully discussed the effects of medication with them.

Many people are understandably frightened by the idea of taking medication that will affect their mind. Taking antidepressants is sometimes considered a sign of weakness by our society, so patients may try to deal with their depression themselves, without medication.

The use of patient information leaflets will help many patients understand the risks and benefits of their treatment, but patients should always be offered the opportunity of discussing their medication with a pharmacist involved in their care as well.

Drug interactions

Many of the drugs used in the treatment of affective disorders have the potential to interact with other drugs that have been prescribed or purchased (see Table 26.2).

Table 26.2 Some important drug interactions		
Drug used in affective disorder	Interacting drug	Effect
Antidepressant		
Tricyclics	Adrenaline (and other directly acting sympathomimetics)	Greatly enhanced effect. Dangerous
	Alcohol	Enhanced sedation
	Anticonvulsants	Lowered seizure threshold and possible lowered tricyclic levels
	MAOIs	Severe hypertension
	Fluoxetine	Increased plasma levels
SSRIs	Anticoagulants	Enhanced effects
	MAOIs	Dangerous
	Lithium	Serotonin syndrome
MAOIs	Alcohol/fermented beverages, tyramine-rich foods	Hypertensive crisis
	Antihypertensives	Increased effect
	Anticonvulsants	Lowered seizure threshold
	Levodopa	Hypertensive crisis
	Sympathomimetics	Hypertensive crisis
Neuroleptics	Anaesthetic agents	Hypotension
	Anticonvulsants	Lowered seizure threshold
Lithium	Non-steroidal anti-inflammatory agents	Enhanced lithium levels
	SSRIs	Enhanced toxicity
	Diuretics	Enhanced lithium plasma levels particularly with thiazides

CASE STUDIES

CASE 26.1

Mrs S. is a 24-year-old woman who presents to her general practitioner with a 2-month history of difficulty in getting to sleep. She has lost interest in most things but does get up and dresses every day. She complains of little energy and spends most of the day sitting in the front room with the television on.

She has a 3-month-old child and feels guilty because she finds it hard to care for the baby.

Q What diagnosis is likely to be given to the patient and what are the important factors to take into account when advising on treatment?

CASE 26.2

Mr D. is a 70-year-old man with a long-standing history of bipolar disorder. He was admitted to an acute psychiatric ward, with a 3-day history of increasing irritability. He had been brought into hospital by the police, who had been contacted by a neighbour, because Mr D. had been standing in the window exposing himself. Mr D. said he felt 'fine, fine all the time' and 'never been better'. He wanted to go home and insisted he was within his rights to go home. He needed to go home as he had important business to deal with. He wouldn't discuss this but said everyone would soon find out.

Mr D's speech was very rapid and it was sometimes difficult to understand what he was saying. He was dressed in a very untidy fashion and had obviously not taken care of his personal hygiene for some time.

On his last admission 18 months ago he was treated with haloperidol.

Q What treatment is appropriate for Mr D.?

CASE 26.3

Mr A. is a 40-year-old salesman who was admitted following an overdose attempt with 20 paracetamol tablets. He felt that everything in his life had gone wrong and there was no point in going on.

Q What course of action would you advise?

ANSWERS TO CASE STUDIES

CASE 26.1

A Mrs S. has a puerperal depressive disorder of moderate severity. She feels guilty at not being able to look after her child.

It should be established that Mrs S. is not a high suicidal risk, the health visitor and other professionals must be consulted to establish that the baby is not at risk. Even though Mrs S. may not be breast feeding it is still important that the mother and child are not separated. Regular professional contact and assesment of Mrs S. should be maintained.

In terms of efficacy, none of the antidepressants is likely to be any more effective than any other in pueperal depression and so the choice of treatment will be determined by other factors.

Although Mrs S. does find it difficult to get off to sleep she still spends most of the day sitting around feeling tired and sleepy. A sedative antidepressant may help sleep initially, but sedative side effects during the day would be a problem.

During the first 1 to 2 weeks of treatment with an antidepressant, Mrs S. will notice an improvement in her sleep pattern. Lofepramine 70 mg twice daily is a suitable choice because of its low side effect profile.

CASE 26.2

A Mr D.'s symptoms of mania need to be brought under control. Haloperdidol would be a suitable choice, in view of his previous response. A medication review should be carried out which would confirm the circumstances of the response to haloperidol during his previous admission.

When Mr D.'s manic symptoms are controlled lithium treatment should be discussed. Renal, thyroid and cardiac function should be assessed and if within normal limits lithium carbonate 400 mg at night may be prescribed.

1 week later a 12-hour standard serum lithium level should be performed and the dose of lithium adjusted to achieve 12-hour levels between 0.4 and 0.8 mmol/L.

Mr D. should be monitored closely for side effects as the combination of neuroleptic and lithium may increase the severity of drug-induced rigidity and tremor.

The side effects and signs of impending toxicity from lithium should be explained to Mr D. He should be warned of the possibility of interaction with drugs he may obtain from doctors or pharmacists in the future.

CASE 26.3

A It is important to use an antidepressant with a low side effect profile and a good safety profile following overdose in this patient. One of the SSRIs would be a suitable choice for Mr A.

He should be told that he is being prescribed a drug that will relieve the symptoms of his depression. While pointing out the benefit of antidepressant treatment, the common side effects should be discussed. Mr A. should be told how long it will take his antidepressant medication to work and that this type of medication is normally prescribed for at least 6 months.

Mr A. should be reassured that his antidepressant is not addictive.

BIBLIOGRAPHY

American Psychiatric Association. Diagnostic and statistical manual of mental disorders, 3rd edn revised. Washington D C: American Psychiatric Association 1987

Cassidy S, Henry J. Fatal toxicity of antidepressant drugs in overdose. British Medical Journal 1987; 295: 1021–1024

Gelder M, Gath D, and Mayou B (eds). Oxford textbook of psychiatry. Oxford Medical Publications 1988

Johnson F N (ed) Depression and mania, modern lithium therapy. Oxford: IRL Press 1987

Rudorfer M V, Potter W Z. Antidepressants a comparative review of the clinical pharmacology and therapeutic use of the newer versus older drugs. Drugs 1989; 37: 713–738

Tyrer P J (ed) Drugs in psychiatric practice. London: Butterworths 1982

Chapter 27

Schizophrenia

D. Branford

The concept of schizophrenia can often be difficult to comprehend. People who do not suffer from schizophrenia can have little idea of what hallucinations and delusions are like. The presentation of schizophrenia can be extremely varied with a great range of possible symptoms. There are also many misconceptions about the condition of schizophrenia which have led to prejudice against sufferers of the illness. Schizophrenics are commonly thought to have low intelligence and to be dangerous. In fact only a minority of patients show violent behaviour with social withdrawal being a more common picture. Up to 10% of schizophrenics commit suicide.

CLASSIFICATION

For the last 100 years there have been frequent attempts to define the illness we now call schizophrenia. Kraepelin in the late 1890s coined the term 'dementia praecox' (early madness) to describe an illness where there was a deterioration of the personality at a young age. Kraepelin coined the terms catatonic (where motor symptoms are prevalent and changes in activity vary), hebephrenic (silly, childish behaviour, affective symptoms and thought disorder prominent), and paranoid (clinical picture dominated by paranoid delusions). A few years later a Swiss psychiatrist called Bleuler introduced the term schizophrenia derived from the Greek words, *skhizo* (to split) and *phren* (mind), meaning the split between the emotions and the intellect.

Schneider (1957) attempted to make diagnosis more reliable by identifying symptoms of first rank importance, but in recent years, two systems of classification have become more widely used. These are DSM III R (American Psychiatric Association) and ICD 10 (World Health Organization).

SYMPTOMS OF SCHIZOPHRENIA

Symptoms common in acute psychotic breakdown

To establish a definite diagnosis of schizophrenia it is important to follow the diagnostic criteria in either DSM III R or ICD10 but symptoms which commonly occur in the acute phase of a psychotic breakdown include:

- Awkward social behaviour, appearing preoccupied, perplexed and withdrawn, or showing unexpected changes in behaviour.
- Initial vagueness in speech which can progress to disorders of the stream of thought or poverty of thought.
- Abnormality of mood such as anxiety, depression, irritability or euphoria.
- Auditory hallucinations, the most common of which are referred to as 'voices'. Such voices can give commands to patients. Some discuss the person in the third person, or comment on their action.
- Delusions of which those relating to control of thoughts are the most diagnostic. For example, patients feel that thoughts are being inserted into or withdrawn from their mind.
- Lack of insight into the illness.

These symptoms are sometimes called positive symptoms.

Factors affecting diagnosis and prognosis

There is a reluctance to classify people as schizophrenic on the basis of one psychotic breakdown, but there are a number of features which lead one to predict whether an acute illness will become chronic.

These features include:

- age of onset which, typically for schizophrenia, is late teenage to age 30 years
- reports of childhood which indicate not mixing or a rather shy and withdrawn personality
- a poor work record
- a desire for social isolation
- being single and not seeming to have sexual relationships
- a gradual onset of the illness and deterioration from previous level of functioning
- grossly disorganized behaviour.

Treatment

There is a wide range of antipsychotic drugs available for the treatment of a psychotic breakdown (see Table 27.1) and the choice of drug will initially depend on the perceived need for sedation. Although all antipsychotic drugs are equally effective in the treatment of psychotic symptoms some individuals do respond better to one drug rather than another.

There is some controversy over how long people should remain on antipsychotic drugs following a first acute breakdown. Some would argue that, if the prognosis is poor, long-term therapy should be advocated. Others would want to see a second breakdown before advocating long-term therapy.

Symptoms common in chronic schizophrenia

60 to 80% of patients who suffer from an acute psychotic breakdown will suffer further breakdowns and become chronically affected. For these patients the diagnosis of schizophrenia can be applied.

As schizophrenia progresses, there may be periods of relapse with acute symptoms but the underlying trend is towards symptoms of lack of drive, social withdrawal and emotional apathy. Such symptoms are sometimes called negative symptoms and respond poorly to drug treatment.

Table 27.1 Neuroleptics/antipsychotics

Drug	Pharmacological properties	Clinical effect
Phenothiazines		
Aliphatic phenothiazines		
Chlorpromazine	Pronounced sedative effects	Drowsiness
	Hypothermia	Low body temperature
	Antiemetic	Useful antinauseant
	Adrenergic blockade	Low blood pressure
		Low rate of metabolism (increased weight gain)
Promazine	As chlorpromazine	As chlorpromazine
	Pharmacological differences compared to chlorpromazine	Clinical significance of differences
Piperidine phenothiazines		
Thioridazine	Moderate sedative effects	
	Marked anticholinergic effects	Increased constipation, dry mouth and blurred vision
Pericyazine	Fewer extrapyramidal effects	Lower incidence of Parkinson-like side effects
Pipothiazine	No antiemetic properties	
Piperazine phenothiazines		
Trifluoperazine	Fewer sedative effects	Higher incidence of Parkinson-like side effects; may require anticholinergic drug
Perphenazine	Fewer anticholinergic effects	
Fluphenazine	More pronounced extrapyramidal side effects	
Prochlorperazine	Antiemetic properties	Useful antinauseant
Thioxanthenes		
Flupenthixol	More extrapyramidal side effects	Provides less sedative alternative at low doses
	Less sedative effect at low doses	
Clopenthixol	More extrapyramidal effects	Similar to fluphenazine, less constipation, dry mouth, etc.
	Fewer anticholinergic effects	
Butyrophenones		
Haloperidol	Less sedating	
	Less hypotensive	Lack of hypothermia and adrenergic effects
	Fewer anticholinergic effects	
	More extrapyramidal effects	
Droperidol	As haloperidol but more depressive	Useful in rapid control of mania: severe depression can result
Benperidol	As haloperidol	Claims to be of value in reducing sexual drive:
Diphenylbutylpiperidines		
Pimozide	Less sedating	Similar to haloperidol
	Few anticholinergic effects	
Benzamides		
Sulpiride	Less sedating at low dosage	
Remoxipride	Few anticholinergic effects	
	Fewer extrapyramidal effects	
Dibenoxazepine tricyclics		
Loxapine	High incidence of extrapyramidal effects	Claims to be of value for paranoid schizophrenia
	Fewer anticholinergic effects	
	Sedating	
Clozapine	Sedating	Licence restricted to treatment-resistant schizophrenic patients
	Low incidence of extrapyramidal effects	
	1% incidence of neutropenia	

Table 27.1 *(cont'd)*		
Drug	Pharmacological properties	Clinical effect
Serotonin-dopamine antagonists Risperidone	5 HT$_2$ receptor antagonist	Low incidence of Parkinson-like effects Improves negative symptoms
	Adrenergic blockade	Low blood pressure

CAUSES OF SCHIZOPHRENIA

Although the cause of schizophrenia remains unknown, there are many theories and models.

Vulnerability model

This model postulates that the persistent characteristic of schizophrenia is not the schizophrenic episode itself but the vulnerability to the development of such episodes of the disorder. The episodes of the illness are time limited but the vulnerability remains, awaiting the trigger of some stress. Such vulnerability can depend on premorbid personality, social network or the environment. Manipulation and avoidance of such stress can abort a potential schizophrenic episode.

Developmental model

The developmental model postulates that there are 'critical periods' in the development of neuronal cells which, if adversely affected, may result in schizophrenia. Two such critical periods are postulated to occur when migrant neural cells do not reach their goal in fetal development and when supernumerary neural cells slough off at adolescence. This model is supported by neuroimaging studies which show structural brain abnormalities in patients with schizophrenia.

Ecological model

The ecological model postulates that external factors involving social, cultural and physical forces in the environment, such as population density, individual space, social–economic status and racial status, influence the development of the disorder. The evidence of such a model remains weak.

Genetic model

There is undoubtably a genetic component to schizophrenia with a higher incidence in the siblings of schizophrenics. However, even in monozygotic twins there are many cases where only one sibling has developed schizophrenia.

Transmitter abnormality model

The suggestion that schizophrenia is caused primarily by an abnormality of dopamine receptors and, in particular, D$_2$ receptors, has largely emerged from research into the effect of antipsychotic drugs. Such a theory is increasingly being questioned.

Other factors involved in schizophrenia

Numerous other factors have been implicated in the development and cause of schizophrenia. These include migration, socio-economic factors, perinatal insult, infections, season of birth, viruses, toxins, and family environment.

In reality all of these factors may influence both the development and progression of schizophrenia. Social, familial and biological factors may lead to premorbid vulnerability and subsequently influence both the acute psychosis and the progression to chronic states. What is then likely is that the illness will feed back to influence social, familial and biological factors, thus leading to future vulnerability.

DRUG TREATMENT IN SCHIZOPHRENIA
Mode of action of antipsychotic drugs

Although the cause of schizophrenia remains an enigma, an understanding of the mode of action of antipsychotic drugs has led to the dopamine theory of schizophrenia. This theory postulates that the symptoms experienced in schizophrenia are caused by an alteration to the level of dopamine activity in the brain. It is based on knowledge that dopamine receptor antagonists are often effective antipsychotics whilst drugs which increase dopamine activity such as amphetamine, can either induce psychosis or exacerbate a schizophrenic illness.

At least six dopamine receptors exist in the brain with much recent activity being focused on the D_2 receptor as being responsible for antipsychotic drug action. Drugs such as pimozide which claim to have a more specific effect on D_2 receptors have less effect on blood pressure and a low risk of anticholinergic side effects but do not appear superior in antipsychotic effect compared to other agents.

The arrival of antipsychotic drugs such as clozapine, sulpiride and remoxipride has caused a change of attention to the mesolimbic system in the brain and to different receptors. Clozapine does not chronically alter striatal D_2 receptors but does appear to affect striatal D_1 receptors. It also appears to have more effect on the limbic system, which may explain its reduced risk of extrapyramidal symptoms.

Rationale and mode of use of drugs

Although a variety of social and psychological therapies are an advantage in the treatment of schizophrenia, drugs form the essential cornerstone. The aim of all therapies is to minimize the level of handicap and achieve the best level of mental functioning. Drugs do not cure schizophrenia. At the same time, benefits have to be balanced against side effects and the need to suppress particular symptoms. For example, if the person has a delusion that he or she is responsible for famine in Africa, but this does not in any way influence the person's behaviour or mood, there would be little point in increasing antipsychotic drug therapy. If, on the other hand, this delusion led to great distress, or violent or dangerous behaviour, then an increase in antipsychotic drugs may be indicated.

It is now accepted that antipsychotic drugs can control or modify symptoms such as hallucinations and delusions which are evident in the acute episode of illness. Except for clozapine and the serotonin-dopamine antagonists, there is little evidence for antipsychotic drugs being of value in the treatment of the negative symptoms, although the matter remains controversial. Antipsychotic drugs increase the length of time between breakdowns and shorten the length of the acute episode in most patients.

Drug selection and dosage

The antipsychotic drugs are listed in Table 27.1, together with their relative adverse effects compared with the standard drug, chlorpromazine. The primary difference between the various agents is their side effect profile. Drug selection may be influenced by iatrogenic problems such as hypotension, extrapyramidal symptoms, anticholinergic effects and sedation. Drug selection should not be based on chemical groupings alone since dosage and individual response to particular drugs is much more important.

Dosage selection should be based on the need for symptom control and titrated against side effects, not based on artificial dosage levels selected from reference books. The publication of upper limits of dosage may lead to polypharmacy as prescribers feel inhibited from prescribing beyond those limits and may resort to prescribing two antipsychotic drugs (or three), in order to achieve the necessary control.

Confusion can also arise between the perceived need in the ward situation for sedation and antipsychotic effects. The sedating side effects of antipsychotic drugs may be evident within hours; they are rapid in onset but may begin to wear off within 2 or 3 weeks. The antipsychotic effects on thought disorder, hallucinations and delusions may take some weeks to appear, although if there has been no response within 2 to 3 weeks a change of antipsychotic drug or increase in dosage is indicated.

The consensus view is that very high doses have not proven beneficial in improving either the speed or the overall level of response in acute psychosis.

Maintenance dosages

Once control of symptoms is achieved, the issue of maintenance dosages then comes to the fore. In particular, concerns about tardive dyskinesia have led to a series of new approaches to maintenance therapy. The aim of maintenance therapy should be to maintain the patient in a state of remission, but at the same time achieve the best possible level of functioning.

A review of the literature up to 1980 found that there was no difference in outcome in patients maintained on doses of neuroleptics above the equivalent of 310 mg chlorpromazine per day compared with those on doses below that level, and there has been no evidence to refute that to date. Patients may also remain stable on reducing doses. Three strategies that have been tried to maintain remission and reduce antipsychotic drug intake are:

Drug holidays. These are no longer advocated as patients become clinically disadvantaged without any reduction in risk of tardive dyskinesia.

Low dose regimens. Trials using low dose regimens of flupenthixol decanoate and fluphenazine decanoate have produced unclear results but indications are that with careful patient selection and good supervision some patients can remain in remission on low doses.

Brief intermittent treatment. Such treatments rely on patient recognition of prodromal symptoms and rapid access to drug therapy. Although some studies have demonstrated encouraging results, others have found such an approach to be associated with a higher rate of both psychotic and dysphoric symptoms.

Neuroleptic equivalence

Although antipsychotic drugs vary in potency, studies on relative dopamine receptor binding have led to the concept of chlorpromazine equivalents as a useful method of transferring dosage from one product to another. Concern has been expressed about the variation between sources for such values, in particular, about the quoted chlorpromazine equivalents of the butyrophenones and the conversion depot doses to oral (see Table 27.2).

Depot antipsychotic drugs

Depot formulations are synthesized by esterification of the hydroxyl group of the antipsychotic drug to a long chain fatty acid such as decanoic acid. The esters which are more lipophilic and soluble are dissolved in an oily vehicle such as sesame oil or a vegetable oil (viscoleo). Once

Table 27.2 Neuroleptic equivalent of antipsychotic drugs to 100 mg chlorpromazine (from Foster 1989)

Drug	Usual dose (mg) equivalent to 100 mg chlorpromazine	Variations in quoted dosage (microgram) equivalents to 100 mg chlorpromazine
Oral antipsychotics		
Promazine	200	100–250
Thioridazine	100	50–120
Trifluoperazine	5	3.5–7.5
Haloperidol	2	1.5–5
Sulpiride	200	—
Depot antipsychotics administered every 2 weeks (all administered as the decanoate)		
Zuclopenthixol	200	80–200
Flupenthixol	40	16–40
Fluphenazine	25	10–25
Haloperidol	20	—

Table 27.3 Comparison of depot antipsychotics (from Jann 1985)

Drug	Ester	Oily vehicle	Time to peak (days)	Half-life (days)
Haloperidol	Decanoate	Sesame	3–9	21
Flupenthixol	Decanoate	Viscoleo	7	17
Zuclopenthixol	Decanoate	Viscoleo	4–7	19
Fluphenazine	Decanoate	Sesame	0.3–1.5	6–9
Pipothiazine	Palmitate	Sesame	10–15	15

the drug is injected into muscle it is slowly released from the oily vehicle. Active drug becomes available following hydrolysis for distribution to the site of the action.

Although the ideal depot antipsychotic should release the drug at a constant rate so that plasma level variations are kept to a minimum, all the available products produce significant variations (see Table 27.3). This can result in increased side effects at the time of peak plasma concentrations and increased patient irritability towards the end of the depot period, as plasma concentrations decline.

In addition to the principles of drug choice and dosage selection which apply with oral drugs, with depot therapy there is also a need to consider the future habitation of the patient. If the patient is to live an independent lifestyle, depot formulations are indicated, but if the person is to remain in staffed accommodation and receive other medicines by routine adminis-tration by nurses, the use of depot formulations may not be logical.

Advantages and disadvantages of depot antipsychotics

Non-compliance with oral medicines is a major problem in patients with psychiatric illnesses and the administration of depot formulations guarantees drug delivery. It has been argued that, although depot injections are expensive, they have economical advantages because they reduce hospital admissions, improve drug bio-availability by avoiding the deactivating processes which occur in the gut and result in more consistent plasma levels of drug.

Depot formulations have the disadvantages of reduced flexibility of dosage, the painful nature of administration and high incidence of both extrapyramidal side effects and weight gain.

Anticholinergic drugs

Anticholinergic drugs are prescribed to counter the extrapyramidal side effects of antipsychotics and at one time were routinely prescribed. It is generally accepted that with the possible excep-

tion of the first few weeks of treatment with antipsychotic drugs known to have a high inci-dence of extrapyramidal side effects, anti-cholinergic drugs should only be prescribed when a need has been shown. A number of studies which have looked at the discontinua-tion of anticholinergic agents have reported re-emergence of the symptoms with up to 62% of patients being affected. 25 to 30% of patients will have a continuing need for anticholinergic drugs.

The anticholinergic drugs are not without problems, having their own range of side effects, including dry mouth, constipation, and blurred vision. Benzhexol, in particular, is renowned for its euphoric effects and withdrawal problems can include cholinergic rebound.

Interactions involving antipsychotic drugs

There are claimed to be many interactions in-volving antipsychotic drugs but few appear to be clinically significant. Propranolol increases the plasma concentration of chlorpromazine, and carbamazepine accelerates the metabolism of haloperidol. When tricyclics are administered with phenothiazines increased antimuscarinic effects can occur and most antipsychotic drugs increase the sedative effect of alcohol.

Adverse effects of antipsychotic drugs

There are a large number of adverse effects associated with antipsychotic drugs. Some of these effects such as sedation, antilibido effect and weight gain, may be considered to be of value with particular patients, but the susceptibility to such adverse effects is often a major factor in determining drug choice.

The major groups of side effects are:

Sedation. Although sedation is greatest with chlorpromazine, it is primarily related to dosage with most other antipsychotics. Products claim-ing to be less sedating can often only substanti-ate such claims for low dosages.

Anticholinergic side effects, such as dry mouth,

constipation, and blurred vision, are particularly associated with piperidine phenothiazines (see Table 27.1).

Extrapyramidal side effects, such as akathisia, dystonia, and Parkinsonian effects occur frequently, particularly with depot antipsychotics, piperazine phenothiazines and butyrophenones. These side effects are reversible by using anticholinergic drugs or by dosage reduction. The common extrapyramidal effects include:

Akathisia, motor restlessness which causes patients to pace up and down, constantly shift their leg position or tap their feet.

Dystonia is the result of sustained muscle contraction. It can present as grimacing and facial distortion, neck twisting and laboured breathing. Occasionally the patient may have an oculogyric crisis in which, after a few moments of fixed staring, the eyeballs move upwards and then sideways, remaining in that position. In addition to these eye movements, the mouth is usually wide open, the tongue protruding and the head tilting backwards.

Parkinson-like side effects usually present as tremor, rigidity and poverty of facial expression. Drooling and excessive salivation are also common. A shuffling gait may be seen and the patient may show signs of fatigue when performing repetitive motor activities.

Hormonal effects are primarily influenced by the effect on prolactin. This may result in galactorrhoea, missed periods and loss of libido.

Postural hypotension and photosensitivity are particularly associated with the aliphatic phenothiazines.

Tardive dyskinesia. Classically the syndrome of tardive dyskinesia affects the tongue, facial and neck muscles but will often also affect the extremities. It is usual to find abnormalities of posture and movements of the fingers in addition to the oral–lingual–masticatory movements.

Epidemiological studies support the association between the prescribing of antipsychotic drugs and the development of tardive dyskinesia. Factors which also appear to be associated are the duration of exposure to antipsychotic drugs, the co-prescribing of anticholinergic drugs, the co-prescribing of lithium, advanced age, prior experience of acute extrapyramidal symptoms and brain damage. Many other factors have been postulated to be associated with tardive dyskinesia such as depot formulations of antipsychotic drugs, gender, dosage of antipsychotic drug, and antipsychotic drugs with high anticholinergic activity, but such associations remain unproven.

Although the mechanism by which tardive dyskinesia arises is unclear, the leading hypothesis is that after prolonged blockade of dopamine receptors a paradoxical increase in the functional activity of dopamine in the basal ganglia occurs. This altered functional state is thought to come about through a phenomenon of disuse supersensitivity of dopamine receptors. The primary clinical evidence to support such a theory is that tardive dyskinesia is late in onset after prolonged exposure to antipsychotic drugs, has a tendency to worsen upon abrupt discontinuation of the antipsychotic drug and that in terms of response to drugs it presents as the opposite of Parkinson's disease, a disease postulated to be caused by a deficiency of dopamine in the caudate nucleus of the brain.

The attempts to treat tardive dyskinesia have been many and varied, but they include dopamine-depleting agents such as reserpine and tetrabenazine, dopamine-blocking agents such as antipsychotic drugs, blockers of catecholamine synthesis such as methyldopa, cholinergic agents such as choline and lecithin, GABA antagonists such as sodium valproate and baclofen and the provision of drug holidays. Such strategies are rarely successful. Most strategies currently involve a gradual withdrawal of antipsychotic drug if at all possible or maintenance of the lowest dosage possible in the hope that symptoms will gradually subside.

CASE STUDIES

CASE 27.1

K. B. was born in the USA and when aged 11 moved to the UK with his father following the death of his mother. As a child he gained a reputation as a loner, being shy, withdrawn and self-conscious. His academic performance was average, although teachers did comment on his strange behaviour and that he seemed uninterested in girls. When he left school at 16 he was employed as an engineering apprentice, but after the first year in employment his performance and attendance began to deteriorate. He was sacked for non-attendance and when interviewed he said he didn't like being watched all the time. At home he would lock himself in his bedroom for days so that others could not spy on him. He refused to communicate with others in the household other than by written messages which were usually irrelevant and incomprehensible. He was admitted to a psychiatric hospital against his will under Section 2 of the 1983 Mental Health Act. This followed an incident where he lay down on the road and refused to move. Upon admission he presented as bewildered with a fixed stare. Upon interview he appeared quite inaccessible at times. He said the reason he stayed in his room was because it was the only safe place where people didn't interfere with his thoughts.

Q1 Outline the drug(s) of choice and the rationale for selection.

Q2 Why is there a poor prognosis?

CASE 27.2

B. P. was born in the Punjab, India, and emigrated to this country with his parents. He first became psychotically ill in his early 20s and was maintained for 8 years on fluphenazine decanoate injections 25 mg every 2 weeks. He lived at home with his parents and was not regarded as suitable for employment.

When he was 30, he became unmanageable at home and was admitted to a psychiatric hospital. The main features were drinking urine, mixing urine with cooking oil and rubbing it into his hair, being aggressive towards his mother, being deliberately incontinent, ignoring his personal hygiene, appearing constantly to be in conversation with a non-existing person and complaining that there was a snake in his stomach which was eating all his food. Upon admission he assaulted a nurse and was subsequently prescribed chlorpromazine 300 mg four times daily.

2 years later he is very quiet and easily managed. He still occasionally hallucinates and believes a snake is in his stomach. He eats huge amounts of food (to feed the snake) and now weighs 23 stones. He appears rather unkempt and dishevelled, has little spontaneity and seems rather flat in mood. His personal hygiene is still poor, he does not involve himself in any ward activities, and is frequently taking to his bed during the day for a quick sleep.

Q1 Is the choice of antipsychotic drug appropriate?

Q2 Is the dosage appropriate?

Q3 Is the formulation appropriate?

CASE 27.3

Joanne, a paranoid schizophrenic, was readmitted to an acute psychiatric ward 2 months ago following an aggressive attack on a member of the public. Attempts to rehabilitate her to live in a community hostel had repeatedly failed and recently she had been refusing to accept her depot antipsychotic injection. 3 weeks ago she was transferred to a secure facility as she could no longer be managed on an acute psychiatric ward. Upon transfer she was prescribed chlorpromazine 300 mg four times daily, zuclopenthixol decanoate 500 mg weekly, haloperidol 10 mg four times daily, procyclidine 10 mg three times daily, carbamazepine 400 mg three times daily, and lithium carbonate 800 mg at night.

Since transfer she has received numerous doses of droperidol in addition to the above in an attempt to curb her violence. As the clinical pharmacist your advice has been sought as to the possible alternatives.

Q1 Would you recommend an increased dosage of antipsychotic drugs?

Q2 Is lithium indicated?

Q3 Is carbamazepine indicated?

Q4 Should clozapine be prescribed?

ANSWERS TO CASE STUDIES

CASE 27.1

A1 The initial choice will often depend upon the need for sedation. If K. B. was aggressive, damaging property or self-injuring, a sedating drug such as chlorpromazine would be the drug of choice. If side effects such as postural hypotension presented a problem, haloperidol is an alternative. If drug refusal was presenting a major problem and frequent injections were proving necessary, a single injection of zuclopenthixol acuphase may provide interim relief.

K. B. is not showing any aggressive features and any antipsychotic drug could be chosen provided the side effects are tolerated.

A2 There are many aspects to K. B.'s history which would indicate a poor prognosis. These include:

- a gradual deterioration in function over many months
- his age, which is typical for the first breakdown in the progression of the illness
- his poor work record
- his strange behaviour when a child and his lack of interest in females
- grossly disorganized behaviour
- his desire for social isolation
- the lack of any obvious precipitant such as drug abuse or life events.

CASE 27.2

A1 No; the choice of chlorpromazine may contribute to the patient's drowsiness and weight problem. It may have been appropriate when he was aggressive upon admission, but now he is easily managed and a less sedating antipsychotic is indicated.

A2 No. He is receiving an unnecessarily large dosage. Such a dosage may have been required on admission but now he is easily managed. His residual symptoms of occasional hallucinations and delusional ideas do not present a management problem.

A3 No. If accommodation in the community is anticipated he is unlikely to comply with a regimen of tablets four times daily and a depot formulation is indicated.

Initial recommendation: flupenthixol decanoate 100 mg weekly with a gradual withdrawal of chlorpromazine over a 3-month period.

CASE 27.3

A1 No; not without a comprehensive study of previous prescribing and the response to it. In Joanne's case, she has had many previous admissions and had responded well to trifluoperazine on two previous admissions. The trifluoperazine was stopped in preference to a depot antipsychotic zuclopenthixol decanoate 6 months ago.

A2 No. Lithium is indicated for the prophylaxis of bipolar affective disorder, the augmentation of tricyclic antidepressants, the treatment of mania, and the control of aggression. There is little evidence to support its being of value in schizophrenia.

A3 No. Carbamazepine is indicated for epilepsy and bipolar affective disorder. Both its value in the treatment of schizophrenia and in the treatment of aggression in people with normal EEGs is unconvincing. In this case it may have led to a deterioration due to an interaction with haloperidol which results in a reduced effect of haloperidol.

A4 If there had been a lack of response to all prescribed antipsychotic drugs, clozapine would be indicated. This case demonstrates the need for a comprehensive drug history before assuming that the patient is drug resistant. The 1 to 2% risk of neutropenia makes weekly blood testing mandatory with clozapine.

BIBLIOGRAPHY

Baldessarani F J, Davis J M. What is the best maintenance dose of neuroleptics in schizophrenia. Psychiatric Research 1980; 3: 115–122

Foster P. Neuroleptic equivalence. Pharmaceutical Journal 1989; 243: 431–432

Gelder M, Gath D, Mayou B. Oxford textbook of psychiatry. Oxford University Press 1988

Jann M W et al. Clinical pharmacokinetics of the depot antipsychotics. Clinical Pharmacokinetics 1985; 10: 315–333

Johnson D A W. Pharmacological treatment of patients with schizophrenia. Drugs 1990; 39(4): 481–488

Kane J. Compliance issues in outpatient treatment. Journal of Clinical Psychopharmacology 1985; 5(3) (Suppl.): 225–275

Chapter 28

Epilepsy

S. Dhillon   J. W. A. S. Sander

An epileptic seizure is a transient paroxysm of uncontrolled discharges of neurones in the brain causing an event which is discernible by the person experiencing the seizure and/or an observer. The tendency to have recurrent attacks is known as epilepsy – by definition a single attack does not constitute epilepsy. Epileptic seizures or attacks are a symptom of many different diseases and the term 'epilepsy' is loosely applied to a number of conditions that have in common only a tendency to have recurrent epileptic attacks.

EPIDEMIOLOGY

There are problems in establishing precise epidemiological statistics for a heterogeneous condition like epilepsy. Unlike most ailments epilepsy is episodic; in between seizures patients may be perfectly normal and have normal investigations. Thus the diagnosis is essentially clinical, relying heavily on eyewitness descriptions of the attacks. In addition, there are a number of other conditions in which consciousness may be transiently impaired and which may be confused with epilepsy. Another problem area is that of case identification. Sometimes the patient may be unaware of the nature of the attacks and so may not seek medical help. Patients with milder epilepsy may also not be receiving ongoing medical care and so may be missed in epidemiological surveys. Furthermore, since there is some degree of stigma attached to epilepsy, patients may sometimes be reluctant to admit their condition.

Incidence and prevalence

Epileptic seizures are common. Incidence (number of new cases per given population per year) has been estimated at between 20 and 70 cases per 100 000 persons, and the cumulative incidence (the risk of having the condition at some point in life) at 2 to 5%. The incidence is higher in the first two decades of life, but falls over the next few decades, only to increase again in late life, due mainly to cerebrovascular diseases. Most studies of the prevalence of active epilepsy (the number of cases in the population at any given time) have estimated figures between 4 and 8 per 1000, and a rate of 5 per 1000 is commonly quoted.

Prognosis of epilepsy

Up to 5% of people will suffer at least one seizure in their lifetime. The prevalence of active epilepsy is, however, much lower and most patients who develop seizures have a very good prognosis. About 70 to 80% of all people developing epilepsy will eventually become seizure free and about half will successfully withdraw their medication. Once a substantial period of remission has been achieved, the risk of further seizures is greatly reduced. A minority of patients (20 to 30%) will develop chronic epilepsy, and in such cases, treatment is more difficult. Patients with symptomatic epilepsy, more than one seizure type, associated mental retardation, or neurological or psychiatric disorders are more likely to have a poor outcome. Of chronic patients, less than 5% will be unable to live in the community or will depend on others for their day to day needs. Most patients are entirely normal between seizures, but in a small minority of patients with severe epilepsy physical and intellectual deterioration may occur.

Mortality

There is an increased mortality in people with epilepsy, especially amongst younger patients and those with severe epilepsy. Most studies have given overall standardized mortality ratios between 2 and 3 times higher than that of the general population. Common causes of death in people with epilepsy include: accidents (e.g. drowning, head injury, road traffic accidents), status epilepticus, tumours, cerebrovascular diseases, pneumonia and suicide. Sudden unexpected death, an entity which remains unexplained, is common particularly in young males.

AETIOLOGY

Epileptic seizures are produced by abnormal discharges of neurones which may be caused by any pathological process which affects the brain. In a significant proportion of cases, however, no cause can be determined; these are known as the idiopathic or cryptogenic epilepsies. Possible explanations for idiopathic epilepsy include as yet unexplained metabolic or biochemical abnormalities and microscopic lesions in the brain resulting from brain trauma during birth or other injury. The term symptomatic epilepsy indicates that a probable cause has been identified.

The likely aetiology of epilepsy depends upon the age of the patient and the type of seizures. The commonest causes in young infants are hypoxia or birth asphyxia, intracranial trauma during birth, metabolic disturbances, congenital malformations of the brain or infection. In young children and adolescents idiopathic seizures account for the majority of the epilepsies although trauma and infection also play a role. In this age group, particularly in children aged between 6 months and 5 years, seizures may occur in association with febrile illness. These are usually short, generalized tonic–clonic convulsions which occur during the early phase of a febrile disease. They must be distinguished from seizures that are triggered by central nervous system infections which produce fever, such as meningitis or encephalitis. Unless febrile seizures are prolonged, focal, recurrent, or there is a background of neurological handicap, the prognosis is excellent, and it is unlikely that the child will develop epilepsy.

The range of causes of adult-onset epilepsy is very wide. Both idiopathic epilepsy and epilepsy due to birth trauma may also begin in early adulthood. Other important causes are head injury, alcohol abuse, brain tumours and cerebrovascular diseases. Brain tumours are responsible for the development of epilepsy in up to a third of patients between the ages of 30 and 50 years. Over the age of 50 years, cerebrovascular disease is the commonest cause of epilepsy and may be present in up to half of the patients.

PATHOPHYSIOLOGY

Epilepsy differs from most neurological conditions as it has no pathognomonic lesion. A variety of different electrical or chemical stimuli can easily give rise to a seizure in any normal brain. The hallmark of epilepsy is a rather rhythmic and repetitive hypersynchronous discharge of neurones, either localized in an area of the cerebral cortex or generalized throughout the cortex and which can be observed on an electroencephalogram (EEG).

A small electrical current is discharged by neurones to release neurotransmitters at synaptic levels to communicate with each other. Neurotransmitters fall into two basic categories: inhibitory or excitatory. Therefore, a neurone discharging can either excite or inhibit neurones connected to it. An excited neurone will activate the next neurone whereas an inhibited neurone will not. In this manner, information is conveyed, transmitted and processed throughout the central nervous system.

A normal neurone discharges repetitively at a low baseline frequency and it is the integrated electrical activity generated by the neurones of the superficial layers of the cortex which is recorded in a normal EEG. If neurones are damaged, injured or suffer a chemical or metabolic insult a change in the discharge pattern may develop. In the case of epilepsy, regular low frequency discharges are replaced by bursts of high frequency discharges usually followed by periods of inactivity. A single neurone discharging in an abnormal manner usually has no clinical significance. It is only when a whole population of neurones discharge synchronously in an abnormal way that an epileptic seizure may be triggered. This abnormal discharge may remain localized or it may spread to adjacent areas recruiting more neurones as it expands. It may also generalize throughout the brain via cortical and subcortical routes including callosal and thalamocortical pathways. The area from which the abnormal discharge originates is known as the epileptic focus. An EEG recording carried out during one of these abnormal discharges may show a variety of atypical signs, depending on which area of the brain is involved, its progression and how the discharging areas project to the superficial cortex.

CLINICAL MANIFESTATIONS

The clinical manifestation of a seizure will depend on the location of the focus and the pathways involved in its spread. An International Seizure Classification scheme based on the clinical features of seizures combined with EEG data is widely used to describe seizure. It divides seizures into two main groups according to the area of the brain in which the abnormal discharge originates. If it involves initial activation of both hemispheres of the brain simultaneously, the seizures are termed generalized. If a discharge starts in a localized area of the brain, they are termed partial or focal seizures.

Generalized seizures

Generalized seizures concur with impairment of consciousness from the onset. There are various types of generalized seizures, among them are:

Tonic–clonic convulsions. Often called grand mal attacks, these are the commonest of all epileptic seizures. Without warning, the patient suddenly goes stiff, falls, and convulses, with laboured breathing and salivation. Cyanosis, incontinence and tongue biting may occur. The convulsion ceases after a few minutes and may often be followed by a period of drowsiness, confusion, headache and sleep. The convulsions consist of both tonic and clonic phases.

Absence attacks. Also known as 'petit mal', these are a much rarer form of generalized seizure. They happen almost exclusively in childhood and early adolescence. The child goes blank and stares; fluttering of the eyelids and flopping of the head may occur. The attacks last only a few seconds and often go unrecognized even by the child having these attacks.

Myoclonic seizures. These are abrupt, very brief involuntary shock-like jerks, which may involve the whole body, or the arms or the head. They usually happen in the morning, shortly after waking. They may sometimes cause the person to fall, but recovery is immediate. It should be noted that there are forms of non-epileptic myoclonic jerks. They occur in a variety of other nerve diseases and may also occur in healthy people, particularly when they are just going off to sleep.

Atonic seizure. These comprise a sudden loss of muscle tone causing the person to collapse to the ground. Recovery afterwards is quick. They are rare, accounting for less than 1% of the epileptic seizures seen in the general population, but much commoner in patients with severe epilepsy starting in infancy.

Partial seizures

Simple partial seizures. In these seizures the discharge remains localized and consciousness is fully preserved. Simple partial attacks on their own are rare and they usually progress to the other forms of partial seizure. What actually happens during a simple partial seizure depends on the area of the discharge and may vary widely from patient to patient, but will always be stereotyped in one patient. Localized jerking of a limb or the face, stiffness or twitching of one part of the body, numbness or abnormal sensations, are examples of what may occur during a simple partial seizure. If the seizure progresses with impairment of consciousness, it is termed a complex partial seizure. If it develops further and a convulsive seizure occurs it is then called a secondarily generalized seizure. In attacks which progress, the early part of the seizure, in which consciousness is preserved, is called the aura.

Complex partial seizures. The patient may present altered or 'automatic' behaviour; plucking his or her clothes, fiddling with various objects and acting in a confused manner. Lipsmacking or chewing movements, grimacing, undressing, performing aimless activities, and wandering around in a drunken fashion may occur on their own or in different combinations during complex partial seizures. Most of these seizures originate in the frontal or temporal lobes and can sometimes progress to secondarily generalized seizures.

Secondarily generalized seizure. These are partial seizures either simple or complex, in which the discharge spreads to the entire brain. The patient may have a warning (the aura), but this is not always the case. The spread of the discharge can occur so quickly that no features of the localized onset are apparent to the patient or an observer, and only an EEG can demonstrate the partial nature of the seizure. The involvement of the entire brain leads to a convulsive attack with the same characteristics as a generalized tonic–clonic convulsion.

DIAGNOSIS

Diagnosing epilepsy can be difficult as it is first necessary to demonstrate a tendency to recurrent epileptic seizures. The one feature that distinguishes epilepsy from all other conditions is its unpredictability and transient nature. The diagnosis of epilepsy is clinical and depends on a reliable account of what happened during the attacks, if possible both from the patient and from an eyewitness, but some investigations may help and the EEG is usually one of them. These investigations cannot, however, conclusively confirm or refute the diagnosis of epilepsy.

There are other conditions which may cause impairment or loss of consciousness that can be misdiagnosed as epilepsy, i.e. syncope, breath-holding attacks, transient ischaemic attacks, psychogenic attacks, etc. In addition, patients may present with acute epileptic seizures as a result of other problems, i.e. drug intake, metabolic dysfunction, infections, head trauma, flashing light (photosensitive seizures). These conditions have to be clearly ruled out before a diagnosis of epilepsy is made. Epilepsy must only be diagnosed when seizures occur spontaneously and are recurrent. The diagnosis must be accurate since the label 'suffering with epilepsy' carries a social stigma which has tremendous implications for the patient.

The EEG is often the only examination required and it aims to record abnormal neuronal discharges. The EEG however has limitations which should be clearly understood. Up to 5% of normal people may have nonspecific abnormalities in their EEG recording while up to 40% of people with epilepsy may have a normal EEG recording between seizures. The diagnosis of epilepsy, therefore, should be strongly supported by a bona fide history of epileptic attacks. The EEG, however, is invaluable in classifying seizures.

The chance of recording the discharges of an actual seizure during a routine EEG, which usually takes 20 to 30 minutes, is slight and because of this ambulatory EEG monitoring and EEG videotelemetry are sometimes required. Ambulatory EEG allows recording in day to day circumstances, using a small cassette recorder. EEG videotelemetry is useful in the assessment of difficult cases. The patient is usually admitted to hospital and remains under continuous monitoring. This is only helpful in a very few cases, and it is best suited for patients who have frequent seizures.

CT (computerized tomography) scan and MRI (magnetic resonance imaging) scan are valuable investigations when structural abnormalities (e.g. stroke, tumour, congenital abnormalities, hydrocephalus) are suspected.

TREATMENT
During seizures

Convulsive seizures may look frightening, but the patient is not in pain, will usually have no recollection of the event afterwards and is usually not seriously injured. Emergency treatment is seldom necessary. Patients should, however, be made as comfortable as possible preferably lying down (ease to the floor if sitting), cushioning the head and loosening any tight clothing or neckwear. During seizures, patients should not be moved, unless they are in a dangerous place, e.g. in a road, by a fire or hot radiator, at the top of stairs or by the edge of water. No attempt should be made to open the patient's mouth or force anything between the teeth. This usually results in damage and broken teeth may be inhaled, causing secondary lung damage. When the seizure stops, patients should be turned over into the recovery position, and the airway checked for any blockage.

Partial attacks are usually less dramatic. During automatisms, patients may behave in a confused fashion and should generally be left undisturbed. Gentle restraint may be necessary if the automatism leads to dangerous wandering. Attempts at firm restraint, however, may increase agitation and confusion. No drinks should be given after an attack, and extra antiepileptic drugs should also not be given. It is commonly felt that a seizure may be life threatening, but this is seldom the case. After a seizure, it is important to stay with the patient and offer reassurance until the confused period has completely subsided and the patient has recovered fully.

If a seizure persists for more than 10 minutes, if a series of seizures occur, or if the seizure is particularly severe, then the intravenous or rectal administration of 10 to 20 mg of diazepam for adults, with lower doses being used in children, is advisable.

Long-term treatment

In most cases, epilepsy can only be treated by long-term regular drug therapy. The objective of therapy is to suppress epileptic discharges, and prevent the development of epileptic seizures. In the majority of cases, full seizure control can be obtained, and in other patients drugs may reduce the frequency or severity of seizures.

Initiating treatment with an antiepileptic drug (AED) is a major event in the life of a patient and the diagnosis should be unequivocal. Treatment options must be considered with careful evaluation of all relevant factors, including the number and frequency of attacks, the presence of precipitating factors, such as alcohol, drugs or flashing lights, and the presence of other medical conditions. Single seizures do not require treatment unless they are associated with a progressive brain disorder or there is a clearly abnormal EEG. If there are long intervals between seizures (over 2 years), there is a case for not starting treatment. If there are more than two attacks which are clearly associated with a precipitating factor, fever or alcohol for instance, then treatment may not be necessary. Therapy is long term, usually for at least 3 years, and depending on circumstances, sometimes for life. Full explanation of all the implications must be given to the patient as agreement with the treatment policy and good compliance are essential. Antiepileptic treatment will fail unless the patient fully understands the importance of regular therapy and the objectives of treatment.

General principles of treatment

Therapy aims at controlling seizures using one drug, at the lowest possible dose and causing the fewest side effects possible. The established AEDs, carbamazepine, clonazepam, ethosuximide, phenobarbitone, phenytoin and sodium valproate form the mainstay of treatment. Acetazolamide, clobazam and primidone are also occasionally used in the treatment of epilepsy. More recently, vigabatrin and lamotrigine have become available and oxcarbazepine may be launched in the near future. The choice of drugs depends largely on seizure type, and so correct diagnosis and classification are essential. Table 28.1 gives the main indications for the AEDs currently available.

Initiation of therapy: newly diagnosed patients

The first line AED most suitable for the patient's seizure type should be introduced slowly, starting with a small dose, as too rapid an introduction may induce side effects which will lose the patient's confidence. For most drugs, this gradual introduction will produce a therapeutic effect just as fast as a rapid introduction and the patient should be reassured about this.

Table 28.1 Choice of antiepileptic drugs (AEDs) for different seizure types

Seizure type	First line	Second line
Partial seizures		
Simple partial	Carbamazepine	Vigabatrin
Complex partial	Phenytoin	Clobazam
Secondary generalized	Valproate	Phenobarbitone
		Acetazolamide
Generalized seizures		
Tonic–clonic	Valproate	Vigabatrin
Tonic	Carbamazepine	Clobazam
Clonic	Phenytoin	Phenobarbitone
		Lamotrigine
Absence	Ethosuximide	Vigabatrin
	Valproate	Clobazam
		Phenobarbitone
		Lamotrigine
Atypical absences	Valproate	Phenobarbitone
Atonic	Clonazepam	Lamotrigine
	Clobazam	Carbamazepine
		Phenytoin
		Acetazolamide
Myoclonic	Valproate	Phenobarbitone
	Clonazepam	Acetazolamide

Maintenance dosage

There is no single optimum dose of any AED which suits all patients. The required dose varies from patient to patient, and from one drug regimen to another. Drugs should be introduced slowly and increased incrementally to an initial maintenance dosage. Seizure control should then be assessed, and the dose of the drug changed if necessary. For most AEDs, dosage increments are constant over a wide range of dosages but with phenytoin more care is needed as the serum level/dose relationship is not linear and small dose changes may result in large serum level changes.

Altering drug regimens

If the maximal tolerated dose of a drug does not control the seizures or if side effects develop, the first drug can be substituted with another first line AED. To do this, the second drug should be added gradually to the first. Once a good dose of the new drug is established, the first drug should then slowly be withdrawn. The withdrawal of individual AEDs should be carried out in a slow stepwise fashion to avoid the precipitation of withdrawal seizures. This risk is particularly great with the barbiturate drugs (phenobarbitone and primidone) and the benzodiazepine drugs (clobazam and clonazepam). If a drug needs to be withdrawn rapidly, for instance if there are life-threatening side effects, then diazepam can be used to cover the withdrawal phase.

Examples of withdrawal programmes (used at Chalfont Centre for Epilepsy, Chalfont St Peter, UK):

- Carbamazepine
  a. 100 to 200 mg every 2 weeks (as part of a drug change)
  b. 100 to 200 mg every 4 weeks (total withdrawal)
- Phenobarbitone
  a. 15 to 30 mg every 2 weeks (as part of a drug change)
  b. 15 to 30 mg every 4 weeks (total withdrawal)
- Phenytoin
  a. 50 mg every 2 weeks (as part of a drug change)
  b. 50 mg every 4 weeks (total withdrawal)
- Sodium valproate
  a. 200 to 400 mg every 2 weeks (as part of a drug change)
  b. 200 to 400 mg every 4 weeks (total withdrawal)
- Ethosuximide
  a. 125 to 200 mg every 2 weeks (as part of a drug change)
  b. 125 to 200 mg every 4 weeks (total withdrawal).

Variations in the above regimen will be used depending on the hospital. The patient should be closely monitored for any changes in fit frequency. The time period of 2 or 4 weeks for each dose reduction may be reduced if the patient is an inpatient.

When to make dosage changes

AEDs tend to have long half-lives, and it may take some time before a change in dose results in a stable blood level. Phenobarbitone, for instance, may take some weeks to produce a stable blood level and for this reason, an assessment of the effectiveness of any dose should be made several weeks after that blood level has been reached.

Follow-up and monitoring of treatment

It is essential to follow up patients in whom AEDs treatment has been started. The reason for this is essentially to monitor the efficacy and side effects of treatment, upon which drug dosage will depend, but also to encourage good compliance. This follow-up is particularly important in the early stages of treatment, when an effective maintenance dose may not have been fully established, when the importance of regular compliance may not have been recognized by the patient, and when the psychological adjustment to regular treatment may not be resolved.

Chronic epilepsy

The drug treatment of patients with established

epilepsy which is uncontrolled despite attempts at therapy is much more difficult than that of newly diagnosed patients. Prognosis is worse, drug resistance may have developed, and there may be additional neurological, psychological or social problems.

Assessment. The diagnosis of epilepsy should be reassessed before assuming the seizures are intractable. A significant proportion of patients may have been incorrectly diagnosed. The aetiology of the epilepsy should also be considered, and the question of a progressive neurological condition addressed. A treatment history should be obtained and notes made of the previous drugs used which were helpful, unhelpful or of uncertain benefit. Also, drugs previously not tried should be identified. Serum level measurements should be obtained.

Choice of drugs and dosage. Treatment should be with one or two AEDs. In the great majority of patients there is no place for therapy with more than two drugs. The choice of drugs should be made according to seizure type and the previous treatment history. Drugs which were helpful in the past or of uncertain benefit, or which had not been used before should be tried, as appropriate to seizure type. The use of sedative AEDs should be minimized where possible.

Intractable epilepsy. It is important to realize that there are limits to AED treatment and that in some patients – albeit a small group – seizure control is not possible with the currently available drugs. In such cases the goal of drug treatment is to reduce medication to minimize toxicity while providing partial control. The sedative drugs, e.g. the barbiturates or benzodiazepine drugs, for instance, should be used only where absolutely necessary. The availability of vigabatrin and lamotrigine for this group of patients should prove beneficial.

Stopping treatment

Withdrawing therapy should be considered in patients who have been seizure free for a considerable period of time. In no individual case, however, can the safety of drug withdrawal be guaranteed, and the risk of relapse on with-drawal of medication in a patient who has been seizure free for more than 2 years is about 40%. The longer the patient has been free of seizures, the lower is the risk of seizure recurrence when drugs are withdrawn. If a patient has a mental handicap, partial seizures or symptomatic epilepsy, or neurological signs or other evidence of cerebral damage, this risk is much higher and in such cases it may be best to continue drug treatment indefinitely. Drug withdrawal should be carried out only very slowly in staged decrements, and only one drug at a time should be withdrawn. The risks of drug withdrawal should be clearly explained to the patient, and the possible medical and social implications taken into account. There may be serious domestic consequences should seizures recur, and the attacks may be subsequently difficult to control, even if the original anticonvulsant regimen is re-established. In the final analysis, the decision to withdraw therapy is an individual one, and a patient should be made aware of the risks and benefits of withdrawal.

Monitoring anticonvulsant therapy

Therapeutic drug monitoring (TDM), i.e. measuring serum anticonvulsant levels and their kinetic interpretation, is an integral component in the management of patients receiving phenytoin and carbamazepine; it is less useful in patients receiving acetazolamide, barbiturates, benzodiazepines, ethosuximide, sodium valproate and vigabatrin.

TDM is indicated:

- at the onset of therapy
- if seizure control is poor
- if toxicity is suspected
- if poor or non-compliance is suspected
- to monitor the time scale of drug interactions.

The frequency of monitoring varies. Routinely, patients may have serum levels checked once or twice a year but more often if one of the above indications is being considered. Clinicians and pharmacists can collaborate to ensure TDM is not misused.

Anticonvulsant drug profiles

A summary of available formulations, doses and target range for each drug is given in Table 28.2. A summary of the pharmacokinetic data of the main AEDs is provided in Table 28.3, common side effects in Table 28.4 and drug interactions in Table 28.5.

Acetazolamide

Acetazolamide, is occasionally used as an AED. It can be prescribed as a second line drug for most types of seizures, but particularly for partial seizures, absence seizures and myoclonic seizures. Its intermittent use in catamenial seizures has also been suggested, these seizures occur in a small proportion of women during the menstrual period. Acetazolamide has only limited use as long-term therapy because of the development of tolerance in the majority of patients. Side effects include skin rashes, weight loss, paraesthesia, drowsiness and depression. Routine TDM is not available for this drug.

Carbamazepine

Carbamazepine, is a drug of first choice in tonic–clonic, tonic, clonic and partial seizures, and may be of benefit in all other seizure types except generalized absence seizures and myoclonic seizures. Tolerance to its beneficial effect does not usually develop. Adverse events may occur in up to a third of patients treated with carbamazepine but only about 5% will necessitate drug withdrawal, usually due to skin rash, gastrointestinal disturbances or hyponatraemia. Dose-related adverse reactions including ataxia, dizziness, blurred vision and diplopia are common. Serious adverse events including hepatic failure and bone marrow depression are extremely uncommon. Carbamazepine shows autoinduction, i.e. it induces its own metabolism as well as inducing the metabolism of other drugs. It should therefore be introduced at low dosage and the dose optimized over a period of 1 month, e.g. in adults start with 100 mg twice daily, increasing to 200 mg twice daily after 1 week up to the desired maintenance dose. This allows for

maximal autoinduction to occur over 3 to 4 weeks.

A relationship between serum carbamazepine levels and clinical effect exists and the most widely quoted therapeutic range is 20 to 40 micromol/L (5 to 10 mg/L). Carbamazepine is metabolized to carbamazepine 10,11,-epoxide which is clinically active; routine monitoring of the epoxide is not required. In patients on polytherapy, however, the epoxide may contribute to clinical toxicity despite therapeutic levels of carbamazepine. Measurement of the epoxide in such circumstances may be useful. In addition, a number of clinically important pharmacokinetic interactions may occur and caution should be used when co-medication is instituted (see Table 28.5). For patients requiring higher doses, the slow-release preparation of carbamazepine has distinct advantages, allowing twice-daily ingestion and avoiding high peak serum concentrations. A chewable tablet (chewtab) formulation is also available and pharmacokinetic studies have shown that chewtabs perform well if inadvertently swallowed whole.

Clobazam

Clobazam is a 1,5-benzodiazepine, which is said to be less sedative than 1,4-benzodiazepine drugs such as clonazepam and diazepam. Although the development of tolerance is common, clobazam is used as an adjunctive therapy to patients with partial or generalized seizures, which have proved unresponsive to other antiepileptic medication. Its intermittent use in catamenial epilepsy has also been suggested. Clobazam may produce less sedation than other benzodiazepines, but otherwise its adverse effects are similar including dizziness, behavioural disturbances and dry mouth. Withdrawal may be difficult.

Clonazepam

Clonazepam, a 1,4-benzodiazepine, is a drug of choice for myoclonic seizures and a second line drug for generalized tonic–clonic seizures, absences, and as adjunctive therapy for partial seizures but as with clobazam effectiveness

Table 28.2 Starting dose, average maintenance dose and contra-indications of anticonvulsants in adults

Drug	Daily starting dose	Average maintenance dose	No. doses per day	Contra-indications
Carbamazepine	200 mg	600–2400 mg	2–4	Previous drug sensitivity to carbamazepine. In patients with severe cardiovascular disease, or with hepatic or renal disorders and in elderly patients the initial dosage should be small and the increments titrated against the patient's condition. Treatment with carbamazepine should be discontinued if the patient developes leucopenia
Clonazepam	0.5 mg	0.5–3 mg	1–2	Hypersensitivity to benzodiazepines; acute pulmonary insufficiency; respiratory depression. The use of clonazepam during pregnancy or lactation should be avoided. Use with caution in patients with chronic pulmonary insufficiency, or with impairment of renal or hepatic function, the elderly, and in debilitated patients
Diazepam	NA	NA	NA	Do not use during pregnancy, especially during the first and last trimesters unless there are compelling reasons. In patients with chronic pulmonary insufficiency, and in patients with chronic renal or hepatic disease, dosage may need to be reduced
Ethosuximide	250 mg	500–1500 mg	1–2	Hypersensitivity to succinimides
Gabapentin	300 mg	900–1200 mg	3	Hypersensitivity. Pregnancy, lactation. Abrupt withdrawal may lead to rebound seizures. May exacerbate absence seizures
Lamotrigine	50 mg (reduced by 50% if on valproate)	100–500 mg (reduced by 50% if on valproate)	2	Hypersensitivity. Use with caution in patients with liver and renal impairment. Should not be used in pregnancy as insufficient data available
Phenobarbitone	60 mg	60–180 mg	1	Use with caution in nursing mothers. Acute intermittent porphyria is an absolute contra-indication
Phenytoin	200–300 mg	200–400 mg	1–2	Hypersensitivity to hydantoins
Primidone	125 mg	500–1500 mg	2	Patients who exhibit hypersensivity or an allergic reaction. Should not be administered to patients with acute intermittent porphyria; use with caution in children, the elderly, debilitated patients or those with impaired renal, hepatic or respiratory function
Sodium valproate	500 mg	2000–4000 mg	1–2	Hypersensitivity. Active liver disease. Women of childbearing age: an increased incidence of congenital abnormalities in offspring born to mothers with epilepsy both untreated and treated has been demonstrated
Vigabatrin	500 mg	2000–4000 mg	1–2	There is inadequate evidence of safety in human pregnancy and lactation. Abrupt withdrawal may lead to rebound seizures. Should be used with caution in patients with a history of psychosis or behavioural problems, in elderly patients or patients with renal insufficiency

Table 28.3   Pharmacokinetic data summary

Drug	% Bio-availability	Tmax (h)	Vd (L/kg)	% Protein binding	t½ (h)	% renal excretion	Active metabolite
Carbamazepine	75–85	1–5 (chronic dosing)	0.8–1.6	70–78	24–45 single 8–24 chronic	< 1	Yes
Clonazepam	80–90	1–2	2.1–4.3	80–90	19–40	2	—
Diazepam	90	1–2	1–2	96	20–95	2	Yes
Ethosuximide	90–95	3–7	0.6–0.9	0	20–60	10–20	No
Gabapentin	51–59	2–3	0.7	0	6	100	No
Lamotrigine	98	2–3	1.2	55	29	7	No
Phenobarbitone	95–100	1–3	0.6	40–50	50–144	20–40	No
Phenytoin	85–95	4–7	0.5–0.7	90–95	9–40 non-linear kinetics	< 5	No
Primidone	90–100	1–3	0.4–1.1	20–30	3–19	40	Yes
Sodium valproate	100	0.5–1	0.1–0.5	88–92	7–17	< 5	No
Vigabatrin	60–80	2	0.6–1.0	0	5–7	100	No

Key: Tmax = time to maximum serum concentration; Vd = volume of distribution; t½ = elimination half-life

Table 28.4   Side effect profile of anticonvulsants

Drug	Dose-related (predictable)	Non-dose-related (idiosyncratic)
Carbamazepine	Diplopia, drowsiness, headache, nausea, orofacial dyskinesia, arrhythmias	Photosensitivity, Stevens–Johnson syndrome, agranulocytosis, aplastic anaemia, hepatotoxicity
Sodium valproate	Dyspepsia, nausea, vomiting, hair loss, anorexia, drowsiness	Acute pancreatitis, aplastic anaemia, thrombocytopenia, hepatotoxicity
Phenytoin	Ataxia, nystagmus, drowsiness, gingival hyperplasia, hirsutism, diplopia, asterixis, orofacial dyskinesia, folate deficiency	Blood dyscrasias, rash, Dupuytren's contracture, hepatotoxicity
Phenobarbitone	Fatigue, listlessness, depression, poor memory, impotence, hypocalcaemia, osteomalacia, folate deficiency	Macropapular rash, exfoliation, hepatotoxicity
Ethosuximide	Nausea, vomiting, drowsiness, headache, lethargy	Rash, erythema multiforma, Stevens–Johnson syndrome
Clonazepam	Fatigue, drowsiness, ataxia	Rash, thrombocytopenia
Vigabatrin	Drowsiness, dizziness, weight gain	Behavioural disturbances, severe psychosis

often wears off with time as tolerance develops. Parenteral clonazepam is useful in status epilepticus. It has an adverse effect profile similar to that of clobazam, but may be more sedating.

Diazepam

Diazepam is used mainly in the treatment of status epilepticus, intravenously or in the acute management of febrile convulsions as a rectal solution – absorption from suppositories or intramuscular injection is slow and erratic. The rectal solution may also be useful in status epilepticus particularly in children if it is not possible to give the drug intravenously.

Ethosuximide

Ethosuximide, is a drug of first choice for generalized absence seizures, and has no useful effect

Table 28.5 Drug interactions

Drug affected	Effect on serum level	Drug implicated	Possible mechanism
Carbamazepine	Increase	Sodium valproate Cimetidine Dextropropoxyphene Propoxyphene Erythromycin Isoniazid Troleandomycin Danazol	Enzyme inhibition
	Decrease	Phenytoin Phenobarbitone	Enzyme induction
Phenytoin	Increase	Sodium valproate Chloramphenicol Isoniazid Disulfirm Fluconazole Flu vaccine	Enzyme inhibition
		Amiodarone	Mechanism unclear
		Fluoxetine	Mechanism unclear (possible inhibition)
	Decrease	Phenobarbitone Rifampicin Carbamazepine	Enzyme induction
		Frusemide	Decreased responsiveness of renal tubules
		Acetazolamide	Increased osteomalacia
Sodium valproate	Increase	Salicylates	Displacement from protein-binding sites and possible enzyme inhibition
	Decrease	Potential enzyme inducers	Enzyme induction
Phenobarbitone	Increase	Sodium valproate	Enzyme inhibition
	Decrease	Rifampicin	Enzyme induction
Ethosuximide	Increase	Sodium valproate	Enzyme inhibition
	Decrease	Carbamazepine	Enzyme induction

against any other seizure types. Tolerance does not seem to be a problem. The most commonly encountered adverse effects are gastrointestinal symptoms, which occur frequently at the beginning of therapy. Behaviour disorders, anorexia, fatigue, sleep disturbances and headaches may also occur. Ethosuximide is started at a dose of 250 mg twice daily and adjusted by 250 mg each week until a maintenance dose (500 to 1500 mg per day in adults) is achieved. At higher doses, increases in daily dose may lead to disproportionately higher increases in average serum concentrations; therefore careful monitoring is indicated. The therapeutic range commonly quoted is between 350 and 700 micromol/L (50 to 100 mg/L) but some patients may require higher concentrations, sometimes as high as 1050 micromol/L (150 mg/L). The bioavailability of the syrup and capsule formulations are equivalent.

Phenobarbitone

Phenobarbitone is a second line drug for the treatment of tonic–clonic, tonic and partial seizures. It may also be used in other seizure types. Its antiepileptic efficacy is similar to that of phenytoin or carbamazepine. Adverse effects on cognitive function, the propensity to produce tolerance and the risk of serious seizure exacerbation on withdrawal make it an unattractive option and it should be used only as a last resort. In addition to sedative and cognitive effects which are often observed, phenobarbitone may cause skin rashes, ataxia, folate deficiency, or osteomalacia in 1 to 2% of patients. Behavioural disturbances are reported particularly in children and an increased risk of connective tissue disorders such as Dupuytren's contracture and frozen shoulder may be observed. The usual adult dose range varies widely from 30 to 240 mg per day. The normal adult target range of 50 to 170 micromol/L (15 to 40 mg/L) should be interpreted with caution due to development of tolerance to some of the pharmacological effects as well as to the antiepileptic action. Decreased elimination is expected in patients with impaired renal and hepatic functions. Once a day dosage is usually adequate in most adults because of the long half-life. However, as steady state is not reached for 2 to 3 weeks the administration of a loading dose is recommended. Routine monitoring is not necessary on initiating therapy as the dose can be adequately titrated according to the clinical response. However, monitoring is indicated if patients do not respond, or exhibit toxicity.

Primidone

Primidone is principally metabolized to phenobarbitone and phenylethylmalonamide (PEMA) in vivo. It has a similar action but a worse side effect profile than phenobarbitone. The drug shows a 'first-dose reaction', i.e. drowsiness, nausea, dizziness and general feeling of being unwell on initiating treatment. This effect diminishes on repeat administration but may last for 24 hours after the first dose. Therapy should be initiated with a small dose, e.g. 62.5 mg at night to avoid this reaction. PEMA is also active; however, it is unclear how much this metabolite contributes to the anticonvulsant effect of primidone. Routine monitoring of primidone is not indicated; however, monitoring phenobarbitone levels may be useful in some patients to assist in dosage optimization. There is nothing to recommend primidone as an AED over phenobarbitone.

Phenytoin

Phenytoin is a drug of first choice for tonic–clonic, tonic, and partial seizures and a second line drug for atonic seizures and atypical absences. It is not effective in typical generalized absences and myoclonic seizures. Tolerance to its antiepileptic action does not usually occur. Phenytoin has non-linear kinetics and a low therapeutic index and in some patients frequent drug serum level measurements may be necessary. Drug interactions are common as phenytoin metabolism is very susceptible to inhibition by other drugs, and it may enhance the metabolism of other drugs. Caution should be exercised when other medication is introduced or withdrawn. Adverse events may occur in up to a half of patients treated with phenytoin but only about 10% will necessitate drug withdrawal, most commonly due to skin rash. Dose-related adverse reactions including nystagmus, ataxia, and lethargy are common. Cosmetic effects such as gum hypertrophy, hirsutism, and acne are well recognized adverse effects and should be taken into account when prescribing for young women and children. The latter effects in some patients may be unacceptable and will require discontinuation of the drug. Improved oral hygiene and regular visits to the dentist may allow continuation of the drug in some patients. Chronic adverse effects include folate deficiency, osteomalacia, Dupuytren's contractures and cerebellar atrophy. Serious idiosyncratic adverse events including hepatic failure and bone marrow depression are extremely uncommon. Most patients require dosages from 250 to 400 mg daily. The rate of drug metabolism of phenytoin is under genetic control hence patients may be slow or fast metabolizers. Slow metabolizers may require doses of 100 to 200 mg a day and fast metabolizers doses of 400 to 600 mg a day. The serum half-life lengthens with increasing serum concentrations. At low serum levels the half-life is about 13 hours and increases to 46 hours at the top end of the therapeutic range. Hence the time to reach steady state varies from 2 to 4 weeks at serum levels within the therapeutic range. The target range for phenytoin is 40 to 80 micromol/L (10 to 20 mg/L) although a number of patients are controlled outside the range. Once patients achieve levels within this range, the majority of patients require once a day dosage.

For the treatment of status epilepticus a loading dose of 15 mg/kg may be indicated. Patients with severe epilepsy may require a loading dose on initiating therapy; a dose of 15 mg/kg or a calculated dose based on volume of distribution 0.65 L/kg can be used. A maintenance dose can then be initiated and serum levels monitored in 2 to 4 weeks to assist in dosage optimization. Phenytoin is available as capsules, tablets, suspension and injection. Phenytoin is usually prescribed to be taken orally although it may be given intravenously.

Oral preparations of phenytoin may present differences in bioavailability (67 to 74%). Patients stabilized on one formulation should continue to receive the same formulation. Care is required when changing from the elixir to the capsule or tablet formulation due to different bioavailability. In addition, care is required in converting from phenytoin to phenytoin sodium: 90 mg phenytoin suspension (30 mg/5 ml or infatabs) is equivalent to 100 mg phenytoin sodium (tablets, capsules or injection).

Intravenous phenytoin should be administered with caution and at a rate not exceeding 50 mg/minute. Intravenous phenytoin may be indicated when patients are nil by mouth or require the drug for status epilepticus. Phenytoin ready mixed parenteral formulation should not be added to intravenous fluids due to a risk of acid precipitation. The drug should never be given intramuscularly because of erratic absorption and pain on injection.

Sodium valproate

Sodium valproate is a drug of first choice for the treatment of generalized absence seizures, myoclonic seizures, and generalized tonic–clonic seizures, especially if these occur as part of the syndrome of primary generalized epilepsy. Tolerance to its antiepileptic action does not usually occur. Drug interactions with other anti-epileptic drugs may be problematic. Phenobarbitone levels increase with valproate co-medication, and a combination of these two drugs may result

in severe sedation. Sodium valproate may also inhibit the metabolism of phenytoin and carbamazepine. Enzyme-inducing drugs enhance the metabolism of sodium valproate, so caution should be exercised when other anti-epileptic drugs are introduced or withdrawn. Up to a third of patients may experience adverse effects but less than 5% will require the drug to be stopped.

Adverse effects include anorexia, nausea, diarrhoea, weight gain, alopecia, skin rash, and thrombocytopenia. Confusion, stupor, tremor and hyperammonaemia are usually dose related.

Serious adverse events including fatal pancreatic and hepatic failure are extremely uncommon. In children under 2 years, on other AEDs and with pre-existing neurological deficit the risk of hepatic failure is 1/500 and in adults on valproate monotherapy the risk is 1/37 000. The usual therapeutic range quoted is 350 to 700 micromol/L (50 to 100 mg/L); however, because of the lack of a good correlation between total valproate concentrations and effect, serum level monitoring of the drug has limited use. TDM should only be performed in cases of suspected toxicity, deterioration in seizure control, to check compliance and to monitor drug interactions. Routine monitoring of this drug is not necessary.

Vigabatrin

Vigabatrin, a suicide inhibitor of GABA transaminase, is a second line drug for partial seizures and generalized tonic–clonic seizures. Vigabatrin may also be useful against other seizure types, with the exception of generalized absences and myoclonus. Up to half of patients with refractory epilepsy showed a > 50% seizure reduction but tolerance may develop in some responders. Vigabatrin does not interact with other drugs apart from decreasing phenytoin levels through an unknown mechanism. Early animal studies with vigabatrin showed intramyelonic oedema and although this has not been seen in humans, this is an area of concern and is the subject of ongoing studies. The commonest adverse events associated with vigabatrin are behavioural disturbances ranging from agitation and confusion to frank psychosis. Other known adverse effects include drowsiness, headaches, ataxia, weight gain, depression and tremor. Careful monitoring for side effects on initiation of therapy is essential. Routine TDM is not necessary for this drug.

Lamotrigine

Lamotrigine, a phenyltriazine drug, is a novel antiepileptic drug which is effective against partial seizures. Recent anecdotal reports, however, suggest that it may be more effective in generalized seizures, particularly in atypical absences. Common adverse effects include skin rash, drowsiness, seizure exacerbation, headache, and diplopia. Some symptoms may, however, have been caused by an interaction with concomitant carbamazepine. Its metabolism is induced by carbamazepine, phenytoin and phenobarbitone. Lamotrigine metabolism is inhibited by sodium valproate and lower doses must therefore be used in this situation. There have

been a few reports of patients taking this drug suffering disseminated intravascular coagulation and sudden death although the significance of lamotrigine in these cases is uncertain.

Oxcarbazepine

Oxcarbazepine is the 10-keto analogue of carbamazepine. It is an inactive pro-drug and is converted in the liver to the active 10-hydroxy metabolite and bypasses the 10,11-epoxide, which is the primary metabolite of carbamazepine. The spectrum of efficacy and side effects is broadly comparable to carbamazepine. The principal advantage of oxcarbazepine over carbamazepine is the lack of induction of hepatic enzymes, with the consequence of lack of autoinduction of the drug's metabolism and less pharmacokinetic interactions. Further, two-thirds of patients who are allergic to carbamazepine can tolerate oxcarbazepine.

CASE STUDIES

CASE 28.1

A 24-year-old man with a history of refractory generalized epilepsy with frequent generalized tonic–clonic convulsions and daily myoclonic seizures since childhood is admitted to hospital for detailed medical review and possible drug changes. At the time of admission his antiepileptic treatment consisted of sodium valproate 3000 mg/day with apparently good compliance. The sodium valproate dose had been progressively increased over the previous 2 years as there had been no effect on seizure frequency and the patient had not complained of any adverse side effects. Within 3 days of admission, the patient became progressively drowsy and confused with episodes of nausea and vomiting.

Q What is the most likely explanation for his sudden deterioration?

CASE 28.2

A 31-year-old man with a history of complex partial seizures and occasional secondary generalization had his last epileptic attack 8 years ago. His seizure disorder started in his middle teens and no aetiology was ever identified. He is still receiving treatment with carbamazepine 800 mg/day and phenytoin 350 mg/day and has no complaint regarding side effects. He attends the outpatient department for a neurological review and the question of withdrawing treatment is raised. He is presently working as a sales person for a computer company and in the course of his work drives an average of 1000 miles a month.

Q What do you advise?

CASE 28.3

Mrs G. S., a 42-year-old Hindu lady was admitted to hospital with suspected tuberculosis. She has a history of tonic–clonic epilepsy. Her medication on admission included phenytoin 300 mg nocte and phenobarbitone 60 mg nocte. Her epilepsy was reasonably well controlled (baseline serum phenytoin level 17.5 mg/L and phenobarbitone 18 mg/L, sample time 15 hours post-dose).

Following admission active pulmonary tuberculosis was confirmed. The patient was commenced on rifampicin 200 mg, isoniazid 300 mg and ethambutol 300 mg daily. Pyridoxine 20 mg daily was added to the regimen.

Q1 What problems may exist for this patient and how would you advise that her therapy is monitored?

2 weeks later the patient is seen by her GP; she has a sudden increase in fit frequency and serum anticonvulsant levels are measured. Serum levels reported are phenytoin 6 mg/L and phenobarbitone 15.5 mg/L.

Q2 Comment on the results; how should the patient be managed for her poor epilepsy control?

CASE 28.4

Mr H. J. is 25 years old and was admitted following a road traffic accident (RTA). The patient is unconscious and requires ventilation. On admission he has a fractured right femur and head injuries. The patient is prescribed a loading dose of phenytoin 15 mg/kg and a maintenance dose of 300 mg daily. The drug is administered by slow i.v. injection (serum phenytoin level on day 5 is 14.5 mg/L). 1 week later the patient is taken off the ventilator. He is now receiving continuous nasogastric feeding and his phenytoin is administered nasogastrically. 2 weeks later the patient's serum phenytoin is measured and reported as 3.5 mg/L.

The dose of phenytoin is increased to 350 mg daily and the serum level monitored 3 weeks later is 4.3 microgram/ml.

Q1 Comment on the loading dose and maintenance dose for phenytoin?

Q2 Comment on the TDM results for this patient. If anticonvulsant treatment is to be continued what advice should be given?

ANSWERS TO CASE STUDIES

CASE 28.1

A This patient had been prescribed a very large dose of sodium valproate on account of a lack of clinical response and the absence of any side effect. On admission to the ward it was decided to observe his seizure pattern before any drug changes were implemented. Within 3 days of admission the patient developed encephalopathy. The possibility of sodium valproate intoxication was raised. An emergency estimate of sodium valproate serum level was carried out and showed a grossly elevated level of 1338 micromol/L (normal range up to 700 micromol/L); and a serum ammonia level of 157 micromol/L (normal range up to 40 micromol/L) confirming the diagnosis. It is likely that this patient had been a chronic non-complier which would explain the lack of response to ever increasing doses and also the absence of any side effects. Indeed on direct questioning, when confronted with the evidence, the patient admitted long-standing erratic drug taking. On follow-up 3 months later the patient (now with his drug taking supervised by his mother) had had no further seizures. One of the commonest causes of AED treatment failure is bad or non-compliance and this should always be throughly checked before assuming that treatment is a failure.

CASE 28.2

A It is good clinical practice to consider drug withdrawal on any patient who has been seizure free for more than 3 years. However, there is always a risk of seizure recurrence on coming off treatment and the decision should not be taken lightly. The pros and cons of continuing and withdrawal of treatment should be clearly explained to the patient. The patient should always be the final arbiter on this issue. The fact that this patient is a professional who depends on holding a driving licence to be able to work makes it unlikely that he will consider coming off all his medication. One seizure would be sufficient to bar him from driving for 2 years as the present regulations stand in the UK. Should he, however, decide otherwise, drug tapering should be done in a very slow fashion in decremental steps with one drug at a time been discontinued.

CASE 28.3

A1 The patient is well controlled clinically and baseline TDM shows adequate serum levels of both drugs. The patient is receiving phenytoin and phenobarbitone, both potent enzyme inducers hence her tuberculosis (TB) therapy needs to be assessed for efficacy. The patient is commenced on recommended doses for the anti-TB drugs. The TB regimen includes rifampicin which is a potent enzyme inducer and isoniazid which is a potent enzyme inhibitor. This regimen will affect the anticonvulsant serum levels. The patient's clinical response should be closely monitored for any changes in fit frequency and weekly serum anticonvulsant levels taken to monitor either enzyme induction effects of rifampicin or inhibition by isoniazid.

A2 The serum anticonvulsant levels are lower than baseline levels taken at the start of anti-TB therapy. Compliance must be assured. The change in the patient's fit frequency is probably due to the enzyme-inducing effects of rifampicin. A cautious 25 to 50 mg increase in the phenytoin dose may be recommended, and serum levels repeated in 2 to 3 weeks. Changes in the phenobarbitone serum levels should be monitored. Further TDM monitoring and assessment of the patient is required since, as the TB therapy progresses, enzyme inhibition due to the isoniazid may be seen and the patient should be closely monitored for drug-induced toxicity. The efficacy of the TB regimen should also be monitored since the patient is receiving anticonvulsants which may affect the TB regimen.

CASE 28.4

A1 The use of anticonvulsants after a road traffic accident (RTA) is controversial and it is important to assess the need for phenytoin in this patient. This should be discussed with the local neurological team.

The patient has received the standard loading and maintenance dose. Standard pharmacokinetic calculations using volume of distribution and aiming for a level of 15 mg/L would give a lower recommended dose. The maintenance dose is a reasonable starting dose for a 70 kg male. Phenytoin shows saturation pharmacokinetics and wide interpatient variation in drug handling. It is advisable to monitor phenytoin serum levels 2 to 3 weeks after initiating treatment to ensure adequate dosing. For prophylaxis following RTA, levels within the therapeutic range 10 to 20 microgram/ml may be desirable. This should be discussed with the local neurologist.

A2 The TDM results for this patient are below the therapeutic range. In addition, a 50 mg increase in dose resulted in a small increase in serum phenytoin level. Phenytoin shows saturation kinetics, hence a 50 mg dosage increase should result in a disproportionate increase in the serum level. Possible explanations are:

- the patient is a rapid metabolizer of the drug
- absorption of phenytoin is impaired by nasogastric feeding
- poor compliance.

The most likely explanation is impaired absorption of phenytoin due to nasogastric feeding, since the i.v. regimen resulted in therapeutic serum levels, and poor compliance can be ruled out.

Nasogastric feeding is known to impair the absorption of phenytoin. Improved absorption is found if the NG feed is stopped 2 hours prior to administration of phenytoin and for 2 hours following administration. If the problem does not resolve it is advisable to use an alternative drug, e.g. sodium valproate.

BIBLIOGRAPHY

Brodie M J. Established anticonvulsants and treatment of refractory epilepsy. Lancet 1990; 336: 350–354

Brodie M J, Porter R J. New and potential anticonvulsants. Lancet 1990; 336: 425–426

Chadwick D, Reynolds E H. When do epileptic patients need treatment? Starting and stopping medication. British Medical Journal 1985; 290: 1885–1888

Commission on Classification and Terminology of the International League Against Epilepsy. Proposal for revised clinical and electroencephalographic classification of epileptic seizures. Epilepsia 1981; 22: 489–501

Dreifuss F E. Valproate: toxicity. In: Dreifuss F E, Mattson R H, Meldrum B S, Penry J K (eds). Antiepileptic drugs, 3rd edn. New York: Raven Press 1989: 643–651

Dreifuss F E, Langer D H, Moline K A, Maxwell J E. Valproic acid hepatic fatalities. II US experience since 1984. Epilepsia 1989; 39: 201–207

Dreifuss F E, Mattson R H, Meldrum B S, Penry J K (eds). Antiepileptic drugs, 3rd edn. New York: Raven Press 1989

Duncan J S. Modern treatment strategies for patients with epilepsy: a review. Journal of the Royal Society of Medicine 1991; 84: 159–162

Duncan J S, Patsalos P N, Shorvon S D. Effects of discontinuation of phenytoin, carbamazepine and valproate on concomitant antiepileptic medication. Epilepsia 1991; 32: 101–116

Editorial. Carbamazepine update. Lancet 1989; ii: 595–597

Editorial. Oxcarbazepine. Lancet 1989; ii: 196–198

MRC Antiepileptic Drug Withdrawal Group. Randomised study of antiepileptic drug withdrawal in patients in remission. Lancet 1991; 337: 1175–1180

Robertson M. Current status of the 1,4- and 1,5-benzodiazepines in the treatment of epilepsy: the place of clobazam. Epilepsia 1986; 27 (Suppl. 1): S527–S541

Sander J W A S, Trevisol-Bittencourt P C, Hart Y M, Patsalos P N, Shorvon S D. The efficacy and long-term tolerability of lamotrigine in the treatment of severe epilepsy. Epilepsy Research 1990; 7: 226–229

Sander J W A S, Duncan J S, Patsalos P N, Shorvon S D. Lamotrigine and generalised seizures. Epilepsia 1991; 32 (Suppl. 1): 59

Sivenius J, Ylinen A, Murros K, Mumford J P, Riekkinen P J. Vigabatrin in drug resistant partial epilepsy: a 5 year follow-up study. Neurology 1991; 41: 562–565

Chapter 29

Parkinson's disease

D. N. Bateman

Parkinson's disease, originally described by James Parkinson in the first half of last century, is a disease which has three cardinal clinical features. These are a tremor, an increase in tone manifested clinically as rigidity, and slowness of movement, akinesia. However, typical features also include a mask-like facial expression with excess salivation, and in more severe cases, a typical gait in which the patient does not swing his or her arms, and in which the steps become gradually shorter with patients sometimes falling forward over their own feet (marche à petit pas).

EPIDEMIOLOGY

In the majority of patients with this condition the epidemiology is unknown. There are some well-documented causes of a parkinsonian syndrome, the commonest being administration of dopamine antagonist drugs such as phenothiazines, butyrophenones and metoclopramide. The condition also followed the epidemic of encephalitis lethargica, caused by an encephalitic virus, which occurred after the First World War, but most patients with post-encephalitic parkinsonism have now died. Other causes of a similar syndrome include cerebrovascular disease, severe anoxia (for example following carbon monoxide poisoning), head injury and poisoning with heavy metals.

The disease is common with a prevelance of approximately 1 in 10 000 but is very much age

433

associated with an increasing incidence over the age of 50 years, and approximately 1 in 200 of patients over the age of 65 years are affected. Studies to identify a viral cause have also been unsuccessful.

AETIOLOGY

The majority of patients with Parkinson's disease have no known predisposing cause. The largest group of patients with an identified aetiology are patients receiving dopamine antagonists (Table 29.1). Susceptibility to drug-induced parkinsonism seems to increase with age. This is probably related to the decline in dopaminergic neurones within the basal ganglia that occurs with ageing.

Another cause of a typical parkinsonian syndrome has been recognized with the toxin MPTP (1-methyl-4-phenyl-1,2,3,6, tetrahydropyridine), a by-product of the illicit manufacture of pethidine. This agent causes specific damage to the basal ganglia and has been used more recently to produce an animal model of the condition.

PATHOPHYSIOLOGY

The fundamental pathological abnormality underlying Parkinson's disease is the degeneration of cells, with loss of pigmented neurones, in the pars compacta of the substantia nigra. These cells project to the caudate nucleus and putamen and their neurotransmitter is dopamine. In Parkinson's disease the degenerating pigmented neurones contain eosinophilic inclusion bodies,

Table 29.1   Common causes of parkinsonian syndrome
Parkinson's disease
Drug-induced parkinsonism:
Neuroleptics, benzamides, methyldopa and reserpine
Post-encephalitic parkinsonism
MPTP toxicity
Heavy metal poisoning
Anoxia (carbon monoxide poisoning)
Post-traumatic
Cerebrovascular disease, (multi-infarct dementia)
Alzheimer's disease

(Lewy bodies), which are characteristic of the disease. These inclusion bodies are also found in about 4% of brains from patients without Parkinson's disease and it is uncertain whether this represents subclinical disease. The origin of these inclusions is unclear.

Although degeneration of the brain stem pigmented nuclei is the crucial feature of the pathology of Parkinson's disease there are often other associated changes, some of which may be typical of the brains of non-parkinsonian, elderly patients. Recent studies suggest that the numbers of dopamine receptors in the human brain fall progressively with age. The original discovery in 1960 by Ehringer & Hornykiewicz that loss of dopamine-containing neurones was the fundamental feature of Parkinson's disease led to the introduction of new treatments with agents that affected these neurones and the receptors they act on. There is, however, evidence of loss of other neurotransmitters as well including 5-hydroxytryptamine and gamma-aminobutyric acid (GABA).

More recent biochemical studies suggest that the remaining neurones actually turn over dopamine more rapidly than those of normal patients. The finding that GABA is also altered in Parkinson's disease may also be relevant since GABA-minergic nerves feed on to dopaminergic nerves modulating the release of dopamine.

Patients may present with Parkinson's disease associated with other specific neurological phenomena. Most commonly recognized are a progressive supranuclear palsy (a lesion of the part of the brain controlling eye movement), often typified by loss of upward gaze, and primary autonomic failure (Shy–Drager syndrome). The latter is often found in younger patients. Autonomic failure may also, however, be a late complication of patients who appear to have otherwise typical Parkinson's disease.

CLINICAL MANIFESTATIONS

The cardinal clinical features of Parkinson's disease are tremor, rigidity, and hypokinesia. The commonest presenting complaint is tremor, and it often occurs initially in one limb or on one side of the body. The tremor is characteristically present at rest and has a rate of approximately 4 to 8 cycles per second. The classical description is of a 'pill-rolling' tremor, which is made worse by nervousness, fatigue and excitement. Voluntary movements will often momentarily inhibit the tremor in the affected part, but concentration on an action in one limb may result in an excess movement in others.

Rigidity, that is a resistance to passive movement of a limb, is another common feature. Again this may initially be unilateral. Increased tone in the muscles of the neck results in a rather forward stooping posture typical of Parkinson's disease. The increase in tone is present throughout the range of movement. It may have both a 'lead-pipe' character or may be 'cogwheel' in type.

Slowness of movement, variably called bradykinesia, hypokinesia or akinesia is often the most disabling feature of Parkinson's disease. This particularly affects initiation of voluntary motor movement, together with a decrease in so-called automatic movements, for example, swinging of the arms when walking. Many other features which are very typical of Parkinson's disease seem to result from akinesia, and these include the mask-like face, the small writing (micrographia), impaired blinking and rather monotonous speech, with in some patients a reduction in speech volume.

The relative dominance of these three symptoms in individual patients varies. In some patients tremor is predominant, whereas in others bradykinesia is the main feature with patients having very little in the way of other features.

Although the classical description by James Parkinson did not describe mental change, a large proportion of patients with Parkinson's disease do have associated disturbance of higher function. In the face of a progressive neurological condition, some patients become depressed although it is unclear whether this is aggravated by concurrent drug therapy with, for example, anticholinergic drugs. In addition intellectual deterioration, sometimes associated with confusional states, hallucinations or frank psychosis may occur. In individual patients it is sometimes

difficult to establish whether these changes are due to the associated drug therapy or to the underlying condition.

A number of other features may be associated with Parkinson's disease. Autonomic abnormalities are quite common, particularly constipation, and changes in blood pressure control. Postural instability is also related to bradykinesia. Drooling of saliva seems, in part, related to difficulties with swallowing (dysphagia) and may be considered another feature of Parkinson's disease, with or without overt complaints of swallowing problems. Perhaps because of difficulty with swallowing, many patients with Parkinson's disease lose weight.

The overall clinical presentation will vary depending upon the duration of illness. Once patients are established on therapy a number of further complications may occur. Some of these relate to adverse effects of the drugs used and include confusion, hallucinations and postural hypotension. Other problems probably reflect a continuing degeneration of the central nervous system.

Initial therapy in a patient with Parkinson's disease is often successful in alleviating symptoms, but these usually begin to recur after a few months or years of therapy. Deterioration in the clinical condition may present as lack of control of symptoms at the end of a dosage interval of the drug (end of dose akinesia) or as severe swings in performance ranging from extra movements (dyskinesia) to complete lack of movement (total akinesia). These swings in performance often do not appear to be directly related to time of drug administration and are termed 'on-off' phenomena or 'yo-yoing'. These manifestations of Parkinson's disease are often very difficult to manage.

INVESTIGATIONS

There are no specific diagnostic tests for Parkinson's disease. It is always important to consider other possible causes of movement disorders. Such causes include a parkinsonian syndrome secondary to toxins or drugs (particularly dopamine antagonists). A proper drug history therefore is important in a patient with suspected Parkinson's disease.

The important differential diagnosis for tremor is that of essential tremor, which is usually first present only on movement, although it may appear later at rest. There is no associated rigidity. This may occur in association with thyrotoxicosis, anxiety states and alcohol and drug withdrawal. Benign essential (familial) tremor is often inherited as an autosomal dominant trait.

In adolescents and young adults, Wilson's disease is an alternative cause of involuntary movements which may be mistaken for parkinsonism. The choreiform movements of Huntington's chorea should not be confused with parkinsonism but rarely Huntington's chorea presents in akinetic form.

It is important to ensure that a patient with Parkinson's disease maintains adequate nutrition, and that he or she has no underlying endocrinological disorders. It is a useful practice to check thyroid function tests, serum electrolytes, blood count and serum albumin.

TREATMENT

The general disorder

Since there is no known cure for Parkinson's disease, treatment is symptomatic. Recent work suggests that the use of selegeline (see below) may perhaps delay progression. This is the first drug with this potential effect, and it is obviously of great interest. All other treatments improve the patient's symptoms but none has any effect on progression. The response of individual patients varies and treatment has to be tailored accordingly. Dosage increase is limited by adverse effects, but in the long term, with deterioration in neurological function, adjustment in dosage frequency with reduction of individual doses may be necessary. Adjustment of therapy will be needed to deal with complications such as the on-off phenomena and other associated problems including autonomic dysfunction and mental changes.

Occasionally patients suffer pain in muscles affected by the condition and this may be particularly difficult to treat.

Involvement of physiotherapists and occupational therapists is often of use, and relatives may need other support. In the UK the Parkinson's Disease Society is another source of support and information for patients and their relatives.

Drug-induced parkinsonism

Treatment with the offending drug should be stopped if possible. In psychiatric patients, where this may not be appropriate, the use of concurrent anticholinergic drugs may be required. Anticholinergic drugs should normally not be used routinely with dopamine antagonists, firstly because not all patients will develop a parkinsonian syndrome, and secondly because they may increase the risk of tardive dyskinesia.

In elderly patients about 30% do not recover after 3 months of stopping dopamine antagonists. At this stage treatment with specific antiparkinsonian drugs should be considered. It is possible that such patients were in a 'pre-parkinsonian' state when started on therapy.

Drug treatment

Parkinson's disease is a long-term degenerative condition without curative therapy. Until recently it was considered that syptomatic therapy was all that was available. However, recent studies on the monoamine oxidase type B inhibitor, selegeline, suggest that it may be possible to affect the progress of the disease, but further work in this area is necessary.

Drug treatment for parkinsonism is based on agents that work through the dopamine or cholinergic system (Table 29.2). It is generally held that dopaminergic receptors act in an inhibitory manner on cholinergic nerves within the basal ganglia. This underlies the use of anticholinergic drugs, which were in fact the first agents used for the management of Parkinson's disease.

Before the discovery of the effectiveness of agents such as levodopa (L-dopa) and dopamine agonists, stereotactic surgery was frequently used for unilateral symptoms in Parkinson's

Table 29.2 Drug therapies for Parkinson's disease		
1. L-dopa preparations: (with peripherally acting dopa decarboxylase inhibitor)		
a. L-dopa with benserazide: co-beneldopa (Madopar)		
Ratio benserazide: L-dopa		*Madopar*
	12.5/50	62.5
	25/100	125
	50/200	250
Slow release	25/100	(Madopar CR)
b. L-dopa with carbidopa: co-careldopa (Sinemet)		
Ratio carbidopa: L-dopa		*Sinemet*
	10/100	110
	25/250	275
	12.5/50	Sinemet LS
	25/100	Sinemet Plus
Slow release	50/200	(Sinemet CR)
2. Anticholinergic drugs		
Benzhexol		
Benztropine		
Biperiden		
Orphenadrine		
Procyclidine		
3. Dopamine agonists		
Bromocriptine		
Lysuride		
Pergolide		
Apomorphine		
4. Monoamine oxidase type B inhibitor		
Selegeline		
5. Miscellaneous		
Amantadine		

Although anticholinergic drugs were at one time considered first line treatment, in general their use as first line agents has been superseded by preparations of L-dopa.

L-*dopa preparations*

L-dopa is the normal physiological precursor of dopamine synthesis, being converted to dopamine by the enzyme dopa decarboxylase. It readily crosses the blood–brain barrier. The enzyme dopa decarboxylase is present in all adrenergic nerve endings and when L-dopa is used alone it is rapidly taken up and metabolized to dopamine by nervous tissue in the periphery, as well as in the brain. This therefore results in an excess of peripheral side effects, particularly cardiovascular and emetic effects, with often little in the way of beneficial effect on a patient's condition. It used to be the case that a slow build up of L-dopa dosage over weeks and even months was required for maximal therapeutic effect. This difficulty in the use of L-dopa was overcome with the introduction of peripherally acting dopa-decarboxylase inhibitors. These are used in combination, in combined tablets, with L-dopa. At present two such products are available containing either carbidopa or benserazide (co-careldopa: Sinemet; co-beneldopa: Madopar).

These combination products have a variety of ratios of L-dopa to peripherally acting dopa-decarboxylase inhibitor, varying from 10:1 to 4:1. In chronic treatment there is no evidence that these differences offer material benefit to the patient. In patients starting on therapy, nausea may be an initial problem. There is some data to suggest that preparations with a higher proportion of decarboxylase inhibitor do produce less nausea in some patients. An alternative approach to this problem is to use a slowly escalating dose of the combination product at the commencement of therapy, and to take the tablets with food to reduce the rate of drug absorption, a major factor in the production of nausea.

L-dopa preparations can be used in the treatment of parkinsonism in all its forms, except acutely in cases that are drug induced. At the

disease. Because the disease is now recognized to be progressive, such surgery is no longer generally held to be useful or appropriate for most patients. Experimental surgical approaches, involving the implantation of adrenal tissue and foetal neurological tissue into the brain, have not been shown to be efficacious in formal studies and cannot be recommended.

The most difficult decision to make in patients with Parkinson's disease is when to commence therapy. This will often depend on the patient's degree of disability, and an empirical decision as to whether therapy is likely to be of benefit. Although some workers consider that early treatment with L-dopa may, in the long term, result in more drug-related adverse effects, this is still a contentious area. There are no good clinical trials demonstrating that a delay in treatment is beneficial to the patient.

commencement of therapy it is sensible to start at a small dose, usually once or twice daily, increasing to the normal three or four times daily regimen over a period of days. The optimum dose for an individual patient varies, and patients will require monitoring, both from the point of view of therapeutic benefit and for adverse effects. The sign of drug overdose is usually dyskinesia, but postural hypotension, nausea and psychological effects, including confusion, hallucinations or frank psychosis, may occur.

L-dopa preparations should not be used in patients receiving standard monoamine oxidase inhibitors, or patients with narrow angle glaucoma.

In the rare patient in whom it is not possible to prevent nausea by gradual dosage increments and taking food with the drug, it may be appropriate to use antiemetic therapy with a drug which does not enter the brain, e.g. domperidone. Centrally acting dopamine antagonist antiemetics such as metoclopramide and prochlorperazine are not suitable for this purpose.

Approximately one-third of patients starting on L-dopa will obtain an excellent response and maintain therapeutic benefit over a 5-year period. Approximately one-third will not respond to L-dopa or other antiparkinsonian medication, and the remainder will show an intermediate level of improvement but with gradual deterioration over the subsequent period of monitoring.

Problems during long-term treatment with L-dopa. It is often difficult to ascertain whether problems that develop during treatment are related to the drugs that patients are receiving (see Table 29.3), or to the underlying condition itself. Nevertheless a number of well-recognized problems occur during long-term therapy. An agitated–confusional state is well-recognized in patients receiving antiparkinsonian medication and some studies suggest that up to 50% of patients will be affected by this after 2 years of therapy. The management of this condition is often difficult but the dosage of L-dopa may need to be reduced.

Loss of therapeutic efficacy is the other principal problem seen in long-term treatment. Loss of efficacy presents in a number of different ways. Initially recurrence of symptoms may respond

Table 29.3 Common adverse effects of antiparkinsonian drugs

L-dopa + decarboxylase inhibitor
  Nausea
  Postural hypotension
  Dyskinesia
  Nightmares
  Psychosis

Bromocriptine
  Nausea
  Postural hypotension
  Dyskinesia
  Nightmares
  Psychosis

Selegeline
  Increases likelihood of adverse effects caused by
  L-dopa or dopamine agonists

Anticholinergic drugs
  Paralysis of accommodation
  Dry mouth (usually beneficial in parkinsonian
  patients with excess saliva)
  Constipation
  Urinary retention
  Confusional state

to a simple dose increase. Subsequently patients will notice that the benefit of treatment wears off between doses, sometimes known as 'end of dose' akinesia. This symptom usually responds well to a change in dosing schedule, perhaps by giving smaller doses of L-dopa more frequently. More disabling, and much more difficult to manage, are sudden unexpected fluctuations in performance, with patients varying from being akinetic to having excess movements (dyskinesias) within a very short period of time, often for no obvious external reason. These variations in performance, known as 'on-off' phenomena or 'yo-yoing' are much more difficult to treat. In some patients they can be controlled by addition of a dopamine agonist, but in the majority they remain resistant to treatment. Fluctuations in physical performance may also be accompanied by fluctuations in mood or behaviour. The abnormal dyskinetic movements seen in these patients may also be accompanied by muscle pain.

L-dopa is absorbed quite rapidly from the upper part of the small intestine, and blood concentrations of L-dopa rise and fall during a dosage interval. This rise and fall in blood concentration may in part relate to the timing of both 'peak dose' dyskinesias and the 'on-off' phenomena. The recently introduced slow-release preparation of L-dopa in combination with benzerazide (Madopar CR) or carbidopa (slow-release Sinemet) is sometimes helpful in the management of patients with peak dose dyskinesia.

Dopamine agonists

Since the primary condition in Parkinson's disease is a loss of dopaminergic neurones, therapy with L-dopa, which depends on conversion to dopamine by these neurones, is a less than ideal solution. For this reason dopamine agonist drugs, which act directly on dopamine receptors, would appear to be a preferable alternative. At present three such drugs are available for oral use, bromocriptine, lysuride, and pergolide. All these three agents are nonselective in pharmacological terms and therefore cause peripheral effects as well as central ones, including postural hypotension. They also can potentially induce psychosis, confusion or vivid dreams. All three probably produce a longer therapeutic action than L-dopa itself, but are generally best reserved for second line management of patients who have developed problems on L-dopa. On present evidence there is little to separate these three dopamine agonists, which are all active orally. Since bromocriptine has been most studied at present' this is the one against which other drugs should be compared.

Dosing with bromocriptine should usually be started at a low dose (e.g. 1 mg two or three times daily) and increased according to the patient's response. Nausea may be a problem early on in treatment, and this can usually be controlled by giving the drug with food to delay the rate of absorption or by prior administration of the antiemetic domperidone. Postural hypotension can be very severe in elderly patients, and this group is also more susceptible to the psychiatric complications of dopamine agonist therapy.

Apomorphine, an alternative dopamine agonist, which is not effective orally, has been used subcutaneously, either by single doses, or by infusion. Its use as an intermittent injection is sometimes useful in patients with 'on-off' phenomena for treatment of 'off' periods. Alternatively, a continuous subcutaneous infusion can be helpful in patients with very frequent fluctuations. Apomorphine is highly emetic, so initial therapy needs to be covered by the antiemetic agent domperidone, which should be started 24 hours prior to apomorphine.

Selegeline

Monoamine oxidase type B is responsible for the breakdown of dopamine within the dopaminergic nerve ending. Selegeline is a selective inhibitor of this enzyme and is of interest for two reasons.

Firstly, because of its effect on monoamine oxidase it increases the amount of dopamine available for release in the nerve endings. Selegeline therefore increases the efficacy of coadministered L-dopa, and may result in an apparent prolongation of the action of L-dopa. Secondly, selegeline prevents the toxic effects of MPTP in experimental animals. This has been used to support the hypothesis that monoamine oxidase type B may be involved in the pathogenesis of Parkinson's disease, by metabolizing environmental toxins to reactive products that cause nerve damage. Recent large trials in the United States of America have suggested that selegeline may diminish the progression of Parkinson's disease when given to patients at presentation. These results are interesting but further confirmation is required. At present therefore selegeline should be used primarily for its potential to reduce the dose of concurrently administered L-dopa (by about 20%) and improve performance swings in patients with 'on-off' phenomena.

Anticholinergic drugs

Anticholinergic drugs were the first treatments used in the management of Parkinson's disease. The history behind their introduction is interesting, since it was noted that patients with Parkinson's disease had excess salivation, and it was known that anticholinergics might therefore be an appropriate treatment for Parkinson's disease. They remained the only drug treatment available for approximately 90 years.

A wide range of anticholinergic drugs are

marketed for the management of Parkinson's disease, but in practice there is little to choose between them. Biperiden, benzhexol and orphenadrine are three examples, usually adminstered two or three times daily. They are sometimes used in addition to preparations containing L-dopa.

Anticholinergic drugs have a moderate effect in reducing tremor but do not have much therapeutic benefit in akinesia. They have a common range of adverse effects, including those due to antagonism of cholinergic receptors outside the brain, e.g. tachycardia, constipation, and micturition problems, and those due to effects within the brain, principally confusion in the elderly.

Occasional patients develop dystonia whilst receiving anticholinergic drugs. This presents as isolated involuntary contractions of the hand, foot or neck and is best managed by withdrawal of the drug.

Tricyclic antidepressants, e.g. amitriptyline, have anticholinergic properties which are normally regarded as a disadvantage in the therapy of depression. However, they are generally longer acting than other anticholinergic drugs and may have a potential benefit in Parkinson's disease, both for their anticholinergic effects and their effects in inhibiting monoamine reuptake at adrenergic nerve endings. A low single dose of a tricyclic antidepressant (e.g. amitriptyline 10 to 25 mg) at night is sometimes useful in alleviating nocturnal akinesia, improving sleep, and improving performance early in the morning.

Amantadine

Amantadine is an antiviral agent which was found to have antiparkinsonian action in clinical trials of its antiviral activity. Its mechanism of action is probably due to a combination of two effects, firstly an increase in the amount of dopamine released during transmission, and secondly inhibition of reuptake of released dopamine into the presynaptic neurone, with consequent increase in duration of effect of released transmitter.

Amantadine has a relatively weak antiparkinsonian activity and has a number of adverse effects, particularly on the brain, occasionally causing confusion or agitation. Its major dis-

advantage is that therapeutic benefit wears off, usually after about 3 months of treatment. It may have a role in patients who are unable to tolerate other forms of therapy, and who have mild parkinsonian symptoms. It is now superseded by other drugs.

A plan for drug treatment is outlined in Figure 29.1.

THE PATIENT

It is apparent that the approach to individual patients will depend upon the duration of their illness, the severity of the disease they have, and the presence of other complicating factors, particularly including autonomic problems and mental changes.

At the start of treatment it is important to explain to the patient the aims of therapy, i.e. that this is symptomatic and not curative. Accurate compliance with the timing of therapy may be particularly important in patients who are beginning to develop the complications of long-term treatment. It is often helpful therefore for patients to keep diary cards when they begin to experience problems with either akinesia or dyskinesia, so that these symptoms can be related to drug and food intake. Careful changes in timing of drug therapy, or meals, may initially be sufficient to reduce variation in performance. Patients will often have periods of the day when activities are more difficult. This is usually first thing in the morning. It may, therefore, be sensible to advise an initial dose of a rapid-acting agent, such as oral L-dopa, to take on first wakening in the morning so that the patient can then get up and dress. Combinations of L-dopa with dopamine agonists, which are more slowly acting, may be useful in patients with 'on-off' problems. Slow-release preparations of L-dopa may be helpful for patients who develop peak dose dyskinesia.

Other factors that need to be considered in patients with Parkinson's disease are the benefits of adequate sleep and rest at night, which may be made more difficult if they have urinary frequency or problems with nocturnal movements, e.g. turning in bed. Judicious use of hypnotic therapy may be appropriate, and a tricyclic anti-

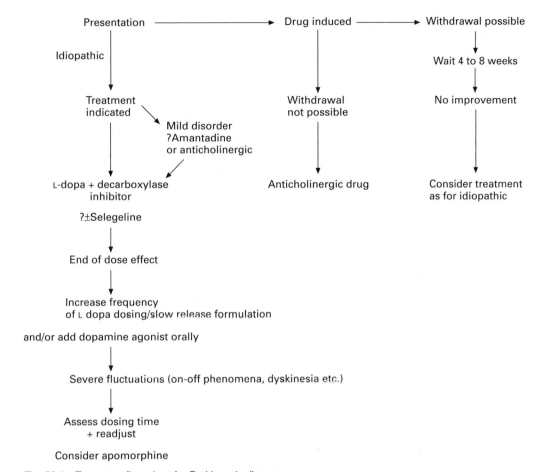

Fig. 29.1 Treatment flow chart for Parkinson's disease.

depressant may offer the dual benefit of sedation with anticholinergic effect. Encouragement of mobility through physiotherapy is also useful.

The treatment of the patient with severe disease, particularly when mental changes become predominant, is the greatest challenge in the management of Parkinson's disease. The use of antipsychotic medication is inappropriate because of the parkinsonian adverse effects that will result. Behavioural disturbances will therefore require discussion with carers and if possible the patient himself/herself. In rare cases it may be necessary to reduce the dose, or even completely withdraw antiparkinsonian therapy in order to control aggressive, sexually demanding or other compulsive behaviour.

Patients' relatives will also need emotional and social support through what can be a very

demanding period. Loss of physical mobility together with a personality change may be very difficult for relatives to cope with. Appropriate use of occupational therapists and social workers in this situation is important.

Most patients can be reassured that they will respond to antiparkinsonian medication and this will give them the ability to lead a relatively normal life for the immediate future. There is a small, but significant, minority, between 25 and 30% of patients, who do not respond to treatment adequately and will require considerable nursing support. They will also require help in adjusting psychologically to a chronic disabling condition.

Other coexisting medical complications that may need attention include disorders of gut motility, which present as constipation or difficulty with swallowing, disturbances of micturition, sometimes presenting as nocturia, and disturbance of autonomic nervous function, presenting as postural hypotension.

Constipation can be managed in the usual way with bulking agents, and if necessary stimulant laxatives and stool-softening agents.

Management of postural hypotension includes assessment of the patient's autonomic function, in order to establish whether this is primarily drug related or associated with autonomic neuropathy. If the patient is dizzy on standing, simple measures such as advice on rising slowly may be adequate. The use of elastic stockings, to reduce pooling of the blood in the lower limbs is sometimes helpful.

Pharmacological approaches primarily involve the use of agents that cause fluid retention, causing a rise in lying blood pressure that results in a less severe postural fall on standing. Fludrocortisone (100 micrograms daily) or the use of a non-steroidal anti-inflammatory drug will often achieve this effect, but care should be taken to avoid precipitation of heart failure. It is also important to consider what other therapies the patient is receiving that might contribute to such symptoms, and to stop these if possible.

Although there is no specific role for drug serum concentration monitoring, compliance monitoring may be appropriate. The use of compliance aids, such as prepackaged therapies may occasionally be of use, particularly in patients with memory impairment.

CASE STUDIES

CASE 29.1

Mr X. is now 75 years old. 4 years ago he developed a tremor of his left hand which responded to co-careldopa 10/100 four times daily. He now notices that his tremor returns before each tablet is due and that he has difficulty getting up to go to the toilet in the middle of the night.

Q What is happening and why? What therapeutic options are there?

CASE 29.2

Mrs Y. attends the outpatient clinic with her husband who says that he is concerned about his wife. 3 months earlier she was started on co-beneldopa 25/100 for newly diagnosed Parkinson's disease. 2 weeks ago bromocriptine 5 mg tablets (one three times daily) were added by a hospital doctor to improve her mobility. Since then she has been increasingly confused and sleeping poorly. When the doctor talks to her she thinks that he is from the police, and he notices she cannot keep her arms by her side, but that they are writhing uncontrollably.

Q What problems can be elicited? What steps should be taken to improve matters?

CASE 29.3

Mrs Z. presents to the outpatient clinic with a history of falls and increasing slowness. Her past history includes hypertension and a severe attack of gastroenteritis 3 months previously.

Q The clinical impression is that she has Parkinson's disease. Is a drug history useful?

ANSWERS TO CASE STUDIES

CASE 29.1

A This patient is demonstrating end of dose problems during the day, and is also probably experiencing the same phenomena during the night. Therapeutic options include:
- increasing the frequency of administration of co-careldopa to 5 times daily
- recognizing the potential problem for increased risk of adverse effects
- addition of a dopamine agonist (e.g. bromocriptine) to produce a background of an agonist effect during the day
- use of selegeline, which will also act to increase the therapeutic efficacy of levodopa both during the day and at night.

CASE 29.2

A This patient is suffering from an overdose of dopamine agonist. This is likely to be due to the addition of the bromocriptine 2 weeks previously. This dose of bromocriptine is a relatively large one, and it would have been sensible to increase the dose more slowly. The particular features which this lady exhibits are psychological (confusion, poor sleeping and paranoid psychosis), and a movement disorder (the writhing arms).

The steps that should be taken are firstly to stop the bromocriptine, and then to reassess. An increase in the dose of co-beneldopa, a more gentle introduction of bromocriptine, or use of alternative therapies including selegeline might be more appropriate.

CASE 29.3

A This history is very typical of drug-induced parkinsonism. The history of hypertension should raise the question of treatment with methyldopa, which rarely can cause parkinsonian symptoms, but it is much more likely that a drug has been introduced to treat the gastroenteritis and perhaps has been continued without further thought. Typical examples of antiemetic drugs that will produce this syndrome are prochlorperazine and metoclopramide. In this situation these drugs should be withdrawn, and the patient observed for a period of a few weeks before other therapies are introduced.

BIBLIOGRAPHY

Hughes A J, Lees A J, Stern G M. Apomorphine test to predict dopaminergic responsiveness in parkinsonian syndromes. Lancet 1990; 336: 32–34

Jankovic J, Calne D B. Parkinson's disease: etiology and treatment. Current Neurology 1987; 7: 193–234

Koller W C, Langston W J (eds). Preclinical detection of Parkinson's disease. Neurology 1991; 41(5) (Suppl. 2)

Langston J W, Ballard P. Parkinsonism induced by 1-methyl-4-phenyl-1,2,3,6 tetrahydropyridine (MPTP): implications for treatment and the pathogenesis of Parkinson's disease. Canadian Journal of Neurological Science 1984; 11: (Suppl. 1) 160–165

Nutt J G, Woodward W R, Hammerstad J P, Carter J H, Andersen J L. The 'on-off' phenomenom in Parkinson's disease. Relationship to levodopa absorption and transport. New England Journal of Medicine 1984; 310: 483–488

Stibe C M H, Lees A J, Kempster P A, Stern G M. Subcutaneous apomorphine in parkinsonian on-off oscillations. Lancet 1988; 1: 403–406

The Parkinson Study Group. Effect of Deprenyl on the progression of disability in early Parkinson's disease. New England Journal of Medicine 1989; 321: 1364–1371

Neurological and psychological disorders

Chapter 30

Migraine

P. Hudgson

The word migraine is derived from *hemicrania*, the term used by the Greek physician Aretaeus of Cappadocia in his writings on the subject in 123 AD, via a number of corruptions including *hemigrania* and megrim, the Anglo-Saxon term for the condition. Aretaeus' description of the clinical features of migraine has never been bettered. In view of the long history of our knowledge of the condition, it is perhaps surprising that the index of suspicion for diagnosing migraine remains low in the medical community and that only a small minority of the afflicted public appreciate the significance of their own symptoms. Many women for instance admit to regular and sometimes intense premenstrual headaches, often with a family history on their mothers' side and deny any knowledge of migraine, clearly regarding their symptoms as part of the 'curse' of everyday life.

CLASSIFICATION OF PAROXYSMAL HEADACHE

No classification of 'vascular' headaches will ever be completely satisfactory (see Table 30.1) and this chapter does not attempt to be all-embracing. In fact, the vast majority of problems seen in practice are encompassed by the first two or three types of migraine and most of the others may be no more than rare variants of the common theme.

Table 30.1 Classification of headaches	
Adult migraine	'Common' (headache without a specific prodrome) 'Classical' (headache preceded or accompanied by prodromal neuro-ophthalmological features)
Childhood migraine	
'Cluster' headaches	(Periodic migrainous neuralgia, Horton's neuralgia, vidian neuralgia)
Chronic paroxysmal hemicrania	
Hemicrania continua	
Hemicrania episodica	
Raeder's syndrome	
Tension headaches	

AETIOLOGY AND PATHOPHYSIOLOGY

The symptoms of migraine were regarded traditionally as being due to sequential vasoconstriction and vasodilatation in the cranial vascular tree, the internal and external carotid circuits and occasionally the vertebrobasilar circuit all being involved. In particular the neuro-ophthalmological prodromes associated with 'classical' migraine have been attributed to vasoconstriction in the intracranial vessels and the headache to vasodilatation of scalp and dural vessels, traditional treatment being directed at reversing the latter phenomenon. This concept has been challenged and the 'spreading depression' theory proposed which explains the neurological prodromes on the basis of waves of electrical silence sweeping through cortical neurones. It has been claimed that reductions in regional cerebral blood flow are secondary to 'spreading depression' which reduce the metabolic requirements of the affected neurones. Nevertheless the vast majority of cerebral blood flow studies show significant reductions in relevant areas of the brain in association with migrainous prodromes. Furthermore, it would be difficult if not impossible to account for the occasional episodes of retinal, cerebral or hindbrain infarction which follow prolonged auras on the basis of 'spreading depression'.

Turning to factors which precipitate attacks in susceptible individuals, there seems to be little doubt that vasoactive amines in some foods act as effective 'triggers' in up to 25% of all cases. The dietary substances quoted most often are cheese, chocolate, bananas, red wine and coffee and some subcontinental dishes. The vasoactive amines incriminated are tyramine and phenylethylamine although there is no certainty about this and the physiological mechanisms involved are unknown. Only cheeses and bananas contain high concentrations of tyramine, chocolate contains low concentrations of tyramine and phenylethylamine and the concentrations of tyramine are roughly the same in red and white wines. Further attempts to provoke attacks in susceptible cases by tyramine challenge, have been unsuccessful in most instances and dietary exclusion of vasoactive amines does not appear to have a preventive effect. However, a recent double-blind study of susceptible individuals showed that red wine precipitated an attack in 9/11 patients whereas a vodka–lemonade mixture with the same alcohol concentration failed to provoke an attack in 8/8 patients suggesting that alcohol alone was unlikely to be the trigger (neither substance induced headache in 8 healthy controls or 5 migraine sufferers who were not intolerant of red wine). It was suggested that the factor responsible in the susceptible patients was the high concentration of phenolic flavonoids in red wine, substances which inhibit the enzyme phenylphosphotransferase. Patients with food-induced migraine are known to have low levels of platelet phenylphosphotransferase, leading to the accumulation of phenolic or monoamine substrates which may in turn precipitate attacks. Red wine intolerance can be transmitted from a susceptible donor to a tolerant recipient via bone marrow transplantation. The mechanism is believed to be transmission of platelets with low phenylphosphotransferase activity. It should be made clear that serotonin (5-hydroxytryptamine, 5HT), does not trigger migraine attacks although high circulating levels of this transmitter have been recorded in patients with common migraine subject to frequent, severe attacks, and some 5HT antagonists are effective migraine prophylactics (see below).

As far as food allergies are concerned, no objective evidence has been obtained to incriminate them in migraine of children or adults. The role of trigger factors in cluster headaches is even less certain, although consumption of only small volumes of alcohol will provoke attacks in some cases.

CLINICAL MANIFESTATIONS

Migraine

Migraine remains underdiagnosed in the community. Any lateralized headache in adolescents or adults (women in the reproductive age range) should be regarded as 'migrainous' or at least 'vascular' in the first instance. The headaches may change sides from time to time (alternating hemicrania) although one side is affected more frequently than the other in the majority of cases. In either classical or common migraine, the headache is usually throbbing in quality, the more observant sufferer noting that the 'throbs' are in strict time with his or her pulse. The headache is almost invariably associated with nausea which may be intense and the paroxysm often ends when the patient vomits. The duration of the paroxysm varies considerably from patient to patient but is seldom less than a few hours and not infrequently lasts as long as a day. In such cases, the patient often takes to his or her bed in a darkened room, relief coming with sleep and the prospect of a better day tomorrow. The response to drug treatment varies considerably from individual to individual and depends to a certain extent on the timing of administration.

Approximately two-thirds of all female patients will report significant deterioration in their headaches immediately before or during their periods and some women only have their attacks during the premenstrual week (catamenial migraine). Most women in the reproductive age range experience deterioration in their headaches when using oral contraceptives (usually the high oestrogen dose combination pill). Conversely most regular sufferers will have 9 months of complete relief during pregnancy although a small minority will have exacerbations whilst others only have attacks during pregnancy. Interestingly some menopausal women who have been plagued with regular attacks during reproductive life and who remit during the climacteric will relapse when they commence regular hormone replacement therapy. This emphasizes the close relationship between migraine and reproductive physiology in women although the mechanisms underlying this relationship have not been identified with precision.

For the clinical neurologist the major interest in migraine rests in the analysis of the neuro-ophthalmological prodromes characteristic of the classical form of the condition. The possibilities in the individual are legion but the commonest prodromes experienced include blurring of vision in one or both eyes, fortification spectra (scintillating coloured or angular figures in the visual fields) and scintillating scotomata (blindspots surrounded by scintilla). The patient will often describe 'flickering lights' in both temporal fields or an appearance like rain running down a window in a similar distribution, the patient often accompanying this description by wiggling his fingers in the air. These symptoms are due respectively to ischaemia in the eye itself and in the occipital lobes. The pure neurological prodromes are usually sensory in nature, numbness and/or paraesthesiae in the circumoral area, often involving the lips and tongue and are a sign of ischaemia in the hind brain. Some patients also experience positive and negative sensory symptoms in their extremeties and, in the upper extremeties particularly, these may march centripetally, the numbness and paraesthesiae which usually start in the fingers defervescing distally as they spread proximally along the upper limbs. Sensory symptoms of this kind (due to ischaemia in the sensory cortex) are not usually accompanied by motor phenomena of any kind although a minority of classical cases may develop transient hemiplegias or ophthalmoplegias, either before or with the onset of headache. In either case, prolongation of the motor phenomena inevitably raises the spectre of an underlying structural cause and predicates further investigation (see below), unless a clear family history is forthcoming. With reference to this, most patients with migraine have a family history (on average 80%, although many will not have recognized this) and a clear family history of hemiplegic migraine will preclude the need for computerized tomographic (CT) brain scanning. Interestingly transmission is usually via the maternal line although the reasons for this are not clear.

Migraine in childhood should not be regarded as a separate entity although it does have some characteristics which set it apart from the adult condition. Cyclical vomiting (i.e. at regular intervals) is probably the commonest manifestation of the tendency in children from the age of 8 to 10 years onwards. However, some children experience severe, throbbing headaches which are undoubtedly vascular in nature and which are accompanied by nausea and vomiting and, in girls, these may have a strict monthly periodicity, anticipating the onset of menstruation. In addition, children not infrequently experience the most interesting prodromal symptoms in a richly varied spectrum. Olfactory hallucinations are well recognized and may occur in adult life as well. Perhaps the most interesting prodromes experienced by children are those involving distortions of body image.

At the end of this section, it would be appropriate to consider the question of loss of consciousness in migraine. There are a priori grounds for assuming that this might occur as part of a migrainous prodrome, namely vasospasm in the perforating vessels originating from the posterior cerebral arteries which perfuse the alerting mechanism in the diencephalon at the back of the third ventricle. However, loss of consciousness occurs only rarely in association with genuine migraine and should alert the observer to the possibility of underlying structural pathology.

Cluster headaches and other forms of acute or chronic paroxysmal hemicrania

In spite of the rapidly expanding literature on the clinical features and treatment of what might be termed the para-migrainous syndromes, little or nothing is known about their pathophysiology. It is accepted that typical periodic migrainous neuralgia is a vascular headache in general terms although this begs the question of the precise mechanisms involved. These remain obscure.

INVESTIGATIONS

The practitioner often has to tell patients with migraine or related conditions (and/or their anxious relatives) that they do not require even screening investigation, provided of course that they respond satisfactorily to the appropriate treatment. This information is often greeted with scepticism, if not hostility. A number of studies have shown that detailed investigation including cerebral angiography of even complicated migraine is not particularly fruitful in most cases. The following criteria identify patients who may be suitable for investigation:

1. Patients with strictly unilateral migraine are more likely to harbour structural (notably vascular) intracranial pathology.

2. Patients with either ophthalmoplegic or hemiplegic migraine should be screened, unless there is a clear-cut family history in the latter.

3. Patients with migraine and epilepsy should be investigated to exclude a cerebral arteriovenous malformation, particularly if there is any clinical hint of a focal lesion.

4. The absence of a family history may be a relative indication for investigation if there are any other suspicious circumstances, especially in late-onset migraine.

5. The presence of fixed neurological deficit between attacks should always be investigated. It will usually turn out to be due to either cerebral or hind-brain infarction consequent upon prolonged vasospasm in either the anterior or posterior circulations although this is clearly a diagnosis of exclusion.

The investigations most likely to be productive in complicated migraine include computerized tomographic scanning of the brain with intravenous contrast and the electroencephalogram, the latter in cases where consciousness has been impaired or the patient has an unusual prodrome, e.g. an olfactory hallucination. In those cases where a definite abnormality is demonstrated, it will be necessary to proceed to cerebral angiography or possibly magnetic resonance angiography.

The investigation of the other syndromes described above is often not worthwhile unless the individual has abnormal physical signs.

TREATMENT

The options for the treatment of migraine attacks seem to be expanding. Unfortunately, the prospects for prophylaxis are not so attractive,

although the agents available are likely to induce some improvement in up to two-thirds of all cases with recurrent attacks. The drugs currently in use for the treatment and prevention of migraine fall into the self-selecting categories described below (see also Table 30.2).

Analgesics

The majority of patients with occasional attacks will self-treat with standard oral analgesics such as codeine, aspirin or paracetamol. In most instances, the individual finds this approach satisfactory unless and until the pattern of the attacks changes for the worse. However, the need

Table 30.2   Major agents used in the treatment and prophylaxis of migraine

Drug	Route of administration	Side effects	Drug interactions	Contra-indications
Ergotamine alkaloids	Sublingual, metered inhalation and subcutaneous injection	Inappropriate vasoconstriction, particularly coronary circulation, abortifacient, vomiting after administration	Erythromycin (ergotism) Beta-adrenoreceptor blockers (enhanced peripheral vasoconstriction) Sumatriptan (CNS toxicity)	Middle-aged patients with asymptomatic ischaemic heart disease, pregnancy
Sumatriptan	Oral, subcutaneous injection	No serious side effects identified	MAOIs and 5HT uptake inhibitors Ergotamine Lithium (enhanced CNS toxicity)	Pregnancy, ischaemic heart disease, hypertension
Antiemetics	Oral	Drowsiness,	Adrenergic neurone blockers, e.g. guanethidine (hypotensive effect antagonized)	Pregnancy in some instances (see text)
Methysergide	Oral	Disequilibrium, chronic fibrosing syndromes, coronary arterial constriction, nausea	Tricyclic antidepressants (hallucinatory experiences)	Ischaemia, heart disease
Pizotifen	Oral	Weight gain (due to direct stimulation of appetite), daytime somnolence	Adreneric neurone blockers, e.g. guanethidine (hypotensive effect antagonized)	No definite contra-indications
Beta-adrenoreceptor blocking drug	Oral	Bronchoconstriction, peripheral vasoconstriction, fatigue	Major interactions include: some calcium channel blockers (increased risk of bradycardia), ergotamine (enhanced peripheral vasoconstriction), sympathomimetics (severe hypertension)	Asthma, cardiac failure, peripheral vascular disease

for these drugs in combination with a variety of antiemetics, and nonspecific stimulants is questionable and may have been obviated by the introduction of the new agent sumatriptan. In addition to orthodox analgesia, there is no doubt that some patients with migraine and with cluster headaches derive significant benefit from other non-steroidal anti-inflammatory agents (NSAIDs), particularly the propionic acid derivatives. This suggests that prostaglandin synthesis and release plays some part in the pathophysiology of both migraine and cluster headaches although the relationship to causation remains unclear.

The use of powerful opiates for the treatment of severe attacks or so-called status migranosus should be deplored. There can be few if any circumstances in which this approach can be justified, the best and simplest first-aid treatment being complete rest in a quiet, darkened room with adequate orthodox analgesics and the use of antiemetic and hypnotic drugs if needed. This can be achieved as easily at home as in hospital although admission may become necessary if the domestic situation is unsatisfactory.

Ergotamine alkaloids

The therapeutic efficacy of ergotamine tartrate has remained untarnished over half a century. However, its regular use is constrained by its vasoconstrictive side effects outside the nervous system. In fact the use of ergotamine tartrate (or dihydroergotamine mesylate, the preferred analogue currently) is confined to otherwise healthy adolescents and young adults, whether administered sublingually, orally or by injection. Certainly these drugs are absolutely contra-indicated in any patient with obliterative vascular disease of any kind, including Prinzmetal angina and Raynaud's phenomenon. They are also absolutely contra-indicated in pregnancy. A further disadvantage of the ergot alkaloids is that they have to be administered during the prodromal phase of the individual attack of migraine to be effective although it is worth trying at any stage of a cluster headache. There is little place for the ergot alkaloids in the preventive treatment of either migraine or cluster headaches.

Antiemetics

Most of the preparations containing ergotamine tartrate include an antiemetic of some kind and antiemetics can be used in isolation to control profuse vomiting. Further details of antiemetic drugs are to be found in Chapter 32.

Sumatriptan

The possibility that 5-hydroxytryptamine (5HT, serotonin) plays a significant part in the pathophysiology of particularly severe attacks of migraine was suggested in the early 1960s and led to the introduction of 5HT antagonists for the prophylactic treatment of the condition. Enthusiasm for these drugs and the underpinning hypothesis has waxed and waned during the ensuing 30 years but interest in the role of 5HT has been renewed by the introduction of a new designer agent, sumatriptan (3-[2-(dimethylamino) ethyl]-N-methylindole-5-methanesulphonamide), a specific and selective agonist of 5HT receptors, notably the $5HT_1$ receptor. Sumatriptan has been introduced for the treatment of both migraine attacks and cluster headaches in doses of 6 mg subcutaneously (maximum 12 mg in any 24-hour period) and has been shown to be effective in large population studies of both conditions. A more recent study indicates that oral administration is likely to be effective as well. It has been suggested that sumatriptan acts by reducing vasodilatation in the intracranial vessel perfusing the brain region geographically related to the site of the headache.

It is too early for an authoritative assessment about side effects to this agent. The contra-indications and precautions are essentially the same as those for the ergot alkaloids. Sumatriptan has not been recommended for prophylactic treatment at this stage.

Migraine prophylaxis

In the light of the personal, domestic and occupational morbidity engendered by migraine and related syndromes it is disappointing that an effective prophylactic agent is not available.

Nevertheless, the advent of the $5HT_2$ antagonists has improved the situation significantly insofar as 60 to 70% of patients treated can expect a reduction in both the frequency and severity of their attacks. The first agent introduced, methysergide, a lysergic acid amide derivative, can induce hallucinations under certain circumstances, particularly with concurrent administration of tricyclic antidepressants. In addition, it shares the vasoconstrictor properties of the ergot alkaloids and it has been associated with several episodes of the onset of myocardial ischaemia and its use should be avoided in patients in middle life and beyond. In view of this, it should be confined to short treatment periods in otherwise healthy adolescents and young adults and then perhaps only as a last resort strategy. Its long-term use has been associated with the occasional development of retroperitoneal fibrosis and obstructive uropathy.

The alternative $5HT_2$ antagonist, pizotifen is reputedly safer than methysergide (chemically unrelated) and has much the same clinical efficacy. Certainly it is prescribed much more often than methysergide and currently enjoys the status of first choice prophylactic agent in both family practice and the hospital service. However, it induces unacceptable daytime somnolence in a proportion of users and a significant number also gain weight at an alarming rate, presumably due to direct stimulation of the hypothalamic appetite centres. This appears to be problematic in female rather than male patients although it can occur in either sex and body habitus is an obvious limiting factor in its prescription.

Beta-adrenoreceptor blocking drugs are useful for migraine prophylaxis. Their reliability in percentage terms is probably less than either pizotifen or methysergide although they remain excellent second line agents for migraine prophylaxis and, in the particular instance of involutional migraine in women entering middle life, they are probably the first choice in combination with a tricyclic antidepressant. It is accepted generally that propranolol (non-cardioselective) is the most effective agent in this situation. Beta-blockade cannot be employed in patients with the relevant cardiorespiratory contra-indications, and many older patients complain that it makes them cold and tired.

The only other drug used on an intermittent basis is clonidine, a central alpha-adrenoreceptor agonist. Some patients claim it is effective as a prophylactic agent.

It has already been suggested that NSAIDs may be helpful in the various cluster headache syndromes and they may well have a preventive as well as a therapeutic value. In the particular case of periodic migrainous neuralgia, both methysergide and pizotifen are well worth at least a trial although the expectation of success is measurably lower in each case than in migraine itself. If these regimens do not help, a trial of lithium carbonate (administered and controlled in the same way as for patients with manic depression) and of oral corticosteroids (prednisolone in rapidly reducing doses from 40 to 60 mg daily over a 4- to 6-week period) may be tried. The rationale for these treatment modalities is yet to be determined with precision.

In conclusion, it is worth bearing in mind that the prophylactic use of aspirin in cerebrovascular disease generally may well be useful in middle-aged and elderly migraine sufferers. Certainly it may be of particular value in those patients with prolonged vasospastic prodromes (in doses of 75 to 150 mg daily).

Herbal remedies

There are a number of herbal remedies which have been recommended for migraine and other headaches over the years, of which feverfew is the most important. The mode of action of the active principle(s) contained in the leaves of feverfew is unknown although there are suggestions that it may share properties in common with the NSAIDs. In addition, substances have been isolated which antagonize both 5HT and histamine. Regular users take feverfew in doses of 1 to 2 large leaves or 2 to 4 small leaves daily, usually encasing the washed leaves in a sandwich containing honey or jam to mask the bitter flavour. No untoward side effects have been reported to date.

CASE STUDIES

CASE 30.1

A middle-aged woman with a family history but no previous history of migraine developed severe, generalized headache accompanied by nausea and occasional vomiting immediately after her menstrual periods. The attacks lasted up to 24 hours at a time and were prostrating. The individual attacks responded in part to treatment with ergotamine tartrate and to long-term treatment with pizotifen although this was withdrawn because of weight gain. The patient also found that ingestion of one glass of red wine induced an exactly similar headache after a few hours (having imbibed in moderation throughout adult life). She still tolerates white wine and spirits.

Q What advice and which drug treatment are appropriate?

CASE 30.2

An 18-year-old male was admitted to hospital with a lateral medullary infarct some hours after a rugby game in which he sustained a minor head injury with transient loss of consciousness. It transpired that he had been subject to regular recurring attacks of migraine with features consistent with hind-brain ischaemia since early adolescence.

Q What would be the treatment plan? How could this incident have been avoided?

CASE 30.3

A middle-aged male developed 'clusters' of severe left parieto-occipital headache without associated symptoms which woke him from sleep at 4 a.m. over a period of 2 weeks. He had a family history of migraine and had occasional attacks of classical migraine with a visual prodrome in adolescence and young adult life but had no regular headaches until the age of 38 years. He found that 'clusters' could be precipitated by consumption of small volumes of alcohol and by stress. The individual attacks were relieved by taking ergotamine tartrate but this was stopped because of paraesthesiae in the extremities.

Q What other drug choices are suitable?

CASE 30.4

Several young women presented with extremely severe alternating hemicrania accompanied by nausea and profuse vomiting in early pregnancy. None had a definite previous history of migraine although some described 'headaches' while using oral contraceptives and others had a clear family history, usually on the maternal side. Clearly, investigation and treatment in these cases had to be limited but each case remitted completely after delivery. One of these women realized she was pregnant for the second time when her headaches recurred.

Q What advice and treatment could be prescribed?

ANSWERS TO CASE STUDIES

CASE 30.1

A This patient suffers from involutional migraine with particular susceptibility to red wine. In view of her age and the difficulty experienced with treatment, a beta-adrenoreceptor blocking drug would be an acceptable alternative (provided there were no cardiorespiratory contra-indications) and sumatriptan may prove to be a suitable preventive agent as well.

CASE 30.2

A This young man suffers from so-called 'basilar' migraine and clearly should have been on migraine prophylaxis of some kind. The catastrophic incident would probably have necessitated months of intensive rehabilitation but probably could not have been prevented. Even trivial head injuries may precipitate attacks of migraine in susceptible sufferers, with unpredictable consequences.

CASE 30.3

A This man has periodic migrainous neuralgia – the middle-aged male's migraine. Ergotamine tartrate-related drugs, e.g. methysergide, should be avoided in males particularly in middle life (because of the risk of coronary vasoconstriction). Beta-adrenoreceptor blockers may well be the treatment modality of choice in the first instance. NSAIDs, lithium carbonate and short courses of corticosteroids are all entirely acceptable alternatives although, once again, sumatriptan may prove to be the definitive prophylactic agent. Acute attacks respond well to sumatriptan by injection.

CASE 30.4

A These women suffer from pregnancy migraine, the only effective preventive measure being safe contraception. Given the unacceptability of this advice in most instances, the treatment options are limited because of the risks of either miscarriage or teratogenesis. The only drugs which can be used with safety in these circumstances are 'orthodox' oral analgesics (and dosage should be monitored strictly) and those antiemetics which have not been incriminated in teratogenetic accidents.

BIBLIOGRAPHY

Dalessio D J. Wolffs headache and other pain. Oxford: Oxford University Press 1972

Friberg L, Olesen J, Iversen K H et al. Migraine pain associated with middle cerebral dilation: reversal by sumatriptan. Lancet 1991; 338: 13–17

Raskin N H. Serotonin receptors and headache. New England Journal of Medicine 1991; 325: 353–354

The Subcutaneous Sumatriptan International Study Group. Treatment of migraine attacks with sumatriptan. New England Journal of Medicine 1991; 325: 316–321

The Subcutaneous Sumatriptan International Study Group. Treatment of acute cluster headaches with Sumatriptan. New England Journal of Medicine 1991; 325: 322–326

Vinken P J, Bruyn G W, Klawans H L (eds), Rose F C (co-ed). Handbook of clinical neurology, revised Series 4. Amsterdam and New York: Elsevier 1986

Chapter 31

Pain

J. E. Charlton   C. Edwards

The International Association for the Study of Pain has defined pain as 'an unpleasant sensory and emotional experience associated with actual or potential tissue damage, or described in terms of such damage.'

Acute pain may be viewed as a symptom of a disease process, serving to allow the patient to avoid or minimize injury. Chronic pain, on the other hand, may be described more as a disease than a symptom.

AETIOLOGY AND NEUROPHYSIOLOGY

The majority of tissues and organs are innervated by special sensory receptors (nociceptors) connected to primary afferent nerve fibres of different diameters. Small myelinated, A delta fibres and unmyelinated C fibres are believed to be responsible for the transmission of painful stimuli. These afferent primary fibres terminate in the dorsal horn of the spinal grey matter.

Pain transmission onward is far more complex and understood less well. The most important parts of this process are the wide dynamic range cells which project to the thalamus and beyond in the spinothalamic tract. Modulation or inhibition also occurs at the level of the spinal cord. This process can be activated by stress or certain analgesic drugs like morphine. When the pain modulation system is active, noxious stimuli produce less activity in the pain transmission pathway. The description of this process is the most significant contribution of the gate theory of pain.

Various neurotransmitters found in the dorsal horn of the spinal cord may be involved in pain modulation. These include GABA, noradrenaline and 5HT. Opioid receptors, particularly the mu receptors and to a smaller extent the kappa receptors are thought to be responsible for the analgesic effect of morphine-like drugs.

ASSESSMENT OF PAIN

Evaluation of pain should include a careful description of the pain and an assessment of its consequences. There should be a full history, psychosocial assessment, medication history and assessment of previous pain problems paying attention to factors which influence the pain. Where necessary, diagnostic tests should be organized. These may include X-rays, various imaging techniques and diagnostic and prognostic nerve blocks.

Pain is a subjective phenomenom and quantitative assessment is difficult. The most commonly used instruments are visual analogue and verbal rating scales. Visual analogue scales are 10 cm long lines labelled with two extremes at each end; usually 'no pain at all' and 'worst pain imaginable'. The patient is required to mark on the scale the severity of his pain between these two extremes. Verbal rating scales use adjectival descriptors such as 'none', 'mild', 'moderate' and 'excruciating'. More elaborate questionnaires such as the McGill Pain Questionnaire help to describe other aspects of the pain, and pain diaries record the influence of activity and medication on pain.

MANAGEMENT

Acute pain results from noxious stimulation, such as injury. It can be managed by analgesic drugs and is often self-limiting.

Chronic pain can be defined as pain which has lasted for 6 months or more. Treatment must be comprehensive and may involve pain clinics, hospices and a multidisciplinary approach to manage medical and behavioural aspects. Non-

medical treatment such as physical therapy and various psychological techniques may form part of the management programme. Pain can be modulated by means other than drugs, such as transcutaneous electrical nerve stimulation (TENS) or invasive procedures such as neurosurgery or neurolytic nerve blocks.

The analgesic ladder

The analgesic ladder forms the basis of many approaches to the use of analgesic drugs. There are essentially three steps: non-opioid analgesics, weak opioids and strong opioids.

The analgesic efficacy of non-opioids such as NSAIDs, aspirin and paracetamol is limited by side effects and ceiling effects (i.e. beyond a certain dose, no further pharmacological effect is seen). Beyond the non-opioids, there are a number of drugs in the mild opioid group such as codeine, dihydrocodeine and dextropropoxyphene, all of which are of some value clinically. There may be some virtue in combining a mild opioid with a non-opioid drug. Strong opioids, of which morphine is the standard, have no ceiling effect and therefore increased dosage gives increased analgesia. The relative potencies of the major opioids are summarized in Table 31.1.

Adjuvant medication

In some types of pain such as the pain of cancer or nerve pain, the addition of non-analgesic drugs to analgesic therapy can enhance pain relief. A list of such adjuvant drugs is given in Table 31.2. It should be remembered that some drugs such as tricyclic antidepressants have intrinsic analgesic activity, perhaps related to their ability to affect 5HT and noradrenergic neurotransmission.

Special techniques

Patient controlled analgesia (PCA)

PCA is a system in which the patient titrates the dose of opioid to suit individual analgesic

Table 31.1 Opioids: potency, oral to parenteral ratios and duration of action (adapted with permission from Thompson J W. In: Doyle D (ed) 1990 Opioids in the treatment of cancer pain. Royal Society of Medicine Services International Congress and Symposium Series no. 146).

Drug	Relative potency	Oral: parenteral ratio	Duration of action (h)
Fentanyl	50	—	1
Buprenorphine	25–50	1.3 (sublingual)	8
Phenazocine	5	2.5 (sublingual)	6
Diamorphine	1.5	0.4	4
Methadone	1 (single dose)	0.5	6
	3–4 (repeated doses)		8
Morphine	1	0.3	4
Papaveretum	0.5	0.3	4
Pethidine	0.125	0.3	2
Dextropro- poxyphene	0.16	0.3	8
Dihydrocodeine	0.1	0.3	4
Codeine	0.08	0.6	4
Pentazocine	0.06	0.25	3

Drugs are listed in order of relative potency, using morphine as a reference

requirements. The drug is contained in a system (usually a syringe attached to either an electronic or non-electronic pump) which delivers a preset dose when activated by the patient depressing a button. A lock-out period, during which the machine is programmed not to respond, ensures that a second dose is not delivered before the previous one has had an effect. Some devices allow an additional background infusion of drug to be delivered continuously. A maximum dose facility ensures that the machine does not deliver more than a preset dose over a given time.

PCA is generally considered to be more efficient than intramuscular administration of opioids and the analgesia obtained is reported to be comparable with that of epidural opioids. The system is convenient and enjoys a high degree of patient acceptability.

Neural blockade

Local anaesthetic drugs injected close to a sensory nerve or plexus will block the conduction of pain impulses. Agents in common use are lignocaine, prilocaine and bupivicaine. Some are given with adrenaline to reduce systemic toxicity and increase the duration of action.

Local anaesthetics can be applied directly to wounds or by local infiltration to produce postoperative analgesia, but will not normally block pain arising from deep internal organs. Continuous infusions via a catheter will permit prolonged analgesia.

More permanent nerve blockade for the control of cancer pain is best achieved by using a neurolytic agent such as alcohol or phenol.

Epidural injection

Epidural injections may be effective in relieving pain arising from non-malignant and malignant disease. They are very effective in postoperative and labour pain. Various combinations of local anaesthetics, opioids or steroids can be introduced into the epidural space near to the level of the pain. Used in this fashion, local anaesthetics will block nerves in the spinal canal serving both superficial and deep tissues. Thus analgesia can be obtained in deep internal organs. Sensory nerves will be blocked, but also sympathetic nerves which maintain smooth muscle tone in

Table 31.2 Adjuvant drugs used in the treatment of pain

Drug class	Type of pain	Example
Anticonvulsants	Neuropathic pain: lancinating pain	Carbamazepine Phenytoin Valproate
Antidepressants	Neuropathic pain: burning pain	Amitriptyline Imipramine Desipramine
Muscle relaxants	Muscle spasm	Baclofen Dantrolene Diazepam
Steroids	Nerve compression, tissue swelling, raised intracranial pressure	Dexamethasone Prednisolone

blood vessels. As a result, vasodilatation can occur which may result in significant hypotension. Epidural catheters allow continuous infusions and long-term therapy by this route. Adverse effects may include muscle weakness in the area supplied by the nerve and rarely, infection and haematomas.

Transcutaneous electrical nerve stimulation (TENS)

TENS machines are portable battery powered devices which generate a small current to electrodes applied to the skin. The electrodes are placed at the painful site or close to the course of the peripheral nerve innervating the painful area and the current is increased until paraesthesiae are felt at the site of the pain.

The current stimulates the large, rapidly conducting (A beta) fibres which close the gating mechanism in the dorsal horn cells and this inhibits the small, slowly conducting fibres (A delta and C). TENS may also exert an additional effect by stimulating endogenous opioids.

TENS is used for trauma, postoperative pain, labour pain and various chronic pains. It offers the patient a simple, non-invasive, self-controlled method of pain relief with few adverse effects.

Analgesic drugs

Strong opioids

Morphine is the standard strong opioid analgesic. It is available as oral, rectal and injectable formulations and has a duration of effect of about 4 hours (sustained-release oral preparations have a longer duration). There is no ceiling effect when the dose is increased. A general protocol for morphine is to begin therapy with an intravenous dose of 5 or 10 mg every 4 hours. This can be given by intermittent bolus or PCA. The aim is to titrate dose against the pain. Where intermittent dosing is used, it may be necessary to double the dose every 24 hours until pain relief is achieved. If the patient can take drugs orally it is appropriate to change to an oral dose, particularly sustained-release preparations which offer twice-daily dosing.

Maximum daily doses of up to 1 or 2 grams of morphine can be achieved if necessary, but few patients require more than about 200 mg daily. Morphine is metabolized in the liver and one metabolite, morphine-6-glucuronide, is pharmacologically active and this should be taken into consideration in patients who have renal failure.

Other opioids such as pethidine and dextromoramide offer little advantage over morphine in that they are generally milder in action with a relatively short duration of action (2 hours). Dipipanone is available only in a preparation which contains an antiemetic (cyclizine) and increasing doses lead to sedation and the risk of developing a tardive dyskinesia with long-term use. Methadone has a long elimination half-life of approximately 24 hours and accumulation may occur in the early stages of use but it has a low side effect profile with long-term use. Some patients who experience serious adverse effects with morphine can tolerate methadone well.

Weak opioids

Drugs of this type are prescribed frequently by primary care physicians either alone or in combination with other analgesics for a wide variety of painful disorders. There are three major drugs in this group: codeine, dihydrocodeine and dextropropoxyphene. They are recommended by the World Health Organization for pain that is not responsive to non-opioid analgesics. Despite this recommendation, there are almost no modern data to show that these drugs are of benefit in the relief of chronic pain.

Codeine. Codeine is suggested as the first choice drug in this group. It is structurally similar to morphine and about 10% of the codeine is demethylated to form morphine and the analgesic effect may be due to this, at least in part. It is a powerful cough suppressant as well as being very constipating. In combination with aspirin-like drugs the analgesic effects are usually additive, but the variability in response is considerable. Its duration of analgesic action is about 3 hours.

Dihydrocodeine. Dihydrocodeine is only available in a few countries and is chemically related to codeine. It has similar properties to codeine when used at the same dosage and is slightly more potent. It has a shorter duration of action than codeine and this makes its value in the management of chronic pain extremely limited.

Dextropropoxyphene. Dextropropoxyphene is prescribed either alone or in combination with other analgesics such as aspirin and paracetamol. There are few hard data on its therapeutic value and at least one major review has concluded that the analgesic efficacy of this drug is less than aspirin and barely more than placebo. At best, dextropropoxyphene has failed to show any superiority over codeine. It has the potential for steadily developing toxicity. Patients with hepatic dysfunction and poor renal function are particularly at risk. It is associated with problems in overdosage, notably a non-naloxone-reversible depression of the cardiac conducting system.

Agonist-antagonist and partial agonists

Most of the drugs in this category are either competitive antagonists at the mu receptor, that is to say they can bind to this site but exert no action; or they exert only limited actions, that is to say they are partial agonists. Those that are antagonist at the mu receptor can provoke a withdrawal syndrome in patients receiving concomitant agonist opioids such as morphine.

Pentazocine. Pentazocine is a benzmorphan derivative which is an agonist and at the same time a very weak antagonist at the mu receptor. This drug became popular in the 1960s when it was thought that it would have little or no abuse potential. This is now known to be untrue, although its abuse potential is less than that of the conventional agonists such as morphine. It produces an analgesia which is clearly different from morphine and probably is due to agonist actions at the kappa receptor. There are no detailed studies of its use in chronic pain, but its short duration of action (about 3 hours) and the high incidence of psychomimetic side effects make it a totally unsuitable drug for such use.

Buprenorphine. This drug is a semisynthetic,

highly lipophilic opioid which is a partial agonist. It undergoes extensive metabolism when administered orally and to avoid this effect it is given sublingually. It has high receptor affinity and, through this property, a duration of action of 6 hours.

A long duration of action and high bioavailability would suggest a role for buprenorphine in the management of chronic pain. However, it is difficult to find any controlled studies in the literature and the high number of adverse effects seems the likely reason. The incidence of nausea and vomiting appears to be substantially higher than with morphine. However, respiratory depression and constipation are less. Patients who can tolerate this drug appear to experience long-lasting effective analgesia.

Adverse effects of opioids

The adverse effects of opioids are nearly all dose-related and tolerance develops to the majority with long-term use.

Respiratory depression. Respiratory depression is potentially dangerous in patients with impaired respiratory function but tolerance is said to develop rapidly with chronic dosing. It can be reversed by naloxone.

Sedation. Sedation is usually mild and self-limiting. Smaller doses, given more frequently may counteract the problem. Rarely, amphetamine has been used to counteract this effect.

Nausea and vomiting. Antiemetics should be co-prescribed routinely with opioids for the first 10 days.

Constipation. Opioids reduce intestinal secretions and peristalsis, causing a dry stool and a hypotonic colon. Stool softeners such as docusate sodium combined with a stimulant laxative such as danthron or senna are needed on a long-term basis when opioids are used.

Tolerance. Chronic drug treatment with opioids often causes tolerance to the analgesic effect. When this occurs the dosage should be increased or alternatively another opioid can be substituted, since cross-tolerance is not usually complete. Addiction is very rare when opioids are prescribed for pain relief.

Smooth muscle spasm. Morphine causes spasm of the sphincter of Oddi in the biliary tract and may cause biliary colic, as well as urinary sphincter spasm and retention of urine. Thus in biliary or renal colic, it is preferable to use another opioid without these effects.

Non-opioid analgesics

The pharmacological actions and use of the conventional non-opioids such as paracetamol, aspirin and non-steroidal anti-inflammatory drugs are well known and will not be discussed further here.

Nefopam is a drug which is chemically related to orphenadrine and diphenhydramine. It is neither an opioid, anti-inflammatory drug nor an antihistamine. The mechanism of analgesic action is unknown. As a non-opioid, it is free from problems of habituation and respiratory depression. The drug has a very high number of dose-related effects in clinical use. These may be linked to the sympathomimetic actions of the drug.

Adjuvant analgesics

To be an analgesic, a drug must relieve pain in animal models of pain and must give demonstrable and reliable pain relief in patients. Drugs such as the opioids and the NSAIDs clearly are analgesics. The evidence is less clear for the drugs in the following section and traditional methods would not classify these drugs as analgesics, but all appear to have given some benefit in the control of chronic pain.

Anticonvulsants

The usefulness of this group of drugs has been established for the treatment of neuropathic pain with a paroxysmal component. Conditions which may respond to anticonvulsants include trigeminal neuralgia, glossopharyngeal neuralgia, various neuropathies, lancinating pain arising from conditions such as post-herpetic neuralgia and multiple sclerosis and similar pains that may follow amputation or back sur-

gery. Carbamazepine is the first line drug for the treatment of these types of condition and about 70% of patients will have significant pain relief. Pain relief is usually rapid in onset. About one third of patients may have intolerable adverse effects. These are generally dose-related and include nausea, dizziness, slurred speech, ataxia, skin rashes, somnolence and rarely, bone marrow depression.

Phenytoin is used widely as an alternative to carbamazepine. Like carbamazepine, the oral absorption is slow, variable and sometimes incomplete. Phenytoin exhibits zero order pharmacokinetics in therapeutic dosage so that a small increment in dose can lead to a substantial rise in plasma level and conversely the circulating concentration can fall by an unexpectedly large amount when the dose is cut back. It may take up to 3 or 4 weeks for steady state to be reached in some patients.

Sodium valproate also is used to manage lancinating pain. There are no well-controlled trials to demonstrate its value but it appears to be effective and has a lower side effect profile than the other drugs in this group. Other anticonvulsants such as clonazepam and vigabatrin have been tried but there is, as yet, no evidence that they offer any clinical advantage over other anticonvulsants in the treatment of pain.

Antidepressants

Persistent chronic pain is accompanied frequently by anxiety and depression. Thus it is not surprising that the use of antidepressants and other psychoactive drugs are part of standard pain management. There is evidence that some of these drugs have analgesic properties that are independent of their psychotropic effects.

The tricyclic antidepressants (TCAs) are frequently used for the treatment of chronic pain conditions and there is a substantial body of literature about their analgesic action. Regrettably, there are few data on mechanisms of action, dosage, interdrug variability or long-term efficacy.

The biochemical activity of the TCAs suggests that their main effect will be on serotonergic and noradrenergic neurones. The TCAs inhibit the reuptake of 5HT and/or noradrenaline, thereby increasing the concentration of neurotransmitter at synapses in the pain neural pathways. This is unlikely to be the sole action responsible for their clinical effect and other possible mechanisms are an antidepressive action or modulation of the activity of other biologically active substances such as the endogenous opioids. Since pain is a common presenting complaint of depression it seems reasonable to assume that some relief of pain will be associated with the reversal of depression. TCAs are effective analgesics in headache, facial pain, low back pain, arthritis, denervation pain and, to a lesser degree, cancer.

Various TCAs have been utilized (amitriptyline, doxepin and desipramine) with or without phenothiazines and anticonvulsants. Drug doses have varied considerably, but most are low, of the order of 25 to 75 mg per day.

Drug dosage and serum levels are sometimes of significance. In some subjects the effect of a therapeutic window has been observed. As dosage increases the pain relieving effect diminishes and vice versa.

The elimination half-lives of the TCAs are long and a therapeutic effect may not be obtained for several weeks. If there is no therapeutic effect with 75 mg daily after 6 to 8 weeks, the dosage may be increased by 25 mg aliquots to a total daily dosage of 150 mg for a further 6 weeks.

If a response occurs, therapy can be maintained for 3 to 6 months. Should there be no response to an adequate trial of one TCA, another with different properties may be tried. For example, if amitriptyline yields no therapeutic result, clomipramine (serotonergic) or maprotiline (catecholaminergic) could be tried.

TCAs have a wide range of adverse effects and these may cause a marked reduction in patient compliance. Studies of newer antidepressant drugs have failed to show any advantages in clinical efficacy, although they may be less likely to produce adverse effects.

Neuroleptics

Phenothiazines, with the exception of methotrimeprazine, have no effect in the treatment of pain. A dose of 15 mg of methotrimeprazine has analgesic activity equivalent to 10 mg intramuscular morphine.

Anxiolytics

Benzodiazepines may be used for pain relief in conditions associated with acute muscle spasm and sometimes are prescribed to reduce the anxiety and muscle tension associated with chronic pain conditions. Many authorities believe that they are antalgesic and reduce pain tolerance. Clonazepam may have a role in the management of neurogenic pain and diazepam can be used to control painful spasticity, due to acute or spinal cord injury.

Antihistamines

These agents were introduced into the management of chronic pain because of their sedative muscle relaxant properties. These actions are non-specific and it is not clear whether the clinical effect is mediated centrally or peripherally. Most clinical studies have been carried out with hydroxyzine, which has shown benefit in acute pain, tension headache and cancer pain.

There is evidence that analgesic combinations of antihistamines, NSAIDs and opioids may yield greater analgesia than that provided by each drug alone.

Skeletal muscle relaxants

Drugs described in this section are used for the relief of muscle spasm or spasticity. It is axiomatic that the underlying cause of the spasticity and any aggravating factors such as pressure sores or infections should be treated. This group of drugs will usually help spasticity, but this may be at the cost of decreased muscle tone elsewhere which may lead to a decrease in the mobility of the patient and thus make matters worse.

The drug of first choice is probably baclofen, which has a peripheral site of action, working directly on the skeletal muscle. Baclofen is a derivative of the inhibitory neurotransmitter, GABA. It is alleged that it is most effective for the treatment of spasticity caused by multiple sclerosis or other diseases of the spinal cord, especially traumatic lesions. There are reports of its use in trigeminal neuralgia and a number of painful conditions including post-herpetic neuralgia.

Diazepam is commonly used in the treatment of spasticity particularly that of spinal cord lesions.

Clonidine

The alpha-adrenergic agonist clonidine has been shown to produce analgesia and there is evidence that both morphine and clonidine produce a dose-dependent inhibition of spinal nociceptive transmission. Which is mediated through different receptors. This may explain why clonidine has been shown to work synergistically with morphine when given intrathecally or epidurally. Clonidine also appears to work when given by other routes or even topically.

Treatment of selected pain syndromes

Herpetic and post-herpetic neuralgia

The pain associated with herpes zoster infection is severe, continuous and often described as burning and lancinating. Antiviral therapy such as acyclovir initiated at the first sign of the rash can reduce the duration of the pain, particularly post-herpetic pain which follows the disappearance of the rash. Analgesics such as non-steroidal anti-inflammatory drugs provide benefit. Tricyclic antidepressants such as amitriptyline are the mainstay of treatment, commencing with a dose of 50 mg at night and increasing to 150 mg if required. They may be combined with anticonvulsants if the pain is lancinating. Carbamazepine (600 mg, increasing to 1200 mg daily) is the standard anticonvulsant used, but phenytoin, valproate and clonazepam have also proved useful. Other treatments of proven value are TENS and appropriate somatic or sympathetic nerve blocks.

Trigeminal neuralgia

Trigeminal neuralgia presents as abrupt, intense bursts of severe, lancinating pain, provoked by touching sensitive trigger areas on one side of the face. The disorder may spontaneously remit for periods of several weeks or months. Anticonvulsants, particularly carbamazepine (600 mg daily in divided doses, increasing as necessary) or phenytoin (commencing at 200 mg daily) have been used successfully. If drug therapy is ineffective, surgical techniques such as glycerol injection or gangliolysis can be of great benefit. If surgery becomes necessary, anticonvulsants should be withdrawn gradually.

Peripheral nerve injury and neuropathy

Damage to, or entrapment of, nerves can cause pain, unpleasant sensations and paraesthesiae. Tricyclics and anticonvulsants have been used with some success to reduce neuropathic pain. A neuroma occurs when damaged or severed nerve fibres sprout new small fibres in an attempt to regenerate. Pain develops several weeks after the nerve injury and is often due to the neuroma growing into scar tissue, causing pain as it is stretched or mobilized.

Sympathetically maintained pain

Causalgia and reflex sympathetic dystrophy are names for an important group of painful conditions that may follow trauma or damage to nerves and which are associated with overactivity of the sympathetic nervous system.

Treatment is directed at blocking sympathetic overactivity, reducing pain and instituting aggressive physiotherapy to facilitate a return to normal function. Sympathetic blockade can be achieved by blocking appropriate nerves using local anaesthetics, or by the technique of intravenous regional sympathetic block (IRSB). This is achieved by isolating the blood supply of the affected limb with a tourniquet and then injecting a dose of guanethidine or phentolamine. This may give a sympathetic block for up to 3 days. Several IRSBs may yield sufficient pain relief to permit physiotherapy and recovery to take place. Other drugs that have been used successfully include oral corticosteroids, both alpha-adrenergic agonists and blockers and calcium channel blocking drugs.

Musculoskeletal (myofascial) pain

Myofascial pain is that arising from muscles and is associated with stiffness and neuralgic symptoms such as tingling and paraesthesiae. It may occur spontaneously or following trauma, such as whiplash injury. Myofascial pain syndrome is also known as myositis, fibrositis, myalgia and myofascitis. Acute muscle injury can be treated by first aid with the application of a cooling spray or ice to reduce inflammation and spasm, followed by passive stretching of the muscle to restore its full range of motion. Injection therapy is used to disrupt sensitive muscle trigger points and may involve injecting local anaesthetic or saline or a form of acupuncture. Chronic myofascial syndromes are managed by a programme of physical therapy.

Post-amputation and phantom limb pain

The majority of amputees suffer significant stump or phantom limb pain for at least a few weeks each year. Pain will be present immediately postoperatively in the stump. This may be caused by muscle spasm, nerve injury and sensitivity of the wound and surrounding skin. As the wound heals, the pain should subside. If it does not, the reason may be vascular insufficiency or infection. Pain occurring some number of years after amputation may be caused by changes in the structure of the bones or skin in the stump, or ischaemia. For instance, reduction in the thickness of overlying tissue with age may expose nerve endings to increased stimuli.

Tricyclic antidepressants may be helpful for stump pain. Standard analgesics can be given and surgery may be necessary to restore the vascular supply or reduce trauma to nerve endings.

Phantom pain is a referred pain which produces a burning or throbbing sensation, felt in the absent limb. Cramping sensations are caused by muscular spasm in the stump. The patient with phantom limb pain is often anxious, depressed and frightened, all of which exacerbate the pain. Analgesic drugs alone are generally not adequate for phantom pain but tricyclic antidepressants and anticonvulsants are useful adjuvants. Other therapy which can be effective includes TENS and sympathetic blockade. These patients frequently require management at specialized pain centres.

Postoperative pain

Although the site and nature of surgery influence the severity of pain, individual variations amongst patients do not allow the amount of pain to be predicted according to the type of operation. However, the majority of patients suffer postoperative pain.

Besides the obvious benefit of relieving suffering, pain relief is desirable for a number of physiological reasons after surgery. For example, poor quality analgesia reduces lung function, increases heart rate and blood pressure and magnifies the stress response to surgery. Patient-controlled intermittent intravenous injections of opioids are used often but can lead to respiratory depression especially when background constant rate infusions are used. Morphine is the drug of choice.

Non-steroidal anti-inflammatory drugs can be used as adjuvants to opioids. Agents such as diclofenac and ketorolac have enjoyed increased usage in recent years. Local anaesthetics may be infiltrated into wounds or infused via catheters to allow intermittent or continuous analgesia.

Headache

The treatment of migraine is dealt with separately (Ch. 30).

Tension headaches are caused by muscle contraction over the neck and scalp. They respond well to TENS and antidepressant drugs such as amitriptyline and doxepin given as a single dose at night. Propranolol and minor tranquillizers have also been used. NSAIDs may be indicated if the headache is associated with cervical spondylosis or neck injury.

Dysmenorrhoea

Dysmenorrhoea is a common cause of pelvic pain. It can be helped by the prescription of oral contraceptives, since pain is absent in anovulatory cycles. Non-steroidal anti-inflammatory drugs are effective because of their action on prostaglandin synthetase.

Burn pain

Patients with burns may require a series of painful procedures such as physiotherapy, debridement or skin grafting. Premedication with a strong opioid before the procedure coupled with intravenous opioids and the use of entonox (premixed 50% nitrous oxide and 50% oxygen) may be necessary to control the pain. Regular, time-contingent opioids such as morphine or methadone may be useful to prevent the pain induced by movement or touch in the burn area.

Pain of malignancy

The pain associated with cancer may arise from many different sources and has the characteristics of both acute and chronic pain. It can be treated both with drugs and other techniques such as radiotherapy and nerve blocks. Drug treatment is based on the analgesic ladder together with the use of adjuvant analgesics. When considering non-opioid analgesics, the NSAIDs have a special role, especially in bone metastases. Some clinicians progress from non-opioid to strong opioid drugs such as morphine, omitting the middle step of the analgesic ladder. Strong opioids are the mainstay for the treatment of cancer pain and virtually every form of cancer pain will respond to some degree. Strong opioids

have no ceiling effects, an increased dose giving increased analgesia.

Morphine is the standard opioid, but if it is not tolerated levorphanol or methadone, both with relatively long half-lives, can be considered. Optimal dosage is determined on an individual basis for each patient by titration against the pain. Methotrimeprazine, a phenothiazine with analgesic activity, is a useful alternative when opioids cannot be tolerated. It causes neither constipation nor respiratory depression and has antiemetic and anxiolytic activity.

Corticosteroids are useful in managing certain aspects of acute and chronic cancer pain. They are particularly useful for raised intracranial pressure and for relieving pressure caused by tumours on the spinal cord or peripheral nerves.

Dexamathasone (16 mg per day) is the most commonly used steroid to ameliorate a raised intracranial pressure in patients with brain tumours. High steroid doses given for 1 or 2 weeks do not require a reducing dosage regimen. They also produce a feeling of well-being, increased appetite and weight gain, although the central effects are usually transient.

Three types of malignant pain are briefly outlined below to indicate various therapeutic approaches.

Cancer of the pancreas. Pain is caused by infiltration of the tumour into the pancreas as well as by obstruction of the bowel and biliary tract and metastases in the liver. Patients will also experience anorexia, nausea, vomiting, diarrhoea and are often depressed. Surgery, radiation and chemotherapy may relieve pain for long periods, as does neurolytic blockade of the coeliac plexus. Opioid analgesics are useful and may be administered intravenously or epidurally either by bolus injection or continuous infusion.

Carcinoma of the lung. Lung cancer causes pain when the tumour penetrates surrounding tissues such as the pleura, chest wall and nerve plexuses. The analgesic ladder should be used first and it should be remembered that any NSAID is useful because inflammation is often a component of the chest wall involvement. Adjuvants such as tricyclic antidepressants or steroids may be helpful. As the tumour progresses, nerve blocks may be necessary and invasion of the vertebrae can lead to nerve root or spinal cord compression. In the latter case, high-dose steroids such as dexamethasone may be given intravenously but radiation is also useful in reducing the size of the tumour.

Metastatic bone pain. Metastatic bone pain is usually treated with courses of chemotherapy and radiotherapy, but analgesics can be used. A prostaglandin-like substance has been isolated from bone metastases and therefore NSAIDs are often used in bone pain. Steroids also interfere with prostaglandin formation and dexamethasone therefore has a role especially where there is nerve root or spinal cord compression.

CASE STUDIES

CASE 31.1

A 45-year-old man presents with intractable low back pain of 10 years' standing. His back was injured in an accident at work and he has had two laminectomies and a spinal fusion. His law suit is now settled and the surgeons say that there is nothing more which can be done. The diagnosis is one of arachnoiditis.

Q Will drug treatment be useful?

CASE 31.2

A 55-year-old lady presents with metastatic cancer of the breast. Her problems include uncontrolled pain in several sites, constipation, poor sleep pattern and malaise. Current medication consists of sustained-release morphine 30 mg twice daily, temazepam 20 mg at night and tamoxifen 20 mg daily.

Q How should her pain be managed?

CASE 31.3

A 78-year-old lady presents with severe pain affecting the upper part of her face. 3 months previously she had an attack of shingles affecting this area of the face. Initially, treatment consisted of acyclovir and paracetamol, followed by a short course of oral steroids. The rash of the shingles has now cleared and she is suffering from a burning, prickling pain with occasional episodes of severe lancinating pain.

Q How should this pain be treated?

ANSWERS TO CASE STUDIES

CASE 31.1

A Management should ensure that adequate trials of simple analgesics have been tried. Opioids are probably inappropriate in this case as arachnoiditis rarely responds to opioid therapy. Other management strategy should focus upon restoration and preservation of function. This can be achieved with the use of stimulation produced analgesia, such as TENS or acupuncture, as well as epidural injections of local anaesthetic steroids such as dexamethasone and centrally acting agents such as tricyclic antidepressants. If the pain has a lancinating or episodic component, the use of anticonvulsants can be considered.

These measures should be coupled with the use of a pain management programme involving prolonged occupational therapy and physiotherapy designed to maximize the patient's physical abilities, pain education classes and the use of psychological techniques designed to increase the patient's coping skills. Life with a disability may lead to profound emotional and social problems and these should be assessed and treated if necessary.

CASE 31.2

A Management should begin with establishing a reason for her pain. Not all pain in cancer patients is caused by cancer. She may have arthritis or other painful conditions. These may respond to non-steroidal anti-inflammatory drugs, as may bony secondaries. Her opioid intake is inadequate and she is taking no laxatives and thus she is receiving poor analgesia and her discomfort is being increased by unnecessary constipation. Initially the patient should be allowed to self-medicate with oral morphine solution in a hospital or hospice environment. This will permit her to obtain pain control quickly. Once stable, the total daily dosage of morphine can be corrected to an equivalent dosage of a long-acting formulation, such as sustained-release morphine. Laxatives should be routinely co-prescribed, since opioid-induced constipation is one adverse effect which does not disappear with prolonged use. During changes in opioid dosage, nausea and sickness may require treatment.

The use of a tricyclic antidepressant at night instead of a benzodiazepine should be considered since benzodiazepines are antalgesic and may reduce the ability to tolerate pain. As her disease progresses, consideration should be given to the use of alternative methods of drug delivery such as intravenous or epidural infusions. Attention should be paid to her emotional and spiritual needs at all times.

CASE 31.3

A Management should initially be directed at reducing the level of her pain and this may be achieved by the serial use of somatic or sympathetic nerve blocks using local anaesthetics. A TENS machine may also yield significant benefit. If the lancinating component continues to be troublesome, anticonvulsant drugs such as carbamazepine and sodium valproate may be useful. The burning component may respond to low doses of tricyclic antidepressants such as amitriptyline (50 mg at night) or desipramine (25 mg twice daily).

The majority of patients who have shingles have severe pain initially which gradually decreases over a period of 6 months to 2 years. Aggressive treatment early in the course of the disease can reduce the period of time that patients have this problem and early referral to seek specialized help is recommended. A small percentage of patients continue to have problems whatever treatment is given.

BIBLIOGRAPHY

Andersson S, Bond M, Mehta M, Swerdlow M (eds). Chronic non-cancer pain. Lancaster: MTP Press 1987

Cousins M J, Bridenbaugh P O (eds). Neural blockade in clinical anaesthesia and management of pain, 2nd edn. Philadelphia: Lippincott 1989

Hanks G W, Justins D M. Cancer pain: management. Lancet 1992; 339: 1031–1036

Melzack R, Wall P D. The challenge of pain, 3rd edn. London: Penguin 1991

Pain mechanisms and management. British Medical Bulletin 1991; 47(3)

Portenoy R K. Cancer pain: pathophysiology and syndromes. Lancet 1992; 339: 1027–1031

Regnard C F B, Tempest S. A guide to symptom relief in advanced cancer, 3rd edn. Manchester: Haigh & Hochland 1992

Thompson J W. Clinical pharmacology of opioid agonists and partial agonists. In: Doyle D (ed) Opioids in the treatment of cancer pain 1990. Royal Society of Medicine Services International Congress and Symposium Series no. 146: 17–38. Royal Society of Medicine Services 1990

Wall P D, Melzack R (eds). Textbook of pain, 2nd edn. Edinburgh: Churchill Livingstone 1989

Wall P D, Jones M. Defeating pain. London: Plenum Press 1991

Chapter 32

Nausea and vomiting

D. N. Bateman   M. Campbell

Nausea and vomiting are common symptoms and are frequently seen in all aspects of medical practice. Nausea is a sensation, whereas vomiting is the physical act of regurgitation of stomach contents. The act of vomiting may actually relieve the sensation of nausea and when assessing patients with these symptoms it should be recognized that the sensation of nausea is often more distressing than the act of vomiting itself.

EPIDEMIOLOGY

The incidence of nausea and vomiting is unknown, but over 4 million prescriptions are written by general practitioners in the UK each year for antiemetic drugs. In the community nausea and vomiting in children is frequently associated with viral infections. In older patients these symptoms often follow dietary indiscretion and overindulgence. They may also be the associated features of migraine, a condition that affects a large proportion of the community. Nausea is common in the early stages of pregnancy, when it results from the physiological changes that are taking place.

In hospitals nausea and vomiting will occur following radiotherapy and the administration of cytotoxic drugs, the incidence depending on the dose of radiotherapy or the type of cytotoxic drug. For example, almost all patients treated with cisplatin will experience nausea and vomiting. The frequency of postoperative nausea and vomiting will depend on a number of factors,

467

including the skill of the anaesthetist, the anaesthetic agent, and the type and duration of surgery. Incidence rates of 10 to 30% are reported after gynaecological procedures, for example.

AETIOLOGY

Outside hospital the commonest causes of vomiting include acute infections (particularly in children), gastroenteritis, labyrinthitis, motion sickness, migraine, pregnancy, diseases of the gastrointestinal tract and nausea and vomiting associated with drug treatment. Within hospital in addition to all these causes patients often suffer vomiting postoperatively, in association with metabolic disorders such as ketoacidosis and uraemia, or in association with raised intracranial pressure, and following radiotherapy or cytotoxic chemotherapy.

PATHOPHYSIOLOGY

The neurological control of nausea and vomiting is complex and precise pathophysiological causes therefore depend on the condition causing the symptom. Within the brain, the vomiting centre, which is situated in the dorsolateral reticular formation close to the respiratory centre, acts as the coordinating centre with information passed to it from a number of other sites. Another important area involved in nausea and vomiting is the chemoreceptor trigger zone (CTZ) which is located on the floor of the fourth ventricle in the area postrema, and is in contact with the blood and the cerebrospinal fluid. It is at this site that many extraneous emetic agents, including drugs and toxins, are thought to act. (See Fig. 32.1.)

Impulses are also passed to the vomiting centre from the higher cortical centres, and these are responsible for the nausea associated with fear, and anticipatory vomiting such as is found in patients undergoing cancer chemotherapy. Other inputs derive from the vestibular apparatus, causing motion sickness, and from the upper parts of the gastrointestinal tract. The pathways from the gut are via vagal and sympathetic nerves.

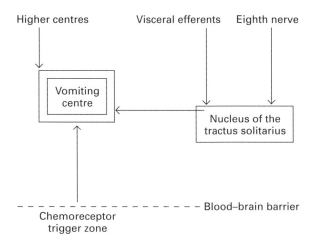

Fig. 32.1 Diagrammatic representation of pathways involved in nausea and vomiting.

CLINICAL MANIFESTATIONS

During the act of vomiting, impulses pass from the vomiting centre via the phrenic, spinal and vagus nerves. These stimuli cause retrograde peristalsis, contraction of the diaphragm and of other skeletal muscles to cause expulsion of gastric contents. There are a number of other features associated with nausea and vomiting which are induced by autonomic stimulation, and these include sweating, pallor and tachycardia.

Although nausea and vomiting are usually self-limiting the metabolic consequences of persistent, repeated vomiting are very serious, due to loss of fluid and electrolytes which can result in acid–base disturbance.

Since there are many pathways involved in the aetiology of nausea and vomiting the pharmacological receptor types implicated also vary. Thus, in motion sickness, excess cholinergic stimulation seems to be particularly important, and sympathetic stimulation of the vomiting centre through a parallel pathway appears to reduce the severity of these effects. In cytotoxic-induced nausea and vomiting recent evidence suggests that, at least for some cytotoxic drugs, stimulation of 5-hydroxytryptamine type 3 ($5HT_3$) receptors is important, and drugs that antagonize these receptors are very effective antiemetics. In the vomiting centre itself there is a wide range of receptor types, but anticholinergic and antihistamine drugs seem to have antiemetic properties in this area of the brain. At the chemoreceptor trigger zone the principal pathway involved in the stimulation of emesis is a dopamine pathway, and dopamine receptor antagonist drugs are very effective at this site. Other drugs that seem to have antiemetic properties include corticosteroids, benzodiazepines and cannabinoids, but the precise site of action of these agents is unclear.

INVESTIGATION

The investigation of the patient with nausea and vomiting will very much depend on the clinical situation. The history may well establish that a patient has an obvious cause for the condition, for example it may be drug-induced or occur during pregnancy. The nausea and vomiting associated with systemic disease may be more difficult to diagnose. The usual approach will be to take a full history and perform a physical examination to exclude associated conditions, for example heart failure with hepatic congestion, secondary liver tumours, lymphadenopathy or gastric and pancreatic masses. In the patient with labyrinthitis it may be possible to induce symptoms by movement of the head, or to demonstrate nystagmus. It is also important to establish the severity of the secondary effects of vomiting by the assessment of blood pressure, pulse and fluid balance both clinically and biochemically. If the patient has been vomiting for some hours measurements of serum electrolytes and urea are important.

DRUG TREATMENT

Antiemetic therapy is inherently symptomatic and may be considered for patients with a very wide spectrum of clinical conditions. Nevertheless, drugs may be given prophylactically, as in motion sickness and postoperative vomiting, or in response to symptoms, such as in labyrinthitis. Antiemetics are widely used, but with the exception of cytotoxic-induced vomiting, there are surprisingly few well-conducted studies in

the published literature; drug selection is therefore often arbitrary, or follows trial and error. Since many antiemetic drugs have multiple pharmacological actions, consideration of their mode of action is only occasionally helpful. The pharmacokinetics of antiemetic drugs are similarly of limited practical use. For the majority of drugs, there is no evidence of a correlation between drug levels and therapeutic effects. In some cases, available pharmacokinetic data are alarmingly incomplete, even for drugs in common clinical use such as prochlorperazine. Pharmacokinetic studies have, however, been useful in determining bioavailability after different routes of administration. In a patient who is vomiting, oral treatment is obviously inappropriate. Subcutaneous, intramuscular or intravenous injections are possible alternatives, but may preclude self-administration. Many antiemetic drugs have been shown to achieve plama levels after rectal administration comparable to those after oral treatment, and this route should be considered if a suitable preparation is available.

In considering drug treatment in this chapter only the following common situations will be addressed, even though nausea and vomiting may occur secondarily to other systemic conditions such as congestive heart failure when treatment of the primary disease will usually result in improvement of these symptoms:

- motion sickness
- postoperative vomiting
- pregnancy
- migraine
- cytotoxic therapy
- labyrinthitis
- drug-induced nausea and vomiting.

Drugs of choice (Table 32.1), pharmacokinetic parameters (Table 32.2), common adverse effects (Table 32.3) and clinically significant drug interactions (Table 32.4) are given in summary form at the end of this section.

Motion sickness

Many drugs with different pharmacological

actions have been shown to be effective at preventing motion sickness and alleviating symptoms already present. However, drugs with dopamine antagonist or 5HT antagonist properties, such as metoclopramide or ondansetron are generally not effective. For drugs with demonstrated efficacy, there is little evidence of superiority between the large number of anticholinergic, calcium channel blocking, or antihistamine drugs available and adverse effects are common. Hence the relative duration of action and available dose form are usually the main criteria for drug selection. Hyoscine is probably the drug of choice, but frequently causes blurred vision and drowsiness, even after transdermal administration. Cinnarizine is also effective and claimed to cause drowsiness less often. In tablet form, both are absorbed from the buccal or sublingual mucosa when chewed, which may facilitate administration, especially in children. Antihistamine drugs are also effective, including cyclizine, promethazine and dimenhydrinate. Treatment should be started before travel; for long journeys, promethazine or transdermal hyoscine may be preferred for their longer duration (24 hours and 3 days respectively). Otherwise, repeated doses will be needed. Cyclizine should probably be avoided because of its abuse potential. Few pharmacokinetic data on anti-motion-sickness drugs are available; there is no evidence of a clear relationship between plasma levels or urinary excretion rate and therapeutic effect.

The most important adverse reaction is sedation, and for anticholinergic drugs, blurred vision, urinary retention and constipation. In laboratory studies, the degree to which these effects impair performance, for example, driving a car, is highly variable, but subjects who take anti-motion-sickness drugs should normally be deemed unfit for such tasks. These centrally acting drugs potentiate the effects of alcohol.

Since motion sickness is an unpleasant and distressing phenomenon, many non-drug treatments have been advocated for alleviation including wristbands, which act on acupuncture points, variously positioned pieces of coloured paper or card, as well as plant extracts such as ginger. Controlled or comparative studies have generally not incorporated any of the wide range of alternative options and, except for the effects of wrist bands, there seems to be no sound basis for their proposed effects. Wrist bands seem to have similar efficacy to the effects of acupuncture, and there is some clinical trial data in support of their efficacy in this condition and in cytotoxic-induced vomiting.

Labyrinthitis

The management of vestibular disorders, as manifested by vertigo, is made difficult by the unpredictable and disabling nature of attacks, and the often progressive nature of some conditions such as Ménière's disease. Dopamine antagonists such as prochlorperazine are probably the best available treatment, though care is needed in the elderly, in whom they may cause drowsiness, hypotension and parkinsonism. Other drugs (cinnarizine, cyclizine) may also be effective for acute attacks. Betahistine, for which there is evidence of a modest prophylactic effect in Ménière's disease, sometimes causes nausea.

Migraine

Nausea and vomiting occur frequently in common migraine, and ergotamine, given for relief of the acute attack, may itself cause nausea. Upper gastrointestinal motility is disturbed early in migraine attacks and oral drugs are poorly absorbed once an attack has started. Metoclopramide, when given parenterally, gives effective symptomatic relief, and has the added potential advantage of reversing the gastric stasis which is a characteristic feature of migraine attacks; hence the absorption of orally administered analgesics is accelerated. Combined preparations of aspirin or paracetamol and metoclopramide (Migravess, Paramax) formulated to give an effervescent solution are often used. There is no evidence of superiority over conventional tablets probably because the metoclopramide is not absorbed and so cannot act once a migraine attack has started. These products are also not suitable for young adults, because of the high risk of drug-induced extrapyramidal effects. If vomiting is severe, prochlorperazine suppositories may be given.

According to clinical trials, prophylaxis of migraine can be achieved by regular aspirin or propranolol in up to 60% of patients. A recent advance in the management of migraine has been the use of the specific $5HT_1$ agonist, sumatriptan, which is available as oral tablets or as a self-administered injection system. Although apparently effective it is expensive and its role in therapy is yet to be established (see Chapter 30).

Postoperative vomiting

Nausea and vomiting are most frequent when patients are emerging from anaesthesia, but so many factors (e.g. type and duration of anaesthesia or operative site) influence the incidence and severity of the symptoms that routine prophylaxis is probably not justified except in procedures involving delicate eye, ear or nose surgery, large visible scars, or where the patient will be unable to clear the mouth of vomitus, for example after jaw wiring. There is little clear evidence of genuine superiority between available drugs in the prevention or treatment of postoperative vomiting. Among drugs with a predominantly anticholinergic action, hyoscine and atropine are both effective though hyoscine is more sedative. Glycopyrrolate appears to have no antiemetic properties. Most phenothiazines are effective but chlorpromazine and promethazine may cause undue sedation and prolong recovery. Perphenazine and prochlorperazine appear best suited for both prophylaxis and treatment. Haloperidol and droperidol are both effective; droperidol has an exceptionally long (up to 24 hours) duration of antiemetic action and can be given in small doses (1.25 mg) with few side effects, even in patients who are awake. Of the antihistamine antiemetics, cyclizine has proven efficacy; it has a short duration of action (4 hours), but is highly effective for the control of established vomiting, with fewer side effects than the phenothiazines. Benzodiazepines are sometimes used as premedication and contribute some antiemetic action, although the precise mechanism of action is not known.

Pregnancy

Nausea and vomiting (morning sickness) are common and troublesome symptoms in early pregnancy. Ideally drugs should not be given in pregnancy. Furthermore, except for the combination of dicyclomine, doxylamine and pyridoxine marketed as Debendox, few drugs have proven efficacy. Debendox was withdrawn in 1983 because of the fear of litigation over claims that it caused congenital malformations. Numerous epidemiological studies have since shown that this risk does not seem to be increased by the use of the preparation. Simple measures, such as small, carbohydrate-rich meals are often enough to control symptoms, and drug treatment is rarely needed. Hyperemesis gravidarum is defined as vomiting occurring before the twentieth week of pregnancy necessitating admission to hospital. Drug treatment may be helpful, with fluid and electrolyte replacement, and rest. For these patients, and other severe cases, there is little comparative safety or efficacy data on which to base drug selection. For severe symptoms in early pregnancy, there is a reasonable body of evidence for the safety of available antiemetics such as cyclizine, dimenhydrinate, metoclopramide, prochlorperazine, and promethazine, and all are likely to be effective. Although some authors have suggested the use of corticosteroids or pyridoxine for this indication, the drugs in the first group should be the treatment of choice.

Cytotoxic and radiotherapy-induced vomiting

Although individual drugs and regimens vary greatly in their emetogenic potential, nausea and vomiting are common effects of cytotoxic drugs and high-dose, intensive X-ray treatment. These symptoms therefore represent serious obstacles to curative or palliative treatment. Chemotherapy regimens containing platinum compounds, etoposide and 5-fluorouracil are the most emetic, and cisplatin causes vomiting in well over 90% of patients unless an antiemetic is used. Virtually all available antiemetics have been tried, singly and in combination, with limited success, but the combination of high-dose metoclopramide, oral or parenteral corticosteroids and a benzo-diazepine, usually lorazepam or diazepam, has become established in recent years as the best available for highly emetogenic drugs. Antihistamines and phenothiazines are commonly used for less emetogenic schedules. The discovery that at high doses metoclopramide (1 to 3 mg/kg) exhibits 5-hydroxytryptamine (5HT) antagonist properties led to the development of specific $5HT_3$ receptor blocking drugs which are potent antiemetics but which do not cause extrapyramidal effects, and recent studies have established their place in treatment. Two drugs, ondansetron and granisetron are licensed for use in the UK. For patients receiving highly emetogenic chemotherapy, ondansetron plus dexamethasone is superior to ondansetron alone, and may be superior to metoclopramide plus dexamethasone. For less emetic regimens, there is no clear evidence of superiority. Granisetron appears to have similar efficacy, but its extended duration of action allows single-dose treatment which has the added benefit of patient convenience.

No one drug or combination appears suitable for all chemotherapy or radiotherapy regimens. It is likely that different cytotoxic drugs give rise to different emetic stimuli, which can in theory be countered by choosing a combination of drugs with the appropriate pharmacological actions. Cytotoxic-induced vomiting is the only clinical condition for which cannabis derivatives are licensed in the UK; nabilone is the only drug available. The use of such agents is limited by variable efficacy against different emetic stimuli, dysphoric reactions and poor solubilility precluding parenteral administration, and they have been superseded by the $5HT_3$ antagonists.

Drug-induced nausea and vomiting

Apart from cytotoxic agents, a variety of drugs are known to cause troublesome nausea and vomiting, either in therapeutic doses or in overdose. Among drugs in common clinical use, cardiac glycosides, dopamine receptor agonists, opiates, theophylline, aminoglycosides, oestrogens (high dose) and ergot alkaloids are frequent causes of nausea.

In the management of poisoning, a number of drugs have been used for their emetic effects. Syrup of ipecacuanha, which contains the alkaloids emetine and cephaeline, is now the preparation of choice, and other emetics should no longer be used. The place of induced emesis is declining because of limited efficacy and the availability of more effective alternatives.

For drugs which cause nausea in therapeutic use, dose alteration or administration with food will often minimize or eliminate the problem. In some cases, tolerance to the adverse effect develops quickly during clinical use. In specific situations, antiemetic prophylaxis may be needed. Nausea and/or vomiting develops in around half of all patients given opiates, and it is commonplace to give a concurrent phenothiazine agent such as prochlorperazine. Tolerance to the emetic effect of opiates develops within 4 to 5 days and therefore patients receiving long-term treatment do not require continuous antiemetic therapy. Fixed dose combinations are therefore inappropriate in such patients.

Antiemetic prophylaxis may also be useful when postcoital contraception is given, since the high dose of oestrogen contained in the normal regimen often causes vomiting. There are no clinical trials to confirm their efficacy, but antihistamines such as cinnarizine appear to reduce the incidence of vomiting in this situation.

THE PATIENT

From the patient's point of view, the appropriate use of antiemetic drugs will depend on the clinical condition being treated. Thus, in situations where nausea and vomiting are to be expected, prophylactic treatment in advance of the event is indicated. The best example of this is the use of antiemetics in cytotoxic-induced vomiting where there is clear evidence of development of a psychological component to vomiting, resulting in anticipatory vomiting in patients who have had previous severe vomiting associated with cytotoxic therapy. There is therefore no justification in allowing patients to suffer vomiting.

In clinical practice the commonest source of vomiting is that associated with acute infections.

Table 32.1   Antiemetic drugs of choice

Condition	Drug(s) of choice
Motion sickness	Antihistamines
	Anticholinergics
Labyrinthitis	Phenothiazines
	Betahistine
Migraine	Metoclopramide
	Prochlorperazine
Postoperative vomiting	Butyrophenones
	Phenothiazines
	Antihistamines
Pregnancy	Antihistamines
	Phenothiazines
	Metoclopramide
Cytotoxic therapy	Phenothiazines
	Metoclopramide
	Corticosteroids
	Benzodiazepines
	5HT$_3$ antagonists

Table 32.2   Selected pharmacokinetic parameters of drugs used as antiemetics

Drug	F	Vd(L/kg)	t$_{1/2}$(hours)
Prochlorperazine	?<10	20	7
Chlorpromazine	?<20	21	30
Metoclopramide	60–80*	3	4
Domperidone	15	6	7.5
Haloperidol	60	10–20	15–25
Hyoscine	?<20	2	2.5
Cinnarizine	?>20		3
Promethazine	25*	13	12
Diphenhydramine	60	3.6	5
Dexamethasone	70–80	0.75–1	3
Methylprednisolone	90	1.5	2
Nabilone	80	Unknown	23
Diazepam	60	2	40
Lorazepam	50	1.5	20
Granisetron	Unknown	2.2–3.3	3–12
Ondansetron	60	2.3	3

*Similar values for rectal administration.
Key: F = bioavailability (%); Vd = volume of distribution (L/kg); t$_{1/2}$ = terminal half-life (hours)

Table 32.3   Adverse effects of antiemetic drugs

Drug/drug group	Adverse drug reactions	Comments
Antihistamines	Sedation	
Anticholinergics	Blurred vision	
	Dry mouth	
Phenothiazines/butyrophenones	Extrapyramidal reactions*	
	Sedation	
Betahistine	Occasionally causes nausea	
Metoclopramide	Extrapyramidal reactions*	
	Sedation	
Corticosteroids		Classic steroid ADRs unlikely, even at high doses
5HT$_3$ antagonists	Headache	
	Constipation	
	Flushing	
Cannabinoids	Sedation	Appear to be better tolerated by younger patients
	Dry mouth	
	Dysphoria	
	Ataxia	

*Extrapyramidal reactions: parkinsonism is more common in the elderly with chronic therapy (usually 2 weeks or more); acute dystonic-dyskinetic reactions occur in the young, and may be more common in females; tardive dyskinesia occurs after months or years of treatment and is more common in the elderly.

These are self-limiting and, particularly in community practice, the use of antiemetic drugs parenterally, certainly on a repeated basis, is practically extremely difficult. The most important factor here is to establish that the patient, particularly if a child, has not become dehydrated. Rehydration is far more important than antiemetic therapy.

Dopamine receptor antagonist drugs, particularly metoclopramide and prochlorperazine, are well known to cause extrapyramidal side effects. These adverse effects are age related,

Table 32.4 Drug interactions with antiemetics

Drug/drug group	Interactions
Antihistamines	Potentiate other CNS sedatives
Anticholinergics	Potentiate other drugs with an anticholinergic action, e.g. tricyclics, phenothiazines
Phenothiazines/	Potentiate other CNS sedatives
Butyrophenones	Potentiate alpha-adrenoreceptor blockers in particular and antihypertensives in general
	Antagonize the action of dopaminergic drugs, e.g. bromocriptine, levodopa
	? Enhance lithium neurotoxicity
Betahistine	No clinically significant interactions reported
Metoclopramide	No clinically significant interactions reported
Corticosteroids	? Increase anticoagulant requirements
	Potentiate potassium when given with diuretics
	Dose may need to be increased when given with drugs which induce liver enzymes (anticonvulsants, rifampicin)
$5HT_3$ antagonists	No clinically significant interactions reported
Cannabinoids	Potentiate other centrally acting drugs

and include acute extrapyramidal reactions, such as dystonia, oculogyric crisis and dyskinesias. They are more common in young adults, particularly with metoclopramide in women under the age of 30 years. The incidence of adverse effects with drugs in this group is in the order of 1 in 80 individuals. In contrast, parkinsonian syndromes, which usually begin 1 or more weeks after the start of therapy are more common in the elderly. Finally chronic treatment with dopamine receptor antagonists may result in tardive dyskinesia, an extremely unpleasant syndrome which is not reversible upon stopping therapy.

In the management of migraine, antiemetic drugs should be taken as early in the attack as possible in the hope that they will be absorbed before a reduction in gastrointestinal tract motility is established. The introduction of self-administered drugs for the management of migraine is a new approach, and the future role of agents such as sumitriptan will, in part, depend upon the cost–benefit analysis of the use of these products.

Since there is no clear general relationship between plasma concentrations of antiemetic drugs and clinical benefits, there is no role for therapeutic drug monitoring. As has been alluded to above, sedation is a common adverse effect of many antiemetic agents, and appropriate counselling with regard to driving and use of machinery will be necessary when prescribing these agents.

CASE STUDIES

CASE 32.1

A 23-year-old female who is 10 weeks' pregnant presents with a history of nausea on waking in the morning, symptoms of reflux and occasional vomiting.

Q What are the therapeutic options?

CASE 32.2

A 45-year-old lady presents with ovarian carcinoma for which she is due to receive a course of cancer chemotherapy.

Q What drugs might be appropriate, when should they be given, and what advice should be given to the patient regarding monitoring of symptoms after treatment with the chemotherapy?

CASE 32.3

A mother presents with a child of 3 years with a 24-hour history of vomiting.

Q What is the appropriate management of this situation?

CASE 32.4

A 50-year-old business man is due to make a transatlantic flight to an important meeting. From past experience he knows that he is likely to suffer from vomiting during the flight.

Q What are the management options and potential adverse effects of treatment.

ANSWERS TO CASE STUDIES

CASE 32.1

A Management of nausea and vomiting in early pregnancy should generally not include drugs. Simple measures such as eating carbohydrate-rich foods, e.g. dry biscuits, first thing in the morning should be tried first. Medical intervention is needed if the patient continues to vomit and therefore becomes fluid and electrolyte deficient. Antiemetics such as cyclizine, dimenhydrinate, metoclopramide, prochlorperazine or perphenazine are likely to be effective and there is little evidence to suggest that they have teratogenic effects.

CASE 32.2

A This lady is likely to receive emetic chemotherapy and therefore should be given prophylactic antiemetics before the start of chemotherapy. The choice of drugs lies between metoclopramide combined with steroids and a benzodiazepine, and one of the newer $5HT_3$ receptor antagonists ondansetron or granisetron. The monitoring of emesis and nausea both within and outside hospital for up to 5 days after treatment is a useful exercise in deciding which patients may need other therapies. It is also important to remember that patients should be given appropriate doses of antiemetics to cover delayed-onset nausea.

CASE 32.3

A Having excluded organic intra-abdominal disease (e.g. appendicitis, intussusception) in a small child presenting with vomiting the most important consideration is fluid replacement. In infants, breast feeding should continue; half-strength feed is usually given to bottle-fed infants. In older children it is usual to withdraw solids until the child's symptoms have settled. Proprietary simple oral rehydration fluids may be given for up to 48 hours after which time they may themselves give rise to loose stools.

CASE 32.4

A Motion sickness responds to a number of drugs, including hyoscine, cinnarizine, cyclizine or promethazine. Of these, cinnarizine may be less likely to cause drowsiness. It would be sensible to ensure that the patient does not suffer this effect by taking a test dose at a time when the effects can be safely monitored. It would also be sensible to avoid alcohol in flight, recognizing the potential additive sedative effect, and it would even be worth considering travelling a day early if nausea and vomiting cannot be controlled by these methods since sedation is very undesirable in the circumstances described.

BIBLIOGRAPHY

Bateman D N. Drug treatment of nausea and vomiting. Prescriber's Journal 1985; 25: 81–86

Bateman D N, Campbell M. Pharmacokinetic optimisation of antiemetic drugs. Clinical Pharmacokinetics 1992; 23(2): 147–160

Hanson J S, McCallum R W. The diagnosis and management of nausea and vomiting: a review. American Journal of Gastroenterology 1985; 80: 210–218

Leatham A M. Safety and efficacy of antiemetics used to treat nausea and vomiting in pregnancy. Clinical Pharmacy 1986; 5: 660–668

Palazzo M G A, Strunin L. Anaesthesia and emesis II: prevention and management. Canadian Anaesthetic Society Journal 1984; 31: 407–415

Perez E A, Hesketh P J, Gandara D R. Serotonin antagonists in the management of cisplatin-induced emesis. Seminars in Oncology 1991; 18: 73–80

Peroutka S J, Snyder S H. Antiemetics; neurotransmitter receptor binding predicts therapeutic effects. Lancet 1982; 1: 658–659

Triozzi P L, Laszlo J. Optimum management of nausea and vomiting in cancer chemotherapy. Drugs 1987; 34: 136–149

Chapter 33

Respiratory infections

S. J. Pedler

Respiratory infections are probably the commonest group of infections seen in the UK. The majority are viral, for which generally there is only symptomatic therapy available, but significant numbers of bacterial respiratory infections do also occur. There is a convenient division, both anatomically and bacteriologically, between upper and lower respiratory tract infections, and upper respiratory tract infections will be considered first.

UPPER RESPIRATORY TRACT INFECTIONS

SORE THROAT (PHARYNGITIS)

Causative organisms

Pharyngitis is a very common condition and most cases never come to medical attention, being treated by simple therapy to relieve symptoms. Many cases are not due to infection, but are caused by other factors such as smoking.

Infection is a very common cause of sore throat and is due in the majority of cases to a virus. Many different viruses may cause pharyngitis. The commonest are the rhinoviruses, which cause the common cold, with a wide variety of other viruses such as coronaviruses, influenza and parainfluenza viruses, and adenoviruses all causing a relatively small number of cases. Epstein–Barr virus (EBV) the cause of glandular fever (infectious mononucleosis) is a less common but particularly important cause of sore throat since clinically it may be confused with streptococcal infection.

By contrast there is only one common bacterial cause of sore throat, *Streptococcus pyogenes*, sometimes referred to as a group A beta-haemolytic streptococcus. Other, less common causes include haemolytic streptococci of groups C and G, *Corynebacterium hemolyticum*, and *Neisseria gonorrhoeae*. Diphtheria is another cause, but is very rare in the UK.

Clinical features

The presenting complaint of pharyngitis is of course a sore throat of varying severity. Many cases will also be associated with fever, which is often mild, and the usual symptoms of the common cold. More severe cases are associated with infection due to EBV or *Strep. pyogenes* and in these patients there may be marked inflammation of the pharynx with a whitish-yellow exudate on the tonsils, plus enlarged, tender cervical lymph nodes. Prior to the widespread use of antibiotics streptococcal infection was frequently accompanied by a macular rash and sometimes considerable systemic illness ('scarlet fever'). This presentation is now very uncommon for reasons that are not clear.

A number of potential complications exist with streptococcal infection. Pharyngeal infection may occasionally give rise to disseminated infection elsewhere, but this is rare. However, otitis media and/or sinusitis are quite frequently seen accompanying streptococcal sore throat. Of greater importance are the non-suppurative complications of streptococcal infection: rheumatic fever and glomerulonephritis. A discussion of these syndromes is outside the scope of this chapter, but occasional cases are still seen after infection due to group A streptococci, and there is some evidence that rheumatic fever is increasing in incidence.

Diagnosis

A bacteriological diagnosis cannot be made in the majority of sore throats and these are presumed to be viral in origin. The aim of any diagnostic procedure is to separate a streptococcal sore throat, which is amenable to antibiotic treatment, from a viral infection which will not respond to antibiotics. Unfortunately glandular fever may be indistinguishable from streptococcal infection and it may not be possible to differentiate between these two on clinical grounds alone. Therefore if streptococcal infection is suspected a throat swab for culture should be taken. If culture is negative, EBV infection should be suspected and a specimen of blood taken for serology.

Treatment

For viral sore throats treatment is symptomatic. Streptococcal sore throat can be treated with antibiotics and therapy should always be given to prevent the development of complications such as rheumatic fever. If streptococcal infection is suspected, treatment may be started before the results of throat swab culture are known; alternatively, it is perfectly acceptable to await culture results and start treatment if a positive culture is obtained. In practice, most busy practitioners would commence treatment empirically.

The most effective treatment is penicillin G (benzylpenicillin), given by intravenous or intramuscular injection. At the present time, resistance to penicillin in group A streptococci has not been described, although occasional strains resistant to erythromycin are seen. To prevent the development of rheumatic fever, the organism must be eradicated from the pharynx and this requires prolonged treatment. For this reason parenteral penicillin G is given only in severe infections while mild or moderate infection can be treated with oral penicillin V (phenoxymethylpenicillin). The usual adult dose is 250 to 500 mg four times daily, taken at least 30 minutes before food, and treatment should continue for 10 days. Shorter courses of treatment are associated with a higher rate of failure to eradicate the organism from the pharynx. In penicillin-hypersensitive patients, erythromycin or cephalexin may be given although it must be remembered that there is a small risk of cross-reactions between the penicillins and cephalosporins in hypersensitive patients.

Penicillin V is poorly absorbed from the gastrointestinal tract with about 50% of a dose being absorbed, or even less when taken concurrently with food, and it is intrinsically slightly less active than penicillin G. Amoxycillin would appear to be a better choice since it is much better absorbed. However, up to 95% of patients with glandular fever develop a rash if given ampicillin or amoxycillin. These agents should never be used to treat sore throats unless proven to be due to streptococci or unless EBV infection has been excluded. In proven streptococcal infection, amoxycillin may be used in patients who fail to respond to penicillin V or who suffer from recurrent infections.

In approximately 20% of patients a 10-day course of penicillin (parenteral or oral) will fail to eradicate the organism from the pharynx. There is a suggestion that beta-lactamase-producing organisms in the pharynx may contribute to such persistence and it is logical to consider using a beta-lactamase stable agent such as cephalexin if a further course of treatment is to be given.

OTITIS MEDIA
Causative organisms

Inflammation of the middle ear (otitis media) is a common condition, seen most frequently in children under the age of 2 years. The majority of cases are due to bacteria, although viruses such as influenza virus and rhinoviruses have been implicated in 25% or more of cases.

Strep. pneumoniae and *Haemophilus influenzae* are the two most frequently encountered bacterial pathogens. *Strep. pyogenes* accounts for a smaller (perhaps 10%) proportion of cases, and other bacteria are only seen rarely.

Clinical features

Classically, otitis media presents with ear pain, which may be severe. If the drum perforates, the pain is relieved and there is often a purulent discharge from the ear. It may be accompanied by a degree of hearing impairment. Non-specific symptoms, such as fever or vomiting, may occur in very young children. Complications of otitis

media include mastoiditis, which is now a very rare condition, meningitis and particularly in the case of *H. influenzae*, septicaemia and disseminated infection.

Diagnosis

The diagnosis of otitis media is essentially made clinically and laboratory investigations have little role to play. For this reason a causative organism is rarely isolated and treatment is given empirically.

Treatment

It has been suggested that because a substantial proportion of cases of otitis media resolve spontaneously, routine antibiotic therapy is not indicated. Treatment, however, is often indicated as it is not possible to predict in which children potentially life-threatening complications will develop.

Antibiotic treatment should be effective against the three main bacterial pathogens, *Strep. pneumoniae*, *H. influenzae* and *Strep. pyogenes*. *Strep. pyogenes* and the pneumococcus are both sensitive to penicillin, but penicillin is much less active against *H. influenzae*. Amoxycillin or ampicillin should be used instead; these two agents are identical in terms of antibacterial activity, but amoxycillin is recommended since it is much better absorbed from the gastrointestinal tract with at least 80% of a dose of amoxycillin being absorbed, compared to 50% of a dose of ampicillin. Pivampicillin, talampicillin and bacampicillin are all esters of ampicillin which are de-esterified in the gut wall or blood. They are all well absorbed but offer no advantages over amoxycillin and are more expensive.

Up to 15% of *H. influenzae* strains are resistant to amoxycillin due to beta-lactamase production. If there is no response to amoxycillin, an alternative agent should be chosen. Both erythromycin and the earlier oral cephalosporins such as cephalexin are insufficiently active against *H. influenzae*, and possible alternatives are co-amoxiclav (a combination of amoxycillin and the beta-lactamase inhibitor clavulanic acid) or co-trimoxazole. Newer oral cephalosporins such as cefixime also possess high activity against *H. influenzae*. Cefuroxime axetil, while very active in vitro, is very poorly absorbed and is associated with a high incidence of diarrhoea.

ACUTE SINUSITIS

Causative organisms

Normally the facial sinuses are sterile and sinusitis occurs following damage to the mucous membrane which lines them. This usually occurs following an upper respiratory tract viral infection, but is sometimes associated with the presence of dental disease. Acute sinusitis is usually caused by the same organisms which cause otitis media but occasionally other organisms such as *Staphylococcus aureus*, viridans streptococci (often but incorrectly known as 'Strep. viridans') and anaerobes may be found. Viruses are occasionally found in conjunction with the bacteria.

Clinical features

The main feature of acute sinusitis is facial pain and tenderness, often accompanied by headache and a purulent nasal discharge. Complications include frontal bone osteomyelitis, meningitis and brain abscess. The condition may become chronic with persistent low grade pain and nasal discharge, sometimes with acute exacerbations.

Diagnosis

As with otitis media this is a clinical diagnosis and obtaining specimens for bacteriological examination is not usually practicable. In patients with chronic sinusitis therapeutic sinus washouts may yield specimens for microbiology.

Treatment

Since the causative organisms are the same as those found in otitis media, the same recommendations for treatment apply. Proximity to the mouth means that anaerobes are implicated quite frequently in acute sinusitis, particularly if associated with dental disease, and in such cases the addition of metronidazole may be worthwhile. Doxycycline has proved popular, parti-

cularly in chronic sinusitis, due to its broad spectrum of activity and once-daily dosage.

LOWER RESPIRATORY TRACT INFECTIONS

CHRONIC BRONCHITIS

Aetiology

A patient with chronic bronchitis can be defined as someone who coughs up sputum on most days for 3 or more consecutive months during 2 or more years. Probably the single most important factor in the aetiology of chronic bronchitis is smoking, with repeated viral or bacterial respiratory infections and dust inhalation being important secondary factors. Not surprisingly therefore chronic bronchitis is extremely common in the UK, where smoking is still common and there is a high incidence of viral respiratory infections. The highest incidence is to be found in miners and other groups where dust inhalation is common.

In chronic bronchitis the bronchial mucosa is thickened due to oedema and inflammation of the bronchi and there is hypertrophy of the mucous glands of the bronchi. This is a response to long-standing irritation and the result is overproduction of mucus and narrowing of the bronchial lumen. Emphysema is often found with chronic bronchitis and the syndrome is frequently referred to as 'chronic obstructive airways disease' (COAD).

Clinical features

The characteristic feature of COAD is cough, which is often worse in the mornings and accompanied by the production of copious sputum. The narrowing of the bronchi leads to dyspnoea and wheezing, and cor pulmonale leading to cardiorespiratory failure may also develop.

Against this background the patient develops acute exacerbations which are generally believed to be of infective origin (but see below). When an exacerbation occurs the cough becomes worse, and sputum production increases, often changing from white to green or yellow, denoting the presence of pus cells. Often dyspnoea also increases and the patient may be tipped over into cardiac failure. Sometimes the condition becomes a frank bronchopneumonia, although the dividing line between a severe exacerbation of COAD and bronchopneumonia is very blurred.

Microbiology of chronic bronchitis

Examination of sputum from chronic bronchitic patients not in an acute exacerbation frequently (in up to 50% of cases) yields potential pathogens, particularly *Strep. pneumoniae* (the pneumococcus) and *H. influenzae*. During an acute exacerbation the same two pathogens are found, and the rate of isolation is not markedly increased. Other organisms which may be detected are *Branhamella catarrhalis*, which is becoming increasingly recognized in this condition, and organisms such as *Staph. aureus*, haemolytic streptococci and Gram-negative bacilli. A considerable proportion (perhaps up to half) of acute exacerbations are associated with viral infections such as colds or influenza.

Since no one pathogen has been unequivocally associated with causing acute exacerbations of COAD, and since the two main suspect organisms are isolated almost as frequently in the absence of an exacerbation, doubt has been cast on the role of bacterial infection in this condition. However, evidence that bacterial infection is important in some cases comes from the presence of fever or a raised peripheral white blood cell count. Nevertheless, antibiotics are now accepted as part of the standard treatment for exacerbations of COAD and it is unlikely that clinical trials comparing antibiotic therapy with a placebo will ever be performed.

Diagnosis

The diagnosis of an acute exacerbation of COAD is made clinically. Where possible a sputum sample should be sent for bacteriology which will at least allow antibiotic sensitivity tests to be performed on potential pathogens. The collection of suitable specimens is difficult in general practice and is not usually done. In patients who have received broad-spectrum agents such as amoxycillin or a cephalosporin, Gram-negative bacilli or staphylococci are frequently isolated from sputum. Care should be taken when interpreting such results as the oropharynx frequently becomes colonized with these organisms due to elimination of the normal upper respiratory flora, without causing a genuine infection.

Treatment

Treatment consists of two main arms, antibiotic therapy and supportive treatment. Supportive treatment consists in the main of physiotherapy to aid coughing up of secretions, bronchodilators, and in some cases a short course of corticosteroids.

Most patients with exacerbations of COAD will be seen by general practitioners and in this case antibiotic treatment will be given empirically. It should be directed against the two main infecting organisms as described above.

The antibiotic sensitivity of the pneumococcus is discussed in the following section. Some strains of *H. influenzae* are capsulated, which is a virulence factor conferring resistance to phagocytosis by polymorphs. Capsulated strains are mainly seen in serious infections in children, such as meningitis or epiglottitis, and often in otitis media as well. By contrast the strains encountered in COAD are non-capsulated. This difference is important because about 15% of capsulated strains are resistant to amoxycillin, due in the majority of cases to beta-lactamase production, whereas only about 7 to 9% of non-capsulated strains are amoxycillin resistant, although this rate is increasing. Beta-lactamase-producing strains are susceptible to co-amoxiclav. Neither erythromycin nor the earlier oral cephalosporins such as cephalexin or cephradine are sufficiently active against *H. influenzae*, although newer agents such as cefaclor and especially cefixime are more active. Most strains are sensitive to trimethoprim or tetracycline. The majority of strains of *B. catarrhalis* are beta-lactamase producers and are therefore resistant to amoxycillin.

Accordingly the following recommendations can be made for the antibiotic treatment of exacerbations of COAD:

- First line:
  — amoxycillin
- Second line:
  — trimethoprim or
  — co-amoxiclav or
  — tetracycline.

There is good evidence that trimethoprim is as effective as co-trimoxazole in this condition, so trimethoprim alone is preferred due to the higher toxicity of co-trimoxazole. Cefixime is another possible alternative, but is very expensive, while ciprofloxacin possesses insufficient activity against the pneumococcus.

PNEUMONIA

Pneumonia is a condition defined as an inflammation of the lung parenchyma (i.e. the alveoli rather than the bronchi) of infective origin and characterized by consolidation. Consolidation is a pathological process in which the alveoli are filled with a mixture of inflammatory exudate, bacteria, and white blood cells, which shows on chest X-ray as an opaque area in the normally clear lung fields.

Because the range of organisms which can cause pneumonia is very large, a classification system is useful. One method of classification is a clinical scheme, in which pneumonia is classified as lobar pneumonia, bronchopneumonia, or atypical pneumonia. This does not correlate entirely with the bacteriological cause, and a better method is to classify pneumonia by place of origin, either community-acquired or hospital-acquired (nosocomial) pneumonia.

Community-acquired pneumonia

The commonest cause of this condition is *Strep. pneumoniae*, the pneumococcus. Classically, this organism causes lobar pneumonia, but nowadays it is more often seen as a cause of bronchopneumonia.

The clinical presentation of lobar pneumonia is with cough, initially dry but later producing purulent or bloodstained sputum, together with dyspnoea, fever and pleuritic chest pain. There is usually a markedly elevated peripheral white blood cell count. Chest X-ray shows consolidation confined to one or more lobes (or segments of lobes) of the lungs and the anatomic boundary between affected segments or lobes is quite distinct. This classical picture is now quite rare perhaps because the early use of antibiotics modifies the natural history of the disease. Patients with lobar pneumonia are usually elderly, and often have an underlying illness of some kind.

Bronchopneumonia on the other hand is a rather ill-defined entity with similar symptoms but with a chest X-ray showing patchy consolidation, usually in the bases of both lungs. It is usually due to the pneumococcus and/or non-capsulated strains of *H. influenzae*. This disease is very common and is typically seen in patients with severe chronic obstructive airways disease or those who are terminally ill.

Another common cause of community-acquired pneumonia is *Mycoplasma pneumoniae*, the most common cause of so-called 'atypical' pneumonia. Patients with atypical pneumonia present with fever, a dry cough and a normal white blood cell count. Chest X-ray shows widespread patchy consolidation scattered over both lung fields. The disease is usually seen in older children and young adults. Most cases are mild and are treated by the general practitioner rather than in hospital. *Chlamydia pneumoniae* (otherwise known as 'strain TWAR') is being increasingly recognized as a cause of community-acquired pneumonia and other, much rarer causes of atypical pneumonia include *Chlamydia psittaci* and *Coxiella burnetii*.

Rare causes of community-acquired pneumonia include *Staph. aureus*, which produces a severe necrotizing pneumonia with lung abscess formation. This is sometimes seen in patients with influenza and has a high mortality rate. *Klebsiella pneumoniae* is very rare as a cause of pneumonia outside hospital in the UK, but is rather more common in the USA. It also produces a severe infection with abscesses, and almost always occurs in patients with chronic underlying disease such as diabetes or alcoholism. Finally, *Legionella pneumophila* is the causative organism of Legionnaire's disease. This infection occurs mainly in outbreaks associated with contaminated air-conditioning or water systems, and is probably a rare cause of sporadic cases of pneumonia. Clinical presentation is very similar to atypical pneumonia but the disease may be rapidly progressive producing very extensive consolidation and eventually respiratory failure.

Hospital-acquired pneumonia

Nosocomial pneumonia accounts for 10 to 15% of all hospital-acquired infections. Patients are predisposed to this condition by a number of factors including mechanical ventilation, chronic lung disease, recent surgery, immunosuppression and previous antibiotics which may have eradicated the normal flora of the oropharynx, allowing replacement with resistant organisms. There is a predominance of Gram-negative bacilli among the causative organisms; these are listed in Table 33.1.

Aspiration pneumonia

One further condition which may be seen either in hospitals or the community is aspiration pneumonia. Risk factors include alcohol, hypnotic drugs, and general anaesthesia – that is, those factors which may make a patient vomit while unconscious. The result is inhalation of stomach contents which are contaminated by bacteria from the mouth. Gastric acid is very destructive of lung tissue; the result is severe tissue necrosis and infection, often with abscess formation. There is usually more than one causative organism, with anaerobic bacteria being particularly common. These are often accompanied by aerobic organisms such as viridans streptococci or (in hospitals) staphylococci and/or Gram-negative bacilli.

Diagnosis

Sputum specimens are the commonest specimen sent for culture but they are sometimes unhelpful as they are often contaminated by mouth flora. If the patient has received antibiotics, the normal mouth flora is often replaced by resistant

Table 33.1 The causative organisms of hospital-acquired (nosocomial) pneumonia
Common organisms
1. Gram-negative bacteria:
Escherichia coli
Klebsiella species
Pseudomonas aeruginosa
2. Gram-positive bacteria:
Streptococcus pneumoniae
Staphylococcus aureus
Less common organisms
1. Gram-negative bacilli:
Enterobacter species
Other 'coliforms'
— *Proteus* species
— *Serratia marcescens*
— *Citrobacter* species
Other *Pseudomonas* species
Legionella pneumophila (and other species)
2. Anaerobic bacteria
3. Fungi:
Candida albicans (and other species)
Aspergillus fumigatus
4. Viruses:
Cytomegalovirus
Herpes simplex virus

organisms such as staphylococci or Gram-negative bacilli, making the interpretation of results difficult.

Techniques have therefore been developed to overcome this problem. In transtracheal aspiration a cannula is inserted into the trachea through the cricothyroid membrane and sputum aspirated with a syringe. This technique is popular in the USA but has never been used widely in the UK because of concern over the dangers of the procedure. Open lung biopsy is sometimes attempted, but is an invasive procedure which has been generally superseded by bronchoscopy with bronchoalveolar lavage. All these procedures obtain material from the lung uncontaminated with bacteria from the mouth.

Other specimens which might be collected include blood cultures, serum for antibodies to *L. pneumophila* or *M. pneumoniae*, and serum or urine for rapid detection of pneumococcal antigen.

Treatment

The antibiotic treatment of pneumonia is dependent on an awareness of the likely infecting organisms in the individual patient. The treatment of choice for pneumococcal pneumonia is benzylpenicillin. Although strains of the pneumococcus with reduced sensitivity to penicillin (which can result in treatment failures in conditions such as pneumonia or meningitis) are known to exist, they are very rare in the UK at the present time. Such strains are commoner in continental Europe and multiresistant strains including resistance to penicillin, erythromycin, and chloramphenicol have been described in Spain. It is likely that these organisms will be seen with increasing frequency as they are imported to the UK by returning travellers. Meanwhile amoxycillin may be substituted for benzylpenicillin when oral therapy is required, and erythromycin may be used in penicillin-hypersensitive patients.

H. influenzae is usually seen in patients with bronchopneumonia, accompanied by the *Pneumococcus*. Its sensitivity to antibiotics has been discussed above. Amoxycillin is the agent of choice with co-amoxiclav or trimethoprim as alternatives.

M. pneumoniae does not possess a cell wall and therefore is not susceptible to the beta-lactam antibiotics which act at this site. A tetracycline or erythromycin is a suitable therapeutic agent. Tetracycline is also effective against *Chlamydia psittaci* and *Coxiella burnetii* which are intracellular bacteria also with no cell wall. Erythromycin is not as effective in these infections but is active against *L. pneumophila*.

Most strains (>90%) of *Staph. aureus* are now resistant to penicillin, but in the UK the vast majority are still susceptible to the penicillinase-resistant antibiotic flucloxacillin and related agents. Staphylococcal pneumonia would usually be treated with flucloxacillin plus another agent such as fusidic acid or gentamicin. Methicillin-resistant *Staph. aureus* (MRSA) is resistant to flucloxacillin and similar agents, the cephalosporins, and often to other antistaphylococcal agents such as tetracycline, erythromycin, and gentamicin. Such strains are fortunately rare in the UK, athough they do cause problems in some hospitals and are very rare in the community.

The treatment of choice for primary *Klebsiella* pneumonia is a cephalosporin such as cefuroxime or cefotaxime, plus an aminoglycoside, e.g. gentamicin. Legionnaire's disease is treated with erythromycin in high doses (1 g four times daily) and there is some evidence that results are improved by the addition of rifampicin. Ciprofloxacin is an alternative to erythromycin but experience in Legionnaire's disease is relatively small.

All the above recommendations presuppose that the infecting organism is known before treatment is commenced. In practice, this is rarely if ever the case and therapy will initially be empiric or 'best-guess' in nature. The choice of empiric therapy is based on the most common infecting organisms, and amoxycillin is therefore a suitable choice. Since *Mycoplasma* infections are common and Legionnaire's disease carries a poor prognosis if untreated, erythromycin is often added. If there is a possibility that the infection may be due to staphylococci or Gram-negative bacilli, cefuroxime, or an equivalent agent such as cefotaxime, should be substituted for the amoxycillin.

The range of organisms which may cause nosocomial pneumonia is very large and therapy must be correspondingly broad spectrum. The patient's underlying condition may give important clues to the infecting organism, such as the possibility of fungi in a neutropenic patient. The choice of antibiotics will be influenced by any preceding antibiotic therapy, and above all by the individual unit's experience with hospital bacteria. The combinations shown in Table 33.2 have all been used at some time and all have advantages and disadvantages. Each combination includes an aminoglycoside and this may not be desirable in all patients. Single-agent therapy is attractive for ease of administration and two agents, ceftazidime and imipenem, have suitably broad spectra of activity. Unfortunately treatment failures have been recorded when cefta-zidime is used alone due to the emergence of resistance while the patient is on treatment. In all cases erythromycin would be added if Legionnaire's disease was suspected and except for the regimen containing clindamycin, metronidazole would be required for suspected anaerobic infection.

Table 33.2 The treatment of nosocomial pneumonia	
Treatment regimen	Comment
1. Ureidopenicillin plus aminoglycoside (e.g. azlocillin or piperacillin plus gentamicin)	Good activity against Gram-negative bacilli, especially *Pseudomonas aeruginosa*, and pneumococci. Some strains of *Escherichia coli*, *Klebsiella* etc. are resistant to azlocillin. Relatively low activity against *Staphylococcus aureus*; poor activity against anaerobes
2. Cephalosporin plus aminoglycoside (e.g. cefuroxime or cefotaxime plus gentamicin)	Good activity against Gram-negative bacilli such as *Esch. coli*, *Klebsiella*, and Gram-positive organisms; relatively low activity against *Ps. aeruginosa*. Poor activity against anaerobes
3. Clindamycin plus aminoglycoside	Good activity against Gram-positive organisms and anaerobes, but much less so against Gram-negative bacteria. This combination is favoured in the United States where metronidazole is unpopular for the treatment of anaerobic infections
4. Ciprofloxacin plus aminoglycoside	Good activity against most Gram-negative bacilli, including *Ps. aeruginosa*. Adequate activity against *Staph. aureus* but poor activity against pneumococci and anaerobes
5. Ceftazidime (alone)	Monotherapy, thus is more convenient and no risk of aminoglycoside toxicity. Very active against Gram-negative bacilli, including *Pseudomonas*, but less so against Gram-positive organisms (especially *Staph. aureus*) and anaerobes
6. Imipenem (alone)	Monotherapy. Very broad spectrum agent but *Legionella* is resistant (this applies to all the above agents as well). Very expensive

CYSTIC FIBROSIS: A SPECIAL CASE

Cystic fibrosis is an inherited disease which at the cellular level is a defect in the transport of ions in and out of cells. In practice this leads to changes in a number of exocrine glands, but in the chest this is manifested by the production of very sticky, tenacious mucus which is very difficult, if not impossible, to clear by the normal mucociliary action. The production of such mucus leads to airway obstruction with resulting infection. Repeated episodes of infection lead eventually to bronchiectasis and permanent lung damage, which in turn further predisposes the patient to infection.

Clinically, cystic fibrosis is characterized by persistent cough with sputum production. At times acute exacerbations occur in which there is fever, increased cough with purulent sputum, and increased dyspnoea. Systemic sepsis, however, is very rare. Eventually, chronic pulmonary infection leads to respiratory insufficiency, cardiac failure and death.

Infecting organisms

In infants and young children *Staph. aureus* is the commonest pathogen, and *H. influenzae* is sometimes encountered. From the age of about 5 years onwards *Pseudomonas aeruginosa* is seen with increasing frequency until by the age of 18 years the majority of patients are chronically infected with this organism. Once present, the organism is never completely eradicated. Occasionally other Gram-negative bacteria such as *Escherichia coli* or *Ps. maltophilia* are seen, and in some centres *Ps. cepacia* has been a particular problem due to its exceptional antibiotic resistance.

An important feature of those *Ps. aeruginosa* strains which infect cystic fibrosis patients is their production of large amounts of 'alginate', a polymer of mannuronic and glucuronic acid. This seems to be a virulence factor for the organism in that it inhibits opsonization and phagocytosis, and enables the bacteria to adhere to the bronchial epithelium, thus inhibiting clearance. It does not confer additional antibiotic resistance. Strains which produce large amounts of alginate have a wet, slimy appearance on laboratory culture media and are termed 'mucoid' strains. Interestingly, other organisms such as *Esch. coli* may also produce alginate in these patients, a characteristic which is otherwise very rare.

Treatment

This section will concentrate mainly on antibiotic therapy, but it should not be forgotten that other means of treatment, such as physiotherapy, also play an important part.

The initial treatment of infection in a cystic fibrosis patient will probably be directed against staphylococci, for which the usual antistaphylococcal antibiotics such as flucloxacillin or erythromycin can be used. In some centres prophylaxis is given with agents such as co-trimoxazole, which may lead to the appearance of unusual resistant strains, for example thymidine-dependent *Staph. aureus*. These are strains which are dependent for growth on the nucleotide precursor thymidine, which completely bypasses the biochemical site of action of the sulphonamides and trimethoprim.

Once the patient is colonized by *Ps. aeruginosa* treatment depends on early and vigorous therapy with antipseudomonal antibiotics. Physiotherapy between exacerbations may help to prevent some episodes of exacerbation, but the role of prophylactic antibiotics is uncertain. *Ps. aeruginosa* can be very antibiotic-resistant, but fortunately there is now a reasonable range of antipseudomonal antibiotics available. These are listed in Table 33.3. At present a combination such as azlocillin plus tobramycin or ceftazidime plus gentamicin is often used; agents such as imipenem or a quinolone are usually reserved for treatment failures or when resistant organisms are encountered. The prolonged use of ceftazidime or ciprofloxacin alone should be avoided if possible since strains of *Ps. aeruginosa* (and some other Gram-negative bacilli) may become resistant to these agents while the patient is receiving treatment. Ciprofloxacin can be given orally and offers the possibility of treatment for less severe exacerbations at home, perhaps after a brief time in hospital for parenteral therapy.

The penetration of antibiotics into sputum may be poor so that the use of inhaled antibiotics

Table 33.3	Antipseudomonal antibiotics
Antibiotic	Comment
Ticarcillin	This penicillin derivative was one of the first beta-lactam agents effective against *Pseudomonas* but is now considered insufficiently active. In combination with the beta-lactamase inhibitor clavulanic acid, it may be active against some ticarcillin- and azlocillin-resistant strains
Ureidopenicillins	Azlocillin and piperacillin are the most active; mezlocillin is relatively inactive against *Pseudomonas*. They should be given in combination with an aminoglycoside, with which these agents are synergistic
Cephalosporins	Ceftazidime is the most active antipseudomonal cephalosporin and is very active against other Gram-negative bacilli. It has rather lower activity against Gram-positive bacteria. One problem is that strains of *Pseudomonas* may develop resistance while the patient is on treatment Cefoperazone also has good antipseudomonal activity but is less active than ceftazidime against other Gram-negative bacilli. It is not licensed in the UK at present Cefsulodin is an unusual agent whose main activity is against *Staphylococcus aureus* and *Ps. aeruginosa*. For this reason it has not proved popular in the UK
Aminoglycosides	Gentamicin and tobramycin have very similar activity; tobramycin is perhaps slightly more active against *Pseudomonas*. Netilmicin is less active than both the above, while amikacin may be active against some gentamicin-resistant strains
Quinolones	Ciprofloxacin can be given orally and parenterally but as with ceftazidime resistance can develop while the patient is on treatment. It is not licensed for use in children
Polymyxins	These peptide antibiotics are too toxic for systemic use but colistin (polymyxin E) can be given by inhalation
Imipenem	This is a very broad spectrum agent with good activity against *Ps. aeruginosa*. Some other species of *Pseudomonas* (notably *Ps. maltophilia*) are resistant

as an adjunct to parenteral therapy has attracted some attention. Colistin is a popular choice for inhaled therapy since if resistance develops it has not caused the loss of an agent used for systemic treatment. However the role and benefits of aerosolized antibiotics remains uncertain at present. Children with cystic fibrosis are admitted to hospital very frequently, sometimes for long periods of time, and it is not surprising that some develop an intense dislike of hospitals. This has encouraged the use of long-term indwelling central venous cannulae to allow administration of intravenous antibiotics at home by the parents, and the use of oral ciprofloxacin and inhaled colistin may also help to reduce the length of admissions.

Interestingly, patients with cystic fibrosis have a more rapid clearance of some antibiotics than other patients. This is particularly noticeable with the aminoglycosides and larger doses are often required to achieve satisfactory serum levels. Despite this, aminoglycoside toxicity is unusual in these patients. It is not unusual to see post-dose levels of gentamicin in the order of 14 to 16 mg/L in cystic fibrosis patients, yet the level 8 hours later (i.e. before the next dose) will still be in the required range of less than 1.5 mg/L.

CASE STUDIES

CASE 33.1

An elderly patient is found collapsed at home. He has been suffering from an acute exacerbation of chronic bronchitis for which he has received amoxycillin from his GP. On admission to hospital, a chest X-ray shows signs of bronchopneumonia and an urgent Gram stain of a sputum sample reveals many pus cells and large numbers of Gram-negative bacilli.

Q1 Why was amoxycillin ineffective? What treatment should he be given?

Q2 The sputum culture next day shows a heavy growth of *Haemophilus influenzae* and *Pseudomonas aeruginosa*. Should therapy be changed?

CASE 33.2

A neonate, delivered at 34 weeks' gestation, is well for 48 hours and then deteriorates rapidly, with hypoxia, severe dyspnoea and apnoeic periods. Chest X-ray shows extensive bilateral consolidation but further, more invasive diagnostic procedures are not indicated due to the baby's poor condition.

Q What treatment should be given?

CASE 33.3

A pregnant woman attends her general practitioner's surgery and is diagnosed as suffering from acute sinusitis. She is given a 7-day course of co-trimoxazole and advised to return if there is no improvement. 5 days later she returns and tells the doctor that the pain is worse. On questioning, she admits that she has only taken two doses, since a friend advised her that co-trimoxazole is harmful in pregnancy.

Q How justified is this fear? What alternative therapy could be given?

ANSWERS TO CASE STUDIES

CASE 33.1

A1 The most likely pathogens in this case are *Streptococcus pneumoniae* and *H. influenzae*. He was given amoxycillin, which may have failed for two potential reasons: beta-lactamase-producing *H. influenzae* are increasing slowly in incidence and secondly *Branhamella catarrhalis* is being increasingly recognized as a pathogen in such patients. Most strains of this organism are resistant to amoxycillin. The best choice in this patient therefore, since he has already received amoxycillin without success, is cefuroxime, which is active against all three of the above organisms, including beta-lactamase producers.

A2 The *Pseudomonas* is probably a red herring, which has colonized the respiratory tract due to the use of a broad-spectrum antibiotic (amoxycillin). Although resistant to cefuroxime, there is no indication to change treatment unless the patient fails to respond or deteriorates. It is more usual to see this organism in patients who have been in hospital for some time, but it is occasionally seen in the community.

CASE 33.2

A Neonatal pneumonia in the first few days after birth is similar in some ways to nosocomial pneumonia, with some important differences. The causative organisms are acquired during passage through the birth canal, and are therefore those which would normally be found in the vagina. This includes Gram-negative bacilli, streptococci and anaerobes. Generally, anaerobic infections are rare in neonatal pneumonia but group B haemolytic streptococci (*Strep. agalactiae*) are important pathogens. *Listeria monocytogenes* is a rare cause of neonatal sepsis but should be included in the spectrum of activity of treatment given. In this case, amoxycillin plus gentamicin is the best combination. Amoxycillin is more active against *Listeria* than penicillin, and the combination is synergistic against streptococci. A cephalosporin would be less appropriate due to lower activity against group B streptococci than amoxycillin and poor activity against *Listeria*.

CASE 33.3

A It has long been known that sulphonamides should not be given to women in the third trimester of pregnancy since these agents may displace bilirubin from its albumin binding sites and cause kernicterus in the neonate. The position of co-trimoxazole or trimethoprim alone in the earlier stages of pregnancy is less certain. In high doses trimethoprim is teratogenic in rats, but there is no evidence of toxicity in humans. Although co-trimoxazole and trimethoprim are not contra-indicated in pregnancy, and indeed have been used for many years in pregnant women, it would seem sensible to avoid these agents at the present time.

Clearly a tetracycline could not be used in a pregnant woman and there are insufficient data concerning the safety in pregnancy of the newer oral cephalosporins with activity against *Haemophilus influenzae*, such as cefixime. In this patient therefore a penicillin such as amoxycillin, or if necessary co-amoxiclav, should be given instead. Metronidazole, if required, is safe for use in pregnancy.

BIBLIOGRAPHY

Cole P. Host–microbial interactions in chronic respiratory disease. In: Reeves D S, Geddes A M (eds) Recent advances in infection: 3. Edinburgh: Churchill Livingstone 1989: 141–151

Donowitz G R, Mandell G L. Acute pneumonia. In: Mandell G L, Douglas R G, Bennett J E (eds) Principles and practice of infectious diseases, 3rd edn. New York: Churchill Livingstone 1990; 540–555

Grayston J T, Campbell L A, Kuo C-C, Mordhorst C H, Saikku P, Thom D H et al. A new respiratory tract pathogen: *Chlamydia pneumoniae* strain TWAR. Journal of Infectious Diseases 1990; 161: 618–625

Grenier B. Use of the new quinolones in cystic fibrosis. Reviews of Infectious Diseases 1989; 11 (Suppl. 5): S1245–S1252

Harrison B D W, Farr B M, Pugh S, Selkon J B, Prescott R J, Connolly C K. Community-acquired pneumonia in adults in British hospitals in 1982–1983: a survey of aetiology, mortality, prognostic factors and outcome. Quarterly Journal of Medicine 1987; 62: 195–220

Jensen T, Pedersen S S, Garne S, Heilmann C, Hoiby N, Koch C. Colistin inhalation therapy in cystic fibrosis patients with chronic *Pseudomonas aeruginosa* lung infection. Journal of Antimicrobial Chemotherapy 1987; 19: 831–838

LaForce F M. Systemic antimicrobial therapy of nosocomial pneumonia: monotherapy versus combination therapy. European Journal of Clinical Microbiology and Infectious Diseases 1989; 8: 61–68

Marrie T J, Durant H, Yates L. Community-acquired pneumonia requiring hospitalization: 5-year prospective study. Reviews of Infectious Diseases 1989; 11: 586–599

Reynolds H Y. Chronic bronchitis and acute infectious exacerbations. In: Mandell G L, Douglas R G, Bennett J E (eds) Principles and practice of infectious diseases, 3rd edn. New York: Churchill Livingstone 1990; 531–535

Shanson D C. Microbiology in clinical practice, 2nd edn. London: Wright 1989

Chapter 34

Urinary tract infections

A. J. Bint

Urinary tract infection (UTI) usually means the presence of microorganisms in the urinary tract together with signs and symptoms of inflammation. It is, however, more precise to use one of the following terms:

• *Significant bacteriuria* which is defined as the presence of $\geqslant 10^5$ bacteria per ml of urine. A quantitative definition like this is needed because small numbers of bacteria are normally found in the anterior urethra, and will be washed out into urine samples. Thus $<10^3$ bacteria per ml are normally considered to be urethral contaminants.

• *Asymptomatic bacteriuria* is significant bacteriuria without causing any symptoms in the patient.

• *Cystitis* means a syndrome of frequency, dysuria, and urgency, and usually suggests infection restricted to the lower urinary tract, i.e. bladder and urethra.

• *Acute pyelonephritis* is acute infection of one or both kidneys; the lower urinary tract is also involved.

• *Chronic pyelonephritis* is difficult to define and usually refers to a particular type of pathology of the kidney, which may or may not be due to infection.

Recurrence of urinary infection in a patient may be either a relapse or a reinfection. A relapse is a recurrence caused by the same organism that caused the original infection. A reinfection is a recurrence caused by a different organism and is therefore a new infection.

EPIDEMIOLOGY

Urinary tract infection is a problem in all age groups, although the prevalence varies markedly. In infants up to the age of 6 months, the incidence is about 2 cases per 1000 live births, and is much more common in boys than in girls. In preschool children the sex ratio reverses and the prevalences of bacteriuria are 4.5% for girls and 0.5% for boys. Infections during these early years are often symptomatic and it is thought that serious renal damage can occur, hence it is very important to treat these infections aggressively and follow up the children for a period of several years if any urinary tract abnormalities are found.

In schoolgirls and schoolboys prevalences of bacteriuria are 1.2% and 0.03% respectively. In girls only about one-third of infections are symptomatic. The occurrence of bacteriuria during childhood appears to lead to a higher incidence of bacteriuria in adulthood.

When women reach adulthood, the prevalence of bacteriuria rises to 3 to 5%. Each year about a quarter of the bacteriuric women clear their bacteriuria spontaneously and are replaced by an equal number of newly infected women (often those with a history of previous infections). At least 10 to 20% of all women will have a symptomatic UTI during their lifetime. In the elderly of both sexes, the prevalence of bacteriuria rises dramatically: 20% for women and 10% for men. In hospitals, a major predisposing cause of UTI is urinary catheterization. If a catheter is left in for longer than 10 days, infection rates rise to 70 to 80%.

AETIOLOGY

In acute uncomplicated UTI in the community, *Escherichia coli* is by far the commonest causative bacterium, causing about 80% of infections. The remaining 20% are caused by other Gram-negative enteric bacteria such as *Klebsiella* and *Proteus*, and by Gram-positive cocci, particularly *Streptococcus faecalis* and *Staphylococcus saprophyticus*. This last organism is almost entirely restricted to infections in young, sexually active women.

In UTI complicated by underlying structural abnormalities such as congenital anomalies, neurogenic bladder, and obstructive uropathy, the frequency of infections with organisms rarely seen in uncomplicated infections, such as *Pseudomonas aeruginosa*, *Enterobacter* and *Serratia*, rises markedly. Such organisms are also more commonly isolated in hospital-acquired urinary infections, including those in patients with urinary catheters. Cross-infection is fairly common in the pathogenesis of hospital-acquired infections. Rare causes of urinary infection are anaerobic bacteria and fungi – when they do occur it is nearly always in association with structural abnormalities or a catheter.

Adenoviruses are thought to cause haemorrhagic cystitis in children.

PATHOGENESIS

There are three possible routes by which organisms can reach the urinary tract and cause infection: ascending, blood-borne, and lymphatic. There is little evidence for the latter route in humans. Blood-borne spread to the kidney can occur in bacteraemic illnesses, most notably *Staph. aureus* septicaemia. However, the most common route by far is the ascending route. In women, urinary tract infections are preceded by colonization of the perineum and periurethral area by the pathogen, most often a strain of *Esch. coli*. These organisms then ascend into the bladder via the urethra. The fact that the female urethra is much shorter than that of the male is probably an important factor in explaining the preponderance of UTI in females. Furthermore, sexual intercourse appears to be important in forcing bacteria into the female bladder. The association of cystitis in women, with intercourse ('honeymoon cystitis') is real.

The organism

Most UTIs are caused by *Esch. coli*. There are many different serogroups of *Esch. coli* but only a few cause most infections. It is therefore thought likely that some strains of *Esch. coli* possess certain virulence factors which enhance their ability to cause infection. Recognized virulence factors include adherence to epithelial cells by bacterial surface structures called fimbriae, resistance to serum bactericidal activity and increased amounts of capsular K antigen. The adhesion properties of *Esch. coli* and other pathogens are thought to be important in initiating infection in the urinary tract.

The host

Although many bacteria can readily grow in urine, the high urea concentration and extremes of osmolality and pH inhibit growth. In addition, there are other defence mechanisms operating against bacterial infection. The flushing mechanism of bladder emptying is protective. Small numbers of bacteria finding their way into the bladder will most likely be eliminated when the bladder is emptied. The bladder mucosa appears to be normally resistant to adherence by bacteria; the substance responsible appears to be a surface mucopolysaccharide. Presumably, large numbers of bacteria with a strong adhesive property can overcome this defence. When the bladder is infected, white blood cells are mobilized to the bladder surface to ingest and destroy invading bacteria.

Because it is known that periurethral colonization precedes infection, it is thought that women who suffer from recurrent infections may have defective local perineal defence mechanisms, but this remains unproven. Although in pyelonephritis the body produces antibodies to several bacterial antigens, and in the urine of such cases IgG and IgA are found, the role of humoral immunity in defence against infection of the urinary tract remains unclear.

Abnormalities of the urinary tract

Any structural abnormalities leading to the obstruction of urine flow increases the likelihood of infection. Such abnormalities include congenital anomalies of the ureter or urethra, renal stones and, in men, an enlarged prostate. All of these lead to stasis of urine. Renal stones can become infected with bacteria, particularly *Proteus* and *Klebsiella* species, and be a source of recurrent infection. Vesicoureteric reflux (VUR) is a condition caused by failure of a physiological valve at the junction of the ureters and the bladder, thus allowing urine to reflux back to the kidneys when the bladder contracts. It is probable that VUR plays an important role in childhood urinary tract infections in leading to chronic renal damage (scarring) and persistence of infection. The presence of abnormal residual urine in the bladder, caused by obstructive lesions like an enlarged prostate, or urethral stricture, predisposes patients to infection.

CLINICAL MANIFESTATIONS

Most UTIs are asymptomatic. When symptoms do occur, in the case of cystitis they are the result of irritation of bladder and urethral mucosa. However, the symptoms of urinary tract infections are very variable and depend on the age of the patient.

Babies and infants

Infections in newborn babies and infants are often overlooked or misdiagnosed because the symptoms are often not referable to the urinary tract. Failure to thrive, vomiting, fever, diarrhoea and apathy may be presenting symptoms.

Children

Above the age of 2 years, children with UTI are more likely to present with some of the classical symptoms. Thus frequency, dysuria and haematuria become likely. However, some children present with acute abdominal pain and vomiting.

Adults

In adults the typical symptoms of lower UTI include frequency, dysuria, urgency and haematuria. Acute pyelonephritis usually causes fever, rigors and loin pain in addition to lower tract symptoms.

Elderly patients

The great majority of elderly patients with UTI are asymptomatic. Symptoms, when present, are not diagnostic because frequency, dysuria, hesitancy and incontinence are fairly common in elderly people without infection.

INVESTIGATION

The key to successful laboratory diagnosis of UTI lies in obtaining an uncontaminated urine sample. Contaminating bacteria can arise from skin, vaginal flora in women and penile flora in men. All patients therefore need to be instructed in how to produce a midstream urine sample (MSU). In very young children, stick-on bags are a useful way of obtaining a urine sample. Occasionally, suprapubic aspiration (SPA) of urine directly from the bladder is necessary.

Microscopy

Microscopy is the first step in laboratory diagnosis of a UTI – it is readily performed in ward siderooms and GPs' surgeries as well as in laboratories, by experienced and skilled personnel. A drop of uncentrifuged urine is placed on a slide, covered with a coverslip and examined under a × 40 objective. More than 5 white cells per high-power field is abnormal. The presence of at least one bacterium per field correlates with $\geq 10^5$ bacteria/ml. Excess white cells are nearly always seen in the urine of patients with symptomatic UTI. Red blood cells are sometimes found in patients with UTI, and white cell casts are suggestive of pyelonephritis.

Culture

Bladder urine is normally sterile. However, when it is passed via the urethra, it is inevitable that some of the urethral bacterial flora will be washed out in the urine. Hence it is important that laboratories quantitate the number of bacteria in urine specimens. Patients with a UTI usually have $\geq 10^5$ bacteria/ml. In patients without infection, the urine count is usually $< 10^3$ bacteria/ml. However, some true infections occur with counts of $< 10^5$/ml. This can occur in symptomatic patients with frequency, causing the bacteria to be washed out, and in infections caused by slow-growing pathogens. Thus counts of 10^4 or even 10^3 of single species, may be significant in symptomatic patients. Most genuine infections are caused by one single bacterial species; mixed cultures suggest contamination.

For general practitioners located at some distance from the laboratory, transport of specimens is a problem. Ordinary MSUs must reach the laboratory within 2 hours, or can be refrigerated; otherwise any bacteria in the specimen will grow and possibly give a false-positive result. Methods of preventing bacterial multiplication in urine are to use a dip-slide, or containers with a small amount of boric acid.

Non-culture methods of detecting urine infection, such as dipstick methods for glucose, nitrite and dehydrogenase are not sufficiently reliable for routine use.

Urethral syndrome

In about 40% of women with dysuria, urgency and frequency, a urine sample has $< 10^5$ bacteria/ml. These patients are said to have the urethral syndrome. Some have a true bacterial infection, but with relatively low counts of bacteria. Others have urethral infection with *Chlamydia trachomatis*, *Neisseria gonorrhoeae*, or a *Mycoplasma* species. In others no known cause can be found. However, most cases of urethral syndrome will respond to a course of a standard antibiotic as used for treating a UTI.

TREATMENT

Any symptomatic UTI needs treatment with an antibiotic to eradicate both symptoms and the pathogen from the urine. Asymptomatic bacteriuria may or may not need treatment depending on factors in the patient. Bacteriuria in preschool children with VUR or other congenital abnormalities, and in pregnant women needs treatment because of the potential serious complications. On the other hand, treatment of non-pregnant bacteriuric adults, without any obstructive lesion, is probably unwarranted if they have no symptoms.

Nonspecific therapy

Advising patients with UTI to drink a lot of fluids is common practice, on the theoretical basis that more infected urine is removed by frequent bladder emptying. However, as there is no evidence that this practice improves the results of antibiotic therapy, such advice is unnecessary.

The activity of some antibiotics is affected by urinary pH. Nitrofurantoin is more active in acid urine. Aminoglycosides and macrolides are more active in alkaline urine. However, most antibiotics used for treating UTI will work at the normal pH of urine, with the exceptions of mandelamine and its mandelic and hippuric acid salts. With these latter agents, it is necessary to acidify the urine with ascorbic acid or methionine. However, this is often difficult to achieve without dietary modification, and is rarely necessary because of the plethora of alternative antibiotics available.

Principles of antimicrobial therapy

There is no evidence that a bactericidal antibiotic is superior to a bacteriostatic one in treating UTI, except perhaps in treating relapsing infections. Blood levels of antibiotics appear not to be important in treating lower UTI – what matters is the concentration in the urine. Blood levels are probably important in treating pyelonephritis, which may progress to septicaemia.

In renal failure, it may be difficult to get adequate therapeutic concentrations of an antibiotic into the urine. There is also the problem of enhanced risk of toxicity of some agents, e.g. aminoglycosides, in renal failure. Penicillins and cephalosporins generally attain satisfactory concentrations in urine, even in renal failure, are relatively non-toxic, and are therefore the agents of choice for treating UTI in the presence of renal failure.

Lower UTI

There is little doubt that for acute, uncomplicated lower UTI, a shorter course than the conventional 7 to 10 days of therapy will work equally well. Whether a single dose or a 3-day course are equally effective is debatable. Single-dose therapy has been used with cure rates of 61 to 100%. It is cheap, achieves good compliance, and has few side effects. However, there may be a poor response if the kidneys are involved, and some antibiotics do not give a good result if used as a single dose. There is some evidence that a 3-day course is superior to one dose, and this is therefore recommended by most experts. Exceptions, which require 7 to 10 days, are infections in males, in patients with symptoms for more than 7 days, in patients with frequent recurrent infections and in suspected upper tract infection. Antibiotics which are suitable for 3-day therapy include trimethoprim, nitrofurantoin, co-trimoxazole, cephalexin, amoxycillin, co-amoxiclav, norfloxacin and ciprofloxacin (see Table 34.1). However, recent trends in resistance patterns mean that not all of these agents are suitable as best-guess therapy. The resistance rate in *Esch. coli*, the commonest UTI pathogen, is 30 to 40% for amoxycillin, and 10 to 15% for trimethoprim and co-trimoxazole. For the other agents mentioned resistance rates are generally <10%. Other factors governing choice include risk of side effects and contra-indications (see Table 34.1).

The preference for best-guess therapy is a choice between macrocrystalline nitrofurantoin, trimethoprim, cephalexin or co-amoxiclav. The quinolones are best reserved for failures and more difficult to treat infections. Overuse of these agents is likely to lead to an increase in resistance.

In the urethral syndrome, it is worth trying a 3-day antibiotic course using one of the agents mentioned above. If this fails, a course of tetracycline (500 mg six-hourly for 7 days) could be tried to deal with possible chlamydia or mycoplasma infection.

Acute pyelonephritis

Patients with pyelonephritis may be severely ill, and if so will require admission to hospital and initial treatment with a parenteral antibiotic.

Table 34.1   Oral antibiotics used for the treatment of lower UTI

Antibiotic	Dose (adult)	Side effects	Contra-indications	Comments
Amoxycillin	250 mg every 8 h	Nausea, diarrhoea, rashes	Penicillin hypersensitivity	30% resistance in *Esch. coli*
Co-amoxiclav	375 mg every 8 h	See amoxycillin Rarely, hepatitis, erythema multiforme	See amoxycillin	
Cephalexin	250 mg every 6 h	Diarrhoea, nausea, allergic reactions	Porphyria	
Co-trimoxazole	960 mg every 12 h	Nausea, vomiting Rarely, erythema multiforme, agranulocytosis	Pregnancy, neonates, renal or hepatic failure	Trimethoprim alone preferable
Trimethoprim	200 mg every 12 h	Nausea, vomiting, pruritus, rashes	Severe renal failure, pregnancy, neonates	
Nitrofurantoin	50 mg every 6 h	Nausea, vomiting. Rarely, pulmonary reactions, peripheral neuropathy	Renal failure, neonates, G6PD deficiency, porphyria	Take with food or milk Turns urine bright yellow Macrocrystalline form causes less nausea
Ciprofloxacin	250 mg every 12 h	Nausea, vomiting, dizziness, headache, rash Rarely, convulsions, hallucinations, hepatitis, photosensitivity, blood disorders	CNS disorders, pregnancy, children, G6PD deficiency	Interacts with theophylline Reserve for difficult to treat UTI
Norfloxacin	400 mg every 12 h	See ciprofloxacin	See ciprofloxacin	See ciprofloxacin

Suitable antibiotics, with good activity against *Esch. coli* and other Gram-negative bacilli, include cephalosporins such as cefuroxime and ceftazidime, some penicillins such as co-amoxiclav, quinolones, and aminoglycosides such as gentamicin (see Table 34.2).

A first choice agent would be parenteral cefuroxime, gentamicin or ciprofloxacin. When the patient is improving, the route of administration may be switched to oral therapy.

Patients who are less severely ill at the outset may be treated with an oral antibiotic. Treatment should be generally for 10 to 14 days. Treatment should be changed if bacteriology shows resistance to the chosen agent, or if the patient is not clinically improving at 48 hours.

In patients with what may be hospital-acquired pyelonephritis, there is a risk that the infecting organism may be a more resistant, hospital type pathogen. In this case it is advisable to start an ultra-broad-spectrum agent such as ceftazidime, imipenem or ciprofloxacin.

Asymptomatic bacteriuria

In children, asymptomatic bacteriuria may have the same bad long-term prognosis as symptomatic infection, and therefore should be treated in the same way. In adults, treatment of asymptomatic bacteriuria is not necessary except in pregnant women and in patients with obstructive structural abnormalities.

Relapsing UTI

The main causes of persistent relapsing UTI are renal infection, structural abnormalities of the urinary tract and, in men, chronic prostatitis. Patients who fail on a 7-to 10-day course should be given a 2-week course, and if that fails a 6-week course can be considered. Structural abnormalities may need surgical correction before cure can be maintained.

A 6-month course of antibiotic may rarely be needed for certain patients with relapsing infec-

Table 34.2 Parenteral antibiotics used for the treatment of pyelonephritis

Antibiotic	Dose (adult)	Side effects	Contra-indications	Comments
Cefuroxime	750 mg i.v. every 8 h	Diarrhoea, nausea, allergic reactions	Porphyria	A first choice agent
Ceftazidime	1 g i.v. every 8 h	See cefuroxime	Porphyria	
Co-amoxiclav	1.2 g i.v. every 8 h	Nausea, diarrhoea, rashes Rarely, hepatitis, erythema multiforme	Penicillin hypersensitivity	
Gentamicin	80–120 mg i.v. every 8 h	Vestibular and hearing damage, nephrotoxicity	Caution in renal failure, pregnancy	A first choice agent Monitoring by serum concentrations mandatory
Ciprofloxacin	200 mg i.v every 12 h	Nausea, vomiting, dizziness, headache Rarely, convulsions, hallucinations, hepatitis, photosensitivity, blood disorders	CNS disorders, pregnancy, children, G6PD deficiency	Interacts with theophylline A first choice agent
Imipenem	500 mg i.v. every 8 h	Nausea, vomiting, diarrhoea, allergic reactions Rarely, convulsions, confusion	Caution in CNS disorders, renal impairment	Reserve for hospital-acquired infection

tions: children, adults with continuous symptoms or who are at risk of progressive renal damage.

It is essential that all long courses (i.e. >4 weeks) of antibiotics are managed under bacteriological control, with monthly cultures.

Prophylaxis for UTI

In some patients, mainly women, reinfections are so frequent that long-term prophylaxis may be indicated. If the reinfections are clearly related to sexual intercourse, then a single dose of an antibiotic after intercourse is appropriate. In other cases long-term, low-dose prophylaxis may be beneficial. One dose of co-trimoxazole (80 mg trimethoprim, 400 mg sulphamethoxazole), trimethoprim (100 mg) or nitrofurantoin (50 mg) at night will suffice. These drugs are unlikely to lead to the emergence of resistant bacteria in the patient.

Bacteriuria of pregnancy

The prevalence of asymptomatic bacteriuria of

pregnancy is about 4 to 7% in pregnant women. In bacteriuric pregnant women there is a 30 to 40% chance of developing acute pyelonephritis during pregnancy. This is the major reason why bacteriuria of pregnancy should be treated. In addition to the definite risk of pyelonephritis, there seems to be statistically significant correlations of bacteriuria with prematurity, low birth weight babies, and maternal hypertension. By treating bacteriuria at an early stage of pregnancy, 50 to 70% of cases of acute pyelonephritis can be prevented. It is therefore necessary to screen all pregnant women at their first antenatal appointment for bacteriuria of pregnancy. All women with bacteriuria are treated with a 7-day course of an antibiotic safe to use in pregnancy (cephalexin, nitrofurantoin, amoxycillin) and followed up at intervals during pregnancy. 3-day courses of antibiotic have not yet been unequivocally shown to be as effective as 7-day courses in bacteriuria of pregnancy.

Catheter-associated infections

In most large hospitals 10 to 15% of patients have

an indwelling urinary catheter. Even with the very best catheter care, the majority of such patients will have infected urine 10 to 14 days after having the catheter inserted. Most of these infections will be asymptomatic. Antibiotic treatment will often appear to eradicate the infecting organism, but as long as the catheter remains, the organism, or another more resistant one, is likely to quickly return. The principles of antibiotic therapy are therefore: do not treat asymptomatic infection; and remove the catheter if at all possible before treating symptomatic infection.

CASE STUDIES

CASE 34.1

A woman aged 35 years presents with frequent episodes of severe cystitis, on average one a month. Radiological examination has shown no urinary tract abnormalities.

Q What would be a reasonable course of action to take?

CASE 34.2

A woman aged 25 years with a recent renal transplant and receiving cyclosporin presents with high fever, rigors and acute loin pain. A MSU cultured a few days previous to this showed *Pseudomonas aeruginosa* at a count of >10⁵/ml.

Q What antibiotic therapy is indicated?

CASE 34.3

A pregnant woman aged 21 years is found to have significant bacteriuria at her first antenatal visit. A fully sensitive *Esch. coli* is isolated from her urine. The patient reports that she had a severe rash when she took ampicillin in the past.

Q What would be appropriate antibiotic therapy for this infection?

ANSWERS TO CASE STUDIES

CASE 34.1

A This patient is a good candidate for long-term low-dose prophylaxis, for a period of perhaps 6 months. Following a full course of therapy with an antibiotic active against the organism, low-dose therapy can be instituted with a daily night-time dose, taken at bedtime, of either trimethoprim 100 mg or macrocrystalline nitrofurantoin 50 mg.

CASE 34.2

A The patient is ill enough to warrant parenteral antibiotic therapy. Antibiotics active against *Ps. aeruginosa* include gentamicin, ceftazidime, ciprofloxacin and ureidopenicillins such as piperacillin and azlocillin. Gentamicin is best avoided in this situation because of its potential nephrotoxicity. Quinolones like ciprofloxacin aggravate the nephrotoxicity of cyclosporin. The best choice is intravenous ceftazidime.

CASE 34.3

A Amoxycillin or ampicillin, cephalexin and nitrofurantoin are all recognized as safe to use in pregnancy. Because of the history of allergy to ampicillin, penicillins and cephalosporins are best avoided. The most appropriate choice is therefore macrocrystalline nitrofurantoin 50 mg q.d.s for 5 or 7 days.

BIBLIOGRAPHY

Kunin C M. Detection, prevention and management of urinary tract infections, 4th edn. Philadelphia: Lea & Febiger 1987

Lambert H P, O'Grady F. Antibiotic and chemotherapy, 6th edn. London: Churchill Livingstone 1992

Pedler S J, Bint A J. Management of bacteriuria in pregnancy. Drugs 1987; 33: 413–421

Shanson D C. Microbiology in clinical practice, 2nd edn. London: Wright 1989

Sobel J D, Kaye D. Urinary tract infections. In: Mandell G L, Douglas R G, Bennett J E (eds) Principles and practice of infectious diseases, 3rd edn. New York: Churchill Livingstone 1990

Chapter 35

Gastrointestinal infections

J. W. Gray   A. J. Bint

Gastrointestinal infections represent a major public health and clinical problem worldwide. Many species of bacteria, viruses and protozoa cause gastrointestinal infection, resulting in two main clinical syndromes. Gastroenteritis is a non-invasive infection of the small or large bowel which manifests clinically as diarrhoea and vomiting. Other infections are invasive, causing systemic illness, often with few gastrointestinal symptoms. The recently recognized pathogen *Helicobacter pylori*, and its association with gastritis and peptic ulceration is discussed in Chapter 9.

EPIDEMIOLOGY AND AETIOLOGY

In western countries the average person probably experiences one or two episodes of infective diarrhoea every year. Infections are rarely severe, and there are relatively few common pathogens. In the UK *Campylobacter*, followed by non-typhoidal *Salmonella* species, are much the commonest causes of bacterial gastroenteritis. Gastroenteritis due to viruses such as rotaviruses, adenoviruses, Norwalk virus, caliciviruses, and astroviruses is also common. In developing countries the incidence of gastrointestinal infection is at least twice as high, and the range of common pathogens is much wider. Infections are often more severe, and represent a major cause of mortality, especially in children.

Gastrointestinal infections can be transmitted by consumption of contaminated food or water,

Table 35.1 Important causes of gastrointestinal infection, their modes of spread, and pathogenic mechanisms

Causative agent	Chief mode(s) of spread	Pathogenic mechanisms
Bacteria		
Campylobacter	Food, especially poultry, milk	Mucosal invasion
		Enterotoxin
Salmonella species other than S. typhi & S. paratyphi	Food, especially poultry, eggs, meat	Mucosal invasion
		Enterotoxin
S. typhi, S. paratyphi	Food, water	Systemic invasion
Shigella	Faecal–oral	Mucosal invasion
		Enterotoxin
Escherichia coli		
Enteropathogenic	Faecal–oral	Mucosal adhesion
Enterotoxigenic	Faecal–oral, water	Enterotoxin
Enteroinvasive	Faecal–oral, food	Mucosal invasion
Enterohaemorrhagic	Meat	Verotoxin
Staphylococcus aureus	Food, especially meat, dairy produce	Emetic toxin
Clostridium perfringens	Food, especially meat	Enterotoxin
Bacillus cereus		
Short incubation period	Food, especially rice	Emetic toxin
Long incubation period	Food, especially meat & vegetable dishes	Enterotoxin
Vibrio cholerae 01	Water	Enterotoxin
V. parahaemolyticus	Seafoods	Mucosal invasion
		Enterotoxin
Clostridium difficile	Uncertain – ? nosocomial	Cytotoxin
		Enterotoxin
Clostridium botulinum	Inadequately heat-treated canned/preserved foods	Neurotoxin
Protozoa		
Giardia lamblia	Water	Mucosal invasion
Cryptosporidium	Water, animal contact	Mucosal invasion
Entamoeba histolytica	Food, water	Mucosal invasion
Viruses	Food, faecal–oral, respiratory secretions	Small intestinal mucosal damage

or by direct faecal–oral spread. The most important causes of gastrointestinal infection and their usual modes of spread are shown in Table 35.1.

In developed countries, the majority of gastrointestinal infections are food-borne. Farm animals are often colonized by gastrointestinal pathogens, especially *Salmonella* and *Campylobacter*, and therefore raw foods such as poultry, meat and eggs are commonly contaminated and must be thoroughly cooked in order to kill such organisms. Raw foods also represent a potential source of cross-contamination of other foods through hands, surfaces or utensils that have been inadequately cleaned. Food can also be contaminated by pathogens carried by food handlers. Asymptomatic faecal carriers of organisms such as *Salmonella*, *Campylobacter* and *Shigella* pose a small risk of contaminating food. However food handlers are the usual source of

Staphylococcus aureus food poisoning. Toxin-producing strains of *Staph. aureus* carried in the nose or on infected skin lesions of food handlers are easily transferred to foods. Food poisoning is often associated with prolonged storage of food at ambient temperature before consumption, which allows many pathogens to multiply.

Water-borne gastrointestinal infection is primarily a problem in countries without a sanitary water supply or sewage system although outbreaks of water-borne cryptosporidiosis have occurred from time to time in the UK.

Spread of pathogens such as *Shigella* or enteropathogenic *Esch. coli* by the faecal–oral route is favoured by overcrowding and poor standards of personal hygiene. Such infections in developed countries are commonest in children, and can cause particularly troublesome outbreaks in nurseries and residential children's homes.

Treatment with broad-spectrum antibiotics

alters the bowel flora, creating conditions that favour superinfection with organisms which cause diarrhoea. *Clostridium difficile* is the only organism that has been found to be commonly associated with antibiotic-associated diarrhoea. *C. difficile* infection can occur in association with any antibiotic, but clindamycin, ampicillin and the cephalosporins are most commonly implicated. The means of transmission of *C. difficile* is unclear: within hospitals patient-to-patient spread can occur, but community-acquired infections are not uncommon.

PATHOPHYSIOLOGY

Development of symptoms after ingestion of gastrointestinal pathogens depends on two factors. First, ingested organisms must survive host defence mechanisms, and second, the pathogen must possess one or more virulence mechanisms in order to cause disease.

Host factors

Healthy individuals possess a number of defence mechanisms which protect against infection by enteropathogens. Therefore large numbers of many pathogens must be ingested for infection to ensue. For example, the infective dose for *Salmonella* is approximately 10^5 organisms. Other species, however, are better able to survive host defence mechanisms; shigellosis can result from ingestion of fewer than 100 organisms.

Gastric acidity

Most microorganisms are rapidly killed at normal gastric pH. Patients whose gastric pH is less acid, e.g. following treatment with antacids or H_2 antagonists, are more susceptible to gastrointestinal infections.

Intestinal motility

Intestinal motility helps to rid the host of enteric pathogens. Therefore antimotility agents are potentially hazardous in the treatment of infective gastroenteritis.

Resident microflora

The resident microflora, largely composed of anaerobic bacteria, helps to resist colonization by enteropathogens.

Intestinal immunity

Phagocytic, humoral and cell-mediated elements are all important in resistance to colonization, clearance of pathogens and neutralization of toxins.

Organism factors

The symptoms of gastrointestinal infection can be mediated by several different mechanisms (Table 35.1).

Toxins

Toxins produced by gastrointestinal pathogens can be classified as enterotoxins, neurotoxins and cytotoxins. Enterotoxins act on intestinal mucosal cells to cause net loss of fluid and electrolytes. The classical enterotoxin-mediated disease is cholera, due to infection with *Vibrio cholerae* 01, but many other organisms produce enterotoxins, including enterotoxigenic *Esch. coli* and *Clostridium perfringens*.

The emetic toxins of *Staph. aureus* and *Bacillus cereus* are neurotoxins which induce vomiting by an action on the central autonomic nervous system. Confusingly, staphylococcal emetic toxins are often referred to as 'enterotoxins' although this is strictly incorrect. The symptoms of botulism are also mediated by a neurotoxin which blocks release of acetylcholine at nerve endings.

Cytotoxins cause mucosal destruction and inflammation (see below). Verocytotoxin produced by enterohaemorrhagic *Esch. coli* causes systemic endothelial cell damage as well as local damage to the gut mucosa.

Mucosal damage

Cytotoxins are important in mediating mucosal invasion, but other mechanisms are also involved. Enteropathogenic *Esch. coli* appears to cause diarrhoea by adhering to, and directly damaging, the small intestine mucosa. Organisms such as *Shigella* and enteroinvasive *Esch. coli* express surface proteins that somehow facilitate mucosal invasion. Diarrhoea due to mucosal damage may be due to reduction in the absorptive surface area, or the presence of increased numbers of immature enterocytes which are secretory rather than absorptive.

Systemic invasion

The mechanism by which *Salmonella typhi* penetrates the gastrointestinal epithelium and invades the bloodstream and lymphatic tissue is poorly understood. The lipopolysaccharide outer membrane and possession of an outer capsule are probably important factors.

CLINICAL MANIFESTATIONS

Many cases of gastrointestinal infection are asymptomatic or cause subclinical illness.

Gastroenteritis is the commonest syndrome of gastrointestinal infection, presenting with vomiting, diarrhoea and abdominal pain. The term 'dysentery' is sometimes applied to infections such as *Shigella* (bacillary dysentery) and *Entamoeba histolytica* (amoebic dysentery), where severe colonic mucosal inflammation causes frequent diarrhoea with blood and pus. Table 35.2 shows the most important causes of gastroenteritis together with a brief description of the typical illness that each causes. However, the symptoms experienced by individuals infected with the same organism can differ considerably.

Esch. coli is present as a harmless commensal in the intestine of almost all individuals. However, certain serotypes of *Esch. coli* possess pathogenic traits that can cause gastrointestinal symptoms. Enteropathogenic *Esch. coli* is an important cause of infantile gastroenteritis, enterotoxigenic *Esch. coli* is the most important cause of traveller's diarrhoea, and enteroinva-

Table 35.2	Characteristic clinical features of various causes of gastroenteritis	
Causative agent	Incubation period	Symptoms syndrome
Campylobacter	2–5 days	Bloody diarrhoea Abdominal pain Systemic upset
Salmonella	6–72 hours	Diarrhoea & vomiting Fever; may be associated bacteraemia (Salmonellosis)
Shigella	1–4 days	Diarrhoea, fever (Shigellosis, bacillary dysentery)
Escherichia coli		
Enteropathogenic	12–72 hours	Infantile diarrhoea
Enterotoxigenic	1–3 days	Traveller's diarrhoea
Enteroinvasive	1–3 days	Similar to *Shigella*
Enterohaemorrhagic	1–3 days	Bloody diarrhoea (Haemorrhagic colitis) Haemolytic uraemic syndrome
Staphylococcus aureus	4–8 hours	Severe nausea & vomiting
Clostridium perfringens	6–24 hours	Diarrhoea
Bacillus cereus		
Short incubation period	1–6 hours	Vomiting
Long incubation period	6–18 hours	Diarrhoea
Vibrio cholerae 01	1–5 days	Profuse diarrhoea (Cholera)
V. parahaemolyticus	12–48 hours	Diarrhoea, abdominal pain
Clostridium difficile	Usually occurs during/just after antibiotic therapy	Diarrhoea, pseudomembranous enterocolitis
Giardia lamblia	1–2 weeks	Watery diarrhoea (often persistent) (Giardiasis)
Cryptosporidium	2 days – 2 weeks	Watery diarrhoea (Cryptosporidiosis)
Entamoeba histolytica	2–4 weeks	Diarrhoea with blood & mucus, abdominal pain, liver abscess (Amoebiasis, amoebic dysentery)
Viruses	1–2 days	Vomiting, diarrhoea

sive *Esch. coli* causes a dysentery-like disease. Enterohaemorrhagic *Esch. coli* is associated with outbreaks and sporadic cases of haemorrhagic colitis and childhood haemolytic uraemic syndrome.

Enteric fever, due to infection with *Salmonella typhi* or *Salmonella paratyphi*, presents insidiously with headache, malaise and abdominal distension after an incubation period of 3 to 21 days. During the first week of the illness the temperature gradually increases but the pulse characteristically remains slow. Without treatment during the second and third weeks the symptoms become more pronounced. Diarrhoea develops in about half of cases. Examination usually reveals splenomegaly, and a few erythematous macules (rose spots) may be found, usually on the trunk. Serious gastrointestinal complications such as haemorrhage and perforation are commonest during the third week. Symptoms begin to subside slowly during the fourth week. In general paratyphoid fever is less severe than typhoid fever.

The clinical spectrum of infection with *C. difficile* ranges from mild self-limiting diarrhoea to life-threatening pseudomembranous colitis (so called because yellow-white plaques or membranes consisting of fibrin, mucus, leucocytes and necrotic epithelial cells are found adherent to the inflamed colonic mucosa).

Botulism typically presents with autonomic nervous system effects, including diplopia and dysphagia, followed by symmetrical descending motor paralysis. There is no sensory involvement.

Gastrointestinal infection is often followed by a period of convalescent carriage of the pathogen. This usually lasts for no more than 4 to 6 weeks, but can be for considerably longer, especially for *Salmonella*.

INVESTIGATIONS

The mainstay of investigation of diarrhoeal illness is examination of the faeces.

Bacterial infections are diagnosed by stool culture. Various selective culture media designed to suppress growth of normal faecal organisms and/or enhance the growth of a particular pathogen are used. When sending specimens to the laboratory it is important that details of the age of the patient, the clinical presentation, and recent foreign travel are provided, so that the appropriate media for the likely pathogens can be selected.

Various other procedures are sometimes useful in investigating patients with suspected bacterial gastroenteritis. Blood cultures should be taken from patients with severe systemic upset. In *Staph. aureus* and *B. cereus* food poisoning the pathogen can often be isolated from vomitus. In cases of likely food poisoning, suspect foods can be cultured. Tests are available for detection in faeces of toxins produced by *C. difficile* and enterohaemorrhagic *Esch. coli*.

Protozoal infections are usually detected by microscopic examination of faeces. Various techniques are available for diagnosis of viral gastroenteritis; electron microscopy is probably the most widely used method.

Sigmoidoscopy is sometimes helpful in evaluating patients with diarrhoea, especially if a non-infective aetiology is thought likely. The findings in infective colitis are nonspecific unless psuedomembranous colitis is seen.

Suspected enteric fever should be investigated by culture of urine, faeces, blood, and sometimes bone marrow. Blood and bone marrow culture are the most sensitive techniques, especially if several blood cultures are taken. Faecal culture is positive in fewer than 50% of cases, and urine culture in fewer still. A serological (Widal) test is available, but is of limited value.

Botulism is diagnosed by demonstration of toxin in serum.

TREATMENT

Many gastrointestinal infections are mild and self-limiting and never reach medical attention. Where treatment is required there are three main therapeutic considerations. Fluid and electrolyte replacement is the cornerstone of treatment of diarrhoeal disease. Most patients can be managed with oral rehydration regimens, but severely dehydrated patients require rapid volume expansion with intravenous fluids. Symptomatic treatment with antiemetics and antidiarrhoeal agents is occasionally prescribed. As has already been alluded to, antidiarrhoeal drugs are not without hazard in infectious diarrhoea. Antimicrobial agents may be useful both in effecting symptomatic improvement and in eliminating faecal carriage of pathogens (and therefore reducing the risk of transmitting infection to others).

Antiemetics and antidiarrhoeal drugs are discussed in Chapter 32 and 11 respectively. This chapter will concentrate on the place of antibiotic therapy in gastrointestinal infections.

Antibiotic therapy

The requirement for antibiotic treatment in gastrointestinal infection depends on both the causative agent and the syndrome that it causes. There is no effective treatment for some gastrointestinal pathogens such as *Cryptosporidium* and viruses. For many other infections, such as *Campylobacter* and *Salmonella*, effective agents are available, but antimicrobial therapy is often not clinically necessary. Serious infections such as enteric fever always require antibiotic treatment.

Conditions for which antibiotic therapy is not available or not usually required

The symptoms of *Staph. aureus* and short incubation period of *B. cereus* food poisoning and botulism are usually caused by ingestion of preformed toxin and therefore antibiotic therapy would not be expected to influence the illness. Pathogens such as *C. perfringens*, *V. parahaemolyticus* and enteropathogenic *Esch. coli* usually cause a brief self-limiting illness that does not require specific treatment. Antibiotics are contraindicated in enterohaemorrhagic *Esch. coli* infection since there is some evidence that exposure of the organism to antibiotics can increase toxin production and possibly worsen the disease. None of the presently available antiviral agents are useful in viral gastroenteritis.

There is no effective anticryptosporidial agent. In healthy individuals cryptosporidiosis is self-limiting, but in the immunocompromised, severe

symptoms persisting for months can occur. If possible, immunosuppression should be stopped. Antidiarrhoeals are rarely effective and their safety is uncertain. A wide variety of antimicrobials have been tried. There are anecdotal reports of success with the macrolide antibiotic spiramycin, but these have not been confirmed in controlled trials. Spiramycin is not licenced in the UK, but is available from the manufacturer on a named patient basis. The recommended dose is 1 g three times daily orally for 14 days or longer in adults, and 50 mg/kg/day in three divided doses for children.

Conditions for which antimicrobial therapy should be considered

The place for antibiotics in the management of uncomplicated gastroenteritis due to organisms such as *Salmonella*, *Campylobacter* and *Shigella* is unresolved. Certain antibiotics are reasonably effective in reducing the duration and severity of clinical illness, and in eradicating the organisms from faeces. However, many microbiologists are cautious about the widespread use of antibiotics in diarrhoeal illness because of the risk of promoting antibiotic resistance. Another difficulty with respect to antibiotic prescribing is that it is not usually possible to determine the aetiological agent of diarrhoea on clinical grounds, and stool culture usually takes at least 48 hours.

It is probably reasonable to limit antibiotic use to patients whose symptoms are severe or worsening at the time a bacteriological diagnosis is established, and to those with severe underlying disease. Antibiotics may also be used to eliminate faecal carriage, for example in controlling troublesome outbreaks in institutions, and in food handlers who may be prevented from returning to work whilst excreting a gastrointestinal pathogen.

Campylobacter **infection.** Some studies have shown that early treatment of *Campylobacter* enteritis with erythromycin can shorten the duration of clinical illness and eliminate the organism from faeces. However, treatment which is commenced more than 72 to 96 hours into the illness is probably of little benefit. The recommended dosage for adults is 250 to 500 mg four times daily orally for 5 to 7 days, and for children, 30 to 50 mg/kg/day in four divided doses. Ciprofloxacin is highly active against *Campylobacter* in vitro, and limited clinical data suggest that it may be at least as effective as erythromycin at a dose of 500 mg twice daily orally for adults.

Salmonellosis. Until recently, there was no effective antibiotic therapy for non-invasive *Salmonella* gastroenteritis. Even agents such as amoxycillin and co-trimoxazole, which have good in vitro anti-salmonella activity, give no symptomatic improvement, and may indeed prolong faecal carriage of the organism. However, there is good evidence that the recently introduced fluoroquinolone antibiotics such as ciprofloxacin are effective in shortening both the symptomatic period and the duration of faecal carriage. The recommended dose of ciprofloxacin is 500 mg twice daily orally for 1 week. Ciprofloxacin, given intravenously at a dose of 200 mg twice daily, is probably also the treatment of choice for *Salmonella* bacteraemia. For patients in whom quinolones are contra-indicated, ampicillin or amoxycillin, co-trimoxazole, or chloramphenicol are effective in invasive infections, although resistance to these agents is not uncommon, especially in imported infections.

Enteric fever. *S. typhi* and *S. paratyphi* cause life-threatening infection for which treatment is always indicated. Chloramphenicol and ampicillin or amoxycillin have been widely used and their efficacies are well established. Resistance to these agents is less common than in other *Salmonella* species although antibiotic-resistant strains are becoming increasingly common, especially from the Indian subcontinent. Ampicillin and amoxycillin may give a slower clinical response, but chloramphenicol carries a risk of serious side effects, and may be associated with a higher relapse rate. The usual dose for chloramphenicol is 50 mg/kg/day in four divided doses for at least 2 weeks, and for ampicillin, 100 mg/kg/day in four divided doses. Although there is much less clinical experience with the fluoroquinolone antibiotics, ciprofloxacin appears to be at least as effective as the traditional

agents, and many would now regard it as the drug of choice in enteric fever, at least in adults. The dose is 200 mg twice daily intravenously, or 500 mg twice daily orally.

Chronic carriers of *Salmonella*. Patients may become chronic carriers after *Salmonella* infection, especially in the presence of underlying biliary tract disease. Oral amoxycillin 3 g twice daily, or ciprofloxacin 500 to 750 mg twice daily continued for up to 6 weeks is often effective in eradicating carriage. In patients with gallbladder disease, cholecystectomy is usually effective when medical treatment fails.

Shigellosis. *Shigella sonnei*, which accounts for most cases of shigellosis in the UK, usually causes a mild self-limiting illness. Other *Shigella* species, however, tend to cause more severe symptoms. Although antibiotic therapy for *Shigella* infection is often not required on clinical grounds, because shigellosis is much more easily transmitted from patient to patient than many other gastrointestinal infections, a strong case can be made for antibiotic treatment in order to eliminate faecal carriage of the organism. A number of antibiotics, including ampicillin or amoxycillin, co-trimoxazole and tetracycline, are effective, but resistance to these agents is common in many developing nations. The fluoroquinolone antibiotics are also highly effective in shigellosis and resistance is rare. However, in the UK most *Shigella* infections occur in children, in whom quinolones are contra-indicated. A quinolone antibiotic, such as ciprofloxacin 500 mg twice daily by mouth for 5 days is the recommended treatment for shigellosis in adults. Alternatives include amoxycillin 250 to 500 mg three times daily in adults or 125 mg three times daily in children, or co-trimoxazole 960 mg twice daily in adults or 60 mg/kg/day in two divided doses for children.

Cholera. Fluid and electrolyte replacement is much the most important aspect of the treatment of cholera. However, antibiotics do shorten the duration of diarrhoea, and therefore reduce overall fluid loss. Tetracycline 250 mg four times daily by mouth for 5 days is the most widely used treatment, but is contra-indicated in childhood and during pregnancy. Other effective agents include ampicillin, co-trimoxazole and ciprofloxacin.

Esch. coli infections. Antibiotic therapy for enterotoxigenic *Esch. coli* infection is usually not necessary, but troublesome symptoms will respond to a short course of a variety of antibiotics, including ciprofloxacin and co-trimoxazole. Ciprofloxacin is probably the treatment of choice for enteroinvasive *Esch. coli* infection. The place for antibiotic treatment of enterohaemorrhagic *Esch. coli* infection has yet to be established.

C. difficile infection. In antibiotic-associated diarrhoea, antibiotic therapy should if possible be stopped. In mild cases that may be all that is necessary. Oral vancomycin, 125 to 500 mg four times daily for at least 1 week is probably the most effective treatment for pseudomembranous colitis. Vancomycin is poorly absorbed from the gut and therefore it is non-toxic, even in patients with renal failure, and high concentrations are achieved in the colonic lumen. Vancomycin can be given by nasogastric tube or enema when conventional oral administration is impossible. The main disadvantage of vancomycin is cost, therefore oral metronidazole 400 mg three times daily is often preferred in patients with less severe *C. difficile* infection. Although most strains of *C. difficile* are sensitive to metronidazole, it is well absorbed from the small gut, and colonic levels may not be sufficient. There is some clinical evidence that metronidazole is less effective than vancomycin.

Recurrence of symptoms occurs in 10 to 20% of patients treated for *C. difficile* infection. Recurrences are probably usually due to germination of spores that have persisted in the colon since the original infection, but may sometimes be due to reinfection. Most recurrences respond to a further course of treatment with vancomycin or metronidazole, but a few patients relapse repeatedly. No reliable means of treating these patients is known, but there are anecdotal reports of success with a variety of regimens, such as long courses of vancomycin or metronidazole followed by gradual tapering of the dose, or several short periods of treatment (5 to 7 days) alternating with similar periods of non-treatment.

Giardiasis. Metronidazole is the treatment of choice for giardiasis. Various oral dosage regimens are effective, e.g. 400 mg three times daily for 7 days, 800 mg three times daily for 5 days, or 2 g/day for 3 days. In children the recommended dose is 7.5 mg/kg three times daily for 7 days. Short-course high-dose regimens may be less effective, and are often poorly tolerated due to nausea and vomiting. Alternative agents to metronidazole include tinidazole 2 g as a single dose, or mepacrine hydrochloride 100 mg three times daily for 5 to 7 days. A single course of treatment for giardiasis has a failure rate of up to 10%. A further course of the same or another agent is often successful. Sometimes repeated relapses are due to reinfection from an asymptomatic family member. In such cases all affected family members should be treated simultaneously.

Amoebiasis. The aim of treatment in amoebiasis is to kill all vegetative amoebae and also to eradicate cysts from the bowel lumen. Metronidazole is highly active against vegetative amoebae, and is the treatment of choice for acute amoebic dysentery and amoebic liver abscess. The dose for adults is 800 mg three times daily for 5 to 10 days and for children, 7.5 mg/kg three times daily. In order to eradicate cysts, metronidazole therapy should be followed by a 5-day course of diloxanide furoate 500 mg three times daily. Asymptomatic excretors of cysts living in areas with a high prevalence of *E. histolytica* infection do not merit treatment because most individuals would quickly become reinfected. However, asymptomatic excretors of cysts in Europe and North America are usually treated with diloxanide fuorate 500 mg three times daily for 5 to 10 days, sometimes combined with metronidazole.

Control of cross-infection

Persons excreting gastrointestinal pathogens are potentially infectious to others. Liquid stools are particularly likely to contaminate the hands and the environment. All cases of gastrointestinal infection should be excluded from work or school at least until the patient is symptom free.

Patients should be advised on general hygiene, and in particular on thorough hand washing and drying after going to the toilet, and before handling food.

In general follow-up stool specimens and screening of asymptomatic contacts of the patient are not clinically necessary, but such samples may be required for other reasons. Doctors have a statutory duty to report all cases of cholera, dysentery, enteric fever, and food poisoning or suspected food poisoning to the public health authorities.

The requirement for contact screening or follow-up clearance stool specimens will normally be judged by public health doctors. For example, certain groups of individuals are at particular risk of transmitting infection, viz. food handlers, health-care and nursery staff, children attending preschool nurseries, and older children or adults who are unable to maintain good standards of personal hygiene, for example because of mental handicap. It may be necessary to demonstrate clearance of the pathogen after infection in individuals belonging to these groups. Similarly, individuals belonging to one of these groups who are household contacts of a case of gastro-intestinal infection may need to be screened in order to ensure that they too are not infected.

CASE STUDIES

CASE 35.1

Three patients in a psychogeriatric ward develop diarrhoea due to *Salmonella typhimurium* which is traced to cold roast beef served at dinner on the previous day. 7 days later another patient develops diarrhoea, from whom the same serotype of *Salmonella* is isolated. Screening of the asymptomatic patients reveals that two are excreting the same organism.

Q1 How do you think the fourth person to develop diarrhoea became infected?

Q2 Do antibiotics have any place in managing this outbreak?

CASE 35.2

An 80-year-old woman is admitted to hospital as an emergency with profuse diarrhoea, fever and abdominal pain. 1 week earlier she had been treated by her general practitioner with cefuroxime axetil for a urinary tract infection. Sigmoidoscopy shows pseudomembranes adherent to the rectal mucosa. She has moderate renal impairment.

Q1 How should she be managed?

Q2 Does her renal impairment influence your choice of antibiotic?

CASE 35.3

A 30-year-old man presents with a 3-day history of abdominal pain, fever and bloody diarrhoea. He has been taking ranitidine for 1 month, after being diagnosed as having a duodenal ulcer. 2 days prior to the onset of symptoms he and his family had dined at a Chinese restaurant where they had all eaten chicken, shellfish and rice. The rest of the family were asymptomatic. A faeces specimen is sent to the laboratory, and 3 days later it is reported that *Campylobacter* has been isolated. By this time the patient's fever and abdominal pain have settled, although his diarrhoea persists.

Q1 Which food was the most likely source of this infection?

Q2 Why might this individual have been infected while the rest of his family remained well?

Q3 Would you recommend antibiotic treatment after receiving the faeces culture result?

ANSWERS TO CASE STUDIES

CASE 35.1

A Environmental soiling due to poor personal hygiene is common in psychogeriatric wards and may lead to cross-infection. In this case it is likely that the fourth person acquired infection from one of the other patients. Quinolone antibiotics such as ciprofloxacin have been shown to be effective in eradicating faecal carriage of *Salmonella*. In this situation it would seem sensible to treat all the patients who are excreting the organism.

CASE 35.2

A The treatment of choice for pseudomembranous colitis is oral vancomycin. If the patient is severely dehydrated, intravenous fluids may be required. Cross-infection with *C. difficile* can occur in hospitals, therefore the patient should be nursed in isolation. Vancomycin is not significantly absorbed from the gastrointestinal tract and can safely be given orally without dose adjustment, even in severe renal failure.

CASE 35.3

A Both shellfish (*V. parahaemolyticus* and viruses) and rice (*B. cereus*) can transmit food poisoning. However *Campylobacter* is most likely to have originated from the chicken. Through taking ranitidine, which inhibits gastric acid production, this individual may have been more susceptible to gastrointestinal infection than the rest of his family. By the time that the faeces culture result was available, the patient had been unwell for 6 days, and he appeared to be recovering. Antibiotic treatment in this instance would be unlikely to give any benefit, and is therefore not indicated.

BIBLIOGRAPHY

Ashkenazi S, Cleary T G. Antibiotic treatment of bacterial gastroenteritis. Pediatric Infectious Diseases Journal 1991; 10: 140–148

Asperilla M O, Smego R A Jr, Scott L K. Quinolone antibiotics in the treatment of salmonella infections. Review of Infectious Diseases 1990; 12: 873–889

Gorbach S L. Bacterial diarrhoea and its treatment. Lancet 1987; ii: 1378–1382

Mandal B K. Modern treatment of typhoid fever. Journal of Infection 1991; 22: 1–4

Mandell G L, Douglas R G Jr, Bennett J E (eds). Principles and practice of infectious diseases, 3rd edn. New York: Churchill Livingstone 1990

Pithie A D, Wood M J. Treatment of typhoid fever and infectious diarrhoea with ciprofloxacin. Journal of Antimicrobial Chemotherapy 1990; 26 (Suppl. F): 47–53

Salam M A, Bennish M L. Antimicrobial therapy for shigellosis. Review of Infectious Diseases 1991; 13 (Suppl. 4): S332–S341

Shanson D C. Microbiology in clinical practice, 2nd edn. London: Wright 1989

Chapter 36

Infective meningitis

H. R. Ingham

The brain and spinal cord are surrounded by three membranes which from without inwards are the dura mater, the arachnoid mater and the pia mater. Between the arachnoid mater and the pia mater, in the subarachnoid space, is to be found the cerebrospinal fluid (CSF) (Fig. 36.1). This fluid, of which there is approximately 150 ml in a normal adult, is secreted by the choroid plexuses, vascular structures which are in the third, fourth and lateral ventricles. CSF passes from the ventricles via communicating apertures to the subarachnoid space whence it flows over the surface of the brain and the spinal cord (Fig. 36.1). The amount of CSF is controlled by resorption into the bloodstream by vascular structures in the subarachnoid space called the arachnoid villi.

Infective meningitis is an inflammation of the arachnoid and the pia mater associated with the presence of microorganisms, including bacteria, viruses, fungi and parasites, in the CSF.

AETIOLOGY AND EPIDEMIOLOGY

Currently there are approximately 2000 cases of bacterial meningitis reported in the United Kingdom per annum (Table 36.1) Over all age groups the commonest causes are *Neisseria meningitidis*, *Haemophilus influenzae* type b and *Streptococcus pneumoniae*. *H. influenzae* type b is the commonest cause of meningitis in children between the ages of 3 months and 5 years. It is very uncommonly incriminated in meningitis in

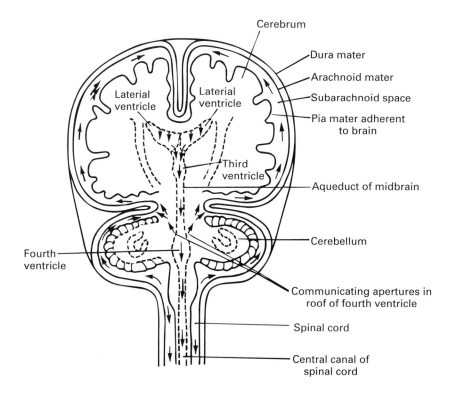

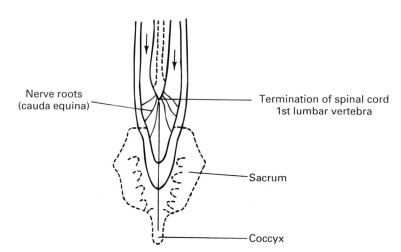

Fig. 36.1 The meninges covering the brain and spinal cord and the flow of cerebrospinal fluid (arrowed). (Modified from Ross & Wilson 1981, by permission of Churchill Livingstone.)

Table 36.1 Laboratory reports of bacterial meningitis in England and Wales 1990 (Information provided by the Public Health Laboratory Service Communicable Disease Surveillance Centre, London NW9 5EQ)

Organism	Number of isolates
Neisseria meningitidis	876 plus 12 clinical (no isolate)
Haemophilus influenzae type b	528 (366)*
Streptococcus pneumoniae	345
Streptococcus group B	72
Other streptococci	40
Staphylococcus aureus	55
Coagulase negative staphylococci	43
Salmonella spp.	3
Listeria spp.	22
Pasteurella spp.	2
Mycobacterium tuberculosis	17
Escherichia coli	46
Other Gram-negative bacilli	48
Aerococcus spp.	1
Bacteroides spp.	1
Capnocytophaga spp.	1
Clostridium spp.	1
Corynebacterium spp.	3
Anaerobic streptococci	1
Propionibacterium spp.	5
	2110

*Proved by serotyping.

adults, presumably due to the development of immunity. Other causative organisms are Group B streptococci, *Staphylococcus aureus*, *Listeria monocytogenes*, *Escherichia coli*, *Mycobacterium tuberculosis* (although this is rare today) and miscellaneous organisms. Even with modern antibiotic therapy some patients still die and up to 50% of survivors have neurological sequelae. The infections due to the commoner causes of meningitis are usually acquired from other individuals who are most often transient carriers.

In many instances meningitis occurs as an isolated event but sometimes there may be secondary cases which in infections due to *N. meningitidis* have resulted in epidemics. Meningitis due to *Strep. pneumoniae* may occur as the result of local spread from infected sites such as the middle ear or paranasal air sinuses or secondary to trauma involving fracture of the base of the skull, in which case it may be recurrent. Many cases of meningitis due to this organism

probably arise as the result of nasopharyngeal colonization with subsequent spread to the meninges or are secondary to septicaemic spread from other infected foci such as the lungs.

Meningitis due to group B streptococci is almost always seen in young infants and results from either infection from the mother who is carrying the organism in her vagina or occasionally from carriers in the environment. Similarly *L. monocytogenes* may cause meningitis in young infants but is also implicated in meningitis in adults, some of whom may be immunocompromised. Meningitis due to *Staph. aureus* may be secondary to trauma, surgery, spread from local infective lesions or metastatic spread, including infective endocarditis. Many organisms which cause meningitis, e.g. *H. influenzae* type b, *N. meningitidis*, *Strep. pneumoniae*, *Esch. coli* K1 and group B streptococci have surface properties and antiphagocytic capsules which allow them to adhere to and penetrate the mucosal surfaces at the primary site of infection and avoid the natural defences of the host.

In the case of tuberculous meningitis the infection either arises as the results of recrudescence of a previous infection in the patient or is contracted from another individual with active tuberculosis who is excreting tubercle bacilli.

Uncommonly meningitis is caused by the yeast *Cryptococcus neoformans*. This organism is present in pigeon droppings and sites inhabited by such birds. It is likely that many people are subject to respiratory exposure to this organism but progressive disease is rare in normal individuals. Those most at risk include patients with underlying malignant disease, those receiving systemic corticosteroids or the immunosuppressed. Cryptococcosis in the latter group has been thrown into prominence by the advent of AIDS.

PATHOPHYSIOLOGY

Bacteria reach the meninges by a number of routes:

- via venous vascular communications from the nasopharynx
- from the bloodstream
- via abnormal communications with the skin

or mucous membranes, e.g. skull fractures, anatomical defects or a meningocoele

- spread from an infected adjacent focus such as a brain abscess, tuberculoma, an infected paranasal air sinus or infection of the middle ear.

Once in the subarachnoid space the infection spreads widely. The cerebral tissue is not usually directly involved although cerebral abscess may complicate some types of meningitis. There is oedema and congestion of the brain and there may be a cortical thrombophlebitis with infarction of the related brain. The presence of exudate may damage cranial nerves and hydrocephalus may result from obstruction of the flow of CSF.

At one time it was thought that the pathophysiological changes seen in meningitis were directly due to virulence factors associated with the causative bacteria. Currently the view is that the host response to the release of toxic bacterial products, which may be increased by exposure to antibiotics, is important in the development of the pathological changes seen in this condition. These toxic products act directly on endothelial cells increasing vascular permeability. Macrophages and microglial cells also release cytokines such as interleukin and tumour necrosis factor which augment the inflammatory response. Other substances such as prostaglandin and platelet activating factor are released by platelets. The net effect of all these processes is disruption of the blood–brain barrier, obstruction of vessels, cerebral oedema, impairment of CSF flow with consequent rise in intracranial pressure, loss of autoregulation of cerebral blood flow and reduced brain perfusion. The microbial products which are concerned in the cytokine cascade include pneumococcal peptidoglycan and teichoic acid, cell wall oligosaccharide from *H. influenzae* and cell wall lipid A (endotoxin) in Gram-negative bacteria. Many features of the inflammatory response can be reproduced by the administration of endotoxin in experimental animals.

CLINICAL MANIFESTATIONS

Sudden onset of fever, generalized headache, vomiting, stiff neck and photophobia are com-

monly seen in acute meningitis. There may be evidence of concomitant infection in primary foci such as the respiratory tract or middle ear. If untreated the condition deteriorates with obtundation and loss of consciousness.

There is usually evidence of meningeal irritation with stiff neck, and a positive Kernig's sign (resistance to extension of the leg when the hip is flexed). There may be seizures, focal cerebral signs such as hemiparesis, difficulty with speech, visual field defects and cranial nerve palsies including loss of hearing. Neurological defects often disappear as the patient recovers but residual damage is seen in some patients.

In infants the physical signs are less specific and include fever, diarrhoea, jaundice, lethargy, feeding difficulties, respiratory distress, seizures, bulging fontanelles and rigidity of the neck.

Bleeding into the skin in the form of either pinpoint lesions – petechiae – or large lesions – purpura or ecchymoses – is most commonly seen with meningococcal meningitis. More rarely, it occurs in other forms of bacterial meningitis.

Although tuberculous meningitis may present with a short onset and signs and symptoms typical of acute meningitis, more commonly the history is longer and there are usually general symptoms such as malaise, apathy and anorexia. As the disease progresses signs more typical of meningitis usually appear.

INVESTIGATIONS

Cerebrospinal fluid is obtained by inserting a needle between the posterior aspect of the 3rd and 4th lumbar vertebrae into the subarachnoid space. Alternatively the sample may be derived by inserting a needle just below the posterior aspect of the base of the skull into an enlargement of the subarachnoid space known as the cisterna magna.

In health the CSF is a clear colourless fluid which in the lumbar region of the spinal cord is at a pressure of 50 to 150 mm of water. There are up to 5 lymphocytes per μL, the protein concentration is up to 0.4 g/L, and glucose is present at a concentration of 2.2 to 4.4 mmol/L (or 60% of the blood sugar). In meningitis the CSF pressure is increased and in the acute pyogenic form of the disease the cell count is usually grossly elevated reaching levels of several hundreds or thousands per µL, nearly all of which are polymorphonuclear leucocytes. The CSF protein is increased and the CSF glucose is reduced to less than half that of a simultaneously obtained blood glucose. Organisms are usually visible in Gram-stained smears and may be present in large numbers. Occasionally in acute pyogenic meningitis the cell count may be only marginally elevated and few or no organisms may be seen. Various methods have been employed for the detection of bacterial antigen in CSF; these include countercurrent electrophoresis, latex particle agglutination and enzyme linked immunosorbent assay. Such techniques have been used with varying degrees of success and are potentially more useful when the patient has received prior chemotherapy which may prevent isolation of the aetiological agent. Culture of the CSF often yields the causative organism. Blood culture, which forms an essential component of the investigation of acute bacterial meningitis, often yields positive results.

Viral meningitis is characterized by a lymphocytic response, an elevated protein and almost invariably a normal glucose level.

In tuberculous and cryptococcal meningitis, and the now very rare syphilitic meningitis, the cell count is not as grossly elevated and there is a mixed cellular response often with lymphocytes predominating. Occasionally in tuberculous meningitis a typical polymorphonuclear response may be seen. In tuberculous and cryptococcal meningitis the CSF protein is elevated and glucose is usually reduced. In tuberculous meningitis organisms may be present in small numbers and not visualized by microscopy but demonstrable by culture. Similarly cryptococci may only be seen in about 50% of cases, diagnosis depending on culture or demonstration of specific antibody and antigen in CSF and serum.

DRUG TREATMENT

The antimicrobial therapy of meningitis requires the attainment of adequate levels of bactericidal agents within the CSF. The passage of antimicrobial agents from the blood into the CSF is affected by the blood–brain barrier. The majority of foreign substances enter the CSF by the choroid plexus but an alternative route is via the capillaries of the central nervous system into the extracellular fluid and thence into the ventricles and subarachnoid space.

The choroidal epithelium is highly impermeable to lipid-insoluble molecules and the passage of antibiotics into the CSF is dependent upon the following:

- lipid solubility
- ionic dissocation at blood pH
- protein binding
- molecular size
- concentration of the drug in the serum
- degree of meningeal inflammation.

Antimicrobials fall into three categories according to their ability to pass into the CSF:

- those that penetrate even when the meninges are not inflamed, e.g. chloramphenicol, metronidazole, isoniazid and pyrazinamide
- those that generally only penetrate when the meninges are inflamed and when used in high dosage, e.g. benzylpenicillin, ampicillin, flucloxacillin, the more recent cephalosporins, the quinolones and rifampicin
- those penetrating poorly under all circumstances, e.g. aminoglycosides, the earlier cephalosporins, erythromycin, clindamycin, fusidic acid and vancomycin.

The chemotherapy of acute bacterial meningitis requires the administration of large doses of appropriate antimicrobials by the intravenous route. The likely microbial pathogen may be indicated by the clinical presentation and the results of examination of a Gram-stained smear of CSF.

Pneumococcal and meningococcal meningitis

In adults the usual treatment of pneumococcal and meningococcal meningitis is intravenous penicillin, initially 1.2 g every 2 to 3 hours, therapy being continued for about 10 days.

A small number of strains of *Strep. pneumoniae* have been reported in various parts of the world which show high-level resistance to benzylpenicillin and chloramphenicol. A number of patients with meningitis due to such strains have shown a high mortality even with high-dose penicillin. Although these strains are relatively uncommon and should therefore not influence the standard therapy of this condition, alternative regimens may be indicated where such strains are encountered, e.g. South Africa and Spain, and certainly need to be employed in any instance where isolates from a patient with meningitis are shown to be resistant. Alternative treatments which have been suggested include vancomycin, the third generation cephalosporins such as cefotaxime and ceftriaxone and rifampicin. Because of concern over limited penetration of vancomycin into the CSF the agent has been given in some patients intrathecally in a dose of 10 to 20 mg daily, apparently without side effects. Resistance to penicillin has also occasionally been reported in *N. meningitidis*. Some of these strains have harboured beta-lactamase-producing plasmids, and thus destroyed penicillin by enzymic action, but most have been beta-lactamase negative and thus inherently resistant to the agent. Alternative therapy in patients infected with such strains has included chloramphenicol or cefotaxime.

Meningitis caused by other organisms

The presence of *Listeria*, as suggested by Gram-positive rods in a stained smear, or as proven by culture, is an indication for the use of ampicillin therapy in large doses, e.g. 2 g, 4-hourly in an adult. There is experimental evidence that the addition of gentamicin to this regimen may be beneficial.

Treatment of meningitis due to other organisms such as *Escherichia coli*, *Proteus* spp., *Pseudomonas* spp. and anaerobic bacteria requires careful clinical and microbiological assessment of the problem in individual patients and the use of appropriate agents. In some instances third generation cephalosporins such as ceftazidime may be indicated, as in meningitis due to *Pseudomonas* spp.; in yet other situations antimicrobial combinations may be required. An example of this is seen in meningitis associated with chronic suppurative otitis media in which a mixture of organisms may be present, often including, *Proteus* spp. and anaerobic bacteria. In this situation an agent active against anaerobes, such as metronidazole, will need to be included in the therapeutic regimen.

Neonates and children

In neonates presenting with meningitis the wide range of organisms which may be encountered, as previously discussed, requires the initial use of broad spectrum chemotherapy. In many centres a standard regimen which has been used in this situation is ampicillin and gentamicin. The use of the latter agent requires monitoring of blood levels both to ascertain adequacy of dosage and to avoid excessive serum concentrations which can cause renal impairment and vestibular damage. Such a regimen is inherently cost effective even when the additional expenditure on assays is taken into account.

Some authorities have employed third generation cephalosporins as alternatives to gentamicin in this age group. Examples of the agents employed are cefotaxime and ceftazidime (Table 36.2). Evidence to date suggests that these new agents are as efficacious as those in routine use. This of course eliminates any risk of toxicity due to the use of gentamicin and the cost of assaying this agent. Disadvantages of prescribing third generation cephalosporins include cost – they are substantially more expensive than standard agents even allowing for the expense of gentamicin assay – and the possibility that their extensive use in the close environment of a neonatal intensive care unit may result in the selection of multidrug-resistant Gram-negative organisms which may pose a cross-infection risk.

The initial blind treatment of meningitis in infants and children up to the age of 3 years must take into account the possible presence of *H. influenzae* type b as this organism is not susceptible to penicillin. Before the introduction of the semisynthetic penicillins the initial therapy

Table 36.2 Recommended antibiotic regimens for initial treatment of meningitis in children of different age groups (modified from Levin & Heyderman (1991) with permission)

Age group	Drug	Dose/day	
		0–7 days	7–28 days
Neonates	Ampicillin	150 mg/kg	200 mg/kg
	and		
	Gentamicin	5 mg/kg	7.5 mg/kg
	or		
	Ampicillin	150 mg/kg	200 mg/kg
	and either		
	Cefotaxime	100 mg/kg	150–200 mg/kg
	or		
	Ceftazidime	60 mg/kg	90 mg/kg
Infants 1 month to 3 months	Ampicillin	200 mg/kg	
	and		
	Cefotaxime	200 mg/kg	
Older infants and children	Ampicillin	300 mg/kg	
	and		
	Chloramphenicol	75–100 mg/kg	
	or		
	Cefuroxime	240 mg/kg	
	or		
	3rd generation cephalosporin:		
	Cefotaxime	200 mg/kg	
	or		
	Ceftriaxone	100 mg/kg	

of choice in this group of patients was chloramphenicol. Subsequently ampicillin was shown to be as effective. With reports of strains of *H. influenzae* type b resistant to ampicillin it became common practice to initiate therapy with a combination of ampicillin and chloramphenicol until the organism and its sensitivity were known. More recently strains of *H. influenzae* type b resistant to both ampicillin and chloramphenicol have been reported. Partly because of this and concern about side effects associated with the use of chloramphenicol, namely marrow aplasia (actually extremely uncommon), and a condition of circulatory collapse known as the 'grey syndrome' in infants, it has been suggested that a third generation cephalosporin be used as the sole initial therapy in these patients (Table 36.2). Table 36.3 shows the CSF concentrations achieved

Table 36.3 CSF concentrations achieved in meningitis and minimum inhibitory concentration of susceptible pathogens to antibiotics (modified from Levin & Heyderman (1991) with permission)

	Peak CSF level (µg/ml) (% penetration)	Minimum inhibitory concentration (µg/ml) (ratio: CSF concentration/MIC)		
		N. meningitidis	*H. influenzae*	*S. pneumoniae*
Penicillin	1.5 (<6%)	0.02 (75)	0.5 (3)	0.02 (75)
Ampicillin	9.9 (15%)	0.02 (495)	0.25 (40)	0.05 (198)
Chloramphenicol	15.0 (65%)	1.0 (15)	1.0 (15)	2.5 (6)
Cefuroxime	18.8 (13%)	0.04 (470)	0.38 (49)	0.03 (627)
Cefotaxime	10.0 (4%)	0.01 (1000)	0.06 (167)	0.25 (40)
Ceftriaxone	13.7 (7%)	0.01 (1370)	0.06 (228)	0.12 (114)
Ceftazidime	7.4 (>15%)	0.01 (740)	0.06 (123)	2.0 (3.7)

in meningitis and the minimal inhibitory concentrations of a range of susceptible pathogens to antibiotics. It can be seen from this table that cefotaxime, ceftazidime and ceftriaxone are the most active in this respect against *N. meningitidis* and *H. influenzae* and cefotaxime and ceftriaxone are also very active against *Strep. pneumoniae*. Cefuroxime, although also very active, appears in clinical trials not to sterilize the CSF as quickly and to give a poorer clinical end result than the third generation cephalosporins. Ceftriaxone, the most potent of these agents, has only recently been licensed for use in the United Kingdom. Gastrointestinal effects are common with this agent.

Antimicrobials were at one time given to some patients intrathecally in the treatment of meningitis with the intention of supplementing levels attained by concomitant systemic therapy, especially of agents such as gentamicin which penetrate poorly into the CSF. This practice gradually waned as it became apparent that systemic therapy alone was as effective as combination treatment. Extension of infection to the ventricles is a much feared complication of meningitis and as intrathecal administration has been shown to produce only low levels in the ventricle, direct administration has been employed. Some studies have produced good results by this method but others have shown that the technique may adversely affect the outcome in the therapy of Gram-negative infections. Despite these conflicting results there is a view that intraventricular therapy has a place in the treatment of certain types of ventriculitis. One instance where this applies is where the infecting organism is only sensitive to agents which do not penetrate well into the CSF, e.g. aminoglycosides and vancomycin. Such organisms include coagulase-negative staphylococci in patients with ventriculo-peritoneal shunts. These shunts are valved tubes which are used as permanent drains in patients with hydrocephalus. They can become colonized with coagulase-negative staphylococci with the resultant development of ventriculitis. The onset of this complication usually requires removal of the shunt. Sometimes this manoeuvre plus systemic chemotherapy is suffi-

cient to eradicate the infection but in other cases local instillation of antimicrobials is necessary. The dosages of various agents which may be given by the intraventricular route are shown in Table 36.4.

Treatment of patients with meningitis due to *N. meningitidis* or *H. influenzae* type b with any of the regimens above discussed does not regularly eradicate nasopharyngeal carriage and therapy should be completed with a course of rifampicin for this purpose.

The role of steroids

In pharmacological doses adrenal corticosteroids regulate many components of the inflammatory response and also lower CSF hydrostatic pressure. The role of these agents in acute non-tuberculous meningitis remains unclear. In one recent study patients with meningitis receiving dexamethasone, in addition to antibiotics, showed higher CSF glucose concentrations and lower concentrations of lactate and protein, lower leucocyte counts at 24 hours and became afebrile sooner than controls not receiving steroids. There was also a reduced incidence of neurological deficits in some of these patients, in particular moderate to severe hearing loss. In a further study no effect was seen on CSF concentrations of lactate and glucose or on the leucocyte count at 24 to 36 hours but mortality was reduced in some patients receiving steroids; again hearing loss was reduced in these patients. A recent recommendation has been that dexamethasone may

Table 36.4 Dose of intraventricular antibiotics			
Antibiotics	Dose(s) in mg daily*		
	Adult	Child	Infant (<2 yr)
Gentamicin	5	2.5	1
Netilmicin	2–3 t.d.s.	†	0.4–0.5 t.d.s.
Amikacin	20	2–3	†
Vancomycin	20	10	10

*All doses are daily doses except where specified three times daily (t.d.s.).
† = Data not available

reasonably be given to those with severe meningitis and in particular those comatose with *H. influenzae* infection.

Antiendotoxin

The role of monoclonal antibodies specifically directed against lipid A of Gram-negative endotoxin is currently being investigated. Preliminary results suggest that the use of one such agent in meningococcal disease, where the patient is in shock, may result in a reduction in mortality.

Chemoprophylaxis

In meningococcal meningitis, spread within families and close contacts is a well-recognized phenomenon and such individuals should receive chemoprophylaxis. The dose of rifampicin in patients over 1 year old is 10 mg/kg 12-hourly for 2 days up to a maximum of 600 mg per dose. For children aged between 3 and 12 months the dose is 5 mg/kg. In adults the dose is 600 mg twice daily for 2 days. Adverse effects include interference with oral contraception, red colouration of urine, sputum and tears. An alternative agent is ceftriaxone in a single dose in adults of 250 mg i.m. and 125 mg i.m. for children under 15 years of age.

More recently chemoprophylaxis has been recommended for all household members where there is an index case of *H. influenzae* type b disease and a child less than 3 years old. Where two or more cases of disease due to *H. influenzae* type b have occurred within 120 days in playgroups, nurseries or crèches, all room contacts (both adults and children) should receive chemoprophylaxis. Exceptions include pregnant or breast-feeding women, any person with severe hepatic dysfunction and children under 3 months old. The dose of rifampicin is 20 mg/kg once daily for 4 days up to a maximum of 600 mg per day.

Tuberculous meningitis

The outcome in tuberculous meningitis, which was always fatal before the introduction of antibacterials, relates directly to the severity of the patient's clinical condition on commencement of therapy. A satisfactory response demands a high degree of clinical suspicion such that appropriate chemotherapy is initiated even if tubercle bacilli are not demonstrated by initial microscopy. Most currently used antituberculous agents achieve effective concentrations in the CSF in tuberculous meningitis. Therapy should be commenced with rifampicin (children 10 to 20 mg/kg/day; adults 10 mg/kg/day; maximum dose in both 600 mg/day), isoniazid (children 10 to 20 mg/kg/day; adults 5 mg/kg/day, maximum dose in both 300 mg/day) and pyrazinamide (children and adults 15 to 30 mg/kg/day, maximum in both 2 g/day) with the duration of therapy being at least 6 months and in some instances up to between 9 and 12 months. An alternative regimen which is recommended by the British Thoracic Society is isoniazid plus rifampicin plus pyrazinamide daily for 2 months, then isoniazid plus rifampicin for 10 months. In the early stages of tuberculous meningitis, ethambutol (children over 6 years and adults 15 to 25 mg/kg/day; maximum 2.5 g/day) and streptomycin (children 20 to 40 mg/kg/day; adults 15 mg/kg/day; maximum in both 1 g/day) diffuse reasonably well into the CSF and may be useful especially if drug resistance is detected. Usually pyrazinamide, streptomycin and ethambutol are stopped after 8 weeks (or earlier if drug toxicity ensues), isoniazid and rifampicin being continued alone. In order to prevent peripheral neuropathy due to isoniazid, pyridoxine 25 to 50 mg/day should be given. In patients with human immunodeficiency virus infection somewhat higher dosages of antituberculous drugs are employed.

If the intracranial pressure is elevated to the extent that there is a risk of brain stem herniation through the point in the skull where the spinal cord exits (the foramen magnum) it is generally conceded that steroid therapy may be beneficial by reducing cerebral oedema. The onset of hydrocephalus which is not relieved by serial lumbar puncture, administration of diuretics and osmotic agents requires surgical intervention in the form of a ventriculo-peritoneal or ventriculo-atrial shunt.

With early diagnosis and appropriate therapy the mortality in tuberculous meningitis varies between 5 to 20%. About one-third of surviving patients have some residual neurological damage such as poor mental state, hemiplegia, paraplegia or cranial nerve damage.

Cryptococcal meningitis

The agent which has most frequently been employed in the therapy of cryptococcal meningitis is amphotericin. This is given intravenously in a dose of 0.4 to 1 mg/kg/day up to a total dose of 2 g. Side effects are common and include fever, nausea, vomiting, local thrombophlebitis, anaemia, hypokalaemia and a rise in blood urea. The latter in particular may cause cessation of treatment. Combination therapy with flucytosine has enabled lower, less toxic doses of amphotericin to be used and has given as good results as treatment with amphotericin alone. Flucytosine cannot be given by itself because of the development of resistance, and when it is used in combination therapy it is necessary to monitor leucocytes and platelets as bone marrow depression may occur; assay of blood levels may be helpful in this situation. Flucytosine may be contra-indicated because in AIDS patients toxic marrow suppression and/or diarrhoea is more likely to occur in this setting. If it is given the dosage must be reduced. A recent advance in the use of amphotericin is the development of liposomal amphotericin which is much less toxic and enables higher doses to be given. A disadvantage of this agent is that it is currently extremely expensive. Occasionally where intravenous amphotericin has failed to produce a therapeutic response the drug has been given by the intrathecal route.

Other new agents include the triazoles, fluconazole and itraconazole. Fluconazole has been used successfully in the treatment of patients with AIDS who have developed cryptococcal meningitis in a dose of 400 mg once daily in adults. A particular advantage of this agent is that it can be given by mouth. It has also proved to be useful as maintenance therapy in patients with AIDS as the relapse rate in cryptococcal meningitis in such patients is very high. Itraconazole has also recently been shown to be effective in the treatment of this condition.

Treatment of cryptococcal meningitis usually needs to be carried on for at least 10 weeks and in certain immunosuppressed patients perhaps longer. The effects of therapy can be followed by serial CSF antigen titres and culture. A successful response is indicated by a reduction in titres to less than 1 in 8 and negative culture results.

CASE STUDIES

CASE 36.1

A 34-year-old woman with a chronically discharging middle ear presents with fever, headache, neck stiffness and a positive Kernig's sign. Lumbar puncture reveals 1500 WBC/μL, 98% of which are polymorphs, a low glucose and an elevated protein, together with the presence of Gram-negative rods. Culture of the CSF yields *Proteus* spp. after 24 hours.

Q How should this patient be managed?

CASE 36.2

A 3-month-old baby is admitted to hospital with suspected meningitis. Ampicillin and chloramphenicol are prescribed.

Q Why is monitoring of chloramphenicol levels desirable?

CASE 36.3

A 15-year-old boy admitted with unequivocal signs of meningitis gives a history of having sustained a head injury 6 weeks earlier and having had an intermittent nasal discharge of clear fluid since that time.

Q What is the likely causative organism and how should this patient be managed?

ANSWERS TO CASE STUDIES

CASE 36.1

A This patient clearly has bacterial meningitis and must be given appropriate 'blind' treatment immediately. Such treatment could be either ampicillin (2 g, 6-hourly), plus gentamicin (80 mg, 8-hourly), chloramphenicol (0.5 to 1 g, 6-hourly) or a third generation cephalosporin such as cefotaxime (1.5 g, 6-hourly). The history of chronic ear infection suggests the possibility of otogenic meningitis and metronidazole 500 mg 8-hourly should be prescribed to cover the possible presence of anaerobic bacteria which are commonly found in chronic suppurative otitis media (CSOM). With this in mind the culture plates should be carefully examined for the presence of anaerobic bacteria.

The presence of *Proteus* spp. in the CSF confirms the impression that the middle ear may be implicated as the source of infection, as this organism is commonly found in CSOM. Because of this great care should be taken to exclude the possibility of a coexisting brain abscess, as this is a commoner complication of CSOM than meningitis alone, and in most instances requires surgical intervention if a successful outcome is to be achieved.

CASE 36.2

A It has been shown that peak serum levels of chloramphenicol above 40 to 50 mg/L may be associated with acute toxicity in this age group. This toxicity is manifest by vomiting and abdominal distension followed by circulatory collapse, hypothermia and an ashen colour which has given rise to the term the 'grey syndrome'. It soon became apparent that the syndrome was a response to dosage with excessive amounts of chloramphenicol. Even when given in recommended dosages chloramphenicol may accumulate especially if there is either liver or kidney failure since it is largely metabolized and a small amount is normally excreted in the urine. Studies have shown that it is extremely difficult to predict the level of chloramphenicol which is achieved in an individual on standard dosage and it is therefore strongly recommended that any newborn or infant receiving such therapy should have chloramphenicol levels regularly monitored. Peak serum levels should be kept between 25 and 50 mg/L and trough levels below 10 mg/L.

It is largely because of this problem that many paediatricians now favour the use of a third generation cephalosporin in the treatment of meningitis as an alternative to chloramphenicol.

CASE 36.3

A This patient almost certainly has a fracture of the base of the skull which has penetrated to the subarachnoid space, the fluid discharge from his nose being escaping CSF. The diagnosis may be confirmed by examination of CSF obtained by lumbar puncture which will show a grossly elevated white cell count (most of the cells being polymorphs) low glucose and raised protein. The organism most commonly implicated in this condition is *Streptococcus pneumoniae*. This organism is rarely resistant to penicillin in the United Kingdom and the treatment of choice is benzylpenicillin 1.2 g every 2 hours. If treated in the early stages of the disease a satisfactory outcome is likely. Where the disease has existed for longer periods of time there is still a significant mortality even with modern chemotherapy. After cessation of therapy it is usually the practice to prescribe chemoprophylactic penicillin V 500 mg every 6 hours. If the CSF leak continues over a period of weeks or if there is a recurrence of meningitis, operative intervention may be required to repair the breach.

BIBLIOGRAPHY

Finch R G, Mandragos C. Corticosteroids in bacterial meningitis. British Medical Journal 1991; 302: 607–608

Holdiness M R. Management of tuberculous meningitis. Practical Therapeutics 1990; 39: 224–233

Iwarson S (ed). Management of bacterial meningitis and septicaemia in children. Role of antibiotics, immunoglobulins and corticosteroids. Scandinavian Journal of Infectious Diseases 1990; (Suppl. 73): 1–56

Kucers A, Bennett N McK. The use of antibiotics, 4th edn. London: Heinemann 1987

Lambert H P (ed). Kass handbook of infectious diseases. Infections of the central nervous system. London: Edward Arnold 1991

Levin M, Heyderman R S. Bacterial meningitis. In: David P J (ed) Recent advances in paediatrics. London: Churchill Livingstone 1991; vol 9: 1–19

Ross J S, Wilson K J W. Revised by Kathleen J W Wilson. Foundations of anatomy and physiology, 5th edn. Edinburgh: Churchill Livingstone 1981; 172–173

Chapter 37

Surgical antibiotic prophylaxis

P. J. Marsh   S. J. Pedler

Postoperative infection constitutes a threat to the successful outcome of a surgical procedure, and the use of antibiotics to prevent infection is the subject of this chapter. Despite extensive research, much remains obscure in this complex and still evolving field.

The vast majority of surgical infections are bacterial and discussion will be confined to these. Wound, urinary and respiratory tract infections all occur and are associated with significant morbidity and even death. Wound infection can delay or prevent healing and is associated with cellulitis, abscess formation, wound dehiscence and septicaemia. Infections of prosthetic materials and devices result in their failure and the result can be catastrophic for the patient. Procedures on the urinary tract and nearby structures may be followed by urinary infection and septicaemia. Postoperative chest infections are related to the use of general anaesthesia and prior respiratory disease, but they have not proven susceptible to antibiotic prophylaxis and will not be discussed further.

The clinical and financial costs are enormous. Antibiotic therapy, surgical intervention or both may be necessary and hospital stay prolonged. Following discharge full recovery may be delayed, and demands on the hospital and community services are consequently increased.

DEFINITIONS, THEORY AND PRACTICE

Surgical antibiotic prophylaxis is intended to

prevent postoperative infection. The term implies the absence of infection prior to surgery but the distinction between extended prophylaxis and treatment can be less than clear cut as in some instances of colorectal or trauma surgery. In the absence of detailed understanding such uncertainty must remain.

A definition of postoperative infection might be given as 'an adverse effect resulting from the action of microorganisms in relation to the performance of a surgical procedure' but in practice the adverse effects must be specified. Definitions and manifestations become synonymous. Some are specific to a given procedure, such as infection of a hip prosthesis, while others are more general, e.g. an abscess in a skin wound. While gross surgical wound infection is unmistakable, milder forms present difficulties. For example, redness of the skin around a wound need not be due to infection. One approach to measuring the impact of postoperative infection is to assess the number and cost of courses of antibiotic therapy, duration of hospital stay, etc. Such information has the advantages of being readily available and numerical in form. In addition, it is independent of diagnostic and therapeutic criteria provided that these are applied uniformly.

PATHOGENESIS

Attention has focused primarily on surgical wound infections, not least because these are most accessible to study. Other forms of postoperative infection are less well understood. In outline, organisms deposited in a wound respond to their new environment and begin to multiply. Local immune defences (complement, immunoglobulins, iron-binding proteins) oppose these activities and act to destroy the organisms. The outcome of the encounter is determined in the first few hours, the 'early decisive period'. The numbers of organisms inoculated and their virulence, including the capacity for synergy between different organisms in mixed infections, are clearly of importance as is the competence of the host defences. Failure of the defences during this time permits the organisms to establish themselves and a clinical wound infection oc-

curs. Rapid growth of a population of virulent organisms manifests itself in a few days, but formation of a biofilm of relatively avirulent organisms on a prosthetic joint surface can take months to become apparent.

Models for some aspects, such as bacterial sensing of the environment, have been described in molecular detail but much remains to be learned of the pathophysiology of wound infection. Despite this basic ignorance, clinically useful observations have been made and these continue to be extended and refined.

RISK FACTORS

A number of factors are associated with an increased risk of surgical wound infection. They pertain to the nature and numbers of microorganisms introduced into the tissues (Table 37.1) or the general (Table 37.2) or local (Table 37.3) ability of the body to deal with them. Some are intrinsic to the patient, some to the surgeon and some to the procedure. Their effects on the probability of surgical wound infection are cumulative.

Table 37.1 Association of wound infections with degree of contamination of a procedure

In the early 1960s a classification of surgical procedures according to the likelihood of contamination by microorganisms was devised. It has been widely used in its original and subsequently modified forms. A simplified version is given here with approximate infection rates in brackets.

Clean
Respiratory, alimentary, biliary and genitourinary tracts not entered; no inflammation encountered (2%)

Clean-contaminated
Respiratory, alimentary, biliary or genitourinary tracts entered without significant spillage and in the absence of infected bile or urine (10%)

Contaminated
Gross spillage from the alimentary tract or entrance into the biliary or genitourinary tract in the presence of infected bile or urine; or non-purulent inflammation encountered (20%)

Dirty
Faecal contamination due to perforated viscus; or pus encountered (40%)

Table 37.2 General risk factors for postoperative infection
Advanced age
Malnutrition
Obesity
Concurrent infection
Diabetes mellitus
Liver impairment
Renal impairment
Immune deficiency states
Length of preoperative stay
Prolonged operation time
Blood transfusion

Table 37.3 Local risk factors for postoperative infection
Ischaemia
Lack of haemostasis
Tissue damage, e.g. crushing with instruments
Presence of necrotic tissue
Presence of foreign bodies including surgical materials

Organisms and sources

A few species are responsible singly or in combination for the majority of infections (Table 37.4) and they are well recognized as pathogens in a number of circumstances. Interestingly, they need not be the most numerous organisms in the initial inoculum. On occasion the occurrence of an unusual organism has required ingenious and painstaking detective work to elucidate the source and route of access.

The type of surgical procedure governs the likely sources and thereby the likely identity of the infecting organisms. Clean operations will be subject primarily to contamination by skin organisms present in relatively low numbers. It is important to remember that at some sites these numbers are higher and include species derived from other parts of the body, e.g. the bacteria of the groin and buttocks include coliforms and other faecal organisms. Skin organisms may originate

Table 37.4 Organisms and their sources
The surfaces of the body, particularly the mucosal surfaces, harbour complex populations. The organisms below are clinically important but not necessarily the commonest or most numerous at the various sites.

Skin

Gram-positive cocci
- *Staphylococcus aureus* – a classic wound pathogen. Found at carriage sites (e.g. nose, axilla, groin) in perhaps 30% of healthy people
- Coagulase-negative staphylococci – less virulent than *Staph. aureus*, particularly associated with low-grade infections of foreign materials. Several species live on man, e.g. *Staph. epidermidis*
- *Streptococcus pyogenes* – another classic pathogen and a common cause of severe wound infection in the pre-antibiotic era. Infrequently carried

Large bowel

Gram-positive cocci
- Enterococci – organisms of relatively low virulence, but may be exceptionally antibiotic resistant. Common cause of urinary infection and occasionally of endocarditis. *Enterococcus faecalis* is most commonly encountered
- Anaerobic cocci – various species of Gram-positive cocci which grow anaerobically. Usually penicillin sensitive

Gram-negative bacilli
- *Escherichia coli* – together with related 'coliforms' (*Klebsiella*, *Proteus*, *Enterobacter* and other genera) possesses a number of beta-lactamases, many carried on plasmids
- *Bacteroides* spp. – the commonest of bowel organisms. Only grow anaerobically; prone to cause intra-abdominal and pelvic abscesses. Some, e.g. *B. fragilis*, are important in producing beta-lactamases

Mouth

- A mixed flora, not as abundant as that of the large bowel but still numerous and not dissimilar for practical purposes. Of note is the general absence of *B. fragilis*. Coliforms are normally sparse but increase greatly in ill-health or following antibiotic therapy

Vagina

- Again shares important similarities with the large bowel in terms of pathogenic species such as *B. fragilis*. After the menopause faecal organisms are more in evidence from the patient or attendants, and skin preparation, sterilization of instruments and aseptic techniques are all designed to minimize the risk from such organisms. However, these measures are imperfect in that organisms can be cultured from most wounds at the end of an operation. On the other hand they are largely successful in that the rate of infection is reduced. Presumably in many cases any contaminating organisms which occur will meet adequate defences.

Members of the abundant mixed flora encountered in contaminated operations are responsible for the majority of wound infections following these procedures. A minority are caused by skin organisms and this possibility must not be overlooked.

THE USE OF ANTIBIOTICS IN THE PROPHYLAXIS OF POSTOPERATIVE INFECTION

Knowledge of the basic epidemiology of postoperative infection has provided the foundation for attempts at control. Surgical skills and techniques are of paramount importance but antibiotics are a valuable adjunct. Few antibiotics have not been examined for their effectiveness in surgical prophylaxis and guidelines for their use have been established over several decades.

Prophylaxis has been considered justified only when the risk of postoperative infection is high or the consequences catastrophic. Examples are wound infection in colonic surgery in the former case and prosthesis infection in the latter. Assessment of the need for antibiotic prophylaxis is becoming more sophisticated as infection rates for different operations are being examined in more detail. Wound infection rates for clean procedures have been found to vary by an order of magnitude and in some cases can warrant prophylaxis.

An ideal antibiotic for prophylaxis must be active against the anticipated infecting organisms, must be rapidly bactericidal and must be unaffected by bacterial resistance mechanisms. There is some evidence that at least partial success can be achieved against mixtures of organisms by killing some component species and thereby disrupting synergistic processes. The

antibiotic chosen must penetrate tissues readily, have an adequate half-life in serum and tissues and be easy to administer. Being given to large numbers of people, many of whom would not, in the event, have needed them, they must be associated with a low incidence of adverse effects. For the same reason they must not readily engender resistance in the organisms exposed to them. In case resistant organisms are selected, antibiotics for prophylaxis should not be those which would be used to treat established infection.

Antibiotics must be present at the site of operation in adequate concentrations before or shortly after inoculation of organisms. That is, they must augment the patient's defences during the 'early decisive period'. Delay reduces efficacy markedly and beyond a very few hours no benefit can be expected. The risk of inoculation is usually present for the duration of the operation, but for certain procedures the period of risk may extend beyond the time of operation.

Several trends are evident in current practice. The preferred method of administration is by the intravenous route. Absorption following intramuscular or rectal administration is slower and less reliable making timing difficult and success uncertain. Antibiotics have been applied to the wound site directly by several means. Injection along the proposed line of incision, application as a powder as the wound is being closed and irrigation of the wound with an antibiotic solution have all been tried. However, infection deep in the wound may not be prevented by such methods and when it is, it seems to be due to systemic absorption from the wound site. Thus there would seem to be no particular advantages in local application, but incorporation of antibiotics into orthopaedic cement may be an exception. Oral antibiotics have been used successfully in colorectal surgery for some years but are being superseded by parenteral regimens.

Antibiotics are usually commenced just before or just after induction of anaesthesia. It may be advantageous for the anaesthetist to give the prophylactic antibiotics just before induction, in that immediate adverse reactions may be easier to observe. In the case of some operations, however, they are best given during the procedure. The earlier practice of commencing antibiotics on the ward prior to transfer to theatre resulted in wide variations in timing in relation to surgery. Any delay could result in inadequate tissue levels at the time of surgery and the consequent failure of prophylaxis.

There has been a steady decrease in the duration of prophylaxis. Early regimens were in effect courses of treatment. Current prophylaxis for many procedures is solely perioperative, but this is not to say that only single doses are used even when prophylaxis is not extended postoperatively. Depending on the duration of the operation and the half-life of the antibiotics, 'top-up' doses may be given intraoperatively. It has been suggested that repeat doses should be given at intervals equal to twice the half-life of the antibiotic during surgery. Unfortunately the behaviour of antibiotics in patients undergoing surgery can differ considerably and unpredictably from that observed in healthy volunteers, and the requirement for intraoperative dosing must ultimately be determined empirically. Brief courses of antibiotics reduce the likelihood of adverse effects (although such events were not frequent even when longer courses were used) and are of course cheaper.

If antibiotics are otherwise similar in effectiveness then comparison of costs is valid. The cost of supply is only one component of the total cost of using an antibiotic. A 30-minute infusion is not only less convenient and flexible than a simple bolus injection but more demanding of medical and nursing time and therefore of money. Intraoperative dosing increases costs. There is considerable debate as to how the true cost of an antibiotic should be calculated.

Currently used antibiotics

Members of several groups of antibiotics are commonly used for surgical antibiotic prophylaxis.

Cephalosporins possess broad-spectrum antibacterial activity. First generation agents (e.g. cephalothin, cephazolin) are active against methicillin-sensitive staphylococci but are limited in their activity against beta-lactamase-producing coliforms. Second generation agents (e.g. cefuroxime, cefamandole) retain antistaphylococcal activity and are more stable to beta-lactamases.

Third generation agents (e.g. ceftazidime) possess greater activity against coliforms and some have activity against *Pseudomonas aeruginosa*. Their antistaphylococcal activity is relatively low. A few cephalosporins (e.g. cefoxitin) have useful activity against anaerobes. None are effective against enterococci.

As a group the cephalosporins are safe and non-toxic and several can be given as an intravenous bolus. The first generation agents have rather short serum half-lives but subsequent generations have adequate and in some cases prolonged half-lives, and have improved tissue penetration. A first or second generation agent is commonly used depending on local coliform sensitivity patterns. Third generation agents are probably best reserved for therapy.

Individual penicillins tend not to possess the same useful breadth of activity as cephalosporins, for example antistaphylococcal penicillins such as flucloxacillin are not active against coliforms. The most widely used are the antistaphylococcal penicillins and those with broad activity against coliforms, such as the ureidopenicillins. The latter are also active against strains of enterococci and many anaerobes. Penicillins have been combined with beta-lactamase inhibitors (e.g. clavulanic acid, sulbactam) to extend the spectrum of activity with some success. Penicillins are in general safe and well tolerated with half-lives comparable to the cephalosporins. A relative disadvantage may be that patients are more likely to claim allergy to penicillins than other antibiotics. As with the cephalosporins, local circumstances often dictate the final choice.

The nitroimidazoles (e.g. metronidazole, tinidazole) are active solely against anaerobes and are extremely effective with few side effects, good tissue penetration and long half-lives. Of note is their activity against *Bacteroides fragilis*, a major pathogen found in the colon and distinguished by its production of a beta-lactamase. In many countries, including the UK, they are the agents of first choice for the treatment of anaerobic infections. They have become available in the USA only relatively recently and research and clinical practice have reflected this. Despite widespread use for both prophylaxis and therapy resistance has rarely been described.

Aminoglycosides are active primarily against coliforms and *Pseudomonas* spp. They are also active against staphylococci but not against streptococci or anaerobes. Nephrotoxic and oto-toxic, they require monitoring of blood levels if several doses are given, which adds to the costs of administration. Toxicity is unlikely with limited doses. Neomycin and kanamycin have been used as components of an oral prophylactic regimen in colorectal surgery. Aminoglycosides are not normally absorbed from the gut but cases of toxicity have been described following absorption through inflamed bowel mucosa.

Of the glycopeptide antibiotics vancomycin has been the most widely used, principally where methicillin-resistant staphylococci have proved troublesome. The drug can only be given by slow infusion. Toxicity and the need for monitor-ing are further disadvantages. Teicoplanin is a much less toxic glycopeptide but is slightly less reliable in its activity against staphylococci.

Clindamycin, erythromycin and tetracycline have all been employed against anaerobes, the latter two in oral regimens in colorectal surgery. Clindamycin is also used for its activity against a wide range of Gram-positive organisms. Rela-tively few problems with pseudomembranous colitis have been described and are probably unlikely when short courses are used.

Trials

The existence of a rational basis for the use of prophylactic antibiotics in a given procedure does not guarantee a satisfactory outcome. Nor does it guarantee, except within broad limits, consistency of regimens between centres, as several surveys have demonstrated. The com-position of a regimen is necessarily arbitrary in the first instance and can only be refined with experience, the ultimate test of any particular prophylactic regimen being in clinical trials.

A number of criteria have been proposed for judging the validity and utility of trials of surgi-cal antibiotic prophylaxis (Table 37.5). Many trials fail by one or more of the accepted criteria, and in particular few recruit adequate numbers. In many studies, it would not be ethical to com-pare patients given prophylaxis with those given only a placebo. Many trials therefore compare two or more regimens.

Trial data can be valid but irrelevant. The agents may not be available or have been super-seded, or there may have been changes in sur-gical practice. It would clearly be unwise to use trial results from one branch of surgery as any-thing more than a guide to possible approaches in another branch of surgery.

Analysis of cases of failure of prophylaxis is important and should be performed whether or not the patient is in a trial. Failure can be due to human error or the presence of resistant organisms, and potentially important differences between regimens have been found on occasion. Otherwise lack of good models of pathogen-

---

Table 37.5 Criteria for judging the validity and utility of antibiotic trials

- A specific question must be formulated and be worth asking.
- Trials must be prospective, blinded and properly randomized with control groups.
- Regimens must be specified and follow the principles established for the proper use of prophylactic antibiotics.
- Outcomes must be specified, defined in detail and judged blind.
- The period of observation is critical. Infections may become apparent after discharge from hospital and extended follow-up is necessary to detect all cases. Failure in this seriously compromises wound infection incidence data.
- Selection and exclusion criteria for patients must be clearly specified.
- The numbers excluded and reasons for doing so must be given, as too high an exclusion rate renders a trial clinically unrealistic.
- If several centres are involved there must be a standard protocol.
- As much raw data as possible must be provided.
- Appropriate statistical analysis must be performed.
- Sufficient numbers of patients must be enrolled to avoid the errors of either assuming a difference when none exists (Type 1 error) or of assuming no difference when one exists (Type 2 error). Greater numbers are required to avoid the latter error.

esis often precludes explanation for failure of prophylaxis.

Current practice

Approaches to surgical antibiotic prophylaxis in a number of fields are outlined below. It will be apparent from the foregoing that at best they are based on incomplete data.

Colorectal surgery

The high incidence of postoperative infection is a result of the extremely high numbers of bacteria in the large bowel. Some spillage of bowel contents at operation is inevitable and any spillage will involve vast numbers of organisms. Good surgical techniques, such as the use of bowel preparation and staple guns, as well as antibiotics are vital to reducing infection in colorectal surgery. Regimens of antibiotic prophylaxis must provide protection against coliforms and anaerobes, ideally without neglecting skin organisms.

Oral antibiotics given from at least the day before surgery have proved effective at reducing wound infection rates. Aminoglycosides, particularly neomycin or kanamycin, have been combined with erythromycin, tetracycline or nitroimidazoles. A significant reduction in the numbers of bacteria in the large bowel is achieved and the latter three agents, which are absorbed from the gastrointestinal tract, are present in the tissues. Oral regimens are relatively cumbersome and expose the patient to antibiotics for a relatively long period with a concomitant risk of adverse effects. By their very nature they will disturb the normal bowel flora. They have retained a degree of popularity until recently comparing favourably with parenteral first generation cephalosporins in several trials. It must be noted that both regimens are superior to a placebo, and given the higher rate of wound infection recorded for the placebo group in many trials it has been considered unethical to include a placebo group in trials in colorectal surgery for some years.

In later trials newer parenteral antibiotic regimens have proven superior. Certain cephalosporins (e.g. cefoxitin) and penicillins combined with beta-lactamase inhibitors are effective against anaerobes, as well as coliforms and skin organisms, and are used on their own. Metronidazole has superior activity against anaerobes and has been successfully combined with a variety of agents active against the other groups of infecting organisms. Local coliform resistance patterns will largely determine the adequacy of a given agent, but second generation cephalosporins maintain a good balance of activity against coliforms and skin organisms.

Reduced regimens are now being examined. Several studies have found single doses of a cephalosporin plus metronidazole to be as effective as several doses given over 24 hours. This is despite the variety in operations (both elective and emergency) and the variation in technical difficulty between left- and right-sided colonic surgery. Contrary reports have indicated that more difficult procedures and those performed for certain conditions such as ulcerative colitis have benefited from regimens of up to several days' duration.

Antibiotics may not need to be given before operation since the major period of contamination follows the opening of the bowel. Administration as the peritoneum is opened so that maximum tissue concentrations coincide more closely with the period of maximum contamination has been advocated. The related issue of a 'top-up' dose to keep tissue concentrations high depends on the duration of operation and the half-life of antibiotics used. Different trials have estimated different safe periods for one dose and this must be examined on an individual basis.

Gastric and small intestinal surgery

Few organisms are present in the normal stomach due to the acidic pH. Those found are usually oral bacteria which have been swallowed. The incidence of wound infection is low if the stomach is not opened as in vagotomy, and not greatly increased if the stomach is entered provided that the gastric pH is low. Several conditions render the stomach less acid and the flora more abundant including malignancy, pyloric stenosis and bleeding peptic ulcer. As a result the risk of wound infection is increased and prophylaxis becomes necessary. First and second generation cephalosporins are effective in reducing the wound infection rate. A mixed aerobic and anaerobic flora is often present but the infecting organisms are usually coliforms or skin organisms. It would not seem unreasonable to include metronidazole.

Operations on the small intestine are relatively infrequent and are commonly performed for obstruction, ischaemia, or Crohn's disease. These conditions increase the moderate microbial count in this part of the gut and it is best to use prophylaxis appropriate to colorectal surgery.

Biliary surgery

Operations on the biliary tract carry a relatively low risk of wound infection provided that the bile is sterile. The presence of bacteria in the bile considerably increases the risk and is associated with certain conditions such as cholangitis and cholestasis. Unfortunately the association is not sufficiently reliable to permit the selective use of prophylaxis, and rapid bacteriological examination of bile obtained at operation is similarly unsatisfactory.

Coliforms are the predominant organisms found in infected bile with few anaerobes encountered. Many different regimens have proved to be effective compared to placebo, and even aminoglycosides which do not penetrate well into bile are effective, suggesting that blood and tissue levels are more important. Once again, cephalosporins have been widely used. A recent meta-analysis of trials found no differences in effectiveness between different cephalosporin regimens. A single dose of a cephalosporin is probably adequate which would permit selection to be based largely on cost. Trials have tended to compare single doses of a second or third generation cephalosporin with several doses of a first generation agent. Therefore, trials of single doses of first generation agents would be needed to confirm equivalence. Whatever trials are performed in the future, the inclusion of a placebo group appears to be unwarranted.

The advent of endoscopic surgery of the biliary tract has provided a more rapid and less hazardous means of dealing with some common problems than open surgery, but if the bile is infected then there is the possibility of septicaemia occurring with manipulation at operation. The choice of antibiotic is based on the considerations outlined for open surgery. Information on the optimum duration of prophylaxis is lacking. A 24-hour or 48-hour course is often used, and sometimes extended if free drainage of the biliary tract is not established. Whether the latter constitutes prophylaxis or treatment of incipient cholangitis is an open question.

Urological surgery

Surgical intervention, including such a common and simple procedure as bladder catheterization, predisposes the patient to urinary infection. Bacteria in the urine may then spread locally, e.g. to produce pyelonephritis. They may also enter the blood where their presence may be transient, even asymptomatic, or result in a life-threatening septicaemia. Entry into the blood may be spontaneous but there is no doubt that surgical manipulations, including catheter insertion and removal, can be the cause.

The problems are illustrated by transurethral resection of the prostate (TURP) and shock-wave lithotripsy. TURP is an extremely common procedure carried out via an endoscope and involving bladder catheterization for several days afterwards. Performed on a patient with sterile urine, TURP may be followed by a simple lower urinary tract infection which is relatively minor and straightforward to treat. However, enlargement of the prostate often causes urinary retention. This may be relieved prior to operation by catheterization, but urinary infection is often present in either case. Preoperative use of antibiotics to treat what is frequently a polymicrobial infection is likely to generate a resistant population of organisms, primarily coliforms. TURP performed on a patient with infected urine causes bacteraemia in about 50% of cases and in a proportion of these clinically apparent septicaemia will result.

In such patients prophylaxis is therefore intended to prevent potentially life-threatening septicaemia. Relief of obstruction and eradication of attendant urinary tract infection constitute treatment, not prophylaxis. Selecting a routine antibiotic is difficult and trials have reported mixed success, no doubt due in part to the variable and considerable resistance of the bacteria involved. One successful approach has been to perform culture and direct sensitivity testing on urine obtained the day before operation, i.e. on admission. The results are available on the day of operation and antibiotics chosen accordingly. Alternatively, first line agents used for serious infections are employed routinely. Aminoglycosides, cephalosporins, penicillins and other beta-lactams in various combinations have been used. Postoperative urine cultures help guide further treatment. Antibiotics are usually given until the catheter is removed unless this is delayed. Infection cannot be eradicated with the catheter in situ and prolonged treatment will promote resistance in the infecting population. It is best to stop therapy and treat subsequent catheter removal as a separate procedure.

Technically advanced procedures such as extracorporeal shock-wave lithotripsy can present additional difficulties. Stones within the urinary tract are shattered by this technique after which the flow of urine flushes them from the body. Bacteria may cause the formation of stones and certainly can colonize them. They can reside within a stone without being present on the surface. Urine may thus be sterile until bacteria are released as the stone is shattered whereupon they may enter the bloodstream. As with TURP a variety of organisms may be responsible. The approach to prophylaxis is essentially the same, with the further handicap that preoperative urine culture is an uncertain guide to the likely pathogens.

Obstetrics and gynaecology

Infection following caesarean section varies considerably in both nature and incidence with the population studied, with both wound and urinary tract infections occurring. Obstetric complications and social class figure prominently as risk factors. The extensive raw area produced in the uterus after delivery is directly exposed to the vaginal flora, and infection at this site (endometritis) is potentially life threatening. The condition of 'febrile morbidity' is also recognized. Its relation to active infection and the need for antibiotic treatment are uncertain although its incidence is reduced by antibiotic prophylaxis.

Wound infections are caused by such skin organisms as *Staphylococcus aureus*, while urinary tract infections are predominantly caused by coliforms. Endometrial infections are usually due to a mixture of aerobic and anaerobic vaginal organisms. Classical pathogens such as *Streptococcus pyogenes* and *Clostridium perfringens* still occur. Given the wide range of organisms encountered it is not surprising that compared to placebo many antibiotics have been found to reduce the incidence of postoperative infections, and a recent meta-analysis confirmed the overall value of antibiotic prophylaxis. Local data must be used in framing patient selection policies. Cephalosporins, broad-spectrum penicillins and metronidazole have all been used individually to reduce infection rates, but combinations of a beta-lactam with metronidazole appear to be no more effective. Antibiotics are given after the umbilical cord is clamped, preventing the baby receiving antibiotics without diminishing maternal protection. A 24-hour course may be more beneficial than a single dose.

Hysterectomy creates a vaginal wound, and a skin wound is also present if the approach is abdominal. Infection at the suture line of the vaginal cuff can extend into the tissues of the pelvis and 'febrile morbidity' is also encountered. *Escherichia coli*, *Staphylococcus aureus* and infections due to mixed vaginal organisms are found. Cephalosporins, broad-spectrum penicillins, penicillins combined with beta-lactamase inhibitors and nitroimidazoles have all been successful and the use of a cephalosporin and nitroimidazole together has been reported to be more effective than either alone. The value of prophylaxis in vaginal hysterectomy is generally accepted, but doubts remain about abdominal hysterectomy. Interestingly, a recent study encompassing the broader aspects of infection such as return to full function, visits by the GP and domiciliary use of antibiotics came to the opposite conclusion. The benefits of prophylaxis accrued to abdominal but not vaginal hysterectomy patients.

Orthopaedic surgery

The insertion of foreign material in clean orthopaedic surgery is attended by a low but significant incidence of infection which can present after a prolonged interval. The significance derives from the fact that infection of the implanted material compromises its function, loosening a joint for example, and usually necessitates its removal. The result is a serious loss of mobility which may be permanent as replacement is not always possible. Such infections are rightly viewed as catastrophic.

A wide variety of organisms can be involved including *Staphylococcus aureus*, other staphylococci, coliforms and anaerobes. The presumed source of these bacteria is the skin.

Several approaches to reducing the rate of infection of prostheses have been explored. The effectiveness of laminar airflow and the use of total body-exhaust suits has been demonstrated, but parenteral antibiotics have a more marked effect. The two methods are additive. Sophisticated airflow control is expensive and not widely available and the discomfort of operating in a 'space suit' is not inconsiderable. Reliance is therefore usually placed on antibiotics. Prophylactic regimens must be broadly active and combinations of a second generation cephalosporin with metronidazole or of an aminoglycoside plus antistaphylococcal penicillin plus metronidazole are used. Where metronidazole has been unavailable or considered unnecessary it has been omitted. The necessary duration of administration is not known but most centres use a relatively short course of 1 to 2 days.

Antibiotics such as gentamicin and cephaloridine have been incorporated into the cement used to anchor joint prostheses to bone. The technique certainly seems to provide prolonged concentrations of antibiotic at this important interface, and animal studies and limited clinical trials have demonstrated a reduction in infection with its use. It is not known if the benefit would be in addition to that derived from parenteral antibiotics. The size and duration of trial required to answer this question probably precludes it being performed and the question must remain unanswered.

Vascular surgery

Postoperative infection in vascular surgery usually takes the form of wound infection or infection of vascular grafts. The risk of infection varies with the site of surgery. Surgery performed on the vessels of the neck and upper limbs carries a low risk of infection and prophylaxis is not considered necessary. Surgery involving the abdominal aorta has a higher rate of infection but the main risk factor is extension of the procedure to the lower limbs. This requires a groin incision and the skin at this site is heavily populated with faecal as well as skin organisms. Prosthetic grafts are commonly used and are more at risk than natural vein grafts.

Wound infections can delay the patient's recovery and discharge while graft infections are literally a threat to life and limb. An infected graft can fail catastrophically. Even when it does not it is likely to require replacement. Insertion of a new graft into a previously infected site is a difficult undertaking and the problem is compounded by the occurrence of graft infections months to years after insertion. Skin wound infections are often due to coliforms and skin organisms such as *Staphylococcus aureus*. These may also be found infecting vascular grafts but low virulence organisms from the skin, such as staphylococci and coryneforms, are common.

Prophylactic antibiotics reduce wound infection and placebo groups would not be warranted in future trials. Unfortunately there is little evidence that they reduce graft infection although as wound infection is a risk factor for graft infection the possibilty of some benefit may exist. Parenteral antibiotics have been used for some time and pioneering work using an early cephalosporin helped set standards for research in other areas of surgery. The range of potential pathogens precludes use of narrow-spectrum agents alone. Aminoglycosides with antistaphyl-ococcal penicillins, several cephalosporins, and penicillins combined with beta-lactamase inhibitors have all been used. A second generation cephalosporin given for 24 hours is regarded as adequate. The view is sometimes taken that antibiotics should be continued until all central vascular cannulae are removed to prevent haematogenous seeding of grafts from infected cannulae. It is doubtful that this practice achieves anything other than predisposition to the acquisition of resistant organisms. The low incidence and occurrence of late infections following seeding at operation mean that thousands of patients would need to be followed for years to refine current approaches further. Improvements in graft materials may offer more hope by creating grafts less prone to infection.

Cardiac surgery

Early trials of antibiotic prophylaxis in cardiac surgery reported unacceptably high rates of postoperative infection in the placebo group. A reluctance to carry out further placebo-controlled trials naturally followed and prophylactic antibiotics have since been used routinely. Advances in technique make it likely that current procedures have a lower intrinsic infection rate than those of some years ago. This is despite the fact that this ostensibly clean surgery involves prolonged operations, the presence of many people in the operating theatre and the use of cardiopulmonary bypass which damages natural defences such as complement. Nevertheless, infections of the sternum or underlying mediastinum, or of synthetic patch grafts or prosthetic heart valves are serious and potentially fatal.

Staphylococci are the predominant pathogens and antistaphylococcal penicillins have been widely used alone or combined with an aminoglycoside. Cephalosporins have also been used to meet the same needs, again sometimes combined with an aminoglycoside. Unless staphylococci resistant to beta-lactams are troublesome vancomycin is not routinely used. Considering that some community and many hospital strains of staphylococci (other than *Staphylococcus aureus*) are resistant to all beta-lactams this re-

flects favourably perhaps on surgical and control of infection techniques. Antibiotics are sometimes continued until central vascular cannulae are removed, but there is no proof of the effectiveness of prolonging regimens beyond 24 hours and as with vascular surgery the practice may be detrimental. Fortunately cannulae are often removed at 24 hours if the patient's progress is satisfactory.

Head and neck surgery

Surgery which does not involve the mucosal surfaces is classified as clean. However mucosal surfaces possess an abundant aerobic and anaerobic flora and there is no doubt that procedures which involve them, especially if a connection is made to the skin, suffer a high incidence of postoperative wound infection. The infections are often polymicrobial reflecting the local flora. *Bacteroides fragilis* is usually absent from this site but coliforms may be present, particularly if the patient has recently received antibiotics for another reason.

Many of the infecting organisms are likely to be susceptible to beta-lactams. Indeed a number of antibiotics including benzylpenicillin have been found to be effective in reducing the incidence of postoperative infection.

A recent meta-analysis suggested that the use of clindamycin for 24 hours perioperatively was probably appropriate although such published evidence as is available slightly favours a more prolonged course of several days. Clindamycin's activity against Gram-positive cocci and anaerobes certainly makes it a reasonable choice. The possible adverse effects may prompt consideration of alternatives where these are available such as metronidazole combined with a second generation cephalosporin. The latter component's activity against coliforms is an added attraction.

Clean surgery

A number of commonly performed operations are categorized as clean and therefore subject to low rates of postoperative infection. They have consequently received much less attention, if any, than those procedures where infection is obviously significant. Despite the lack of studies some surgeons do use prophylactic antibiotics against skin organisms in clean procedures. Recent trial data has supported this use, such clinically beneficial effects as a reduction in staphylococcal wound infections being obtained. Hundreds of thousands of such operations are performed annually and the economic significance of infection rates is undoubted. Further studies are to be expected.

Selecting a regimen

That a standard regimen is used for the individual patient reflects the imprecise nature of the data available. It is not possible to predict risk and need in each case. An attempt to optimize prophylaxis at each institution can nevertheless be made in the light of the relevant literature. Local information is vital and clinical audit will play a central role. Patient population, types of surgery, prior infection rates, antibiotic sensitivity patterns and so on must all be taken into consideration. The process may well result in agreement with Oscar Wilde that truth is rarely pure, and never simple.

CASE STUDIES

CASE 37.1
A patient is to undergo colonic surgery.

Q What form of antibiotic prophylaxis might be employed?

CASE 37.2

A patient is admitted to hospital for total hip joint replacement.

Q What perioperative measures might be employed to prevent postoperative infection?

CASE 37.3

The vascular surgeons in a hospital are preparing an antibiotic policy.

Q How does the site of a vascular surgical procedure influence antibiotic prophylaxis and what antibiotic regimens might be employed?

ANSWERS TO CASE STUDIES

CASE 37.1

A Colonic surgery carries a high risk of postoperative infection due to mixed aerobic and anaerobic bowel organisms. Skin organisms constitute an additional threat. A broad-spectrum cephalosporin such as cefuroxime together with metronidazole are commonly given intravenously at induction of anaesthesia. A cephalosporin with antianaerobic activity such as cefoxitin or a combination of a penicillin and beta-lactamase inhibitor have also been used.

CASE 37.2

A Hip joint replacement is regarded as a clean procedure with an intrinsically low incidence of infection. However, as infection of a prosthesis is a serious matter prophylactic measures are vital. The types of organisms involved are varied and include staphylococci, coliforms and anaerobes.

The provision of ultra-clean air in the operating theatre with or without body-exhaust suits for individuals is of proven value but expensive and cumbersome. A 48-hour course of antibiotics is the most widely used approach. A second generation cephalosporin or the combination of an aminoglycoside with an antistaphylococcal penicillin are used. Metronidazole may be added depending on the perceived threat of anaerobes. Addition of antibiotics such as aminoglycosides or cephalosporins to the bone cement is also used and is thought to be of value.

CASE 37.3

A The neck and upper limbs are sites with a low incidence of infection and are not currently thought to warrant antibiotic prophylaxis. The risk of wound infection increases for abdominal and lower limb sites. Incisions in the groin in particular involve a site with an abundance of both skin and faecal organisms. Second generation cephalosporins, aminoglycosides and antistaphylococcal penicillins or combinations of a penicillin with a beta-lactamase inhibitor have all been employed with success. The use of grafts, particularly prosthetic materials, is an additional risk factor but the benefits of antibiotic prophylaxis with regard to graft infection are uncertain.

BIBLIOGRAPHY

Evans M, Pollock A V. Trials on trial. Archives of Surgery 1984; 119: 109–113

Howie P W, Davey P G. Prophylactic antibiotics and caesarean section. British Medical Journal 1990; 300: 2–3

Kaiser A B. Antimicrobial prophylaxis in surgery. New England Journal of Medicine 1986; 315 (18): 1129–1138

Kaiser A B. Surgical-wound infection. New England Journal of Medicine 1991; 324(2): 123–124

Kernodle D S, Classen D C, Burke J P, Kaiser A B. Failure of cephalosporins to prevent *Staphylococcus aureus* surgical wound infections. JAMA 1990; 263(7): 961–966

Murray G D. Meta-analysis. British Journal of Surgery 1990; 77: 243–244

Platt R, Zaleznik D F, Hopkins C C, Dellinger E P, Karchmer A W, Bryan C S et al. Perioperative antibiotic prophylaxis for herniorrhaphy and breast surgery. New England Journal of Medicine 1990; 322(3): 153–160

Wenzel R P. Preoperative antibiotic prophylaxis. New England Journal of Medicine 1992; 326(5): 337–339

Chapter 38

Endocarditis

F. K. Gould

Endocarditis can be defined as an inflammation of the endocardial surface of the heart, usually, but not always, as the result of an infective process. It occurs most frequently on the surface of heart valves, natural or prosthetic, but can also arise on other areas of the mural endocardium or on foreign bodies such as the patches used to repair or create shunts.

EPIDEMIOLOGY

Endocarditis has been recognized worldwide, but there is no accurate information available regarding its incidence or prevalence. Reported hospital admission rates vary strikingly from centre to centre, which could be due to local variations in the incidence of the disease, although differences in reporting criteria seem more likely. However, a reasonable estimate would be an incidence of 33 cases per million of population per year. Most authorities agree that the condition occurs at least twice as often in males as in females and that the average age at presentation is currently about 50 years, although this has been rising steadily over the past 40 years. This can be explained to some extent by changes which have occurred in the prevalence of the predisposing conditions.

AETIOLOGY AND PATHOPHYSIOLOGY

Endocarditis commonly develops as a complication of other forms of heart disease, which have in some way altered the normal blood flow within the heart resulting in turbulence. Any thrombus overlying the myocardium then acts as a focus on which microorganisms can adhere. Rheumatic heart disease used to be the most frequent predisposing factor, accounting for more than 60% of all cases of endocarditis in the 1950s. The decline in the incidence of rheumatic fever has been offset by the advances in cardiac surgery, and the frequency of calcific aortic stenosis seen in our increasingly numerous geriatric population. Social factors have also played a part, since recurrent right-sided endocarditis is a well-recognized complication of intravenous drug abuse. Endocarditis secondary to congenital heart disease has remained constant at 5 to 15% of all cases of endocarditis.

In order for microorganisms to cause endocarditis they must be present in the circulation in sufficient numbers and for an adequate duration. Transient bacteraemia has been demonstrated in normal individuals following such diverse manoeuvres as defaecation and tooth brushing. More sustained bacteraemia, of the sort felt likely to result in endocarditis in susceptible individuals, can occur following dental trauma in patients with chronic periodontal disease. The ability of an organism to adhere to mural thrombi is also an important factor, and may reduce the required inoculum, and this accounts for the association between different organisms and the type of endocarditis. For example, alpha-haemolytic streptococci which form part of the normal flora of the mouth are most frequently associated with native valve endocarditis. Coagulase-negative staphylococci, on the other hand, many of which produce extracellular slime allowing them to adhere easily to plastics, are encountered more frequently with intracardiac prostheses. Some organisms, particularly *Staphylococcus aureus* and *Streptococcus pneumoniae* can adhere even to normal endocardium if present in the circulation in sufficient numbers. Table 38.1 summarizes the range of organisms usually implicated in infective endocarditis.

Historically endocarditis has been classified as either 'acute' or 'subacute' depending on the clinical course of the disease or the virulence of the infecting organism. These differences have become less important since the advent of antimicrobial chemotherapy.

The characteristic pathological feature of endocarditis is infected thrombotic vegetations, usually situated on, or beneath valve leaflets. The base of these lesions often contains granulation tissue, suggesting a nonspecific chronic inflammatory host response. These friable lesions may break off and embolize into the circulation producing distant sequelae. In addition, in common with other chronic infections, circulating antigen/antibody complexes can cause glomerulonephritis or vasculitis.

CLINICAL MANIFESTATIONS

The presenting features of endocarditis can vary widely between patients. Some individuals, particularly those with *Staph. aureus* endocarditis can be critically ill, whereas others remain well throughout their entire clinical course. Symptoms can be attributed to the infection itself and to its cardiac and non-cardiac complications. However, the classical presenting triad of fever,

Table 38.1 Causative organisms implicated in endocarditis

Streptococci	Staphylococci	Fungi	Others
Alpha-haemolytic 'viridans' esp. *Strep. sanguis*	C-ve staphylococci esp. *Staph. epidermidis*	Yeasts	*Coxiella burneti*
		Aspergillus Mucor	Corynebacteria Enterobacteriaceae
Beta-haemolytic esp. Group B (*Strep. agalactiae*) Enterococci	*Staphylococcus aureus*		*Pseudomonas* sp.

heart murmur – often changing – and anaemia should alert the clinician to the potential diagnosis. Cardiac complications are usually due to destruction of the affected valve precipitating congestive cardiac failure. Local extension of the infection or abscess formation can lead to interruption of the conduction system resulting in heart block or arrhythmias.

Non-cardiac complications are generally the result of embolic or immunological phenomena. Examples of immunological manifestations include the microscopic haematuria of glomerulonephritis and petechiae. Splinter haemorrhages, Osler's nodes (transient, painful, erythematous lesions on the palms or soles probably due to a hypersensitivity reaction) and Roth spots (varicose degeneration of nerve fibres in the retina) although frequently sought, in practice rarely occur. Large emboli may break off from vegetations causing infarcts in the brain, limbs and gut in left-sided endocarditis, and predominantly lung infarcts in right-sided disease, although paradoxical emboli may occur in patients with septal defects.

INVESTIGATIONS

Diagnosis of endocarditis is usually confirmed by the identification of the infecting organism and demonstration of vegetations by echocardiography.

Bacteraemia is usually detected by conventional blood culturing techniques although the incubation period may need to be prolonged to recover some of the more slow-growing pathogens. Despite this, in up to 30% of all cases of endocarditis, blood cultures may prove negative. There are a number of explanations for this, the most likely being that the numbers of bacteria present in the circulation are too low to be picked up by conventional means. This occurs in cases of endocarditis due to enterococci, or in right-sided endocarditis where the majority of bacteria have been filtered out by the lungs before they reach the peripheral circulation. In some circumstances this difficulty can be overcome by increasing the volume of blood cultured. Fastidious organisms such as *Brucella* spp. and *Neisseria gonorrhoeae* may not grow well in conventional media. *Coxiella burnetii*, the cause of Q-fever endocarditis, cannot be cultured using artificial media, and so the diagnosis must be made serologically.

Non-infective endocarditis (murantic endocarditis) can be indistinguishable from bacterial endocarditis in terms of clinical presentation and the presence of vegetations on echocardiography. This form of endocarditis usually occurs in patients suffering from connective tissue disorders or malignancy.

Although advances in echocardiography techniques have improved the resolution of intracardiac imaging, vegetations may be difficult to demonstrate early in the clinical course of the disease, on prostheses and in patients with septal defects. Vegetations may also 'disappear' following major emboli.

DRUG TREATMENT

The aim of the antimicrobial therapy of endocarditis is to eliminate the infecting organism. These organisms are protected from the hosts defence mechanisms, being situated deep within a vegetative thrombus, so the antibiotics used must be bactericidal. Since heart valves are largely avascular the antibiotic has to diffuse into the vegetation from the blood passing over it, necessitating an adequate diffusion gradient from serum to tissue. Early animal models demonstrated that the serum concentration of antibiotic had to be at least eight times the minimum bactericidal concentration (MBC) of the infecting organism to penetrate the vegetation and effect a cure. It is for this reason that large doses of antibiotics may be required for a prolonged period.

Where clinically appropriate, therapy should be withheld until the infecting organism has been identified, since the majority of patients with endocarditis have been unwell for many months. Management protocols for choice of antibiotic and duration of therapy vary between centres, and according to the type of organism isolated. Most authorities now agree that with a few exceptions treatment should be continued for a total of 4 to 6 weeks, 2 weeks of which are usually by the intravenous route. Although it is very tempting to administer the antibiotics with the help of a central venous catheter, especially in patients with poor venous access, this should be avoided if at all possible. Intravenous cannulae quickly become colonized with staphylococci, and may continuously shed organisms over an already damaged heart valve. If these infections are then treated with other broad-spectrum antibiotics there is a real probability of the patient succumbing to candida septicaemia. If the use of such a cannula is essential, the risk of colonization may be reduced by the prophylactic use of sodium metabisulphite flushes, which has been shown to decrease the incidence of canula colonization. With the introduction of newer and better-absorbed oral agents there is every hope that in the future parenteral antibiotics may be unnecessary in the majority of cases.

It is essential for adequate treatment that accurate measurement is made of both minimum inhibitory concentration (MIC) and MBC for the chosen antibiotic against the infecting organism. This is because some organisms can demonstrate 'tolerance' to certain antibiotics, particularly beta-lactams and glycopeptides. In these instances the MBC exceeds the MIC by at least a fourfold difference, and another antibiotic which is synergistic, usually an aminoglycoside, needs to be added to the treatment regimen to produce a bactericidal combination. MIC and MBC testing is a highly specialized procedure which is not frequently performed in most diagnostic laboratories. Although medical treatment effects a cure in the majority of cases of endocarditis, the presence of a very large vegetation, destruction of the valve by the infection, or the presence of intracardiac suppuration may require surgical intervention. Aortic valve endocarditis and *Staph. aureus* infection may have a rapid progression and may require urgent surgery. An outline of recommended treatment regimens can be seen in Table 38.2.

Streptococci

If the isolate is sensitive the 'gold standard' for the therapy of streptococcal endocarditis is penicillin. Some centres prefer to use ampicillin (or

Table 38.2 Therapeutic regimens for common causes of endocarditis

Streptococci		
Penicillin non-tolerant	Ampicillin/amoxycillin 2 g i.v. 6-hourly	14 days
	Then	
	Amoxycillin 500 mg orally 6-hourly	14 days
Penicillin tolerant	Above regimen	14 days
	Plus	
	Gentamicin 80 mg i.v. or i.m. 12-hourly*	
Ampicillin resistant, penicillin allergy or lack of synergy with gentamicin	Rifampicin 600 mg 12-hourly orally	28 days
	Plus	
	Gentamicin 80 mg 12-hourly i.v. or i.m.	
	Or	
	Vancomycin 1 g i.v. 12-hourly*	28 days
	Plus if tolerant	
	Gentamicin 80 mg i.v. 12-hourly*	
Staphylococci		
Methicillin sensitive	Flucloxacillin 2 g i.v. 6-hourly	14 days
	Then	
	Flucloxacillin 1 g orally 6-hourly	28 days
Methicillin resistant or penicillin allergy	Rifampicin 600 mg 12-hourly orally	
	Plus	
	Erythromycin 500 mg 6-hourly orally	
	Or	
	Vancomycin 1 g i.v. 12-hourly	42 days

*Or less – according to renal function.

amoxycillin). Not only does the latter have better activity against enterococci, but it is less toxic in the large doses required to treat endocarditis. For example, it is not neurotoxic in patients with impaired renal function and, perhaps more importantly, it contains less sodium in the intravenous form than penicillin and so will not precipitate congestive cardiac failure in this susceptible group of patients.

Tolerance occurs more frequently in streptococci than in other species of bacteria, and so initial treatment should consist of a penicillin–aminoglycoside combination until the results of MIC, MBC and synergy testing are available. It is important to note that gentamicin is the only aminoglycoside which will reliably produce synergy in the treatment of enterococci, and the dosage required to produce this synergistic effect is much less than the therapeutic dosage required to, say, treat a Gram-negative septicaemia. This lower dosage should reduce the incidence of toxic side effects, but dosages must still be adjusted in patients with renal impairment and trough levels should be monitored on a regular basis to ensure that there has not been an accumulation of the drug.

Patients with a definite history of allergy to penicillin can be desensitized by rapidly inducing tolerance with increasing doses of penicillin given over 24 hours. However, in practice alternative antibiotics are usually employed, according to the sensitivity pattern of the isolate. In particularly resistant isolates, a glycopeptide such as vancomycin can be used, although these organisms are usually tolerant necessitating the addition of an aminoglycoside, producing an unavoidably nephrotoxic combination. If vancomycin is used, serum levels should be regularly monitored.

Staphylococci

The antibiotic of choice for the treatment of staphylococci is flucloxacillin. Some authorities recommend that it should be combined with an aminoglycoside for optimal therapy, but there is good evidence that the combination fails to improve failure rates and increases the incidence of renal dysfunction. Patients with penicillin allergy, or those infected with resistant organisms may be treated with antibiotic combinations which include rifampicin, or glycopeptides.

Fungi

Fungal endocarditis carries a high mortality, both because it frequently produces large emboli, and because it is difficult to treat successfully by medical means alone. The 'gold standard' for therapy is intravenous amphotericin B combined with 5-flucytosine in yeast infections. The toxic side effects of both agents are well recognized and it is hoped that the newer formulations such as liposomal amphotericin B or new agents such as the triazoles will improve the morbidity associated with therapy.

Other organisms

The choice of antimicrobial agent will depend on the sensitivity pattern of the infecting organism, and whether adequate serum bactericidal levels can be reached. Generally speaking if an organism is sensitive to penicillin or ampicillin this should be used in preference to other agents, but may need to be combined with an aminoglycoside to produce bactericidal activity.

Treatment of endocarditis due to *Coxiella burneti* (Q Fever) may require prolonged therapy, sometimes up to a year in total. This is because the organism is an obligate intracellular pathogen, and there may be multiorgan involvement, particularly the liver. Therefore the antibiotics selected must have both adequate intracellular bactericidal activity, and achieve good serum levels. One favoured antibiotic combination is rifampicin plus trimethoprim, and since both agents are well absorbed from the gut, therapy can be by the oral route from the outset.

PATIENT MONITORING

Since the success or failure of an antibiotic to eradicate the infecting organism in bacterial endocarditis depends on an adequate diffusion gradient between serum and vegetation it is logical to give the intravenous antibiotics where possible as a bolus injection to ensure an optimal peak serum level. Similarly, antibiotics should be administered at strictly equal time intervals throughout the 24-hour period. For example, in the treatment of endocarditis, an 8-hourly dosage regimen cannot be interpreted as 'breakfast, lunch and tea'. It is also sensible to arrange the timing of antibiotic administration to enable monitoring of levels to be carried out at sociable hours.

Table 38.3 outlines the possible adverse effects which may be encountered during therapy. Gastrointestinal upset, hypersensitivity and superinfection with other bacteria or fungi can occur during any antibiotic therapy, and with the exception of hypersensitivity are not usually severe

Table 38.3	Adverse drug reactions
All agents	Sensitivity reactions, e.g. skin rashes, candida, phlebitis, gastrointestinal disturbances
Penicillins	Neurotoxicity Sodium overload
Aminoglycosides	Nephrotoxicity Otoxicity
Vancomycin	Nephrotoxicity 'Red man' syndrome
Rifampicin	Induction of hepatic enzymes Drug interactions

enough to warrant a change of therapy. In addition to measuring trough and peak levels of potentially toxic antibiotics it is also important to ensure that adequate bactericidal activity has been reached in the serum of the patient undergoing therapy. This can be done in the laboratory by taking a serum specimen collected 1 hour after intravenous antibiotics (or 2 hours with oral agents), making double dilutions in broth or serum and challenging with the patient's infecting organism. This test is said to be satisfactory if the serum is bactericidal to a titre of at least 1:8.

This so-called 'serum cidal level' or 'back titration' can be very helpful in the patient's management. If it is unsatisfactory and the patient remains pyrexial a change of antibiotic may be indicated.

If it is satisfactory, and the patient is pyrexial, other causes should be sought. A sustained pyrexia in an otherwise well patient may be due to 'beta-lactam' fever, a form of penicillin allergy, and may resolve when therapy is converted from the intravenous to oral route. Isolated spikes of temperature are commonly associated with embolization, and if the patient remains well between these attacks they can usually be ignored. A continued spiking temperature which never returns to normal associated with a raised peripheral neutrophil count suggests abscess formation which could be intra- or extracardiac. These abscesses usually only resolve after formal surgical drainage.

The therapy of Q-fever endocarditis can be monitored by measuring the patient's antibody titre, although no significant change should be expected during the first 3 months of therapy.

PREVENTION OF ENDOCARDITIS

Although endocarditis can occur in a previously normal heart, it is more frequently seen in patients with a pre-existing cardiac lesion, either congenital or acquired. For this reason, patients known to have such lesions, or prostheses, should be given general advice about reducing the risk of sustained bacteraemia. Since periodontal sepsis is a likely source, patients should be encouraged to make regular visits to their dental practitioner. All invasive medical, surgical or dental procedures should be covered by an appropriate antibiotic. Specific and current guidelines for the choice and route of administration are regularly updated in the British National Formulary. Early prosthetic valve endocarditis occurs within 3 months of implantation of a prosthetic valve, and usually occurs as a result of intraoperative bacterial contamination. The incidence of this condition has been reduced dramatically with the use of prophylactic antibiotics in cardiac surgery. Since the most likely contaminating organisms are staphylococci, flucloxacillin has been successfully used and the incidence of early prosthetic valve endocarditis has remained below 2% of all operations. Other agents such as cephalosporins, aminoglycosides, or a combination of both have also been employed with varying success.

CASE STUDIES

CASE 38.1

A 55-year-old lady with a prosthetic mitral valve is admitted to hospital for investigation of a pyrexia.

Q What investigations would be advised to confirm or exclude endocarditis?

CASE 38.2

A 75-year-old man with calcific aortic stenosis has *Staphylococcus aureus* isolated from two sets of blood cultures.

Q What antibiotic therapy would be advised?

CASE 38.3

A 22-year-old man is undergoing therapy for staphylococcal endocarditis with flucloxacillin. Despite a resolution of his pyrexia when antibiotics were commenced, he is now spiking temperatures up to 39°C, and his peripheral white cell count is rising.

Q Should his antibiotic therapy be changed?

CASE 38.4

A patient with a prosthetic mitral valve has been referred for upper gastrointestinal endoscopy following indomethacin-induced renal failure.

Q What antibiotic prophylaxis should he receive?

CASE 38.4

A Under normal circumstances the patient would receive intravenous amoxycillin plus gentamicin, or vancomycin if the patient was allergic to penicillin. However, the use of a glycopeptide or an aminoglycoside may not be appropriate in a patient whose renal function is compromised. A clinical decision, weighing up the risk of endocarditis and incurring a possible 4-week course of aminoglycoside, has to be balanced against the risk of precipitating acute renal failure. In most cases amoxycillin alone may suffice, clindamycin being used in the penicillin-allergic patient. Teicoplanin, a newer glycopeptide, reputed to be less nephrotoxic than vancomycin, may have a role in this situation.

ANSWERS TO CASE STUDIES

CASE 38.1

A A series of blood cultures should be collected, and serum sent for Q-fever antibodies. A specimen of urine should be microscoped or dip-tested for the presence of red blood cells. Vegetations may be seen on echocardiography.

CASE 38.2

A *Staph. aureus* septicaemia is a life-threatening condition and antibiotic therapy should be commenced immediately. If there is no history of penicillin allergy, flucloxacillin 2 g i.v. 6-hourly should be commenced.

CASE 38.3

A It is very tempting in this situation to ascribe the pyrexia to a failure of antibiotic therapy; however this is rarely the case, and many patients are eventually referred to regional cardiothoracic centres on their third or fourth different antibiotic combination. If results of MIC and MBC testing suggest that the organism is sensitive and non-tolerant to methicillin, and the serum bactericidal levels are 1:8 or greater, then the problem lies with the patient and not the antibiotic. Staphylococci have a propensity to form abscesses, and these should be excluded by ultrasonography or CT scanning. Occasionally patients develop a 'beta-lactam' fever which resolves when the antibiotic is converted from intravenous to oral administration, although this syndrome is rarely associated with a raised white cell count.

BIBLIOGRAPHY

Bisno A L. Treatment of infective endocarditis. New York: Grune & Stratton 1981

Bisno A L et al. Antimicrobial treatment of infective endocarditis due to viridans streptococci, enterococci and staphylococci. JAMA 1989; 261: 1471–1477

Horstkotte D, Bodnar E. Infective endocarditis. London: ICR publishers 1991

Kaye D. Infective endocarditis. Baltimore University Park Press 1976

Rahimtoola S H. Infective endocarditis. New York: Grune & Stratton 1978

Sande M A, Kaye D, Root R K. Contemporary issues in infectious diseases. Volume 2: Endocarditis. Edinburgh: Churchill Livingstone 1984

Chapter 39

Tuberculosis

P. J. Baker

Tuberculosis almost always occurs as a result of infection with *Mycobacterium tuberculosis*. After the initial infection, which often passes unnoticed, the disease can follow a variety of clinical courses, sometimes lying dormant for months or years before reactivating. Active clinical disease, although chiefly associated with the lungs, can occur in many other organs.

EPIDEMIOLOGY

Distinction should be made between tuberculous infection and tuberculous disease. In the former, tubercle bacilli are established in the host but there are no symptoms or detectable evidence of disease. In tuberculous disease one or more body systems show clinical, bacteriological or radiographic evidence of disease. During the last century, both incidence and death rates have been steadily declining, probably due to improved social conditions, less overcrowding and better nutrition. In the last few decades treatment, vaccination and case-finding programmes have speeded up this decline such that tuberculosis is now much less of a public health problem. In the undeveloped world, where control measures have not yet resulted in the same rates of decline, tuberculosis remains a large problem.

The incidence of tuberculosis is dependent on a variety of factors such as race, age, social conditions and geography. In the UK, tuberculosis is a notifiable disease and consequently incidences are known, but in the developing world, they can only be estimated. The incidence in England and Wales in 1988 was 8.6 per 100 000 per year. This overall figure masks large variation. The incidence in Indian and Pakistani immigrants to the UK is 126 per 100 000 per year whilst that of the white ethnic group is 4.6 per 100 000 per year. In the Indian sub-continent incidences as high as 2000 per 100 000 per year have been quoted.

Risk factors that increase an individual's chance of tuberculous disease are shown in Table 39.1.

AETIOLOGY

Tuberculous infection is caused by tubercle bacilli. The mycobacteria are a large group of bacteria but only three species are recognized as causing tuberculosis. *Mycobacterium tuberculosis* is by far the most common infecting organism. *M. bovis* is now uncommon due to the virtual eradication of bovine tuberculosis from cattle. *M. africanum* is very rare in Britain occurring, as its name suggests, mainly in Africa. Other pathogenic mycobacteria are not tubercle bacilli and do not cause tuberculosis.

None of the mycobacteria take up microbiological stains very readily but when they do they are hard to decolourize. When stained with the Zeil–Nielson stain, they do not decolourize with either acid or alcohol and are therefore called acid-fast or acid-alcohol-fast bacilli (AFB or AAFB).

Tuberculous infection occurs almost invariably as a result of the inhalation of infected droplets. Droplets coughed up by an infected person can remain viable for days. Their size enables them to reach the alveoli where they are deposited. Therefore, the primary focus of infection is almost always the lung. It is possible to become infected through ingestion of bacilli, but large numbers would have to be ingested to be sure that viable organisms passed the gastric acid barrier. Ingestion of *M. bovis* in milk used to cause infection.

Although extremely rare, it is possible for tuberculosis to be transmitted by direct inoculation. This may occur in laboratory staff or following BCG vaccination (usually in immuno-compromised individuals).

PATHOPHYSIOLOGY

The initial primary infection is often widespread. Within the first few days of infection, before the onset of an acquired immune response, bacilli are taken up into macrophages but continue to multiply intracellularly. They are transported to the regional lymph glands and may enter the bloodstream from where they may infect other organs, principally other areas of the lung, the kidney, and the bones. It is during this time that the characteristic lesions of tuberculosis, tubercles, appear in the lungs. At this stage there is no cavitation and the patient would still be tuberculin negative. Over the next few days and weeks, a delayed hypersensitivity response does occur making the patient tuberculin positive.

Usually the primary infection is quickly contained by the immune system and the lesions heal. However, viable bacilli often remain in the body and the infection may recur, sometimes many years later. Sometimes the primary infection may not be fully controlled and progressive disease occurs. This may occur in organs infected with mycobacteria early after infection, or rarely, as a generalized miliary infection. Miliary disease is not common but is more frequent in young children (particularly in the first few months of life) and in those with impaired immune systems.

Post-primary tuberculosis can occur at any time after primary infection, usually within the

Table 39.1 Risk factors for tuberculosis
Close contact with a smear-positive patient
Originating from or living in a country where tuberculosis is common
Age (especially those under 5 years and middle-aged men)
HIV infection
Diabetes
Poor social conditions (malnutrition, poverty, vagrants, those living in lodging houses/hostels)

first 1 or 2 years. Anything that affects the body's immune response, e.g. malignancy, HIV infection, old age or malnutrition, makes reactivation more likely. Post-primary tuberculosis is usually localized resulting from the reactivation of one or more primary lesions. There is usually no further dissemination at this stage.

SIGNS AND SYMPTOMS
Primary tuberculosis

Primary tuberculosis is usually symptomless and passes unnoticed and undiagnosed. If a diagnosis is made it is usually after a routine chest X-ray or Mantoux test, often as part of the system of tracing contacts of known sufferers or during pre-employment health screening. Occasionally the primary infection may cause a mild febrile illness, with or without cough, of about 1 week in duration. Medical help is not usually sought and the symptoms resolve spontaneously.

Post-primary tuberculosis

The clinical course of post-primary tuberculosis can vary greatly. The disease can present in an insidious or an acute way. The lung is by far the most common site but any of the organs seeded during the primary infection may be involved.

The onset of pulmonary post-primary tuberculosis is usually insidious with no specific symptoms. It is often diagnosed by chance after a routine chest X-ray. It is a disease with many varieties. When patients become symptomatic, they often complain of nonspecific symptoms such as malaise, fever, weight loss and night sweats. The most commonly presenting pulmonary feature is cough which may be either dry or purulent and blood-stained. Haemoptysis is rare and usually a sign of more advanced disease. It is not unusual for the diagnosis to be delayed because the presenting symptoms are ascribed to something else, for example smoker's cough or bronchitis. A chest X-ray is, however, usually diagnostic.

Miliary tuberculosis is rare in the UK. It usually presents insidiously in the elderly, who may have a negative Mantoux test. In younger patients the onset is usually acute. It is a serious illness and is almost always fatal if left untreated. Generally, symptoms are nonspecific including fever, weight loss, malaise and weakness. In both age groups there may be meningeal signs if it is accompanied by meningeal tuberculosis.

Tuberculosis of other sites usually present with symptoms suggestive of the area infected such as back pain in spinal tuberculosis. Non-pulmonary disease is not common in the UK but should be considered especially in Asian and African patients.

INVESTIGATIONS

For control of the disease to be successful, it is important not only to diagnose tubercular disease, but also to identify those with asymptomatic infection, who may require treatment if they are not to infect others. Three main investigations used are:

- chest X-ray
- tuberculin testing
- bacteriological examination.

Chest X-ray

Chest radiography is very important in the diagnosis of tuberculosis. In primary tuberculosis the chest X-ray will characteristically show lesions in the lower or middle lobes of the affected lung. It is rare for both lung fields to be affected at this stage. In children local lymph nodes may also show lesions. In post-primary tuberculosis the number of lesions seen may be greater and they may be bilateral. As lesions heal they become more visible as they calcify. It is possible to see numbers of lesions at different stages on the same film. Miliary tuberculosis usually shows a fine mottling throughout both lung fields.

Tuberculin testing

Tuberculin testing is usually used to confirm

infection with tubercle bacilli. There are two main types of test performed today. Both tests use solutions of tuberculin purified protein derivative (PPD). The tine test is not recommended.

The Heaf (multiple puncture) test is both quick and simple. It is usually used in areas where many tests are performed, e.g. school clinics. A concentrated solution (100 000 units/ ml) of tuberculin PPD is applied and an instrument with six needles arranged in a circle is used to puncture the skin. The result is read at 7 to 10 days. Four grades of response are recognized:

- grade 1 – four or more discrete papules
- grade 2 – confluent papules forming a ring
- grade 3 – a disc of induration
- grade 4 – induration of greater than 10 mm.

In the UK, grades 3 and 4 are recognized as indicating likely tuberculosis infection.

The Mantoux test is more time consuming and requires greater skill to administer but does not require any special equipment. A solution of tuberculin (PPD) is injected intradermally into the forearm. An area of inflammation and oedema greater than 5 mm in diameter after 2 to 4 days is regarded as a positive result. Initially 1 unit of tuberculin PPD in 0.1 ml is injected. If this gives a negative result, the test is repeated with a 0.1 ml injection containing 10 units in 0.1 ml.

Traditionally the strength of tuberculin PPD was quoted as a dilution of the concentrated Heaf test solution. Nowadays it is described in units of tuberculin PPD per ml. Thus the weakest available solution is now described as containing tuberculin PPD 10 units per ml. This same strength used to be described as 1 in 10 000.

Tuberculin testing is a quick method of finding both infected contacts of an index case and those who are non-immune and therefore require vaccination. Unfortunately, both false negative and false positive results do occur. Infection with non-tubercle bacilli may occasionally give a positive result. False negative results may occur in some patients. This is usually due to recent infection or immunosuppression, e.g. HIV infection, malignancy, immunosuppressive drugs. Sometimes the elderly respond poorly, especially if they have miliary tuberculosis.

Bacteriological examination

Demonstration of tubercle bacilli gives absolute proof of infection or disease. A negative result does not exclude tuberculosis. In primary tuberculosis, there is seldom sputum to culture. In non-pulmonary tuberculosis, bacilli are often demonstrable from other locations, e.g. bone marrow, gastric washings or urine, depending on the site of infection.

TREATMENT

The goals of treatment are the eradication of infection in an individual and the control of the spread of disease. The latter is achieved by contact tracing and treatment. In the developed world, tuberculosis is almost invariably curable with combination antitubercular chemotherapy if the patient complies with treatment. Non-compliance is by far the biggest cause of treatment failure.

Traditionally, tuberculosis was treated with bed rest, isolation and open spaces in sanitoria. Although this treatment may have had some effect in non-cavitary cases, it was less effective in more advanced disease.

Tuberculosis had started to decline in the UK before the advent of chemotherapy, probably due to improved nutrition and social conditions in the population. With the advent of effective antitubercular chemotherapy it became apparent that patients no longer needed sanitorium treatment. Isolation was no longer needed as effective treatment meant that patients rapidly became non-infectious. Results with regimens containing isoniazid together with para-aminosalicylate (PAS) or ethambutol and, sometimes, streptomycin gave excellent results. Treatment was required for 18 to 24 months if relapse was to be prevented. The availability of pyrazinamide and, more importantly, rifampicin made shorter courses of treatment a possibility.

Most regimens in the developed world now

contain isoniazid, rifampicin and pyrazinamide, possibly with another agent such as ethambutol or streptomycin. Regimens containing these drugs when taken correctly by the patient for 6 to 9 months are as effective, but no more so, than the older 18- to 24-month regimens.

In order to eradicate infection in an individual, combination antitubercular chemotherapy is always used. The choice of drug regimen is based on a number of factors, e.g. reducing the risk of resistance emerging or improving patient compliance.

In most developed countries there are firm guidelines for the treatment of tuberculosis and the treatment of contacts. Guidelines for both the treatment of tuberculosis and the treatment of tubercular contacts have been recently published in the UK by the Joint Tuberculosis Committee of the British Thoracic Society.

Antimicrobial resistance

Prevention of drug resistance is one reason why combination chemotherapy is used. The chances of an organism being spontaneously resistant to more than one antibiotic is extremely low. All populations of bacteria will contain mutants that are resistant to one or other of the therapeutic agents. A large population such as that found in a pulmonary cavity will contain many thousands of resistant bacilli. If such a population were exposed to inadequate chemotherapy, (e.g. isoniazid alone), the drug-sensitive organisms would be suppressed allowing the resistant organisms to repopulate the cavity. The patient may then infect others who would then have primary isoniazid-resistant tuberculosis.

In practice, primary resistance usually occurs because patients are not prescribed adequate treatment or they do not comply adequately with the prescribed treatment. The levels of primary resistance varies enormously around the world. In Britain, resistance is very rare in white patients, but up to 6% of patients from the Indian sub-continent will be resistant to isoniazid. In areas where tuberculosis is endemic and treatment regimens are poor, the amount of resistance is greater. It must be stressed, however, that the usual reason for treatment failure is non-compliance.

Bacterial characteristics

There are four environments in which tubercle bacilli live. The abilities of antitubercular agents in these environments will influence the choice of regimen. Open pulmonary cavities have a plentiful supply of oxygen and will have large numbers of rapidly growing organisms. However, bacilli in closed lesions will be oxygen starved and therefore slow growing or dormant. Intracellular tubercle bacilli will be slow growing due to the low intracellular pH and lack of oxygen. There may also be some bacilli that are growing intermittently as their environment changes around them. The antitubercular agents differ in their abilities to kill these different populations of bacilli. Isoniazid, rifampicin and streptomycin are most effective against continually growing bacilli. Pyrazinamide is most effective against intracellular organisms and rifampicin against intermittently dividing bacilli. Dormant bacilli are usually in closed lesions hidden from the effects of both the body's immune system and the effects of drugs and are usually eradicated by encapsulation and fibrosis over time.

Treatment of pulmonary tuberculosis

In Britain, the regimen recommended by the Joint Tuberculosis Committee is a 6-month regimen consisting of rifampicin, isoniazid, pyrazinamide and ethambutol for the initial 2 months followed by a further 4 months of rifampicin and isoniazid. In patients with a low risk of resistance to isoniazid (previously untreated patients in Britain), the ethambutol may be omitted. The doses of all drugs which should be given in a single daily dose, are shown in Table 39.2. Although considered a first line agent, streptomycin is now rarely used in uncomplicated pulmonary tuberculosis due to its toxicity and the inconvenience of having to administer it by injection.

Table 39.2   Dosages of first line antitubercular agents*

Drug	Forms available	Dosage			Reduce dose in	
		Adults daily	Adults intermittent (doses per week)	Children daily	Renal failure	Liver failure
Rifampicin	Capsules 150 mg, 300 mg†	450 mg (<50 kg)				Only in severe liver impairment
	Liquid 100 mg in 5 ml Injection for infusion 300 mg	600 mg (>50 kg)	600–900 mg (3)	10 mg/kg	No	
Isoniazid	Tablets 100 mg† Injection 100 mg Mixture‡	300 mg	15 mg/kg (3)	10 mg/kg	Only in severe renal impairment	In patients with acute or chronic liver disease
Ethambutol	Tablets 100 mg, 400 mg† Mixture‡	25 mg/kg§	30 mg/kg (3) 45 mg/kg (2)	As adult dose	Yes	No
Pyrazinamide	Tablets 500 mg	1.5 g (<50 kg) 2.0 g (>50 kg)	2.5 g (3)¶ 3.5 g (2)¶	35 mg/kg	Yes	No
Streptomycin	Injection 1 g	750 mg (<50 kg)‖ 1 g (> 50 kg)	750 mg – 1 g‖	15–20 mg/kg	Yes	No

* Some of the dosages quoted are not licensed but have been recommended by the British Thoracic Society (see bibliography).
† Also available as combined oral preparations (see BNF).
‡ Mixture may be prepared extemporaneously.
§ Reduce dose to 15 mg/kg/day if used for longer than 2 months.
¶ Doses refer to patients over 50 kg. Reduce by 500 mg for patients weighing less than 50 kg.
‖ Drug levels should be monitored to prevent toxicity.

These regimens are often too expensive for many developing countries where tuberculosis is rife and money for public health services is short. Many regimens are used but the duration of treatment is usually increased to 12 to 18 months if rifampicin is not used. In spite of its unpleasant toxic effects, para-aminosalicylate (PAS) is still used in a number of countries as it is cheap. Using unpleasant, less effective regimens leads to non-compliance which leads to recurrence of disease, possibly with resistant organisms, which makes treatment that much more difficult.

Intermittent regimens

For short course regimens to be effective, patients must comply with treatment. If this is found to be a problem, or is thought likely to be so, treatment may be given intermittently, two or three times weekly. In this way treatment can be fully supervised ensuring that compliance is complete. This may be useful for certain groups in whom compliance is likely to be a problem, e.g. vagrants and alcoholics. In the developing world, intermittent regimens may also be of use in an attempt to overcome non-compliance. Strong consideration should be given to the use of an intermittent directly supervised regimen if there are serious doubts about compliance.

A number of trials of intermittent regimens have shown that a short course of therapy is as effective if given intermittently as when given daily. Regimens may be fully or partially intermittent. In the latter, four drugs (isoniazid, rifampicin, pyrazinamide and either ethambutol or streptomycin) are given daily for 2 months followed by rifampicin and isoniazid two or three times weekly for the subsequent 4 months.

For most drugs the doses are increased when given intermittently and are shown in Table 39.2.

Treatment of non-pulmonary tuberculosis

There have been relatively few comparative trials of treatments for non-pulmonary disease. It is thought, however, that regimens used for pulmonary tuberculosis are effective in extra-pulmonary disease. However, the duration of treatment may need to be extended for certain sites.

Tuberculous meningitis

Tuberculous meningitis has been treated effectively with rifampicin and isoniazid for 12 months together with pyrazinamide for the first 2 months. Streptomycin or ethambutol may also be used in the first phase of treatment but they only reach the CSF through inflamed meninges. Tuberculous meningitis is a serious disease and treatment must be started promptly. The factor that most affects the prognosis is the stage at which the disease is diagnosed and treatment started. In view of this it is often justified to start a therapeutic trial of antituberculous drugs in the absence of a definite diagnosis.

Tuberculosis of the lymph glands

This is the most common form of non-pulmonary tuberculosis and has responded well to a 9-month regimen of rifampicin and isoniazid with ethambutol for the first 2 months. It is possible that the duration could be reduced to 6 months if pyrazinamide was used.

Bone and joint tuberculosis

Bone and joint tuberculosis is treated effectively with standard agents for 9 months. The spine is the most common site for bone tuberculosis and, occasionally, surgery may also be needed to either relieve spinal cord compression or correct spinal deformities that may have occurred.

Miliary tuberculosis

Generalized (miliary) tuberculosis must be treated promptly as there is still appreciable mortality from delayed diagnosis and treatment. Standard regimens containing both isoniazid and rifampicin are used. If the patient is severely ill or hypoxaemic, then corticosteroids may also be used (see below).

Treatment of tuberculosis in special circumstances

Tuberculosis in children

Treatment is very similar to that of adults. The doses of the drugs used are shown in Table 39.2. Various doses of rifampicin and isoniazid have been published in the literature but in the UK a dose of 10 mg/kg/day for both drugs is recommended. Ethambutol should not routinely be used in young children who would be unable to report visual toxicity if it occurred. However, it may have to be used if toxicity or resistance to other agents occurs.

Pregnancy

Pregnant women should be given standard therapy, although streptomycin should not be used as it may be ototoxic to the fetus. Although the other first line drugs have not been shown to be teratogenic, they are either contra-indicated or the manufacturers' data sheets urge caution. It is considered safe for mothers to breast feed whilst taking antituberculous agents.

Renal disease

Patients with renal disease may be given isoniazid, rifampicin and pyrazinamide in standard doses as these drugs are eliminated by predominantly non-renal routes. Ethambutol is predominantly renally excreted and dose reduction is therefore needed. Some authors have suggested monitoring serum concentrations; however, in many centres this service is not readily available. Streptomycin must be used with considerable caution if toxicity is to be prevented and is best avoided in renal failure. Rifampicin may be given in standard doses to patients on dialysis. The doses of the other agents need to be modified. A number of different regimens have been suggested.

Liver disease

In patients who present with liver failure or in alcoholics, monitoring of liver enzymes is recommended as rifampicin, isoniazid and pyrazinamide are all known to be potentially hepatotoxic. However, increases in transaminases at the start of antituberculous treatment occur frequently. These are usually transient and not a reason for stopping treatment unless frank jaundice or hepatitis develop, in which case all drugs should be stopped. It is usually possible to restart treatment when values have returned to pretreatment levels.

Immunocompromised patients

Patients who are immunocompromised, including those with AIDS, should be treated with normal first line agents. Theoretically these patients have a greater risk of relapse and may need to be treated for longer than the normal 6 months.

Steroids

Corticosteroids have long been used in the treatment of tuberculosis, chiefly for their anti-inflammatory properties. They may be of benefit and a dose of around 60 to 80 mg prednisolone has been used. Steroids probably find their greatest use in pleural disease where they cause rapid resolution of symptoms, and in genito-urinary tuberculosis where they help reduce the symptoms of cystitis and obstruction. In tuberculous meningitis corticosteroids are said to improve survival and reduce sequelae. Their use in other types of tuberculosis is unproven but they may well be tried in patients who are gravely ill, irrespective of the site of infection.

Drug resistance

Drug resistant tuberculosis is a considerable problem worldwide, but is not often seen in Britain. Isoniazid is the most usual agent to which resistance is seen. At least three agents to which the organisms are sensitive should be given. The UK guidelines recommend a four-drug regimen. If multiple resistance is encountered, specialist advice on treatment is usually required and treatment is based on the sensitivities of the infecting organisms. If rifampicin is not included in the regimen, then the duration of treatment will have to be increased to 12 to 18 months.

It is rarely necessary to resort to second line agents, some of which are becoming difficult to obtain in Britain. The doses and side effects of the second line agents are shown in Table 39.3.

Table 39.3 Dosages and adverse effects of second line drugs			
Drug	Adult dose and route	Major adverse effects	Comments
Para-aminosalicylate (sodium salt) (PAS)	10–12 g per day in divided doses (oral)	Gastrointestinal upset, rash, hepatitis	Very unpalatable, still used in Third World due to cost. May cause sodium overload. No licensed source in UK
Ethionamide/ Prothionamide	750 mg–1 g per day (oral)	Gastrointestinal upset	Neither licensed in UK. Importation may be possible
Capreomycin	1 g per day (i.m. injection)	Hypersensitivity (urticaria + rash), ototoxicity (e.g. tinnitus)	May cause pain at injection site. Use in caution with other ototoxic drugs
Cycloserine	250–500 mg twice daily (oral)	Headache, dizziness	Some sources suggest assessment of mental status should be carried out

Some workers have tried some of the newer broad-spectrum antibacterial agents in patients with drug resistance. The fluoroquinolones, especially ciprofloxacin and ofloxacin have been used as has rifabutin (ansamycin).

Monitoring treatment

In pulmonary tuberculosis, sputum examination and culture are the most sensitive markers of the success of treatment. Patients taking regimens containing rifampicin and isoniazid should be non-infective within 2 weeks. If a patient does not become culture negative, it may be due to either drug resistance or non-compliance, the latter being most likely. Chest X-rays only provide limited information as to the progress of treatment.

Good compliance is essential if treatment is to be successful. Compliance checking is not easy,

especially where a patient is being uncooperative. Rifampicin will colour the urine red within about 4 hours of a dose.

Drugs used and toxicities

In this country the first line drugs for the treatment of tuberculosis are rifampicin, isoniazid, pyrazinamide, ethambutol, and streptomycin. Other agents such as capreomycin, para-amino-salicylate (PAS) and cycloserine are reserved for use when first line agents fail, usually due to resistance. Ethionamide and prothionamide are no longer available in Britain, but it is possible to import the latter.

The actions and pharmacokinetics of the first line agents are shown in Table 39.4. Their major adverse effects and toxicities are shown in Table 39.5.

With the exception of streptomycin, the first

Table 39.4 Pharmacokinetics of first line antitubercular drugs

Drug	Site of action	Half-life (hours)	Reduce dose in Renal impairment	Reduce dose in Liver impairment	Penetration into CSF	Method of elimination
Rifampicin	Bactericidal. Inhibits DNA-dependent RNA polymerase	1.5–5 (mean 2.8)	No	Yes	About 30% of serum levels with inflamed meninges	Extensive first-pass effect. Partially active metabolite formed by deacetylation in liver undergoes enterohepatic recirculation. 50–60% excreted in faeces; 10–15% as unchanged drug in urine
Isoniazid	Bactericidal. Inhibits production of cell wall components	0.5–1.5 (2–4)*	No	Yes	About 20% serum levels (more with inflamed meninges)	Acetylated in liver. Metabolites (inactive) excreted in urine
Ethambutol	Bacteriostatic. Uncertain action. Possibly RNA antimetabolite	4–6	Yes	No	Up to 54% serum levels with inflamed meninges	Nearly all recovered in urine after 24 hours, predominantly as unchanged drug
Pyrazinamide	Bactericidal. Uncertain action	12–24	Yes	Yes	Up to 100% serum levels with inflamed meninges	Metabolized to inactive metabolites which are excreted in urine
Streptomycin	Bactericidal. Ribosomal inhibition	5	Yes	No	Little	Renal elimination of unchanged drug

* Figures in brackets refer to slow acetylators.

Table 39.5 Major adverse reactions and interactions of major antituberculous agents

Drug	Adverse reactions	Interactions	Comments
Rifampicin	Gastrointestinal disturbance Subclinical hepatitis is common but frank jaundice less so*. (Patients with pre-existing liver disease at greater risk) 'Flu like' syndrome, especially with intermittent or irregular dosing	Rifampicin is a potent inducer of the hepatic mixed function oxidase system and reduces the concentration of many drugs. Those with the most clinical significance are: • Warfarin (& analogues) — the effect can last for a week after rifampicin is stopped • Oral contraceptive pill – additional methods of contraception need to be used • Corticosteroids – doses may need to be doubled while rifampicin is being taken.	Patients should be warned that rifampicin will stain body fluids including urine, sweat and tears an orange/red colour. They should be reassured that this is quite normal and also harmless. Patients should be asked about the use of contact lenses and advised not to use soft lenses as they may be permanently stained. Gas-permeable and hard contact lenses should not be affected
Isoniazid	Subclinical hepatitis* (rare in the young, incidence increases with age) Peripheral neuropathy which can be prevented by administration of pyridoxine. (Alcoholics, the malnourished and those with renal impairment, diabetes & liver disease are especially at risk and should be offered pyridoxine)	Inhibits the metabolism of both carbamazepine and phenytoin, which may lead to increased toxicity of the anticonvulsants. Patients may need to be monitored for overdosage when both drugs are given together and for underdosage when isoniazid is discontinued The frequency of liver toxicity is increased in patients also taking rifampicin	Patients, especially those not taking pyridoxine, should be asked to report any numbness or tingling in their hands or feet to their doctor Be aware of risk of overt hepatitis, especially in those also taking rifampicin and/or pyrazinamide
Ethambutol	Ocular toxicity is the most serious but is rare at recommended doses. Those with impaired renal function are most at risk. It is reversible if the drug is stopped promptly but may take time to resolve Increases uric acid levels – may precipitate gout	No serious interactions	Patients should be asked to report any changes in vision, especially blurred vision, reduction of visual field or colour vision
Pyrazinamide	Although less common with lower doses used today, hepatotoxicity may range from asymptomatic derangement of liver function tests to severe hepatitis May cause increased concentration of uric acid but only rarely precipitates gout. If gout occurs, the drug should be withdrawn May cause gastrointestinal intolerance and rashes	No serious interactions	Be aware of risk of overt hepatitis, especially in those also taking rifampicin and/or isoniazid
Streptomycin	Ototoxicity usually vestibular and less often auditory, related to serum levels can occur. Older patients and those with poor renal function are at greater risk Streptomycin is less toxic to the kidneys than other aminoglycosides	May potentially cause additive renal and ototoxicity when given together with other renal & ototoxic drugs such as amphotericin B, loop diuretics, or other aminoglycosides	May cause hypersensitivity both in patients and in those handling the drug

* Derangement of liver function tests is common at the start of treatment for both isoniazid and rifampicin and even more common when both drugs are given.

line agents are usually administered orally. For patients who cannot take tablets or capsules, there is a liquid preparation of rifampicin. There are no commercial sources of liquid isoniazid, ethambutol or pyrazinamide in Britain at present although there is a BPC formulation for isoniazid elixir. Extemporaneous formulations for all three drugs have been used. The manufacturers or local drug information centres are probably the best sources of information about these individual formulations. Rifampicin may also be given intravenously and isoniazid by the intravenous and intramuscular routes in patients who are severely ill and cannot take oral medication. Although not commercially available, ethambutol injection has been used and may be available on request from the manufacturer.

Rifampicin, isoniazid and pyrazinamide are all potentially hepatotoxic. Transient increases in transaminases and bilirubin commonly occur at the start of treatment. However, there is no need to monitor liver function routinely in patients with normal liver function at the start of treatment. If frank jaundice or hepatitis occurs, all drugs should be stopped and liver function allowed to return to normal, at which time treatment should be recommenced one drug at a time. Clinical hepatitis is rare but pharmacists should be aware that patients may complain of vague symptoms such as abdominal pain and malaise which may indicate impending hepatitis.

Isoniazid may also cause a dose-dependent peripheral neuropathy, probably due to depletion of vitamin B_6. This reaction is rare in recommended doses but certain patient groups, e.g. the poorly nourished, alcoholics, diabetics, uraemic patients and pregnant women, are at greater risk and should receive pyridoxine supplementation at a dose of 10 to 20 mg per day.

Hypersensitivity reactions or rashes may occur with any of the drugs although the most important is that due to rifampicin, which, although rare, can be quite severe. It is more prevalent during intermittent treatment and presents as a 'flu-like' syndrome sometimes with abdominal pain and respiratory symptoms. This usually resolves on reverting to a daily dosage. However, if more serious effects such as renal impairment or haematological abnormalities occur, the drug should be stopped and never restarted. Rashes can occur with isoniazid, pyrazinamide and streptomycin.

Ocular toxicity is by far the most important toxicity of ethambutol. It occurs in less than 2% of patients at the usual dosage of 15 mg/kg but is more common in the elderly and the renally impaired. Patients may complain of changes in colour vision or visual field which may appear suddenly. The effect is usually reversible on discontinuation but permanent damage may occur if the drug is continued. It is important that visual acuity is checked before treatment. It has been recommended that regular visual checks should be performed. However, as the majority of patients only receive the drug for 8 weeks, many clinicians do not feel that this is necessary, preferring to counsel patients to report any changes in visual acuity. This precludes its use in those who are unable to report such changes such as young children and the severely ill.

DISEASE CONTROL AND PREVENTION

In order to control the spread of tuberculosis, vigorous efforts are made to trace contacts of infectious cases so that they can be screened. Other groups, notably health service, school and nursing home employees, and immigrants from countries where tuberculosis occurs frequently are also often screened. Investigation is usually by inquiry about past vaccination and Heaf test.

Chemoprophylaxis is routinely offered to the following groups:

- children under 16 years old with Heaf grade 2–4 and no history of BCG
- children under 5 years old in close contact with smear-positive adult.

It may be considered in:

- children under 16 years old with strongly positive (grade 3–4) Heaf who have had BCG
- adults who have recently converted to tuberculin positivity
- Asian adult contacts under 35 years old

either Heaf positive (grade 3–4) or Heaf positive (grade 2) and no BCG
- Heaf positive HIV patients.

Prophylaxis is usually with isoniazid alone for 6 to 12 months or rifampicin and isoniazid for 3 months. Both regimens are equally effective.

Vaccination against tuberculosis is carried out routinely in Britain at about 13 years of age. BCG intradermal contains a live attenuated strain of *M. bovis* and should be administered by strict intradermal injection. After vaccination, there is usually a local reaction within 2 to 6 weeks. Very occasionally, this may progress to a shallow, discharging ulcer which should be covered with a dry dressing. Isoniazid powder has been used but is not recommended. More serious injection site reactions are largely due to incorrect injection technique or vaccination of a tuberculin-positive patient.

The need for vaccination for all is under constant review due to the declining incidence of tuberculosis. However, it is likely to be continued for some time especially as the AIDS epidemic may cause the incidence to rise again. Patients receiving isoniazid prophylaxis may in some cases be vaccinated. They should receive isoniazid-resistant BCG vaccine. If they are given the normal vaccine, it will be killed by the isoniazid.

THE PATIENT

It is possible to cure virtually all patients with tuberculous infection or disease provided that an adequate regimen is prescribed and that the patient complies with treatment. By far the largest cause of treatment failure is non-compliance by the patient, which may occur willfully or through ignorance. Non-compliance has serious consequences, treatment may fail and disease may relapse, in some cases with resistant organisms. If a non-compliant patient remains infectious he will also be a public health hazard.

Factors affecting compliance

A number of studies have shown that compli-ance falls as the number of tablets to be taken per day increases, and that compliance falls further if doses have to be taken frequently through the day. Ideally, the least number of tablets should be given.

Patients may fail to comply because they feel better and do not appreciate the need to continue with their medication. Lack of clarity of instructions, written, verbal or otherwise may compromise compliance, particularly if the patient is being confused by being given conflicting advice by different health-care professionals. Finally, adverse effects or symptoms perceived to be adverse effects may reduce compliance.

Improving patient compliance

Antituberculous therapy should be prescribed once a day using as few tablets as possible. Single daily dosing enables patients to fit their medication into their daily routine. Rifampicin and isoniazid are both well absorbed when taken on an empty stomach. However, absorption is reduced and delayed when taken with or after food. It is therefore recommended that both are taken ½ to 1 hour before food to achieve rapid high blood levels. It is usually recommended that patients take their antituberculous medication before breakfast. Cueing tablet taking to a regular activity such as brushing the teeth may improve compliance in some patients.

The number of tablets to be taken each day may be reduced by using combination preparations. These also have the advantage of reducing the possibility of monotherapy and consequent resistance. There are a number of combination preparations available. Some of the preparations, for example Rifater, contain ratios of drugs that differ slightly from the dosages recommended by the British Thoracic Society. This slight difference in dosage is probably not clinically significant and is far more preferable than potential undertreatment due to non-compliance. Mynah is a preparation available in a number of different ratios to facilitate reasonably accurate calculation of the dose of ethambutol.

Combination preparations may not be suitable for use in children as their dosage recommendations differ from those of adults.

Patient education

Patient education is an area where pharmacists can perform a useful role and can confirm the information that the patient has already received. Written instruction and/or patient information leaflets may be offered in addition to verbal counselling if there is any doubt as to the patient's understanding. It should be emphasized that the disease will be cured but that this will take some months and that the tablets should continue to be taken as prescribed even if the patient feels better. Some patients will comply initially while they are unwell, but will fail to comply later as they begin to feel better.

The occurrence of some adverse effects may require discontinuation of a drug, but others are harmless. The patient should be told which side effects to expect and which require referral back to their doctor. Again written instructions may be helpful.

A number of Asian patients with tuberculosis have a poor command of English. It may still be possible to give written instructions on dosage as some pharmaceutical companies are able to provide pictorial material and dosage sheets in a number of languages.

Counselling points

Patients taking rifampicin should be told that the drug will cause a harmless discolouration of their urine and other body fluids, for example sweat and tears. The staining of tears is important if the patient uses soft contact lenses as these may be permanently stained. Gas-permeable and hard lenses are unaffected. Female patients using the oral contraceptive pill should be advised to use other non-hormonal methods of contraception for the duration of treatment with rifampicin and for one cycle afterwards.

Although ocular side effects are rare when ethambutol is taken in normal dosages, patients should be warned of this potentially serious side effect. They should be advised to stop the drug and report to their doctor if they notice any changes in their vision, e.g. reduction in visual acuity or changes in colour vision. This is especially important because visual changes are usually reversible on discontinuation of the drug but may be permanent if the drug is not stopped.

CASE STUDIES

CASE 39.1

Mr H. E. is a 34-year-old HIV positive homosexual man who presents at the HIV clinic complaining of weight loss, shortness of breath, night sweats and productive cough. A chest X-ray reveals consolidation of the left upper and middle lobes. His sputum is found to be smear positive for acid–alcohol-fast bacilli (AAFB) which were shown later on culture to be *M. tuberculosis*. A diagnostic Mantoux test was therefore not required. Treatment was started with rifampicin 450 mg, isoniazid 300 mg, pyrazinamide 2 g and ethambutol 800 mg.

Q1 Was Mr H. E. commenced on the correct treatment?

Q2 For how long should treatment be continued?

Q3 Can tuberculosis be prevented in HIV positive patients?

CASE 39.2

Mrs C.D. is a 30-year-old lady with pulmonary tuberculosis. She is at present taking rifampicin and isoniazid but was on a four-drug regimen consisting of rifampicin, isoniazid, pyrazinamide and ethambutol until last week. She now thinks that she may be pregnant as a home test has given a positive result.

Q The doctor wishes to know whether her therapy should be stopped or changed and whether the pregnancy should be continued or termination offered.

CASE 39.3

Mr A. B. is a 58-year-old Indian gentleman who has been resident in Britain for about 20 years. He has recently returned from a visit to his family in India. He had been to see his general practitioner 2 weeks ago complaining of malaise and headaches for which he was prescribed co-dydramol, 1 or 2 tablets when necessary. Subsequently his symptoms had worsened and he complained of increasing headache, malaise, night sweats, abdominal pain and vomiting as well as a non-productive cough. At this time his doctor arranged admission to hospital.

On examination Mr A. B. was found to be slightly confused and drowsy. In view of his meningeal symptoms he was sent for an urgent CT scan which showed no abnormality. A lumbar puncture was performed and showed increased white blood cells (especially lymphocytes) and a low CSF glucose. A chest X-ray showed evidence of previous pulmonary tuberculosis which, together with the CSF results raised the possibility of tuberculous meningitis. Mr A. B. was investigated for tuberculous infection and commenced on a therapeutic trial of antituberculous medication.

Q1 Which drugs should be used and are they given intrathecally?

Q2 Is there a place for corticosteroids?

ANSWERS TO CASE STUDIES

CASE 39.1

A1 In the absence of adverse sensitivity data, treatment should be commenced with standard drugs (four are recommended in Britain). Mr H. E.'s therapy is therefore correct. The response to treatment is usually excellent.

A2 The optimum duration of treatment is not known but it may be expected that treatment may need to be prolonged. It has been suggested that treatment should be continued with rifampicin and isoniazid for at least 6 months after sputum becomes culture negative and that prophylaxis be offered to prevent recurrence of disease.

A3 To prevent tuberculosis, HIV positive patients should ideally be given a Mantoux test. If the test is positive and active disease has been ruled out, the patient may be offered isoniazid prophylaxis (300 mg daily). The duration of prophylaxis is not known but is likely to be prolonged, possibly for life. There is a significant false negative response to the Mantoux test and therefore a negative result does not rule out infection. BCG vaccine is not recommended for HIV positive patients as the vaccine is live and reports of active disease following vaccination have been reported.

CASE 39.2

A Treatment should be continued as her disease may recur if it is stopped. This would put both her and her unborn child at risk, as well as the community around her if she became infectious. Untreated tuberculosis is a far greater danger to both mother and unborn child than is the treatment of the disease. A number of studies have investigated tuberculosis treatment during pregnancy and have concluded that, with the exception of streptomycin, the first line agents are all safe to use. This is reflected in the advice of both the British and American Thoracic Societies.

Both rifampicin and isoniazid cross the placenta but in small concentrations. They have both been implicated in causing birth defects but no study has proven either drug to be a teratogen. There is a risk that isoniazid may cause neuropathy in the fetus as well as the mother so pyridoxine prophylaxis may be offered.

Mrs C. D. has previously received ethambutol and pyrazinamide. Ethambutol also crosses the placenta but, as for rifampicin and isoniazid, it has not been shown to be a teratogen. Concern has been expressed at the possibility of optic damage but at present the risks, if any, are unknown. Very little is known about the use of pyrazinamide in pregnancy although it would be expected to cross the placenta. However, no reports linking its use to birth defects have been published.

Streptomycin is an aminoglycoside and has been associated with auditory nerve and vestibular apparatus damage. In cases where damage occurs the effects are variable but often consist of hearing loss above normal speech frequencies. Children are often not handicapped by this. The drug should, however, be avoided in all stages of pregnancy.

The first line drugs all appear in breast milk in low concentrations but breast feeding need not be discouraged as toxicity does not usually occur in the baby.

CASE 39.3

A1 Isoniazid and pyrazinamide both pass into the CSF well, CSF drug levels of up to 100% those of serum having been quoted in some studies. Rifampicin penetrates less well but as with ethambutol and streptomycin, CSF drug levels are increased in the presence of inflamed meninges. All the first line agents penetrate the CSF well enough to make intrathecal treatment unnecessary.

There is little information on which to base treatment guidelines as there have been relatively few trials of treatment for tuberculous meningitis. Treatment with rifampicin and isoniazid for 18 to 24 months has been recommended as it is known that response to treatment is often slow. As with other forms of tuberculosis, attempts have been made to shorten treatment and it is now recommended that rifampicin and isoniazid are given for up to 12 months together with pyrazinamide for at least 2 months. Either ethambutol or streptomycin may be used if a fourth drug is required. Standard doses are normally used. Because of the difficulty in diagnosing tuberculous meningitis, treatment is often started on an empiric basis as soon as the disease is suspected.

A2 The role of corticosteroids in the treatment of tuberculous meningitis remains controversial. In spite of a lack of conclusive data to support their use they are sometimes used in severe disease, where there is a general consensus that they may be of benefit. Prednisolone in a dose of around 60 mg per day (1 to 3 mg/kg/day in children) is normally used.

BIBLIOGRAPHY

Allen M B, Cooke N J. Corticosteroids and tuberculosis. (Editorial), British Medical Journal 1991; 303: 871–872

American Thoracic Society. Treatment of tuberculosis and tuberculosis infection in adults and children. American Review of Respiratory Disease 1986; 134: 355–363

Citron K M, Girling D J. Tuberculosis. In: Weatherall D J, Ledingham J G G, Warrell D A (eds) The Oxford textbook of medicine, 2nd edn. London: Oxford University Press 1988; 5.278–5.299

Des Prez R M, Heim C R. Mycobacterium tuberculosis. In: Mandell G L, Douglas R G, Bennett J E (eds) Principle and practice of infectious diseases, 3rd edn. New York: Churchill Livingstone 1990; 1877–1906

Farrar K. Tuberculosis and its treatment. Pharmaceutical Journal 1988; 240: 149–151

Ormerod L P. Chemotherapy and management of tuberculosis in the United Kingdom: recommendations of the Joint Tuberculosis Committee of the British Thoracic Society. Thorax 1990; 45: 403–408

Sarosi, G A (ed). Seminars in respiratory infections. 1989; 4(3): 155–242

Stratton M A, Reed M T. Short course drug therapy for tuberculosis. Clinical Pharmacy 1986; 5: 977–987

Subcommittee of the Joint Tuberculosis Committee of the British Thoracic Society. Control and prevention of tuberculosis in Britain: an updated code of practice. British Medical Journal 1990; 300: 995–999

The management of extra-pulmonary tuberculosis. Drug and Therapeutics Bulletin 1991; 29: 26–28

Chapter 40

Sexually transmitted diseases

P. G. Watson

BACKGROUND AND EPIDEMIOLOGY

The total number of conditions diagnosed in English NHS genitourinary medicine clinics rose steadily to 1986 (647 359) and there was a slight fall in 1987 (620 266). Many patients are found not to have a sexually transmitted disease (STD), often attending through worry or because they may have been in contact with a STD.

Over the last 10 years there has been a change in the type of diagnosis seen in the UK with the venereal diseases syphilis and gonorrhoea becoming less common and viral infections, particularly genital warts and genital herpes, more common. In 1987 the commonest male and female STDs were nongonococcal urethritis and chlamydial cervicitis, respectively, followed by genital warts in both sexes. In both sexes the great majority of STDs occur in the 15 to 34 year old age group.

CLINICAL ASPECTS

A full history, including a sexual history, is taken from patients and the anogenital region is examined together with other regions as indicated. Specimens should be collected to explain the clinical features and, with the aid of microscopy, often a working diagnosis can be made at the patient's first attendance. In addition, specimens should be taken to exclude treatable infections which commonly are asymptomatic – chlamydial infection and gonorrhoea in women and syphilis in both sexes.

Patients should be given adequate treatment in regimens which are easy to take and they should be educated about the illness, its sexual transmission and the risks of re-infection. After treatment, patients should be reviewed to assess the response.

Without attempting to cover fully the wide range of clinical presentations seen in genito-urinary medicine clinics, it is practical to consider:

• gonorrhoea, *Chlamydia trachomatis* infection and nongonococcal urethritis
• causes of vaginal discharge
• causes of genital ulceration
• genital warts
• arthropod infestations.

Human immunodeficiency virus (HIV) infection and viral hepatitis are covered in other chapters.

Gonorrhoea, nongonococcal urethritis and *C. trachomatis* infection

Aetiology and investigations

In men these conditions usually cause an anterior urethritis with symptoms of dysuria or a urethral discharge of pus or both. When an anterior urethritis is not caused by *Neisseria gonorrhoeae* it is termed nongonococcal urethritis. Sexually transmitted causes of nongonococcal urethritis include *C. trachomatis* infection in up to 50% of cases and the other causes are not identified. Not all causes of nongonococcal urethritis are STDs and include:

• urinary tract infection
• bacterial prostatitis
• urethral obstruction to urinary outflow
• instrumentation of the urethra.

Uncommonly, infection of the male urethra with *N. gonorrhoeae* or *C. trachomatis* is asymptomatic.

When a man presents with symptoms of urethritis, material should be obtained from the urethra, smeared on to a microscope slide and Gram stained. On microscopy the presence of pus cells will confirm the urethritis and the presence or absence of *N. gonorrhoeae*, seen as Gram-negative diplococci, allows a working diagnosis of gonor-

rhoea or nongonococcal urethritis, respectively, to be made (sensitivity and specificity both 95%). Urethral material should also be sent for culture of *N. gonorrhoeae* to confirm or exclude gonorrhoea and for antibiotic sensitivity testing of isolated *N. gonorrhoeae*. Orogenital or anal intercourse may lead to, usually asymptomatic, infection of the throat or rectum with *N. gonorrhoeae* and specimens can be taken from those sites for culture.

C. trachomatis is too small to be seen on light microscopy. Urethral specimens may be obtained to isolate it in cell culture or detect it by enzyme-linked immunosorbent assay (ELISA) or immunofluoresence microscopy.

In women *N. gonorrhoeae* and *C. trachomatis* primarily infect the cervix or urethra. Usually they are asymptomatic infections but may cause vaginal discharge, dysuria or altered menstrual bleeding. Specimens should be taken from the endocervix and urethra for microscopy and culture to exclude gonorrhoea. The sensitivity of microscopy in the diagnosis of female gonorrhoea is only about 50%. Specimens can also be taken from the throat and rectum for culture. Endocervical specimens should be taken for the detection of *C. trachomatis*.

Treatment

Uncomplicated gonorrhoea will respond well to a single oral or parenteral dose of an antibiotic (Table 40.1). Gonorrhoea is often treated at the patient's first attendance on the basis of microscopy and before the sensitivities of the organism are known. *N. gonorrhoeae* is sensitive to a number of antibiotics. The choice of first line treatment should be guided by knowledge of the usual sensitivities of strains of *N. gonorrhoeae* isolated in the geographical area where the infection was acquired. Strains of beta-lactamase (penicillinase) producing *N. gonorrhoeae* are common in Africa and Asia and beta-lactamase-stable antibiotics should be used for infections acquired in those areas.

Oropharyngeal gonorrhoea may respond poorly to single-dose oral treatments. Alternative treatments are given in Table 40.2.

Table 40.1   Single-dose treatments for uncomplicated anogenital gonorrhoea

Antibiotic	Dose	Route	Comments
Penicillin			
Ampicillin	2 g	p.o.*	Inexpensive
Bacampicillin	1.6 g	p.o.*	
Talampicillin	1.5 g	p.o.*	
Amoxycillin	3 g	p.o.*	
4-Quinolones			
Ciprofloxacin	250 mg	p.o.	Beta-lactamase
	(500 mg	p.o.)†	stable
Acrosoxacin	300 mg	p.o.	
Enoxacin	400 mg	p.o.	
Ofloxacin	400 mg	p.o.	
Cephalosporins			
Cefoxitin	2 g	i.m.	Beta-lactamase
Cefuroxime	1.5 g	i.m.	stable
Cefuroxime axetil ester	1.5 g	p.o.*	Expensive
Cefaclor	3 g	p.o.*	
Ceftizoxime	500 mg	i.m.	
Ceftriaxone	250 mg	i.m.†	
Other			
Spectinomycin	2 g	i.m.†	Beta-lactamase stable Expensive

* With probenecid 1 g p.o.
† World Health Organization recommended first line treatment.

Table 40.2   Treatment regimens for uncomplicated oropharyngeal gonorrhoea

Antibiotic	Regimen
Ampicillin or talampicillin	250 mg p.o. four times daily for 5 days
Cefuroxime	1.5 g i.m. daily for 3 days
Ceftriaxone	250 mg i.m. once
Co-trimoxazole	9 tablets (3600 mg sulphamethoxazole, 720 mg trimethoprim) as a single dose daily for 5 days

The treatment of uncomplicated *C. trachomatis* infection in men or women requires at least 7 days of a tetracycline preparation or erythromycin stearate. The new macrolide preparation, azithromycin, produces very high tissue levels with a long half-life, and a single dose of azithromycin 1 g has been shown to be effective in uncomplicated genital *C. trachomatis* infection (Table 40.3). No drugs have been found to be more effective than tetracycline preparations or erythromycin stearate in the treatment of sexually transmitted nongonococcal urethritis not due to *C. trachomatis*. The results of treatment of nongonococcal urethritis are variable. Relapse after treatment often occurs especially when the causative organism is not *C. trachomatis*.

Non-sexually transmitted nongonococcal urethritis should be treated appropriately.

Side effects from single dose treatments are uncommon and the risks of drug interactions minimal because most genitourinary medicine patients are not on other medication. Side effects and drug interactions to consider are detailed in Tables 40.4 and 40.5.

Patients who have been treated for gonor-

Table 40.3   Treatment regimens for uncomplicated *Chlamydia trachomatis* infection and nongonococcal urethritis

Antibiotic	Regimen	Comments
Oxytetracycline	250 mg p.o. four times daily for 7 days	Inexpensive but four times daily regimen
Deteclo	One tablet twice daily for 7 days	More expensive Contains demeclocycline which is slowly excreted
Doxycycline	200 mg p.o. then 100 mg p.o. daily for 7 days	Well absorbed and slowly excreted allowing once-daily regimen Expensive
Erythromycin stearate	500 mg p.o. twice daily or 250 mg four times daily for 7 days	The twice-daily regimen may cause more GI side effects
Azithromycin	1 g p.o. as a single dose	Produces high tissue concentrations with a long half-life Very expensive

Table 40.4 Points to consider in the treatment of gonorrhoea, nongonococcal urethritis and *Chlamydia trachomatis* infection

Drug	Points to consider
Broad-spectrum penicillins	Avoid in glandular fever Use cautiously if there is a history of allergy Discontinue treatment if a rash develops
Probenecid	Contra-indicated in porphyria and if there is a history of blood disorders or nephrolithiasis
4-Quinolones	Not recommended for pregnant or lactating women or for those still growing Use cautiously where there is a history of epilepsy
Cephalosporins	Contra-indicated in porphyria Use cautiously if there is a history of penicillin allergy
Co-trimoxazole	Contra-indicated in pregnancy and for infants less than 6 weeks old and in renal or hepatic failure and blood disorders Not recommended for lactating women Commonly causes skin rashes especially in HIV infected patients
Tetracyclines	Swallow tablets or capsules whole with plenty of fluid and while sitting or standing Contra-indicated in pregnancy and for children less than 12 years old, in systemic lupus erythematosus and severe renal failure Not recommended for lactating women Risk of photosensitivity Absorption decreased by dairy products
Erythromycin	Contra-indicated in porphyria, and estolate preparation contra-indicated in liver disease Larger doses may cause nausea and vomiting and diarrhoea
Azithromycin	See under Erythromycin Use cautiously in renal impairment and in pregnant or lactating women

rhoea, nongonococcal urethritis or *C. trachomatis* infection should be reviewed after treatment to ensure cure and to exclude other STDs. Men with urethral gonorrhoea often also have nongonococcal urethritis and this can be diagnosed only after the gonorrhoea has been treated. Sexual partners should attend a genitourinary medicine clinic.

Complications of gonorrhoea and particularly *C. trachomatis* infection in men and women include acute epididymitis and acute pelvic inflammatory disease. As both these conditions can lead to a reduction of fertility, it is most important that they are managed by experts who will make an accurate diagnosis, isolate the infecting organism and give appropriate treatment. Treatment should be started before microbiological results are available and therefore the antibiotic(s) should be aimed at the likely causes and reviewed as results become available. Patients with these conditions may require admission to hospital and parenteral antibiotics ini-

tially. Treatment should be given for at least 2 weeks until complete recovery occurs. Sexual partners should be seen.

Less commonly *N. gonorrhoeae* causes disseminated gonococcal infection, often producing a systemically ill patient with skin lesions, tenosynovitis and migratory polyarthritis. *C. trachomatis* infection may cause Reiter's syndrome – urethritis, arthritis and conjunctivitis or iritis. These require expert management often with hospital admission.

The newborn child of a mother infected with *N. gonorrhoeae* or *C. trachomatis* at delivery may develop conjunctivitis, which will require expert management. The child's mother and her sexual partner(s) must be investigated.

Vaginal discharge

Aetiology

The causes of an altered vaginal discharge include:

Table 40.5 Drug interactions with drugs used in the treatment of gonorrhoea, nongonococcal urethritis and *Chlamydia trachomatis* infection

Drug	Interactions
Broad-spectrum penicillins	Action of oral anticoagulants may be enhanced
Probenecid	Effect reduced by aspirin Reduces excretion of non-steroidal anti-inflammatory agents, e.g. indomethacin, ketoprofen and naproxen; antibiotics, e.g. cephalosporins, cinoxacin, dapsone, nalidixic acid, nitrofurantoin and penicillins; antiviral agents, e.g. acyclovir and zidovudine, captopril, methotrexate
4-Quinolones	Absorption of some reduced by antacids, oral iron and sucralfate Action of oral anticoagulants enhanced by some Plasma theophylline concentration increased by some
Cephalosporins	Excretion reduced by probenecid
Co-trimoxazole	Action of oral anticoagulants and sulphonylureas enhanced Increases the antifolate effects of phenytoin, pyrimethamine and methotrexate
Tetracyclines	Absorption reduced by antacids and ulcer-healing drugs, e.g. bismuth chelate and sucralfate, calcium, magnesium, and zinc salts and oral iron Absorption of zinc salts and oral iron reduced Metabolism of doxycycline increased by antiepileptics, e.g. carbamazepine, phenobarbitone, phenytoin and primidone Action of oral anticoagulants may be enhanced
Erythromycin	Enhances effects of oral anticoagulants and digoxin Increases plasma concentrations of alfentanil, disopyramide, carbamazepine, triazolam, cyclosporin and theophylline
Azithromycin	Absorption reduced by antacids and adsorbents May enhance the effects of warfarin and digoxin Ergotism possible if given with ergotamine

- vaginal infections
  - — vulvovaginal candidosis
  - — trichomoniasis
  - — bacterial vaginosis
- cervical infections with *C. trachomatis* or *N. gonorrhoeae*
- chemical irritation
- intravaginal foreign bodies
- toxic shock syndrome.

In managing a vaginal discharge, it is important properly to examine and investigate the patient. Her description of the symptoms may be misleading.

Vulvovaginal candidosis. Usually in vulvovaginal candidosis or thrush, there is a thick, white discharge associated with vulval irritation. On examination there are reddened and swollen mucosal surfaces and skin, sometimes with fissuring, and adherent plaques of discharge are seen in the vagina. It is caused by *Candida* spp.,

usually *Candida albicans* and these fungi may be seen on microscopy or isolated on culture of a high vaginal swab. The detection of commensal vaginal *Candida* spp. without symptoms is common and should not be diagnosed as vulvovaginal candidosis. The sexual partner of a woman with candidosis may develop an itchy penile rash but it is not commonly sexually transmitted.

Treatment. The standard treatment of vulvovaginal candidosis is the topical vaginal application of an imidazole – clotrimoxazole, econazole, ketoconazole or miconazole – as vaginal tablets, ovules, coated tampons or creams. Slow-release preparations, requiring only a single insertion, produce results comparable to preparations which are inserted each night for up to 7 doses. The polyene antibiotic, nystatin, is effective but requires the daily insertion of vaginal tablets for at least 14 days. When vulvitis is marked the preparation used should also be applied as a cream to the vulval skin and mucosa. An imidazole cream is suitable for men with penile thrush.

Side effects from topical preparations are uncommon although local irritation may result.

The newer triazole preparations, fluconazole and itraconazole, may be preferred by some patients. They are taken orally, fluconazole in a single dose of 150 mg and itraconazole as two doses of 200 mg in a single day. Studies suggest that oral triazoles are as effective as topical imidazoles in the treatment of vulvovaginal candidosis but the hope that they would prevent recurrent episodes has not been realized. Treatment points and drug interactions with fluconazole and itraconazole are shown in Tables 40.6 and 40.7.

Trichomoniasis. Infection with the flagellate protozoon *Trichomonas vaginalis* can be asymptomatic but usually causes a thin, grey, malodorous vaginal discharge with intense symptoms of vulval irritation, and vulvitis and vaginitis are obvious on examination. The organism can be seen on microscopy of the discharge, grown on culture or seen on a smear taken for cytology. Trichomoniasis is a STD and although sexual partners rarely develop symptoms, commonly they are infected with the organism. Co-existing STDs are common.

Treatment. The 5-nitroimidazole, metronidazole, is the drug of choice for trichomoniasis and tinidazole is an alternative. A single oral dose of 2 g of metronidazole has been found to be as effective as a 7-day course of 400 mg twice daily and does not depend on patient compliance. As discussed above, sexual partners should be treated but if that is not possible, the 7-day course of treatment may protect a woman against reinfection. Treatment points and drug interactions with metronidazole and tinidazole are shown in Tables 40.8 and 40.9.

Table 40.6 Points to consider when prescribing triazole antifungal drugs

Drug	Points to consider
Fluconazole	Use with caution in pregnancy, renal failure, children and lactating women May cause common GI side effects, abnormal liver function tests or a rash (indication for stopping treatment)
Itraconazole	Contra-indicated if there is a history of liver disease Use with caution in pregnant or lactating women May cause GI side effects or headache

Table 40.7 Drug interactions with triazole antifungal drugs

Drug	Interactions
Fluconazole	Metabolism accelerated by rifampicin Serum concentrations of phenytoin, sulphonylureas, and cyclosporin increased Effects of oral anticoagulants enhanced
Itraconazole	Metabolism accelerated by rifampicin Absorption decreased by antacids

Table 40.8 Points to consider when prescribing metronidazole or tinidazole

Drug	Points to consider
Metronidazole	Use with caution in hepatic failure and in pregnant or lactating women May cause nausea, vomiting, unpleasant taste, furred tongue, GI disturbances, rashes, headache, drowsiness, dizziness, ataxia
Tinidazole	As metronidazole Contra-indicated in porphyria

Table 40.9 Drug interactions with metronidazole and tinidazole

Drug	Interactions
Metronidazole	Disulfiram-like reaction with alcohol Effects of oral anticoagulants enhanced Increases plasma phenytoin concentration Plasma metronidazole concentration decreased by phenobarbitone Plasma metronidazole concentration increased by cimetidine
Tinidazole	Disulfiram-like reaction with alcohol

After treatment, patients should be reviewed to show that the organism has been eliminated. Causes of treatment failure include:

- treatment not taken
- reinfection
- metronidazole-inactivating vaginal bacteria
- metronidazole-resistant *T. vaginalis*.

Giving metronidazole together with a broad-spectrum antibiotic has proved a successful treatment when vaginal bacteria are capable of inactivating metronidazole. The management of infection with metronidazole-resistant *T. vaginalis* can be very difficult. Other successful treatment regimens which have been reported include:

- intravenous metronidazole
- intravaginal metronidazole suppositories
- clotrimazole vaginal tablets
- natamycin vaginal tablets
- Povidone-iodine vaginal tablets
- vaccination with inactivated *Lactobacillus acidophilus* (Gynatren)
- acetarsol vaginal ovules.

Bacterial vaginosis. The cause of bacterial vaginosis is not fully understood. It is probably not a STD but may mask the presence of STDs which should be excluded in making the diagnosis. Bacterial vaginosis is diagnosed when a patient complains of a vaginal discharge, which is usually thin, grey and malodorous and at least two of the following criteria are met:

- microscopy of the vaginal discharge shows epithelial cells surrounded and obscured by a common vaginal commensal bacterium, *Gardnerella vaginalis* (these are termed clue cells)
- the vaginal pH is greater than 4.5
- the addition of 5 to 10% potassium hydroxide to the discharge will increase the ammoniacal odour.

A risk factor for developing bacterial vaginosis is the presence of an intrauterine contraceptive device. Sexual partners of women with bacterial vaginosis do not develop symptoms and their treatment is not indicated.

Treatment. The standard treatment is oral metronidazole 400 mg twice daily for 1 week. Recurrences are common.

Genital ulceration

The differential diagnosis of genital ulceration includes:

- infections
  - genital herpes
  - syphilis
  - chancroid
  - lymphogranuloma venereum
  - granuloma inguinale
- other causes
  - Crohn's disease
  - Behcet's syndrome
  - Stevens–Johnson syndrome
  - malignant tumours
  - trauma.

In developed countries, infection with either type of herpes simplex virus (HSV), HSV-1 or HSV-2, is the commonest cause of genital ulceration, and syphilis the second commonest. Chancroid, lymphogranuloma venereum and granuloma inguinale are largely diseases of the tropics and subtropics. It is important not to rely only on the appearance of genital ulceration in making a diagnosis but to exclude possible causes.

Genital herpes. Close physical contact with HSV in lesions or body fluids, allows inoculation of the virus on to a susceptible mucosal surface or into broken skin.

After 3 to 9 days small vesicles develop at the site of inoculation and these quickly break down to form usually multiple, very superficial, painful and tender ulcers. Without treatment these will gradually resolve, healing usually being complete within 3 weeks. Genital herpes, particularly first attacks, may be associated with tender inguinal lymphadenopathy, 'flu-like symptoms and herpetic cervicitis. Complications include extragenital lesions and, less commonly, neurological manifestations.

Asymptomatic infection with HSV is common as is asymptomatic excretion of HSV in saliva and genital secretions.

At the time of the first infection, HSV ascends nerve fibres and establishes a latent infection in the nerve root ganglia. Many patients experience recurrent infections, some very frequently. Recurrences are usually less severe and of shorter duration than the first attack. Sometimes recurrences are preceded by prodromal symptoms, e.g. mild tingling or severe shooting pains.

Genital herpes in pregnancy is associated with spontaneous abortion and premature delivery. The symptomatic or asymptomatic shedding of HSV at delivery can lead to neonatal infection which carries a high mortality rate.

The diagnosis may be supported by using cell culture, immunofluorescence microscopy or electron microscopy to demonstrate HSV in vesicular fluid or early ulcers. Particularly in recurrent genital herpes, often it is not possible to isolate HSV.

Treatment. As there is no uniform presentation in genital herpes, so there is no uniform treatment. In severe attacks and particularly in attacks with constitutional symptoms, patients should be advised to take bed rest as required. Patients should be educated about the condition, and how it can be spread to sexual partners and from a mother to a fetus during pregnancy or to a neonate at delivery. They should be given advice about measures which they can take to obtain local relief of symptoms, e.g. frequent warm baths and micturition in the bath, which lessens external dysuria.

Acyclovir is a specific anti-HSV drug, which lessens the severity of symptoms and shortens the duration of symptoms and viral shedding and the time taken to healing. It does not prevent the establishment of latent HSV infection. Infections with acyclovir-resistant HSV mutants have been described in immunocompromised patients.

Oral acyclovir 200 mg five times daily for 5 days has been shown to be of benefit in both first and recurrent attacks. In recurrences some workers have found acyclovir 5% cream applied topically five times daily for 5 days to be as effective and much cheaper than the oral preparation. When acyclovir is used, it is important that treatment is started as early as possible (with the onset of prodromal symptoms in recurrences) since the drug is of less value later in the attack. Some patients should be provided with a course of acyclovir to enable them to start treatment at the first sign of a recurrence.

There is debate about the best management of genital herpes in pregnancy but there have been reports of acyclovir being used in late pregnancy without harmful effects. Data are needed to determine whether giving acyclovir to a pregnant mother for some days before delivery will prevent excretion of HSV and thus prevent neonatal infection.

When recurrences are very frequent or cause a patient significant physical or psychological harm, their frequency can be reduced by giving acyclovir prophylactically in a regimen of 400 mg orally twice daily. This may be done continuously or intermittently to cover important life events. The ideal duration of continuous prophylaxis is not known but many would advise withdrawing it after 6 to 12 months.

Syphilis. The causative organism is *Treponema pallidum* and after an incubation period of 10 to 90 days, a chancre (primary syphilis) develops at the site of inoculation. Although a classical chancre is a single, firm, painless, non-tender, ulcerated papule, which does not bleed easily but from which, on pressure, a serous fluid exudes, 50% of chancres are atypical and they may be multiple. Usually within 3 to 7 days of the chancre appearing, there is painless, rubbery enlargement of the draining lymph nodes. Secondary infection of a chancre may cause the chancre and the lymphadenopathy to be painful. A chancre may not be noticed by the patient and without treatment, it will disappear in 2 to 8 weeks, leaving no sign of its presence.

Some 6 to 8 weeks after the chancre develops, the patient develops signs of secondary syphilis, which can involve most body systems. The more common clinical features include 'flu-like symptoms, a non-itchy skin rash, hair loss, hoarseness and generalized lymph node enlargement. Again without treatment the lesions of secondary syphilis will resolve and the patient becomes asymptomatic, non-infectious to sexual partners and is said to have latent syphilis.

Some patients with untreated syphilis will remain well but many years later a proportion will develop neurological or cardiovascular disease or gummas – destructive lesions of the skin, bones, mucous membranes or other organs.

Syphilis in pregnancy is associated with spontaneous abortion, stillbirth, perinatal death and congenital syphilis.

It is not practical to culture *T. pallidum* but in primary and secondary syphilis the organism can be seen on dark-ground microscopy of material obtained from the chancre or other lesions. In addition serological tests for syphilis can be performed. In latent and late stage syphilis, it is not possible to obtain material containing *T. pallidum* and the diagnosis is based on the serological test results. Serological tests for syphilis include inexpensive screening tests, e.g. the Venereal Disease Research Laboratory (VDRL) test, where false positive results are common, and confirmatory tests such as the *Treponema pallidum* haemagglutination assay and the fluorescent treponemal antibody absorbed test. Newer ELISAs are being introduced. The interpretation of the results of serological tests for syphilis requires experience but all health care workers should understand that a positive VDRL does not diagnose syphilis but must be confirmed by other tests. After effective treatment some or all of the serological tests will remain positive.

Treatment. The drug of choice for syphilis is penicillin. The recommended treatment regimens depend on how long the patient has had syphilis and differ on opposite sides of the Atlantic. Some of the regimens have not been assessed adequately. Coexisting HIV infection or HIV infection acquired at a later date may compromise the treatment of syphilis or lead to the reactivation of treated syphilis.

In the UK, the treatment regimen for early syphilis (infected for less than 1 year) is to give daily, intramuscular procaine penicillin 900 mg to 1.2 g for 14 consecutive days. If it will be difficult to give injections at weekends, it is acceptable to replace the Saturday and Sunday doses of procaine penicillin with an intramuscular injection of benethamine penicillin 570 mg, to be given on Friday in addition to the Friday dose of intramuscular procaine penicillin.

In the USA it is popular to treat early syphilis with a single dose of intramuscular benzathine penicillin, a preparation that is not available in the UK. The recommended regimen is benzathine penicillin 2.4 million units (1.836 g) intramuscularly at a single session.

It is known that in early syphilis, abnormalities of the cerebrospinal fluid (CSF) are common although symptoms of neurological involvement are rare. The standard treatment for early syphilis will reverse the CSF changes and there is no risk of the later development of neurosyphilis. If the duration of syphilis is greater than 1 year and if there is neurological involvement, it is believed that giving the standard treatment may not prevent the development of neurological disease and that penicillin should be given in higher doses. Therefore patients who have had syphilis for more than 1 year should have their CSF examined to exclude neurological involvement. If neurosyphilis is diagnosed, there is debate about what is the optimum treatment. In the UK many physicians would treat neurosyphilis with 21 consecutive, daily, intramuscular injections of procaine penicillin 1.2 g together with oral probenecid 500 mg four times daily for 21 days. Probenecid raises CSF levels of penicillin by reducing renal excretion of penicillin, causing higher serum levels, and by blocking active transport of penicillin out of the CSF. However, as probenecid may reduce the accumulation of penicillin in brain tissue, it may be better to give higher doses of penicillin rather than probenecid. Treatment regimens in the USA for the management of neurosyphilis include:

- intravenous benzylpenicillin 2 to 4 million units (1.2 to 2.4 g) every 4 hours for 10 days followed by three intramuscular injections of benzathine penicillin 2.4 million units (1.836 g) given at weekly intervals; or

- intramuscular procaine penicillin 2.4 million units (2.378 g) daily and oral probenecid 500 mg four times daily, both for 10 days followed by three intramuscular injections of benzathine penicillin 2.4 million units (1.836 g) given at weekly intervals.

Gummatous syphilis can be treated with a 21-day course of daily, intramuscular injections of procaine penicillin 1.2 g and cases of cardio-vascular syphilis should be managed by a cardiologist.

Patients who are allergic to penicillin can be given oral tetracycline hydrochloride or oxy-tetracycline or erythromycin (stearate, succinate or base) 500 mg four times daily for 15 days for early syphilis, and for 30 days for syphilis of more than 1 year's duration. However, these treatments have not been assessed properly and patients who are thought to be allergic to penicillin should have the allergy confirmed before treating syphilis with another drug.

After treatment patients with early syphilis should be followed up for 2 years with regular estimation of the VDRL titre which should become progressively weaker, often becoming negative. Patients not treated with penicillin should be followed for life. Retreatment should be considered if the VDRL titre fails to fall significantly or rises. Patients with treated neurosyphilis are often followed for life, repeat

Table 40.11 Drug interactions with acyclovir or procaine penicillin

Drug	Interactions
Acyclovir	Serum acyclovir concentration increased by probenecid Extreme lethargy reported when i.v. acyclovir given with zidovudine
Procaine penicillin	Plasma penicillin concentration increased by probenecid

analysis of the CSF usually being done 6 months after treatment.

Sexual partners should be seen.

Tables 40.10 and 40.11 detail side effects from and drug interactions with acyclovir and procaine penicillin.

Genital warts

Anogenital warts are caused by certain types of the human papilloma virus (HPV) which infect anogenital skin and mucosa. Infection is transmitted by skin to skin contact during sexual intercourse.

Usually the diagnosis is made clinically although occasionally biopsy and histology are necessary.

Women who develop genital warts should have a specimen taken for cervical cytology as there is an association between cervical HPV infection and abnormal cervical smears.

Methods of treatment include awaiting spontaneous regression, which is not guaranteed, and the use of cytotoxic or destructive agents. All methods carry a high recurrence rate.

The main cytotoxic agent used is a 5 to 20% preparation of podophyllum resin or its main active agent, podophyllotoxin 0.5%. Podophyllum resin preparations should be applied sparingly to the wart(s) for up to 6 hours, usually at weekly intervals, protecting the surrounding skin. Podophyllotoxin 0.5% should be applied in a similar way but twice daily for 3 days. Treatment may be repeated after a week. Fluorouracil as a 5% cream has been tried mainly for male urethral

Table 40.10 Points to consider when prescribing acyclovir or procaine penicillin

Drug	Points to consider
Acyclovir	Use with caution in renal impairment or pregnancy May cause skin rashes, GI side effects, elevated levels of bilirubin, liver enzymes, urea or creatinine, decreased haematological indices, headache, neurological reactions, fatigue
Procaine penicillin	Use with caution in renal impairment or when there is a history of allergy May cause sensitivity reactions

Table 40.12   Points to consider in the treatment of genital warts with cytotoxic agents

Drug	Points to consider
Podophyllum resin preparations or podophyllotoxin	May damage normal skin or mucosa Do not use in areas where the preparation cannot be confined to the wart Do not use where scarring is unacceptable, e.g. urethral meatus Contra-indicated in pregnancy Application of large amounts may cause serious illness and peripheral neuropathy
Fluorouracil	May damage normal skin or mucosa Contra-indicated in pregnancy

Table 40.13   Points to consider in the treatment of pubic lice or scabies

Drug	Points to consider
Lindane 1% Malathion 0.5%	Use aqueous lotions which provide better coverage than creams and irritate the genitalia and excoriated skin less than alcoholic lotions Avoid contact with the eyes Use malathion for children and pregnant or lactating women

warts. It offers few advantages. Side effects from and contra-indications to the use of cytotoxic agents are detailed in Table 40.12.

Destructive methods of treating genital warts include the application of trichloroacetic acid, scissor excision or electocautery under local or general anaesthesia, and cryotherapy using liquid nitrogen.

Arthropod infestations

Pubic lice. The pubic louse, *Pthirus pubis*, is usually confined to the pubic and perianal hair although it can be found on any body hair including the eyelashes.

The transmission of *P. pubis* occurs during sexual intercourse but, as lice can survive for 24 hours off the host, it is possible through sharing clothing.

The adult lice and eggs are easily visible to the naked eye and the infestation is often diagnosed by the patient. Sensitivity to louse bites varies and therefore so does the degree of itching experienced. Louse bites may cause small blue spots on the skin.

Treatment. An aqueous lotion of malathion 0.5% or lindane 1% should be applied to all hairy parts of the body for 12 hours and reapplied 7 days later to kill lice emerging from surviving eggs. Crab lice on eyelashes are rare but can be treated with aqueous malathion lotion.

Scabies. The transmission of the itch mite, *Sarcoptes scabiei*, requires close physical contact and therefore in sexually active young adults, sexual transmission is common.

The infestation causes itching which is worse at night. Skin burrows with vesicles near their ends are seen commonly on the wrists and hands, between the fingers, on the elbows, around the nipples in women and in the natal cleft. The mite may be visible in burrows. Other skin changes include urticarial papules remote from the mites, itchy, indurated nodules on the trunk and genitalia and eczematous changes due to scratching. The differential diagnosis includes most pruritic dermatoses so the diagnosis is best confirmed by visualizing a mite microscopically.

Treatment. Aqueous preparations of lindane 1% or malathion 0.5% should be used for scabies, applying treatment once for 24 hours to the whole body, especially the webs of the fingers and toes and under the ends of the nails. All household contacts should be treated. (Malathion should be used in preference to lindane for children and pregnant or nursing mothers.) Separate antipruritic treatment, e.g. with calamine preparations, may be necessary.

Comments on lindane 1% and malathion 0.5% are given in Table 40.13.

CASE STUDIES

CASE 40.1

A 20-year-old man presented with a urethral discharge and dysuria which started 4 days after he had unprotected sexual intercourse locally with a woman whom he does not know. Pus cells and Gram-negative diplococci were seen on microscopy of the discharge. Urethral and throat specimens were sent for culture of *N. gonorrhoeae* and blood was obtained for serological tests for syphilis. He was treated with a single dose of amoxycillin 3 g and probenecid 1 g for his presumed gonorrhoea and was advised to abstain from sexual intercourse and to return in a week. When he is reviewed he complains that his symptoms persist.

Q Outline your further management.

CASE 40.2

A 30-year-old woman complains that she has experienced a malodorous vaginal discharge since having an intrauterine contraceptive device fitted over a year ago. She has consulted her general practitioner many times and although she has been given various vaginal and oral preparations for thrush, her discharge has not been helped.

Q Outline your management.

CASE 40.3

A 25-year-old woman presents with a 2-day history of painful genital ulceration. Having examined the patient, specimens are taken which exclude other causes of genital ulceration and a clinical diagnosis of genital herpes is made. The patient was treated with a 5-day course of oral acyclovir 200 mg five times daily and the symptoms resolved. Subsequently HSV-2 was isolated from one of the ulcers.

Now, 3 months later, the patient presents with a second recurrence of similar, although less severe, symptoms, which this time she has had for 6 days. She had some difficulty arranging to see the doctor and seems depressed by the recurrence of symptoms.

Q Describe what can be offered to this patient.

ANSWERS TO CASE STUDIES

CASE 40.1

A By now it will be known whether *N. gonorrhoeae* was isolated from the two specimens and there should be information about the organism's sensitivities to antibiotics. Although unlikely, it is possible that the working diagnosis of gonorrhoea was incorrect and amoxycillin will have been an inappropriate treatment for nongonococcal urethritis.

Information about the antibiotic sensitivities of the isolated *N. gonorrhoeae* will be valuable. Although amoxycillin may have been found to be effective in locally acquired gonorrhoea, there is no information about the presumed source of this infection. It may be that the woman has visited parts of the world where she has been at risk of becoming infected with a beta-lactamase-producing strain of *N. gonorrhoeae*.

Assuming that the laboratory tests confirm the patient was infected with a penicillin-sensitive strain of *N. gonorrhoeae*, information is required about whether he has been at risk of reinfection with gonorrhoea. He is not likely to have had further sexual intercourse with the presumed source of the infection but he may well have had intercourse with his regular girlfriend (despite the instruction!) and it is possible that gonorrhoea was transmitted to her before the patient was treated and then back to him after he received treatment. The patient should be re-examined to confirm that the discharge does persist and obtain specimens for repeat microscopy and culture. If microscopy shows pus cells without Gram-negative diplococci, this would strongly suggest the patient originally had both gonorrhoea and nongonococcal urethritis. Only the gonorrhoea has been treated and now the doctor should give him treatment for the nongonococcal urethritis and arrange to review him.

The result of culture of the throat swab will indicate whether the patient requires additional treatment for oropharyngeal gonorrhoea.

It must be impressed upon the patient that his regular girlfriend should be screened for STDs.

CASE 40.2

A Although the patient's history suggests a diagnosis of bacterial vaginosis she must be examined and specimens collected to allow a diagnosis to be made and to exclude STDs and other causes of a vaginal discharge. If bacterial vaginosis is confirmed, the patient should be given a 7-day course of oral metronidazole 400 mg twice daily. She should be reviewed to ensure that the treatment has been successful and that STDs have been excluded.

The presence of an intrauterine contraceptive device is known to predispose to bacterial vaginosis. However, as this patient has only now had appropriate treatment for her first attack of bacterial vaginosis and as she may never have a recurrence, there is no need yet to consider removing the device.

CASE 40.3

A Unfortunately this woman is suffering relatively frequent attacks of recurrent genital herpes. It is important that she understands that she will remain infected with the herpes simplex virus for the rest of her life although it is to be hoped that with the passage of time the recurrences will become less frequent.

The use of acyclovir early in a recurrence has been shown to be of benefit but the length of time since the onset of this recurrence means that acyclovir has little to offer now. As the patient had difficulty arranging to see the doctor this time, he may wish to provide her with an acyclovir preparation to keep at home for any further recurrence. She could be given a 5-day course of oral acyclovir 200 mg five times daily to keep at home and to start at the first sign of a further recurrence. Less convenient but also less expensive would be acyclovir 5% cream to be applied five times daily for 5 days at the first sign of a recurrence.

If having immediate access to a treatment regimen does not allow the patient to come to terms with her infection, prophylactic treatment with oral acyclovir in a dose of 400 mg twice daily could be offered. The doctor and patient should agree on the proposed duration of prophylaxis and the patient should understand that she is likely to suffer further recurrences when the prophylactic acyclovir is stopped.

BIBLIOGRAPHY

Adler M W. ABC of sexually transmitted diseases, 2nd edn. London: British Medical Journal 1990

Department of Health. New cases seen at NHS genito-urinary medicine clinics in England, 1988 annual and December figures, summary information from form KC60

Easmon C S F. The changing pattern of antibiotic resistance of *Neisseria gonorrhoeae*. Genitourinary Medicine 1990; 66(2): 55–56

Easmon C S F, Hay P E, Ison C A. Bacterial vaginosis: a diagnostic approach. Genitourinary Medicine 1992; 68(2): 134–138

Holmes K K, Mårdh P-A, Sparling P F, Wiesner P J (eds). Sexually transmitted diseases, 2nd edn. New York: McGraw-Hill Information Services 1990

Robertson D H H, McMillan A, Young H. Clinical practice in sexually transmissible diseases, 2nd edn. Edinburgh: Churchill Livingstone 1989

Woolley P D. Recent advances in non-gonococcal urethritis: pathogenesis, investigation and treatment. International Journal of STD and AIDS 1990; 1(3): 157–160

Chapter 41

HIV infection

S. Knight

Acquired immunodeficiency syndrome (AIDS) is the state of profound immunosuppression produced by chronic infection with human immunodeficiency virus (HIV).

EPIDEMIOLOGY

In June 1981, the Centers for Disease Control (CDC) reported the cases of five homosexual men in California who had acquired *Pneumocystis carinii* pneumonia (PCP). Other reports quickly followed, linking cases of unusual infections and tumours, notably Kaposi's sarcoma. All patients had a marked impairment of cellular immune response. These were the first reports of AIDS.

HIV infection is now epidemic in the western world and in Africa. The CDC estimate the number of AIDS cases worldwide to be 1.5 million. In the UK and USA the first wave of the epidemic occurred in homosexual men. The second and current wave is among intravenous drug misusers and it is via this group that the heterosexual spread of the virus is occurring. In Africa, the male to female ratio of cases is virtually 1:1. Previous classifications of 'high' or 'low' risk populations are now seen as obsolete.

CAUSES

HIV is not easily transmitted from person to person. The virus has been isolated from blood, semen, vaginal secretions, saliva, breast milk, tears, urine, serum and cerebrospinal fluid. The isolation of the virus from a body fluid does not, however, necessarily mean that the fluid is important in transmission.

The most common mode of transmission of HIV throughout the world is sexual intercourse. There is no consistent relationship between seropositivity, the number of sexual encounters or specific sexual practices for a given individual. This suggests that individual host susceptibility factors, variations in infectivity among viral strains, or both may be important. Other modes of transmission include the sharing of unsterilized needles and syringes, the infusion of contaminated blood or blood products, and organs donated for transplantation. Health-care workers can be infected through needle-stick injuries and by mucosal exposure to infected body fluids and blood.

HIV may be transmitted from infected women to their offspring by three possible mechanisms: to the fetus through the maternal circulation, to the infant during labour and delivery, and after birth through infected breast milk. The precise rate of perinatal transmission is not known and recent estimates range from 25 to 40%.

PATHOPHYSIOLOGY

HIV is a retrovirus which was first identified in 1983. Retroviruses possess the enzyme reverse transcriptase and have a lipid-containing membrane surrounding the capsid. Another retrovirus, HIV-2 which is structurally different from HIV, but produces a similar clinical syndrome is uncommon outside West Africa.

HIV is surprisingly fragile. It is easily inactivated by physical and chemical agents including household bleach in a 1:10 dilution, hydrogen peroxide, glutaraldehyde, ethyl and isopropyl alcohols and heat (56°C for 10 minutes).

After gaining entry into a cell, the reverse transcriptase enzyme converts viral RNA to DNA using nucleosides. The viral DNA then incorporates itself into the host cell DNA. When the host cell is stimulated to replicate, production of

HIV occurs. The newly manufactured virus then buds out of the host cell and destroys it in the process.

HIV is immunosuppressive because it has an affinity for a particular subset of lymphocytes. The main target of the virus is a subset of thymus-derived (T) lymphocytes, the helper/inducer cells. These carry on their surface a glycoprotein receptor called CD4 which has been shown to bind with the outer glycoprotein coat of the HIV virus. Monocytes and macrophages may have CD4 receptors in low densities and can also be infected.

Helper/inducer T-lymphocytes have a central role in the immune response. When these cells are stimulated by contact with an antigen, they respond with cell division and the production of lymphokines, such as interleukin-2 and interferons. These act as local hormones to affect the growth and function of monocytes, macrophages and other lymphocytes.

The hallmark of disease progression, in addition to the development of clinical symptoms, is a fall in the number of helper/inducer CD4 lymphocytes. As disease progresses the function of T-lymphocytes, including production of lymphokines, becomes increasingly abnormal. The ability of monocytes and macrophages to kill intracellular parasites is also impaired. Consequently, many opportunistic viral, fungal, mycobacterial and protozoal infections occur which are normally suppressed.

CLINICAL MANIFESTATIONS

Infection with HIV produces a varied clinical picture ranging from asymptomatic seroconversion to full-blown AIDS many years later. The CDC defines the stages of HIV infection into four groups (Table 41.1).

Acute infection (CDC group I) is asymptomatic for the majority of individuals. For others, a glandular-fever-like illness (fever, malaise, myalgia, lymphadenopathy) has been described at the time of seroconversion. Acute reversible encephalopathy, meningitis, myelopathy and neuropathy have also been reported.

Table 41.1 Summary of CDC classification system for human immunodeficiency virus

Group I	Acute infection
Group II	Asymptomatic infection
Group III	Persistent generalized lymphadenopathy
Group IV	Other disease
Subgroup A	Constitutional disease (fever > 1 month, weight loss > 10% baseline, diarrhoea > 1 month)
Subgroup B	Neurological disease
Subgroup C	Secondary infectious diseases
	C1 Specified secondary infectious diseases listed in CDC definition of AIDS
	C2 Other specified secondary infectious diseases
Subgroup D	Secondary cancers
Subgroup E	Other conditions

The asymptomatic phase (CDC group II) is now believed to average 8 to 10 years. Patients will remain well with no signs other than alterations in prognostic markers.

Approximately 5 to 25% of individuals develop a persistent, symmetrical swelling of the lymph nodes (CDC group III). This is termed persistent generalized lymphadenopathy (PGL). Other possible causes such as infection or malignancy must be excluded before a diagnosis of PGL is made.

Weight loss of greater than 10% baseline, persistent fever or diarrhoea of greater than 1 month's duration signals symptomatic progression (CDC group IV, subgroup A). This period is sometimes referred to as AIDS-related complex (ARC). Whether any cofactors trigger or enhance progression is unknown.

The diagnosis of AIDS in an adult requires the individual to be HIV-antibody positive, and have a recognized opportunistic infection, a secondary malignancy or a neurological syndrome (CDC group IV, subgroups B, C or D).

The CDC identifies separate criteria for the definition of AIDS in children. Presence of the virus must be confirmed as detection of antibodies may reflect passive maternal transfer. Lymphoid interstitial pneumonitis is an AIDS-defining illness in addition to the same subgroup headings of CDC group IV for adults.

INVESTIGATIONS

Specific immune responses to HIV are mounted following exposure. Antibody production results, but this does not confer immunity. Since becoming commercially available in 1985, the sensitivity and specificity of HIV antibody assays have improved. Blood samples are normally used but assays using urine or saliva are available. Tests detect antibodies formed to both HIV-1 and HIV-2. The two common assays used for diagnosis in patients are the western blot and ELISA tests. In most countries, a sample must show a positive result to both tests before a patient is informed. Individual pre-and post-test counselling is a vital requirement in HIV testing because of the social and medical implications of a positive result. This is best done by a trained counsellor. Confidentiality at all stages of the process must be maintained.

Also present in the serum are viral antigens, in particular the main HIV core antigen (p24). Detection and monitoring of the p24 antigen may assist in the diagnosis of early infection and in recognition of infection in infants. The effect of antiretroviral therapy can also be monitored by changes in p24 antigen titres.

Prognostic markers can indicate whether an HIV-infected patient is at increased risk of progression from asymptomatic infection to ARC or AIDS. Prognostic tests used in HIV infection include measurements of β_2-microglobulin, erythrocyte sedimentation rate, haemoglobin, and p24 antigen. The most extensive clinical experience however, is with T-lymphocyte counts.

There are three interrelated measurements of T-lymphocytes: the CD4 count (the number of T-lymphocytes carrying the CD4 surface receptor), the CD4 per cent and the ratio of CD4 to CD8 (T-suppressor) cells. Measurements of T-lymphocytes are imprecise. They vary from day to day, at different times of the day, and on reanalysis of the same sample. Results are seen consequently as being within a certain range.

TREATMENT

Chronic HIV infection results in an insidious

weakening of the immune system for which there is currently no cure. The treatment of HIV aims to slow the rate of disease progression, manage the complications of immunosuppression and provide symptomatic control to maintain patient quality of life as long as possible.

Patients with AIDS appear more susceptible to drug-induced side effects than other populations taking the same drugs. As the disease progresses, polypharmacy develops and the potential for drug interactions therefore increases.

Many therapies for patients with AIDS are experimental and extrapolated from the treatment of similar conditions in patients without AIDS. Thus, treatments can vary considerably in different medical centres. Legal accountability must also be considered as many treatments are not licensed. Table 41.2 indicates the legal status of therapies in the UK at the time of writing.

Drug treatment

Opportunistic infections in adults with AIDS do not normally occur with CD4 cell counts greater than $200/mm^3$ (normal adult level $> 700–1200/mm^3$). As individuals approach $200/mm^3$, they are at increased risk of opportunistic infection. Primary prophylactic drug therapies are being investigated as a way of preventing acute opportunistic infections that commonly occur in AIDS.

Protozoal infections

Pneumocystis carinii pneumonia (PCP). This extracellular protozoon exists as trophozoite and cyst forms within the pulmonary alveoli. Patients with PCP typically describe a prolonged history (6 to 8 weeks) of symptoms. Respiratory symptoms are a non-productive cough, breathlessness, and an inability to take a deep breath. Fever, anorexia, weight loss and lymphopenia may be non-respiratory symptoms. Chest X-rays show a diffuse interstitial shadowing pattern. Diagnosis is normally by Grocott's methenamine silver stain of sputum (often sputum must be induced by prior use of a hypertonic saline nebulizer). Cultures for bacteria, mycobacteria and fungi, to exclude mixed infection are normally performed. Measurement of arterial oxygenation is essential for early detection of hypoxia and its treatment with oxygen.

The two treatments predominantly used for PCP are co-trimoxazole and pentamidine (Table 41.2). Studies have shown both agents to be equally efficacious and both have a similar incidence of side effects. However, pentamidine's side effect profile is potentially more serious. Consequently, unless the patient has a known allergy to sulphonamides, co-trimoxazole is used as first line therapy. Oral dosing with co-trimoxazole has the advantage that mild cases of PCP may not require hospitalization. The two components of co-trimoxazole (trimethoprim and sulphamethoxazole) both work by preventing the formation of tetrahydrofolic acid, the metabolically active form of folic acid.

Co-trimoxazole injections must be adequately diluted as solutions of less than 1:25 may not be stable for the required 1.5- to 3-hour infusion period. Both the infusion bag and line should be periodically checked for precipitation. Fluid overload can occur with intravenous treatment, so patients should be changed to tablets when appropriate. Nausea, vomiting (dose related) and skin rashes (often to the sulphonamide component) are the most common side effects and concurrent antiemetics and antihistamines may be required. Other adverse effects include drug fever, neutropenia and anaemia.

The exact mechanism of action of pentamidine in PCP has not been established. It may act as a folate antagonist, inhibit protozoal replication or inhibit protozoal glucose metabolism. Intravenous infusion of pentamidine may cause postural hypotension, the patient should, therefore, be supine and the drug infused over at least 1 hour. Alterations in blood glucose can occur and pentamidine is well known to be nephrotoxic in approximately 25% of patients. This is usually mild and reversible. Patients with pre-existing renal disease, or those receiving other nephrotoxic drugs must be closely monitored.

For mild cases of PCP pentamidine may be nebulized daily. A suitable nebulizer unit should be used to produce a particle size of less than 5 microns to ensure uniform distribution and

Table 41.2 Drugs used to treat opportunistic infections in HIV disease

Drug	Indication	Dosage, route, frequency, duration	Side effects	Interactions	Monitoring	Comments
Acyclovir	Herpes simplex	5 mg/kg i.v. three times daily for 5–10 days 200–400 mg p.o. five times daily for 5–10 days	Skin rash, increased LFTs, extravasation i.v.	Probenecid	Renal function	i.v. infusion diluted to 0.5% w/v & infused over at least 1 hour
	Herpes zoster	10 mg/kg i.v. three times daily for 5–10 days 800 mg p.o. five times daily for 7 days				
	Prophylaxis/ suppression of herpes infections	200–400 mg p.o. twice daily continuously				
Amphotericin	Cryptococcal meningitis other severe fungal infections	0.25–1.0 mg/kg i.v. once daily for up to 6 weeks	Non-infusion related: nephrotoxicity, hypokalaemia, anaemia	Nephrotoxic drugs, anti-neoplastics, corticosteroids	Renal function FBC U + Es	Start with lower dose and gradually increase
	Oral candida	One lozenge sucked four times daily	Infusion related: fever, chills, nausea & vomiting, myalgia, thrombophlebitis			Dilute in buffered dextrose
Clarithromycin	Atypical *Mycobacterium* infections (MAC)*	1 g p.o. twice daily continuously	Nausea, vomiting, abdominal pain, rash	Theophylline, warfarin, digoxin, carbamazepine	FBCs Renal function	
Clindamycin	Treatment of PCP*	450–900 mg i.v./ p.o. three or four times daily for 14–21 days	Diarrhoea, gastrointestinal disturbance. Rarely, pseudo-membranous colitis	Care with neuromuscular blocking agents	LFTs FBCs Diarrhoea	Taken with primaquine
	Toxoplasmosis treatment*	300–600 mg p.o. four times daily for 4–6 weeks				Taken with pyrimethamine
	Toxoplasmosis maintenance*	600 mg p.o. daily in divided doses				
Co-trimoxazole	Treatment of PCP	120 mg/kg i.v./p.o. in two to four divided doses for 14–21 days	Rash, nausea & vomiting, neutropenia, increased LFTs, anaemia, Stevens–Johnson syndrome, drug fever	Bone marrow suppressive therapy, sulphonylureas, phenytoin	FBC Renal function LFTs Rash	Infusion given in two doses and diluted 1:25, infused over 1.5–3 hours
	Prophylaxis against PCP	960 mg p.o. once or twice a day continuously				
Dapsone	Prophylaxis against PCP*	100 mg p.o. daily continuously	Rash, gastrointestinal disturbance, anaemia, leucopenia, methaemoglobin-aemia	Rifampicin, probenecid, nitrofurantoin	FBC U + Es LFTs	Tests for G6PD in patients of African or Mediterranean origin

Table 41.2 (*cont'd*)

Drug	Indication	Dosage, route, frequency, duration	Side effects	Interactions	Monitoring	Comments
Didanosine[†]	Antiretroviral agent	167–375 mg p.o. twice daily	Pancreatitis, peripheral neuropathy, diarrhoea, rash	Should not be taken within 2 hours of any other drug	Amylase U + Es	Needs neutral environment for absorption
Fluconazole	Oropharyngeal candidiasis Cryptococcal meningitis treatment Cryptococcal meningitis prophylaxis*	50–100 mg p.o. daily for 7–14 days 400 mg i.v./p.o. daily for 6 weeks 200–400 mg p.o. daily continuously	Gastrointestinal disturbance, rash	Anticoagulants, hypoglycaemics, phenytoin, rifampicin	Renal function	
Foscarnet	Cytomegalovirus retinitis treatment Cytomegalovirus retinitis maintenance*	Up to 200 mg/kg/day i.v. according to serum creatinine, as continuous infusion for 14–21 days 80–120 mg/kg i.v. once daily over 2 hours for 5–7 days of each week	Nephroxicity, alterations in serum calcium, anaemia, headache, thrombophlebitis, penile ulceration	Nephrotoxic drugs, pentamidine	Renal function Serum calcium FBC	Licensed only for treatment of CMV retinitis resistant to ganciclovir Patients must be well hydrated
Ganciclovir	Cytomegalovirus infection treatment Cytomegalovirus retinitis maintenance	5 mg/kg i.v. twice daily for 14–21 days 5 mg/kg i.v. once every day or 6 mg/kg i.v. once daily for 5 days of each week	Neutropenia, thrombocytopenia, abnormal LFTs, CNS effects	Zidovudine, imipenem, bone marrow suppressive agents	FBC Renal function LFTs	Give over 1 hour, preferably via central i.v. access
Itraconazole	Oropharyngeal candidiasis	200 mg p.o. daily for 15 days	Nausea, abdominal pain, headache	Rifampicin, phenytoin, H_2 antagonists, antacids	LFTs	With or after food
Ketoconazole	Oropharyngeal candidiasis	200 mg p.o. twice daily for 7–14 days	Abnormal LFTs, gastrointestinal disturbance, rash	Rifampicin, phenytoin, H_2 antagonists, antacids, oral anticoagulants	LFTS Adrenal function	With or after food
Nystatin	Oral candidiasis	1–2 ml suspenion p.o. or 1 pastille sucked four times daily	Rarely, nausea, vomiting, diarrhoea		Not required	Combine with strict dental hygiene
Pentamidine isethionate	PCP treatment Mild PCP treatment PCP prophylaxis	4 mg/kg i.v. once daily for 14–21 days 600 mg nebulized daily for 21 days 300 mg nebulized every 4 weeks	Intravenous: nephrotoxicity, postural hypotension, leucopenia, hypo/hyperglycaemia Nebulized: bronchospasm, cough	Nephrotoxic drugs, foscarnet	Renal function Blood glucose Blood pressure U + Es LFTs	Infuse over 1 hour, with patient supine Pretreat with bronchodilator if nebulized
Primaquine	PCP treatment*	15–30 mg p.o. daily for 14–21 days	Methaemoglobinaemia, haemolytic anaemia, nausea	Bone marrow suppressive drugs	FBC	Tests for G6PD in patients of African or Mediterranean origin

Table 41.2 (cont'd)

Drug	Indication	Dosage, route, frequency, duration	Side effects	Interactions	Monitoring	Comments
Pyrimethamine	Toxoplasmosis treatment*	25–75 mg p.o. once daily for 4–6 weeks	Anaemia, rash, bone marrow suppression	Bone marrow suppressive drugs	FBC	Combined with sulphadiazine or clindamycin Consider use of folinic acid
	Toxoplasmosis maintenance*	25 mg p.o. once daily continuously				
Rifabutin†	Atypical *Mycobacterium* infections (MAC)	300–450 mg p.o. once daily with other drugs; 300 mg daily if <50 kg or abnormal LFTs	Abnormal LFTs, bone marrow suppression	Unknown	LFTs	Combine with two or three other drugs for MAC
Spiramycin†	Cryptosporidial diarrhoea	500–1000 mg p.o. three to four times daily for 1–4 weeks	Gastrointestinal disturbance, rash	Unknown	LFTs	Macrolide related to erythromycin
Sulphadiazine	Toxoplasmosis treatment*	1–2 g i.v./p.o. four times daily for 4–6 weeks	Rash (including Stevens–Johnson syndrome), bone marrow suppression, nausea, vomiting, renal failure	Bone marrow suppressive drugs	Renal function LFTs FBC	Use with pyrimethamine Use folinic acid 15 mg i.v./p.o. during treatment phase
	Toxoplasmosis maintenance*	2 g p.o. daily in divided doses				
Zidovudine	Antiretroviral agent	Adults with CD4 cell count <500/mm^3: 500–1500 mg p.o. daily in two to five divided doses Children >3 months: 180 mg/m^2 p.o. four times daily	Anaemia, neutropenia, nausea, headache, rash, myopathy	Ganciclovir, glucuronidated drugs, probenecid	FBC	Viral resistance, optimal dose and length of treatment to be established

* Unlicensed treatment indication (relates only to the UK and at the time of writing).
† Unlicensed drug (relates only to the UK and at the time of writing).
Key: p.o. – oral dose; U + Es – urea and electrolyte determinations; FBC – full blood count; LFTs – Liver function tests; MAC – *Mycobacterium avium* complex; PCP – *Pneumocystis carinii* pneumonia

alveolar penetration. Bronchospasm may be avoided by pretreating with a bronchodilator. Patients may find the fine mist difficult to inhale, and its metallic taste unpleasant, but nebulized therapy shows minimal systemic blood levels, and many side effects can be avoided.

A combination of clindamycin and primaquine may be used in patients who either do not respond, or who have side effects to co-trimoxazole or pentamidine. Recent data suggest that it may be increasingly used as first line therapy.

Adjunctive corticosteroid therapy may reduce the likelihood of death, respiratory failure or further deterioration in patients with moderate to severe PCP. Prednisolone or equivalent doses of methylprednisolone can be used, and should

be initiated within 24 to 72 hours of initial PCP therapy.

Primary PCP prophylaxis is initiated when patients begin to show signs of immunosuppression (CDC group IV, subgroup A) or have CD4 cell counts of approximately 200/mm^3. Secondary prophylaxis must be started immediately following acute treatment. Treatments include co-trimoxazole, nebulized pentamidine and dapsone. The optimal drug, dose and regimen of these agents has not yet been established but guidelines for both adults and children have been published by the CDC.

Toxoplasmosis. *Toxoplasma gondii* is the most commonly diagnosed cause of central nervous system (CNS) lesions in patients with AIDS. In cerebral toxoplasmosis, severe headaches, confusion, neurological abnormalities, seizures and sometimes fever, developing over 1 to 2 weeks, are characteristic presentations. Computed tomography (CT) scan shows solitary or multiple ring-enhancing lesions often with surrounding oedema.

Toxoplasmosis responds well if treatment is started early. A combination of pyrimethamine and sulphadiazine for 4 to 6 weeks followed by lifelong lower dose maintenance is the treatment of choice. Both drugs are folate antagonists and interfere with the biosynthesis of tetrahydrofolic acid, which is an essential co-factor in the pathway of nucleic acid synthesis. Both drugs can cause bone marrow suppression. This can be prevented by the addition of folinic acid to the treatment regimen. Folinic acid will not interfere with the antibacterial or antiprotozoal action of the folic antagonists since it cannot be utilized by toxoplasma protozoa but can be used by man for cell production.

Side effects, such as rash, may require the sulphadiazine to be stopped and substituted with clindamycin. Short course corticosteroids, particularly dexamethasone, may be used in severe cases to reduce cerebral oedema.

Cryptosporidiosis. Cryptosporidiosis is a protozoal parasitic infection of the gastrointestinal tract. Symptoms include epigastric cramping, nausea, vomiting, anorexia, weight loss and diarrhoea. The diarrhoea can be severe and debilitating (upto 10 L per 24 hours). Stool testing for cryptosporidium oocysts is the most common method of diagnosis.

The response to treatment of *Cryptosporidium* has been very poor among AIDS patients. Symptomatic treatment with antidiarrhoeal drugs permits fluid and electrolyte reabsorption, thus decreasing stool volume and allowing stools to become more formed. Morphine (10 to 30 mg as sustained-release tablets twice a day) may be used in patients who are refractory to maximum doses of first line agents (codeine up to 60 mg four times daily, loperamide up to 16 mg in 24 hours, diphenoxylate up to 10 tablets daily).

Of the drugs under investigation for the treatment of cryptosporidiosis, the macrolide group of antibiotics appears to be the most efficacious. Spiramycin has little toxicity, and marked improvements in symptoms have been reported despite patients continuing to shed oocysts in their stools. Erythromycin may be tried in normal therapeutic doses and the aminoglycoside paromomycin has shown promising results.

Somatostatin analogues have been investigated and inhibit intestinal secretions rather than affecting immune status or attacking the organism. Total parenteral nutrition has been used in patients with very severe diarrhoeal illness and malabsorption due to persistent cryptosporidiosis, but its usefulness remains to be evaluated.

Bacterial infections

Bacterial pneumonias are frequent and normally involve *Streptococcus pneumoniae* or *Haemophilus influenzae*. Skin infections and *Salmonella* infections may also occur in AIDS, and normally respond to appropriate antibiotics.

Mycobacteria. *Mycobacterium tuberculosis* and other mycobacterioses are well recognized complications of immunosuppression. HIV infection is now an important risk factor for tuberculosis. For HIV-antibody-positive intravenous drug misusers, tuberculosis is the second most common opportunistic infection after PCP. Reactivation of a latent tuberculosis rather than acute infection is thought to be the main mechanism. Patients with HIV infection with a tuberculin test greater than 5 mm induration, are often given prophylactic isoniazid (300 mg daily) irrespective of their Bacillus Calmette–Guérin (BCG) vaccination status.

Conventional therapy for treatment is used (see Ch. 39) but the emergence of drug-resistant tuberculosis in patients with HIV infection has been reported. In patients who comply, therapy results in the rapid sterilization of sputum, radiographic improvements, and low rates of relapse.

Atypical mycobacteria found in AIDS include *M. xenopi*, *M. kansasii* and *Mycobacterium avium* complex (MAC). MAC is seen in 60% of patients at autopsy, but it appears to contribute little to overall morbidity and mortality of patients with AIDS. Signs and symptoms of disseminated MAC include fever, night sweats, weight loss, diarrhoea and persistent anaemia.

There is no standardized treatment for MAC infection and MAC tends to show in vitro resistance to traditional antituberculous drugs. Responses reported to multiple drug regimens (at least three drugs) are often poor and frequently short lived.

Drugs commonly used in the management of patients with MAC include rifabutin (an analogue of rifampicin), ciprofloxacin, clofazimine, ethambutol and amikacin. Significant skin staining can occur with both rifabutin and clofazimine and patients should be counselled. Recent trials suggest that clarithromycin or azithromycin may also be used.

Fungal infections

Candidiasis. Oropharyngeal candidiasis is the most common fungal infection in patients with HIV and is predictive of progressive immunosuppression. Oral candidiasis is characterized by creamy curd-like patches on the tongue and buccal mucosa. Topical nystatin given as an oral suspension or as a pastille at least four times a day remains the mainstay of treatment. Topical amphotericin lozenges, syrup or miconazole gel may also be used.

Candida oesophagitis is more serious and can cause dysphagia, nausea, epigastric pain and patients may develop anorexia and weight loss. Severe cases may lead to perforation and haemorrhage. Systemic antifungals are indicated and ketoconazole is used initially. Liver function tests should be monitored throughout treatment as ketoconazole has been associated with hepatotoxicity. Ketoconazole's drug interactions should also be considered (see Ch. 42). The newer triazole compounds, fluconazole and itraconazole, are also used but are not regarded as first line treatments in patients with AIDS because therapeutic superiority has not been demonstrated and they are considerably more expensive.

Maintenance therapy for candidiasis is sometimes used, but breakthrough or resistance may occur, leading to increased doses or alternative drugs (e.g. intravenous amphotericin) being required for treatment. Disseminated candidiasis can occur in AIDS, but is quite rare.

As other oral complications such as gingivitis (treated with 0.2% chlorhexidene mouthwash) frequently occur together with candidiasis, dental hygiene is encouraged for all patients.

Cryptococcosis. *Cryptococcus neoformans* is an encapsulated yeast-like fungus. It is acquired by inhalation from the environment. In contrast to immunocompetent hosts, patients with AIDS invariably develop disseminated disease, with 85% having meningeal involvement. Of these, nearly 60% of patients die from this infection. Signs and symptoms are typical of meningitis (headache, fever, nausea, vomiting, blurred vision, stiff neck), but the course is often more acute than in non-AIDS patients.

Intravenous amphotericin is the first line treatment. Amphotericin's adverse effects can be related to drug administration (thrombophlebitis, shaking, chills or rigors) or more chronic adverse reactions related to organ toxicities (anaemia, nephrotoxicity). Whether combination therapy with 5-flucytosine is more efficacious, or less toxic than amphotericin used alone (in higher doses), is unknown. 5-flucytosine may not be appropriate for patients with AIDS as it may produce leucopenia and thrombocytopenia. A liposomal formulation of amphotericin showing reduced nephrotoxicity is available.

Fluconazole is an alternative treatment which can be administered orally or intravenously. Cerebrospinal fluid levels reach 50 to 70% of plasma levels in normal individuals, with increased penetration in patients with meningitis. Fluconazole, however, does not appear to offer a therapeutic advantage over amphotericin in patients who are at risk of early deterioration. Adverse effects to fluconazole are generally mild and infrequent. Numerous injectable agents (including ceftazidime, piperacillin and erythromycin) have been shown to be incompatible with intravenous fluconazole.

After completing primary therapy, all AIDS patients with cryptococcal disease should be commenced on lifelong suppressive therapy. Oral fluconazole is effective and preferable to weekly intravenous amphotericin. Clinical efficacy with itraconazole as maintenance therapy has also been shown.

Viral infections

Cytomegalovirus. Cytomegalovirus (CMV) is a herpes virus which can cause life-threatening viral infection in immunocompromised patients. CMV retinitis is the most common manifestation and is seen in approximately 25% of patients with AIDS. Symptoms include decreased visual acuity, visual field defects, and complaints of 'floaters'. Typically there is no pain. Retinal involvement is usually unilateral at first but can become bilateral. Prompt treatment is required to prevent rapidly progressive blindness. Other sites of infection by CMV include the gastrointestinal tract, lungs, liver, central nervous system and adrenal glands.

Ganciclovir and foscarnet are two antiviral agents that have shown significant activity against CMV in vitro and in vivo. Superior clinical efficacy in the acute treatment of CMV disease has not be shown with either agent.

Ganciclovir is an analogue of 2'-deoxyguanosine and is structurally related to acyclovir. In virus-infected cells ganciclovir triphosphate competitively inhibits DNA polymerase, resulting in inhibition of DNA synthesis and termination of DNA elongation. Oral absorption is poor and parenteral solutions are alkaline (pH 9 to 11) and can cause thrombophlebitis. Its most serious dose-limiting adverse effect is neutropenia, which is seen in approximately 40% of patients. Potential risk factors for neutropenia include ganciclovir dose, a low baseline neutrophil count, and concomitant use of bone marrow suppressive agents including zidovudine. It is therefore generally recommended that patients on zidovudine temporarily stop dosing whilst receiving acute ganciclovir treatment. Ganciclovir may impair fertility and is potentially teratogenic.

Foscarnet (trisodium phosphonoformate) is a pyrophosphate analogue with in vitro activity against all human herpes viruses and HIV. It inhibits viral replication by non-competitive inhibition of viral DNA polymerase.

Recent data suggest that for patients with AIDS and CMV retinitis, treatment with foscarnet may result in patients living several months longer compared to patients who receive ganciclovir. This is possibly because of foscarnet's antiretroviral action. This effect requires further investigation particularly as patients may not tolerate foscarnet as well as ganciclovir. The choice of drug therefore, will often depend upon individual patient factors.

Like ganciclovir, foscarnet is administered by parenteral routes. There is a direct correlation between plasma foscarnet clearance and renal function, so doses are calculated according to serum creatinine levels.

Foscarnet may produce an acute tubular necrosis, and an increase in serum creatinine of at least 25% over baseline in 66% of patients. Concomitant use of other nephrotoxic drugs is an important risk factor. Maintaining a high level of hydration (approximately 2 L per day of intravenous fluids) throughout the course of foscarnet therapy can prevent clinical renal damage. Serum creatinine should always be monitored for an upward trend. Other adverse effects with foscarnet include alteration in serum calcium (both hypo- and hypercalcaemia have been reported), anaemia and rash.

CMV retinitis usually shows a favourable clinical response with reduction in retinal inflammation and some improvement in visual acuity. Because relapse is common, prolonged maintenance therapy is required. Permanent central intravenous access is therefore required. Septicaemia from contamination of the catheter may sometimes occur. Patients who have had zidovudine therapy stopped because of acute ganciclovir treatment may have zidovudine restarted, with close monitoring of haematological parameters occurring.

Herpes simplex/herpes zoster. Herpes simplex virus (HSV) infections are frequent in patients with HIV infection. In homosexual patients the most frequent site of infection is the perianal area but perioral, vulval and skin lesions occur commonly. Rarely there may be neurological involvement with signs and symptoms of meningitis or encephalitis.

Acyclovir is used in standard doses and maintenance therapy (200 to 400 mg twice daily) is used to reduce recurrent herpetic attacks. HSV is known to become resistant to acyclovir following prolonged therapy. The HSV becomes deficient in thymidine kinase activity and can no longer phosphorylate acyclovir to the active compound acyclovir triphosphate. Foscarnet (unlike acyclovir and ganciclovir) does not require phosphorylation by cellular kinase for activity and can be used for patients with acyclovir-resistant HSV strains.

Herpes zoster has long been recognized as a sign of immunosuppression. Herpes zoster infections in patients with AIDS may show a high frequency of trigeminal nerve involvement, recurrent episodes and chronic cutaneous lesions. Acyclovir is used, and duration of therapy depends on clinical improvement. Adverse effects of acyclovir are generally rare but skin rashes, abnormal liver function tests, renal, haematological and neurological reactions can all occur. The intravenous injection can cause thrombophlebitis.

Cancers

AIDS-related Kaposi's sarcoma. Before the recognition of AIDS, Kaposi's sarcoma (KS) was seen in some elderly patients of Jewish or East European origin, in parts of Africa, and in patients receiving immunosuppressive therapy.

The lesions of AIDS-related KS often begin as small flat dusky red or violet areas of skin discolouration, progressing in weeks or months to raised painless firm nodules and plaques. The tumour may be seen on the trunk, arms, legs and face. In most patients with AIDS, KS never becomes life threatening. However, gastrointestinal or pulmonary dissemination may result in debilitation, and life-threatening haemorrhage. Treatment should be tailored to the form of the disease.

Cutaneous manifestations respond well to local radiotherapy. Dosing may be fractionated over several weeks, particularly with oral lesions because of the risk of severe mucositis. Rapidly progressive KS may be treated with chemotherapy or immunotherapy. Six to seven fortnightly cycles of systemic vincristine 2 mg plus bleomycin 30 mg are often used because they cause little myelotoxocity, nausea and vomiting. Hair loss may occur whilst undergoing vincristine therapy and this is important when one considers that the aim of treatment in part is cosmetic. The total dose of bleomycin is limited to 300 mg because of the risk of progressive pulmonary fibrosis (bleomycin lung). Vinblastine, epirubicin and etoposide may be used as single agents. Side effects include leucopenia, neutropenia, nausea, lethargy and stomatitis.

Immunotherapy utilizes the antiproliferative action of interferon alpha. A combination of zidovudine plus interferon alpha in patients with a relatively intact immune system (CD4 count of $>200/mm^3$ and no constitutional symptoms) gives the best results. Doses are high (30 million i.u./m^2 given subcutaneously three times a week) and can cause side effects of shivering, fevers and malaise. Average time to reponse is 2 months and maintenance dosing is required. Due to their expense and the low mortality rate associated with external KS, interferons are not being used extensively outside clinical trials. Zidovudine may slow the development of new KS lesions, and flatten existing lesions.

Malignant lymphomas. Although various types of malignant lymphoma have been described in patients with HIV infection, most AIDS-related lymphomas are extranodal high grade B-cell lymphomas. Sites of infiltration include the central nervous system, gastrointestinal tract (including the rectum), bone marrow and liver.

Standard chemotherapy is used as for non-Hodgkin's lymphoma (see Ch. 48). Patients with asymptomatic HIV infection at the time of diagnosis have the best treatment results, but median survival time is usually less than 1 year. Multiple chemotherapy regimens such as cyclophosphamide, doxorubicin, vincristine and prednisolone (CHOP) or bleomycin, cyclophosphamide, vincristine, and prednisolone (BACOP) have resulted in complete remission, but there is a high relapse rate and poor response to second line therapy. Intrathecal methotrexate plus bleomycin, doxorubicin, cyclophosphamide, dexamethasone and leucovorin (M-BACOD) is used but is associated with significant risk of opportunistic infection. Clinical trials are underway to evaluate the efficacy of lower-dose chemotherapy regimens.

Whole brain radiotherapy may be of some use in primary cerebral lymphoma although survival tends to be very poor.

Clinical judgement and patient preference must shape treatment decisions.

Neurological manifestations

Neurological symptoms may be due to opportunistic infections, tumours, or the primary neurological effects of HIV.

About one-third of patients with AIDS develop subacute encephalitis. Major cognitive symptoms include forgetfulness, loss of concentration, and slowness of thought. Other findings include withdrawal, gait ataxia, and leg weakness. The illness may progress in some patients to severe dementia (AIDS–dementia complex), the patient eventually becoming bedridden and incontinent. It has been suggested that the syndrome is due to direct effects of HIV on the brain. The incidence of AIDS–dementia complex appears to have declined since patients began taking zidovudine treatment. But the minumim dose of zidovudine that inhibits HIV replication and thus protects against subacute encephalitis is not known.

An unusual demyelinating disease, sometimes seen in patients with AIDS is progressive multifocal leucoencephalopathy (PML). It may cause aphasia, blindness, hemiparesis and ataxia. Some response with cytarabine (a potent immunosuppresant used for treating acute leukaemias) has been seen. HIV may also have a directly degenerative effect on the spinal cord producing leg weakness, ataxia, paraesthesia and urinary incontinence. Carbamazepine or analgesics may be used for symptomatic nerve pain and zidovudine may have some effect in assisting recovery from a neurological deficit, but overall the response is poor.

Antiretroviral therapy

Antiretroviral therapy is of paramount importance since it is the continued HIV replication that contributes to the progression of the disease. Theoretically, inhibition of viral replication will slow the rate of disease progression and may also allow some recovery of immune function. Various potential targets for antiretroviral treatment have been identified based on the replicative cycle and molecular biology of HIV. To date only one drug in the UK, zidovudine, is licensed as an antiretroviral agent.

Nucleoside analogues. The nucleoside analogues, of which zidovudine (3'azido-3'deoxythymidine) is an example, are potent inhibitors of HIV replication in vitro.

An essential step in the replication cycle of HIV is the formation of a viral DNA transcript which can become integrated into the host cell DNA. The formation of the transcript is mediated by the enzyme reverse transcriptase and requires the presence of nucleosides such as thymidine. Zidovudine triphosphate (phosphorylation occurring within the cell) acts as a false thymidine, with the drug becoming bound into the DNA transcript. Replication is halted because the malformed DNA transcript cannot integrate into the host cell.

Zidovudine has 60% bioavailability when given by mouth; and crosses the blood–brain barrier with a level in the cerebrospinal fluid that is 50 to 60% of that in serum. The drug is mainly inactivated by glucuronidation in the liver, but 25% is excreted unchanged in the urine. Its short plasma half-life of about 1 hour prompted a 4-hourly dosing schedule initially, but the need for such frequent dosing is uncertain.

The clinical benefit of zidovudine was first demonstrated in a placebo-controlled trial in adults with AIDS or severe ARC, in which mortality and the frequency and severity of opportunistic infections were significantly decreased.

During the first months of therapy, patients may also show weight gain, remission of fever, modest improvements in CD4 lymphocyte counts, and reduction of about 90% in serum p24 antigen levels. These changes, however, may be transient and by 6 months can return to pre-treatment levels. Some cases of HIV-related encephalopathy, neuropathy, psoriasis, cryptosporidiosis and Kaposi's sarcoma have improved.

Side effects commonly seen early during treatment include nausea, insomnia, myalgia and severe headache. Rashes, vomiting and fever result in interruption of treatment in 1 to 2% of patients. Bone marrow toxicity will often limit the long-term dose and duration of zidovudine therapy. The non-folate or vitamin B_{12} dependent anaemia that can develop is corrected with repeated blood transfusions or zidovudine dose reduction. Neutropenia may develop before 6 weeks and although platelet counts rise initially, thrombocytopenia may recur.

Giving zidovudine to asymptomatic patients with CD4 cell counts less than $500/mm^3$ may result in delayed progression to symptomatic illness. The decline in the count of CD4 cells is slowed, and p24 antigen levels are suppressed. Zidovudine is also better tolerated compared to patients with more advanced disease.

The long-term benefits of early intervention to delay clinical progression and thus potentially prolong survival are not known. The development of in vitro resistance to zidovudine, which is related to duration of therapy, occurs although its importance has not been determined. Thus, the ideal moment – perhaps occurring between CD4 cell counts of 200 and $500/mm^3$ – when efficacy may be maximized, toxicity minimized, and the most durable benefit ensured is not yet known.

Other promising nucleoside analogues include didanosine (dideoxyinosine, DDI) and dideoxycytidine (DDC). Both drugs have a similar mechanism of action to zidovudine and act as false inosine and cytidine substrates respectively. Didanosine does not have the haematological toxicity of zidovudine. Patients currently receiving didanosine have normally already been treated with zidovudine. In these patients didanosine has shown a transient modest increase in CD4 lymphocyte counts, but a reduction in disease progression or mortality has yet to be reported.

Combination therapy of antiretrovirals or immunostimulants may give a synergistic action, or diminuation of drug toxicity.

Terminal care

Eventually, either the patient or clinician will decide that further active management is no longer appropriate. Active therapy will be stopped but symptomatic drug treatment is used to maintain the patient's quality of life. The principles of care for the terminally ill apply directly to patients with AIDS.

THE PATIENT

HIV disease affects a wide variety of patient populations. Each particular group will present with unique challenges. In intravenous substance misusers for example, liver impairment, drug compliance, and substances of abuse mimicking neurological symptoms, may be troublesome. Newly developed drugs such as zidovudine have not been used extensively in women and paediatrics and the long-term adverse effects are not yet known.

Table 41.2 lists some of the biochemical and haematological parameters that require monitoring during therapy with a particular drug. Many patients also use therapies such as homeopathy, acupuncture, aromatherapy and special diets. Discussion with the patient can be beneficial in determining if any interactions or risks are present.

Prevention strategies are a key resource in controlling the spread of the epidemic. Behavioural changes and a reduction in HIV transmission rates in the initially targeted population of homosexual men have occurred but studies show that education must be continual. National campaigns have increased public awareness but many people require more detailed information.

Individual counselling backed with practical sound information is the most likely mechanism to achieve education and behavioural change. Clinical vaccines are in development. These are typically non-infectious glycoprotein fragments derived from HIV. Efficacy of vaccines will be difficult to prove as transmission rates are changing and alternative methods of prevention (for example 'safe sex') cannot be discouraged. It will be many years before a vaccine is in widespread use.

CASE STUDIES

CASE 41.1

Mrs A. J. is a 38-year-old, 55 kg, female, diagnosed HIV-antibody positive 3 years ago. She has presented to her regular outpatient appointment with a 2-week history of shortness of breath, lethargy, fevers, weight loss and night sweats. 3 months ago she was transfused in the day clinic with four units of blood for a haemoglobin of 8.4 g/dl. Drug therapy so far has been zidovudine 250 mg four times daily for the last 18 months. Her CD4 cell count has been 231 and 197/mm³ for the last two readings respectively.

Q1 What is the likely cause of Mrs A. J.'s persistent anaemia and what are the treatment options?

Q2 What is the significance of her current symptoms and CD4 counts?

CASE 41.2

Mr P. N. is a 31-year-old, 75 kg, homosexual male who presented to the hospital casualty department with a 3-week history of dry non-productive cough, fever, tachycardia and severe shortness of breath. He has already been to his general practitioner, and had a course of amoxycillin, but this has not helped his 'chest infection'. Investigations show a chest X-ray of bilateral diffuse interstitial shadowing and other results are PO_2 of 8.1 kPa, temperature 39.5°C, pulse 109 per minute. He is admitted and commenced on 4 co-trimoxazole 480 mg tablets four times a day for 3 weeks and cefuroxime injection 750 mg three times a day for 7 days.

Q1 What diagnosis has been made and what tests are required for confirmation?

Q2 What would you monitor with regard to his co-trimoxazole therapy?

Q3 If side effects occur, what are the treatment options?

CASE 41.3

Mr M. B. is a 55-year-old, 63 kg, male AIDS patient. He has a previous medical history of PCP 1 year ago (his AIDS-defining illness), recurrent genital herpes and oral candidosis. He presented with painless, persistent blurring of vision in his left eye only, of 5-days' duration. His current drug therapy is: zidovudine 100 mg five times a day, dapsone 100 mg daily, acyclovir 200 mg twice a day and amphotericin lozenges when required. Recent biochemical results revealed CD4 cell count 75/mm³, haemoglobin 10.7 g/dl and serum creatinine 95 µmol/L. He was admitted, and after investigations, a permanent central intravenous line was surgically inserted and ganciclovir 300 mg in 100 ml normal saline over 1 hour, twice daily for 3 weeks prescribed.

Q1 What is the diagnosis?

Q2 What drug interaction is there between the ganciclovir and Mr M. B.'s current drugs?

Q3 What is the alternative therapy and how is it different?

CASE 41.4

Mr A. G. is a 49-year-old, 59 kg, male AIDS patient. Kaposi's sarcoma was diagnosed 2 years ago and there are now extensive lesions on the trunk, legs and face for which he has received radiotherapy. Further courses for his facial KS are unlikely because it has produced local ulceration. Other problems are recurrent oesophageal candidosis and recently he has shown neurological symptoms of forgetfulness, loss of concentration and lethargy. He received zidovudine for 5 months but developed a painful muscle weakness and tenderness with elevated serum creatinine kinase levels which all reversed upon stopping zidovudine. Current drug therapy is pentamidine 300 mg nebulized monthly for PCP prophylaxis, fluconazole 50 mg daily, miconazole cream for fungal skin infections of the genitals and feet, and dihydrocodeine for occasional headaches and diarrhoea. CD4 cell count is 104/mm³.

Q1 Is Kaposi's sarcoma a significant cause of mortality in HIV disease?

Q2 What are the treatments for Karposi's sarcoma?

Q3 What are possible causes of his neurological symptoms?

ANSWERS TO CASE STUDIES

CASE 41.1

A1 Mrs A. J.'s anaemia is probably due to zidovudine therapy. Other possible causes such as *Mycobacterium avium* complex should be considered, and investigations may be warranted. The mechanism of zidovudine's bone marrow toxicity has not been established and it may also cause neutropenia, leucopenia and thrombocytopenia. Risk factors for developing myelotoxicity include prolonged therapy, high doses (1200–1500 mg/day), patients with advanced disease, and CD4 counts of less than 100/mm³.

The treatment normally used for zidovudine-related anaemia is blood transfusion. If the need for transfusions becomes regular then dosage reduction to 500 mg/day would occur. If neutrophil counts are low, temporary stopping of therapy for 2 weeks will normally allow recovery. Mrs A. J. could also be changed to the other nucleoside analogue, didanosine, which does not appear to have the haematological side effects of zidovudine.

A2 Opportunistic infections in adults with AIDS do not normally occur with CD4 cell counts above 200/mm³. Mrs A. J.'s current levels, the presence of fevers, night sweats, and loss of weight would indicate that she is at risk of disease progression.

Because of the risk of opportunistic infection, particularly *Pneumocystis carinii* pneumonia (PCP), Mrs A. J. should be commenced on primary PCP prophylaxis. The choice of drug should be determined by discussion with the patient who, for example, may prefer nebulized pentamidine monthly to daily co-trimoxazole or dapsone tablets.

CASE 41.2

A1 The presumptive diagnosis is PCP. This is based upon the patient's non-response to conventional treatment for bacterial pneumonia, chest X-ray typical of PCP, presence of a dry cough and shortness of breath. The patient's sexuality in this setting does contribute to the presumptive diagnosis, but both ethically and scientifically, cannot be used as the significant or sole factor.

Sputum should be cultured for *Pneumocystis* and screened for mixed flora. The cefuroxime may be stopped if no bacteria are isolated but mixed infection can commonly occur. Based on these results the patient may need to be counselled regarding a possible HIV test. Patients must consent before a test can be done, and both pre- and post-test counselling must occur. Confidentiality and sensitivity will be extremely important.

A2 The dose of co-trimoxazole used in the treatment of PCP is significantly higher than for bacterial infections. Nausea and vomiting occur very commonly and antiemetics should be co-prescribed. If extrapyramidal side effects occur with either metoclopramide or prochlorperazine, domperidone can be used (the suppository formulation being useful) as it does not cross the blood–brain barrier. Skin rashes and pruritus may occur following several days' therapy and respond to chlorpheniramine. Serious skin reactions such as Stevens–Johnson syndrome require immediate change of treatment. Anaemia due to folic acid deficiency may also occur. If fever persists, but other parameters improve, drug-related fever due to sulphamethoxazole should be suspected. Substitution of the sulphamethoxazole with dapsone 100 mg per day and continuing the trimethoprim component at the same dose is sometimes used. Full blood counts, urea and electrolyte determinations, and liver function tests should be routinely performed.

A3 Alternatives for treatment are intravenous or nebulized pentamidine, or clindamycin plus primaquine. If skin rash due to the sulphonamide component develops towards the end of the treatment course, regular chlorpheniramine may sometimes be prescribed, and therapy continued to 'treat through' the allergy. Following acute treatment for PCP, secondary prophylaxis must be initiated.

CASE 41.3

A1 Cytomegalovirus retinitis. A diagnosis can be made if characteristic funduscopic haemorrhages or exudates are present and the virus is isolated from another site (throat, urine, blood). Treatment followed by maintenance therapy is required to prevent further retinal deterioration and recurrent viraemia.

A2 Approximately 40% of patients receiving ganciclovir develop neutropenia. Concomitant administration of other bone marrow suppressive drugs such as zidovudine should therefore be avoided during acute treatment. Reintroduction of zidovudine might be considered once Mr M. B. is on maintenance ganciclovir. Careful monitoring of Mr M. B.'s neutrophils will be required as levels below 1 × 10⁹/L increase his risk of infection.

A3 Foscarnet does not use cellular kinase for activation and cytomegalovirus resistance to foscarnet has not yet been reported. Its side effect profile does not include white blood cells but anaemia can occur. Renal function must be monitored and hydration maintained. Because foscarnet distributes into bone, alterations in serum calcium levels may also occur.

CASE 41.4

A1 For the majority of patients, Kaposi's sarcoma is only external and not life threatening. Prognosis is dictated by the underlying immune deficiency. But symptoms of cough with haemoptysis, or melaena and rectal obstruction may indicate pulmonary or gastrointestinal lesions respectively. At these sites, extensive tissue damage and massive haemorrhage may occur.

A2 The main alternative to radiotherapy is chemotherapy. A combined decision between Mr A. G. and his clinician will need to be made regarding the respective risks and benefits in his particular case. A combination of bleomycin and vincristine administered fortnightly may flatten existing lesions and reduce facial oedema if present. Immunotherapy may not be appropriate because interferons, when used in KS in patients with AIDS, are most effective when combined with zidovudine (which Mr A. G. cannot tolerate) and in patients at an earlier stage of HIV disease.

Many patients obtain benefit from the use of cosmetic camouflaging creams for facial lesions.

A3 Neurological manifestations may be due to opportunistic infections (cytomegalovirus, herpes simplex, atypical mycobacteria), space-occupying lesions (toxoplasma), tumours or by HIV itself. His late stage of disease progression, and lack of antiretroviral therapy might also suggest HIV-related encephalitis. Computed tomography (CT) scan, and examination of cerebrospinal fluid will be needed to eliminate some of the possible causes.

BIBLIOGRAPHY

Adler M W (ed). ABC of AIDS, 2nd edn. London: British Medical Journal 1991

Centers for Disease Control. Guidelines for prophylaxis against pneumocystis carinii pneumonia for persons infected with human immunodeficiency virus. Journal of the American Medical Association 1989; 262: 335–339

Fischl M A, Richman B D, Grieco M H et al. The toxicity of azidothymidine (AZT) in the treatment of patients with AIDS and AIDS-related complex: a double blind, placebo controlled trial. New England Journal of Medicine 1987; 317: 185–191

Friedland G H, Klein R S. Transmission of the human immunodeficiency virus. New England Journal of Medicine 1987; 317: 1125–1135

Glatt A E, Chirgwin K, Landesman S H. Treatment of infections associated with human immunodeficiency virus. New England Journal of Medicine 1988; 318: 1439–1448

Green J, McCreanor A, (eds). Counselling in HIV infection and AIDS. London: Blackwell Scientific Publications 1989

Pau A K, Pitrak D L. Management of cytomegalovirus infection in patients with acquired immunodeficiency syndrome. Clinical Pharmacy 1990; 9: 613–631

Rathbun R C, Martin E S, Eaton V E, Mathew E B. Current and investigational therapies for AIDS associated mycobacterium avium complex disease. Clinical Pharmacy 1991; 10: 280–291

Volberding P A, Lagabos S W, Koch M A, Pettinelli C, Myers M W, Booth D K et al. Zidovudine in asymptomatic human immunodeficiency virus infection: a controlled trial in persons with fewer than 500 CD4-positive cells per cubic millimeter. New England Journal of Medicine 1990; 322: 941–949

Youle M, Clarbour J, Wade P, Farthing C. AIDS: therapeutics in HIV disease. London: Churchill Livingstone 1988

Chapter 42

Fungal infections

S. J. Pedler

Fungi are extremely common organisms which are widely distributed in nature. Fortunately, only a tiny minority cause human disease. Such infections fall conveniently into two groups: superficial infections of skin or mucosal surfaces and deep (or systemic) infections. Generally speaking, fungi can be conveniently classified as either yeasts or moulds. Yeasts have round or oval cells while the moulds, or filamentous fungi (such as those which grow on decaying organic material), produce long, branching tubular structures called hyphae. The true yeasts include such common yeasts as baker's yeast, while the yeast-like fungi are similar to yeasts but occasionally produce hyphae-like structures as well. This group includes the commonest human fungal pathogen, *Candida albicans*. Finally, there is a group of 'dimorphic' fungi which can exist either as yeasts (at 37°C in the body) or as moulds.

SUPERFICIAL INFECTIONS

SUPERFICIAL *CANDIDA* INFECTIONS

Epidemiology

C. albicans and related fungi such as *C. glabrata* are very common yeast-like fungi which form part of the normal flora of the gastrointestinal tract of virtually all healthy individuals. When infection occurs it is usually endogenous (i.e. the source of the organism is the patient's own flora) although cross-infection leading to outbreaks of candidiasis have been described in hospitals.

Superficial candidiasis usually presents as an oral mucositis or as a vaginitis (oral and vaginal thrush) although skin infection and occasionally nail infection may also occur. Predisposing factors for oral candidiasis include the presence of dentures and the use of inhaled steroids for the treatment of asthma. AIDS patients also have a high incidence of oral candidiasis. Antibiotics (which remove the normal vaginal flora, allowing colonization by *Candida*), diabetes mellitus, pregnancy and the oral contraceptive pill are predisposing factors for vaginal thrush. Candidiasis of the skin usually occurs in moist areas such as in 'nappy rash', the perianal region, and intertriginous areas such as skin folds and under the breasts.

Clinical presentation

The usual presentation of oral thrush is a sore mouth, particularly on eating. Examination shows white patches of the fungus on the oral mucosa and tongue (the presence of milk curds in babies' mouths may be similar in appearance); these can be removed leaving a raw, tender, often bleeding surface behind. Vaginal candidiasis usually presents as a vaginal discharge which classically is thick and creamy in nature, often accompanied by itching, which may be severe. Infection of the sexual partner may occur which may be asymptomatic or lead to a balanitis (inflammation of the glans penis).

Infection of the skin causes an inflamed, itching area of skin with pustules and maceration and fissuring of the skin. Nail involvement may present as infection of the subcutaneous tissue around and under the nail (*Candida* paronychia), which is often seen in people whose hands are frequently immersed in water, or as infection of the nail itself (onychomycosis).

Diagnosis

The diagnosis of oral or vaginal candidiasis is usually made clinically but can be confirmed readily by taking a swab of the affected area. Microscopy of the specimen shows large numbers of yeast cells and hyphae, and culture will readily yield the organism. Skin and nail infections may be confused with other infections and conditions such as eczema, and culture should always be performed.

Treatment

Until recently the treatment of thrush was only possible by the topical application of antifungal agents. The drugs currently available for topical use fall into two groups, the polyenes (of which only amphotericin and nystatin are used clinically) and the imidazoles, of which several are available including econazole, clotrimazole and miconazole. The two triazoles (fluconazole and itraconazole) can be given systemically by mouth. Skin infections may also be treated topically but nail infections are unlikely to respond to a topical antifungal agent and may need systemic treatment.

Topical treatment

The polyenes are broad-spectrum antifungal agents which are virtually insoluble in water and which are not absorbed from the gastrointestinal tract or from skin or mucous membranes. Both nystatin and amphotericin (but particularly nystatin) are available in a wide range of formulations including pessaries, creams, gels, tablets, pastilles, etc. The choice of formulation clearly depends on the site of infection. Nystatin is also available in combination with steroids (which may be useful in relieving associated inflammation and itching in skin infections) and antibiotics such as tetracyclines and bacitracin.

Very little in the way of unwanted effects occurs with these agents, but in mixed formulations the effects of the other components must also be taken into account. They are safe for use in pregnancy.

The imidazoles also have a broad antifungal spectrum and are active against some Gram-positive bacteria. Once again, they are available in a wide variety of formulations and may be combined with steroids. Absorption when taken by mouth or from mucosal surfaces is minimal, but detectable serum levels are present after oral administration (particularly with miconazole). Unwanted effects are few; the imidazoles are fetotoxic in high doses in laboratory animals but this has never been shown to occur in pregnant women.

Is there any clinical difference between the polyenes and the imidazoles? For the therapy of oral thrush, the two groups seem equally efficacious. In vaginal candidiasis, although there are no direct comparisons in clinical trials, the imidazoles seem to be more effective (cure rates of 90% versus 80% for the polyenes have been quoted).

Systemic treatment

Two new triazole agents have recently been licensed for the treatment of oral and vaginal candidiasis. These compounds, fluconazole and itraconazole, are discussed in detail later.

Fluconazole is effective in vaginal candidiasis giving similar cure rates to topical therapy. However, many patients find oral administration preferable to topical therapy particularly as it is given as a single dose of 150 mg. In oral candidiasis, fluconazole therapy would usually be considered after failure of topical therapy or in difficult clinical conditions such as patients with human immunodeficiency virus (HIV) infection. Typical doses would be 50 to 100 mg daily for 7 to 14 days. Itraconazole is also effective in vaginal candidiasis, given as two oral doses of 200 mg 12 hours apart.

DERMATOPHYTOSIS
Epidemiology and causative organisms

This condition is caused by the three genera of dermatophyte fungi, *Trichophyton*, *Epidermophyton* and *Microsporum*. Unlike *Candida* these are filamentous fungi (moulds) which have a predilection for keratinized tissue (i.e. skin, nail and hair). These fungi are extremely widely distributed throughout the world and may be acquired

from the soil, from animals or from humans infected with the fungus.

Clinical features

The classical clinical presentation of dermatophyte infection of the skin is 'ringworm', a circular, inflamed lesion with a raised edge and scaling. However, presentation is influenced by the site of infection and by the actual species of fungus causing the infection. In general, less severe lesions are produced by human fungal strains, while those acquired from animals can produce quite intense inflammatory reactions.

Dermatophytosis of the nail results in thickened, discoloured nails while in the scalp infection presents with itching, skin scaling and inflammation, and patchy hair loss (alopecia).

Diagnosis

The diagnosis of dermatophyte infection is confirmed by collecting appropriate specimens such as material from infected nails and skin. The fungi can be seen microscopically after the material is 'cleared' in 10% potassium hydroxide. Specimens may also be cultured.

Treatment

As with superficial *Candida* infections, dermatophytosis can be treated either topically or systemically.

Topical therapy

This is most appropriate for small or medium areas of skin infection. Larger areas, or nail or hair infection should be treated with a systemic agent. The most commonly used agents are the imidazoles, such as clotrimazole, econazole, miconazole and sulconazole. There is nothing to choose between these agents all of which are usually applied twice daily, continuing for perhaps 2 weeks after the lesions have healed. Side effects are uncommon and usually consist of mild skin irritation. Other topical agents include benzoyl peroxide and tolnaftate.

Systemic therapy

The first orally administered treatment for dermatophytosis was griseofulvin, which has now been available for over 30 years. Griseofulvin is active only against dermatophyte fungi; it is inactive against all other fungi and bacteria. In order to exert its antifungal effect it must be incorporated into keratinous tissue (where levels are much greater than serum levels) and therefore has no effect if used topically.

The usual adult dose is 500 to 1000 mg daily, given in one dose or divided doses if required. Griseofulvin is well absorbed and absorption is enhanced if taken with a high-fat meal. In children it may be given with milk. A 1000 mg dose produces a peak serum level of about 1 to 2 mg/L after 4 hours, with a half-life of at least 9 hours. There is also an ultrafine preparation of griseofulvin which is almost totally absorbed and permits the use of lower doses (typically 330 to 660 mg daily). This preparation is not available in the UK. Elimination is mainly through the liver, and inactive metabolites are excreted in the urine. Less than 1% of a dose is excreted in urine in the active form but some active drug is excreted in the faeces.

The main drug interactions with griseofulvin are shown in Table 42.1, and side effects in Table 42.2. Griseofulvin is teratogenic in animals and is contra-indicated in pregnancy and in severe liver disease.

The duration of treatment with griseofulvin is dependent entirely on clinical response. Skin or hair infection usually requires 4 to 12 weeks of therapy but nail infections respond much more slowly; 6 months' treatment is often required for fingernails, a year or more for toenail infections. Unfortunately the rate of treatment failure or relapse in nail infection is high, and may reach up to 60%.

Because of this high failure rate, other agents have been sought. Ketoconazole is an alternative to griseofulvin, but concern about side effects such as hepatotoxicity and interference with testosterone synthesis is leading to its replacement by itraconazole, which has been shown to be an

Table 42.1 Interactions of antifungal agents with other drugs

Drug	Interaction with:	Result
Griseofulvin	Warfarin	Reduces anticoagulant effect (induces liver enzymes which metabolize warfarin)
	Oral contraceptives	Reduces contraceptive efficacy (induces liver enzymes which metabolize the oral contraceptive)
Amphotericin	Any nephrotoxic drug (e.g. aminoglycosides)	Enhanced nephrotoxicity
Miconazole	Warfarin	Enhanced anticoagulant effect (may displace warfarin from serum albumin binding sites and inhibit metabolism of warfarin)
	Sulphonylureas	Enhanced effects of sulphonylureas
	Phenytoin	Enhanced effect of phenytoin
Ketoconazole	Warfarin	As miconazole
	Phenytoin	As miconazole; plus possibly reduced ketoconazole levels
	Cyclosporin	Elevated serum cyclosporin levels (due to reduced cyclosporin metabolism)
	Rifampicin	Reduced serum ketoconazole levels (rifampicin induces more rapid ketoconazole metabolism)
Fluconazole	Warfarin	As miconazole
	Sulphonylureas	As miconazole
	Phenytoin	As miconazole
Itraconazole	Rifampicin	Reduced itraconazole levels (reason as for ketoconazole)
	Cyclosporin	As ketoconazole

Table 42.2 Side effects of antifungal agents	
Drug	Side effects
Griseofulvin	Mild: headache, gastrointestinal side effects. Hypersensitivity reactions such as skin rashes, including photosensitivity Moderate: exacerbation of acute intermittent porphyria; rarely, precipitation of systemic lupus erythematosus. Contra-indicated in both these conditions
Amphotericin	Immediate reactions (during infusion) include headache, pyrexia, rigors, nausea, vomiting, hypotension. Occasionally these can be severe. Thrombophlebitis after the infusion is very common Nephrotoxicity Mild: anaemia due to reduced erythropoiesis Peripheral neuropathy (rare) Cardiac failure (this is exacerbated by hypokalemia due to nephrotoxicity) Immunomodulation (the drug can both enhance and inhibit some immunological functions)
Flucytosine	Mild: gastrointestinal side effects (nausea, vomiting). Occasional skin rashes Moderate: myelosuppression. Hepatotoxicity
Miconazole	Mild: nausea and vomiting, skin rashes, febrile episodes, thrombophlebitis Moderate: anaphylactic reactions and cardiac arrhythmias – these can be avoided by infusing the solution over at least 30 minutes; anaemia; rouleaux appearance in blood films and hyperlipidemia (both probably due to the lipid carrier cremophor EL)
Ketoconazole	Mild: nausea, vomiting; occasional skin rashes Moderate: reduced testosterone levels; reduced plasma cortisol levels (but this may not be clinically significant) Severe: hepatotoxicity, although usually confined to elevated liver enzymes, can lead to frank jaundice and possibly fatal hepatotoxicity
Fluconazole:	Mild: nausea, vomiting and occasional skin rashes
Itraconazole:	Mild: nausea and abdominal pain

effective, well-tolerated treatment for dermatophyte infections including those in which griseofulvin therapy has failed. A new class of antifungal agents, the allylamines, are under development of which terbinafine is the first to become available.

DEEP-SEATED FUNGAL INFECTIONS

Most deep-seated or systemic fungal infections seen in the UK are the result of some breakdown in the normal body defences, whether this is due to disease or medical treatment. There are, however, a group of fungi (often referred to rather misleadingly as the 'pathogenic fungi') which are able to cause systemic infection in a previously healthy person. These infections, which include diseases such as histoplasmosis, blastomycosis, and coccidioidomycosis, are rare in the UK but rather more common in the USA and some other parts of the world. They will not be discussed further in this chapter.

FUNGAL INFECTIONS IN THE COMPROMISED HOST
Epidemiology and predisposing factors

There are a large number of conditions which may predispose the individual to systemic or deep-seated fungal infection. These are summarized in Table 42.3. Fungal urinary tract infection is particularly common in catheterized patients who have received broad-spectrum antibiotics, while total parenteral nutrition (TPN) is also strongly associated with fungaemia, sometimes with unusual fungi such as *Malassezia furfur*, a lipophilic skin yeast associated with the use of intravenous lipid infusion. Most cases of fungal infection, however, are associated with some defect in the patient's immune system, and the nature of the organisms encountered is often related to the nature of the immunosuppression. Neutropenia for example is usually associated with *Candida* species, *Aspergillus* and mucormy-

Table 42.3 Conditions predisposing to systemic or deep-seated fungal infection

Infection	Predisposing conditions
Systemic candidiasis	Neutropenia from any cause (disease or treatment) Use of broad-spectrum antibiotics which eliminate the normal body flora Indwelling intravenous cannulae, especially when used for total parenteral nutrition Hematological malignancy Organ transplantation AIDS (particularly associated with severe mucocutaneous infection) Intravenous drug abuse Cardiac surgery and heart valve replacement, leading to *Candida* endocarditis Gastrointestinal tract surgery
Aspergillosis	Neutropenia from any cause, especially if severe and prolonged Acute leukaemia Organ transplantation Chronic granulomatous disease of childhood (defect in neutrophil function) Pre-existing lung disease (usually leads to aspergillomas – fungus balls in the lung – rather than invasive or disseminated infection)
Cryptococcosis	AIDS Systemic therapy with corticosteroids Renal transplantation Hodgkin's disease and other lymphomas Sarcoidosis Collagen vascular diseases
Mucormycosis	Diabetic hyperglycaemic ketoacidosis Severe, prolonged neutropenia

cosis, while defects of cell-mediated immunity (e.g. HIV infection) are strongly associated with *Cryptococcus* infection.

Causative fungi

Many different fungi have been described as causing systemic fungal infection but the commonest organisms encountered are listed in Table 42.4 and of these *Candida* and *Aspergillus* are by far the most common.

Clinical presentation

Deep-seated fungal infection can present in a large number of different ways. The most common presentation is as a fungaemia, with fever, low blood pressure, and the other features of septic shock. Relatively low-grade fungaemias (for example, those associated with TPN) often present only with fever. Both *Candida* and *Aspergillus* infection may present as fungal pneumonia, while the usual presentation of mucormycosis is with rhinocerebral infection leading to encephalitis. Cryptococcosis most frequently presents

with a chronic, insidious meningitis and occasionally as pneumonia. Disseminated infection, particularly in candidiasis and aspergillosis, is quite common and multiple organ systems may be involved.

Diagnostic measures

Unfortunately the diagnosis of deep-seated fungal infection is difficult and is often only made post-mortem. Systemic candidiasis may be diagnosed by isolation of the organism from blood culture and culture of other appropriate specimens. *Cryptococcus neoformans* grows readily on laboratory media and can be isolated from blood and cerebrospinal fluid; a simple test for the detection of cryptococcal antigen in CSF and serum is also available. Aspergillosis is rarely, if ever, diagnosed from blood culture but the organism can occasionally be isolated from sputum; however, bronchoalveolar lavage is the best technique for the diagnosis of pulmonary aspergillosis. Mucormycosis is most readily diagnosed by histological examination of tissue biopsies since

Table 42.4 The common causes of systemic and deep-seated fungal infection

Organism	Common clinical presentations
Candidiasis *(Candida albicans,* *C. glabrata,* *C. tropicalis,* other *Candida* species)	Fungaemia Colonization of intravenous cannulae *Candida* pneumonia *Candida* meningitis Bone and joint infections Endocarditis Endophthalmitis Peritonitis in chronic ambulatory peritoneal dialysis
Aspergillosis *(Aspergillus fumigatus,* *A. flavus,* other *Aspergillus* species)	Invasive pulmonary aspergillosis Aspergilloma Disseminated aspergillosis Endocarditis
Cryptococcosis *(Cryptococcus neoformans)*	Meningitis Pneumonia
Mucormycosis (various species of the genera *Rhizopus, Absidia* and *Mucor*)	Rhinocerebral disease Pulmonary mucormycosis
Malassezia furfur	Fungaemia associated with total parenteral nutrition

the organism is rarely cultured from clinical specimens.

Drug treatment

The difficulties in making the diagnosis of systemic fungal infection are accompanied by a paucity of effective antifungal agents. At the present time only six agents are routinely available, and of these, two (miconazole and ketoconazole) are now considered obsolescent.

Amphotericin

Amphotericin is a member of the polyene group of antibiotics, which are obtained from various species of *Streptomyces*. There are a number of different polyenes but for various reasons (lack of stability or solubility, or excess toxicity) only amphotericin is used systemically. Nystatin is only used topically.

The chemical structure of amphotericin is that of a macrolide carbon ring containing 37 carbon atoms and closed by a lactone bond. The molecule contains seven carbon-to-carbon double bonds (hence the name 'polyene' for this group

of compounds) which are all situated on one side of the molecule while the other side contains seven hydroxyl groups. The molecule is therefore amphipathic (or amphoteric) in nature and this may be of some importance in the mode of action of the polyenes. All the polyenes have very limited solubility in water and organic non-polar solvents, but will readily dissolve in organic polar solvents such as dimethylsulphoxide. In water, amphotericin forms a colloidal suspension of micelles, which is rendered more stable if a surfactant such as sodium desoxycholate is added.

The mode of action of the polyenes is to increase the permeability of the cytoplasmic membrane leading to leakage of the cell contents and eventually death. This action is dependent on binding of the antibiotic to sterols present in the cell membrane and organisms (such as bacteria) which do not contain sterols are inherently resistant to the polyenes. The different polyenes have differing affinities for sterols, and amphotericin has a higher affinity for ergosterol (present in fungal cytoplasmic membranes) than cholesterol, which is found in mammalian cell membranes. This fact presumably explains the selective toxicity of amphotericin for fungal cells.

Acquired resistance to amphotericin is not a clinical problem.

Amphotericin is active against virtually all the fungi which cause systemic mycoses. It is synergistic in vitro with other agents such as flucytosine and rifampicin and in some cases (e.g. amphotericin plus flucytosine in candidiasis) the synergistic interaction appears to be of clinical significance. The results of combination with the imidazoles is less certain, and both synergy and antagonism have been described.

The pharmacokinetics of amphotericin are unusual. A 50 mg dose produces a peak serum level of 0.5 to 3.5 mg/L, but the level cannot be related to clinical response. Amphotericin penetrates poorly into CSF and is heavily (99%) protein bound. Initial elimination of the drug occurs with a half-life of 24 to 48 hours, but after several days this is followed by very slow elimination (half-life about 2 weeks) and the drug may take several weeks more to disappear completely. This may result from strong binding to cell membranes with a gradual elution over a period of weeks. Repeated doses of the drug do not cause accumulation in serum. A small fraction (perhaps 3%) of a dose is excreted in the urine, so that renal dysfunction does not affect serum levels, and the rest appears to be inactivated in the body.

Amphotericin is administered by slow intravenous infusion. If the drug is added to electrolyte solutions or solutions with a low pH it will precipitate out, so it must always be given in buffered 5% dextrose. Several different dosage schedules have been suggested; the two schedules given in Table 42.5 have been used successfully. The doses shown are for adults and would need to be modified for children. In each case a 1 mg test dose should be given in 250 ml of 5% dextrose over a 2- to 4-hour period and the patient monitored for serious side effects (such as fever, rigors and hypotension), during that time. If the patient tolerates the test dose, there are two options. The first is designed to minimize serious

Table 42.5 Suggested dosage schedules for amphotericin B

Regimen 1: for use in a patient with a non-life-threatening, deep-seated infection

Dose	Volume of 5% dextrose	Day	Duration of infusion
1 mg (test dose)	250 ml	1	2 hours
10 mg	500 ml	1	6 hours
20 mg	1000 ml	2	6 hours
30 mg	1000 ml	3	6 hours
40 mg	1000 ml	4	6 hours
50 mg	1000 ml	5 et seq.	6 hours

Regimen 2: for use in a compromised patient with a life-threatening infection

Dose	Volume of 5% dextrose	Day	Duration of infusion
1 mg (test dose)	250 ml	1	2 hours
24 mg	1000 ml	1	6 hours
		6-hour interval	
25 mg	1000 ml	1	6 hours
50 mg	1000 ml	2 et seq.	6 hours

Notes:
1. 50 mg represents a dose of about 0.7 mg/kg for a 70 kg adult. It may not be possible to achieve this dose, depending on the side effects. In this case the highest dose which does not produce unacceptable side effects should be given.
2. In very ill patients the daily dose can be increased up to a maximum of 1.5 mg/kg.
3. Alternate day treatment with a higher unit dose (up to a maximum unit dose of 1.5 mg/kg) may be given. This has the advantage of allowing the patient to attend for outpatient therapy. If the patient is still in hospital it will reduce the amount of time needed for amphotericin administration, which otherwise makes heavy use of intravenous access time that may be needed for other purposes.

side effects by a gradual build-up to the usual maximum daily dose of 50 mg. This is satisfactory if the infection is not immediately life threatening but would be inappropriate for fulminating infections. Here the dose is increased rapidly with careful monitoring of the patient by medical staff.

It is also possible to give amphotericin intrathecally in very small doses (25 to 50 micrograms). In catheterized patients with fungal urinary tract infection treatment is usually not indicated unless the patient is symptomatic, but if required amphotericin can be given as a bladder washout in a concentration of 50 mg/L.

Amphotericin is associated with a long list of toxic effects, which are given in Table 42.2. It is possible to try to minimize the immediate side effects (during the infusion) by adding 50 mg of hydrocortisone to the infusion bag, and antiemetics and an antihistamine may also be given. Nephrotoxicity is the most serious side effect of amphotericin, and is almost invariable in patients given a full course of treatment. Renal function should be monitored regularly (at least every other day) and if the serum urea exceeds 17 mmol/L or the creatinine exceeds 170 µmol/L the drug should be discontinued until the urea or creatinine level falls below this limit. Hypokalaemia is also a problem and may be severe, necessitating replacement therapy. Fortunately renal function returns to normal in most patients unless very large total doses have been given.

The duration of therapy is guided by clinical response. There is some evidence that the total dose administered is of some importance in determining response, and for an established deep-seated infection a total dose of 1.5 to 2 g would be appropriate. This represents about 4 weeks of therapy at 50 mg/day. The patient may be well enough to attend for treatment on an outpatient basis, in which case the drug can be given in a higher unit dose on alternate days. However, the maximum daily dose of 1.5 mg/kg should not be exceeded. For fungaemia due to infected intravenous cannulae the main therapeutic action is removal of the cannula, the use of antifungal agents being less important. However, they should still be given to prevent disseminated infection elsewhere in the body. There is no consensus about the length of therapy in such patients but one week's treatment (full dose) has been suggested.

In an attempt to produce a less toxic form of amphotericin, a methyl ester was developed. Unfortunately this was associated with neurological side effects and is therefore currently unavailable in the UK. The most promising development has been the delivery of amphotericin in liposomes in which the amphotericin is contained in 'vesicles' composed of a phospholipid bilayer. The advantages of this method of delivery are that a higher unit dose may be given and there is a reduction in toxic effects. It appears likely that due to the high cost of the liposomal form it will be reserved for patients who fail to respond to conventional amphotericin (in whom higher doses might be effective) or those who suffer severe side effects from conventional therapy.

Flucytosine

Another useful agent for systemic fungal infection is flucytosine (5-fluorocytosine), a synthetic fluorinated nucleotide analogue. The mode of action is twofold. Following uptake by the cell, which is dependent on the presence of cytosine permease, flucytosine is deaminated to 5-fluorouracil by cytosine deaminase. This in turn is incorporated into fungal RNA in place of uracil, leading to impairment of protein synthesis. Further metabolism of 5-fluorouracil leads to a metabolite which inhibits the enzyme thymidylate synthetase, in turn leading to inhibition of DNA synthesis. Mammalian cells have absent or weak cytosine deaminase activity which accounts for the selective toxicity of flucytosine.

For all practical purposes flucytosine is only active against yeasts and yeast-like fungi. Primary resistance occurs in perhaps 10% of clinical isolates of *Candida* species and resistance develops rapidly if the drug is used alone. There are several resistance mechanisms some of which result from a single-step mutation giving a high frequency of secondary resistance in organisms exposed to the drug. For this reason flucytosine should always be given in combination with another agent such as amphotericin, with which it is synergistic.

Flucytosine is highly soluble in water and over 90% of an oral dose is absorbed from the gastrointestinal tract. Virtually all of the absorbed dose is excreted unchanged in the urine by glomerular filtration. The elimination half-life is about 4 hours, but this is greatly prolonged in renal failure, and dosage modification will be required in patients with renal dysfunction. The degree of protein binding is very low and flucytosine penetrates well into all tissues including the aqueous humour of the eye (where about 10% of the serum level is achieved) and the CSF (about 80% of the serum level).

Flucytosine is given orally or by a short intravenous infusion and the dose by either route in patients with normal renal function is 150 to 200 mg/kg/day in 4 divided doses. This must be reduced in renal failure, but the degree of reduction depends on the degree of renal impairment and it is obligatory to monitor the serum levels of flucytosine. It must be remembered that flucytosine is often given in conjunction with amphotericin which will probably cause some degree of renal dysfunction. To avoid dose-related marrow toxicity (see below) the peak serum level (obtained at 1 hour after an intravenous dose or 2 hours after an oral dose) should be maintained in the range 25 to 50 mg/L and should not be allowed to exceed 80 mg/L. Hemodialysis readily removes flucytosine and patients on dialysis can be treated by giving a single dose of 25 mg/kg after each episode of dialysis.

The side effects of flucytosine are given in Table 42.2. The most important toxic effect is a dose-related myelosuppression with neutropenia and thrombocytopenia. This is usually reversible and can be avoided by monitoring serum levels of flucytosine and adjusting the dose accordingly. Hepatotoxicity is also probably a result of high serum levels, and liver function tests should be performed regularly. The drug is teratogenic in some animals and is not recommended in pregnant women for relatively trivial infections such as fungal urinary tract

infection. In cases of life-threatening fungal infection (very rare in pregnancy) the potential benefits of flucytosine must be weighed against the possible risks.

Imidazoles

There are currently two imidazole compounds (miconazole and ketoconazole) available in the UK for the treatment of systemic fungal infection (plus others used only for topical therapy) but both have been superseded to a great extent by the newer triazoles. The basic chemical structure of the imidazoles is the azole ring, a five-membered ring containing two nitrogen atoms. (The triazoles also contain the azole ring but with three nitrogen atoms.)

The main mode of action is by inhibition of the synthesis of ergosterol, which is an important component of the cytoplasmic membrane in fungal but not in mammalian cells. One of the nitrogen atoms of the azole ring binds to the iron atom of cytochrome P450 and inhibits its activation. Ergosterol synthesis is dependent on cytochrome P450 activation and as a result its production is impaired. The imidazoles also damage the cytoplasmic membrane directly but this is only achieved at higher concentrations.

The imidazoles have a broad spectrum of action, including most yeasts and yeast-like fungi, the dimorphic fungi and the dermatophytes. Filamentous fungi causing systemic infection are variable in sensitivity and in vitro activity is not always accompanied by an in vivo response. Naturally occurring resistance is very rare but it can occasionally develop in patients given the drug.

Miconazole and ketoconazole are only slightly water soluble but are soluble in organic solvents. Miconazole is poorly absorbed from the gastrointestinal tract and therefore must be given intravenously. It is heavily protein bound (about 90%). Due to its low solubility in water it is supplied in 'cremophor EL', a polyethoxylated castor oil base, which causes some of the side effects of systemic miconazole. Most of a dose of miconazole is metabolized in the body; about 1% is excreted unchanged in the urine. The initial elimination half-life is short, about 30 minutes, but this is followed by a much longer elimination phase (half-life about 20 hours). The half-life is not affected by renal function and the dose need not be altered in patients with renal failure. The usual adult dose is 600 mg three times daily, given by adding the drug to 200 ml of physiological saline or 5% dextrose which is then administered by a short infusion.

Ketoconazole is only available in an oral preparation. It is not soluble in water unless the pH is less than 3, and the presence of gastric acid is therefore required for optimal absorption. The concomitant use of antacids or H_2 antagonists will reduce the absorption of ketoconazole. The drug is lipophilic and absorption is improved if taken with food. As with miconazole, protein binding is high (99%) and since only a small amount is excreted in the urine dose adjustment in renal failure is not required. The elimination half-life is about 8 to 10 hours. Most of a dose (over 50%) of ketoconazole is excreted in the faeces as active drug and inactive metabolites. The standard adult dose is 200 mg once daily, but this can be increased to 400 mg daily if required.

The side effects of these two drugs are listed in Table 42.2. Some of the side effects of miconazole appear to be due to the cremophor base, including hyperlipidaemia, anaemia and thrombophlebitis. The most important side effect of ketoconazole is hepatotoxicity. Abnormalities of liver function tests (LFTs) are quite common in patients receiving ketoconazole but frank hepatitis (which may be fatal) is less common (perhaps 1 in 12 000 cases). Therapy of more than 14-days' duration is more frequently associated with hepatotoxicity and for this reason all patients receiving long courses of ketoconazole should have their LFTs monitored prior to treatment and at regular intervals thereafter. Treatment should be stopped if the LFTs show a progressive rise or if clinical hepatitis develops. Ketoconazole can inhibit the synthesis of testosterone and this may lead to the development of gynaecomastia in males on long-term, high-dose therapy.

Triazoles

The triazoles, fluconazole and itraconazole, have a similar mode of action to the imidazoles, but differ substantially from one another in their physical properties and in vivo activity. Itraconazole is a lipophilic, poorly water-soluble compound which is well absorbed (>90% of a dose) from the gastrointestinal tract; like ketoconazole, absorption is improved by food. It has a half-life of about 17 hours and most of a dose is metabolized in the body, less than 1% appearing as active drug in the urine. It is heavily (99%) protein bound and penetration into CSF is poor. Conversely, fluconazole is hydrophilic and water soluble. It is also well absorbed (about 85%) when taken orally, but this is not affected by food. It has a long half-life of 22 hours, but protein binding is low (about 11%) and it penetrates well into CSF, reaching 60% of the serum level. It is excreted mainly in the urine as unchanged drug and therefore the dose must be adjusted in renal failure.

Itraconazole is available in an oral form only, while fluconazole can be given orally or intravenously as a short infusion. The main side effects of these agents are listed in Table 42.2.

Choice of treatment

Which antifungal agent should be used in the treatment of systemic fungal infection? Until recently the 'gold standard' was amphotericin, combined with flucytosine in infections due to yeasts, but this is now changing. As alternatives to amphotericin, the usefulness of miconazole and ketoconazole is now seen to be diminishing due to insufficient efficacy and relatively high toxicity, and they are being replaced by the triazoles. A possible alternative in yeast infections is fluconazole, particularly for cryptococcosis, and fluconazole has also been found effective in the prevention of relapses of cryptococcal infection in AIDS patients. There is less experience of itraconazole in systemic candidiasis and

Table 42.6 The choice of antifungal agents for common systemic infections

Condition	1st line therapy	2nd line therapy
Candidiasis	Amphotericin plus flucytosine	Fluconazole
Aspergillosis	Amphotericin. The addition of flucytosine is recommended by some but there is no evidence from controlled trials to support this	Itraconazole
Cryptococcosis	Amphotericin plus flucytosine The position of these two regimens may be reversed in the future. Fluconazole is said to be more effective than amphotericin in AIDS patients and this may prove to be the case in non-AIDS patients in the future	Fluconazole
Mucormycosis	Amphotericin	None

Notes:
1. In fungaemia due to colonized intravenous cannulae the removal of the cannula is at least as important as the administration of an antifungal agent.
2. Surgery to remove necrotic tissue is an important component of the treatment of mucormycosis.

cryptococcosis but this agent has been used with success in treating infections due to the 'pathogenic' fungi. There are also potentially exciting results of the use of itraconazole in aspergillosis but the numbers of patients are small at present. Finally, investigation is now underway of the use of fluconazole and itraconazole in the prophylaxis of fungal infection in immunocompromised patients. The choice of antifungal agent in selected conditions is summarized in Table 42.6.

CASE STUDIES

CASE 42.1

A 35-year-old male with acute myeloid leukaemia undergoing induction therapy resulting in profound neutropenia develops systemic candidiasis. He is treated with amphotericin and flucytosine (50 mg/kg four times daily) but his renal function worsens and after 1 week's treatment his flucytosine levels are 54 mg/L predose and 95 mg/L post-dose.

Q Does his therapy need modification, and if so how?

CASE 42.2

A 46-year-old woman has recently had a renal transplant and presents with meningitis, subsequently found to be due to *Cryptococcus neoformans*. Her renal function is very poor as the transplant is not functioning well.

Q What is the most appropriate treatment?

CASE 42.3

A 10-year-old boy with aplastic anaemia has recently undergone a bone marrow transplant. Several days post-transplant he develops a pneumonia unresponsive to antibiotics and invasive aspergillosis is diagnosed. Amphotericin is commenced but he is unable to tolerate treatment, because of hypotension and severe rigors.

Q What other options are available?

ANSWERS TO CASE STUDIES

CASE 42.1

A From the point of view of dose-related toxicity the peak level is the significant value. This should be kept below 100 mg/L (preferably below 80 mg/L). The predose level indicates that the patient is clearly accumulating flucytosine; with normal renal function the level of flucytosine 6 hours after this dose would be expected to be below 30 mg/L. The dose must be adjusted therefore to avoid exceeding the 100 mg/L limit. The individual unit dose however is satisfactory, producing a difference between pre- and post-dose levels of 41 mg/L. The most appropriate course of action would be to lengthen the dosage interval, for example to 50 mg/kg three times daily rather than four times daily, or even to twice daily if renal function is continuing to worsen.

CASE 42.2

A Although amphotericin would normally be used (in conjunction with flucytosine) it may not be wise to use such a nephrotoxic agent in this patient, for fear of worsening renal function still further. Fluconazole has achieved good results in AIDS patients with cryptococcosis, but has the disadvantage that since it is excreted almost entirely by the kidney, dose adjustment will be necessary. Although itraconazole penetrates poorly into CSF good results have been obtained in cryptococcosis (again in AIDS patients) and this might be considered preferable in this patient since modification of the dose is not necessary. Unfortunately as a renal transplant recipient the patient will probably be receiving cyclosporin which interacts with itraconazole but not fluconazole (see Table 41.1)! This problem illustrates the difficulty of choosing a suitable antifungal when so few effective agents are available. In this patient the need to adjust cyclosporin levels might be thought undesirable, even though a major adjustment to the dose of fluconazole will be needed, but the choice is to a great extent a matter of personal preference. One last point is that studies of the efficacy of both fluconazole and itraconazole in cryptococcosis have been performed to a great extent in AIDS patients and it is not known if these results are applicable to other groups of patients.

CASE 42.3

A There are three possibilities. It may be possible to counter the side effects of amphotericin with hydrocortisone and antihistamines. If this is unsuccessful then a change of treatment must be considered. In this case either liposomal amphotericin or itraconazole would be potential alternatives (fluconazole or an imidazole would not be useful due to lack of activity against the infecting organism). Amphotericin is still considered to be the treatment of choice for *Aspergillus* infections and the liposomal form has been used in patients who cannot tolerate the standard preparation. It has also been shown to be useful in those patients whose infection does not respond to standard amphotericin, and these patients appear to benefit from the much higher doses which can be given using the liposomal form. Only if the patient cannot tolerate even the liposomal preparation should itraconazole be used since comparable efficacy to amphotericin has not yet been demonstrated and aspergillosis is associated with a high mortality rate in neutropenic patients.

BIBLIOGRAPHY

Denning D W, Tucker R M, Hanson L H, Stevens D A. Treatment of invasive aspergillosis with itraconazole. American Journal of Medicine 1989; 86: 791–800

Gallis H A, Drew R H, Pickard W W. Amphotericin B: 30 years of clinical experience. Reviews of Infectious Diseases 1990; 12: 308–329

Kucers A, Bennett N McK. The use of antibiotics, 4th edn. London: William Heinemann 1987

Lopez-Bernstein G, Bodey G P, Fainstein V, Keating M, Frankel L S, Zeluff B et al. Treatment of systemic fungal infections with liposomal amphotericin B. Archives of Internal Medicine 1989; 149: 2533–2536

Saag M S, Dismukes W E. Azole antifungal agents: emphasis on new triazoles. Antimicrobial Agents and Chemotherapy 1988; 32: 1–8

Speller D C E (ed). Antifungal chemotherapy. Chichester: John Wiley & Sons 1980

Stern J J, Hartman B J, Sharkey P, Rowland V, Squires K E, Murray H W et al. Oral fluconazole therapy for patients with acquired immunodeficiency syndrome and cryptococcosis: experience in 22 patients. American Journal of Medicine 1988; 85: 477–480

Sugar A M, Saunders C. Oral fluconazole as suppressive therapy of disseminated cryptococcosis in patients with acquired immunodeficiency syndrome. American Journal of Medicine 1988; 85: 481–489

Warnock D W, Richardson M D (ed). Fungal infection in the compromised patient, 2nd edn. Chichester: John Wiley & Sons 1991

Chapter 43

Thyroid and parathyroid disorders

J. Cantrill

HYPOTHYROIDISM

Hypothyroidism is the clinical state which results from decreased production of thyroid hormones, or, very rarely, from their decreased action at tissue level.

EPIDEMIOLOGY

Comparison of studies of the prevalence and incidence of hypothyroidism is difficult due to the variation in definitions and population samples. Using a uniform set of diagnostic criteria, the prevalence of previously undiagnosed, spontaneous, overt hypothyroidism has been estimated to be between 2 and 4 per 1000 total population worldwide. However, if all cases of previously diagnosed hypothyroidism, previous thyroid surgery and radio-iodine treatment are included, this prevalence rises to approximately 10 per 1000. The prevalence of overt hypothyroidism in the UK is 14 per 1000 for females and around 1 to 2 per 10 000 for males. The question of widespread population screening for hypothyroidism is unsettled, but is probably not cost effective unless incorporated into a screening programme for other conditions.

Although the disease may occur at any age, most patients present between 30 and 60 years of age.

AETIOLOGY

Hypothyroidism can be induced by a variety of

structural or functional abnormalities. The condition can be classified in several ways. The principal classification is: primary, secondary, tertiary and peripheral. Primary hypothyroidism accounts for more than 95% of adult cases and is due to a failure of the thyroid gland itself. Secondary disease is due to hypopituitarism and tertiary disease is due to failure of the hypothalamus. Peripheral hypothyroidism is due to tissue insensitivity to the action of thyroid hormones. A more extensive classification is shown in Table 43.1.

In approximately 20% of patients, hypothyroidism results from destruction of the gland as a result of treatment for hyperthyroidism. Several other disorders are associated with primary hypothyroidism but are not directly causal. These include Addison's disease, pernicious anaemia and diabetes mellitus. Occasionally, hypothyroidism may be drug induced (Table 43.2).

Hypothyroidism can also be classified as nongoitrous or goitrous. Goitre is the term used for enlargement of the thyroid gland. This occurs as a direct result of excessive stimulation by thyroid-stimulating hormone (TSH) in response to low levels of circulating thyroid hormones. The commonest cause of goitre is Hashimoto's thyroiditis. This is characterized by diffuse enlargement and lymphocytic infiltration of the gland. This is an immunological disorder with measurable titres of circulating antibodies against the thyroid gland.

Goitres may also result from the use of certain drugs with antithyroid activity. Drugs used therapeutically in the treatment of hyperthyroidism may produce goitre if used in excessive doses.

Iodides may produce hypothyroidism in certain patients who are extremely sensitive to their ability to block the active transport pump of the thyroid gland. Iodine absorption from topical

Table 43.1 Classification of hypothyroidism
Primary hypothyroidism
Congenital hypothyroidism
Antithyroid drugs
Hashimoto's thyroiditis
Postpartum hypothyroidism
Spontaneous hypothyroidism in Graves' disease
Postoperative hypothyroidism
Hypothyroidism after radioactive iodine
External radiation
Secondary hypothyroidism
Hypopituitarism
Selective TSH deficiency
Tertiary hypothyroidism
Hypothalamic disorders
Peripheral hypothyroidism

Table 43.2 Drug-induced thyroid disease		
Drug	Effect	Comments*
Amiodarone	A. Hypothyroidism Blocks conversion of T_4 to T_3 Compensatory ↑ in TSH	Affects 2–20% of patients Treatment with conventional thyroxine replacement Monitor underlying cardiac disease
	B. Hyperthyroidism Due to iodine content of the drug	Drug may mask clinical features of hyperthyroidism: may remit spontaneously within 6 months May be treated with carbimazole, corticosteroids or a combination of thioamide and potassium perchlorate.
Lithium	A. Hypothyroidism Inhibits iodine uptake and thyroid hormone release	Affects 5–15% of patients on long-term treatment Treat with conventional thyroxine replacement
	B. Hyperthyroidism Paradoxical effect Mechanism unknown	Rare
* Suggested management assumes the drug cannot be discontinued.		

iodine-containing antiseptics has been shown to cause hypothyroidism in neonates. This is potentially very dangerous at a critical time of neurological development in the newborn infant. Transient hypothyroidism may be seen in 25% of iodine-exposed infants.

PATHOPHYSIOLOGY

The thyroid gland consists of 2 lobes and is situated in the lower neck. The gland synthesizes, stores and releases two major metabolically active hormones; thyroxine (T_4) and triiodothyronine (T_3). Regulation of hormone synthesis is by the secretion of TSH from the anterior pituitary. In turn, TSH is regulated by hypothalamic secretion of thyrotropin-releasing hormone (TRH). Low circulating levels of thyroid hormones initiate the release of TSH, and possibly also of TRH. Rising levels of TSH promote increased iodide trapping by the gland with a subsequent increase in synthesis. The increase in circulating hormone levels feeds back on the pituitary and hypothalamus shutting off TSH, TRH and further hormone synthesis.

Both T_4 and T_3 are produced within the gland. Dietary inorganic iodide is trapped by the gland and oxidized by the enzyme peroxidase to iodine. The next step is the incorporation of iodine with tyrosine molecules to form monoiodotyrosine (MIT) and diiodotyrosine (DIT). Subsequently the formation of T_4 occurs as a result of the coupling of two DIT residues and of T_3 by coupling a DIT and a MIT residue. The hormones are then stored within the gland until their release into the circulation by enzymatic cleavage.

The ratio of T_4:T_3 secreted by the thyroid gland is approximately 10:1. Consequently the gland secretes approximately 80 to 100 micrograms of T_4 and 10 micrograms of T_3 per day. However, only 20% of circulating T_3 is derived from direct thyroidal secretion, the remaining 80% is produced by peripheral conversion from T_4. Thyroxine can therefore be considered a prohormone which is converted in the peripheral tissues (liver, kidney and brain) either to the active hormone T_3 or the biologically inactive reverse T_3 (rT_3). In the circulation, the hormones exist in both the active free and inactive protein-bound forms. Thyroxine is 99.98% bound with only 0.02% circulating free. Triiodothyronine is slightly less protein bound (99.8%), resulting in a considerably higher circulating free fraction (0.2%). Details of protein binding are shown in Table 43.3.

The hormones are metabolized in the periphery (kidney, liver and heart) by deiodination. T_4 and T_3 are also eliminated by biliary secretion of their glucuronide and sulphate conjugates (15 to 20%). The half-life of T_4 in plasma is about 6 to 7 days and that of T_3 24 to 36 hours in euthyroid adults. The apparent volume of distribution for T_4 is about 10 litres and for T_3 about 40 litres.

CLINICAL MANIFESTATIONS

The symptoms of hypothyroidism can affect multiple body systems and are usually nonspecific and gradual in onset (Table 43.4). Symptoms,

Table 43.3 Protein binding of thyroid hormones		
	T_4	T_3
Thyroid-binding globulin (TBG)	70%	77%
Thyroid-binding prealbumin (TBPA)	10%	8%
Albumin	20%	15%

Table 43.4 Signs and symptoms of hypothyroidism	
Skin and appendages	Dry, cool, flaking skin Faint yellow colour Puffy facies and eyes Coarse, brittle hair
Nervous system	Slow speech Poor memory Somnolence Carpal tunnel syndrome Psychiatric disturbance Hearing loss Depression
Muscle	Muscle pain and weakness Delayed deep tendon reflexes
Gastrointestinal	Weight gain with decreased appetite Abdominal distension Constipation
Cardiovascular	Reduced cardiac output Bradycardia Cardiac enlargement

especially in the early stages, are frequently vague. It is not uncommon, particularly in the elderly, for symptoms to be attributed incorrectly, by patients and their relatives, to increasing age. The most common symptoms reported by patients are weakness, lethargy, cold intolerance, slowness, memory loss and weight gain (without eating more). The skin becomes dry, hair 'lifeless' and the patient may have noticed a change in voice with deepening or gruffness. The commonest conditions with which hypothyroidism are confused are obesity and depression.

Effusions may occur into pericardial, pleural, peritoneal or joint spaces. Mild anaemia of a macrocytic type is quite common and responds to thyroxine replacement. Pernicious anaemia is a frequent concomitant finding in hypothyroidism. Other, organ-specific autoimmune diseases such as Addison's disease may be associated.

Myxoedema coma

Myxoedema coma is a rare but potentially fatal complication of severe, untreated hypothyroidism. Loss of consciousness is often associated with hypothermia. Coma can be precipitated by cold weather, stress, infection, trauma and certain drugs. Respiratory depressants of any kind which are metabolized slowly in the hypothyroid patient can precipitate coma. These include anaesthetic agents, narcotics, phenothiazines and hypnotics. The condition should be treated rapidly and aggressively.

The term myxoedema used to be synonymous with hypothyroidism. It is now reserved for advanced disease in which there is undue swelling of the skin and subcutaneous tissues.

INVESTIGATIONS

In most cases, laboratory investigation of thyroid disorders is extremely simple, due to specific radioimmunoassays for T_3, T_4, TSH and, where relevant, assay methods for TBG. Usually clinical assessment, combined with a single estimation of thyroid hormones and TSH, is sufficient to make the diagnosis of hypothyroidism. In primary disease, T_4 and T_3 are low and the TSH

rises markedly. However, in the early stages or in patients who have had a subtotal thyroidectomy, the T_4 and T_3 may be normal with only a modest elevation of TSH.

A diagnosis of secondary or tertiary hypothyroidism is suspected on the basis of a low T_4 and low TSH levels. Elevation of TSH occurs early in the course of thyroid failure and may be present before overt clinical manifestations appear. It is important to appreciate that hypothyroidism is not one disease, but a whole spectrum. Hypothyroidism can be graded according to the degree of clinical and laboratory abnormalities.

In the case of overt hypothyroidism there are clear clinical features as well as characteristic abnormalities of T_4 and TSH. This rarely presents a diagnostic problem.

Mild hypothyroidism

The symptoms are less obvious and may be as nonspecific as lack of energy. The results of thyroid function tests may be equivocal but a normal TSH excludes the diagnosis. T_4 is probably more reliable than T_3 for early cases, because T_3 can often be decreased as a nonspecific consequence of illness.

Although there are a large range of other thyroid function tests available they are only rarely required to make the diagnosis of hypothyroidism. When interpreting the results of thyroid function tests caution may be required if the patient has other disease states and/or is taking other drugs (Table 43.5).

A chest X-ray may detect the presence of effusions and an ECG is useful especially in patients with angina or ischaemic heart disease.

TREATMENT

The aims of treatment with thyroxine are to ensure that patients receive a dose which will restore well-being and return the TSH to within the normal range. It is important to avoid both under- and over-treatment. All patients with symptomatic hypothyroidism require replacement therapy. Thyroxine is usually the treatment of choice except in myxoedema coma where T_3

Table 43.5 Drugs and disease states affecting thyroid function tests	
1. Oestrogens Combined oral contraceptive Clofibrate	↑ Serum TBG concentration
Heroin addiction Pregnancy Acute and chronic active hepatitis	↑ Total T_4 and T_3 (free concentration unchanged)
2. Androgens Anabolic steroids Glucocorticoids	↓ Serum TBG concentration
L-asparaginase Nephrotic syndrome	↓ Total T_4 and T_3
3. Phenytoin High dose salicylates 5-fluorouracil	Displacement of T_4 and T_3 from TBG ↓ Total T_4
4. Glucocorticoids Old age Acute and chronic systemic illness	Impairs peripheral conversion of T_4 to T_3 Normal or ↑ Total T_4 ↓ Total T_3

TBG = Thyroid binding globulin

may be used. Before commencing thyroxine replacement the diagnosis of hypopituitarism must be excluded in order to prevent precipitation of an Addisonian crisis. If in doubt, hydrocortisone replacement should be given concomitantly until cortisol deficiency is excluded.

Drug treatment

Once the diagnosis has been established, treatment should be commenced. The condition is very rarely life threatening and adverse effects may result from overzealous treatment. The initial dose of T_4 will depend on the patient's age, the severity and duration of disease and the coexistence of cardiac disease.

In young healthy patients with disease of short duration, T_4 may be commenced in a dose of 100 to 150 micrograms daily. As the drug has a long half-life it should only be given once daily. The most convenient time is usually in the morning. After 4 to 6 weeks on the same dose, thyroid function tests should be checked. The TSH concentration is the best predictor of the euthyroid state and this should be used for further dosage adjustment. Clearly a raised TSH concentration

indicates either inadequate treatment or poor compliance. The majority of patients will be controlled with doses of 100 to 200 micrograms daily, with few patients requiring more than 200 micrograms. In adults the median dose required to suppress TSH to normal is 125 micrograms daily.

In elderly patients, particularly those with ischaemic heart disease, treatment should be introduced more cautiously. Some 5% of patients with long-standing hypothyroidism either complain of angina at presentation or develop it during treatment with thyroxine. Exacerbation of myocardial ischaemia, infarction and sudden death are all well-recognized complications of thyroxine replacement therapy. Patients with ischaemic heart disease may be unable to tolerate full replacement doses because of palpitations, angina or heart failure. Treatment should be started with 25 micrograms daily and increased slowly by 25 micrograms every 4 to 6 weeks. Some authorities recommend starting with 5 micrograms of T_3. The proposed advantage is that if adverse effects occur, these will be alleviated more rapidly due to the shorter half-life of T_3. During this time the patient's clinical progress should be carefully monitored. In some patients thyroxine may be better tolerated if a beta-adrenoreceptor blocking drug such as propranolol is given concomitantly.

There has been considerable recent interest in the risks of over-treatment with thyroxine. Although thyroxine exerts an effect on many organs and tissues, it is probably the effect on bone which gives the greatest cause for concern. There is evidence that bone density may be reduced in patients taking thyroxine replacement therapy. In order to minimize the risk of development of osteoporosis the dose should be carefully tailored to the needs of each individual patient.

Treatment of myxoedema coma

The treatment of myxoedema coma has been poorly studied and the optimal regimen remains to be defined. Thyroid hormone replacement should be commenced by giving 5 to 10 micrograms of T_3 parenterally twice daily. Possible adrenal underactivity should be treated with parenteral hydrocortisone 100 mg three times daily. Heart failure and arrhythmias should be treated if they arise.

Sources of infection should be actively sought, particularly chest or urinary infections and treated aggressively. The body temperature should be monitored rectally and allowed to rise slowly by keeping the patient in a warm room in a 'space blanket' which retains heat. Urea, electrolyte and haematological assessments must be made and corrected as necessary. Even with this kind of management approach, the mortality rate exceeds 50%.

THE PATIENT

The treatment of hypothyroidism requires life-long treatment with thyroxine. Patients on long-term drug therapy are well recognized to be poor compliers and these patients are no exception. Treatment with thyroxine is often terminated because patients feel well and think that treatment is no longer required.

Prevention

At present nothing can be done to prevent thyroid failure from developing; however, much can be done to ensure early detection and treatment.

Careful follow-up of patients who have undergone I^{131} treatment or subtotal thyroidectomy is essential. The earliest biochemical change is an increase in TSH with normal concentrations of T_3 and T_4. These should be used to diagnose hypothyroidism before the patient becomes symptomatic.

HYPERTHYROIDISM

Hyperthyroidism is defined as the production and secretion of excessive amounts of thyroid hormones.

EPIDEMIOLOGY

The most common cause of hyperthyroidism in the western world is Graves' disease, accounting for 90% of cases. This form of hyperthyroidism may affect any age group but it is uncommon in childhood and most frequent in the third to fifth decades. Females are affected about 10 times more often than males. In the United Kingdom the prevalence of overt hyperthyroidism is 20 per 1000 females and 2 per 1000 males.

AETIOLOGY

Hyperthyroidism is a disorder of various aetiologies. The hyperthyroidism and goitre of Graves' disease are thought to result from the action of thyroid-stimulating antibodies which mimic the effect of TSH. An uncertain proportion (perhaps 20%) of these patients will spontaneously become hypothyroid if followed for a long period of time. These immunoglobulins are now known to be antibodies to the TSH receptor on the thyroid gland. Many patients with Graves' disease have distinctive eye signs. It seems likely that these are a manifestation of a parallel but distinct immunological mechanism involving ophthalmogenic immunoglobulins. Graves' disease is a familial condition and many studies suggest that there is a genetic predisposition to the disease.

Toxic nodular goitre is another form of hyperthyroidism. For reasons that are not clear, diffuse or focal autonomous nodule formation develops in the enlarged thyroid, with associated thyrotoxicosis which is generally of a relatively mild degree. Thyroid growth is probably stimulated by a growth-receptor-stimulating antibody. Growth of new follicles outstrips local blood supply resulting in necrosis in the centre of the growth, followed by repair and fibrosis with the formation of multiple nodules. Hyperthyroidism may also be caused by autonomous thyroid adenomas. These are benign well differentiated tumours that secrete excessive amounts of thyroid hormones.

Hyperthyroidism of any aetiology usually suggests excessive levels of T_4. However, approximately 5% of patients will have the syndrome of T_3 toxicosis which is probably due to preferential secretion of T_3 by the thyroid gland.

Occasionally, hyperthyroidism may be drug induced (Table 43.2).

CLINICAL MANIFESTATIONS

Hyperthyroidism is characterized by increased metabolism of all body systems due to excessive quantities of thyroid hormones. There is a wide spectrum of clinical thyroid hormone excess. The clinical signs and symptoms reflect increased adrenergic activity, especially in the cardio-vascular and neurological systems (Table 43.6).

Not all manifestations will be seen in every patient. The classical presentation is a patient, usually female, complaining of palpitations, ex-cessive sweating, fine tremor and weight loss in spite of a good or increased appetite. She may be intolerant of heat and almost invariably admits to a preference for cooler weather.

The diagnosis of hyperthyroidism in the elderly may not be so easily made. Signs and symptoms of cardiovascular strain tend to pre-dominate. Atrial fibrillation is frequent and the patient may be in congestive cardiac failure. Un-explained heart failure after middle age should always arouse suspicion of hyperthyroidism. Also suggestive is failure of standard doses of

digoxin to control the rapid heart rate. Other less common presentations include: muscle weak-ness, diarrhoea, amenorrhoea and osteoporosis. A goitre may be noted and complained of, especially if the gland is large and vascular.

Graves' disease is characterized by the typical signs and symptoms of hyperthyroidism, eye signs and, rarely, localized myxoedema. The eye signs comprise swelling of the eyelids, irritation of the conjunctivae, exophthalmos (proptosis), lid retraction and ophthalmoplegia. They may occur alone or in combination. Exophthalmos refers to the characteristic protrusion of the eyeball. Ophthalmoplegia is paresis of one or more of the extraocular muscles and usually causes diplopia. Another extrathyroid abnormality of Graves' disease, occurring in about 5% of patients, is lo-calized (pretibial) myxoedema. There is swelling, and sometimes tissue overgrowth, affecting the front of the shins which may extend to the dorsum of the feet and toes.

INVESTIGATIONS

In any patient with suspected hyperthyroidism it is good practice to document the diagnosis with at least two sets of thyroid function tests. If the diagnosis is in doubt, treatment should be with-held. Hyperthyroidism can usually be safely ob-served while investigations are carried out. Plasma total T_4 is clearly elevated in more than 90% of patients with hyperthyroidism. It should be noted that oestrogens promote hepatic synthesis of thyroid-binding globulin (TBG) and other hormone-binding proteins (Table 43.5). During pregnancy or treatment with a combined oral contraceptive, an increase in total T_4 concentra-tion is seen, but when the increase in TBG is taken into account the free T_4 concentration is usually normal. A low TSH level can also be helpful in making the diagnosis of hyperthyroidism.

In the majority of patients the combination of the clinical findings and these simple investiga-tions, is sufficient to make a firm diagnosis. If the diagnosis is still equivocal the clinical findings should be reassessed and particular attention paid to the patients' drug history. There are a number of drugs which may modify the clinical

Table 43.6	Signs and symptoms of hyperthyroidism
Skin and appendages	Warm, moist skin Thinning or loss of hair Prominence of eyes, lid retraction Increased sweating Heat intolerance Pretibial myxoedema
Nervous system	Insomnia Irritability, nervousness Symptoms of an anxiety state Psychosis (rarely)
Musculoskeletal	Osteoporosis Muscle weakness Rapid deep tendon reflexes Tremor
Gastrointestinal	Weight loss with increased appetite Diarrhoea
Cardiovascular	Palpitations, tachycardia Shortness of breath on exertion Angina Atrial fibrillation

features or interfere with the tests. If there is still doubt, it is usual to assess the response of TSH to the intravenous administration of 200 micrograms of TRH. A normal response excludes hyperthyroidism. An absent or impaired response would support the diagnosis. Other diagnostic techniques may be required including isotope scan with ^{99}Tc, ultrasound and needle aspiration.

TREATMENT

Numerous factors need to be considered when choosing the most appropriate form of therapy for an individual patient (Table 43.7).

After giving due consideration to these factors, there may be more than one therapeutic option available and the patient should be involved in the decision making. The decision may also be influenced by physician preference, which, in turn, will depend in part on the facilities available to him. Three standard forms of therapy are available: antithyroid drugs, surgery (partial thyroidectomy) and radioactive iodine. There is no general agreement as to the specific indications for each form of therapy, and none of them is ideal, each being associated with both short- and long-term sequelae. One commonly agreed principle is that surgery should not be undertaken, nor ^{131}I given, while the patient is grossly thyrotoxic. The patient should first be rendered euthyroid with antithyroid drugs because there is a risk of precipitating a thyrotoxic 'storm' (the abrupt onset of symptoms of thyrotoxicosis) with ^{131}I or surgery when the patient is still thyrotoxic.

Table 43.7 Factors influencing choice of treatment of hyperthyroidism
Large goitre causing obstruction
Severe heart failure
Pregnancy, puerperium
Neonate
Iodide exposure
Concurrent amiodarone therapy
Previous drug side effect
Poor compliance
Severity of symptoms
Age
Existence of complications

Surgery may be difficult in children and the complication rate is higher. Radioiodine is contra-indicated because of the potential for development of thyroid malignancy. Operation should be avoided in pregnancy if the disease can be controlled with drugs. Doses should be kept as low as possible, especially in the last 2 months of pregnancy, as excessive treatment may produce goitre in the fetus. Radioiodine therapy is absolutely contra-indicated since the thyroid gland of the fetus can concentrate iodide from the third month onwards.

In patients with small goitres, relapse after a course of antithyroid therapy is less common than in those with significant gland enlargement.

If surgery is contra-indicated the patient should be treated medically. If operative treatment is selected, all patients should be rendered euthyroid prior to surgery. In patients who relapse after previous partial thyroidectomy, surgery results in distortion of local anatomy making further operations hazardous.

Drug treatment

The thioamides, propylthiouracil (PTU), methimazole and its precursor carbimazole, are the mainstay of pharmacological treatment for hyperthyroidism. In the United Kingdom, carbimazole is usually used. These drugs prevent thyroid hormone synthesis by inhibiting the oxidation binding of iodide and its coupling to tyrosine residues. PTU, but not carbimazole, inhibits the peripheral deiodination of T_4 to T_3. In addition, the thioamides are also thought to have an immunosuppressive mechanism of action. Potassium perchlorate, which interferes with the gland's iodine binding, is rarely used due to the high incidence of serious adverse reactions, notably aplastic anaemia and nephrotic syndrome.

The most common side effects of antithyroid treatment are reversible leucopenia, which occurs in approximately 1% of patients, and skin rashes (macular or papular and itchy), occurring in 5% of patients. Both of these side effects usually occur during the first 6 weeks of treatment. Cross-sensitivity between carbimazole and propylthiouracil is rare and the patient can usually be safely changed to the alternative agent. During this time the white cell count should be checked every 2 weeks or if a sore throat develops. Other very rare adverse effects are: lymphadenopathy, splenomegaly, cholestatic jaundice, arthropathy, polyarteritis nodosa and polyneuritis (Table 43.8).

Carbimazole is usually given initially in high doses of 40 to 60 mg daily. It can be given as a single daily dose in order to aid compliance. Although the plasma half-life is short (4 to 6 hours) the biological effect lasts longer (up to 40 hours). After 3 to 4 weeks of treatment the dose is usually decreased to a maintenance dose of 5 to 30 mg daily. Some authorities feel that this tapering regimen may not be necessary. An alternative policy is to start immediately with the likely maintenance dose (higher for patients with gross thyrotoxicosis or a large vascular gland) and to titrate against symptoms of hyperthyroidism and gain in weight. Thyroid function tests can be difficult to interpret. The T_4 is lower than expected when the patient is euthyroid because the drug-blocked gland secretes relatively more T_3. Failure to respond to antithyroid drugs can only mean that the initial diagnosis was incorrect or that the patient is not taking the medication.

It is important to appreciate that there is a lag of 1 to 2 weeks between the achievement of biochemical euthyroidism and that of clinical euthyroidism. If this is overlooked, the patient may be over-treated resulting in biochemical hypothyroidism with clinical thyrotoxicosis. For this reason, some centres routinely give initial high doses of carbimazole in combination with replacement doses of T_4.

The optimal duration of antithyroid treatment is usually 12 to 18 months. However, less than 50% of patients remain in permanent remission after an 18-month course of carbimazole. Now that there is evidence that the drugs act in part by exerting an immunosuppressive effect on the thyroid gland, this may help to prevent relapse and provide an argument for prolonged treatment. Adverse effects are usually seen in the first few weeks of treatment and there does not appear to be any additional risk from long-term maintenance.

Beta-adrenoreceptor blockers give symptomatic relief and can therefore be usefully employed

Table 43.8	Adverse effect of thioamides	
	Adverse effects	Comments
Skin	Pruritic, maculopapular rash.	Most common in first 6 weeks May disappear spontaneously with continued treatment Change to alternative agent Occurs in 5% of patients
	Rash with systemic symptoms, i.e. fever, arthralgia.	Discontinue drug Alternative treatment required
Haematological	Agranulocytosis	Most common in first 6 weeks Incidence increases with age Discontinue drug Reversible Consider change to alternative agent (but 50% cross-sensitivity) Consider alternative treatment Occurs in 0.5% of patients
	Leucopenia	Transient Continue treatment Does not predispose to agranulocytosis
Other	Hepatitis Vasculitis Hypoprothrombinaemia Aplastic anaemia Thrombocytopenia	Rare Discontinue drug

as an adjunct to carbimazole in the first few weeks of therapy. They are also useful in the management of patients with severe thyrotoxicosis who are awaiting surgery or radioactive iodine therapy. Small doses of a non-selective agent are usually adequate, e.g. propranolol 20 to 40 mg two to four times daily. This usually results in relief of palpitations, anxiety, sweating, tremor and diarrhoea. More severely toxic patients may require higher doses. Beta-adrenoreceptor blockers are not recommended for long-term use as they do not affect the underlying cause of the condition.

Patient counselling

Patients should be advised of the importance of regular clinic attendance. This is necessary to monitor both therapeutic outcome and the development of adverse effects. The development of skin rashes, mouth ulcers or a sore throat should be immediately reported to a doctor and a full blood count performed. Pharmacists should be aware that it may be dangerous to treat these symptoms with over-the-counter medication without referring for further investigation. If a patient presents with these symptoms, the pharmacist should enquire into their medication history.

It is important for the patient to understand the difference between specific antithyroid therapy and symptomatic treatment. The patient should also be advised about the timing of doses to aid compliance (Table 43.9).

Following completion of a course of treatment it is important for the patient to appreciate that relapse may occur and he or she should seek medical help if the initial symptoms reoccur.

Table 43.9 Counselling points for patients on antithyroid drugs

1. Carbimazole can be given as a single daily dose
2. Anticipated duration of treatment
3. Tapering to maintenance dose
4. Use of adjuvant therapy, e.g. beta-adrenoreceptor blockers
5. Report skin rashes, sore throat or mouth ulcers
6. Need for regular review
7. Management of relapse

Surgery

The hyperthyroid patient to be treated surgically should first be rendered euthyroid. This may require a combination of antithyroid drugs, iodide and beta-adrenoreceptor blockers.

Potassium iodide exerts a transient inhibitory effect on the gland's ability to trap iodide. In a dose of 5 mg three times daily, potassium iodide also has the effect of reducing the vascularity of the gland. Lithium has been used in patients who are hypersensitive to iodides. In doses of 800 to 1200 mg/day lithium has actions similar to iodides. Lithium levels should be monitored to minimize toxicity. The dose of beta-adrenoreceptor blockers should be titrated to reduce the pulse rate to below 80 beats per minute. This is usually continued for 1 week postoperatively. It is imperative that treatment is given right up to the time of operation since the operation will be deferred if the pulse rate is not adequately controlled. Inadequate pretreatment can result in the occurrence of thyroid 'storm' within the first day or two of operation. The pulse rate is rapid, dehydration occurs and atrial fibrillation and heart failure may develop.

Hypoparathyroidism may arise postoperatively due to interference with the blood supply to the parathyroids or their inadvertent removal during surgery. Tetany will begin shortly after the operation and treatment should be initiated with intravenous calcium gluconate. All patients who have undergone partial thyroidectomy should have a serum calcium estimation 3 months after operation since the development of hypoparathyroidism can be delayed.

Later complications of thyroidectomy include hypothyroidism and recurrent hyperthyroidism. The incidence of hypothyroidism is about 20% and is related to the amount of gland removed and the extent of lymphoid infiltration of the gland. The prevalence of recurrent hyperthyroidism is usually less than 5%.

Radioactive iodine

Radioiodine therapy is easy to administer and effective. The difficulty lies in calculating the minimum dose required to render the patient euthyroid. Although there has been concern over the complications of radioiodine therapy, accumulated experience has not demonstrated any discernible genetic risk or increase in thyroid malignancy or leukaemia.

The commonest complication is the development of hypothyroidism, the incidence depending on the dose given. Using doses to deliver 8000 to 10 000 rad to the thyroid, about 10% of patients become hypothyroid within 1 year and about 40% at 10 years, with subsequent yearly increments of about 3%. To reduce this risk some centres use lower doses, e.g. 3500 rad.

If antithyroid drugs have been used they should be withdrawn 1 week before radioiodine is given and, if necessary, reinstituted 1 week afterwards. Drug therapy can then be withdrawn at 3 to 6 months to assess the effects of the radioiodine.

Treatment of complications

Treatment of eye signs

In most patients with Graves' disease no specific treatment is required for the eyes. The commonest complaint is of 'grittiness' which can be treated with hypromellose eye drops. If lid retraction is severe the inadequate lid closure can result in early morning soreness. This can be alleviated by the short-term use of 5% guanethidine eye drops instilled each night and morning. The eyes should be monitored for any signs of infection and treated appropriately.

Fortunately, severe eye involvement occurs in less than 2% of patients with Graves' disease. Progressive ophthalmopathy producing severe complications from proptosis, diplopia or visual failure should be treated with high-dose steroid therapy (prednisolone 60 mg daily) until symptoms resolve. Failure to respond is an indication for orbital irradiation or surgical decompression. Cyclosporin has proved beneficial in some patients with ophthalmopathy, but its precise role remains to be defined.

Treatment of localized myxoedema

Myxoedema is usually localized to small areas and is asymptomatic. More extensive disease causes difficulty in walking and considerable discomfort. Probably the most effective therapy is the nightly topical application of steroid creams, e.g. betamethasone under occlusive polythene dressings.

HYPOPARATHYROIDISM

Hypoparathyroidism is the clinical state which may arise either from failure of the parathyroid glands to secrete parathyroid hormone (PTH), or from failure of its action at tissue level.

EPIDEMIOLOGY

The most common cause of hypoparathyroidism is related to surgical excision or exploration of the neck. In experienced hands, the incidence of permanent hypoparathyroidism is less than 1% for all thyroid and parathyroid surgery.

AETIOLOGY

Hypoparathyroidism due to PTH deficiency can arise in a number of different ways, either as an idiopathic isolated autoimmune disorder or as part of a multiple endocrine deficiency. The latter is an autosomal recessive disorder characterized by hyposecretion of endocrine glands. Postoperative hypoparathyroidism is common and follows thyroid surgery, parathyroid surgery and other neck operations. Transient hypoparathyroidism with symptomatic hypocalcaemia can occur in neonates.

PATHOPHYSIOLOGY

Most individuals possess four parathyroid glands situated along the posterior surface of the thyroid. Ionized plasma calcium levels regulate the secretion of PTH, increased levels suppressing secretion and low levels stimulating it. PTH is an 84 amino acid residue, straight chain polypeptide which acts on hormone-specific receptors on target tissue cells.

PTH acts on the renal tubular transport of calcium and phosphate and also stimulates the renal synthesis of 1,25-dihydroxycholecalciferol.

PTH increases distal tubular reabsorption of calcium and decreases proximal and distal tubular reabsorption of phosphate. The effects of PTH on bone are complex. The two major cell types in bone are osteoblasts and osteoclasts. Osteoblasts are responsible for the synthesis of extracellular bone matrix and the priming of its subsequent mineralization. Osteoclasts decalcify and digest the protein matrix of bone, liberating calcium. PTH stimulates osteoclast-mediated bone resorption in addition to anabolic effects on bone, with an increase in osteoblast number and function.

PTH, calcitonin, vitamin D and related preparations all act to maintain plasma calcium levels within the normal range. The long-term use of phenytoin and phenobarbitone stimulates the hepatic conversion of cholecalciferol and 25-hydroxycholecalciferol to biologically inactive metabolites. This increases the risk of malabsorption of calcium and development of hypocalcaemia. The risk is highest in patients on long-term therapy, those with low dietary calcium intake and patients with little sunlight exposure.

CLINICAL MANIFESTATIONS

Many of the clinical features of hypoparathyroidism are due to hypocalcaemia. The decrease in plasma calcium levels leads to increased neuromuscular excitability. The major signs and symptoms are shown in Table 43.10.

INVESTIGATIONS

Hypocalcaemia associated with undetectable or low plasma PTH levels is consistent with hypoparathyroidism. Total plasma calcium levels should always be corrected for any abnormality in the plasma albumin concentration. Hyperphosphataemia is often present.

It should be noted that there are many other causes of hypocalcaemia (Table 43.11).

Pseudohypoparathyroidism is easily distinguished as it is associated with excessive PTH secretion and reduced target organ responsiveness. Drugs which may produce hypocalcaemia include; calcitonin, plicamycin (formerly mithra-

Table 43.10   Signs and symptoms of hypocalcaemia
Numbness and tingling in extremities
Numbness and tingling around mouth
Muscle spasm
Irritability
Cataracts (prolonged hypocalcaemia)
Positive Chvostek's sign
Positive Trousseau's sign

Table 43.11   Causes of hypocalacaemia
Pseudohypoparathyroidism
Vitamin D deficiency
Acute and chronic renal failure
Intestinal malabsorption
Hypomaganesaemia
Drug-induced
Acute pancreatitis
Medullary carcinoma of the thyroid
Hypoproteinaemia

mycin), phosphate, bisphosphonates, phenytoin, phenobarbitone and cholestyramine.

TREATMENT

Severe, acute hypocalcaemia with tetany should be treated with intravenous calcium gluconate. Initially, 10 ml of 10% calcium gluconate is given by slow intravenous injection, preferably with ECG monitoring. If the patient can swallow, oral therapy should be commenced. If further parenteral therapy is required, 20 ml of 10% calcium gluconate should be added to each 500 ml of intravenous fluid and given over 6 hours. The plasma magnesium level should always be measured in patients with hypocalcaemia and, if low, magnesium therapy instituted.

For chronic treatment, PTH therapy is not currently a practical option. The hormone has to be administered parenterally and the current high cost is prohibitive. Maintenance treatment for hypoparathyroidism is with a vitamin D preparation to increase intestinal calcium absorption, often in conjunction with calcium supplementation. Details of the preparations available are given in Tables 43.12, 43.13 and 43.14. Calciferol (vitamin D_3) can be difficult to use. It has a long pharmacological and biological half-life, takes

Table 43.12 Vitamin D preparations

Drug	Preparations
Ergocalciferol (calciferol, vitamin D₂)	Calciferol injection BPC 7.5 mg (300 000 units) per ml Strong calciferol tablets BP 1.25 mg (50 000 units) High strength calciferol tablets BP 250 micrograms (10 000 units) Calcium and ergocalciferol tablets (2.4 mmol of calcium + 400 units vitamin D)
1α-hydroxycholecalciferol	Alfacalcidol 250 nanograms and 1 microgram
1,25-dihydroxycholecalciferol	Calcitriol 250 nanograms and 500 nanograms
Dihydrotachysterol	Dihydrotachysterol oral solution 250 micrograms per ml Dihydrotachysterol tablets 200 micrograms

Table 43.13 Comparison of vitamin D preparations

Preparations	Activity	Kinetics	Dose
Calciferol	Requires renal and hepatic activation	Long t₁/₂ Slow elimination Duration 3–6 months	50–100 000 units/day
1α-hydroxycholecalciferol	Requires hepatic activation		0.5–1 microgram/day
1,25-dihydroxycholecalciferol	Active	Rapid onset, 1–3 days t₁/₂ 1–2 hours	0.5–2 microgram/day
Dihydrotachysterol	Requires hepatic activation	Rapid onset Duration 1–2 weeks Short t₁/₂	0.2–2.5 mg/day

Table 43.14 Oral calcium supplements

Preparation	Calcium content (mmol)
Calcium gluconate tablet	1.35
Calcium gluconate tablet effervescent	2.25
Calcium lactate tablet	1.00
Cacit	12.6
Calcichew	12.6
Calcium – 500 (calcium carbonate)	12.5
Calcium – Sandoz	2.7/5 ml
Citrical	12.6/sachet
Ossopan	4.4/tablet
Sandocal – 400	10.0
Sandocal – 1000	25.0

4 to 8 weeks to restore normocalcaemia and its effect persists for 6 to 18 weeks following withdrawal. In contrast, 1,25-dihydroxycholecalciferol and its synthetic analogue 1α-hydroxycholecalciferol are much easier to use. 1α-hydroxycholecalciferol restores normocalcaemia within 1 week and its effect only persists for 1 week following withdrawal, permitting greater flexibility in dosage manipulation. The usual daily dose is 0.5 to 2 micrograms. Initially patients will need to be closely monitored until stable normocalcaemia is achieved. Occasionally dihydrotachysterol is used. This is a synthetic compound which is an analogue of 1,25-dihydroxycholecalciferol.

HYPERPARATHYROIDISM

Hyperparathyroidism is the clinical state which results from increased production of PTH by the parathyroid gland.

EPIDEMIOLOGY

Recent studies in the USA and Europe indicate an incidence rate for primary hyperparathyroidism of 25 cases per 100 000 population per year. The incidence is two to three times higher in women than in men and the disease most commonly presents between the third and fifth decades.

AETIOLOGY

The aetiology of primary hyperparathyroidism is unknown. It may occur as part of a group of familial conditions, the multiple endocrine neoplasia (MEN) syndromes.

There are several conditions associated with secondary hyperparathyroidism including chronic renal failure and vitamin D deficiency. In these conditions the excess PTH is required for a compensatory purpose. Chronic renal failure is the commonest cause and in the early stages of the disease a rise in plasma phosphate causes a decrease in plasma calcium concentration with compensatory stimulation of PTH. In the later stages reduced renal 1α-hydroxylase activity and reduced intestinal calcium absorption, lead to further stimulation of the parathyroid glands. Tertiary hyperparathyroidism is the term used to describe a further stage in the development of the secondary type where autonomy of the parathyroids occurs.

PATHOPHYSIOLOGY

Primary hyperparathyroidism can result from a parathyroid adenoma, hyperplasia or carcinoma. Solitary adenoma is the commonest, occurring in over 80% of cases. Carcinoma is rare, occurring in approximately 2 to 3%. Metastases are relatively rare and tend to occur in the lymph nodes, liver or bone marrow.

CLINICAL MANIFESTATIONS

With increasingly early recognition of the biochemical abnormalities of primary hyperparathyroidism, largely due to automated measurement of plasma calcium, the clinical spectrum of the disease has moved towards mild or asymptomatic cases. Overt bone disease and renal stones are now relatively uncommon manifestations of the disease. Recent studies indicate that over 50% of cases are asymptomatic at the time of diagnosis. The clinical features of primary hyperparathyroidism are shown in Table 43.15.

Although radiological evidence of bone disease

Table 43.15 Signs and symptoms of hyperparathyroidism

Anorexia, weight loss
Nausea, vomiting
Constipation
Fatigue
Proximal myopathy
Polydipsia, polyuria
Mental changes
Pruritus
Renal stones
Conjunctival and corneal deposits
Bone pain and deformity
Pathological fractures

is now rare in these patients, measurement of bone mineral content usually indicates that bone loss is accelerated. Thus, the risk of osteoporotic fractures later on in life may be increased.

INVESTIGATIONS

Fasting hypercalcaemia is the primary biochemical abnormality in primary hyperparathyroidism. It should be noted that there are many other causes of hypercalcaemia, including: malignancy, drugs (thiazides, excess vitamin D), thyrotoxicosis, immobilization and sarcoidosis.

The most common cause of symptomatic hypercalcaemia is that associated with malignancy, and this diagnosis must always be excluded.

In primary hyperparathyroidism the plasma phosphate levels are often normal in mild cases but are decreased in patients with more advanced disease. PTH levels are usually elevated.

Various techniques may be required for localization of parathyroid tumours, including isotope and CT scanning.

TREATMENT

Following the diagnosis of primary hyperparathyroidism early surgery is normally indicated. However, the natural history of primary hyperparathyroidism is not fully documented. Some studies have indicated that over 50% of untreated patients with primary hyperparathyroidism show no deterioration over 5 years; but the longer-term effects on renal function and bone mass remain unknown.

The main indications for surgical treatment are persistent hypercalcaemia (>2.75 mmol/L), symptomatic hypercalcaemia, renal impairment, recurrent renal stones and evidence of hyperparathyroid bone disease. In the postoperative period, temporary hypocalcaemia occurs in 20% of patients, particularly if there is bone involvement. In patients with bone disease, treatment with 1α-hydroxycholecalciferol should be started on the day before the operation. Approximately 10% develop permanent hypoparathyroidism. There is no ideal pharmacological substitute for surgery. Several treatment modalities are available for the treatment of hypercalcaemia but their usefulness in primary hyperparathyroidism varies (Table 43.16).

Hypercalcaemia can be corrected by inhibiting bone resorption, increasing calcium excretion, or decreasing calcium absorption. General therapeutic measures will depend on the degree and severity of the hypercalcaemia but may include adequate hydration, mobilization, restriction of dietary calcium and avoidance of thiazide diuretics which can decrease urinary calcium excretion. The use of hormone therapy has been suggested in patients who either cannot or will not undergo definitive surgical treatment. The limited data currently available suggests that normalization of serum calcium is more likely to occur with oestrogen than with progestagen treatment. Hormone therapy will have the added benefit of providing skeletal protection. Several agents have been specifically investigated for the medical management of hyperparathyroidism. Beta-adrenoreceptor blockers have been investigated because catecholamines have been shown to stimulate PTH secretion. However, propranolol has been ineffective suggesting that the abnormal glands may lose their responsiveness to catecholamine. Histamine has also been shown to stimulate PTH release, leading to the use of cimetidine. Although, one study found cimetidine effective, most have found it to be ineffective.

Table 43.16 Treatment of hypercalcaemia

Treatment	Efficacy in hyperparathyroidism	Comments
Inhibition of bone resorption		
Plicamycin	Yes	Parenteral only Severe toxicity with repeated doses
Calcitonin	No	—
Oestrogens	Yes	Skeletal protection
Increase calcium excretion		
Hydration	Yes	Use 0.9% saline
Frusemide	Yes	Require large doses Monitor electrolytes
Decrease calcium absorption		
Phosphates	Yes	i.v. causes hypotension, renal failure Orally causes GI disturbance
Other mechanisms		
Steroids	No	—
Bisphosphonates	Yes	Impair function of osteoclast
Indomethacin	No	—
Dialysis	Yes	Temporary – rebound effect seen

CASE STUDIES

CASE 43.1

E. A. is a 66-year-old lady who has recently been complaining of tiredness, lethargy and weight gain. Her general practitioner performed routine thyroid function tests and diagnosed primary hypothyroidism.

She had a myocardial infarction 5 years ago and has suffered from exertional angina for 7 years.

Her current drug therapy is:

- Isosorbide mononitrate 20 mg at 8 a.m. and 2 p.m.
- Glyceryl trinitrate 500 micrograms sublingually as required
- Aspirin 150 mg at 8 a.m.

Her doctor now wishes to commence her on thyroxine replacement therapy.

Q1 What are the therapeutic objectives in this patient?

Q2 How should thyroxine therapy be instituted?

Q3 How should the replacement therapy be monitored?

CASE 43.2

A. N. is a 43-year-old lady who has had insulin-dependent diabetes mellitus (IDDM) for 15 years. On a recent routine appointment at the diabetic clinic she was noted to be anxious and tearful. She is also concerned that over the last 2 months her total daily insulin requirements have increased from 50 units to 72 units. In addition, she has lost 6 kg in weight over the last 6 weeks.

She carries out regular home blood glucose monitoring. Physical examination was unremarkable except for a pulse rate of 110 beats per minute. An ECG carried out at that time showed a sinus tachyarrhythmia.

Thyroid function tests later reveal that she has hyperthyroidism. Her current drug therapy is:

- Human Insulatard insulin 42 units a.m. and 30 units p.m.
- Diazepam 2 mg as required.

She is now to be commenced on carbimazole 20 mg daily.

Q1 Why might Mrs A.N.'s insulin requirements have increased?

Q2 What will happen to her blood glucose following treatment with carbimazole?

CASE 43.3

E. H. is a 55-year-old lady who has been attending the anticoagulant clinic for several years. She is on long-term anticoagulant therapy following a prosthetic heart valve replacement 3 years ago. Recently, her anticoagulant control has been difficult and she has required decreasing doses of warfarin to maintain a therapeutic INR.

Other recent symptoms include diarrhoea and weight loss which have been investigated by her GP; as a result of which she has been found to have hyperthyroidism.

Her current drug therapy is:

- Warfarin 2 mg daily
- Loperamide 2 mg as required.

Q1 How may thyroid disease influence warfarin dosage?

Q2 What will happen to Mrs E. H.'s warfarin requirements when her hyperthyroidism is treated?

CASE 43.4

M. L. is a 48-year-old gentleman who suffered an anterior myocardial infarction 6 months ago. Subsequent management was complicated by the development of ventricular arrhythmias which were only responsive to amiodarone therapy.

For the first 2 weeks he was prescribed amiodarone 600 mg daily; this was subsequently decreased to 400 mg daily.

He is now complaining of irritability, sweating, diarrhoea and weight loss despite having a normal appetite.

Q1 What might be the cause of Mr M. L.'s new symptoms?

Q2 How might this problem be managed?

ANSWERS TO CASE STUDIES

CASE 43.1

A1 The therapeutic objectives should be to relieve the symptoms (tiredness, lethargy and weight gain) of hypothyroidism without producing an exacerbation of Mrs E. A.'s ischaemic heart disease.

A2 Thyroxine replacement therapy should be introduced very cautiously in this patient. Most newly diagnosed patients with hypothyroidism have a long-standing deficiency and the rapid introduction of replacement therapy can only do more harm than good. The low circulating levels of thyroid hormones actually protect the heart from any increased metabolic demands which might result in an exacerbation of angina or a myocardial infarction.

Mrs E. A. should be commenced on thyroxine 25 micrograms daily. If this is well tolerated, the dose can be gradually increased every 4 to 6 weeks. In older patients the daily maintenance dosage of thyroxine is usually 100 micrograms or less, which is lower than that for younger patients.

It has been suggested that triiodothyronine (T_3) should be used as replacement therapy in patients with cardiac disease. T_3 has a shorter half-life than thyroxine and therefore if adverse effects do develop, the effect will last for a shorter period of time. However, T_3 is more biologically active than T_4 and therefore potentially more cardiotoxic.

A3 Thyroxine replacement therapy should be monitored both clinically and biochemically. Symptomatic improvement of hypothyroidism should occur within 2 to 3 weeks of starting therapy, but maximal benefit may take considerably longer. The clinical assessment should include symptoms of both hypothyroidism and ischaemic heart disease, of which the most critical is the latter.

The patient should be questioned about the frequency and severity of angina attacks and about GTN usage. If there is a clear exacerbation of the angina, the thyroxine should be discontinued or the dose reduced. If there are no contra-indications, beta-adrenoreceptor blockers may be used to provide cardiac protection from the stimulant effect of thyroxine.

CASE 43.2

A1 Hyperthyroidism can exacerbate hyperglycaemia and occasionally unmask previously undiagnosed diabetes mellitus. Also of note is that thyroid disorders (both hypo- and hyperthyroidism) occur more frequently in diabetic patients and their first degree relatives than in the non-diabetic population.

There have been several proposed mechanisms for the hyperglycaemia, of which an increase in basal hepatic glucose production and altered insulin metabolism are the most likely. Although insulin degradation takes place at a number of sites in the body, the most active are the liver and the kidney.

Hyperthyroidism results in increased insulin degradation without a corresponding increase in the rate of insulin production. This inevitably will decrease the rate of peripheral glucose utilization.

In a patient with diabetes this can increase exogenous insulin requirements dramatically. The symptom of weight loss can easily be ascribed to poorly controlled diabetes and the diagnosis of hyperthyroidism can be overlooked. The other symptoms that Mrs A. N. has (tachycardia and emotional liability) could be thought to be a consequence of anxiety.

A2 Following the initiation of antithyroid therapy it usually takes approximately 8 weeks to achieve euthyroidism. During that time it could be anticipated that Mrs A. N.'s insulin requirements will gradually decline, and the patient can be advised to carry out regular home blood glucose monitoring and adjust the dose of insulin as often as is necessary.

This patient may also require symptomatic treatment with beta-adrenoreceptor blockers. In some patients with IDDM beta-adrenoreceptor blockers may mask the warning symptoms of hypoglycaemia. It is important that patients are aware of this, particularly at a time when insulin requirements are falling and they are prone to hypoglycaemia.

Patients should also be counselled about the possibility of future relapse of hyperthyroidism and to seek prompt medical attention if symptoms recur or if there is a marked increase in insulin requirements.

CASE 43.3

A1 Thyroid dysfunction can alter the metabolism of both oral anticoagulants and vitamin K dependent clotting factors. An enhanced anticoagulant response is seen due to an increase in clotting factor catabolism caused by hyperthyroidism. This effect is apparently greater than any induced effect on warfarin metabolism.

It can be predicted that patients with hyperthyroidism will require less warfarin to produce a therapeutic INR than euthyroid patients.

A2 When Mrs E. H.'s hyperthyroidism is treated her warfarin requirements will increase. The time to stabilization will depend on which form of treatment is used. Warfarin requirements would be expected to change quickly after surgery. If drug therapy is used it usually takes about 2 months to achieve euthyroidism but if radioactive iodine therapy is used this time period could be much longer.

Regardless of which form of treatment is used, frequent tests of anticoagulant control will need to be performed and the dose of warfarin adjusted accordingly.

CASE 43.4

A1 The clinical picture is highly suggestive of amiodarone-induced hyperthyroidism. Each tablet contains 75 mg of iodine, approximately 6 mg of which is released during the metabolism of the drug. This is 100 times in excess of normal daily dietary intake. Amiodarone is now the commonest cause of the clinical entity of iodine-induced hyperthyroidism(Jod–Basedow syndrome). A large excess of iodine usually inhibits thyroid hormone synthesis and release, but in some subjects it has the opposite effect and produces hyperthyroidism. This is more likely to occur in patients who have pre-existing thyroid abnormalities. Thyroid function tests should be carried out and will usually reveal a suppressed TSH, but total T_4 may be normal or increased. Likewise, T_3 may be increased or may be normal, the latter due to the suppression seen in many acute and chronic non-thyroidal illnesses.

Amiodarone may mask some of the clinical features of hyperthyroidism due to its nonspecific adrenergic blocking properties. In such cases symptoms of tiredness and weight loss usually predominate.

A2 Discontinuation of amiodarone usually leads to spontaneous euthyroidism, but only after several months due to the long half-life of the drug (40 to 100 days). However, many patients require the drug for the control of refractory arrhythmias and in those circumstances it is not possible to discontinue it. Occasionally, the thyroid abnormality will remit spontaneously despite continuing amiodarone.

Surgery or radioactive iodine therapy are usually not indicated unless there is an underlying thyroid abnormality. Surgery is also not desirable in patients with severe cardiac disease. As with other causes of iodine-induced hyperthyroidism, thioamides in conventional doses are less effective than in patients with spontaneous hyperthyroidism. Carbimazole may be used to produce a euthyroid state without discontinuing the amiodarone. Combination therapy with methimazole (40 mg daily) and potassium perchlorate (1 g daily) has also been shown to be effective. However, potassium perchlorate has the potential to produce serious adverse reactions. Corticosteroid therapy (prednisolone 60 mg daily) has also been effective in the management of amiodarone-induced hyperthyroidism. Its mechanism of action is unclear.

In each individual case the patient should be carefully evaluated and the need for amiodarone reassessed before further management is decided upon.

BIBLIOGRAPHY

Consensus Development Conference Panel. Diagnosis and management of asymptomatic primary hyperparathyroidism: Consensus Development Conference Statement. Annals of Internal Medicine 1991; 114(7): 593–596

Davies P H, Franklyn J A. The effect of drugs on tests of thyroid function. European Journal of Clinical Pharmacology 1991; 40: 439–451

Greenspan F S (ed). Thyroid diseases. Medical Clinics of North America 1991; 75(1)

Sheppard M C. Thyroid. In: Sheppard M C, Franklyn J A (eds). Clinical endocrinolgy and metabolism. Churchill Livingstone 1988; 37–60

Stockigt J R, Topliss D J. Hyperthyroidism. Current drug therapy. Drugs 1989; 37(3): 375–381

Endocrine disorders

Chapter 44

Diabetes mellitus

J. Cantrill

Diabetes mellitus is a heterogeneous group of disorders characterized by varying degrees of insulin hyposecretion and/or insulin insensitivity. Regardless of cause, it is associated with hyperglycaemia.

EPIDEMIOLOGY

There are major ethnic and geographical differences in the prevalence and incidence of insulin-dependent diabetes mellitus (IDDM). Figures are highest in Caucasians whilst the disorder is rare in the Japanese and in the Pacific. In northern Europe the prevalence is approximately 0.3% in those under 30 years of age. There is currently evidence that the prevalence is increasing. IDDM may present at any age but there is a sharp increase around the time of puberty and a decline thereafter. Approximately 50 to 60% of patients with IDDM will present before 20 years of age.

Non-insulin-dependent diabetes mellitus (NIDDM) is much commoner than IDDM, accounting for 75 to 95% of all diabetics in most populations. It usually only occurs in patients over the age of 40 years. In the United Kingdom, diabetes affects approximately 750 000 people, of whom 600 000 have NIDDM. The incidence of NIDDM increases with age and with increasing obesity. As with IDDM, there are major ethnic and geographical variations. In general, in non-obese populations the prevalence is 1 to 3%. In the more obese societies, there is a sharp increase in prevalence with figures of 6 to 8% in the USA increasing to values as high as 30% in Hindu Tamils in South Africa. Diabetes is 5 times more common among Asian immigrants in the United Kingdom than in the indigenous population. World studies of immigrants have suggested that the chances of developing NIDDM are between 2 and 20 times higher in well fed populations than in lean populations of the same race.

AETIOLOGY

Before considering the aetiology it is necessary to understand the classification of diabetes. The World Health Organization classification was last refined in 1985 (Table 44.1). The two main types of diabetes are IDDM and NIDDM. These are also referred to as Type 1 and Type 2 respectively.

The aetiology of IDDM is currently the subject of considerable research. Genetic factors are

---

Table 44.1 Classification of diabetes mellitus and allied categories of glucose intolerance (WHO 1985)

A. CLINICAL CLASSES
Diabetes mellitus (DM)
Insulin-dependent diabetes mellitus (IDDM)
Non-insulin-dependent diabetes mellitus (NIDDM)
(a) Non-obese
(b) Obese
Malnutrition-related diabetes mellitus (MRDM)
Other types of diabetes associated with certain conditions and syndromes:
(1) pancreatic disease; (2) disease of hormonal aetiology; (3) drug-induced or chemical-induced conditions; (4) abnormalities of insulin or its receptors; (5) certain genetic syndromes; (6) miscellaneous.
Impaired glucose tolerance (IGT)
(a) Non-obese
(b) Obese
(c) Associated with certain conditions and syndromes
Gestational diabetes mellitus (GDM)

B. STATISTICAL RISK CLASSES (Subjects with normal glucose tolerance but substantially increased risk of developing diabetes)
Previous abnormality of glucose tolerance
Potential abnormality of glucose tolerance

---

important but do not explain fully the development of IDDM. There is a strong immunological component to IDDM and a clear association with many organ-specific autoimmune diseases. Circulating islet cell antibodies (ICA) are present in more than 70% of IDDM at the time of diagnosis. Family studies have now shown that the appearance of ICA often precedes the onset of clinical diabetes by as much as 3 years. IDDM has been widely believed to be a disease of sudden onset, but the development now appears to be a slow process of progressive immunological damage. However, it is not currently possible to use screening methods to identify patients who will develop diabetes in the future. The final event, which precipitates clinical diabetes, may be caused by sudden stress such as an infection when the mass of the beta-cells of the pancreas falls below 5 to 10%. Studies have been carried out in which patients with newly diagnosed IDDM have been treated with immunosuppressive therapy, notably cyclosporin. Although some patients do benefit and no longer require insulin therapy, such treatment is not a safe option for long-term control.

NIDDM has a much stronger genetic relationship than IDDM. Identical twins have a concordance rate approaching 100%. This suggests relative importance of inheritance over environment. If a parent has NIDDM, the risk of a child eventually developing NIDDM is 5 to 10% compared to 1 to 2% for IDDM. The clearest association of NIDDM is with obesity. Obesity is associated with hyperinsulinaemia and marked insulin insensitivity and a decrease in the number of insulin receptors. It has also been suggested that there is a selective defect in the beta-cell secretory mechanism which prevents it from responding normally to glucose. On average patients with NIDDM retain approximately 50% of their beta-cell mass. Circulating insulin levels are normal or raised when compared with normal subjects, but are inappropriately low for the degree of hyperglycaemia present.

The last WHO report included malnutrition-related diabetes mellitus (MRDM) as a new class of diabetes. MDRM is found in tropical developing countries in patients who are grossly under-weight and who have a history of malnutrition in childhood. The aetiology is far from clear, but one hypothesis is the high consumption of foods containing cyanogenic glycosides resulting in pancreatic damage.

PATHOPHYSIOLOGY

The islets of Langerhans are the endocrine component of the pancreas, and they constitute 1% of the total pancreatic mass. Insulin is synthesized in the pancreatic beta-cells. It is synthesized initially as a polypeptide precursor – preproinsulin. The latter is rapidly converted in the pancreas to proinsulin, which, through the removal of 4 amino acid residues forms equal amounts of insulin and C-peptide. Insulin consists of 51 amino acids in two chains connected by two disulphide bridges. In the islets, insulin, C-peptide (and some proinsulin) are packaged into granules. Insulin associates spontaneously into a hexamer which contains two zinc ions and one calcium ion.

Glucose is the major stimulant to insulin release. The response is triggered both by the intake of nutrients and the release of gastro-intestinal peptide hormones. Following an intra-venous injection of glucose there is a biphasic insulin response. There is an initial rapid response in the first 2 minutes, followed after 5 to 10 minutes by a second response which is smaller in magnitude but sustained over 1 hour. The initial response represents the release of stored insulin and the second phase reflects discharge of newly synthesized insulin. Glucose is unique; other agents, including sulphonylureas, do not result in insulin biosynthesis, only release. Once released from the pancreas, insulin enters the portal circulation. It is rapidly degraded by the liver and only 50% reaches the peripheral circulation. In the basal state, insulin secretion is at the rate of approximately 1 unit per hour. The intake of food results in a prompt 5- to 10-fold increase. Total daily secretion is approximately 40 units.

Insulin circulates free as a monomer, has a half-life of 4 to 5 minutes and is primarily metabolized by the liver and kidneys. In the kidneys insulin is filtered by the glomeruli and reabsorbed by the tubules which also degrade it. In both renal and hepatic disease there is a decrease in the rate of insulin clearance which may necessitate dosage adjustment. Peripheral tissues such as muscle and fat also degrade insulin, but this is of minor quantitative significance.

Many tissues contain receptors which are highly specific for insulin and to which it binds reversibly. The biological response to insulin can be altered by either a change in the receptor affinity for insulin, or a change in the total number of receptors. Changes in the number of receptors occur in two important clinical situations; obesity and chronic exposure to high insulin levels. Both lead to a decrease in the number of receptors, i.e. downregulation. In obese patients, calorie restriction is associated with an increase in receptor numbers even before weight loss occurs.

The interaction of insulin with the receptor on the cell surface sets off a chain of messengers within the cell. This opens up transport processes for glucose, amino acids and electrolytes.

Acute deficiency of insulin leads to unrestrained hepatic glycogenolysis and gluconeogenesis with a consequent increase in hepatic glucose output. Glucose uptake is decreased in insulin-sensitive tissues and hyperglycaemia ensues. Either as a result of the metabolic disturbance itself or secondary to infection or other acute illness, there is increased secretion of the counter-regulatory hormones glucagon, cortisol, catecholamine and growth hormone. All of these will further increase hepatic glucose production. At the same time the normal restraining effect of insulin on lipolysis is removed. Non-esterified fatty acids are released into the circulation and taken up by the liver which produces acetyl CoA. The capacity of the tricarboxylate (TCA) cycle to metabolize the acetyl CoA is rapidly exceeded. Ketone bodies, acetoacetate and hydroxybutyrate are formed in increased amounts and released into the circulation. This results in the clinical picture known as diabetic ketoacidosis (DKA).

CLINICAL MANIFESTATIONS

IDDM

The main symptoms of IDDM include polyuria and polydipsia which are a consequence of osmotic diuresis secondary to sustained hyperglycaemia. Another consequence of the hyperosmolar state is blurred vision which often develops as the lenses and retinae are exposed to hyperosmolar fluids. Weight loss despite normal or increased appetite is a common feature.

Lowered plasma volume produces dizziness and weakness due to postural hypotension. Total body potassium loss and the general catabolism of muscle protein contribute to the weakness. When insulin deficiency is severe and of acute onset, all of these symptoms progress in an accelerated manner. Ketoacidosis exacerbates the dehydration and hyperosmolality by producing anorexia, nausea and vomiting. As the plasma osmolality rises, impaired consciousness ensues. With progression of the acidosis, deep breathing with a rapid ventilatory rate (Kussmaul respiration) occurs as the body attempts to correct the acidosis. The patients breath may have the fruity odour of acetone.

NIDDM

The clinical presentation of NIDDM may occur in a number of different ways. The classic symptoms of polyuria, polydipsia, blurred vision and fatigue are manifestations of hyperglycaemia and are therefore common to both types of diabetes.

However, many patients with NIDDM have an insidious onset of hyperglycaemia and they may have few or no symptoms. This is particularly true in obese individuals, whose diabetes may only be detected after glycosuria or hyperglycaemia is detected during routine investigation. Chronic skin infections are common, as sustained hyperglycaemia can result in severe impairment of phagocyte function. Generalized pruritus and symptoms of vaginitis are frequently the initial complaints of women with NIDDM.

Occasionally patients will present when the complications of sustained hyperglycaemia have already developed. Retinopathy may be detected on routine ophthalmological examination or the combination of neuropathy, peripheral vascular disease and infection may manifest as foot ulceration or gangrene.

INVESTIGATIONS

The diagnosis of diabetes mellitus is usually straightforward. Once the diagnosis is suspected on clinical grounds, measurement of blood glucose on two separate occasions is usually adequate to confirm the diagnosis. A fasting whole blood glucose of >6.7 mmol/L or a random value of >10 mmol/L is deemed diagnostic. Blood glucose measurement for diagnostic purposes should be performed in a biochemical laboratory which takes part in a recognized quality assurance scheme. Test strips should only be used if no other method is available. In clinical practice a glucose tolerance test is rarely required and is reserved for borderline cases. Urine testing is currently being investigated as a screening tool for diabetes. It should be carried out using a reagent strip which is glucose specific. One limitation of urine testing is the wide interindividual variation in renal threshold, between 6 and 15 mmol/L. However, a positive urine test should be followed by a laboratory blood glucose estimation.

The biochemical diagnosis of ketoacidosis is usually made at the bedside and confirmed in the laboratory. Urinalysis will show heavy glycosuria and significant ketones. A blood glucose test strip will usually show a blood glucose of >22 mmol/L. Formal laboratory measurement of glucose, urea, creatinine, electrolytes and arterial pH, PO_2 and PCO_2 (to determine the extent of the acidosis) should be carried out. Two potentially misleading laboratory results are white blood cell count and serum sodium. The former will always be raised but correlates with the ketone body level and is not therefore a guide to infection. The serum sodium will often be low due to the osmotic effect of glucose draining from the cells and diluting the sodium. Sodium will also be spuriously low if there is marked hyper-lipidaemia.

TREATMENT

Treatment aims initially to relieve the immediate signs and symptoms of diabetes (thirst and polyuria, weight loss, ketoacidosis). In the longer term, the main aim of treatment is to prevent the development of or slow the progression of the long-term complications of the disease. Treatment should also aim to minimize the occurrence of hypoglycaemia.

The theoretical target for control is normoglycaemia but in practice this is unattainable. The target should be modified to provide each individual with the best possible blood glucose control which is compatible with an acceptable lifestyle. Attention should also be given to other risk factors for the development of complications; including hypertension, hyperlipidaemia and smoking.

Persistent hyperglycaemia is believed to be the major controllable factor which influences the development of diabetic complications. These can be divided into those caused by microvascular disease and those secondary to macrovascular disease. The main sites and forms of tissue damage are discussed below. Although they may all occur in all types of diabetes, the spectrum of incidence is different. Renal failure due to severe microvascular nephropathy is the major cause of death in IDDM, whereas macrovascular disease is the leading cause in NIDDM. Although blindness may occur in both types, the aetiology is often different. Similarly, although neuropathy is common in both types, severe autonomic neuropathy is much more common in IDDM. In countries for which there are adequate data, diabetes is the commonest cause of blindness before the age of 65 years. Where renal transplantation is offered to patients below the age of 70 years with progressive renal failure, diabetes accounts for 20 to 25% of referrals. Peripheral vascular disease causing ulceration or gangrene in the lower limbs is the major cause of hospital bed occupancy by diabetic patients.

It is worthwhile considering in a little more detail the impact of some of these chronic complications.

Eye disease

Blurring of vision is usually a benign occurrence associated with rapid changes in blood glucose control. It is most commonly reported in newly treated patients. They should be warned that this may occur and reassured that it is temporary.

Open angle glaucoma is more common in diabetics than in the general population, for reasons that are unclear. Management is the same as for a non-diabetic. Cataracts are also common in diabetic patients past middle age.

In any population of adults with diabetes, retinopathy will be present in between 10 and 50%. It is closely related to the duration of the disease. In the early stages retinopathy may not interfere with the patient's vision, and therefore should be actively screened for. Once detected careful attention should be paid to blood glucose and blood pressure control. Some forms of retinopathy can be treated using laser photocoagulation. In advanced disease, surgery may be required.

Diseases of the urinary tract

Urinary tract infections are common in diabetes. Management is no different to that in the non-diabetic population except that recurrence is common. The role of prophylactic antibiotics in preventing chronic renal damage is unclear.

Nephropathy is one of the potentially life-threatening complications of diabetes. Poor control of diabetes is associated with enlargement of the kidneys and a high glomerular filtration rate. These features are often present at diagnosis and resolve with effective treatment. Patients who go on to develop microalbuminuria are at risk of developing frank albuminuria and renal failure in later years. Once the serum creatinine rises above normal, it usually increases linearly if a reciprocal plot against time is produced. When end-stage renal failure develops, standard therapy is used to treat symptoms. Continuous ambulatory peritoneal dialysis (CAPD) carries a risk of peritonitis, and blood glucose must be carefully monitored and controlled. Insulin may be given in the peritoneal infusate to cover the high carbohydrate load administered.

Nerve damage

Neuropathy can affect patients with diabetes in many different ways. The most common peripheral neuropathy is of the distal sensory type which often affects the feet. It is most prevalent in elderly patients with NIDDM, but may be found with any type of diabetes, at any age beyond childhood. Painful diabetic neuropathy can be one of the most disabling of all diabetic complications, and is a cause of considerable morbidity.

In diabetic proximal motor neuropathy, there is rapid onset of weakness and wasting, principally of the thigh muscles. Muscle pain is common and may require opiate analgesia.

Autonomic neuropathy may affect any part of the sympathetic or parasympathetic nervous systems. The commonest manifestation is diabetic impotence. Bladder dysfunction usually takes the form of loss of bladder tone with a large increase in volume. Diabetic diarrhoea is uncommon, but can be troublesome through its tendency to occur at night. Gastroparesis may cause delayed gastrointestinal transit and variable food absorption causing difficulty in the insulin-treated patient, or it may cause vomiting. Postural hypotension due to autonomic neuropathy is uncommon, but can be severe and disabling. Disorders of the efferent and afferent nerves controlling cardiac and respiratory function are more common, but rarely symptomatic.

Cardiac disease

Myocardial infarction is the major cause of death in diabetes. Peripheral vascular disease is also common, and accounts for much of the morbidity associated with foot problems. Cerebrovascular events occur at an increased frequency when compared with the non-diabetic population.

Hypertension is common, in association with both macrovascular and microvascular disease. In some populations of NIDDM, the prevalence may be as high as 50%.

The diabetic foot

Foot problems in diabetes cause more inpatient hospital bed occupancy than all the other medical problems put together. They may be, at least in part, preventable by education. Foot ulcers can be divided into three categories. Classical neuropathic ulceration which occurs on the sole of the foot. The ulcers can be deep but are usually painless. Ischaemic ulcers are classically painful, usually occur on the distal ends of the toes, and are associated with signs of peripheral vascular disease and ischaemia. The most common lesions are infected foot ulcers. There are usually a number of factors involved; vascular disease, neuropathy, poor hygiene and poorly controlled diabetes.

Infections

Many infections are seen more frequently in diabetes, and are an indication of poor diabetic control. There is some evidence that leucocyte function is impaired by blood glucose levels above 10 to 13 mmol/L.

Other

There is a whole spectrum of rare complications which can also occur in diabetes. These include musculoskeletal problems, e.g. Dupuytren's contracture and Charcot arthropathy; and dermatological conditions, e.g. acanthosis nigricans and necrobiosis lipoidica.

In addition to all of these chronic complications, the patient with diabetes may also be at risk of experiencing the acute complications; hypoglycaemia, diabetic ketoacidosis and non-ketotic hypoglycaemic coma.

THERAPY

From a management standpoint, patients with diabetes fall into three broad groups:

1. The obese and mainly middle-aged or elderly patient in whom carbohydrate and total calorie restriction are sufficient to cause weight loss and produce normoglycaemia. The overweight should be advised to restrict energy intake to lose weight and achieve a body mass index below 27. The diabetes cannot be regarded as cured; it may reappear in times of stress or if dietary control is lost. In this group of patients, dietary adherence, appropriate exercise and education may avoid the need for pharmacological intervention.

2. If after 2 months of dietary restriction the patient with NIDDM remains symptomatic or persistently has a blood glucose of >10 mmol/L, oral hypoglycaemic agents will be required. Some patients will require this intervention at an earlier stage if the blood glucose levels are markedly elevated.

3. All patients with IDDM require a diet containing controlled amounts of carbohydrate, and insulin therapy.

Dietary therapy

Dietary control is the mainstay of treatment for NIDDM, and plays an integral part in the management of IDDM. The principles of dietary management are basically the same for all diabetic patients, but in insulin-treated patients there are additional considerations of matching carbohydrate intake to insulin delivery. Dietary recommendations have undergone a considerable change in recent years, in both diabetic and non-diabetic populations. Nutritional advice is now the same for both groups and there is no need for a 'special' diabetic diet.

Carbohydrate

The blood glucose level is closely affected by carbohydrate intake. Daily intake should be kept fairly constant and the amount given should be appropriate to the level of physical activity. Most active young people will require 180 g of carbohydrate per day whereas 100 g may suffice for an elderly person. If fibre-rich foods such as wholemeal bread, jacket potatoes etc. are eaten, the carbohydrate content of the diet may make up to 50 to 55% of the calories. A man engaged in heavy physical activity may require more carbohydrate, e.g. 260 g. Sugar should be avoided, including sweets, jams, cakes and pastries. Advice has to be tailored to the individual patient. Some patients on insulin prefer to manage their carbohydrate intake by working in 'exchanges'. One 'exchange' or 'portion' refers to a 10 g unit of carbohydrate. Using this system, the patient can vary their diet but keep the carbohydrate intake constant. This system is far from perfect as the absorption of carbohydrate varies according to its type and the other food that is eaten with it.

Fat

One major reason for increasing the proportion of calories as carbohydrate is to reduce fat intake. Since there is an increased risk of death from coronary artery disease in diabetics, it is wise to restrict saturated fats and to substitute unsaturated fats. Furthermore, obesity is a major problem in diabetes, and fats contain more than twice the energy content per unit weight than either carbohydrate or protein. About 30% or less of the total daily calorie intake should be provided by fat.

Fibre

Dietary fibre has two useful properties. Firstly, it is physically bulky and increases satiety. Secondly, fibre delays the digestion and absorption of complex carbohydrates, thereby minimizing hyperglycaemia. The intake of fibre in an urbanized society is limited by tolerability, but 30 g daily is recommended.

Insulin therapy

All patients with IDDM require treatment with insulin. Some patients with NIDDM who initially respond to diet and/or oral hypoglycaemic agents will eventually require insulin therapy. There is now a wide variety of different insulin preparations available. These may differ

Table 44.2 Insulin preparations

Preparation	Origin*	Onset (h)	Peak (h)	Duration (h)
Neutral insulin				
Human Actrapid (pry)	H	0.5	2–5	8
Human Velosulin (emp)	H	0.5	1–3	8
Humulin S (prb)	H	0.5	1–3	7
Hypurin Neutral	B	1	2–6	8
Velosulin	P	1	1–3	8
Pur-In Neutral (emp)	H	0.5	1–2	5–8
Biphasic insulin				
Human Actraphane (pry)	H	1	2–12	24
Human Initard (emp)	H	1	4–8	24
Human Mixtard (emp)	H	1	4–8	24
Humulin M1 (prb)	H	0.5–1	2–10	18
Humulin M2 (prb)	H	0.5	1–10	16
Humulin M3 (prb)	H	0.5	1–9	14
Humulin M4 (prb)	H	0.5	1–8	14
Initard	P	1	4–8	24
Mixtard	P	1	4–8	24
Rapitard	B+P	2	4–12	20
Penmix (pyr)	H	1	2–12	24
Pur-In Mix 50/50 (emp)	H	0.5	1–2	10–16
Pur-In Mix 25/75 (emp)	H	0.5	1–2	12–18
Pur-In Mix 15/85 (emp)	H	0.5	3–5	11–20
Insulin zinc suspension (amorphous)				
Semitard	P	2	5–10	16
Isophane insulin				
Human Insulatard (emp)	H	1	4–12	24
Human Protaphane (pyr)	H	2	4–12	24
Humulin I (prb)	H	1	2–8	20
Hypurin Isophane	B	2	6–12	24
Insulatard	P	2	4–12	24
Pur-in Isophane (emp)	H	0.5–1.5	4–6	11–24
Insulin zinc suspension (mixed)				
Human Monotard (pyr)	H	3	6–14	22
Humulin Lente (prb)	H	2	4–16	24
Hypurin Lente	B	2	5–12	30
Lentard	B+P	3	6–14	22
Insulin zinc suspension (crystalline)				
Human Ultratard (pyr)	H	4	8–12	28
Humulin Zn (prb)	H	3	6–14	24
Protamine zinc				
Hypurin Protamine Zinc	B	4	10–20	36

* Insulin preparations classified as being of human (H), beef (B) or pork (P) origin.
Key: emp = enzymatically modified pork; prb = proinsulin recombinant bacteria; pyr = precursor yeast recombinant

in species, onset of action, time to peak effect and duration of action (Table 44.2).

Species. There are three species of insulin available; beef, pork and human. Beef insulin differs from human insulin in three amino acids. The slightly different chemical structure does give rise to some pharmacokinetic differences. Beef insulin is more slowly absorbed after subcutaneous injection and has a longer duration of action when compared to an 'equivalent' pork or human formulation. Porcine insulin differs from human insulin in only one amino acid at the end of the B chain. This substitution has only minimal effect on the molecular structure of the protein, with the result that the body is much less likely to mount an antibody response to pork insulin than to beef insulin. Human insulin has been available for 10 years but has not yet been proven to be clinically superior to pork insulin. Human insulin can be prepared by chemical substitution of the single differing amino acid of pork insulin. This type of insulin is referred to as enzymatically modified pork (emp). Human insulin has the distinction of being the first commercial pharmaceutical to be prepared by genetic engineering. This process can involve the production of proinsulin by *Escherichia coli* (prb) or a recombinant technique using baker's yeast (pyr). Human insulins remain slightly antigenic on subcutaneous injection, probably through the formation of certain insulin derivatives during purification, packing and storage. However, this does not appear to pose a clinical problem.

In recent years it has become almost standard practice to commence all patients newly requiring insulin on human insulin. This has recently been re-examined in the light of alleged reports of patients developing hypoglycaemic unawareness after transfer from animal to human insulin. Although there is currently little or no scientific evidence to support this concern some patients have requested that they be changed back to pork insulin. Although it may be argued that there is no proven clinical need for any insulin other than human, equally there is no proven benefit of human over pork insulin.

Purity. For many decades insulin formulations were purified after extraction by recrystallization only. Modern insulin preparations are now further purified by gel filtration and ion exchange chromatography. These procedures remove nearly all contaminants producing formulations of such purity that does not usually give rise to clinical problems.

Insulin preparations. The onset of action, peak effect and duration of action are determined by both the insulin species and the physical and chemical form of the insulin.

Neutral insulin is the quickest and shortest acting of all the available insulins. It is also commonly referred to as soluble insulin. After subcutaneous injection neutral insulin appears in the circulation within 10 minutes. The concentration rises to a peak after about 2 hours and then declines over a further 4 to 8 hours. This absorption curve can be contrasted with the physiological insulin concentration curve, where peak concentrations are reached 30 to 40 minutes after a meal, and decline rapidly to 10 to 20% of peak levels after about 2 hours. Consequently in diabetic patients, the subcutaneous injection must be given 30 minutes before the meal if a rapid rise in blood glucose concentrations is to be avoided.

Isophane insulin is a complex of salmon or trout protamine with insulin. The onset of action is usually 1 to 2 hours with the peak effect being seen at 4 to 8 hours. There is considerable interpatient variation in the duration of action but it usually requires twice daily administration. Isophane and neutral insulin do not interact when mixed together. As a result there are now a wide range of biphasic insulins available which contain varying proportions of isophane and neutral insulin.

Lente insulin is an insulin zinc suspension which is a 30:70 mixture of an amorphous insulin and a crystalline zinc–insulin complex in suspension. Lente insulin has a slower onset of action than isophane insulin, and a longer duration of effect at the same dose. In order to maintain the integrity of the insulin crystals, all insulin zinc suspensions contain significant amounts of free zinc in solution. If mixed with neutral insulin some of the latter may be precipitated into a loose complex if they remain in contact for any length of time. Consequently it is recommended that if these two insulins are mixed, they should be injected immediately.

Ultralente insulin is the crystalline form of an insulin zinc suspension. This is very slowly absorbed from subcutaneous tissue and has a very variable bioavailability.

Insulin delivery

The subcutaneous route is the one of choice for the majority of insulin-requiring diabetics. Its main advantages are accessibility and that it allows most patients to administer their own insulin. However, this route cannot be regarded as physiological as it delivers insulin to the systemic rather than the portal circulation. In recent years most patients have used disposable plastic syringes and insulin from a vial as their means of insulin administration. There are now an increasing number and variety of pen injection devices being marketed for insulin administration. The devices are compact and do away with the need to draw up insulin from a vial. The most recent advance in insulin delivery has been the introduction of a disposable (but biodegradable) pen. The pen devices are not in themselves a means to improve diabetic control, but are a convenience which may ultimately aid compliance. Insulin can be injected into the thigh, abdominal wall, buttocks or upper arm.

Intravenous delivery should be used in the management of ketoacidosis. The short half-life of insulin means that changes in the rate of the infusion have a rapid effect on insulin action. This is not generally a satisfactory route for long-term administration.

Insulin regimens

Once-daily therapy can usually only be employed where it is accepted that good blood glucose control is not an important target of treatment. The exception may be in some patients with NIDDM who still have the ability to mount an adequate insulin response to food if the basal glucose level is maintained by a long-acting insulin preparation. In this circumstance it may be appropriate to give the injection in the evening or at bedtime. Twice-daily injection is the most commonly used regimen in the UK. This may involve the use of intermediate-acting insulin alone or in combination with neutral insulin. The injections are usually given half an hour before breakfast and half an hour before the evening meal. The ratio of short- to intermediate-acting preparations, and the split between morning and afternoon doses varies from patient to patient. In the newly diagnosed patient who is not acutely ill, it may be simpler to start therapy at home with an intermediate-acting insulin alone, adding in the short-acting if and when indicated by self-monitoring.

Multiple-injection regimen is the term which refers to the use of neutral insulin to cover the three main meals, and an intermediate- or long-acting preparation for the overnight period. Injection of neutral insulin before each meal allows greater flexibility of insulin dosage and eating habits. The injections before meals are usually given using a pen device and the basal insulin injected via a conventional syringe.

Adjusting the insulin dose

The information on which insulin dosage adjustment is based is derived from self-monitoring of blood glucose, and the incidence and timing of hypoglycaemia. On twice-daily rapid- and intermediate-acting insulin regimens, the neutral insulin may be considered as acting up to the next meal or to bedtime, while the extended-acting insulins act up to the next injection. The glucose concentration at the end of the period can be taken as a measure of the appropriateness of the relevant dose. For most patients, adjustments of insulin dose will be up or down 2 to 6 units at a time.

Storage of insulin

Insulin formulations are stable if kept out of light, and they are not subject to freezing or extremes of heat. Loss of potency of 5 to 10% occurs in vials kept at high ambient room temperatures for 2 to 3 months. Insulin should therefore be stored in a domestic refrigerator except for the vial(s) in current use. When a pen injector device is being used this should never be stored in a refrigerator.

Adverse effects of insulin

Systemic allergic reactions rarely occur with the

current use of highly purified insulins. Though not usually species-specific it is worthwhile trying insulin of a different species if allergy occurs.

The commonest injection site problem is thickening of subcutaneous tissues as a result of recurrent injection in a small area (lipohypertrophy). This may result in impaired and erratic insulin absorption. The solution is to rotate injection sites. Bruising is usually a sign of superficial injections. Localized skin reactions occasionally occur but usually resolve even with continued use of the same insulin preparation.

Hypoglycaemia is a major, physiological complication of insulin therapy and is often a source of great anxiety to patients. The signs and symptoms produced by hypoglycaemia fall into two groups; those due to adrenaline release and those due to neuroglycopenia. The manifestations may occur at different blood glucose levels in different individuals. In some diabetic patients they may occur with concentrations above 2.2 mmol/L, especially if the blood glucose falls rapidly. The release of adrenaline may result in palpitations, tremor, tachycardia, hunger and sweating. Some patients treated with beta-adrenoreceptor blocking agents may lose these adrenergic warning signs, with the exception of sweating which may increase. As the neuroglycopenia ensues, restlessness and mental instability may be present as well as irritability, obstinacy and agitation. Patients also commonly complain of perioral numbness and tingling.

Oral hypoglycaemic agents

For the patient with NIDDM, if dietary measures and exercise do not produce adequate glycaemic control, oral hypoglycaemic therapy will be required.

In the UK, seven sulphonylureas are currently available and one biguanide.

Sulphonylureas

Mode of action. The major actions of this class of drug rely on the ability of the pancreas to secrete insulin. All sulphonylureas lower blood sugar by increasing pancreatic beta-cell sensitivity to glucose, so that more insulin is released for any given glucose load. Sulphonylurea therapy is also associated with an increased tissue sensitivity to insulin, resulting in improved insulin action.

Recent studies have also suggested that sulphonylureas may promote an increased systemic bioavailability of insulin due to reduced hepatic extraction of the insulin secreted from the pancreas. Several reports have suggested that sulphonylureas, and in particular gliclazide, may reduce platelet aggregation. However, it is likely that the antiplatelet effects are secondary to the improvement in blood glucose concentrations produced by these drugs. There is no convincing evidence that gliclazide is superior to any other sulphonylurea with regard to antiplatelet effects.

Pharmacokinetics. The pharmacokinetic parameters of the oral hypoglycaemic agents are shown in Table 44.3. Chlorpropamide is the slowest- and longest-acting agent. Following the development of an improved assay, glibenclamide has been shown to have a short elimination half-life. However, it has a prolonged biological effect which may be explained by slower distribution and the existence of a deep compartment, possibly the islet cells. All sulphonylureas are metabolized by the liver to some degree and some have active metabolites.

Choice of drug. There are many factors which may influence the choice of sulphonylurea. These may relate to the drug itself, the patient or the prescriber (Table 44.4). There are few well-controlled long-term clinical comparisons between sulphonylureas. It would appear that when dosage is individualized and governed by the effect on fasting blood glucose, there is little or no difference in clinical efficacy between the different agents. In general, if a patient is not well controlled on maximum dosage of one sulphonylurea, it is not worthwhile changing to another one, except possibly for tolbutamide.

Adverse effects. The frequency of adverse effects from sulphonylureas is low. They are usually mild and reversible on withdrawal of the drug (Table 44.5). The most common adverse

Table 44.3 Pharmacokinetic properties of oral hypoglycaemic agents

Drug	Route of elimination	Elimination half-life (h)	Duration of action (h)	Daily dose range	Doses per day
Sulphonylureas					
First generation					
Tolbutamide	Hepatic	4–25	6–10	1–2 g	1–3
Chlorpropamide	Hepatic (80%) Renal (20%)	24–48	24–72	100–500 mg	1
Tolazamide	Hepatic Active metabolite	Parent 7 Metab.?	12–18	0.1–1 g	1–2
Second generation					
Glibenclamide	Hepatic Biliary	2–4	16–24	2.5–15 mg	1–2
Glipizide	Hepatic	1–5	6–24	2.5–40 mg	1–3
Gliquidone	Hepatic	1–2	6–24 (?)	15–180 mg	2–3
Gliclazide	Hepatic	6–15	12–24	40–320 mg	1–2
Biguanides					
Metformin	Renal	1–4.5	5–6	1–3 g	2–3

effect is hypoglycaemia. This may be profound and long-lasting, occasionally leading to permanent neurological damage or death. Hypoglycaemia due to sulphonylureas is often misdiagnosed, particularly in the elderly. The major risk factors for the development of hypoglycaemia are: use of a long-acting agent, increasing age, inadequate carbohydrate intake and renal or hepatic dysfunction.

Other adverse effects are rare; blood dyscrasias occur in 0.1% of patients and rashes in 3%. Chlorpropamide can produce troublesome

Table 44.4 Factors influencing the choice of sulphonylurea

The drug
• potency
• duration of action
• route of elimination
• number of daily doses required
• cost

The patient
• age
• renal function
• hepatic function
• ability to comply

The doctor
• experience
• personal preference

flushing after ingestion of alcohol, and about 5% of patients develop hyponatraemia due to its effect on increasing renal sensitivity to antidiuretic hormone (ADH). Most patients are asymptomatic with this problem but occasionally severe hyponatraemia is observed. It is not widely appreciated that patients treated with sulphonylureas often gain weight. This is unfortunate as it will exacerbate their resistance to insulin and to the sulphonylureas themselves.

Sulphonylurea dosage. The dosage should be individualized for each patient and the lowest possible dose used to attain the desired levels of blood glucose, without producing hypoglycaemia. Treatment should start with a low dose and be increased approximately every 2 weeks. For many agents the maximum effect is seen if the dose is taken half an hour before a meal, rather than with or after food. The number of daily doses required will depend on the agent used and the total daily dose. For several drugs it becomes necessary to administer the drug two or three times daily when the dose is increased.

Drug interactions. Several drugs can interfere with the efficacy of sulphonylureas, by influencing either their pharmacokinetics or pharmacodynamics, or both. Tables 44.6 and 44.7 show some drugs which can have a direct influence

Table 44.5 Adverse effects of sulphonylureas

Adverse effect	Comments
Gastrointestinal	Affects approximately 2% Most commonly nausea and vomiting Dose related Advise patient to take with or after food

Dermatological	Affects 1–3%
	Usually occur within the first 2–6 weeks
	Most commonly:
	    generalized photosensitivity
	    pruritus
	    maculopapular
	May require discontinuation of drug
	Cross-sensitivity between sulphonylureas is common
	Rare cases of severe allergic reactions, e.g. erythema multiforme, Stevens–Johnson syndrome

Haematological	Rare cases of fatal agranulocytosis or pancytopenia Other haematological effects usually reversible on discontinuing drug Some reports of reversible haemolytic anaemia
Hepatic	Mild, reversible elevation of liver function tests Cholestatic jaundice Usually a hypersensitivity reaction associated with fever, rash and eosinophilia Possible excess of cardiovascular mortality in patients treated with tolbutamide not proven
Hypothyroidism	Association not proven May be rare cases
Alcohol flush	Rarely seen with sulphonylureas other than chlorpropamide Change to another agent or 'pretreat' with aspirin
Syndrome of inappropriate ADH (SIADH)	Chlorpropamide and, to a lesser extent, tolbutamide enhance the effect of ADH on the kidney Results in hyponatraemia Risk factors are: increasing age, CCF and diuretic therapy
Hypoglycaemia	The most common adverse effect and may be severe and prolonged Highest incidence with chlorpropamide and glibenclamide All sulphonylureas have been implicated Risk factors include: increasing age, impaired renal or hepatic function, reduced food intake and weight loss Either decrease dose, change to a shorter-acting agent or discontinue sulphonylurea therapy

Table 44.6 Drug interactions with sulphonylureas – potentiating agents

Drug	Mechanism	Comments

Common or predictable interactions
  Beta-adrenoreceptor blocking agents
  Alcohol
  Salicylates
  Fibric acid derivatives
	Decreased hypoglycaemic awareness
	Decreased hepatic gluconeogensis
	Increased insulin secretion
	Increased insulin sensitivity
	Decreased glycogen secretion
		See also Table 44.7
		
		Only in high doses (4–6 g/day)

Uncommon or case reports only
  Chloramphenicol
  Cimetidine/ranitidine
  Quinine/quinidine
  ACE Inhibitors
  Chloroquine
  Disopyramide
	Inhibition of hepatic metabolism
	Inhibition of hepatic metabolism
	Increased insulin secretion
	Increased peripheral glucose utilization
	Inhibits insulin degradation
	Uncertain
		Rare reports

Table 44.7 Drug interactions with sulphonylureas – antagonising agents

Drug	Mechanism	Comments
Common or predictable interactions		
Beta-adrenoreceptor blocking agents	Decreased insulin secretion	Occasional hypoglycaemia due to decreased hepatic gluconeogenesis
Thiazide diuretics	Decreased insulin secretion	Dose related
	Increased insulin resistance	? Exacerbated by hypokalaemia
Loop diuretics	As for thiazide diuretics	Less common than with thiazide diuretics
Glucocorticoids	Increased hepatic gluconeogenesis	Dose related
	Increased insulin resistance	
Oral contraceptive	Increased cortisol secretion	Use lowest dose possible
	Increased insulin resistance	
Uncommon or case reports only		
Beta-adrenoreceptor agnoists	Increased hepatic gluconeogenesis	Only reported with high dose
Calcium channel blocking agents	Decreased insulin secretion	? Dose related
Amiodarone	Uncertain	
Octreotide	Decreased insulin secretion	Also rare hypoglycaemia
Theophylline	Increased catecholamine release	Only in overdosage
Phenytoin	Decreased insulin secretion	In overdosage or long-term high-dose treatment
Pentamidine	Destruction of pancreatic islet cells	May be preceded by hypoglycaemia
Phenothiazines	Uncertain	

on blood glucose concentrations. There is much written in the literature about displacement interactions with sulphonylureas; however, their clinical significance is doubtful. Many reported cases involve first generation agents which have a different protein-binding site to the second generation agents. The first generation agents are readily displaced from albumin by other acidic drugs, e.g. aspirin, whereas the second generation agents bind in a nonionic fashion and are not readily displaced. Ingestion of alcohol can cause hypoglycaemia in itself and can also prolong the hypoglycaemic effect of sulphonylureas.

Biguanides

Metformin is the only biguanide available in the UK. The mechanism of action of biguanides is still poorly understood, but many theories have been proposed. These include: reduced gastrointestinal absorption of carbohydrate; inhibition of hepatic gluconeogenesis; stimulation of tissue uptake of glucose; and increased insulin receptor binding. Of these probably the most important is the effect on hepatic gluconeogenesis. The action

of metformin does not involve stimulation of pancreatic insulin secretion. The major advantages of metformin over sulphonylureas are that it does not cause either hypoglycaemia or weight gain.

Metformin has a short duration of action and is not bound to plasma proteins. It is not metabolized and is totally renally eliminated.

Adverse effects. The most common adverse effects of metformin result from gastrointestinal disturbance. These include anorexia, nausea, abdominal discomfort and diarrhoea. These effects are usually transient and can be minimized by starting with a low dose, increasing the dose slowly and administering the drug with food. Despite these precautions a few patients are genuinely intolerant of the drug.

A rare, but potentially life-threatening adverse effect is lactic acidosis. The patients at most risk are those with renal insufficiency in whom the drug accumulates, those with coexisting conditions in which lactate accumulates and those who are unable to metabolize lactate. In practice metformin should not be prescribed to patients who have renal impairment, liver disease, alcoholism, uncontrolled cardiac failure or severe pulmonary insufficiency. It should also be withdrawn in a patient who develops a severe intercurrent illness, e.g. acute myocardial infarction or septicaemia.

Role of metformin. Metformin is useful in the obese diabetic as it does not cause weight gain. If there are no contra-indications it can be used in conjunction with diet as second line therapy in patients not adequately controlled on diet alone. As it has a different mode of action to the sulphonylureas, it can be valuable when prescribed in conjunction with them.

Insulin therapy in NIDDM

Patients who respond initially to oral hypoglycaemic agents for 1 month or longer, and who subsequently relapse, are referred to as 'secondary failures'. The rate of secondary failure varies from 3 to 30% in different series. These patients require treatment with insulin. Although these patients are often reluctant to change to insulin therapy, doing so can often result in a considerable improvement in well-being.

α-Glucosidase inhibitors

The α-glucosidase inhibitors are a new group of oral agents developed to treat diabetes mellitus. Acarabose was the first α-glucosidase inhibitor to be developed. It inhibits disaccharides being split into monosaccharides in the gut and consequently delays the formation of monosaccharides, and hence absorption, and results in lower postprandial blood glucose levels. The α-glucosidase inhibitors have the potential to be used in combination with insulin or oral hypoglycaemics.

THE PATIENT

Diabetes is a chronic, incurable condition which has considerable impact on the life of each individual patient, whatever his or her age or type of diabetes. Patient involvement is paramount for the successful care of the patient with diabetes. The principal task of the health-care team is to give each patient knowledge, self-confidence and support.

The way in which education is delivered will depend upon the individual patient and the availability of local resources. Individual tuition is desirable in the early stages after diagnosis. This type of education is usually delivered by a diabetes specialist nurse. The educational aspect of care is a gradual and ongoing process. At a later stage, group education can be effectively used, especially in NIDDM. Many such programmes are multidisciplinary and may involve doctors, nurses, dietitians, pharmacists and chiropodists. It is also essential to involve the patient's family and carers in the educational process. Patients can also obtain support and information from specialist organizations and their literature, e.g. The British Diabetic Association (BDA). The BDA also organizes a network of local support groups providing a forum for patients to exchange ideas and problems.

Patients require education and information about a wide range of subjects (Table 44.8). In

Table 44.8 Patient education in diabetes

1. The disease
  • signs and symptoms
2. Hyperglycaemia
  • signs, symptoms and treatments
3. Hypoglycaemia
  • signs, symptoms and treatments
4. Exercise
  • benefits and effect on blood glucose control
5. Diet
6. Insulin therapy
  • injection technique
  • types of insulin
  • onset and peak actions
  • storage
  • stability
7. Urine testing
  • glucose
  • ketones
8. Home blood glucose testing
  • technique
  • interpretation
9. Oral hypoglycaemic agents
  • mode of action
  • dosing
10. Foot care
11. Management during illness
12. Cardiovascular risk factors
  • smoking
  • hypertension
  • obesity
  • hyperlipidaemia
13. Regular medical and ophthalmologic examinations

particular, pharmacists should be able to give appropriate advice about the use of over-the-counter medication, foot care products and 'diabetic' food products.

Monitoring

Patients with IDDM. All patients treated with insulin should, wherever possible, undertake home blood glucose monitoring (HBGM). After the capillary blood has been applied to the reagent strip a colour reaction occurs. The result can either be visually compared to a colour chart or measured using a battery operated reflectance meter. Whether the extra precision of a meter is worthwhile is largely a matter of personal preference. Strips read visually are perfectly adequate for most situations although the extra accuracy may be desirable in pregnancy. HBGM has the additional benefits that it can detect hypogyclaemia and, unlike urine tests, in which glycosuria may only be detected some time after changes in blood glucose have occurred, it enables more accurate calculations of insulin doses.

Patients with IDDM, who are by definition ketosis prone, should also know how and when to test their urine for ketones. This test need not be carried out as part of routine monitoring, but is essential at times of intercurrent illness.

Patients with NIDDM. For most patients with NIDDM who are treated with diet alone or oral hypoglycaemic agents, urine glucose monitoring is adequate. This is a simple non-invasive test which can detect hyper- but not hypoglycaemia. HBGM is used by some patients with NIDDM, particularly if control is poor or if they are being treated with insulin.

Clinic monitoring

There are several ways in which diabetic control can be monitored in the clinic or general practitioner's surgery. Careful monitoring of weight change is important. In the obese patient with NIDDM weight loss may be the only form of treatment required. Unexpected weight loss may indicate poor control. In the young patient with

diabetes it is essential to ensure that normal growth and development is maintained.

The use of random blood glucose measurements in the clinic has largely been superseded by the monitoring of glycosylated proteins. Glycosylation of minor haemoglobin components occurs in the blood and the extent depends on both the amount of glucose present and the duration of exposure of the haemoglobin to glucose. Estimates of glycosylated haemoglobin provide an index of average diabetic control over the preceding 3 to 6 weeks. Serum fructosamine represents the glycosylation of all serum proteins and gives information about control over 3 weeks. As albumin is the major serum protein, the albumin concentration must be known for interpretation of fructosamine levels.

Patients should also have a comprehensive annual review and examination to look for the development of complications. In patients who already have complications, they will need to be reviewed more frequently.

CASE STUDIES

CASE 44.1

W. E. is a 61-year-old gentleman who has had NIDDM for 13 years. He has been treated with oral hypoglycaemic agents and diet. He carries out home urine glucose monitoring, but not on a regular basis. Over the past 3 months he has developed a severe burning pain in both feet. It is now progressing and is particularly intense at night. Sometimes this can be so severe that he is unable to tolerate the bedclothes touching his feet. His GP has prescribed several different analgesics, but none have been very effective. He has now been referred to the diabetic clinic for assessment.

In the clinic he is found to have a glycosylated haemoglobin of 11.5%.

His current drug treatment is:

- **Glipizide 10 mg daily**
- **Co-dydramol 1 or 2 when required**
- **Ibuprofen 400 mg three times daily.**

Q1 What may be the cause of Mr W. E.'s foot pain?

Q2 What action should be taken?

CASE 44.2

H. I. is a 72-year-old lady who has recently been found to have glycosuria when screened by her general practitioner. The diagnosis of diabetes was subsequently confirmed.

Mrs H. I. was given an appointment to see the dietitian, commenced on glibenclamide 5 mg daily and taught how to carry out urine glucose monitoring at home. She is not taking any other medication. The dietitian gives general dietary advice and a reduced calorie diet as she has a body mass index of 29. 4 weeks later she returns to see her GP. She is now complaining that she has had two episodes of shaking and dizziness in the last week.

Q1 What might be the cause of Mrs H. I.'s current symptoms?

Q2 How might these symptoms be alleviated?

CASE 44.3

A. I. is an 8-year-old boy who has developed an ear infection and has been prescribed a course of antibiotics by his GP. He has had IDDM for 3 years and is currently being treated with Humulin (prb) 22 units in the morning and 12 units in the evening. His mother brings the prescription into the pharmacy and also mentions that he is 'off his food' and she is having difficulty in getting him to eat. She is unsure what she should do about his insulin injections.

Q1 What advice should the pharmacist give to the patient's mother about his insulin treatment?

Q2 What advice should the pharmacist give about maintaining food intake?

CASE 44.4

O. P. is a 42-year-old lady who has had IDDM for 14 years. Initially her glycaemic control was poor and she showed little interest in her disease. However, in recent years she has become much more involved in her own diabetes management. In spite of the improved control she has had proteinuria for several months. This is being closely monitored by the diabetic clinic. On the last two occasions she has attended the clinic her blood pressure has been 160/95 mmHg and 155/90 mmHg. Today it is 165/95 mmHg. Mrs O. P. does not smoke, is not overweight and eats a healthy, balanced diet. It is decided to commence her on antihypertensive treatment.

Q1 Why is the management of hypertension of particular importance in diabetes?

Q2 Which drug(s) would be appropriate for the management of her hypertension?

CASE 44.5

W. T. is a 75-year-old gentleman who has had NIDDM for 17 years. His current treatment for his diabetes is:

- Glipizide 15 mg twice daily
- Metformin 850 mg three times daily.

He frequently has glycosuria and the last two glycosylated haemoglobin concentrations have been 11.3% and 12.0%. He is feeling generally unwell and lethargic.

His doctor suggests to him that the only way to adequately control his diabetes is by insulin injections. However, in view of the fact that he lives alone and has poor eyesight, it is suggested that the district nurse comes in to give his insulin injections.

Mr W. T. has always been proud of his independence and is reluctant to agree to this suggestion.

Q1 Why does Mr W. T. require insulin therapy?

Q2 How might the difficulties over insulin administration be overcome?

Q3 What kind of insulin regimen would be appropriate?

ANSWERS TO CASE STUDIES

CASE 44.1

A1 Mr W. E. is describing the classical symptoms of painful peripheral neuropathy. The pain, which can be severe and incapacitating, does not usually respond to conventional analgesics, including opiates.

There are two main hypotheses for the causation of diabetic neuropathy: depletion of myo-inositol and sorbitol accumulation. Depletion of myo-inositol may affect nerve conduction via membrane Na/K ATPase. Many cells contain an enzyme aldose reductase which, at high glucose concentrations, converts glucose to sorbitol. Sorbitol therefore accumulates in poorly controlled diabetes and may induce damage by either an osmotic or direct toxic action.

A2 The high glycosylated haemoglobin concentration indicates that Mr W. E.'s diabetic control has recently been poor and the first step should be to optimize glycaemic control. This could be achieved by checking dietary compliance and by either increasing the dosage of glipizide or by a period of treatment with insulin. A bed cradle can be used to remove the pressure of bedclothes at night.

For pain relief, a trial of tricyclic antidepressants could be initiated. These have been used to manage chronic, severe nerve pain of various aetiologies and are thought to enhance central inhibition of sensory input. It should be made clear to the patient that they are not being used as antidepressant therapy. In many patients pain relief occurs within 48 to 72 hours, a time course which differs from the antidepressant action. Imipramine or amitriptyline can be used in an initial dosage of 25 mg at night, increased every 3 days to the maximum tolerated dose or 150 mg daily. The patient should be carefully monitored for the development of side effects; Mr W. E. is an elderly male and is at risk of developing urinary retention due to the anticholinergic activity of these drugs.

Other treatments which have been tried with some success include: combination tricyclic and phenothiazine therapy; carbamazepine; phenytoin; and intravenous lignocaine. Drugs have been developed which inhibit aldose reductase and hence prevent tissue accumulation of sorbitol. In clinical trials, these agents have shown some improvement in the symptoms of peripheral neuropathy, but objective assessments have shown little or no improvement.

CASE 44.2

A1 The most likely cause of Mrs H. I.'s symptoms is sulphonylurea-induced hypoglycaemia. This is the commonest side effect of these drugs for which the incidence increases with age, decreased carbohydrate intake and renal or hepatic dysfunction.

Hypoglycaemia can be induced by all sulphonylureas, but the agents most likely to cause it are those with a long duration of action; notably glibenclamide and chlorpropamide. The hypoglycaemia can be severe and prolonged. It is particularly dangerous in an elderly patient who is living alone.

There is considerable interpatient variability with regard to the symptoms, which can be nonspecific. The classical symptoms include: blurred vision; sweating; tremor; hunger; confusion; odd behaviour; anxiety; and perioral tingling.

This case highlights the dangers for the newly diagnosed patient with NIDDM who adheres to a diet, loses weight and continues to take a sulphonylurea. Unless the degree of hyperglycaemia is severe at the time of diagnosis, the patient should initially be managed with dietary manipulation alone and pharmacological therapy only added if this proves unsuccessful.

A2 The clinical situation should be reassessed, in particular the need for pharmacological therapy. Glibenclamide should be avoided in elderly patients due to the risks of hypoglycaemia. If a sulphonylurea is required, it is more appropriate to use a shorter-acting agent such as glipizide or tolbutamide. If there are no contra-indications to its use, metformin should be considered as it cannot cause hypoglycaemia.

It is also important to note that most patients treated with oral hypoglycaemic agents carry out urine glucose monitoring, not blood glucose monitoring. Urine monitoring cannot detect hypoglycaemia. A negative test result cannot distinguish between a normal and a low blood glucose concentration. For this reason there is an increasing tendency for patients on oral hypoglycaemic agents to carry out home blood glucose monitoring. If the patient experiences symptoms but their is doubt about whether they can be attributed to hypoglycaemia, the patient should be advised to eat glucose, e.g. three glucose tablets or two sweet biscuits. If hypoglycaemia is the cause, the symptoms should resolve within 5 minutes.

CASE 44.3

A1 The pharmacist should advise the patient's mother that insulin should never be omitted unless advised to do so by a doctor. He will certainly require his normal dose of insulin and may even require more. It is a common mistake made by patients and relatives to decrease or discontinue insulin in these circumstances; action which may result in the development of diabetic ketoacidosis.

Insulin requirements usually increase in the presence of an infection, acute illness or stress. This is due to the increase in the amount of circulating counter-regulatory hormones (glucagon, cortisol, growth hormone, adrenaline and noradrenaline), which oppose the action of insulin. The patient's mother should be advised to carry out regular blood glucose tests every 3 to 4 hours and to give more insulin if required. Patients who are not on regular injections of quick-acting (neutral) insulin are usually advised to keep a supply at home for use in emergencies. This can be used to supplement the normal insulin and to treat hyperglycaemia rapidly. If a patient is unwell and has hyperglycaemia he should be advised to test his urine for ketones. If ketones are persistently present he must seek medical attention. As the infection resolves the insulin requirements should decline.

The management of illness at home is a very important part of the education of diabetic patients and their families. It is also important that all health-care professionals understand these principles of management.

A2 Of equal importance to the insulin therapy is fluid and carbohydrate intake. Fluid is essential if dehydration is to be avoided. The patient will lose a considerable volume of fluid as a result of glycosuria and, if present, through vomiting. If carbohydrate intake is inadequate, the body will respond by breaking down muscle and fat, predisposing the patient to ketoacidosis. The patient should be encouraged to drink regular quantities of fluid. If the patient does not feel like eating this could be in the form of milk with sugar, fruit juice or any glucose-containing drink or food supplement.

CASE 44.4

A1 Hypertension is two to three times more common in people with diabetes than in the general population. Both hypertension and diabetes are risk factors for coronary artery disease, cerebrovascular accidents, peripheral vascular disease and congestive cardiac failure. In addition, complications such as nephropathy and retinopathy are also accelerated in the presence of hypertension. The postulated mechanisms for the synergy between these two conditions are many and various but include: sodium homeostasis and fluid volume abnormalities; hyperinsulinaemia; abnormal renin–angiotensin–aldosterone axis; and abnormal noradrenaline levels.

Hypertensive diabetic patients are at especially high risk of developing the serious complications of diabetes. It is now widely recognized that control of blood glucose is not the only factor to be considered in diabetes management. Attention must also be paid to the other risk factors, including hypertension.

A2 Drug therapy should only be considered when appropriate non-pharmacological measures have failed. These include: exercise; weight reduction; decreasing salt intake; stopping smoking; and decreasing alcohol intake. When selecting an antihypertensive agent, consideration should be given to any potential for adverse effects on carbohydrate and lipid metabolism. Antihypertensive agents can also produce side effects which could exacerbate the complications of diabetes: compromised peripheral blood flow; sexual dysfunction; orthostatic hypotension; and adverse effects on renal function. For these reasons, the conventional use of thiazides and beta-adrenoreceptor blockers as first line therapy in diabetes is controversial.

Angiotensin converting enzyme (ACE) inhibitors and calcium channel blockers can be regarded as metabolically neutral, producing no adverse effects on blood glucose or lipid profiles. In addition, these drugs, and in particular ACE inhibitors, may exert beneficial effects on renal function. In view of her persistent proteinuria, an ACE inhibitor, may be an appropriate choice for Mrs O. P. Before commencing therapy it is essential to rule out the coexistence of renal artery stenosis, and after starting treatment to monitor renal function and potassium concentrations carefully. Calcium channel blockers provide a useful alternative.

CASE 44.5

A1 The glycosylated haemoglobin estimations indicate that Mr W. T. has chronic, poor diabetic control. In addition he has nonspecific symptoms (feeling generally unwell and lethargic) which are often attributed to old age or other medical conditions, but are actually characteristic of chronic, mild hyperglycaemia. The dose of glipizide could be increased to a maximum of 40 mg daily, but few patients achieve improved glycaemic control through this increase and in those that do the improvement is often only short-lived.

A2 In elderly patients with NIDDM who have been treated with oral hypoglycaemic agents for many years, there is often extreme, but understandable reluctance to start insulin therapy. Some perceived barriers to insulin therapy in the elderly include lack of motivation, poor eyesight and impaired manual dexterity. Potentially the most serious complication of insulin therapy in this group is hypoglycaemia.

Patient's reservations about insulin therapy can usually be overcome by offering them a 'trial' of insulin. At the end of the trial period the patient can be given the choice of continuing insulin therapy or going back onto tablets. In practice, patient well-being often improves dramatically on insulin therapy and they choose to remain on it.

Use of a pen-injector device does away with the need for drawing up insulin and can facilitate correct dosage administration in patient with visual impairment. With many pen devices, the insulin dose can be dialled up by the use of an audible click, allowing the dose to be counted without visual confirmation. The degree of manual dexterity required is much less than for a conventional insulin injection technique.

A3 The insulin regimen should be as simple as possible with the aim of relieving Mr W. T.'s symptoms and improving well-being. This may be achieved with a single daily injection of an intermediate-acting insulin. Conventionally this has been given in the morning but can also safely be given as an evening or bedtime dose, without significant danger of nocturnal hypoglycaemia. Some elderly patients will require twice-daily injection to control hyperglycaemia. If the patient requires the addition of a neutral insulin, there is a wide range of fixed mixtures of isophane and neutral insulins available.

BIBLIOGRAPHY

Chan J C N, Cockram C S. Drug-induced disturbances of carbohydrate metabolism. Adverse Drug Reactions and Toxicology Reviews 1990; 10(1): 1–29

Dornan T (ed). Diabetes care: a problem solving approach. London: Heinemann Professional Publishing 1988

Hill R D. Diabetes health care. A guide to the provision of health services. London: Chapman & Hall 1987

Kennedy F P. Recent developments in insulin delivery techniques. Current status and future potential. Drugs 1991; 42(2): 213–227

Marchetti P, Navalesi R. Pharmacokinetic–pharmacodynamic relationships of oral hypoglycaemic agents. An update. Clinical Pharmacokinetics 1989; 16(2): 100–128

Melander A, Bitzen P-O, Faber O, Groop L. Sulphonylurea antidiabetic drugs. An update of their clinical pharmacology and rational therapeutic use. Drugs 1989; 37(1): 58–72

Tattersall R B, Gale E A M (eds). Diabetes – clinical management. Churchill Livingstone 1990

Chapter 45

Anaemia

C. Acomb

Anaemia is a reduction from normal of the quantity of haemoglobin in the blood. It results in a corresponding decrease in the oxygen carrying capacity of the blood.

Anaemia can result from a number of different pathologies.

EPIDEMIOLOGY

Anaemia is possibly one of the most common conditions in the world and results in significant morbidity and mortality.

Iron deficiency anaemia

Iron deficiency anaemia (worldwide, the commonest form of anaemia) may be present in up to 20% of the world's population. A diet deficient in iron, parasitic infestations e.g. hookworm (causing blood loss), and multiple pregnancies contribute to a high prevalence of iron deficiency anaemia in underdeveloped countries. Even in western societies it has been reported that as many as 20% of menstruating females show a rise in haemoglobin on iron therapy.

Sideroblastic anaemia

Hereditary sideroblastic anaemia is a rare sex-linked recessive disorder which presents in males in childhood. Some of the acquired forms are relatively common with as many as 30% of alcoholics admitted to hospital having sideroblastic anaemia.

Folic acid deficiency anaemia

Much of the world's population has a marginal dietary intake of folate. Body stores are low and as soon as there is a decrease in dietary intake or there is increased folate demand, deficiency readily occurs.

Vitamin B$_{12}$ deficiency anaemia

Pernicious anaemia (reduced vitamin B$_{12}$ absorption due to a lack of intrinsic factor) is found most commonly in people of northern European descent. In Britain the incidence is about 120 per 100 000. Pernicious anaemia is usually a disease of the elderly the average patient presenting at 60 years of age. Strict vegans (e.g. Hindus) commonly have low vitamin B$_{12}$ levels due to their dietary deficiency.

Glucose-6-phosphate dehydrogenase deficiency anaemia

There are more than 100 different forms of glucose-6-phosphate dehydrogenase (G6PD) deficiency only some of which cause anaemia. The most common form of G6PD deficiency is found in 15% of black Americans. It causes anaemia when the individual is exposed to a trigger factor. A more severe form is the Mediterranean variant of G6PD deficiency. Some of these individuals may have chronic haemolytic anaemia even in the apparent absence of exposure to a precipitating factor.

AETIOLOGY

Anaemia results from two different mechanisms:

- reduced haemoglobin synthesis which may be due to lack of nutrient or bone marrow failure
- increased haemoglobin loss due to haemorrhage (red cell loss) or haemolysis (red cell destruction).

It is not unusual to find more than one cause in a patient.

Iron deficiency anaemia

In western societies the commonest cause of iron deficiency is due to blood loss. In women of child-bearing age this is most commonly due to menstrual loss. Amongst adult males the most likely cause is gastrointestinal bleeding. A loss of 100 ml of blood represents the amount of iron normally absorbed from a western diet over 40 days. The daily requirement varies with age (Table 45.1).

Sideroblastic anaemia

This consists of a number of disorders which include: those inherited; those associated with other disorders; and those acquired following ingestion of agents such as alcohol or isoniazid (Table 45.2). Regardless of the cause there is usually impaired haem synthesis despite adequate nutrition.

Folic acid deficiency anaemia

Folate is readily available in a normal diet. Fruit, green vegetables and yeast all contain relatively

Table 45.1 Typical daily requirements of iron	
Adult male	0.9 mg
Postmenopausal female	0.9 mg
Menstruating adult	2.0 mg
Adolescent male	1.8 mg
Adolescent female	2.4 mg
Pregnancy	3–5 mg

Table 45.2 Types of acquired sideroblastic anaemia
Associated with other disorders
Myelodysplastic syndromes
Myeloid leukaemia
Myeloma
Collagen diseases
Associated with drugs and toxins
Isoniazid
Cycloserine
Pyrazinamide
Alcohol
Lead

large amounts of folate. Despite this relative abundance of folate in many foods, dietary deficiency is common, either as the sole cause of the folic acid deficiency anaemia or in conjunction with increased folate utilization.

Vitamin B$_{12}$ deficiency anaemia

The only dietary source of vitamin B$_{12}$ (cyanocobalamin) is from food of animal origin. It is present in meat, fish, eggs, cheese and milk. Cooking does not usually destroy vitamin B$_{12}$. Daily requirements are between 1 and 3 micrograms. Deficiency arises either from inadequate intake over a prolonged period or more commonly, in the West, from impaired absorption.

G6PD deficiency anaemia

G6PD deficiency can under certain circumstances result in haemolytic anaemia. There are various other causes of haemolytic anaemia (see Table 45.3) of which only G6PD deficiency will be discussed here. Haemolytic anaemia occurs when the survival of mature red blood cells is shortened and the bone marrow cannot compensate for their decreased lifespan.

PATHOPHYSIOLOGY

To understand how the various anaemias arise it is necessary to outline normal erythropoiesis (red cell production). It is thought that white cells, red cells and platelets are all originally derived from a common cell known as a pluripotent stem cell found within the bone marrow. The bone marrow produces cells that progressively become committed to a specific cell line (see Fig. 45.1).

Erythropoietin, a hormone produced by the kidney, stimulates the proliferation and differentiation of the CFU-E. The cells mature through various stages during which time the cells synthesize haemoglobin, DNA and RNA. Reticulocytes are found in the peripheral circulation for 24 hours before maturing into erythrocytes. Reticulocytes are released into the peripheral circulation prematurely during times of increased erythropoiesis.

Each day approximately 2×10^{11} erythrocytes enter into the circulation. Normal erythrocytes survive in the peripheral circulation for about 120 days. Abnormal erythrocytes have a shortened lifespan. At the end of their lifespan the red cells are destroyed by the cells of the reticulo-endothelial system found in the spleen and the bone marrow. Iron is removed from the haem component of haemoglobin and transported back to the bone marrow for reuse. The pyrole ring from globin is excreted as conjugated bilirubin by the liver and the polypeptide enters the body's protein pool.

Table 45.3 Common forms of haemolytic anaemia
Inherited forms
Glucose-6-phosphate dehydrogenase deficiency
Hereditary spherocytosis
Hereditary elliptocytosis
Pyruvate kinase deficiency
Sickle cell anaemia
Thalassaemia
Acquired forms
Autoimmune haemolytic anaemia
Isoimmune haemolytic anaemia
Drug-induced immune haemolytic anaemia
Hypersplenism
Toxins, e.g. chemical, infection, drugs

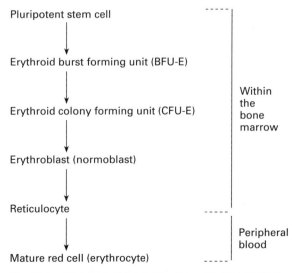

Fig. 45.1 Simplified diagram of some of the stages within erythropoiesis.

Iron deficiency anaemia

The major causes of iron deficiency are listed in Table 45.4. The elimination of iron is not controlled physiologically so the homeostasis is maintained by controlling iron absorption.

Iron is absorbed mainly from the duodenum and jejunum. Absorption itself is inefficient; iron bound to haem (found in red meat) is better absorbed than iron found in green vegetables. Malabsorption of iron may occur in patients with coeliac disease, and in 50% of patients following partial gastrectomy.

During pregnancy there is an increase in red cell mass but there is also a proportionally bigger increase in plasma volume which results in a physiological dilutional anaemia. It is thought that the gut increases its ability to absorb iron during pregnancy to meet the additional demands of fetal red cell production. Some of the increased demand is met by stopping of menstruation. If, however, there is inadequate iron absorption, then anaemia may result.

Sideroblastic anaemia

In sideroblastic anaemia some of the erythroblasts in the bone marrow have iron granules surrounding the cell nucleus. These cells are known as ring sideroblasts. The disorder is often acccompanied by a number of metabolic abnormalities including defects in one or more steps of haem synthesis, which result in hypochromic, microcytic red cells; decreased red cell production; and an increase in serum iron and transferrin saturation.

Reduced levels of delta-amino laevulinic acid (ALA) synthetase are found in hereditary and primary acquired forms of sideroblastic anaemia. It is a key enzyme involved in haem synthesis and requires pyridoxine as a co-enzyme. It often responds to treatment with large doses of pyridoxine.

Folic acid deficiency anaemia

The folate found in food is mainly conjugated to polyglutamic acid. Enzymes found in the gut convert the polyglutamate form to monoglutamate which is readily absorbed. During absorption the folate is methylated and reduced to methyltetrahydrofolate monoglutamate. This travels through the plasma and is transported into cells via a carrier specific for the tetrahydrofolate form. Within the cell the methyl group is removed (in a reaction requiring vitamin B_{12}) and the folate is reconverted back to a polyglutamate form (Fig. 45.2). It has been suggested that the polyglutamate form prevents the folate leaking out of cells. The folate eventually acts as a co-enzyme involved in a number of reactions including DNA and RNA synthesis.

Defective DNA synthesis mainly affects cells with a rapid turnover, e.g. gastrointestinal cells, red blood cells, hence the sore tongue and anaemia, seen in folic acid deficiency. During DNA synthesis the folate co-enzyme is oxidized

Table 45.4   Major causes of iron deficiency anaemia
Inadequate absorption
Dietary deficiency
Malabsorption
Increased physiological demand
Loss through bleeding

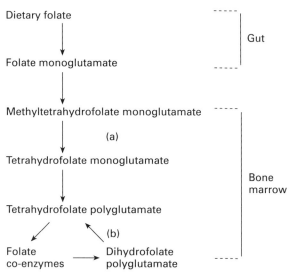

Fig. 45.2 Simplified pathway of folate metabolism. Key: (a) vitamin B_{12} is required as co-enzyme for this reaction; (b) the enzyme dihydrofolate reductase converts inactive dihydrofolate back to the active tetrahydrofolate.

to the dihydrofolate form, which is inactive and has to be reactivated by the enzyme dihydrofolate reductase. This is the enzyme inhibited by methotrexate and to a lesser extent by trimethoprim and pyrimethamine.

Vitamin B$_{12}$ deficiency

Absorption of vitamin B$_{12}$ is mainly by an active process. Enzymes in the stomach release vitamin B$_{12}$ from protein complexes. One molecule of vitamin B$_{12}$ then combines with one molecule of a glycoprotein called intrinsic factor. The intrinsic factor protects the vitamin B$_{12}$ from breakdown by microorganisms. There are specific receptors in the distal ileum for the intrinsic factor–vitamin B$_{12}$ complex. The vitamin B$_{12}$ enters the ileal cell and is then transported through the blood attached to transport proteins. Intrinsic factor does not appear in the blood.

Malabsorption occurs if the distal ileum is removed, it may also occur with certain intestinal pathologies, particularly stagnant loop syndrome, tropical sprue and fish tapeworm infestation. Passive absorption does take place in the jejunum but this is very inefficient and usually accounts for less than 1% of an oral dose.

Pernicious anaemia is probably autoimmune in origin and is one form of vitamin B$_{12}$ deficiency anaemia. Patients typically have a gastric atrophy and no (or virtually no) intrinsic factor secretion. Two different intrinsic factor antibodies have been found in the serum of patients with pernicious anaemia. Gastric parietal cell antibodies are found in 90% of adult pernicious anaemia patients.

Since intrinsic factor is only produced by the gastric parietal cells, a total gastrectomy always leads to vitamin B$_{12}$ deficiency. Approximately 10 to 15% of patients who have had a partial gastrectomy also develop deficiency. The onset of anaemia is usually delayed because the body typically has stores of 2 to 3 mg which is sufficient for 2 to 3 years.

Vitamin B$_{12}$ is a co-enzyme for the removal of a methyl group from methyltetrahydrofolate. Lack of vitamin B$_{12}$ traps the folate as methyl-tetrahydrofolate and prevents DNA synthesis (Fig. 45.2).

The exact mechanism by which vitamin B$_{12}$ deficiency causes neuropathy is not clear but may be due to a defect in the methylation reactions needed for myelin formation.

G6PD deficiency

There are a large number of variants of G6PD activity found in different populations and ethnic groups. G6PD is an enzyme that is indirectly involved in the production of reduced glutathione. Glutathione is produced in response to, and protects red cells from, oxidizing reagents. If there is a deficiency in G6PD and hence glutathione, in the presence of an oxidizing reagent the red cell membrane becomes damaged, the haemoglobin becomes oxidized and forms what are known as Heinz bodies. Some of the red cells haemolyse and others have their Heinz bodies removed by the spleen to form 'bite cells'.

CLINICAL MANIFESTATIONS

In its mildest form, anaemia results in tiredness and lethargy while at its most severe it results in death unless treated. There is some suggestion that even mild anaemia may inhibit physical exercise and result in reduced mental performance.

The various forms of anaemia are best separated clinically into three types depending on the average size of the red cells in the circulation, i.e. mean corpuscular volume (MCV). Care must be taken since the MCV indicates the average size of the cells. If there are two concurrent pathologies, where one causes large cells and the second causes small cells, the MCV may appear normal or be misleading.

Iron deficiency anaemia

In addition to the general symptoms of anaemia various other features may be present (Table 45.5).

The colour of the skin is very subjective and often unreliable. Patients at risk of heart failure may present with breathlessness when anaemic. Koilonychia, dysphagia and pica are found only after chronic iron deficiency and are relatively rare.

Table 45.5   Features of iron deficiency anaemia
Pale skin and mucous membranes
Painless glossitis
Angular stomatitis
Koilonychia (spoon-shaped nails)
Dysphagia (due to pharyngeal web)
Pica (unusual cravings)
Atrophic gastritis

Table 45.6   Clinical features of megaloblastic anaemia
Glossitis (sore, pale, smooth tongue)
Angular stomatitis
Altered bowel habit (diarrhoea or constipation)
Anorexia
Mild jaundice
Insidious onset
Sterility
Bilateral peripheral neuropathy (vit B_{12} deficiency only)
Melanin skin pigmentation (rare)

Sideroblastic anaemia

Many patients are stable and asymptomatic for long periods of time but others become progressively anaemic. In congenital sideroblastic anaemia many of the cells in the peripheral blood are microcytic and hypochromic. Despite this there are frequently increased iron stores in the bone marrow. The serum iron and serum ferritin are also high and the total iron binding capacity (TIBC) is saturated. There is often splenomegaly which may lead to mild thrombocytopenia.

The acquired forms vary a little in their manifestation but the common finding in both hereditary and acquired forms is the presence of sideroblasts in the marrow.

When sideroblastic anaemia is associated with the disorders in Table 45.2, the clinical picture is dominated by the underlying disease rather than the anaemia.

Folic acid deficiency anaemia

In addition to the general features of anaemia, megaloblastic anaemia (of which folic acid deficiency and B_{12} deficiency anaemia are the two most common examples) has certain characteristics (Table 45.6).

Alcoholics and the elderly are particularly prone to nutritional deficiency. Elderly people living alone on tea and toast are typical of at-risk patients. Alcoholics develop deficiency due to their poor diet; although some beers contain small amounts of folate, spirits contain none.

A number of drugs have been implicated in causing folic acid deficiency (Table 45.7). Actual megaloblastic anaemia is uncommon and the exact mechanism(s) has not always been established.

Serious malabsorption can occur in tropical sprue and coeliac disease. Reduced absorption is seen in Crohn's disease and following partial gastrectomy and jejunal resection.

There is a physiological increase in folate utilization during pregnancy. There may be an increased utilization in various pathological conditions, in association with inflammation or in a number of chronic haemolytic anaemias, particularly thalassaemia major, sickle cell disease and autoimmune haemolytic anaemia.

Vitamin B_{12} deficiency anaemia

Vitamin B_{12} deficiency causes megaloblastic anaemia and therefore has similar features to folic acid deficiency (Table 45.6). In addition to the macrocytosis, anisocytosis and poikilocytosis there is often mild thrombocytopenia. The spleen may be slightly enlarged and there may be a slight fever. Mild jaundice may be present due to the increased breakdown of haemoglobin found in the abnormal red cells. The onset is slow and insidious so patients often present late or are diagnosed during other investigations.

Table 45.7   Drugs implicated in causing folic acid deficiency
Malabsorption ?
Phenytoin
Barbiturates
Sulphasalazine
Cholestyramine
Oral contraceptives
Impaired metabolism
Methotrexate
Pyrimethamine
Triamterene
Pentamidine
Trimethoprim

The feature that separates vitamin B_{12} deficiency from the other megaloblastic anaemias is progressive neuropathy. It is symmetrical and affects the legs rather than the arms. Patients notice a tingling in their feet and a loss of vibration sense. Occasionally patients have difficulty in walking or experience frequent falls.

G6PD deficiency anaemia

Clinically the two most important types of G6PD deficiency occur in the Negro population and in people originating from the Mediterranean. The Negro population has a milder form which results in an acute self-limiting haemolytic anaemia following exposure to an oxidizing agent, e.g. infection, acute illness, fava beans or drugs (Table 45.8). The haemolytic anaemia is self limiting because the young cells produced by the bone marrow have higher levels of G6PD activity than old cells. Following exposure to the oxidizing agent, the old cells are haemolysed but the new cells produced in response are more capable of tolerating the insult (until they grow old). In the Mediterranean form the enzyme activity is very low, haemolysis is not usually self limiting and indeed some patients have a chronic haemolytic anaemia despite the absence of an obvious causative factor.

Patients with acute haemolytic anaemia commonly complain of malaise, fever, abdominal pain, dark urine and jaundice. They have haemoglobulinaemia, hyperbilirubinaemia, reticulocytosis and increased urobilinogen levels in the urine. Patients with chronic haemolytic anaemia also usually have splenomegaly. Their anaemia is usually normochromic and normocytic.

INVESTIGATIONS
General

In most patients with anaemia the blood volume remains constant and the anaemia is a consequence of a reduced concentration of haemoglobin in each red cell and/or a reduced number of red cells in the peripheral blood. Blood volumes may be increased in pregnancy or congestive heart failure and blood haemoglobin concentrations may appear falsely low. On the other hand patients with an acute reduction in blood volume (e.g. burns or following vigourous diuresis) may appear to have a high haemoglobin concentration.

In addition to the actual numbers of red cells present in a full blood count the morphology is equally important. The size, shape and colour all contribute to the investigation. Following on from this baseline other investigations may be required. Bone marrow examinations by either aspiration or trephine may be needed to make a diagnosis.

Iron deficiency anaemia

A full blood count is an essential screening test. The cells of the peripheral blood are microcytic and hypochromic with poikilocytes (often pencil shaped) and occasional target cells (abnormal thin erythrocytes which when stained show a dark centre and peripheral ring).

Three parameters help establish the iron status of the patient; the serum iron, the total iron binding capacity (TIBC) and the serum ferritin.

The serum iron exhibits diurnal variation, being higher in the morning. Iron is transported around the body bound to a serum protein called transferrin. Normally this protein is only one-third saturated with iron. The parameter

---

Table 45.8 Common drugs implicated in causing haemolysis in G6PD deficiency
Drugs to be avoided in all variants
Ciprofloxacin (and probably other quinolones)
Dapsone
Methylene blue
Primaquine (reduced dose may be used in milder variants)
Nalidixic acid
Nitrofurantoin
Sulphonamides (including co-trimoxazole)
Drugs to be avoided in more severe variants
Aspirin (low dose used under supervision)
Chloramphenicol
Chloroquine (acceptable in acute malaria)
Menadione
Probenicid
Quinidine
Quinine (acceptable in acute malaria)

TIBC is the sum of the serum iron and the unsaturated iron binding capacity (UBIC) of the iron transport proteins in the blood. The serum iron and TIBC vary with iron status (Fig. 45.3).

The serum ferritin is low in iron deficiency anaemia and markedly raised in iron overload.

Sideroblastic anaemia

The findings in the peripheral blood vary slightly depending on the form of sideroblastic anaemia. In hereditary forms the peripheral blood may show a hypochromic, usually microcytic picture, similar to iron deficiency but in sideroblastic anaemia the serum iron is raised and the TIBC saturated. In primary acquired sideroblastic anaemia the peripheral blood is dimorphic with some hypochromic cells and a raised MCV. In both cases examination of the bone marrow is often essential and shows erythroid hyperplasia, a large number of sideroblasts and a large excess of iron.

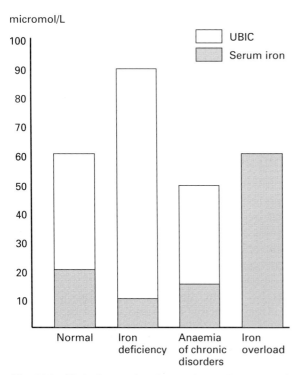

micromol/L

UBIC
Serum iron

Normal / Iron deficiency / Anaemia of chronic disorders / Iron overload

Fig. 45.3   Typical examples of serum iron and unsaturated iron binding capacity (UBIC).

Folic acid deficiency anaemia

Many patients are symptomless initially and the diagnosis is made following a full blood count carried out for another reason. The peripheral blood reveals large oval red cells. Anisocytosis and poikilocytosis are common. Some of the neutrophils are hypersegmented and thrombocytopenia may be present. Red cell folate accurately reflects folate stores and is a more preferable parameter than serum folate which is subject to changes in diet and does not correlate as closely with anaemia.

Vitamin B_{12} deficiency anaemia

Following the recognition of megaloblastic anaemia from the full blood count, one of the first investigations will be the determination of the serum vitamin B_{12} level. The red cell folate or serum folate is normally done at the same time. The serum vitamin B_{12} is low in mild anaemia and may be very low if there is marked megaloblastic anaemia or neuropathy. If there is no concurrent folate deficiency the serum folate level tends to be raised whilst the red cell folate falls (possibly due to a failure of folate polyglutamate synthesis in cells).

Oral vitamin B_{12} absorption can be measured by a number of techniques, the most common test being the Schilling test. The test is based on giving a radiolabelled oral dose of vitamin B_{12} and an unlabelled parenteral dose which saturates the vitamin B_{12} binding proteins. The amount of labelled vitamin in the urine gives a measure of absorption. The test can be repeated by giving the radiolabelled oral dose with intrinsic factor. The absorption should now be approaching normal if the patient has intrinsic factor deficiency but remains low if there is ileal disease.

Although 90% of patients with pernicious anaemia have parietal cell antibodies their presence is not diagnostic because 50% of patients with gastric atrophy without pernicious anaemia also have the antibodies present.

G6PD deficiency anaemia

The history and the clinical findings steer the

diagnosis which is then confirmed by measuring G6PD activity. Care must be taken during the acute phase since there are increased numbers of young cells with higher levels of activity which may be misleading. The increased numbers of young cells result from the selective destruction of older cells and the increased production of reticulocytes.

THERAPY

Since anaemia is a sign of a disease rather than a diagnosis, there is no general treatment for anaemia. Correct diagnosis is vital before proceeding with specific therapy.

Occasionally anaemia can be 'cured' by stopping a causative drug or toxin. More usually drugs are used to manage the condition and reduce symptoms. With careful thought, prophylaxis is possible in a number of conditions.

Iron deficiency anaemia

The aim of treatment is to correct the anaemia and to replenish iron stores. Although the treatment of iron deficiency anaemia is relatively simple it should not be embarked upon lightly. It is important to resolve the underlying cause as far as possible. Over-the-counter sales of iron should be discouraged except in those patients who have been fully investigated. It is not unknown for patients to be given iron unnecessarily resulting in iron overload. On the other hand giving iron therapy to a patient who is continuing to bleed from their gastrointestinal tract, is not helping to resolve the underlying problem.

Prophylaxis of iron deficiency anaemia is used in pregnancy (together with folic acid), menorrhagia and after partial gastrectomy.

Oral iron in the ferrous form is cheap, safe and effective in most patients. Depending on the state of the body's iron stores it may be necessary to continue treatment for up to 6 months to both correct the anaemia and replenish body stores. The standard treatment is ferrous sulphate 200 mg three times a day. It typically takes between 1 and 2 weeks for the haemoglobin to rise 1 g/dl. An earlier indication of response can be seen by looking at the reticulocyte count which should start to rise 2 to 3 days after starting effective treatment. Some patients receiving iron are troubled by nausea, abdominal pain or a change in bowel habit. Giving the iron with food makes it better tolerated but tends to reduce the amount absorbed. Alternative salts of iron are sometimes tried; these tend to have fewer side effects simply because they contain less elemental iron (Table 45.9). Taking fewer ferrous sulphate tablets each day would have the same effect. During the early stages of treatment the body absorbs iron better. Absorption is commonly around 15% of intake for the first 2 to 3 weeks but falls off to an average of 5% thereafter.

There are two preparations of parenteral iron: iron dextran which may be given intravenously or intramuscularly and iron sorbitol which is only for intramuscular injection. Parenteral therapy is rarely needed and should be reserved for use in patients where oral therapy has failed or is not possible. The rate of haemoglobin rise is the same for equivalent doses of oral and parenteral iron. The most common situation where parenteral iron is tried is in patients with severe vomiting during pregnancy.

The major problems with parenteral administration are that patients may require a series of painful intramuscular injections (usually 10 injections) or if iron dextran is given intravenously there is a significant risk of anaphylaxis. Patients receiving intravenous iron infusions should be given a test dose and closely monitored throughout the infusion period and for 1 hour afterwards. Intravenous infusions are contra-indicated in asthmatics.

Table 45.9 Elemental iron content of common preparations	
Preparation	Approximate iron content
Ferrous sulphate tablet 200 mg	65 mg
Ferrous gluconate tablet 300 mg	35 mg
Ferrous fumarate tablet 200 mg	65 mg
Ferrous fumarate syrup 140 mg in 5 ml	45 mg
Ferrous glycine sulphate syrup 141 mg in 5 ml	25 mg
Ferrous succinate elixir 106 mg in 5 ml	37 mg
Sodium ironeditate 190 mg in 5 ml	28 mg

There are a number of modified-release oral preparations available. They have no clear therapeutic advantage over ferrous sulphate and are not recommended. Indeed the modified-release characteristic may cause the oral iron to be carried into the lower gut which is much poorer at absorbing iron than the duodenum. Modified-release preparations may be more likely to exacerbate diarrhoea in patients with inflammatory bowel disease.

Patients who have lost blood acutely may require blood transfusions.

Sideroblastic anaemia

Although the peripheral blood cells in sideroblastic anaemia are frequently microcytic and hypochromic the condition is associated with increased iron stores and so iron therapy should be avoided. The drugs and toxins listed in Table 45.2 tend to cause a reversible sideroblastic anaemia. Removing the offending agent usually resolves the anaemia.

In patients with a hereditary form, large doses of pyridoxine (200 mg daily) reduce the severity of the anaemia. Patients with an acquired form occasionally respond to high dose pyridoxine and a 2- to 3-month trial may be helpful in symptomatic patients. The response tends to be slow and only partial. When there is an increased marrow cell turnover, folate supplements may also be necessary. In patients who require frequent transfusions there is a risk of iron overload. Desferrioxamine therapy which chelates and removes iron from the body is often required.

Folic acid deficiency anaemia

Folic acid deficiency is usually managed by replacement therapy. The duration of the treatment depends on the cause of the deficiency. Changes in dietary habits or removal of any precipitating factor should also be considered.

The normal daily requirement of folic acid is approximately 100 micrograms a day; despite this the usual treatment doses given are 5 to 15 mg a day. Even in malabsorption states, because of these large doses, sufficient folate is usually absorbed. Therefore parenteral folic acid treatment is not normally required. Treatment for 4 months will normally be sufficient to ensure that folatedeficient red cells are replaced.

In pregnancy the daily requirement rises to approximately 300 micrograms a day and it is usual to give a combination iron and folic acid product. These products contain 350 to 500 micrograms of folic acid and must only be used for prophylaxis during pregnancy and never for the treatment of other megaloblastic anaemias.

Large doses of folic acid can produce a partial haematological response in patients with B_{12} deficiency. The blood picture appears nearly normal but the neurological damage due to the vitamin B_{12} deficiency continues. Folic acid therapy should not be started until vitamin B_{12} deficiency has been excluded. It has also been suggested that patients on long-term folic acid therapy should have their vitamin B_{12} levels checked at regular intervals (e.g. yearly).

Vitamin B_{12} deficiency

The majority of patients with vitamin B_{12} deficiency require lifelong replacement therapy. Occasionally specific therapy related to the underlying disorder may be all that is necessary (e.g. treatment of fish tapeworm).

It is necessary to establish whether the patient with pernicious anaemia has vitamin B_{12} deficiency or folic acid deficiency or both. Treatment of vitamin B_{12} deficiency with folic acid may lead to the resolution of the haematological abnormalities but does not correct the neuropathy which continues to deteriorate.

Since the anaemia has developed slowly the cardiovascular system does not tolerate blood transfusions very well and is easily overloaded. Transfusions should not normally be given. In severe cases where emergency transfusion is deemed necessary, packed cells may be given slowly whilst blood (mainly plasma) is removed from the other arm. Diuretics may also need to be given especially if the patient has congestive heart failure and poorly tolerates fluid overload. If it is not possible to delay until a definitive diagnosis is made, both folic acid and vitamin B_{12} may be given.

For most patients a definite diagnosis is made before treatment is started. The standard treatment is hydroxocobalamin 1 mg intramuscularly repeated five times at 2- to 3-day intervals to replenish body stores. This is followed by a maintenance dose; usually 1 mg intramuscularly every 3 months. American texts recommend cyanocobalamin rather than hydroxocobalamin because of the fear that some patients appear to develop antibodies to the vitamin B_{12} transport protein complex in the serum. In the UK hydroxocobalamin is the treatment of choice. It is retained in the body longer than cyanocobalamin and reactions to it are very rare. The haematological response to both is probably identical.

Hypokalaemia develops in some patients during the initial haematological response. (Potassium is an intracellular ion and is used in the production of new cells.) Potassium supplements may be needed in the elderly and patients receiving diuretics or digoxin. The serum iron also falls as it is incorporated into haemoglobin. The more severe the anaemia the more likely it is to see a fall in serum potassium or iron.

Not only is it very gratifying to follow the response to treatment it is also important to monitor the response to ensure that the patient returns to normal without any attendant problems. There is often a subjective improvement before an objective one. Typically the patient feels better within 24 to 48 hours and yet there may be no discernible haematological response. The first haematological change in the peripheral blood is a rise in the reticulocyte count starting around day 3 or 4 and peaking after 7 to 8 days. The more severe the anaemia the higher the peak reticulocyte count. The reticulocyte count should remain raised whilst the haematocrit is less than 35%. Failure to remain raised during this time indicates the need for further evaluation. The arrest or slowing down of erythropoiesis may be due to inadequate stores of other essential factors (e.g. iron) or may be due to coexisting disease such as hypothyroidism or infection.

The red cells return to normal and the platelet count rises to normal (or even higher) after 7 to 10 days. The haemoglobin takes much longer to return to normal. It should rise by approximately 2 to 3 g/dl each fortnight.

Neurological damage may be irreversible. Peripheral neuropathy of recent onset often partially improves but any spinal cord damage is irreversible even with optimum therapy.

G6PD deficiency anaemia

In cases of acute haemolytic anaemia the causative oxidizing agent should be stopped and general supportive measures adopted. In chronic haemolytic anaemia most patients become reasonably well adjusted to their anaemia. They need to avoid known precipitating factors to prevent acute episodes occurring on top of their chronic haemolytic anaemia.

There is no specific drug treatment. During acute episodes the patient should be kept well hydrated to ensure good urine output (to prevent haemoglobin damaging the kidney). Blood transfusions may be necessary. In chronic haemolytic anaemia folic acid supplements may help erythropoiesis. Vitamin E (an antioxidant) appears to have little clinical benefit in preventing haemolysis.

THE PATIENT

Much of the therapy for anaemia is either prophylactic or long term. Patients therefore have to be well informed and motivated otherwise poor compliance may result.

Iron deficiency anaemia

It is usual practice to advise patients to take iron products with or after meals as this probably reduces the incidence of nausea. Patients should be told that their faeces may become darker and that this is nothing to worry about. This is important in patients who have had malaena since they may associate their dark stools with the bleed and worry that they are still bleeding from the gastrointestinal tract.

The length of treatment and compliance should be discussed and an explanation given that iron stores need to be replenished and that this takes time.

Sideroblastic anaemia

Few patients have completely reversible anaemia. In those patients who show an improvement on pyridoxine the progress is very slow. Patients need to be aware that therapy may take several months before there are any signs of improvement.

Folic acid deficiency anaemia

In patients who have a dietary component to their deficiency, appropriate nutritional advice should go alongside their folic acid therapy. If the cause of the deficiency has been eliminated patients can expect to receive folic acid for approximately 4 to 6 months. In patients with a continuing requirement (e.g. haemolytic anaemia) patients can expect lifelong treatment. Those starting out on folic acid therapy can anticipate feeling better after a few days but should be informed that their blood picture will take much longer to return to normal.

Vitamin B$_{12}$ deficiency anaemia

Patients feel subjectively better very shortly after their first hydroxocobalamin injection. They can be told that their sore tongue will start to improve within 2 days and be back to normal after 2 to 4 weeks. Patients need to be informed that they need regular injections, usually every 3 months. Surprisingly some patients say that they feel they are ready for this injection as they approach their appointment time and feel better after their injection. Compliance is not usually a problem.

G6PD deficiency anaemia

Since drug therapy does not play a large part in the management of these patients, pharmacists do not often become involved in patient education. Patients can be given a list of drugs to avoid but since most of these drugs are prescription-only medicines it is important that patients remind health care professionals of their condition.

CASE STUDIES

CASE 45.1

Mr H. A., a 62-year-old, single, unemployed man, was admitted to hospital for investigation of anaemia. He presented with a 6-month history of lethargy, chest pain, dizziness and falls, and a past history of having a partial gastrectomy 16 years ago. The drug history taken by the junior doctor showed that Mr H. A. was taking diazepam and a GTN spray on admission. Review of systems revealed no vomiting and no melaena. He complained of some indigestion after meals and reported his appetite as 'fine if someone else cooks'. On examination he was pale, with a BP of 140/80, a pulse of 90 and a haemoglobin level of 2.5 g/dl (normal range 13.5 to 18.0 g/dl). A gastroscopy was normal and a biopsy showed no evidence of coeliac disease. A barium enema was normal and faecal occult bloods (FOBs) were negative.

Over the first 3 days he was transfused with 8 units of blood and was given frusemide 40 mg with alternate bags. On day 7 he was started on ferrous sulphate 200 mg three times a day, folic acid 5 mg twice daily and ascorbic acid 200 mg three times daily.

Q1 How might a full drug history taken by a pharmacist help this patient?

Q2 Comment on the use of vitamin C in Mr H. A.

Q3 How long should Mr H. A. remain on ferrous sulphate?

CASE 45.2

Mr W. K., a 46-year-old mechanic, was referred to hospital by his GP. He gave a history of diarrhoea and vomiting a week ago and now was complaining of headaches and feeling 'lousy'. His GP had given him metoclopramide and ferrous sulphate. Mr W. K. did not appear jaundiced although he said he had noticed his urine was unusually dark a few days ago. On examination he was obese with a BP of 120/80 mmHg, and a pulse of 80. Rectal examination revealed black stools. He had a normal gastroscopy and three negative FOBs. His serum biochemistry showed a normal level of alanine transaminase and a slightly raised total bilirubin. Mr W. K.'s reticulocyte count was 13.5% (normal range 0.5 to 1.5%). Mr W. K. was diagnosed as having glucose-6-phosphate dehydrogenase (G6PD) deficiency probably triggered by an infection.

Q1 How do you explain Mr W. K.'s dark urine and dark stools?

Q2 Would Mr W. K. benefit from any medication following his admission?

Q3 Why would it be necessary to repeat his red cell G6PD after 2 months?

CASE 45.3

Miss P. R., a grey-haired, 58-year-old lady, was admitted from casualty. She had fallen over and bruised herself but had not broken any bones. The casualty officer thought Miss P. R. appeared pale with possibly a lemon-yellow tinge to her skin, she was slightly confused and had paraesthesiae of the feet and fingers. She had a past history of heart failure and was taking frusemide and amiloride. She was admitted for investigation and discovered to have a macrocytic anaemia. Pernicious anaemia was suspected. Folate levels, vitamin B_{12} levels and a Schilling test were carried out before commencing treatment.

Q1 What are the features that may lead you to consider pernicious anaemia as a diagnosis?

Q2 Can Miss P. R. have a blood transfusion after samples have been taken for folate and vitamin B_{12} levels?

Q3 The red cell folate is reported as 150 mg/L (reference range 160 to 640 mg/L). Would Miss P. R. benefit from folate therapy?

CASE 45.4

Mrs G. N., a 76-year-old retired textile factory worker, was seen by her GP, complaining of tiredness. She had been seen 2 months earlier and started on ferrous sulphate for a microcytic anaemia. Initially she had felt better but the tiredness soon returned. A bone marrow aspiration revealed increased erythropoiesis, iron stores and red cell precursors.

A diagnosis of sideroblastic anaemia was made and it was decided to give her monthly transfusions. She was also started on pyridoxine 50 mg three times a day in addition to the ferrous sulphate.

Q1 What are the potential problems of Mrs G. N.'s treatment?

Q2 After 3 months there appeared to be little benefit to show from the pyridoxine. How might the management be improved?

CASE 45.5

Mrs R. O., a 70-year-old retired teacher, presented with a history of increasing tiredness over the last 6 weeks. She had a past history of a partial gastrectomy 4 years ago. On questioning, her relevant symptoms include 'pins and needles' in her toes and loose bowels. She said that she had never been a good eater but ate red meat twice a week.

Q1 Why was it 4 years after her gastrectomy before Mrs R. O. developed vitamin B_{12} deficiency?

Q2 How long will it take for Mrs R. O. to respond to treatment?

Q3 What long-term therapy will Mrs R. O. require?

ANSWERS TO CASE STUDIES

CASE 45.1

A1 The house officer who clerked in Mr H. A. probably documented all his prescribed drugs, but it is possible that Mr H. A. was taking purchased medication. On admission he complained of indigestion over the last 3 months and on questioning revealed that he was self-medicating with aluminium hydroxide mixture. From a theoretical point of view, antacids may reduce the amount of iron absorbed by increasing the pH of the stomach and by reducing the solubility of ferrous salts. It is unlikely that this contributed significantly to the development of his anaemia, but if he intends to continue using an antacid after discharge it would be better not to take a dose of antacid within 1 to 2 hours of his ferrous sulphate. It would be also worth checking to see if he has been self-medicating with a purchased aspirin- or ibuprofen-based product; both drugs have been implicated in causing gastrointestinal blood loss, though in this case his gastroscopy was normal and FOB negative.

A2 Ascorbic acid slightly increases the absorption of iron in some patients. It probably keeps iron in solution either in the ferrous form or by forming a soluble chelate with the ferric form. In most patients this is of little clinical benefit. It may have an advantage in Mr H. A. since he appears to have had a poor diet and may be vitamin C deficient, he may also benefit from a short course of multivitamins.

A3 Mr H. A. needs to continue iron therapy until he has at least replenished his iron stores. This may take up to 6 months, after which time he should be reassessed taking into account whether he is now having a suitable diet. In practice since his haemoglobin was dangerously low on admission it may be quite reasonable to leave him on iron for the rest of his life.

CASE 45.2

A1 Mr W. K.'s dark urine was a consequence of his haemolytic anaemia. Bilirubin is a breakdown product of haemoglobin which is transported to the liver and conjugated before being excreted in the bile. Bacteria in the intestine convert this to urobilinogen most of which is excreted in the stool. Small amounts of urobilinogen are reabsorbed and some of this appears in the urine. Urobilinogen is oxidized to urobilin which is coloured. During episodes of haemolysis, erythrocytes are destroyed faster than normal and hence there is an increase in the formation of bilirubin and increased excretion of urobilinogen in the urine. Also during haemolysis free haemoglobin may be released into the blood. If the haemolysis is severe enough the normal mechanism for removing haemoglobin from the circulation is overcome and haemoglobin may appear in the urine.

Dark stools may indicate melaena and upper gastrointestinal bleeding. In Mr W. K.'s case his gastroscopy was normal and he had three negative FOBs. His dark stools were due to the ferrous sulphate prescribed by his GP prior to admission.

A2 His raised reticulocyte count indicates he is rapidly replacing his lost red cells. Erythropoiesis consumes folate and iron and since his folate is towards the lower end of the reference range it may be worth giving him a short course of folate supplements.

A3 Young red cells tend to have higher levels of enzyme activity than more mature cells. Determining G6PD levels during the acute phase may be misleading since there is a relatively high proportion of young cells. Mr W.K.'s result 2 months later would more accurately represent his normal state.

CASE 45.3

A1 Macrocytic anaemia and paraesthesiae are typical features (though not diagnostic) of pernicious anaemia. Patients may be mildly jaundiced which is often described as lemon-yellow in colour. Interestingly pernicious anaemia is more common in women than men and is associated with blue eyes and early greying of the hair. Miss P. R. may have other features of pernicious anaemia which include glossitis, angular stomatitis and altered bowel habit.

A2 Patients with pernicious anaemia develop their anaemia over a long period of time and tend not to tolerate increases in blood volume very well. A transfusion may result in fluid overload and precipitate heart failure. Miss P. R. already has heart failure so, unless she becomes severely compromised by the anaemia, a transfusion should not be given. In patients who have such a pronounced anaemia that an urgent transfusion is required, an exchange transfusion of a small volume of packed cells may be appropriate.

A3 In vitamin B_{12} deficiency, folate tends to leak from cells and the red cell folate is often low (serum folate is sometimes raised). Many patients initially require both folate and vitamin B_{12}, although the folate can usually be stopped after a short course. Folate therapy must never be given to patients who have not been fully investigated for vitamin B_{12} deficiency. If vitamin B_{12} deficient patients are given large doses of folate without hydroxocobalamin, the full blood count can appear to improve but the peripheral neuropathy from the vitamin B_{12} deficiency progresses.

CASE 45.4

A1 Mrs G. N.'s bone marrow aspiration and serum ferritin showed that she had high levels of stored iron. Repeated monthly transfusions will also contribute to further iron accumulation. In sideroblastic anaemia the bone marrow appears to be inefficient at incorporating iron into haem. The administration of iron leads to iron overload which may result in damage to the heart, liver and endocrine organs. The ferrous sulphate must be stopped. If iron accumulation remains a problem, desferrioxamine therapy may be tried.

A2 Pyridoxine does not always improve the blood picture in patients with sideroblastic anaemia. Doses up to 400 mg a day have been used. In the case of Mrs G. N. an increase in dose should be tried. Patients with sideroblastic anaemia often do not realize that pyridoxine is not just a simple vitamin but a specific treatment for anaemia. Counselling the patient may improve compliance. Some patients also benefit from folate and this should be tried especially if Mrs G. N.'s serum folate was found to be low.

CASE 45.5

A1 Vitamin B_{12} requires intrinsic factor produced by the stomach for absorption. Patients who have had a total gastrectomy, and some with a partial gastrectomy, malabsorb vitamin B_{12}. Most patients have good body stores and even with no new vitamin B_{12} entering the body (e.g. following a total gastrectomy) it takes at least 2 years to deplete the stores.

A2 Many patients feel better within days of starting hydroxocobalamin and before a change in their haemoglobin concentration can be detected. Mrs R. O.'s blood picture may take a number of weeks to return to normal but the 'pins and needles' may be a sign of peripheral neuropathy which is frequently irreversible and may not respond to the hydroxocobalamin treatment.

A3 Mrs R. O. will need lifelong replacement therapy with hydroxocobalamin. This is usually given at a dose of 1 mg i.m. every 3 months.

BIBLIOGRAPHY

Barnard D L, McVerry B A, Norfolk D R. Clinical haematology. Mainstream Medicine Series. Oxford: Heinemann Medical Publications 1989

Beck W S (ed). Hematology, 5th edn. Boston: MIT Press 1991

Hoffbrand A V, Lowis S M. Postgraduate haematology, 3rd edn. Oxford: Heinemann Medical Publishers 1989

Hoffbrand A V, Pettit J E. Essential haematology, 2nd edn. Oxford: Blackwell Scientific 1984

Chapter 46

Drug-induced blood disorders

P. Magee   L. Beeley

Many drugs are used therapeutically to modify haematological functions such as coagulation and immune response. If such drugs are used in overdose they normally produce a Type A adverse reaction which is predictable from the known pharmacology of the drug. However, most drug-induced blood dyscrasias are not predictable and are classified as Type B adverse drug reactions. This chapter will deal largely with those drugs which induce Type B blood disorders.

The exact incidence of drug-induced blood dyscrasias is difficult to assess, but they are among the more common serious adverse effects of drug therapy, having a high morbidity and mortality. The high incidence of blood dyscrasias with some drugs has necessitated their withdrawal from the market, e.g. amidopyrine. With others such as mianserin it is recommended that routine blood screening be carried out during drug therapy.

Patients with a drug-induced blood dyscrasia usually present acutely with dramatic clinical symptoms. The problem can often only be detected at an earlier stage if regular blood screens are performed. It is important to confirm a diagnosis as quickly and accurately as possible since withdrawal of the drug is often followed by prompt recovery if there are no associated complications. An exception is aplastic anaemia, which may not be reversible, may progress after drug withdrawal and can result in considerable morbidity and mortality.

The diagnosis of a drug-induced blood dyscrasia is made clinically and by blood tests. A drug cause is implicated by:

- previously reported associations between the drug and the dyscrasia
- the pattern of clinical association, e.g. dose, history of administration
- other manifestations of drug sensitivity
- the absence of other causes.

BONE MARROW DEPRESSION

A list of drugs causing marrow depression is shown in Table 46.1.

APLASTIC ANAEMIA

This term describes the anaemia that results from a panmyelopathy where there is suppression of red cells, white cells (agranulocytosis) and platelets (thrombocytopenia). Drug-induced aplastic anaemia occurs less commonly than agranulocytosis or thrombocytopenia but in contrast to the latter, aplastic anaemia persists and often becomes more severe after withdrawal of the drug, resulting in a high incidence of mortality and protracted morbidity in those patients who survive.

Aplastic anaemia can be congenital but most cases are induced by myelotoxic drugs or chemicals. In situations where it is not possible to identify a cause for the anaemia, the condition is termed idiopathic.

Clinical presentation

Drug-induced aplastic anaemia produces a clinical picture indistinguishable from the idiopathic form, both being characterized by suppression of each cellular component. Severity depends on the degree of suppression.

Red cell aplasia gives symptoms of pallor, weakness, fatigue and breathlessness. Thrombocytopenia can produce haemorrhage into the skin, and bleeding from the gums and gastrointestinal tract. Menorrhagia is a feature in female patients. Death can occur from cerebral haemorrhage. Agranulocytosis presents with the signs and symptoms of infection, sore throat, ulceration of the mouth and pharynx, fever with rigors and infections of the skin and mucous membranes.

Secondary infection with candida is common. Pneumonia and septicaemia are frequent causes of death.

Drug-induced aplastic anaemia can be either acute or, more commonly, chronic. Acute cases present with severe bleeding and sometimes with infection. When the onset is insidious, the symptoms of red cell aplasia predominate with general lassitude, headache and increasing pallor. Symptoms of agranulocytosis and thrombocytopenia are less evident although a decrease in leucocytes and platelets is usually found on a blood screen. Signs of chronic anaemia occur over weeks or months following drug exposure.

Mechanisms of drug induction

Drugs can induce aplastic anaemia in one of two ways:

- a direct, dose related effect on cell division in the bone marrow (Type A)
- an unpredictable sensitivity reaction which may be genetically determined (Type B).

Type A

The classic example of drugs causing the first type of reaction is cytotoxic agents. All drugs that interfere with cell division that are used in the treatment of malignancies will depress bone marrow in a dose-related manner. Their effect is immediate and reversible on drug withdrawal. Cytotoxic agents used as immunosuppressants will also have this effect and although these agents are used in 'low' doses, patients require regular blood screens.

Type B

The 'sensitivity' type of reaction can be more serious because its onset may be delayed, sometimes not becoming apparent until several

Table 46.1 Drugs reported to have caused aplastic anaemia, agranulocytosis or thrombocytopenia

Group	Examples	Type of dyscrasia most commonly reported
ACE inhibitors	Captopril	Agranulocytosis Thrombocytopenia
Antiarrhythmics	Digitoxin Disopyramide Quinidine Procainamide	Agranulocytosis Thrombocytopenia
Antibacterials	Cephalosporins Chloramphenicol (including eye preparations) Semisynthetic penicillins Streptomycin Sulphonamides Tetracycline Vancomycin	Aplastic anaemia Agranulocytosis Thrombocytopenia
Anticonvulsants	Carbamazepine Ethosuximide Phenytoin Primidone Valproate	Aplastic anaemia Agranulocytosis
Antihistamines	Chlorpheniramine H_2 receptor blockers	Aplastic anaemia Agranulocytosis Thrombocytopenia
Antimalarials	Chloroquine Mepacrine Pyrimethamine Quinine	Aplastic anaemia Agranulocytosis Thrombocytopenia
Antirheumatics	Allopurinol Aspirin Colchicine Gold salts Ibuprofen Indomethacin Naproxen Oxyphenbutazone Penicillamine Phenylbutazone	Agranulocytosis Thrombocytopenia
Antithyroid drugs	Carbimazole Potassium perchlorate Propythiouracil	Aplastic anaemia Agranulocytosis
Antivirals	Ganciclovir Zidovudine	Aplastic anaemia Agranulocytosis
Cytotoxics	Alkylating agents Antimetabolites Vinca alkaloids	Aplastic anaemia
Diuretics	Acetazolamide Frusemide Thiazide	Agranulocytosis Thrombocytopenia
Psychotropics	Meprobamate Phenothiazines Tricyclic antidepressants Mianserin	Agranulocytosis
Sulphonylureas	Chlorpropamide Tolbutamide	Agranulocytosis

months after the drug has been stopped. Although rare this reaction has a high risk of mortality.

Some drugs, such as chloramphenicol, phenytoin and propylthiouracil can produce both types of reaction but not in the same patient.

Chloramphenicol-induced aplastic anaemia. Chloramphenicol produces a mild reversible bone marrow depression in all patients when given in large doses. The red cell series is primarily involved but there is some reduction of the white cells and platelets.

The reported incidence of the Type B reaction induced by chloramphenicol varies from 1 in 10 000 to 1 in 50 000. This form of aplastic anaemia is more serious, frequently irreversible and ultimately fatal. It is not related to dosage or duration of treatment and is usually detected 2 weeks to 5 months after therapy has stopped. It is an unpredictable reaction which cannot be prevented by regular blood monitoring or drug withdrawal. There is some evidence to suggest a genetic propensity to this type of reaction.

Aplastic anaemia has been reported with the use of chloramphenicol eye drops and eye ointment.

Treatment and monitoring

Drug-induced aplastic anaemia is a serious condition with a mortality rate of approximately 70%, with partial recovery in 20% and full recovery in only 10% of cases.

Treatment is essentially supportive and aimed at prolonging survival until remission occurs. In all cases the causative drug should be stopped and if the aplastic anaemia is of the dose-related type, Type A reaction, then the prognosis is better.

Regular blood transfusion is the most important therapy. When neutropenia is marked, reverse barrier nursing is indicated together with antibiotic therapy. Antibiotic combinations are used to offer the widest possible cover. Granulocyte infusions can be used if the neutrophil count continues to fall. Granulocyte colony stimulating factor (G-CSF) has been used, although this is not a licensed condition for it. Corticosteroids can be used to control purpura resulting from the thrombocytopenia but the role of androgenic steroids in promoting marrow regeneration is uncertain, although oxymetholone is often used.

Bone marrow transplantation now offers the best hope for patients with irreversible drug-induced aplastic anaemia.

AGRANULOCYTOSIS

Drugs can cause a leucopenia, that is a decrease in the total white cell count involving monocytes and lymphocytes as well as granulocytes, but more often they induce a selective neutropenia or agranulocytosis.

Agranulocytosis and neutropenia occur more frequently than aplastic anaemia. The incidence is highest in elderly females and the risk is higher with some of the causative drugs than with others.

Clinical presentation

In neutropenia and agranulocytosis, the body's ability to fight infection is compromised and the clinical presentation is one of infection.

In acute neutropenia, common first symptoms are fever, sore throat and painful mucosal ulcers. Candida infections are also common particularly in the mouth and pharynx. Without treatment, fatal sepsis will occur.

Mechanisms of drug induction

Drugs can selectively induce agranulocytosis in one of three ways:

- the destruction of neutrophils by drug antibodies (allergic reactions)
- the development of a lupus-like syndrome
- toxic depression of bone marrow.

Allergic reaction

When agranulocytosis is induced by drug allergy, the onset of symptoms is abrupt, although the time of onset varies between a few days and several weeks from the start of drug therapy. It can occasionally occur later than this. With-drawal of the drug may be followed by complete recovery in 2 to 3 weeks; however, it is impor-tant to note that the patient has been sensitized to the drug and any further administration will result in prompt recurrence. The classic example of a drug which induces agranulocytosis by an immune mechanism is amidopyrine, an anal-gesic which is no longer available, for which antibodies directed against granulocytes have been demonstrated. Other drugs which can cause the condition include the sulphonamides, antithyroid agents, phenothiazines and the sulphonylureas.

Development of lupus-like syndrome

Agranulocytosis can also develop when drugs induce a syndrome similar to systemic lupus erythematosus such as occurs with isoniazid, hydralazine, and procainamide. The fall in the granulocyte count is accompanied by fever, arthropathy, butterfly rash on the face, lym-phadenopathy and a positive test for nuclear antibody. Generally the syndrome is produced by large and repeated doses of drugs and is reversible on cessation of treatment.

Toxic depression of bone marrow

Toxic depression of the granulocyte cell line in the marrow is related to the cumulative dose of a drug. The phenothiazines, in particular chlor-promazine, are a common cause of this type of reaction. It is directly related to the total drug dose (for chlorpromazine, 5 to 30 g) and the duration of treatment (for chlorpromazine, 10 to 30 days). If the phenothiazine has been used for over 3 months without any adverse effect, agranulocytosis is unlikely to develop but can occasionally do so. On drug withdrawal, the granulocyte count returns to normal and, if there is no suitable alternative, a phenothiazine may be reintroduced, at a lower dose, without a fall in the white cell count. The tricyclic antidepres-sants are also believed to depress granulocyte production selectively in this way.

Treatment and monitoring

Patients receiving drugs known to induce agran-ulocytosis frequently (e.g. mianserin, penicilla-mine, gold, clozapine and cytotoxic agents) should undergo regular blood screens (see data sheets). However, blood counts do not always correlate with progression to agranulocytosis which can occur acutely between blood screens. There are no specific guidelines for predicting the development of agranulocytosis and there-fore patient counselling to ensure self-referral at the first signs of pharyngitis and fever is essential for those taking a high risk drug.

If agranulocytosis does occur, withdrawal of the drug responsible is usually followed by restoration of adequate neutrophil counts within several days to several weeks. Corticosteroid therapy has been suggested to promote recovery but its value is uncertain and it may further compromise the patient's immune system. Anti-biotic cover should be given while the neutro-phils are low and any infections treated promptly. The prognosis for patients with re-versible agranulocytosis is good, provided that there is appropriate antibiotic, antifungal and antiviral therapy. However, death from over-whelming infection occurs in approximately 10% of patients.

THROMBOCYTOPENIA

Examples of drugs causing thrombocytopenia are shown in Tables 46.1 and 46.2.

Thrombocytopenia is a reduction in the plate-let count to below 150×10^9 per litre although symptoms of haemorrhage are unlikely to occur unless the count falls below 100×10^9 per litre.

Thrombocytopenia is possibly the most com-mon drug-induced blood dyscrasia. It is associ-ated with a lower mortality than aplastic anaemia.

Table 46.2 Drugs associated with thrombocytopenia only

Digitoxin
Heparin
Paracetamol
Rifampicin

Clinical presentation

Haemorrhage is the main clinical feature of thrombocytopenia and is characterized by a prolonged bleeding time, but normal clotting. The skin is the most common site of haemorrhage which results in many small purple blotches termed 'purpura'. The small bleeding points are called petechiae. Other sites include the gastrointestinal and genitourinary tracts and rarely other internal organs. Cerebral haemorrhage is the most common cause of death in thrombocytopenic patients. The clinical picture varies with the severity of the thrombocytopenia and, if an immune reaction is responsible, there will also be signs of drug allergy which often precedes the purpura, e.g. fever and chills.

Mechanisms of drug induction

Drugs induce thrombocytopenia by one of two mechanisms:

- selective bone marrow suppression
- an immune mechanism where antibody production causes platelet agglutination.

Bone marrow suppression

Drugs which can induce aplastic anaemia through generalized marrow toxicity will sometimes produce thrombocytopenia selectively. This could be because the platelet precursors are more vulnerable than other stem cells to cytotoxic agents. This generally occurs 7 to 10 days after drug administration (e.g. thiazide diuretics).

Immune mechanism

The immune mechanism of drug-induced thrombocytopenia is often an IgG-mediated response with the platelet count falling weeks to years after therapy has been initiated (e.g. quinine, hydrochlorothiazide, imipramine, heparin, paracetamol).

Treatment and monitoring

Withdrawal of the responsible drug is usually followed by restoration of adequate platelet counts within several days. Recovery is quickest when the drug is rapidly excreted particularly if the thrombocytopenia is of the immune type as the drug is no longer available to participate in drug–antibody reactions.

If the platelet count is very low, platelet transfusions can be used. Corticosteroids may be beneficial if drug allergy is involved. Aspirin and non-steroidal anti-inflammatory drugs should be avoided as they decrease the effectiveness of the remaining platelets and may cause gastrointestinal bleeds.

Drug-induced thrombocytopenia is not predictable but when it has occurred, steps can be taken to avoid it in the future. In vitro agglutination tests can be performed to test for cross-sensitivity with drugs of a similar chemical structure. The drug allergy should be entered in the patient's notes and the patient counselled to inform medical staff of the allergy and to avoid exposure to over-the-counter preparations that may contain the drug. Quinine and heparin are worth highlighting. Quinine is found in OTC preparations, tonic water and soft drinks. If parenteral anticoagulation is unavoidable, a suitable alternative to heparin will be required such as snake venom or prostacyclin. Low molecular weight heparin may be safe for some patients but tests for cross-sensitivity should be carried out first.

HAEMOLYTIC ANAEMIA

Haemolysis involves the destruction of red blood cells with lysis of the cell membrane and the removal of red cell contents by phagocytosis. The life span of the red cell is shortened and anaemia results when bone marrow production can no longer compensate for the red cell destruction.

Drug-induced haemolytic anaemia occurs less frequently than agranulocytosis or thrombocytopenia.

Clinical presentation

Haemolytic anaemia can be either acute or chronic.

If acute the symptoms of anaemia will be severe with fatigue, weakness and breathlessness and may be accompanied by chills, fever and back pain. The increased destruction of the red cells will overwhelm the liver's ability to remove haemoglobin. Jaundice will occur and, when the plasma haemoglobin level is above 1 g per litre, haemoglobin will be excreted in the urine (haemoglobinuria).

In pronounced haemoglobinuria the urine will be black and renal failure can occur.

If haemolysis is due to an antibody–antigen reaction there may be symptoms of anaphylaxis.

Chronic haemolysis will present with mild to moderate anaemia unless the bone marrow compensates with a sufficient increase in red cell production, in which case the only evidence of chronic haemolysis will be a reticulocytosis and an enlarged spleen.

Mechanisms of drug induction

The severity and morbidity of haemolytic anaemia will depend on the mechanism of its induction. Drugs induce haemolytic anaemia by one of two basic mechanisms:

- a direct effect on the metabolic processes of the red cell
- an immune mechanism involving both the drug and the red cell.

Metabolic mechanism

Oxidative drugs cause damage to the cell membrane by denaturing haemoglobin and forming unstable complexes, which are seen on blood films as Heinz bodies (abnormal cell inclusions). Dapsone has this effect at high doses in all individuals but most drugs require a defect in red cell metabolism which is a genetically determined trait such as glucose-6-phosphate dehydrogenase (G6PD) deficiency, glutathione synthetase deficiency, glutathione reductase deficiency and glutathione peroxidase deficiency. The last three conditions are very rare but G6PD deficiency is common in certain ethnic groups, notably American Negroes and Mediterranean races.

Table 46.3 Drugs reported to induce haemolytic anaemia in patients with G6PD deficiency

Antimalarials: chloroquine, primaquine
Aspirin
Chloramphenicol
Dapsone
Nalidixic acid
Nitrofurantoin
Probenecid
Sulphonamides, sulphasalazine
Vitamin C
Vitamin K – water-soluble preparations

The disorder is transmitted by a sex-linked gene (X chromosome) of intermediate dominance. The clinical picture of this type of anaemia varies with the race of the subject and the nature and dose of the drug. Drugs causing haemolysis in G6PD deficiency are shown in Table 46.3.

Immune mechanism

There are two ways in which drugs can induce haemolytic anaemia by an immune mechanism:

Immune haemolysis: antibodies are formed against the drug. The antibodies, generally the IgM or IgG type, are formed during initial exposure to the drug. On further administration, a drug–antibody complex forms and absorbs on to the red cells where it activates the complement mechanism at the cell membrane, leading to cell lysis. Examples of drugs inducing this type of haemolysis appear in Table 46.4.

Table 46.4 Drugs which induce haemolytic anaemia by immunological mechanisms

Immune mechanism
  Cephalosporins
  Cimetidine
  Insulin
  Isoniazid
  Penicillins
  Quinine, quinidine
  Rifampicin
  Sulphonamides

Autoimmune mechanism
  Azapropazone
  Levodopa
  Mefenamic acid
  Methyldopa

A Coombs' test, which detects antibody, will only be positive whilst the drug is present in the serum, as the antibody will only react with the red cell membrane in the form of a drug–antibody complex.

Autoimmune haemolysis: antibodies are directed against components of the red cell membrane. This haemolysis is more common than the immune type and methyldopa is the commonest drug involved. The Coombs' test usually becomes positive after 3 to 6 months but it may be delayed for up to 3 years. It will always be positive, even in the absence of the drug. This is because the antibody is directed against the cell membrane and does not form a complex with the drug. Drugs involved through this mechanism appear in Table 46.4.

Treatment and monitoring

In patients with a known G6PD deficiency, all drugs that have been reported to cause haemolytic anaemia should be avoided. If drug-induced haemolysis does occur, on drug withdrawal the lysis will cease within a matter of days and the haemoglobin will return to normal.

Immune haemolytic anaemia presents acutely, often with haemoglobinuria and in some cases with evidence of renal failure. Only a small dose of drug is required to induce haemolysis but there is usually a history of previous administration. On drug withdrawal, haemolysis ceases and the blood picture returns to normal in 2 to 3 weeks. The patient may require general supportive measures such as dialysis. Haemolytic anaemias of the immune type respond well to treatment with corticosteroids.

With an autoimmune haemolysis not all patients with a positive Coombs' test will show signs of haemolysis. In those that do, withdrawal of the drug will produce a rapid reversal of the anaemia but the Coombs' test only becomes negative after 1 or 2 years.

MEGALOBLASTIC (MACROCYTIC) ANAEMIA

Megaloblastic anaemia occurs when DNA syn-

Table 46.5   Drugs reported to induce megaloblastic anaemia
Acyclovir
Anticonvulsants
Cycloserine
Methotrexate
Oral contraceptives
Pentamidine
Pyrimethamine
Sulphasalazine
Triamterine
Trimethoprim

thesis in the bone marrow is inhibited but RNA synthesis continues. Defective 'macrocytic' red blood cells are formed. The mechanism involves an interference with vitamin B_{12} or folate metabolism.

Megaloblastic anaemia is the least common drug-induced major haematological disorder. Table 46.5 lists examples of drugs implicated.

Clinical presentation

Megaloblastic anaemia presents insidiously with general signs of anaemia: weakness, fatigue, weight loss and glossitis. Neurological and mental changes are also common with peripheral neuropathy, irritability, depression and rarely acute psychosis (megaloblastic madness).

Mechanisms of drug induction

Drugs can induce megaloblastic anaemia in one of two ways:

- by inhibiting the absorption or utilization of B_{12} or folic acid
- by directly inhibiting DNA synthesis without depleting folate or B_{12} (cytotoxic agents).

Treatment and monitoring

Normal doses of folate reductase inhibitors such as co-trimoxazole and pyrimethamine will not usually induce megaloblastic anaemia but may aggravate pre-existing folate or B_{12} deficiencies. Methotrexate induces megaloblastic anaemia in a dose-related manner and, when large intravenous doses are used, 'rescue' with calcium leucovorin must be employed.

The anticonvulsant drugs such as phenytoin are associated with a low incidence of megaloblastic anaemia. The mechanism is believed to be a disturbance of folate metabolism and can be treated by giving folic acid supplements.

CASE STUDIES

CASE 46.1

G. S. is a 50-year-old male who developed acute renal failure following an emergency laparotomy which required haemodialysis. His platelet count fell to 14×10^9 per litre, at which time his drug therapy was: omeprazole, phenytoin and cisapride. His WCC and RBC were normal.

Q What are the possible causes of the thrombocytopenia and how should it be treated?

CASE 46.2

A heart transplant patient receiving triple immunosuppression; cyclosporin, azathioprine and prednisolone initially has weekly blood counts.

2 months post-transplant the white cell count falls to $2 \times 10^9/L$ with a neutrophil count of $0.5 \times 10^9/L$.

Q Why are weekly blood counts performed and what is the likely cause of the neutropenia?

ANSWERS TO CASE STUDIES

CASE 46.1

A Mr G. S. was suffering from severe thrombocytopenia (platelet count $<100 \times 10^9/L$) with nose bleeds and melaena. The possible causes were:

- consumptive haematoma
- drug-induced thrombocytopenia.

A drug-induced thrombocytopenia was the most likely cause. A consumptive haematoma (bleeding into the tissues) had been eliminated by assessing the uptake and survival of radiolabelled platelets. However, omeprazole and cisapride have not been reported to induce thrombocytopenia and phenytoin has only rarely been implicated.

It had been overlooked that the patient was receiving heparin during dialysis, as this was not recorded on the drug chart.

A diagnosis of heparin-induced thrombocytopenia was made using a platelet aggregation test. The heparin was stopped and it was possible to dialyse using low molecular weight heparin, which was negative for platelet aggregation in this patient.

CASE 46.2

A One of the reasons regular blood counts are performed is to monitor the toxic effect of the azathioprine on bone marrow. In this case the azathioprine has induced a neutropenia which will severely compromise the patient's ability to deal with infection.

The azathioprine must be stopped and antibiotic prophylaxis may be necessary. Once the white cell count returns to normal the azathioprine may be reintroduced but at a lower dose, since the bone marrow suppression is dose related.

BIBLIOGRAPHY

Beeley L, Drury V W M (eds). Treatment: a handbook of drug therapy. Edinburgh: Churchill Livingstone 1978

Davies D M (ed). Textbook of adverse drug reactions, 4th edn. Oxford: Oxford Medical Publications 1991
De Gruchy G C. Drug-induced blood disorders. Oxford: Blackwell Scientific Publications 1975
Girdwood R H (ed). Blood disorders due to drugs and other agents. Amsterdam: Excerpta Medica 1973

Chapter 47

Leukaemia

M. Nicolson   P. S. Warrington

Leukaemia, together with lymphoma are the main haematological malignancies. Although rare, they are of particular interest in that dramatic improvements in the prognosis for patients with these tumours have been achieved through the use of chemotherapy, and cure is now a possibility in a significant number of patients.

Many forms of leukaemia exist but they are all characterized by the production of excessive numbers of abnormal white blood cells.

The leukaemias can be broadly divided into 4 groups:

- acute myeloid leukaemia (AML)
- acute lymphoblastic leukaemia (ALL)
- chronic myeloid leukaemia (CML)
- chronic lymphoid leukaemia (CLL).

The leukaemias were originally defined as acute or chronic, on the basis of the patient's life expectancy. They are now classified on the basis of cell morphology and maturity. The adjective *myeloid* or *lymphoid* refers to the predominant cell involved and the suffix *cytic* or *blastic* to mature or immature cells respectively.

EPIDEMIOLOGY

Together the haematological malignancies account for only 5% of all cancers and of these CLL is the most common form of leukaemia in Europe and the United States (Table 47.1). CLL mainly affects an older age group; 90%

Table 47.1 Incidence of leukaemia in the UK (1984–1988)*

	New cases/year	Incidence per 100 000 of the population
CLL	3500	6.15
CML	650	1.05
ALL	650	1.02
AML	2000	3.35

* Reference: Leukaemia and lymphoma. An atlas of distribution within areas of England and Wales 1984–1988. Leukaemia Research Fund 1990.

of patients are over the age of 50 years and nearly two-thirds of patients are over 60 years. It rarely occurs in young people and is twice as common in men as in women. CML is primarily a disease of middle age with the median onset in the 40- to 50-year age group, but it can occur in young people.

Acute leukaemia is rare, with a total annual incidence of approximately 4 per 100 000 of the population. The more common form of the disease is AML, which accounts for 75% of cases of acute leukaemia. The incidence of AML rises steadily with age, occurring only rarely in young children. In contrast ALL is predominantly a childhood disease, with the peak incidence in the 3- to 5-year age group, and is the most common childhood cancer.

AETIOLOGY

In common with other cancers, leukaemia is thought to result from a combination of factors but its aetiology is not yet full understood. A number of specific risk factors for the development of leukaemia have, however, been identified from epidemiological studies.

Radiation

An increased incidence of leukaemia was noted as early as the 1940s in radiologists following occupational exposure. The association between ionizing radiation and the development of leukaemia is evident from nuclear disasters such as Hiroshima and more recently

Chernobyl. Long-term follow-up of survivors of Nagasaki and Hiroshima show an increase in all forms of leukaemia other than chronic lymphoid leukaemia, which appears to be dose related. The link is also apparent from patients who received radiotherapy for the treatment of non-malignant conditions such as ankylosing spondylitis. However, the effect of chronic low level exposure to radiation is less certain.

Exposure to chemicals and cytotoxic drugs

There is a small but definite risk of acute leukaemia occurring in patients successfully treated for other malignancies with cytotoxic and immunosuppressive agents. The combination of chemotherapy, especially alkylating agents such as cyclophosphamide, and radiotherapy presents the highest risk. This has practical implications as an increasing number of patients achieve a 'cure' as a result of combination therapy, whilst occupational exposure of health professionals to these agents is also an area of concern. Occupational exposure to paint, insecticides and solvents, in particular the aromatic solvent benzene, have all been associated with the development of leukaemia.

Viruses

Although a link between retroviruses and animal leukaemia is well recognized, no link has been found between viruses and the development of leukaemia in humans in the West. In the West Indies and Japan human T-cell lymphotrophic virus, an RNA retrovirus, has been linked to a rare T-cell leukaemia/lymphoma.

Genetic factors

Down's syndrome, an inherited chromosomal disorder, is associated with an increased risk of developing leukaemia. Other disorders that predispose to chromosomal breaks such as Fanconi's anaemia are also associated with an increased risk of developing acute leukaemia. Possibly these alterations allow for the expression of oncogenes which are genes capable of promoting malignant transformation.

PATHOPHYSIOLOGY

The leukaemias are characterized by excessive accumulation in the bone marrow and peripheral blood of immature blood cells which are, to a variable extent, functionally useless.

In leukaemia the normal process of haematopoiesis is altered (Fig. 47.1). Transformation to malignancy appears to occur in a single cell, usually at the pluripotential stem cell level, but sometimes it occurs in a committed stem cell with capacity for more limited differentiation. Accumulation leads to progressive impairment of the normal bone marrow function, and ultimately bone marrow failure.

Acute leukaemias

In acute leukaemia the normal bone marrow is replaced by a malignant clone of immature blast cells derived from the myeloid (AML) or lymphoid (ALL) series. More than 50% of the cellular elements of the bone marrow are replaced with blast forms and this is usually associated with the appearance of blasts in the peripheral circulation. Particularly with ALL, the blasts infiltrate the lymph nodes and frequently other tissues, such as liver, spleen, testis, and the walls of subarachnoid veins. AML may be subdivided according to the French–American–British (FAB) classification, depending on the predominant differentiation pathway and the degree of maturation (Table 47.2). For the M1, M2 and M3 classifications, granulocytic

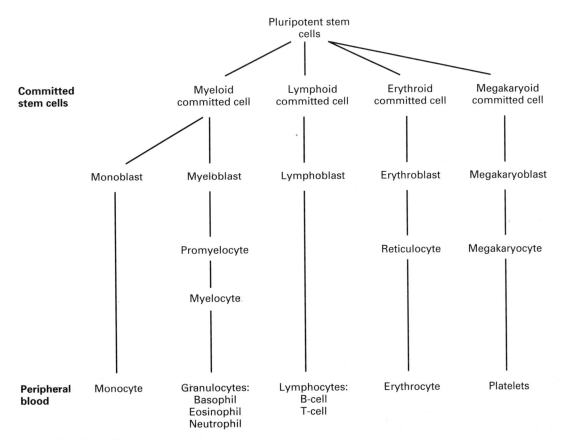

Fig. 47.1 Haematopoiesis.

Table 47.2 French–American–British (FAB) classification of AML

Classification	Leukaemia type	Adult distribution %
M1	Myeloblastic (undifferentiated)	20
M2	Myeloblastic	30
M3	Promyelocytic	10
M4	Myelomonocytic	25
M5	Monoblastic	10
M6	Erythroleukaemic	5
M7	Megakaryoblastic	<1

differentiation is predominant; for M4, differentiation is mixed granulocytic and monocytic; for M5 monocytic; for M6 erythroid; and for M7 differentiation is predominantly the megakaryocytic lineage. Although the clinical presentation may vary between types, no definite prognostic difference has yet been identified between the seven groups. An FAB classification based on cell morphology also exists for ALL but the disease is usually classified immunologically, based on the presence or absence of B-cell or T-cell markers (Table 47.3). Each subtype displays different clinical presentations, response to treatment and ultimately, prognosis, with c-ALL having the best prognosis and B-ALL the worst.

Chronic leukaemias

Chronic leukaemias are described as being lymphocytic (CLL) or myelocytic (CML). CLL is characterized by the appearance of apparently mature long-lived lymphocytes which accumulate in peripheral blood and give rise to a leucocytosis which may be very marked. In the majority of patients these lymphocytes have B-cell characteristics, but occasionally a T-cell type is seen. Eventually lymphocytes accumu-

late in lymph nodes and spread to other lymphoid tissue. The liver and spleen become moderately enlarged and the bone marrow is progressively infiltrated The cells appear morphologically normal but they are unable to secrete immunoglobulin or differentiate into plasma cells.

The characteristic feature of CML is the predominance of granulocytic cells in blood, bone marrow, liver, spleen and other organs. Different types of CML have been identified (Table 47.4). Chronic granulocytic leukaemia (CGL) is the most common form and further discussion will mainly refer to this form of CML, although the terms are often used interchangeably. CML was the first cancer to be associated with a specific chromosomal abnormality: the Philadelphia chromosome translocation (Ph[1]) seen in over 90% of cases. This is a translocation of genetic material between the long arms of chromosome 22 and chromosome 9. As a result an abnormal gene transcription occurs which may affect growth regulation.

Proto-oncogenes are normal genes with the potential to become oncogenes. The Ph[1] translocation results in the transposition of a proto-oncogene from its usual site on chromosome 9 to chromosome 22. A new oncogene is formed. This gene produces a protein which is associated with triggering growth factor receptors and it may be responsible for the uncontrolled growth of the leukaemic cells. Other oncogenes have also been implicated in CML.

CLINICAL MANIFESTATIONS

Most of the clinical manifestations of acute leukaemia are related to bone marrow failure, causing infection and bleeding, and the effects of infiltration of organs by the malignant cell

Table 47.3 Classification of ALL

Common ALL	Possessing the common ALL antigen; c-ALL
T-cell type	T-ALL
B-cell type	B-ALL or Burkitt's type
Null	Non-B, non-T and lacking c-ALL antigen

Table 47.4 Chronic myeloid leukaemias

Chronic granulocytic leukaemia (CGL)
Philadelphia negative CGL
Chronic myelomonocytic leukaemia (CMML)
Juvenile CML
Chronic neutrophilic leukaemia
Chronic eosinophilic leukaemia

population. The most common presenting symptoms of acute leukaemia include progressive weakness, lethargy and pallor due to anaemia. Approximately one third of patients will present with a serious skin or respiratory tract infection. Bleeding may be in evidence with purpura, bruising, bleeding mucous membranes and menorrhagia. The disease commonly presents with a short history, and left untreated it is rapidly fatal.

The involvement of other tissues such as spleen, liver and lymph nodes is more common in ALL than AML. Involvement of the CNS gives rise to headaches, vomiting and irritable behaviour. CNS disease is rare at presentation, but develops in up to 75% of children with ALL unless specific prophylactic treatment is given. Less commonly patients present with features of hypermetabolism, hyperuricaemia or bone pain.

Chronic leukaemia

In the case of CGL patients commonly present with nonspecific symptoms, such as malaise, weight loss and night sweats, or with symptoms of anaemia like fatigue, shortness of breath and pallor. The main physical sign is an enlarged spleen which may give rise to abdominal discomfort which worsens with progressive disease. Hepatomegaly is also detected in approximately 40% of newly diagnosed cases, but lymphadenopathy is less common. Neutropenia and thrombocytopenia are uncommon in the initial stage of disease. Thus, unlike the acute leukaemias, patients with CML rarely present with symptoms of infection or haemorrhage. In up to 30% of cases patients are asymptomatic and the disease is detected as a result of a routine blood test performed for other reasons.

The course of CGL may be divided into three phases. The initial chronic phase may last from several months to 10 years; the median is around 3 years. During this time treatment can alleviate symptoms and reduce the white blood count (WBC) and spleen size, allowing patients to lead near normal lives. An accelerated phase eventually occurs where the disease becomes more aggressive with progressively worsening symptoms, unexplained fevers, bone pain, anaemia, thrombocytopenia or thrombocytosis. Finally, after a period of weeks or months a blast crisis occurs, resembling fulminating acute leukaemia. In a small percentage of patients this occurs abruptly without warning.

As in CML, a proportion of patients are diagnosed as having CLL by chance. Presenting complaints may again be nonspecific: fatigue, anorexia, weight loss and shortness of breath. At diagnosis, findings usually include generalized lymphadenopathy and some enlargement of the liver and spleen. The course of CLL is variable; in some patients the disease may remain indolent for many years whilst others experience a steady deterioration in their health. The median survival varies from 2 to 7 years depending on the extent of disease. Patients are immunocompromised with granulocytopenia and a reduction in serum gamma globulin and are at increased risk of bacterial, viral and fungal infections. There may be an increased susceptibility to autoimmune disease such as immune haemolytic anaemias, thrombocytopenia and vasculitis. With progressive disease, anaemia and thrombocytopenia may become apparent resulting in incapacitating fatigue and bleeding episodes, and the disease becomes less responsive to treatment. Patients with CLL also have an increased risk of developing a second and even third malignancy, which may be attributed to impaired immune surveillance.

INVESTIGATIONS

Examination of peripheral blood and bone marrow are the key laboratory investigations carried out in cases of suspected leukaemia. However, some additional investigations can help in the diagnosis and classification of this group of diseases. Some of the main findings at diagnosis are presented in Table 47.5.

In acute leukaemia, leukaemic blast cells are usually found in the peripheral blood film unless the WBC is markedly reduced. The blasts of ALL and AML are distinguished using cytochemical stains. In CML the principal feature is

Table 47.5   Findings at diagnosis in leukaemia

	AML	ALL	CGL	CLL
WBC	↑ in 60%, may be N or ↓	↑ in 50%, may be N or ↓	↑, commonly 100–250 × 10⁹/L	Commonly ↑
Differential WBC	Many myeloblasts	Many lymphoblasts	Granulocytes ↑↑, esp. basophils and eosinophils <10% blasts present	Lymphocytes >10 × 10⁹/L
RBC	Severe anaemia	Severe anaemia	Anaemia common, esp. when spleen enlarged	Anaemia in about 50% of patients, generally mild
Platelets	↓	↓	Usually ↑, may be N or ↓	↓ in 20–30%
Bone marrow aspiration and trephine			Hypercellular. >15% blasts suggests transformation	Shows infiltration by lymphocytes
Cytogenic analysis			Presence of Ph¹ chromosome	
NAP score			↓ or zero	
Lymphadenopathy	Occasional	Common	Infrequent	Common
Splenomegaly	50%	60%	Usual and severe	Usual and moderate
Other features			Serum B₁₂ and B₁₂ binding protein ↑↑, serum uric acid and alkaline phosphatase ↑	Serum uric acid generally ↑, serum immunoglobulin ↓

Key: N – normal; ↓ – reduced; ↑ – increased

a leucocytosis with WBC ranging from 30–250 × 10^9/L comprising the complete spectrum from blasts to mature polymorphonuclear cells. The presence of >20% blast cells suggests impending blast transformation. In CLL it is lymphocytes in particular which are increased with levels exceeding 10×10^9/L. As with CML and the Philadelphia chromosome, non-random chromosome abnormalities are increasingly being identified in patients with leukaemia. The information obtained from cytogenic analysis of bone marrow or peripheral blood cells can be used to confirm the diagnosis and classification of leukaemia and may provide a guide to the likely response to treatment and prognosis.

TREATMENT

Although radiotherapy may be used to treat localized disease, the nature of leukaemia necessitates the use of systemic chemotherapy. Bone marrow transplantation increasingly has a role in the management of this disease. In the treatment of acute leukaemias the aim is to eradicate the disease and to restore normal bone marrow function. For the majority of patients with chronic leukaemia such intensive therapy carries greater risk without a corresponding increase in survival and thus the aim is to palliate the disease. Although significant progress has been achieved in the treatment of leukaemia, efforts are continually being made to bring about further improvements. This is largely done by evaluating changes in therapy through clinical trials. Studies are frequently carried out on a national basis and some of the main studies are coordinated by the Medical Research Council (MRC).

In addition to the specific antileukaemia treatment, general supportive therapy is needed, both to manage the disease and to manage the complications of therapy.

Acute leukaemia

At the outset, intensive combination chemotherapy is given in the hope of achieving a complete remission (CR). This initial phase of treatment is termed induction or remission induction chemotherapy. A complete remission can only be achieved by virtual ablation of the bone marrow, followed by recovery of normal haematopoiesis. If 2 to 3 cycles of therapy fail to induce CR an alternative drug regimen can be used. If this is unsuccessful it is unlikely that CR will be achieved. The subsequent duration of the first remission is closely linked to survival.

Remission is defined as the absence of all clinical and microscopic signs of leukaemia, less than 5% blast forms in the bone marrow and return of normal cellularity and haematopoietic elements. Despite achieving CR, occult residual disease may persist and further intensive therapy is given in an attempt to sustain the remission. This post-remission therapy may be

chemotherapy, or the combination of chemotherapy, radiotherapy and bone marrow transplantation.

Acute lymphoblastic leukaemia

The approach to therapy for adults with ALL has evolved along similar lines to that successfully employed in children although the results are generally less favourable (Table 47.6). The combination of vincristine and prednisolone will induce complete remission in about 85% of children with ALL. In adults, or children at high risk (patients under 2 years or over 9 years of age or with high blast cell counts), an anthracycline, l-asparaginase or both are included in the treatment, achieving a CR of 80% in adults. Other active drugs in the treatment of ALL include methotrexate, 6-mercaptopurine, cyclophosphamide, and mitoxantrone.

Patients with ALL are at a high risk of developing metastatic disease in the central nervous system. Cytotoxic drugs penetrate poorly into the central nervous system which thus acts as a sanctuary for leukaemic cells. Therefore all

Table 47.6 Treatment of ALL (adapted from MRC protocol)

	Dose	Route	Regimen
Induction (4 weeks)			
Vincristine	1.5 mg/m^2	i.v.	Weekly for 4 weeks
Prednisolone	40 mg/m^2	oral	Daily for 4 weeks
L-asparaginase	6000 u/m^2	i.m.	3 × weekly for 3 weeks
Daunorubicin	45 mg/m^2	i.v.	Daily for 2 days
Intensification (1 week)			
Vincristine	1.5 mg/m^2	i.v.	1 dose
Daunorubicin	45 mg/m^2	i.v.	Daily for 2 days
Prednisolone	40 mg/m^2	oral	Daily for 5 days
Etoposide	100 mg/m^2	i.v.	Daily for 5 days
Cytarabine	100 mg/m^2	i.v.	2 × daily for 5 days
Thioguanine	80 mg/m^2	oral	Daily for 5 days
CNS prophylaxis (3 weeks)			
Cranial irradiation	24 Gy		
Methotrexate	i.t. weekly for 3 weeks also given during induction and intensification		
Maintenance therapy (2 years)			
Methotrexate	20 mg/m^2	oral	Weekly
6-mercaptopurine	75 mg/m^2	oral	Daily
Prednisolone	40 mg/m^2	oral	5 days/month
Vincristine 1.5 mg/m^2 i.v.	Monthly		

Key: i.t. – intrathecal

patients with ALL who achieve complete remission receive some form of central nervous system prophylaxis. Cranial irradiation plus intrathecal methotrexate or high-dose systemic methotrexate have all been used. Craniospinal irradiation without intrathecal methotrexate is equally effective but substantially more myelotoxic.

With ALL, maintenance treatment is also given in an attempt to sustain a complete remission. It is usually gentler than induction or consolidation chemotherapy, but is carried on for at least 18 months. Treatment usually consists of weekly methotrexate and daily 6-mercaptopurine, although a variety of schedules are employed. Most schedules also include regular prednisolone and vincristine at 8 to 12 week intervals, often in association with further daunorubicin or cyclophosphamide.

The treatment of relapsed disease varies with the site of relapse. Isolated central nervous system or testicular relapse may be successfully treated with radiation and reinduction therapy, and cure can still be achieved for some patients. Bone marrow relapse is much more difficult to cure, even if it occurs late.

Acute myeloid leukaemia

The initial approach to the treatment of AML is similar to ALL. However, with AML the chemotherapy regimens used to achieve remission are much more myelotoxic, and patients require intensive supportive care to survive periods of bone marrow aplasia (Fig. 47.2). The pyrimidine analogue cytarabine has formed the basis of treatment for AML for 20 years. The addition of daunorubicin, probably the most effective single agent in AML, and oral thioguanine has achieved a CR rate of 75% in patients under the age of 60 years, and around 50% in those over 60 years. The precise dose and scheduling of these agents is continually being refined in order to improve the response rates. Amsacrine, etoposide and mitozantrone also show activity in AML and the place of these newer agents in the management of the disease is under investigation. Despite the numbers of patients who

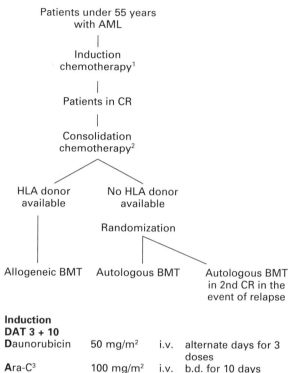

Induction			
DAT 3 + 10			
Daunorubicin	50 mg/m²	i.v.	alternate days for 3 doses
Ara-C³	100 mg/m²	i.v.	b.d. for 10 days
Thioguanine or	100 mg/m²	i.v.	b.d. for 10 days
ADE 10 + 3 + 5			
Ara-C	100 mg/m²	i.v.	b.d. for 10 days
Daunorubicin	50 mg/m²	i.v.	alternate days for 3 doses
Etoposide	100 mg/m²	i.v.	daily for 5 days
Consolidation			
MACE			
Amsacrine (**M**-amsa)	100 mg/m²	i.v.	daily for 5 days
Ara-C	200 mg/m²	i.v.	continuous infusion for 5 days
Etoposide	100 mg/m²	i.v.	daily for 5 days
MidAC			
Mitozantrone	10 mg/m²	i.v.	daily for 5 days
Ara-C	1 g/m²	i.v.	b.d. for 3 days

Fig. 47.2 Treatment of AML (adapted from MRC trial). Key to superscript numerals: 1 – more than one course of chemotherapy may be needed to induce remission; 2 – one to three courses of consolidation chemotherapy are given at approximately 4- to 6-week intervals depending on the speed of recovery of peripheral blood counts; 3 – Ara-C is cytarabine.

achieve CR following induction therapy, the majority of patients relapse, with only about 25% of patients becoming long-term disease-free survivors. Thus, in common with ALL, additional post-remission therapy is required. Consolidation with similar courses of chemotherapy, as used in induction, appears to offer little or no advantage. However, more intensive consolidation chemotherapy with high-dose cytarabine and daunorubicin or amsacrine appears to improve survival rates to approximately 50% after 3 years, with even more encouraging results being obtained in patients under 25 years of age. There is no clear role for maintenance therapy in AML. Similarly central nervous system prophylaxis is not routinely indicated although a relapse in the central nervous system may become more of a problem in AML if prolonged remissions are increasingly being attained.

An alternative approach to post-remission therapy is bone marrow transplantation. In patients under 40 years of age allogeneic bone marrow transplantation has resulted in disease-free survival of 45 to 65% at 5 years post-transplant, with these patients probably having achieved cure of their disease. However, only about 10% of patients are suitable for allogeneic bone marrow transplants, and it may be that, taking into account the age and generally better prognosis of this population of patients, intensive consolidation produces comparable results. Autologous bone marrow transplantation has also been performed in AML although it is still too early to draw conclusions on its success. Current MRC research is looking at the place of both autologous and allogeneic bone marrow transplantation in combination with intensive consolidation in the post-remission treatment of AML.

Chronic leukaemia

Chronic granulocytic leukaemia

The management of CGL continues to pose major problems. Progress has been very slow in comparison to the acute leukaemias and the prognosis remains poor with an average survival of 40 to 50 months. Treatment is essentially palliative, producing modest increases in survival, but with the main aim of keeping patients asymptomatic by maintaining the WBC below

$50 \times 10^9/L$. Hydroxyurea and busulphan are the most widely used drugs in the management of CGL in the chronic phase. Treatment with hydroxyurea is initiated at a dose of 1.5 to 2 g/day and usually brings the WBC under control within 1 to 2 weeks. The dose can then be reduced to a maintenance dose of 0.5 to 2 g/day. Withdrawing or reducing the dose abruptly can cause a rebound increase in WBC. The side effects of hydroxyurea are generally mild but include rashes and gut disturbances. Busulphan can be given either at a low daily dose of 2 to 6 mg or as a single dose of 50 to 100 mg at 4- to 6-week intervals. The main adverse effect of busulphan is myelosuppression, and treatment should be discontinued when the WBC falls to $20 \times 10^9/L$. In a few patients, myelosuppression is irreversible and its use must be closely monitored. Other side effects of busulphan include pulmonary fibrosis, sterility and cutaneous pigmentation.

The place of interferon in the management of CGL is currently under investigation.

Interferon can control symptoms of CGL and in contrast to conventional chemotherapy, it has also been shown to suppress the population of Ph^1 cells in approximately 20% of patients. This may be due to suppression of the oncogene. Another development has been the use of allogeneic bone marrow transplantation in selected patients under 50 years of age for whom a suitable donor can be found. There is a high risk of mortality with this procedure (20%) and 5 to 10% of patients relapse within the first 3 years, but there are now a number of long-term survivors who can be considered cured.

Transformation of CGL into acute leukaemia can be treated in the same manner as de novo acute leukaemia, in an effort to achieve a second chronic phase. Treatment is slightly more successful if transformation is lymphoid rather than myeloid but in general is less successful than the treatment of de novo leukaemia. Again allogeneic bone marrow transplantation can be attempted although the median duration of a second chronic phase is short and the mortality and risk of relapse are much worse than in chronic phase CGL.

Chronic lymphoid leukaemia

Although CLL is the most prevalent adult leukaemia, current therapy is unable to cure this disease. In view of the age of most sufferers with CLL and the indolent nature of the disease most patients are given no active treatment in the early stages of disease. Treatment is initiated in cases of:

- increasing or troublesome lymphadenopathy
- systemic symptoms
- marrow failure
- autoimmune complications.

The aim is to control the symptoms of progressive disease and improve the patient's quality of life. The alkylating agents, chlorambucil and cyclophosphamide, are commonly used. Prednisolone can reduce the lymphocyte count without contributing to myelosuppression and is given for autoimmune phenomena such as haemolytic anaemia and immune thrombocytopenia. Continued use of corticosteroids can increase the likelihood of infection and, wherever possible, treatment should be tailed off and discontinued within 6 to 8 weeks. Severe hypersplenism can be very painful as well as sequestering platelets and may necessitate splenic irradiation or splenectomy. Radiotherapy can also be used to control painful splenomegaly and localized lymphadenopathy. Combination chemotherapy, such as CHOP (Ch. 48) used in lymphoma may be beneficial in advanced disease. The new antimetabolite fludarabine also shows activity in the management of CLL.

An important aspect of the management of CLL is the treatment of intercurrent infections to which these patients are particularly prone. Herpes zoster for example can rapidly become generalized and requires prompt treatment with i.v. acyclovir.

Bone marrow transplantation

The potential role of bone marrow transplantation is increasingly being explored in the management of all types of leukaemia. This technique provides a means of overcoming the potentially lethal effects on the bone marrow of ablative therapy given in an attempt to eradicate all traces of disease (Fig. 47.3). The conditioning regimen most commonly used is a combination of high-dose cyclophosphamide and total body irradiation. Other conditioning regimens include high-dose melphalan, etoposide or cytarabine.

2 to 3 days elapse following administration of chemotherapy, to allow its elimination from the body, then previously harvested bone marrow is reinfused peripherally. The stem cells will return to and repopulate the marrow, hopefully restoring normal haematopoiesis. Harvested bone marrow is usually obtained from an HLA-matched donor and carried out under general anaesthetic. This is known as an allogeneic bone marrow transplantation or allograft. Under certain circumstances in the absence of a matched sibling donor, an autologous bone marrow transplantation or autograft can be performed. Following conditioning, the patients receive their own cryopreserved marrow which was previously harvested from them while in complete remission. Autologous bone marrow transplantation also allows the used of aggressive, high-dose chemotherapy to be given in the treatment of solid tumours. However, there is a potential risk that marrow obtained in this way may contain undetected, residual disease. Various methods have been explored of ridding the marrow of disease in vitro.

Following bone marrow transplantation, normal haematopoiesis and peripheral blood counts recover in 4 to 6 weeks. Throughout this time patients require intensive supportive care and the procedure, particularly allogeneic bone marrow transplantation, causes significant morbidity and has a mortality rate of 5 to 20%. The place of bone marrow transplantation in the management of a particular form of leukaemia depends very much on the prognosis of patients treated with conventional chemotherapy (Table 47.7). For example, the results of intensive chemotherapy in children with ALL are good and bone marrow transplantation is generally only considered for children who have relapsed and in whom a second remission can be achieved. However, treatment of adults is less successful and

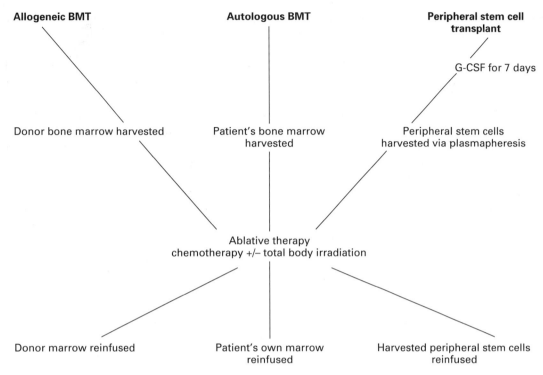

Fig. 47.3 Bone marrow transplantation.

allogeneic bone marrow transplantation may be offered to adults in first remission.

Peripheral stem cell transplantation

A new technique for rescuing bone marrow following ablative therapy, peripheral stem cell transplantation, is currently under investigation. Patients receive the haematopoietic growth factor G-CSF for a period of 7 days. This stimulates the release of stem cells into the peripheral circulation. Stem cells are then harvested from the peripheral circulation by a process of plasmapheresis. The harvested cells can then be reinfused into the patient following conditioning therapy. Peripheral stem cell transplantation offers some potential advantages over conventional bone marrow transplant techniques; collection of peripheral stem cells is simpler to carry out and it has also been found that the recovery period following transplantation is shortened by 10 to 14 days.

THE PATIENT
Supportive care

The treatment of CLL and CGL is largely carried out on an outpatient basis, with patients taking oral medication in the home, or attending outpatient clinics on a weekly or monthly basis for injections of chemotherapy. Patients are routinely monitored to follow the progress of disease and to observe treatment-related side effects. Supportive therapy such as blood transfusions can

Table 47.7 Indications for autologous bone marrow transplantation in leukaemia	
AML	First remission*
CGL	Chronic phase
ALL	First remission in adults*
	Second remission in children
CLL	Not appropriate
* Autologous BMT may be considered in acute leukaemia in the absence of a suitable donor.	

also be given on an outpatient basis. In contrast, the intensity of induction and consolidation regimens used in the management of patients with acute leukaemia, renders them pancytopenic. Therapy is usually given on an inpatient basis with patients remaining in hospital following treatment for 3 to 4 weeks until their bone marrow recovers sufficiently. This is in contrast to therapy for most solid tumours where, following administration of treatment, patients are well enough to remain at home until their next cycle of chemotherapy is due.

Advanced leukaemia, bone marrow transplants and aggressive chemotherapy for acute leukaemia, all result in pancytopenia. The life span of red blood cells is considerably longer than platelets or neutrophils and hence anaemia is usually the last sign to develop. Packed red cell transfusions are given to patients to maintain their haemoglobin above 8 to 9 g/dl. Evidence of bleeding includes petechial haemorrhages in skin and mucous membranes, and patients receiving aggressive treatment must be checked daily for any of the above signs. Platelet concentrates are given to patients who have signs of bleeding and may be given prophylactically should platelets fall below 20×10^9/L. The probability of infection developing rises as the WBC, specifically the neutrophil count, falls. With an absolute neutrophil count of below 0.5×10^9/L, patients are at high risk of infection developing; below 0.1×10^9/L, infection is almost inevitable, particularly if neutropenia is prolonged.

Chapters 48 and 49 will examine many of the non-haematological toxicities which result from the use of cytotoxic drugs, but in the management of acute leukaemia, infection is the major cause of morbidity and mortality.

Infection in the immunocompromised patient

A number of intrinsic and extrinsic factors all contribute to the risk of infection in this vulnerable group of patients (Fig. 47.4).

Whilst cross-infection can occur via staff, other patients or contaminated objects, the main

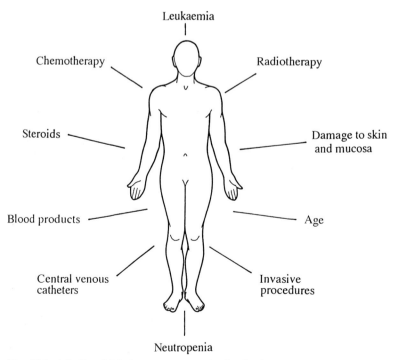

Fig. 47.4 Infection risk in immunocompromised patients.

sources of infection in this group of patients are endogenous, arising from commensal gut and skin organisms. The normal host defences to infection are broken down; damage to mucous membranes and the gut occur due to chemotherapy, especially the anthracyclines, and radiotherapy allows entry to the bloodstream of infecting organisms. Most infections in neutropenic patients arise from three main sites: the gastrointestinal and respiratory tracts, and the skin. Table 47.8 lists the main pathogens responsible for infection in this group of patients.

Preventive measures

Strenuous efforts must be made to minimize the risks of infection occurring.

Oral hygiene. Mouth care is important in all patients receiving chemotherapy but particularly neutropenic patients. Patients should receive regular chlorhexidine or povidone iodine antiseptic mouthwash every 2 to 4 hours and prophylactic antifungal therapy. Although it is important to avoid any sort of trauma to the oral mucosa, teeth should be cleaned regularly using a soft toothbrush. Attention must also be paid to the care of dentures. Patients require careful counselling on mouth care, stressing the importance of oral hygiene.

Prophylactic anti-infectives. In general, prophylactic antibiotics should be avoided because of the possible development of resistant organisms, but they may have a place in the management of periods of prolonged immunosuppression following chemotherapy for ALL and bone marrow transplantation. Prophylactic antifungal agents are routinely given and patients undergoing bone marrow transplantation and therapy for ALL require prophylaxis against cytomegalovirus and *Pneumocystis carinii* (Table 47.9).

Gut decontamination. Gut decontamination using a combination of non-absorbable oral antibiotics and antifungal agents reduces the population of potentially pathogenic organisms in the intestine. One such combination includes neomycin sulphate, colistin sulphate, nystatin and amphotericin. However, opinions are divided over this practice, as it can lead to the overgrowth of resistant organisms.

Growth factors. An exciting development in the care of patients with leukaemia has been the production of haematopoietic growth factors using recombinant DNA technology. The first of these, granulocyte colony-stimulating factor (G-CSF), given daily by subcutaneous injection or intravenous infusion after completion of chemotherapy, stimulates neutrophil production and reduces the duration of neutropenia by up to 7 days. The cost of these compounds is a major issue but their use may prove cost effective if the incidence of serious infection is reduced.

Table 47.8 Pathogens commonly causing infection in neutropenic patients	
Gram-negative bacteria	*Pseudomonas* species *Escherichia coli* *Klebsiella* species *Enterobacter* species *Proteus* species *Serratia* species *Legionella pneumophilia*
Gram-positive bacteria	*Streptococcus* species *Staph. epidermidis* *Staph. aureus*
Anaerobes	*Clostridium difficile* *Clostridium perfringens* *Bacteroides* species
Fungi	*Candida* species *Aspergillus* species
Viruses	Herpes simplex Herpes zoster Cytomegalovirus Hepatitis
Protozoa	*Pneumocystis carinii*

Table 47.9 Prophylactic anti-infectives	
Gram-negative bacteria	Co-trimoxazole Ciprofloxacin
Candidiasis	Ketoconazole Nystatin Fluconazole
Herpes simplex	Acyclovir
Cytomegalovirus	Co-trimoxazole
Pneumocystis carinii	Co-trimoxazole

Aseptic technique. Careful attention should be paid to the care of intravenous cannulae, particularly central venous catheters. The increased incidence of staphylococcal infection in immunocompromised patients can largely be attributed to their use. Invasive procedures, such as venepuncture, must be carried out using strict aseptic technique. Similarly, urinary catheters are a major source of infection and their use should be avoided if at all possible.

Protective isolation. Reverse barrier isolation during periods of neutropenia, and nursing in strict sterile environments have been used in an attempt to reduce infection rates. This is extremely demanding for staff and patients alike and is generally only appropriate with high-dose chemotherapy and following bone marrow transplantation.

Treatment of infection

Commonly, neutropenic patients show no signs of focal infection, e.g. they are unable to form pus. The only clinical manifestations of septicaemia might be general malaise or fever. A patient's condition can deteriorate very rapidly, collapse occurring within hours of the first signs of infection and so treatment should be instigated immediately. Following a febrile episode (temperature 38°C or more for 2 hours or 39°C or more for a single reading) cultures are taken immediately but intravenous antibiotics must be started empirically. Standard empirical therapy may involve the combination of an aminoglycoside with an antipseudomonal penicillin such as pipericillin to provide broad-spectrum bactericidal cover. In penicillin-allergic patients cefuroxime or cefotaxime may be substituted, but local resistance patterns are of paramount importance. Antibiotics with a broad spectrum of activity, such as ciprofloxacin, have been used as single agents, but further studies are required to support their use.

Vancomycin may be prescribed if an infected central venous catheter is suspected, to provide additional cover for staphylococci. Similarly metronidazole should be added to the antibiotic regimen to cover anaerobes if the clinical presentation suggests the source of the infection may be oral, perineal or gut. Therapy is subsequently modified on the basis of cultures but in the majority of neutropenic patients a causative organism is never identified.

If the pyrexia persists for more than 5 days in spite of adequate therapy, if cultures are repeatedly negative or if the patient's condition is deteriorating, systemic fungal infection should be suspected. Intravenous amphotericin is generally the first choice to ensure *Aspergillus* and *Candida* are covered. The main limitation of amphotericin is its toxicity, in particular nephrotoxicity. A new formulation of liposomal amphotericin may be appropriate in patients with pre-existing renal impairment or in cases where conventional amphotericin has induced nephrotoxicity. It also allows the dose of amphotericin to be escalated in those patients with life-threatening fungal infection who have failed to respond to conventional amphotericin.

Complications of bone marrow transplantation

Allogeneic bone marrow transplantation is associated with a very high mortality rate, approaching 20 to 25% in the 3- to 4-month period post-transplant.

Infection is almost inevitable in patients undergoing bone marrow transplantation. Other significant complications include interstitial pneumonitis and hepatic veno-occlusive disease but the major life-threatening complication is acute graft-versus-host disease (GVHD). The likelihood of GVHD occurring increases with age, with the result that allografts are largely restricted to patients under 45 years of age. GVHD is caused by T-lymphocytes in the donated marrow reacting to host tissues. The severity of the reaction ranges from a mild maculopapular rash to multisystem organ failure, with a high mortality rate. Acute GVHD occurs within 100 days of the bone marrow transplantation and typically presents with fever, rash, diarrhoea and liver dysfunction. Prophylactic therapy is routinely given with methotrexate or cyclosporin, alone or in combination, for 6 to 12 months post-transplant. Should an acute GVHD develop, high-dose methylprednisolone, cyclosporin, antithymocyte globulin and more recently, monoclonal antibodies have been used to treat the condition.

Chronic GVHD can occur in the 3 to 6 months following bone marrow transplantation. It is a multisystem disorder, with associated chronic hepatitis and profound immunosuppression. Treatment is succesful in approximately 50% of patients and consists of immunosupression with azathioprine and prednisolone together with prophylactic antibiotics; cyclosporin can also be used. The main cause of death is infection.

CASE STUDIES

CASE 47.1

Miss N. B. is a 22-year-old patient with ALL. A complete remission was obtained with chemotherapy and she went on to receive CNS prophylaxis with intrathecal methotrexate.

Q1 Why is methotrexate administered intrathecally?

Q2 How is this administration performed?

Q3 What precautions must be taken to avoid any adverse effects when administering intrathecal chemotherapy?

CASE 47.2

Mrs R. Y. is a 40-year-old woman undergoing an allogeneic bone marrow transplant for CGL. Post-transplant she experienced severe mucositis and gastrointestinal toxicity. She was unable to eat and take in adequate nutrition and in view of this was commenced on total parenteral nutrition. On day 16 she spiked a temperature and antibiotic therapy was initiated with gentamicin and piperacillin. 72 hours later the fever had not resolved and blood cultures remained negative. Daily blood counts taken to monitor the fall and recovery of her peripheral blood count revealed she was still pancytopenic. In patients such as Mrs R. Y. with persistent fever not responding to adequate antimicrobial therapy, there is a high possibility of systemic fungal infection, most commonly with *Candida* species. In light of this, therapy was commenced with intravenous amphotericin B.

Q1 What advice would you give to nursing and medical staff on the preparation and administration of amphotericin?

Q2 How might the need for venous access be met?

CASE 47.3

An order is received from the haematology ward to prepare the following chemotherapy for Mr K. B., a 33-year-old patient with ALL:

- Daunorubicin 90 mg
- Vincristine 3 mg.

Daunorubicin and vincristine have been prescribed as part of the following induction chemotherapy regimen for ALL:

Induction (4 weeks)
- Vincristine 1.5 mg/m^2 i.v.
- Daunorubicin 45 mg/m^2 i.v.
- Prednisolone 40 mg/m^2 oral daily for 4 weeks
- L-asparaginase 6000 units/m^2 i.m. three times weekly for 3 weeks

Mr K. B.'s height and weight were documented on admission to be 180 cm and 80 kg respectively giving him a body surface area of 2 m^2.

Q1 What further steps should be taken to ensure that the treatment given to Mr K. B. is optimal?

CASE 47.4

Mr T. G. is a 67-year-old man with a history of CLL. He has progressive disease with worsening symptoms and his treatment was changed to CHOP combination chemotherapy. The cytotoxic drugs were administered by slow intravenous injection in the hospital outpatient department and Mr T. G. was given a prescription for prednisolone to take to his pharmacy.

CHOP chemotherapy
- Cyclophosphamide 600 mg/m^2 i.v. on day 1
- Doxorubicin 30 mg/m^2 i.v. on day 1
- Vincristine 1.4 mg/m^2 i.v. on day 1
- Prednisolone 40 mg p.o. on days 1 to 5

Q1 What is the purpose of the prednisolone in this regimen?

Q2 How should the prednisolone be administered?

Q3 What advice would you give to Mr T. G. regarding the prednisolone?

Q4 Should Mr T. G. be supplied with a steroid warning card?

ANSWERS TO CASE STUDIES

CASE 47.1

A1 CNS penetration of most cytotoxic agents is very poor. Following an intravenous dose of 50 mg of methotrexate the peak CSF levels achieved are less than 0.1% of the corresponding plasma levels. Therefore in order to reach sanctuary sites in the CNS methotrexate may be injected directly into the subarachnoid space. The usual dose is 12 mg/m² to a maximum of 15 mg.

A2 Injection into the CSF is usually done by lumbar puncture. The patient lies horizontally in a fetal position to widen the vertebral spaces. The procedure is carried out under local anaesthetic. Distribution into the cisternae and ventricles can be improved with larger injection volumes. For most adults convenient volumes range from 5 to 15 ml. This is generally well tolerated if an equivalent amount of CSF is first removed or used as the diluent. When frequent access to the CNS is required, this may be achieved by the use of an Ommaya reservoir. This is a subcutaneous depot inserted in the scalp which allows direct intraventricular access.

A3 Administration of intrathecal methotrexate has been associated with a range of neurotoxic effects ranging from headache and blurred vision to motor dysfunction, convulsions and even coma. Toxicity is greater when intrathecal methotrexate is combined with cranial irradiation.

In order to avoid adverse effects from this procedure a number of precautions must be taken.

- Solutions must be preservative free, isotonic and preferably physiological.
- Strict aseptic technique is essential to prevent the introduction of infection into the spinal canal. The injection should be prepared aseptically and must be free from any particulate matter.
- Extreme care must be taken to avoid inadvertent intrathecal injection of other drugs which may have fatal consequences. Only methotrexate, cytarabine and hydrocortisone are likely to be given by intrathecal injection in the management of this group of patients.
- The patient is closely monitored for signs of raised intracranial pressure following injection.
- The patient is advised to lie flat for approximately 4 hours to minimize headache. Simple analgesia such as paracetamol may be prescribed.

CASE 47.2

A1 Amphotericin injection should be reconstituted with water for injection and added to glucose 5% infusion. It must not be administered with sodium chloride as solutions containing electrolytes will disrupt the colloidal suspension. The glucose should have a pH greater than 4.2 and phosphate buffer may be added to ensure this. The infusion should pass through an in-line filter with a mean pore diameter greater than 1 μm to retain any aggregates of amphotericin which may form. It should also be protected from light. A final concentration less than 0.1 mg/ml reduces the chance of aggregate formation and minimizes thrombophlebitis. Nephrotoxicity is the most serious adverse effect of amphotericin therapy and the dose of amphotericin is increased gradually to minimize this problem. A number of dosing schedules have been adopted, but in a critically ill patient such as Mrs R. Y. treatment may be started with 0.5 mg/kg/day and increased each day by 0.25 mg/kg to a maximum dose of 1 mg/kg/day. Hypersensitivity reactions can also occur and a test dose of 1 mg may be administered prior to starting treatment. Other acute toxicities of amphotericin include fever, chills, nausea, vomiting, headache, myalgia and arthralgia. If fever does occur patients can be given hydrocortisone and chlopheniramine prior to subsequent doses. Toxicity is also minimized by administering the drug over at least 6 hours.

Mrs R. Y.'s renal function and electrolytes must be carefully monitored throughout the course of treatment with amphotericin. The risk of renal toxicity is increased when other nephrotoxic agents, such as aminoglycosides, are prescribed concurrently. Patients frequently develop hypokalaemia during amphotericin therapy and potassium levels must be carefully monitored and oral or parenteral potassium supplements are commonly required.

New formulations of amphotericin have been developed to overcome the toxicity of the existing amphotericin preparation. Liposomally encapsulated amphotericin, enables much higher doses of amphotericin to be administered without the usual toxicities, especially nephrotoxicity. This allows the use of amphotericin in patients with pre-existing renal disease or patients who have experienced amphotericin-induced nephrotoxicity. The new formulations also permit the dose to be escalated over 1 mg/kg in cases of life-threatening infection which could not be eradicated with conventional doses.

A2 For most patients with acute leukaemia, venous access eventually becomes a problem. Peripheral veins become thrombosed with repeated injections of chemotherapy and other agents. Patients can also become increasingly distressed by repeated venepunctures. At the outset of treatment most patients will have a central venous catheter inserted. The tip of the catheter is inserted into the superior vena cava, via the cephalic vein and exits through a subcutaneous tunnel in the chest wall. This is usually performed under a general anaesthetic. The line can have up to 3 lumens and this allows the administration of drugs, parenteral nutrition, blood products and access for sampling blood. Provided the line is placed correctly, vesicant drugs can also be safely given via a central line without fear of them causing soft-tissue damage. The major complication with central venous lines is the risk of infection; local soft-tissue infection of the subcutaneous tunnel or more serious bacteraemia or septicaemia. To lessen this risk, local policies should be implemented which lay down specific procedures for catheter care. Infection rates are minimized by reducing manipulation of the line. Handling of central venous catheters is frequently restricted to designated, trained personnel. Where appropriate, patients may be trained to look after their lines themselves.

CASE 47.3

A Presciptions for cancer chemotherapy are often complex involving combinations of both parenteral and oral cytotoxic drugs, intravenous fluids and other supportive therapies. To effectively monitor and check prescribing, the pharmacist must recognize and anticipate a whole range of potential problems.

Initially it must be determined if the therapy forms part of an established regimen or clinical trial protocol. Doses of cytotoxic drugs must be individually calculated for each patient on the basis of weight or more commonly, on body surface area.

Mr K.B.'s surface area was found to be 2 m², confirming the dose of daunorubicin; however, the maximum dose of vincristine which should be given to any patient regardless of his or her surface area is 2 mg.

The regimen also contains the drugs prednisolone and asparaginase. Particular attention must be paid to oral therapy such as prednisolone where the stop date should be clearly indicated on the prescription sheet to ensure that it is not continued inadvertently.

The protocol should be checked to confirm the scheduling of the chemotherapy. Vincristine is to be given weekly for 4 weeks and daunorubicin is given on 2 consecutive days. When treatment is being prepared, steps must be taken to find out when it is intended to administer the chemotherapy to ensure that the drug will be used within its expiry time. Some agents such as melphalan are unstable and must be administered soon after they are prepared. In situations such as this, arrangement for the preparation and administration of the drug must be carefully coordinated.

This chemotherapy regimen will give rise to myelosuppression and the effects on Mr K. B.'s peripheral blood counts need to be carefully monitored throughout treatment. In general a course of chemotherapy would be delayed in patients with a white cell count below 3000/mm³ or a platelet count below 100 000/mm³ to ensure that the bone marrow had sufficient reserve to withstand treatment. However, in patients with acute leukaemia it is more important to initiate treatment without any delay despite the fact that they may present with deranged peripheral blood counts.

All cytotoxic drugs have a low therapeutic index and doses of the drug may require adjustment in the presence of renal or hepatic impairment to ensure that delayed excretion does not result in toxicity.

Vincristine and daunorubicin are eliminated via hepatic metabolism and it is generally recommended that the doses of both drugs should be reduced if there is evidence of impaired liver function. Mr K. B.'s liver function tests should be examined, but again unlike the situation with many solid tumours, it may be more important to initiate treatment aggressively in this disease with full doses of chemotherapy unless his liver function tests were grossly deranged. Asparaginase can give rise to elevated liver enzymes and these should be monitored throughout treatment.

The routes of drug administration should be confirmed and advice given on appropriate infusion fluids or dilution, or the rate of infusion should this be necessary. Both vincristine and daunorubicin are administered as an intravenous bolus injection and are capable of causing severe local tissue necrosis in the event of extravasation. If the drugs are being administered into a peripheral vein, then a fast-running intravenous infusion of sodium chloride should be established. The cytotoxic drugs are then slowly administered via the injection port of the drip tubing. Many patients being treated for acute leukaemia will have had a central venous line inserted and vesicant chemotherapy can be safely given directly in this way.

Appropriate supportive therapy should be prescribed for the patient. In the case of Mr K. B. the prescribed combination of chemotherapy is likely to give rise to some degree of nausea and/or vomiting and prophylactic antiemetics will be required. Allopurinol should also be prescribed to avoid the risk of precipitating gout caused by elevated uric acid levels associated with the death or breakdown of large numbers of cells.

Prohylactic anti-infectives may be required depending on local policies, in particular the patient should be started on an oral hygiene regimen to avoid the mouth becoming a source of infection. Prophylactic therapy with the growth factors G-CSF or GM-CSF again may be considered.

Finally, every effort should be made to ensure that all treatment is clearly and accurately documented in the patient's case notes. This is particularly important with agents such as daunorubicin where toxicity is related to the total cumulative dose delivered throughout the entire treatment period.

CASE 47.4

A1 In the case of Mr T. G., prednisolone forms part of his anticancer therapy.

The uses of corticosteroids in oncology and haematology are many and varied. They have a role in the management of complications arising from therapy, such as the use of dexamethasone in the management of chemotherapy-induced nausea and vomiting, and also in managing complications of disease, such as spinal cord compression. In patients with lymphoma, leukaemia, breast cancer and brain tumours the glucocorticoids play a part in the treatment of the disease itself. The discovery of the tumour-suppressing activity of corticosteroids was arrived at empirically and the exact mechanism that results in cell lysis remains unknown although knowledge of steroid effects on gene expression and cell growth is increasing rapidly.

A2 The prednisolone can be taken as a single daily dose or in divided doses. Whether or not the enteric-coated preparation actually reduces the risk of peptic ulcer is unproven; despite this many clinicians favour the use of enteric-coated preparations of prednisolone which are only available in strengths of 2.5 and 5 mg. Use of 25 mg prednisolone tablets would considerably reduce the number of tablets Mr T. G. has to take each day.

A3 A number of points concerning the use of corticosteroids need to be emphasized;

- Patients often have misconceptions over the use of steroids and it is important to stress that the steroids form part of the active therapy for CLL.
- Ensure that the patient is aware of the correct dose. Mr T. G. may be taking up to 8 tablets in a single dose and he should be reassured that this is correct.
- Treatment is to be stopped after 5 days of therapy. There is potential for confusion if the information supplied to the GP is inadequate, resulting in treatment with prednisolone being continued inadvertently. Therefore Mr T. G. should be fully informed as to the number of days on which he has to take the prednisolone and that treatment should be stopped after that time.

Mr T. G. should be aware of potential side effects and given advice on how to minimize the risk of these developing. Prednisolone should be taken with food to minimize gastrointestinal disturbance and Mr T. G. should be alerted to the need to inform his doctor should any GI symptoms develop.

Euphoria and an increase in appetite are often seen with steroids and may not be a disadvantage in patients with neoplastic disease. This may, however, give rise to insomnia or disturbed sleep. These problems can be aggravated if patients take the medication last thing at night. Patients should be advised to take the dose of prednisolone no later than 6 p.m. Administration in the morning is preferable as the effect on cortisol secretion is least at this time.

More severe psychiatric disturbances can occur, with patients becoming emotionally labile, undergoing personality changes and even experiencing major psychosis.

A4 While the majority of the information contained in the steroid warning card is consistent with the advice given to Mr T. G., the statement that steroids should not be stopped abruptly may cause confusion. Perhaps the most appropriate course of action is to design an information leaflet specifically for this group of patients.

BIBLIOGRAPHY

Bunch C. Bone marrow failure. Medicine International 1992; 97: 4032–4034

Cranfield T, Bunch C. Acute leukaemias. Medicine International 1992; 97: 4038–4044

Goldman J M, James N D. Leukaemia and bone marrow transplantation. In: Sikora K, Halnan K E (eds) Treatment of cancer, 2nd edn. London: Chapman & Hall 1990

Henke Yarbro C (ed) Adult leukaemia. Seminars in Oncology Nursing. 1990; 6: 1–88

Jones L, Goldman J M. Mangement of chronic leukaemias. Medicine International 1992; 97: 4045–4049

Leukaemia and lymphoma. An atlas of distribution within areas of England and Wales 1984–1988. Leukaemia Research Fund 1990

Parr M D, Messino M J, McIntyre W. Allogeneic bone marrow transplantation: procedures and complications. American Journal of Hospital Pharmacy 1991; 48: 127–137

Singer C R J. Bone marrow transplantation. Medicine International 1992; 97: 4054–4057

Souhami R, Tobias J. Leukaemia. In: Cancer and its management. Oxford: Blackwell Scientific Publications 1986

Whittaker J A, Delamore I W (eds). Leukaemia. Oxford: Blackwell Scientific Publications 1987

Malignant disorders

Chapter 48

Lymphomas

C. A. Stevens   M. C. Maclean   S. M. Kelsey

The lymphomas are malignant tumours of lymph nodes or other lymphatic tissues. The primary cancerous cell of origin is the lymphocyte; as a result there is often considerable overlap between lymphomas and lymphoid leukaemias. The lymphomas are divided into two major groups, namely Hodgkin's disease and the non-Hodgkin's lymphomas.

HODGKIN'S DISEASE

Hodgkin's disease, described by Thomas Hodgkin in 1832, has an incidence in the United Kingdom of 2 per 100 000 population. It is predominantly a disease of young adults, having a peak incidence between the ages of 15 and 40 years. Males are affected more often than females (ratio approximately 1.5:1). The aetiology is unclear although both a genetic susceptibility and an underlying viral infection, possibly the Epstein–Barr (glandular fever) virus, have been proposed as causative factors. There is an increased incidence of the disease of up to seven times in blood relatives of affected persons.

Clinical features

Hodgkin's disease usually presents with painless enlargement of lymph nodes, often in the neck. This may be associated with symptoms such as fever, night sweats and weight loss. These have prognostic significance and are designated 'B' symptoms. Others include malaise, itching or pain at the site of enlarged nodes after drinking alcohol. Bone pain may result from skeletal involvement. Primary involvement of the gut, central nervous system or bone marrow is rare. Laboratory findings include anaemia, a raised erythrocyte sedimentation rate and eosinophilia. There is often a disturbance of immune function. The diagnosis is made by lymph node biopsy.

Histopathology

The diagnostic feature of Hodgkin's disease is the identification of the giant binucleate Reed–Sternberg cell. The disease is subclassified into four histological types:

- nodular sclerosing, which is the commonest type in the UK and commoner in women
- lymphocyte predominant
- mixed cellularity, which is commoner in older males and carries a poor prognosis
- lymphocyte depleted.

Investigations and staging

Once the diagnosis has been made on a biopsy, further investigations are needed to assess disease activity and the extent of its spread through the lymphoid system or other body sites. This is called 'staging' (Table 48.1) and has considerable prognostic significance with cure rates for localized tumours (stage I or II) being much higher than those for widespread disease (stage IV). The most effective ways of staging are by chest X-ray and computerized tomographic (CT)

scanning. Other useful tests include erythrocyte sedimentation rate, serum lactate dehydrogenase and liver function tests. Rarely, a laparotomy with liver biopsy and splenectomy is required for accurate staging.

NON-HODGKIN'S LYMPHOMA

The non-Hodgkin's lymphomas are a heterogeneous group of lymphoid malignancies ranging from indolent, slow-growing tumours to aggressive, rapidly fatal disease. Paradoxically, the more aggressive non-Hodgkin's lymphomas are more susceptible to anticancer therapy. The overall incidence of non-Hodgkin's lymphoma in the United Kingdom is 7 per 100 000. The disease is rare in subjects less than 30 years old and increases steadily in incidence with increasing age. Childhood non-Hodgkin's lymphoma is commoner in developing countries than in developed nations.

The aetiology is unclear although immunosuppression, such as following organ transplantation, may predispose to the development of lymphoma, possibly in association with Epstein–Barr virus infection. Infection with the human immunodeficiency virus (HIV-1) is associated with an increased incidence of lymphoma and there is an increased risk amongst survivors of atomic explosions. There is some evidence that Burkitt's lymphoma, an aggressive B-cell lymphoma common in West African children, is caused by an interaction between Epstein–Barr virus infection and malaria.

Non-Hodgkin's lymphoma usually presents as enlargement of lymphoid tissue, although extranodal presentation or spread is more common than in Hodgkin's disease. The gut, bone marrow or nervous system are not uncommon sites of presentation. 'B' symptoms may be present but lack prognostic significance. T-cell lymphomas commonly present with skin infiltration. Laboratory examinations may reveal anaemia, a raised erythrocyte sedimentation rate and raised serum lactate dehydrogenase. There may be reduction in circulating immunoglobulins and a monoclonal paraprotein may be seen in a small number of cases. The immune disruption caused

Table 48.1 The Ann Arbor staging classification for Hodgkin's disease	
Stage I	Involvement of a single lymph node region
Stage II	Involvement of two or more lymph node regions on the same side of the diaphragm
Stage III	Involvement of lymph node regions on both sides of the diaphragm
Stage IV	Diffuse or disseminated involvement of one or more extralymphatic organs

Note: suffix a = without B symptoms e.g. stage Ia; suffix b = with B symptoms e.g. stage Ib.

by the disease may also result in an increased susceptibility to viral infection or autoimmune haemolytic anaemia or thrombocytopenia.

Histopathology and classification

There have been many attempts to classify the non-Hodgkin's lymphomas into histological categories which have clinical significance. In addition to histological appearance, the lymphocyte subtype from which the tumour is thought to be derived is also taken into consideration. Approximately 90% of true non-Hodgkin's lymphomas are of B-cell origin while a minority are of T-cell origin or are unclassifiable. Probably the most useful classification is the Kiel classification which divides them into high grade lymphomas and low grade lymphomas (Table 48.2). The Working formulation of 1980 adds a third group, intermediate grade.

Chromosomal abnormalities may also be of diagnostic importance; for instance, African Burkitt's lymphoma is invariably associated with a specific translocation between chromosomes 8 and 14. In future more sophisticated techniques, such as new immunological markers and detection of rearrangements of the immunoglobulin or T-cell receptor genes, may facilitate more accurate subclassification.

Table 48.2 Kiel classification of the non-Hodgkin's lymphomas	
High grade	Composed of blast-like, immature cells which usually give rise to an aggressive tumour. May be B-cell or T-cell. Subgrouped into either: (a) centroblastic (b) lymphoblastic (c) immunoblastic (d) unclassified
Low grade	Composed of more mature cells usually giving rise to a slower-growing tumour. Again may be either B-cell type or T-cell type. Subgrouped into either: (a) lymphocytic lymphoma (which includes the T-cell tumours, mycosis fungoides and Sézary syndrome, and may also include chronic lymphocytic leukaemia) (b) lymphoplasmacytoid lymphoma

Investigations and staging

The non-Hodgkin's lymphomas can be staged according to the Ann Arbor classification used for Hodgkin's disease but without the use of the A (without 'B' symptoms) or B (with 'B' symptoms) suffixes. Nodal enlargement can be assessed by computerized tomography. Bone marrow trephine biopsy will detect bone marrow involvement which is more common than in Hodgkin's disease. Erythrocyte sedimentation rate, serum lactate dehydrogenase and serum beta$_2$-microglobulin levels may indicate disease activity and can be of prognostic importance.

COMPLICATIONS OF HODGKIN'S DISEASE AND THE NON-HODGKIN'S LYMPHOMAS

The complications of the lymphomas can be divided into those of the disease itself and those of the treatment. Complications of therapy are discussed later. The disease itself may present with large nodes which have a direct compressive effect on other organs such as the trachea or bronchi. Direct involvement of extralymphatic tissues may occur. Infiltration of the bone marrow may lead to bone marrow failure. Spinal cord compression may occur as a presenting feature while involvement of the brain is more often a feature of lymphoma relapsing after therapy. Lung involvement may be associated with development of pleural effusions and has a poor prognosis. Other complications of the lymphomas include disturbance of the immune system with increased susceptibility to infection and, occasionally, autoimmune haemolytic anaemia or thrombocytopenia.

PROGNOSIS

Hodgkin's disease and high grade non-Hodgkin's lymphomas are aggressive diseases which are rapidly fatal if untreated. The objective of therapy is to achieve eradication of the disease and thus affect a cure, which is reflected clinically as long-term disease-free survival. The prognosis for Hodgkin's disease, if treated optimally, depends predominantly on the stage of the disease at diagnosis, the presence of B symptoms and the histological subtype. Stage Ia disease has an extremely good prognosis with 5-year disease-free survival in the region of 95%. By contrast the 5-year disease-free survival rate for those with IVb disease may be as low as 40%. Males, and those of older age, tend to have a poorer prognosis. The prognosis for high grade non-Hodgkin's lymphoma depends largely upon age and histological subtype. Overall, with optimal therapy, 2-year disease-free survival is about 50%.

Low grade non-Hodgkin's lymphomas are difficult to eradicate with anticancer therapy. The indolent nature of the disease may mean that therapy is not required for some years until symptoms or complications develop. Treatment, when required, is aimed at controlling the disease rather than eradication. The low grade lymphomas may be consistent with long-term survival of 10 to 15 years from diagnosis.

TREATMENT

The management of Hodgkin's disease (HD) and non-Hodgkin's lymphoma (NHL) is different and will therefore be discussed separately. In both cases the appropriate treatment is determined by the stage and grade of disease. The various treatments are subject to much research and controversy with new data being published all the time. As information to determine the optimum treatment is being investigated, many patients diagnosed with a lymphoma in the UK will be entered into one of the ongoing national clinical trials. Groups such as the BNLI (British National Lymphoma Investigation), NCI (National Cancer Institute, USA) and the ICRF (Imperial Cancer Research Fund) co-ordinate large national and international multicentre studies comparing different treatment strategies.

Hodgkin's disease

Hodgkin's disease is, in general, sensitive to radiotherapy and cytotoxic chemotherapy. The aim of treatment is to obtain complete remission.

This is defined as a complete disappearance of all tumour and symptoms, with a return to normal activity by the patient.

Localized disease

Localized disease which has been clinically staged as I or II is usually treated by radiotherapy alone, unless the patient exhibits B symptoms when more aggressive therapy is required. Where the disease is confined to above the diaphragm the mantle field is used (Fig. 48.1). The inverted Y field is employed when the disease is confined to below the diaphragm (Fig. 48.1). The adjacent organs such as the lungs and gonads are shielded from the radiation by the use of specially moulded lead blocks so that only the radiation field is exposed. The field is irradiated with X-rays, delivered as daily fractions over 3 to 4 weeks. Most studies using mantle field radiation on localized disease report that 40% of patients relapse within 10 years of treatment. Relapse usually

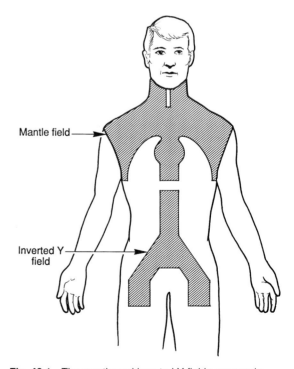

Fig. 48.1 The mantle and inverted Y fields commonly employed in the treatment of Hodgkin's disease.

occurs below the diaphragm and it is then assumed that the disease is widespread. Combination cytotoxic chemotherapy then becomes the
treatment of choice. Research investigating the
use of combination chemotherapy in localized
disease has not shown any significant overall
advantages. The additive toxicities, particularly
bone marrow suppression and nausea and vomiting, are generally more severe. Most centres,
therefore, use radiotherapy for localized disease
and then use combination chemotherapy to
treat any subsequent relapse.

Advanced disease

Patients with stage IIb or greater are treated
with chemotherapy. It is uncommon to obtain
a complete remission with a single cytotoxic
agent and these responses tend to be short-lived.
Subsequent relapses tend to be less responsive
to further chemotherapy. Combination chemotherapy is, therefore, the treatment of choice.

Most regimens are based on the MOPP regimen which was introduced in the late 1960s.
It comprises mustine (alkylating agent), vincristine, procarbazine and prednisolone (Table 48.3).
The cycle is repeated every month until six
cycles have been administered. The results of
one 10-year follow-up study of 188 patients
treated with MOPP showed that 84% of patients
achieved complete remission with 66% remaining disease free at 10 years. MOPP causes severe
nausea, vomiting and myelosuppression and is
likely to cause sterility which may be permanent.
Because many patients are young, sperm bank-
ing is recommended for males before treatment
commences. There have also been reports of
secondary malignancies, particularly leukaemias,
associated with MOPP. Most of the side effects
can be attributed to the mustine.

Most of the recent research has been aimed
at comparing new regimens with MOPP in
order to find a combination which is as effective
but with fewer side effects. One study comparing
MOPP with LOPP (chlorambucil used instead
of mustine) has shown no significant difference in response rates but with significantly
less myelosuppression, emesis and secondary
malignancies with the LOPP combination.

The outlook for patients who fail to respond
to MOPP is poor (Fig. 48.2). The addition of an
anthracycline (e.g. doxorubicin) in EVAP (Table
48.3) has been shown to improve complete response rates. The use of alternating regimens
such as LOPP/EVAP is being investigated in
patients who have relapsed or are refractory to
conventional chemotherapy. The role of intensive chemotherapy followed by bone marrow
transplantation is also the subject of current
research.

Table 48.3 Combination chemotherapy regimens which have been used in the treatment of advanced Hodgkin's Disease

Regimen	Dose & route	Frequency
MOPP (28-day cycle)		
M Mustine	6 mg/m^2 i.v.	Day 1 & 8
O Vincristine (Oncovin)	1.4 mg/m^2 (max. 2 mg) i.v.	Day 1 & 8
P Procarbazine	100 mg/m^2 (max. 200 mg) oral	Days 1–14
P Prednisolone	40 mg/m^2 oral	Days 1–14
LOPP (28-day cycle)		
L Chlorambucil (Leukeran)	10 mg oral	Days 1–10
O Vincristine	1.4 mg/m^2 (max. 2 mg) i.v.	Day 1 & 8
P Procarbazine	100 mg/m^2 (max. 200 mg) oral	Days 1–14
P Prednisolone	25 mg/m^2 oral	Days 1–14
EVAP (28-day cycle)		
E Etoposide	150 mg/m^2 oral	Days 1–3
V Vinblastine	6 mg/m^2 (max. 10 mg) i.v.	Day 1 & 8
A Doxorubicin (Adriamycin)	25 mg/m^2 i.v.	Day 1 & 8
P Prednisolone	25 mg/m^2 oral	Days 1–14

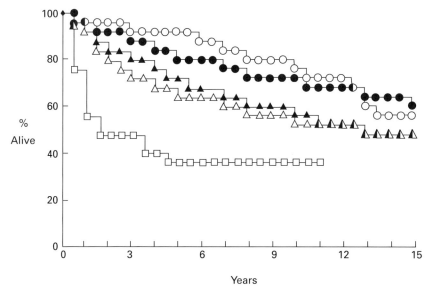

Fig. 48.2 Overall survival in non-Hodgkin's lymphomas divided according to histological type (BNLI). *Key:* ○ LP, 149; ● NSI, 1225; △ NSII, 671; ▲ MC, 482; □ LD, 41; LP, lymphocyte predominant; NSI, nodular sclerosis: low grade; NSII, nodular sclerosis: high grade; MC, mixed cellularity; LD, lymphocyte depleted. (Reproduced with permission from Linch D C, Vaughan-Hudson B 1988 The management of Hodgkin's disease and Non-Hodgkin's lymphomas. In: Hoffbrand A V (ed) Recent advances in haematology. Churchill Livingstone, Edinburgh).

Non-Hodgkin's lymphoma

The management of NHL is dependent upon whether the disease is high grade or low grade. Comparing studies from different centres is difficult due to varying study entry criteria and the fact that many patients are elderly. Other diseases may therefore have an impact on survival data. Low grade NHL runs a slow but indolent course. The advanced stages, which tend to be less responsive to treatment, are eventually fatal to the patient. The high grade lymphomas are more aggressive but are generally more responsive to treatment. The survival curves for low and high grade disease therefore cross at around 10 years (Fig. 48.3).

Low grade non-Hodgkin's lymphoma

When the lymphoma is localized (stages I and II), radiotherapy alone is generally used. An extended field, such as the mantle, has no proven advantage. Only the involved field is therefore irradiated. Some centres prefer to use chemotherapy to treat stage II disease. The use of adjuvant chemotherapy (i.e. chemotherapy combined with radiotherapy) has shown conflicting results making its role controversial.

Where the disease is more advanced there is much controversy as to the appropriate treatment. Most current research is aimed at comparing single agent alkylating agents with combination chemotherapy. The BNLI are comparing CHOP (Table 48.4) with chlorambucil in the treatment of stage III and IV low grade NHL. Results analysed to date, after 148 patients, showed complete remission with CHOP (53%) to be significantly greater than with chlorambucil (35%). The overall survival rate in these patients at 2 years, however, is not significantly different. Since most patients are elderly, chlorambucil is more commonly used as it is better tolerated than CHOP. Some centres adopt a 'wait and see' policy and treat symptomatically. The overall aim is to maintain a good quality of life

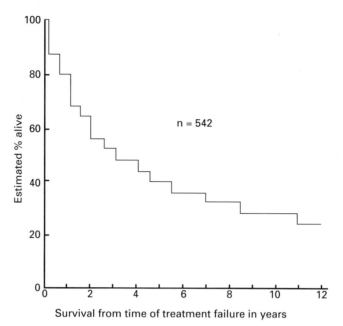

Fig. 48.3 Actuarial survival of patients with Hodgkin's disease failing MOPP type chemotherapy, all ages.
(Reproduced with permission from Linch D C, Vaughan-Hudson B 1988 The management of Hodgkin's disease and non-Hodgkin's lymphomas. In: Hoffbrand A V (ed) Recent advances in haematology. Churchill Livingstone, Edinburgh).

in these patients. With young patients, however, many centres would opt to use combination chemotherapy.

The use of alpha-interferon is being investigated both as a single agent and in combination with chemotherapy in the treatment of low grade NHL.

High grade non-Hodgkin's lymphoma

In contrast to low grade NHL, the treatment of high grade NHL is aimed at curing the patient. First line therapy is combination chemotherapy, with CHOP being the regimen most commonly used. It combines cyclophosphamide (alkylating agent), doxorubicin (anthracycline), vincristine (vinca alkaloid) and prednisolone (Table 48.4). This cycle is repeated monthly for six cycles. Complete remission rates of 44 to 70% have been reported with about 30% of patients disease-free at 5 years. Current research is aimed at increasing cure rates by comparing new regimens with CHOP.

Patients who do not respond or relapse after first line therapy are treated with aggressive 'salvage' chemotherapy regimens with varying

Table 48.4 CHOP regimen used in the treatment of NHL		
Drug	Dose & route	Frequency
CHOP (28-day cycle)		
C Cyclophosphamide	750 mg/m² i.v.	Day 1 & 8
H Doxorubicin (Hydroxydaunorubicin)	25 mg/m² i.v.	Day 1 & 8
O Vincristine (Oncovin)	1.4 mg/m² (max. 2 mg) i.v.	Day 1 & 8
P Prednisolone	50 mg/m² oral	Days 1–8

degrees of success. In general, the outlook is poor in patients who have relapsed. Lymphomas which are still sensitive to chemotherapy may respond to intensive regimens followed by an autologous bone marrow transplant. This type of treatment is discussed in more detail in Chapter 47.

Monitoring the patient receiving chemotherapy

The regimens used to treat HD and NHL (Table 48.5) are usually administered on an outpatient basis with the patient visiting the clinic regularly for assessment and treatment. The interval between each cycle of chemotherapy enables normal body cells to recover prior to further treatment. Myelosuppression is usually the dose-limiting factor with chemotherapy, and recovery is monitored by carrying out full blood counts prior to therapy. If the white blood count is too low the dose may be reduced or delayed by a week. Patients are examined clinically for evidence of response and for other side effects. Both the patient, and the medical and nursing staff must be vigilant for signs of infection. This is further discussed below. Once the course of chemotherapy has been completed the patient is reinvestigated fully for signs of disease and his or her response classified.

Table 48.5 Current strategies in the treatment of the lymphomas

Disease	Stage	Strategy
Hodgkin's disease	Ia, IIa	Extended field radiotherapy
	IIb and above	Combination chemotherapy
Non-Hodgkin's lymphoma		
Low grade	I, II	Involved field radiotherapy
	II, III, IV	Single agent chemotherapy
		Combination chemotherapy
		Alpha-interferon
High grade	I	Involved field radiotherapy
	I, II, III, IV	Combined chemotherapy
		Intensive chemotherapy with bone marrow transplant

Table 48.6 Adverse effects of CHOP regimen with concurrent risk factors

Drug	Adverse effects	Risk factors
Cyclophos-phamide	Myelosuppression Alopecia Haemorrhagic cystitis	Underlying infection Renal dysfunction
Doxorubicin	Cardiomyopathy	History of heart disease
	Myelosuppression Alopecia Mucositis	Underlying infection
Vincristine	Peripheral neuropathy	Inherited peripheral nerve disease Hepatic dysfunction
Prednisolone	Immunosuppression	Underlying infection
	Decreased glucose tolerance	Diabetes

THE PATIENT

Prior to treatment with chemotherapy, the patient should be counselled by a specialist nurse or physician. He or she will explain how the chemotherapy is to be given and discuss both potential and inevitable side effects. Counselling, an essential part of the care of the cancer patient, involves more than the explanation of drug therapy and investigations and includes the psychological support of the patient and his or her family.

As discussed in an earlier section, the choice of therapy depends on the histology and stage of disease. Once appropriate therapy has been selected, individual patient factors have to be considered. These include the patient's age, renal and hepatic function and underlying medical conditions, e.g. heart disease, diabetes or chronic pulmonary disease. The patient's tolerance of side effects and complications of treatment may then be predicted. The probability of successful treatment must be weighed against the prospect of serious and life-threatening adverse effects. The decision is based on an understanding of the clinical pharmacology of the drugs being used as well as the condition of the patient. An example of these considerations for a patient receiving CHOP is shown in Table 48.6. The pharmacist can provide advice on potential problems in patients on concurrent medication for underlying medical conditions, dosage alterations in impaired hepatic and renal function and pharmaceutical aspects of administration.

During a course of chemotherapy the patient requires supportive care to minimize the adverse effects of treatment. The adverse effects common to the chemotherapy regimens discussed in this chapter are outlined in Table 48.7. These will occur to varying degrees depending on the combinations of drugs and the doses used as well as individual patient factors. Those in which the pharmacist has a role will be discussed with regard to how the patient is monitored, any supportive drug therapy and patient education needs.

Table 48.7 Adverse effects associated with chemotherapy regimens used in the lymphomas with supportive measures and counselling points

Adverse effect	Cytotoxics implicated	Supportive measures	Counselling points
Bone marrow suppression	Chlorambucil Cyclophosphamide Doxorubicin Mustine Prednisolone	Blood transfusion Platelet transfusion Mouth care Gut decontamination Antibiotic therapy for febrile episodes	Expect tiredness Report bleeding or unusual bruising Importance of good personal hygiene Adhere to mouth care & gut decontamination regimens Avoid people with infection Monitor temperature Report febrile episodes or signs of infection **immediately**
Nausea & vomiting	Cyclophosphamide Doxorubicin Mustine Procarbazine	Antiemetic therapy	Emphasize regular use – a short course is more effective than 'as required' Take before meals Report episodes of vomiting (especially with oral cytotoxics)
Mucositis	Doxorubicin Methotrexate	Mouthcare regimen Analgesia if painful	Importance of good oral hygiene, stress importance of regular use of mouthwashes as prescribed & describe how mouthwashes should be used
Tumour lysis syndrome	If tumour load is high and is sensitive to chemotherapy regimen	Hydration Allopurinol	Stress importance of regular therapy until appropriate to discontinue Drink plenty of fluids
Alopecia	Cyclophosphamide Doxorubicin Etoposide Mustine	Provision of wig	Pharmacist not usually involved
Impaired gonadal function	Alkylating agents Procarbazine Doxorubicin* Methotrexate*	May be reversible, depends on regimen used	Pharmacist not usually involved
Neuropathy	Vincristine	Clinical assessment Discontinue use or substitute with vinblastine	
Cardiomyopathy	Doxorubicin	Monitor ECG & cardiac function	
Lung fibrosis	Bleomycin	Lung function tests	

*To a lesser degree.

Bone marrow suppression

The patient is monitored by full blood counts carried out before each cycle of chemotherapy and at the 'nadir' between cycles. The nadir is when the blood count is at its lowest point, usually 10 to 14 days after the chemotherapy has been given. Dose reductions are made or treatment is delayed if the patient is too myelosuppressed.

Anaemia is treated with blood transfusions as necessary and thrombocytopenia with platelet transfusions. Prolonged thrombocytopenia is not usually a problem with the regimens described in this chapter.

Neutropenia is the most life-threatening toxicity; the neutropenic patient is at constant risk from infections. Seemingly minor infections such as cold sores can spread rapidly and infections not seen in the normal population such as systemic fungal infections can occur. Supportive measures involve reducing the risks and the aggressive treatment of any infectious episodes. The patient is counselled to avoid contact with people with infections or who may be carriers. Most infections, however, are from an endogenous source such as the gut or skin. The patient is educated on the importance of good personal hygiene, mouth care, how to monitor body temperature and to report any febrile episodes immediately. Selective gut decontamination with antibiotics such as co-trimoxazole (960 mg b.d.) is used with regimens where neutropenia is likely to be prolonged.

A febrile episode in the neutropenic patient is an indication for immediate treatment with broad-spectrum intravenous antibiotics. The patient is assessed to determine, if possible, the site of infection. Blood cultures and any other appropriate cultures are taken and then antibiotic therapy is commenced. Gram-negative septicaemia is probable in this situation and therefore first line therapy is usually with an aminoglycoside with either a third generation cephalosporin or an antipseudomonal penicillin. If the patient does not respond to this combination within 48 hours, second line therapy with a Gram-positive bias is substituted. If positive microbiological cultures are found the appropriate antibiotic should be prescribed. The infecting organism is often not isolated as only one-third of suspected infections are ever confirmed. Renal function and aminoglycoside levels should be monitored.

Nausea and vomiting

Nausea and vomiting following chemotherapy is the most distressing and most feared adverse effect of chemotherapy. Its effect on the patient cannot be underestimated and is therefore an important part of supportive care. The severity will depend on the combination of drugs used. For example, oral chlorambucil is generally well tolerated by almost all patients and requires no antiemetic cover. Regimens such as CHOP and EVAP are moderately emetic and will make most patients vomit if no antiemetics are given. The control of chemotherapy-induced nausea and vomiting is discussed in Chapter 32. The pharmacist can advise on suitable regimens for specific chemotherapy combinations and counsel the patient on the use of antiemetics.

Mucositis

Mouth care should be instituted with myelosuppressive regimens. Bacteria and fungi present in the mouth will have easier systemic access in the patient with mucositis. Local infections can spread rapidly. Mouth care involves good oral hygiene and the regular use of an antiseptic mouthwash such as 0.2% chlorhexidine or 0.1% hexetidine and antifungal mouthwashes, usually nystatin or amphotericin. These are used more frequently and (for the antifungals) at higher doses than standard.

Tumour lysis syndrome

If the tumour load is high and is sensitive to the chemotherapy regimen used, the resulting lysis of cells will lead to hyperuricaemia and may result in urate nephropathy. The patient should be encouraged to maintain a high fluid intake.

Renal function and serum urate levels should be monitored. Allopurinol is usually commenced prior to chemotherapy and continued until the tumour load has reduced and urate levels are normal. The patient should be counselled on the importance of a high fluid intake and regular allopurinol therapy until told to stop by the doctor.

The support available to the cancer patient, to help cope with both the illness and its treatment, has improved dramatically in recent years. Multidisciplinary teams working within specialized units have become skilled in anticipating the problems of lymphomas and their treatment. The oncology pharmacist is an important member of these teams. Also, many charities provide care, support and advice, e.g. BACUP (British Association of Cancer United Patients) provides information and support by telephone and letter and produces information booklets on chemotherapy, individual cancers and other topics related to treatment.

CASE STUDIES

CASE 48.1

Miss A. is 20 years old and is receiving a course of LOPP/EVAP for stage IIb Hodgkin's disease. She has no other medical problems and has normal renal and hepatic function. She received her first cycle of LOPP 4 weeks ago and was prescribed metoclopramide (20 mg three times daily when required) to take home. She has now come to the chemotherapy clinic for a cycle of EVAP. Her full blood count has recovered sufficiently for her to receive this cycle.

She tolerated the LOPP combination reasonably well complaining only of mild nausea which started 2 days after starting the course and continued while she was taking the oral cytotoxics. She took the metoclopramide initially but experienced jaw spasm which resolved when she stopped taking the tablets.

Q1   Comment on the use of metoclopramide in this patient.

Q2   What antiemetic regimen would you recommend with the EVAP she is to receive this visit?

Q3   What antiemetic regimen would you recommend for future courses of LOPP?

CASE 48.2

Mrs B. is a 72-year-old widow who has been newly diagnosed with low grade NHL. She has been seen in the outpatient haematology clinic and has brought a prescription to the pharmacy for:

- **Chlorambucil 10 mg daily for 14 days.**

When she hands in her prescription she expresses concern about the side effects of the tablets. The doctor who saw her had spent a lot of time talking to her about her treatment but she feels confused with all the information given.

Q1   What are the side effects of chlorambucil?

Q2   How would you counsel this patient?

CASE 48.3

Mr C. is 56 years old and was diagnosed with stage III high grade NHL over 10 weeks ago. Since then he has received three cycles of CHOP and has come up to the hospital for his nadir blood count. He complains of painful mouth ulcers and a sore throat. On examination he has mucositis and oropharyngeal candidiasis. He has a white blood cell count of 3.2 (normal range 3.5 to 11 $\times$ 10^9/L) with 25% neutrophils (normal range 30 to 75%). When questioned about mouth care he revealed that he had been prescribed 0.2% chlorhexidine (10 ml four times daily) and nystatin (1 ml four times daily) and has been using these regularly as counselled.

Q1   How would you treat this patient's *Candida* infection?

Q2   Would you alter the mouth care regimen?

Q3   How would you counsel the patient?

CASE 48.4

Mr D., 38 years old with stage IV high grade NHL, is admitted to the haematology ward as an emergency from clinic. He was due to receive week 10 of his chemotherapy regimen but had a temperature of 39°C, has vomited twice that morning and feels very unwell. The regimen he has been receiving is PACE-BOM, which is as follows:

Day 1:
- Cyclophosphamide 300 mg/m^2
- Doxorubicin 35 mg/m^2
- Etoposide 150 mg/m^2

Day 8:
- Methotrexate 100 mg/m^2 (with folinic acid rescue)
- Vincristine 1.4 mg/m^2 (max. 2 mg)
- Bleomycin 10 mg/m^2
  These two cycles are repeated six times (i.e. 12-week course).
- Prednisolone 50 mg daily for 4 weeks then alternate days for 8 weeks.

On admission he is taking the following medication:

- Allopurinol 300 mg daily
- Co-trimoxazole 960 mg twice daily
- Prednisolone 50 mg alternate days
- 0.2% chlorhexidine mouthwash 10 ml four times daily
- Nystatin mouthwash 4 ml four times daily

The house officer takes blood cultures and prescribes gentamicin 80 mg three times daily and piperacillin 4 g four times daily to be commenced immediately. Blood biochemistry results are normal, his full blood count was Hb 10.8 (normal range 13.5 to 18.0 g/dl for males), WCC 3.1 with 28% neutrophils (normal range 3.5 to 11 × 10^9/L with 30 to 75% neutrophils), platelets 190 (normal range 150 to 400 × 10^9/L). Mr D. weighs 80 kg and is 186 cm tall.

Q1 Comment on the antibiotic therapy.

Q2 How would you monitor this patient?

CASE 48.5

Mrs E. is 52 years old and has just been diagnosed with stage III high grade NHL. She is a non-insulin-dependent diabetic stabilized on glibenclamide 10 mg daily. She is prescribed her first course of CHOP (Table 48.4) as an inpatient. She is 161 cm tall and weighs 78 kg giving a surface area of 1.85 m^2. Her prescription chart is as follows:

- Cyclophosphamide   1390 mg i.v. days 1 and 8
- Doxorubicin   46 mg i.v. days 1 and 8
- Vincristine   2 mg i.v. days 1 and 8
- Prednisolone   90 mg once daily for 8 days
- Allopurinol   300 mg once daily
- Glibenclamide   10 mg once daily
- Metoclopramide   20 mg four times daily

Q1 Discuss potential drug interactions. Which would you discuss with the medical staff?

Q2 How could Mrs E.'s diabetes be controlled?

ANSWERS TO CASE STUDIES

CASE 48.1

A1 Metoclopramide is the most widely used antiemetic in cancer chemotherapy; however, it can cause disturbing dystonic reactions, drowsiness, restlessness and diarrhoea. Patients under 30 years of age and women are more likely to experience dystonic reactions. The jaw spasm Miss A. described is one form of dystonic reaction. Because of her age and sex it is not surprising that she was unable to tolerate the metoclopramide. Severe dystonic reactions can be reversed with an intravenous anticholinergic agent such as procyclidine.

A2 Doxorubicin is moderately emetogenic; etoposide and vinblastine are rarely emetic. Half an hour before administration of the intravenous doses Miss A. should be given dexamethasone 4 mg and domperidone 20 mg orally. The antiemetics should continue with domperidone 20 mg four times daily and dexamethasone 2 mg three times daily regularly for 2 to 3 days. Domperidone, like metoclopramide, is a dopamine antagonist but does not readily cross the blood–brain barrier. Dystonic reactions, therefore, are rare.

Miss A. should be counselled to take the antiemetics regularly and complete the course as this is the most effective way of controlling the sickness. She should inform the hospital if she vomits and is unable to keep down her etoposide and antiemetics. A 5HT$_3$ antagonist should be considered if this antiemetic regimen fails.

A3 Procarbazine often causes nausea and occasionally vomiting. For future courses of LOPP Miss A. should be prescribed a regular antiemetic such as domperidone 20 mg four times daily for the duration of the regimen. She should be advised to take the doses 30 minutes before meals and at night. If she vomits she should inform the hospital.

CASE 48.2

A1 Chlorambucil, an alkylating agent, is generally well tolerated. The major side effect is bone marrow suppression. Other side effects are uncommon and include nausea and vomiting, mucositis and diarrhoea. Hepatotoxicity and jaundice have been reported. Mrs B. is an elderly patient and is more likely to experience toxicity because of deteriorating renal and hepatic function and underlying medical conditions.

A2 Mrs B. may be distressed by her diagnosis and may not have been able to absorb all the information she was given in the clinic. She may also be seeking confirmation of information. Although pharmacists are not usually involved in counselling patients on their chemotherapy we can give reassurance and reinforce information.

Mrs B. should be counselled to complete the course of tablets as prescribed. She should be told that she will probably feel tired and be more prone to infection because the tablets lower the blood count and resistance to infection. She should be advised to inform the haematologists if she feels unwell. Chlorambucil is unlikely to make her feel nauseous but if this occurs, she should inform the doctor who will be able to prescribe an antiemetic.

CASE 48.3

A1 Mr C. has an absolute neutrophil count (ANC) of $0.8 \times 10^9/L$ (25% of WCC) and is therefore neutropenic (ANC $< 1.5 \times 10^9/L$). Localized candidal infections can spread rapidly in the immunosuppressed patient so local therapy with an antifungal mouthwash will be inadequate therapy. A course of fluconazole (100 mg daily for at least 7 days) should be prescribed. Therapy should continue for a further 7 days if Mr C. is still neutropenic or if the thrush has not completely resolved.

A2 Chlorhexidine mouthwash should be continued as before. The nystatin dose should be increased to 4 ml to ensure the oropharynx is entirely coated with the mouthwash. As Mr C. is complaining of pain an analgesic should be added. Benzydamine mouthwash, a locally acting analgesic, could be prescribed initially. If this does not give adequate pain relief then systemic analgesics should be given.

A3 Regular mouth care reduces the risk of infection but does not entirely remove it. It is not necessarily a reflection of how well the patient has adhered to his mouth care regimen. Mr C. should continue his mouth care regimen as before. Chlorhexidine mouthwash should be used first, held in the mouth as long as possible ensuring the entire mucosa is covered before spitting out. The nystatin should then be used in the same manner but swallowed. The reason for increasing the nystatin dose should be explained. The mouthwashes should be used after meals and at bedtime. He should not eat or drink for at least half an hour after using the mouthwashes.

The benzydamine should be used before meals as Mr C. will probably find eating painful. He should be advised to eat 'soft' foods and to avoid hot and spicy dishes. He may be reassured that once his blood count recovers his mouth ulcers should resolve and that the fluconazole should relieve his sore throat.

CASE 48.4

A1 As Mr D. is neutropenic on admission (28% of WCC gives an ANC of 0.87) the combination of gentamicin and piperacillin is appropriate first line empiric therapy. It provides broad-spectrum cover with a Gram-negative bias. The co-trimoxazole is for gut decontamination and can be discontinued while the patient is receiving intravenous antibiotics. Mr D. should have received a loading dose of gentamicin and, as he is a large man with normal renal function, will probably require a higher dose to maintain adequate levels

A2 The patient's blood biochemistry – creatinine, urea and electrolytes – should be monitored daily to detect any deterioration in renal function. Gentamicin levels should be checked every 3 days and at steady state after any dose alterations. Microbiology reports should be checked and antibiotics reviewed if any microorganisms have been cultured. Treatment often remains empiric as the infecting organism is isolated in only one-third of cases. If the patient remains febrile on the gentamicin and piperacillin combination they should be substituted after 48 hours with appropriate second line therapy. This should include broad-spectrum Gram-positive cover with vancomycin or teicoplanin. The course of antibiotics should continue for at least 5 days. Patients often improve as their neutrophil count recovers.

CASE 48.5

A1 There are three documented drug interactions: a corticosteroid with a hypoglycaemic agent; cyclophosphamide with a hypoglycaemic agent; and allopurinol with cyclophosphamide.

The hypoglycaemic effect of glibenclamide will be opposed by the hyperglycaemic action of prednisolone. Intermittent courses of prednisolone will affect Mrs E.'s diabetic control. Cyclophosphamide has been reported to cause both acute hypoglycaemia and induce diabetes. It is unlikely that these are clinically significant but would warrant close monitoring of the diabetic patient receiving cyclophosphamide. Allopurinol has been reported to increase the incidence of severe bone marrow depression with cyclophosphamide. The evidence for this interaction is controversial. In clinical practice the two drugs are often prescribed together. Patients receiving chemotherapy are closely monitored for signs of bone marrow suppression, as a routine. The risk of tumour lysis syndrome outweighs the risk from this interaction.

Only the interaction between glibenclamide and prednisolone needs to be discussed with the medical staff. It is important that Mrs E. receives the prednisolone which is part of the chemotherapy regimen and also that her diabetes is controlled.

A2 The high dose of prednisolone and intermittent use will make control of Mrs E.'s diabetes with an oral hypoglycaemic difficult. It will probably be necessary to convert this patient to insulin therapy while on chemotherapy. Dose requirement can be titrated using an intravenous insulin infusion. Mrs E. required 180 units per day while on prednisolone. On completion of each course of prednisolone the dose of insulin required decreased gradually and stabilized in a matter of days. The patient monitored blood glucose daily and altered insulin dose accordingly.

BIBLIOGRAPHY

Cartwright R A, McKinney P A, Barnes N. Epidemiology of lymphoma in the United Kingdom: recent developments. In: McElwain T J, Lister T A (eds) Bailliere's clinical haematology: the lymphomas. Baillière Tindall 1987; 59–76

Chabner B A. Clinical strategies for cancer treatment: the role of drugs. In: Chabner B A, Collins J M (eds) Cancer chemotherapy: principles and pratice. Philadelphia: Lipincott 1990; 1–15

Crowther D, Wagstaffe J. Management of high grade non-Hodgkin's lymphoma in adults. In: McElwain T J, Lister T A, (eds) Bailliere's clinical haematology: the lymphomas. Baillière Tindall 1987; 157–184

Desforges J F, Rutherford C J, Piro A. Hodgkin's disease. New England Journal of Medicine 1979; 301: 1212–1222

Linch D C, Vaughan-Hudson B. The management of Hodgkin's disease and the non-Hodgkin's lymphomas. In: Hoffbrand A V (ed) Recent Advances in Haematology 1988

Longo D L, Young R C, Wesley M et al. Twenty years of MOPP therapy for Hodgkin's disease. Journal of Clinical Oncology 1986; 4: 1295–1306

Souhami R, Tobias J. Cancer and its management. Oxford: Blackwell Scientific Publications 1986

Chapter 49

Solid tumours

P. S. Warrington   M. Nicolson

The term cancer refers to a group of diseases including the leukaemias, lymphomas and solid tumours.

This chapter outlines the management of solid tumours and their treatment with chemotherapy. A solid tumour can affect any organ and represents a population of cells which have a growth regulatory defect. There are a large number of different tumour types and specific problems are posed by each type. Lung and breast cancer will be used to illustrate many of the management aspects which are applicable to other tumour types.

EPIDEMIOLOGY

Cancer is second only to heart disease as the most common cause of death in the United Kingdom. Table 49.1 shows the common cancers and the approximate numbers of deaths per year.

Table 49.1 Common solid tumours: approximate deaths/year in UK (1988)			
	Male	Female	Total
Lung	28 000	12 000	40 000
Bowel (colon & rectum)	9500	10 000	19 500
Breast	—	15 000	15 000
Prostate	8000	—	8000
Ovary	—	5000	5000
Cervix	—	4500	4500

AETIOLOGY

For most patients the cause of their malignancy is unknown. However, more than three-quarters of human cancers are thought to have an environmental cause, e.g. exposure to carcinogens such as asbestos, irradiation and specific chemicals. Some people are more susceptible to carcinogens than others and this variation in susceptibility is a major area of research. Some cancers emerge from a precancerous state which can be identified from cell changes.

Smoking causes 90% of all lung cancer deaths and nearly a third of all cancer deaths in Britain. A smaller but unknown percentage of lung tumours is caused by passive smoking. Smoking is also a well-established risk factor for other cancers including stomach and cervical cancers. Cervical cancer is twice as common in women who smoke regularly compared to those who are non-smokers. It has been suggested that smoking may either alter the immune function of the cervical epithelium or it may act as a carcinogen.

Cervical cancer is a disease of sexually active women. The risk of cervical cancer increases with the number of partners. Two viruses, the human papilloma virus (HPV) and to a lesser extent the herpes simplex virus type 2, have been associated with the development of cervical cancer.

There can be a genetic predisposition to the development of some solid tumours. A woman's risk of developing breast cancer is increased if her mother, sister or daughter has had premenopausal or bilateral breast cancer. Occasionally ovarian cancer runs in families as an autosomal dominant trait.

TUMOUR GROWTH

A solid tumour represents a population of dividing and non-dividing cells. Within a single solid tumour the variation in cell population can be infinite. Tumour growth depends on the cell cycle time, the cell loss and the growth fraction. The growth fraction is the ratio between the number of cycling cells and the total number of cells in the tumour. In most solid tumours the cell cycle times are variable and the growth fraction is low.

The time taken for the tumour to double in volume may be constant and measurable and is therefore termed exponential growth. This form of growth is seen in aggressive childhood tumours and some leukaemias. However, in most solid tumours the growth rate is very rapid initially and then slows as the tumour increases in size and age, a phenomenon referred to as Gompertzion growth.

As a primary tumour grows and invades normal tissue, malignant cells can infiltrate blood vessels and the lymphatic system. Malignant cells are thereby transported to other organs of the body and can subsequently form secondaries (metastasis). The pattern of spread tends to be predictable for different tumour types. Breast cancer usually metastasizes to the lungs and central nervous system whilst prostate cancer tends to metastasize to bone, in particular to the lumbar spine.

CLINICAL MANIFESTATIONS

The clinical features of cancer vary with tumour type. However, patients most commonly present with nonspecific complaints which include weight loss, bleeding, malaise, pain or the presence of a painless lump. Solid tumours are usually clinically detectable when there are approximately 10^8 to 10^9 tumour cells present. The patient is usually in the terminal stages of the disease when there are 10^{12} cells present. This means that unless a tumour is detected during a routine physical examination, presentation is usually late in the disease process.

ASSESSMENT OF THE PATIENT

At the time of presentation each patient must undergo a thorough assessment to establish an accurate diagnosis, the extent of the disease and his or her well-being. These factors will influence treatment choice and help give a guide to prognosis.

An accurate diagnosis is usually made from a sample of tissue. This sample may be obtained invasively, for example during bronchoscopy when lung cancer is suspected, or it may involve a non-invasive approach and, for the patient presenting with a breast lump, aspiration through a fine needle is possible. Tumours vary in their sensitivity to chemotherapy and so precise histology is important. For example, within the four main types of lung cancer, squamous cell carcinoma, small cell carcinoma, adenocarcinoma and large cell carcinoma, the squamous cell carcinoma is unresponsive to chemotherapy in contrast to small cell lung cancer which is chemosensitive.

Performance status

The patient's general level of fitness at the time of diagnosis is often a good prognostic indicator and helps determine which patients are likely to withstand intensive treatment. A number of physical rating scales have been devised to assess the patient's 'performance status'. Of these the most widely used are the Karnofsky performance index and the World Health Organization performance scale.

Staging

Frequently the tumour has disseminated by the time of presentation. Patients may undergo staging investigations to establish the extent and nature of the disease spread. Staging strongly influences the form of treatment offered to the patient. Investigations can include clinical examination, blood tests, radiological examination and for some patients, surgery. Most tumours are classified into three or four stages. In general the higher the stage the more advanced the disease and the poorer the prognosis.

Tumour marker

There are some specific tests which can help confirm the diagnosis of particular tumours. Measurement of the 'tumour markers', alpha-fetoprotein and human gonadotrophin, is useful in patients suspected of having testicular tumours. In addition to helping establish the diagnosis, tumour markers can help monitor response to chemotherapy and may be the first sign of relapsing disease.

TREATMENT

After the diagnosis of cancer has been confirmed and the staging investigation has been completed,

a decision is made by the clinician whether to give potentially curative treatment, palliative or symptomatic treatment. The decision is influenced by the natural history of the disease, the efficacy of available treatments, the extent of the disease the performance status of the patient and importantly, the patient's wishes.

Patients are said to be cured of cancer when they are completely disease free and have a normal life expectancy. The smaller the tumour bulk when treatment is given, the greater the opportunity of achieving cure.

Palliative treatment may be given when cure is unlikely, with the intention of giving symptomatic relief and hopefully achieving a worthwhile increase in survival time. The possibility of cure or long-term survival justifies aggressive treatment but with palliation it is particularly important that the toxicity of treatment is carefully weighed against the potential benefits.

Failure to achieve cure or long-term survival with chemotherapy commonly results from resistance within the tumour cell population. Clones of cells can be inherently resistant, with the fraction of cells killed reducing with each successive course of treatment. Other tumour cells appear to acquire resistance. In the laboratory, malignant cells have demonstrated a variety of methods of resisting the effect of cytotoxic drugs. Cells may develop the ability to reduce intracellular concentrations of cytotoxic drug via a membrane pump, the p-glycoprotein. Some cells show the ability to deactivate the drug enzymatically. In other instances the cells develop a mechanism for repairing damaged DNA.

Small-cell lung cancer and ovarian cancer illustrate the problem of drug resistance. In most patients these tumours do respond initially to chemotherapy but they often fail to respond to treatment when relapse occurs. This may involve resistance to more than one drug, when it is termed cross-resistance or multidrug resistance. One approach to overcoming multidrug resistance is to alternate treatment with non-cross-resistant drug combinations. This technique has produced reasonable success in lymphoma but disappointing results in solid tumours.

Three main options are available for the treatment of patients with solid tumours; surgery, radiotherapy and chemotherapy. Each modality has a number of roles, either alone or in combination. Ideally, decisions on treatment choice should be based on an approach which has shown the best results in clinical trials.

Childhood malignancies and aggressive tumours in adults are most responsive to chemotherapy and for a small group of diseases, including teratoma and Wilms' tumour in children, patients with advanced disease potentially can be cured. Other solid tumours, e.g. non-small-cell lung cancer and melanoma, are generally unresponsive to chemotherapy. In approximately 70% of patients treated with chemotherapy, cure or prolonged survival is unlikely but may be palliative (Table 49.2).

Adjuvant and neo-adjuvant chemotherapy

Traditionally, surgery and radiotherapy have been used to treat apparently localized tumour while chemotherapy has been used for treating recurrent or advanced disseminated disease.

One problem with this approach is that despite seemingly adequate local treatment, tumour recurs as metastatic disease. Recurrence may be attributed to the presence of undetectable micrometastatic disease at diagnosis. Adjuvant therapy, where chemotherapy is combined with the best local therapy, allows for the early treatment of metastatic disease. In breast cancer, chemotherapy following surgery and radiotherapy has achieved an increased survival for

premenopausal women who have disease involving up to three axillary nodes.

Neo-adjuvant chemotherapy, where chemotherapy is given before local therapy, can reduce tumour size and facilitate surgical removal. The use of neo-adjuvant chemotherapy allows children and adolescents with Ewing's sarcoma, one of the most common bone tumours, to have limb-sparing surgery as an alternative to amputation. It may be some weeks following surgery before the patient is fit for chemotherapy. Neo-adjuvant chemotherapy allows presurgical treatment of metastatic disease and gives improved 5-year survival rates in Ewing's sarcoma.

The main disadvantage of adjuvant and neo-adjuvant therapy is that it exposes to chemotherapy a proportion of patients who could have been cured without it.

Combination chemotherapy

Chemotherapy was formerly administered as a single agent on a continuous basis until cure, drug resistance or unacceptable toxicity occurred. In the mid 1950s combination therapy was developed with two or more drugs being used for additive or synergistic effects. Drugs used in combination should ideally have efficacy established as single agents, different mechanisms of action and differing toxicity profiles to allow their use at optimal doses.

After chemotherapy, malignant cells repair and repopulate less effectively than normal cells and treatment is now generally given in pulses at 3- or 4-week intervals, allowing the normal cell population a chance to recover. Damage to normal cells occurs shortly after chemotherapy is received, and rapidly proliferating tissue, e.g. bone marrow, is at most risk. With many myelosuppressive cytotoxic drugs, the white blood cell count is at its lowest level or 'nadir' around 10 days after treatment. Recovery generally occurs by day 20 post-treatment, and therefore treatment is repeated every 3 to 4 weeks. Recovery is delayed with agents such as melphalan and mitomycin where blood cells do not fully recover for 42 to 50 days following treatment.

Dose reductions and delays in treatment are

Table 49.2 Response to chemotherapy		
Possible cure	Possible increase in survival	Generally unresponsive
Ewing's sarcoma Testicular cancer Choriocarcinoma	Small cell lung cancer Breast cancer Cervical cancer Ovarian cancer	Non-small cell lung cancer Gastric cancer Colorectal cancer Renal cell carcinoma Bladder cancer Melanoma

necessary when bone marrow does not recover sufficiently between courses of treatment. A reduction in dose intensity, the dose of cytotoxic delivered for unit time, is associated with reduced response rate and survival.

The understanding of cell cycle kinetics helps when combining cytotoxic drugs and scheduling treatment. Within a solid tumour a proportion of non-dividing cells will die while others remain in a resting phase of growth. Since dividing cells are most responsive to chemotherapy, resting cells should ideally be encouraged into the cell cycle, a process called recruitment. Recruitment may follow an initial reduction in the tumour cell population and should increase the proportion of cells killed by successive courses of treatment.

Some cytotoxic drugs are phase specific in that they affect cells at defined stages in the cell cycle. Treatment should ideally be scheduled to allow tumour cells to be in the drug-sensitive phase of the cell cycle. For example, vincristine, a vinca alkaloid, is phase specific and affects mitosis. Continuous infusions of phase-specific agents with a short half-life should have the advantage of inducing a higher cell kill and this approach is currently being investigated in patients with breast cancer and gastric cancer.

High-dose chemotherapy

In vitro studies have demonstrated a clear dose-response relationship for chemotherapy-sensitive tumours. The profound toxicity of chemotherapy is the major obstacle to exploiting this phenomenon.

Potentially lethal myelosuppression has been reduced using autologous bone marrow transplantation where marrow is removed and re-infused following the administration of high-dose chemotherapy.

Drug administration

Admission to hospital is influenced by a number of factors: the predictable acute toxicity of the regimen, the route of administration and the schedule of drug delivery.

Cisplatin toxicity, requiring prolonged hydra-tion with intravenous fluids and aggressive use of antiemetics, favours inpatient treatment especially when the protocol requires therapy to be given on successive days. Complex administration techniques, e.g. isolated limb perfusion, are used to achieve high concentrations of cytotoxic drug at the tumour site. These techniques require the close supervision afforded by inpatient treatment.

Providing toxicity is acceptable, day care or outpatient chemotherapy is possible for regimens where cytotoxics are given by intravenous bolus or injection at 3- or 4-week intervals.

Oral cytotoxic drugs can be taken at home but consideration must be given to potential poor compliance and reduced bioavailability from impaired absorption or vomiting.

Parenteral therapy can be given at home. Many patients cope well with self-administered subcutaneous injections of interferon. The availability of central venous catheters has enabled patients at home to receive continuous ambulatory chemotherapy via a portable pump. The disposable drug cassettes must be filled aseptically, requiring cooperation between hospital and community services.

Toxicity

Successful treatment can be compromised by toxicity. Most cytotoxics have been selected because of their effect on dividing cells and therefore rapidly proliferating normal tissue is at risk. Table 49.3 shows the World Health Organization's standardized scale for rating the predictable acute side effects of chemotherapy. The scale allows comparisons between published reports.

Myelosuppression is frequently dose limiting and thrombocytopenia and neutropenia place patients at risk of bleeding and life-threatening infection. Cardiotoxicity, nephrotoxicity and pulmonary toxicity, which are specific to the chemotherapeutic agent or class, may depend on total dose exposure, the schedule of administration and previous therapy.

Doxorubicin has activity in many solid tumours. Its acute side effects include bone mar-

Table 49.3 WHO grading of acute and subacute toxicity to chemotherapy

Toxicity	Grade 0	Grade 1	Grade 2	Grade 3	Grade 4
Nausea/vomiting	None	Nausea	Transient vomiting	Vomiting, requiring therapy	Intractable vomiting
Diarrhoea	None	Transient <2 days	Tolerable, but >2 days	Intolerable, requiring therapy	Haemorrhagic dehydration
Constipation	None	Mild	Moderate	Abdominal distention	Distention and vomiting
Oral	No change	Soreness/erythema	Erythema, ulcers; can eat solids	Ulcers; requires liquid diet only	Alimentation not possible
Leucocytes (1000/mm^3)	>4.0	3.0–3.9	2.0–2.9	1.0–1.9	<1.0
Platelets (1000/mm^3)	>100	75–99	50–74	25–49	<25
Haemoglobin (g/100 ml)	>11.0	9.5–10.9	8.0–9.4	6.5–7.9	<6.5
Hair	No change	Minimal hair loss	Moderate, patchy alopecia	Complete alopecia, but reversible	Non-reversible alopecia

row suppression, alopecia and severe mucositis. However, most commonly its use is limited by a cumulative dose-dependent cardiomyopathy. A number of other factors including treatment schedule, patient, age and pre-existing cardiac disease have been implicated but dose is the most important. The maximum recommended cumulative dose of doxorubicin is 550 mg/m^2 and this is reduced to 400 mg/m^2 for patients who have received previous radiotherapy to the mediastinum.

There has been progress in the ability to minimize the toxicity of chemotherapy. One approach has been to develop analogues of existing agents. Carboplatin, an analogue of cisplatin, is not associated with the severe nephrotoxicity and neurotoxicity which is seen with the parent compound.

The administration of a specific antidote, mesna, which is a sulfydryl-containing compound, has reduced the incidence of haemorrhagic cystitis associated with ifosfamide and high dose cyclophosphamide.

Biological response modifiers

The interferons, interleukins and tumour necrosis factors are endogenous polypeptides. These cytokines produced by various cell types have been shown to play an important role in the body's defence against cancer. The mechanism by which these biological response modifiers exert antitumour effects are complex. For example, the interferons have antiviral, antiproliferative and immunomodulatory activities, but the exact mechnism by which they achieve their cytotoxic effect remains unknown.

Advances in genetic engineering have led to commercial production of the biological response modifiers and current research is exploring their use alone or in combination both with each other and with conventional cytotoxics.

Biological response modifiers have produced responses in a range of solid tumours resistant to conventional chemotherapy. While their place in therapy requires to be established, their use is limited by toxicity or major cost implications.

Response to treatment

The response to treatment must be closely monitored so that if first line therapy proves ineffective an alternative can be introduced without delay. Response is monitored by clinical examination, X-ray, laboratory blood tests or tumour markers. In clinical trials more extensive investigations may be carried out to document the response formally. Additional information can be obtained from ultrasound or CT scans carried out after a predetermined number of cycles. As with staging investigations, accurate assessment of response is limited by the sensitivity of the tests. Standard definitions of response have been developed and allow for comparison of results between different studies.

However, although clinical response indicates tumour sensitivity, it may not necessarily predict long-term survival. The risk of late relapse, e.g. in breast cancer, requires long-term follow-up and assessment of the patient.

The response to palliative therapy is difficult to assess objectively. Tumour shrinkage does not automatically give symptom relief and toxicity may be unjustifiable if symptom relief is limited. Performance scales can be used to measure a response to palliative therapy; however, their value is limited in that they assess general physical condition, ignore specific symptoms and rely on an observer's assessment. Quality of life measurements, used to quantify the subjective benefits of treatment, are becoming increasingly important in evaluating new treatment strategies.

THE PATIENT

Discussion and counselling are essential in the care of patients with solid tumours. The physician will discuss with the patient the aim of treatment, what is involved and the possible side effects.

Table 49.4 shows the clinical pharmacy monitoring required for patients receiving chemotherapy. The treatment protocol is selected according to the factors discussed above. The exact details of a regimen may vary according to the protocol and the pharmacist should confirm the regimen with the prescriber.

Appropriate investigations must be carried out to confirm that the patient is fit for treatment. In particular, bone marrow, renal and hepatic function should be investigated usually by routine blood analysis. Drug doses are based on surface area or weight but may require modification in the presence of renal or hepatic impairment (Table 49.5) ensuring reduced or delayed excretion does not cause toxicity. Surface area will require to be recalculated where there is appreciable weight loss between courses of treatment.

A medication review will identify potential drug interactions. Care is required when assessing the clinical significance of potentially harmful interactions. A documented interaction does

Table 49.4 Clinical pharmacy: monitoring chemotherapy	
Diagnosis Protocol Regimen Weight/height	Is prescription in accordance with treatment protocol/ established regimen/standard dose? Calculate body surface area Confirm dose

Clinical factors:
   Age
   Bone marrow function
   Renal function
   Liver function
   Underlying disease
   Allergy
	Is dose adjustment required?
	Contra-indications

Route of administration	Is route appropriate? Suitable venous access Appropriate scheduling
Interactions	With concurrent medication? Pharmaceutical interactions with i.v. drugs or infusion fluids
Supportive care	Anticipate side effects Ensure appropriate supportive therapy is prescribed Ensure appropriate monitoring is carried out
Documentation	Ensure therapy is accurately documented

Table 49.5 Cytotoxics requiring dosage adjustment with organ dysfunction		
	Dosage adjustment required	
	Renal dysfunction	Hepatic dysfunction
Bleomycin	√	
Carboplatin	√	
Cisplatin	√	
Cyclophosphamide	√	√
Daunorubicin		√
Doxorubicin		√
Epirubicin		√
Etoposide		√
Fluorouracil		√
Idarubicin	√	√
Ifosfamide	√	
Methotrexate	√	√
Mitozantrone		√
Nitrosoureas	√	
Vinca alkaloids		√

immediately report pain or a stinging sensation at the injection site.

Myelosuppression is common and for some patients profound. The risk of systemic infection can be reduced by good mouth care using antiseptic mouthwashes and antifungal prophylaxis (prophylactic antibiotics are generally not indicated). Patients should immediately report symptoms of infection and bruising. Platelets may be required and life-threatening infection must be promptly treated with broad-spectrum intravenous antibiotics.

Careful counselling is required to encourage patient compliance with oral chemotherapy. In order to avoid confusion, they should be aware of precisely which drugs prescribed for them are the cytotoxic agents. Clear instructions are required on the duration of all medication to avoid treatment being continued inadvertently.

not necessarily imply that drugs should not be used together but requires close monitoring of the patient. Interactions can be avoided by specifying infusion fluids and supportive therapy.

Nausea and vomiting are probably felt by most patients to be the most distressing side effects of chemotherapy and poor symptom control can result in patients refusing further treatment. Antiemetic selection depends on the incidence, time to onset, severity and duration of symptoms associated with a particular drug or regimen. Symptoms can vary with schedule and dosage.

The route of administration for antiemetics requires careful consideration for outpatient and home chemotherapy. Continuous infusions or intermittent injections are impractical in the home. Thus oral antiemetics are best suited for outpatients, with bolus doses being preferred in the clinic. When vomiting occurs, sublingual or rectal administration can be considered. Because of the risk of bleeding, the rectal route should be avoided when patients are thrombocytopenic.

The accidental leakage of irritant cytotoxic drug into the extravascular compartment (extravasation) can cause severe local necrosis, and extreme care must be taken when administering these drugs. The patient should be asked to

CASE STUDIES

CASE 49.1

Thirty-year-old Mr W. is admitted to the Medical Oncology Unit for treatment of his advanced malignant teratoma. Investigations prior to admission have confirmed stage IV disease and full blood count and biological investigations are normal except for the following:

- Human chorionic gonadotrophin (HCG) 1026 i.u./ml (normal <5)
- Alpha-fetoprotein (AFP) 364 i.u./ml (normal 2–6)

Mr W. is to have combination chemotherapy with the BEP regimen:

- Bleomycin 30 mg intravenously on days 2, 9 and 16
- Etoposide 120 mg/m² intravenously on days 1–3
- Cisplatin 20 mg/m² intravenously on days 1–5.

The following additional medication was prescribed for Mr W.:

- Allopurinol 300 mg orally
- Ondansetron 8 mg intravenously
- Dexamethasone 20 mg intravenously.

Q1 What are the indications for each additional medicine and what are the special administration requirements for ondansetron and dexamethasone?

Q2 What medication will Mr W. require to take home?

CASE 49.2

Mrs M., a 64-year-old woman with advanced breast cancer, received outpatient treatment with six courses of cyclophosphamide, doxorubicin, vincristine and prednisolone. Nausea and vomiting were severe despite combination antiemetic therapy. By course three she had complete hair loss and felt sick on entering the clinic.

Q1 Which cytotoxic drugs were responsible for Mrs M.'s alopecia?

Q2 What measure can be taken to prevent or minimize hair loss?

Q3 Would the above measure have been appropriate for Mrs M.?

Q4 Why did Mrs M. feel sick before she had her chemotherapy?

Mrs M. completed chemotherapy 7 months ago and her hair has completely regrown. The following medication has been prescribed:

- **Chlorambucil 12 mg daily for 14 days**
- **Prednisolone 20 mg daily for 14 days.**

Q5 What questions might Mrs M. ask?

Q6 What advice should be given to Mrs M. about her current therapy?

CASE 49.3

Mr S., a 55-year-old man with extensive small cell lung cancer, is admitted to the ward for his first course of CAV chemotherapy. Pretreatment blood count, renal and hepatic function tests are normal and he is receiving no medication.

CAV *regimen:*
- Cyclophosphamide 1 g/m^2 intravenously on day 1
- Doxorubicin (Adriamycin) 50 mg/m^2 intravenously on day 1
- Vincristine 1.4 mg/m^2 (maximum 2 mg) intravenously on day 1
- Cycle frequency on 21 days.

Q1 What steps can be taken to minimize the risk of extravasation while the drugs are being administered?

The injection of cyclophosphamide is given uneventfully; however, whilst receiving vincristine Mr S. complains of pain and a stinging sensation at the injection site. The doctor suspects vincristine is extravasating into the surrounding tissue.

Q2 What immediate steps should be taken?

CASE 49.4

Miss D., a 20-year-old woman with operable osteosarcoma, is to be treated with adjuvant chemotherapy.
The regimen prescribed is:

- Vincristine 1.5 mg/m^2 (maximum 2 mg) intravenously on day 1
- Methotrexate 8 g/m^2 intravenously on day 1
- Folinic acid 12 mg/m^2 intravenously, 6-hourly for 5 doses
- Folinic acid 15 mg/m^2 orally, 6-hourly for 5 doses.

Q1 What measures can be taken to reduce the nephrotoxicity associated with high-dose methotrexate?

Q2 Why was folinic acid prescribed?

Q3 A decision is made to discharge Miss D. with three doses of oral folinic acid to be taken at home at 8 p.m., 2 a.m. and 8 a.m. What advice should the patient receive?

CASE 49.5

Mr K., a 63-year-old farmer with renal cell carcinoma, is recovering from surgical removal of his left kidney. He has been prescribed interferon to treat metastatic lung disease according to the following schedule:

- Interferon alfa-2a (rbe)
  — 3 million i.u. daily on days 1 to 3
  — 9 million i.u. daily on days 4 to 6
  — 18 million i.u. daily on days 7 to 9

Stabilized on a maintenance dose of 18 million i.u. by subcutaneous injection three times a week, Mr K. will be assessed monthly at outpatient clinic. The consultant has asked the clinical nurse specialist and the pharmacist to help the patient prepare for self-administration of interferon at home.

Q1 What arrangements should be made for Mr K. to go home and what information does he require?

Q2 What are the specific counselling points for interferon?

ANSWERS TO CASE STUDIES

CASE 49.1

A1 Mr W. is prescribed allopurinol to avoid hyperuricaemia and possible urate nephropathy following the lysis of malignant cells.

Dexamethasone and ondansetron are being prescribed as combination antiemetic therapy.

Cisplatin, which is probably one of the most emetogenic cytotoxic drugs used in the treatment of cancer, causes severe emesis (WHO grade 3 or 4) in greater than 90% of patients. Symptoms begin within 6 hours of starting treatment. Bleomycin and etoposide have a low emetic potential, with <30% incidence of severe emesis.

Treatment with one antiemetic does not provide reliable control of symptoms caused by severely emetogenic drugs. Antiemetics used in combination should preferably have different sites of action. Ondansetron blocks 5-hydroxytryptamine type 3 ($5HT_3$) receptors in the small intestine and in the chemoreceptor trigger zone. Dexamethasone has an uncertain mechanism of action. A suitable alternative regimen is a combination of dexamethasone with high-dose metoclopramide (1 to 10 mg/kg). Metoclopramide is thought to act by inhibiting dopamine receptors at these high doses. The new $5HT_3$ antagonists, ondansetron and granisetron, are free of the extrapyramidal side effects associated with metoclopramide.

Mr W. is administered a single dose of dexamethasone sodium phosphate 15 minutes before starting chemotherapy. Dexamethasone administered as a 15-minute infusion avoids the perineal discomfort associated with a bolus injection. Ondansetron 8 mg can be administered as a slow intravenous injection immediately before chemotherapy, followed by a further two doses of 8 mg given by slow intravenous injection, 4 hours apart.

A2 Mr W. requires allopurinol to take home and serum urate should be closely monitored.

Antiemetic therapy may also be required. Late nausea and vomiting have been reported in 20 to 70% of patients receiving cisplatin. Symptoms continue for 1 to 14 days after treatment. The treatment of cisplatin-induced delayed emesis is unclear but oral dexamethasone and metoclopramide have been found to be a useful combination.

CASE 49.2

A1 Doxorubicin and cyclophosphamide cause severe hair loss. Anthracyclines and alkylating agents cause alopecia through the cytotoxic effect on rapidly dividing cells of the hair follicle.

A2 Scalp cooling is used to reduce drug uptake into the hair follicle. Cooling should start 20 minutes before giving chemotherapy. The response to cooling is variable, depending on the dose, terminal half-life and combination of cytotoxic drugs administered. Cooling frequently causes headache and discomfort. The risk of alopecia increases with dose and cooling should only be considered for drugs with a short elimination half-life. Patients need to be psychologically prepared for losing their hair with information and advice. They should be reassured hair will regrow on completing treatment and given advice on obtaining a wig.

A3 Breast cancer can metastasize to skin. Scalp cooling, by preventing cytotoxic drug uptake into tumour cells, may provide a 'sanctuary site' for metastasis. Cooling would not be offered to Mrs M.

A4 Anticipatory nausea is worsened by poor emetic control. Anticipatory nausea and vomiting can be helped by prescribing the benzodiazepine, lorazepam. Lorazepam has sedative, anxiolytic and amnesic properties which are useful in this situation although it has limited activity as an antiemetic.

A5 Nausea, vomiting and alopecia are the most distressing side effects for the majority of patients receiving chemotherapy. Mrs M. will be concerned that these effects may recur with the new regimen. Reassurance should be given that chlorambucil will not cause hair loss and rarely causes nausea and vomiting.

Mrs M. is at more risk of developing nausea and vomiting having had previous exposure to chemotherapy where symptom control was poor. For this reason prophylactic antiemetics could have been prescribed.

A6 The advice should include:

- Chlorambucil tablets should be kept in the fridge and taken with food.
- Prednisolone is being given as part of chemotherapy and is only to be used for a short course of treatment. A further supply should not be obtained from the General Practitioner.
- If Mrs M. is sick after taking her tablets, she should contact the doctor.
- As the patient is potentially at risk of infection due to bone marrow suppression she should contact the doctor if she feels unwell.

CASE 49.3

A1 Safe administration of cytotoxics is critical as little can be done to minimize the damage of extravasation or to promote healing.

Specific measures to ensure safe administration include:

- Chemotherapy should be administered via the distal veins of the dorsum of the hand. The antecubital fossa should be avoided.
- Vein patency must be established using a free-flowing infusion of saline or glucose.
- The infusion or slow intravenous bolus should be given through the injection port of the giving set. Known vesicants should be given as a short injection wherever possible to ensure constant monitoring at the injection site during administration.
- On completion of each injection the line should be flushed with saline or glucose.

A2 Doxorubicin and vincristine are both vesicants causing severe local necrosis if extravasated. On suspecting extravasation the injection or infusion should be stopped, leaving the needle in place to allow drug aspiration.

There are two approaches to management. One is to apply dry heat to allow spread or dilution of the vesicant. The other involves localizing the vesicant using an ice-pack followed by administration of an antidote at the extravasation site.

Recommendations for vincristine are to:

- inject hyaluronidase locally
- apply moderate heat to the area of leakage.

After these measures have been taken, the drip should be resited and doxorubicin administered.

The extravasation site should be closely monitored. Early surgical intervention may be necessary.

CASE 49.4

A1 Acute tubular necrosis caused by the precipitation of methotrexate in the renal tubules is likely when urine pH approaches 5.4, the pKa value for methotrexate. The risk of toxicity can be reduced by hydration to ensure a minimum output of 2 L/m^2 in 24 hours and urine alkalinization, with oral administration of sodium bicarbonate to maintain a urine pH greater than 7. Intravenous sodium bicarbonate may be necessary for patients who are vomiting or if urine pH falls below 7.

The use of other nephrotoxic drugs should be avoided. Vincristine is not nephrotoxic and Miss D. is prescribed no other medication.

A2 High-dose methotrexate can cause severe gastrointestinal toxicity, mucositis, nephrotoxicity and myelosuppression.

At methotrexate doses above 100 mg/m^2 normal cells must be 'rescued' by the administration of folinic acid. Methotrexate inhibits the enzyme dihydrofolate reductase interfering with purine and pyrimidine synthesis. Folinic acid overcomes this effect in normal cells to a greater extent than in tumour cells.

Folinic acid rescue should be started around 24 hours from the start of methotrexate therapy; given earlier it may compromise the activity of the methotrexate.

At doses of 1 g/m^2 serum concentrations of methotrexate must be measured to ensure that folinic acid rescue is adequate. Levels are generally measured at 24 hours to ensure that the dose of folinic acid is sufficient, then again at 48 hours. Therapy is required until methotrexate concentrations fall below 0.1 micromol/L. Generally this occurs within 24 to 48 hours of completion of methotrexate therapy, but severe late toxicity can occur due to persistent low concentrations of methotrexate.

Concentrations should also be measured if there is any evidence of renal impairment or the presence of ascites or pleural effusion which can act as a 'third space' reservoir from which methotrexate can slowly leech into the circulation maintaining serum concentrations.

A3 The timing of the folinic acid dose is very important and Miss D. must be advised to set her alarm for the 2 a.m. dose. She should contact the doctor for advice if she is sick after her medication.

CASE 49.5

 Home chemotherapy with cytotoxic drugs or biological response modifiers depends on close collaboration between doctor, nurse, pharmacist and patient. A comprehensive training programme should be agreed covering storage, preparation and administration of interferon. Additional information should be given on the disposal of unused medication, needles and syringes. The training programme should be accompanied by concise written information and, on completion of training, Mr K. 's technique should be assessed to assure his competence.

Continuity of supply must be assured through the hospital or community pharmacy, providing an opportunity for the community and oncology pharmacists to work together and exchange information. Home care packs containing medication, syringes and needles are commercially available for interferon.

This approach gives the patient the required support and confidence to cope with self-administration.

A2 Mild flu-like symptoms, including mild fever, chills and myalgia, are the most common adverse effects with interferon. Mr K. can be advised to take two 500 mg paracetamol tablets before his injection. Further doses can be repeated 4- to 6-hourly, to a maximum of 8 tablets in 24 hours. Symptoms usually subside after a few weeks of treatment. Symptoms of lethargy and fatigue are common but do not resolve and many patients prefer night-time administration.

Hair thinning occurs in some patients, with total hair loss being rare. Hair growth recovers on stopping treatment.

White blood cell production may be depressed and it should be explained to Mr K. that he will be more at risk of infection. A high temperature should not always be attributed to the interferon. The times of the elevated temperature and the injection should be noted and the doctor informed.

BIBLIOGRAPHY

Allwood M, Wright P. The cytotoxic handbook. Oxford: Radcliffe Medical Press 1990

Committee of Specialty Practice in Oncology, Society of Hospital Pharmacists of Australia. Patient counselling for antineoplastic drugs: a pharmacist's guide to advisory labels and patient information. Australian Journal of Hospital Pharmacy 1990; 20: 458–460

Devita V T, Hellman S, Rosenberg S A. Cancer principles and practice of oncology, 3rd edn. Philadelphia: J B Lippincott 1989

Koren G, Beatty K, Seto A, Einarson T R, Listner M. The effects of impaired liver function on the elimination of antineoplastic agents. Annals of Pharmacotherapy 1992; 26: 363–370

Nicolson M, Warrington P S. Cancer chemotherapy, Parts 1 and 2. Pharmaceutical Journal 1992; 248: 804–806, 842–844

Priestman T. Cancer chemotherapy: an introduction, 3rd edn. Berlin: Springer-Verlag 1989

WHO handbook for reporting results of cancer treatment. Geneva: WHO Offset Publications 1979

Chapter 50

Rheumatoid arthritis and osteoarthritis

E. A. Kay

RHEUMATOID ARTHRITIS

Rheumatoid arthritis (RA) in its fully developed form is a symmetrical, inflammatory disease of the synovial lining of peripheral joints characterized by potentially deforming polyarthritis and a wide spectrum of extra-articular features (Table 50.1).

EPIDEMIOLOGY

RA occurs throughout the world in all ethnic groups and all climates, although people living in the developed world are more severely affected. It is the most common chronic inflammatory disease of the joint. There are reports of population frequency differences with prevalence varying from 0.1% in black South Africans

Table 50.1 The extra-articular features of rheumatoid arthritis	
Common	Uncommon
Anaemia	Pleural effusion
Nodules	Pulmonary fibrosis
Muscle wasting	Pericarditis
Dry eyes	Scleritis
Depression	Systemic vasculitis
Episcleritis	
Osteoporosis	
Carpal tunnel syndrome	
Leg ulcers	
Lymphadenopathy	
Nail-fold vasculitis	
Peripheral sensory neuropathy	

to 3% amongst caucasians. Comparative studies amongst urban and rural populations suggest that environmental factors associated with modern urban life may be important.

The prevalence of definite RA increases with age in both sexes with 2% of males and 5% of females affected over the age of 55 years. The age of onset reaches its peak in the fourth decade. The overall female to male ratio is 3:1, although when the onset is under 60 years the sex ratio is 5:1, and 2:1 when the onset is at an older age.

AETIOLOGY

The cause of RA is unknown. It is possible that many different arthritogenic stimuli activate the immune response in the immunogenetically susceptible host. The incidence of seropositive RA is more common in people with HLA DR4 (60%) than in the normal control population (15%). There is no evidence that trauma, climate, diet, stress, metabolic or endocrine factors are involved.

The similarity of RA to other arthritides such as Lyme disease for which an infectious agent has been identified has prompted the search for similar candidates. Epstein–Barr virus has been linked to RA for over 10 years. 80% of patients with RA have a circulating antibody directed against antigens specific for Epstein–Barr virus and the autoantibody response in RA enhances the response to these antigens. Parvoviruses are small DNA viruses that cause disease in many species and parvovirus B19 has been linked to RA. Mycobacteria have also been linked to RA because these bacteria express heat-shock proteins which are the arthritogenic factors of adjuvant arthritis in rats.

PATHOPHYSIOLOGY

Antigen-presenting cells (macrophages or dendritic cells in the synovial membrane) are the first to be involved in the immune response. These cells ingest, process and present foreign protein antigens to T-lymphocytes which initiate a cellular immune response and stimulate differentiation of B-lymphocytes into plasma cells that secrete antibody.

The central event is the formation within the joint of immune complexes. These activate complement, and attract polymorphs into the synovial fluid. Phagocytosis occurs and lysosomal enzymes are released along with chemotactic factors and other chemical mediators of inflammation. There is a paucity of CD8 positive suppressor T-lymphocytes, and natural killer cells, whose function it is to 'turn-off' the immune response, and there is a deficiency of lymphokines (e.g. interleukin 2) which suggests that both the humoral and cellular response is incomplete. The initiating antigen thus triggers an aberrant response, which becomes self-perpetuating, long after the offending antigen has been cleared.

Sustained inflammation leads to hypertrophy of the synovium and the formation of 'pannus' which spreads over the surface of the joint causing erosive destruction of the cartilage and bone. The presence of persistent synovitis causes an effusion consisting of synovial fluid rich in proteins and inflammatory cells. The extra-articular features of the disease may be due to systemic circulation of these immune complexes.

CLINICAL MANIFESTATIONS

The diagnosis of RA is based on criteria first developed by the American Rheumatism Association in 1958, and subsequently modified in 1988 (Table 50.2). These criteria were designed principally for disease classification, and differences in their interpretation may partly explain variable incidence figures.

The course of RA is highly variable and although it is primarily a disease of the synovial joints it can affect many organ systems. The disease is characterized by flares and remissions. Approximately 20% of patients achieve remis-

---

Table 50.2 Diagnostic criteria for rheumatoid arthritis

Arthritis of three or more joint areas
Arthritis of hand joints
Symmetrical swelling (arthritis) of same joint areas
Serum rheumatoid factor
Radiographic features of RA

sion after a short illness with no further disease activity, 25% obtain remission with mild residual disease, 45% have persistent activity with variable progressive deformity, and 10% progress to complete disability.

Early symptoms of RA are nonspecific and consist of fatigue, malaise, diffuse musculoskeletal pain and stiffness. Joint pain, stiffness and loss of function are the most obvious symptoms of RA. The peripheral joints of the hands and feet are usually involved first and symmetrically. The metacarpophalangeal and proximal interphalangeal joints of the hands and the metatarsophalangeal joints of the feet are affected, but the distal interphalangeal joint is usually spared. Ultimately any of the diarthrodial joints can be affected. Synovial hypertrophy and effusion cause swelling and the affected joints are warm and tender. Affected joints cannot be fully extended or fully flexed due to tenosynovitis. Erosive changes give rise to joint instability and subluxation. Characteristic deformities include ulnar deviation, swan neck and Boutonnière deformities (Fig. 50.1). Patients usually experience prolonged morning stiffness, which improves during the day, only to return at night.

The extra-articular features of RA (Table 50.1) occur in approximately 75% of seropositive patients and these are usually associated with a poor prognosis.

INVESTIGATIONS

The diagnosis of RA is made on presenting signs and symptoms and some biochemical investigations. The most useful of these are the erythrocyte sedimentation rate (ESR) and the rheumatoid factor test. A raised ESR simply confirms the presence of an inflammatory condition and is present in many disease states. A normal ESR does not preclude active disease. Rheumatoid factors are autoantibodies directed against the host gammaglobulin. Routinely performed tests only detect IgM rheumatoid factor. This is present in approximately 80% of patients with RA and 5% of normal subjects. However, approximately 25% of those with RA are seronegative. Antinuclear antibodies are present in 30% of patients with RA but the DNA binding is not elevated. Other abnormal laboratory tests include elevated C-reactive protein, elevated alkaline phosphatase, elevated platelet count, decreased serum albumin, and a normochromic, normocytic anaemia.

X-rays, mainly of the hands and feet, are used to establish the diagnosis of RA and to follow its progression. Erosions can be seen at the joint margins and loss of joint space due to erosion of cartilage and bone may be identified. In severe long-standing disease the dominant features include subluxation and deformity.

The synovial fluid is not routinely analysed to establish the diagnosis of RA but typically it is yellow, watery and turbid due to a high white blood cell count, and has a low glucose content.

TREATMENT

The goals of management of RA are to relieve pain and inflammation, to prevent joint destruction and to preserve or improve a patient's functional ability.

The treatment of RA is empirical as the cause of the disease is unknown. A combination of rest, exercise, occupational therapy, psychological support and drugs is used. Exercise, through physiotherapy, aims to preserve a range of joint movement and to improve muscle tone. Surgery has an important role, particularly for the feet to enable patients to wear shoes, and through joint replacements especially of the knee. The foundation supporting the treatment of RA is education of the patient and his or her family. Education

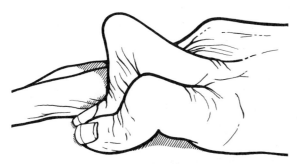

Fig. 50.1 Typical Boutonnière deformity with flexion of the PIP joint and extension of the DIP joint.

should provide basic information about the disease and reinforce the importance of compliance with all aspects of the treatment plan.

The treatment for each patient is individualized and based on factors such as the age, occupation and family responsibilities. Other considerations include the degree of disease activity and joint function, and the patient's response to previous therapy.

Rheumatoid arthritis is a disease with a variable prognosis which can impair the duration as well as the quality of life. Epidemiological, genetic and natural history studies have helped to identify patients who are at risk of the devel-

Table 50.3 Drugs used in the treatment of RA

First line agents
    Analgesics
    Non-steroidal anti-inflammatory agents

Second line agents
    Antimalarials
    Gold – parenteral and oral
    Penicillamine
    Sulphasalazine

Third line agents
    Azathioprine
    Methotrexate
    Cyclophosphamide

Other agents
    Corticosteroids – parenteral or oral

Table 50.4 Pharmaceutical parameters of NSAIDs

Drug	Adult daily dose range for rheumatoid arthritis	Dosage forms
Acetic acids		
Diclofenac	75–150 mg in 3 doses	EC tablet, SR tablet, dispersible tablet, injection, suppository
Tolmetin	1.2–2.0 g in 3–4 doses	Capsule
Anthranilic acids		
Mefenamic acid	1500 mg in 3 doses	Capsule, tablet, dispersible tablet, suspension
Indole/indene acetic acids		
Etodolac	200–600 mg in 2 doses	Capsule, tablet
Indomethacin	50–200 mg in 3 doses	Capsule, SR capsule, SR tablet, suppository, suspension
Sulindac	300–400 mg in 2 doses	Tablet
Propionic acids		
Fenbufen	600–1000 mg in 2 doses	Capsule, tablet, effervescent tablet
Fenoprofen	2.4–3.2 g in 4 doses	Tablet
Flurbiprofen	150–300 mg in 2–4 doses	Tablet, suppository, SR capsule
Ibuprofen	1.2–3.2 g in 3–4 doses	Tablet, SR capsule, syrup
Ketoprofen	150–300 mg in 3 doses	Capsule, SR capsule, suppository, injection
Naproxen	500–750 mg in 2 doses	Tablet, capsule, suppository, suspension, granules/sachet
Tiaprofenic acid	600–1200 mg in 3 doses	Tablet, SR capsule, granules/sachet
Butanone		
Nabumetone	1–1.5 g in 1–2 doses	Tablet, suspension
Oxicams		
Piroxicam	20 mg in 1 or 2 doses	Capsule, suppository, dispersible tablet
Tenoxicam	20 mg daily	Tablet
Pyrazolidinediones		
Phenylbutazone	300–400 mg in 3–4 doses	EC tablet
Azapropazone	1.2 g in 2–4 doses	Capsule, tablet
Salicylates		
Aspirin	3–6 g in 4–6 doses	Dispersible tablet, EC tablet, SR tablet
Benorylate	4–8 g in 2–3 doses	Tablet, suspension, granules/sachet
Choline magnesium trisalicylate	2–3 g in 1–2 doses	Tablet
Diflunisal	1.0 g in 2 doses	Tablet
Salsalate	3.0 g in 2–3 doses	Capsule

opment of more serious disease. These include female patients who are under 50 years old with gradual disease onset, upper extremity polyarthritis, systemic disease (particularly vasculitis), seropositivity, decreased serum IgM levels, bony erosions occurring early and the presence of HLA DR4 and DR1.

A recent trend in the drug treatment of RA is to commence disease-modifying antirheumatic drugs (DMARDs) at an early stage. This is particularly important in those patients with factors suggesting a poor prognosis.

The drug management for RA should proceed in a stepwise manner (Table 50.3).

First line agents

The major pharmacological agents for the relief of pain and inflammation in rheumatic diseases are the non-steroidal anti-inflammatory drugs (NSAIDs). These agents have replaced the use of high-dose aspirin as they are less toxic, longer

acting and thus have better compliance. These agents have attracted much adverse publicity due, principally, to serious adverse reactions. Many NSAIDs have been withdrawn, although one, ibuprofen, has been made available for sale from pharmacies. The agents available are shown in Table 50.4.

The inflammatory mediators upon which NSAIDs have an inhibitory effect include prostaglandin and leukotriene synthesis, neutrophil function, lymphocyte activation, oxygen radical formation and cytokine production. Although the NSAIDs differ in chemical structure, they all have similar pharmacological properties (antipyretic, anti-inflammatory, and analgesic actions), adverse effect profiles and pharmacokinetics (Table 50.5).

Patient response to NSAIDs is highly variable and therapeutic trials with several NSAIDs may be necessary to determine the best agent. From a choice of four different NSAIDs approximately 60% of patients will gain some symptom control

Table 50.5   Pharmacokinetic parameters of non-steroidal anti-inflammatory drugs

Drug	Tmax (h)	Vd L/kg	$t_{1/2}$ (h)	% renal excretion
Short half-life				
Aspirin	1–2	0.15	0.25	<2
Diclofenac	1–3	0.12	1.1	<1
Etodolac			3	
Fenoprofen	1–2	0.10	2.5	2–5
Flufenamic acid	1.5–6		9.0	<1
Flurbiprofen	1–2	0.10	3–4	<15
Ibuprofen	0.5–1.5		2.1	1
Indomethacin	1–2	0.12	4.6	<15
Ketorolac	1	0.11–0.33	4–6	50–60
Ketoprofen	0.5–2	0.11	1.8	<1
Tiaprofenic acid			3	
Tolmetin			1	
Long half-life				
Azapropazone	3–6	0.16	15	62
Diflunisal	1–2	0.10	5–20	<3
Fenbufen	1–2		11	4
Nabumetone	3–6	0.11	26	1
Naproxen	1–2	0.10	14	<1
Phenylbutazone	2	0.17	50–100	1
Piroxicam	2	0.12	38	10
Salicylate	2	0.17	2–30	2–30
Sulindac	1		7 (sulindac) 16 (active sulphide)	7
Tenoxicam	1–2	0.12	60	<1

Key: Tmax = time to maximum serum concentration; Vd = volume of distribution; $t_{1/2}$ = elimination half-life but approximately 10% will not find any agent beneficial. A 2-week trial is usually sufficient to assess efficacy. This variability in response to NSAIDs may be partly explained by their differing individual effects on the inflammatory pathways although other factors are clearly important. Patient preference and compliance are the best indicators of success. The factors which should be considered in choosing a specific NSAID are relative efficacy, toxicity, concomitant drugs, concurrent disease states, patient's age, renal function, dosing frequency and cost.

There is no evidence of synergism or reduced toxicity with the use of more than one NSAID. Only one agent should usually be prescribed at a time, although a short-acting drug may be used during the day with a longer-acting preparation at night.

The NSAIDs can be broadly divided into those with a long or short plasma half-life. The site of action for NSAIDs is assumed to be within the joint space and thus synovial fluid pharmacokinetics may be more important for efficacy than plasma kinetic profiles. However, in synovial fluid, prostaglandin concentrations remain suppressed long after an NSAID becomes undetectable. Studies on synovial fluid kinetics demonstrate that drug concentrations are more sustained and show less variability than plasma concentrations. This means that many short half-life NSAIDs need only be given twice daily to reduce pain and stiffness, whilst many long half-life NSAIDs take more time to reach steady state and remain in the synovial fluid longer after treatment withdrawal. The half-lives of NSAIDs are shown in Table 50.5.

Adverse effects

The most important adverse effects of NSAIDs are gastrointestinal bleeding and perforation. Patients may complain of nausea and indigestion while taking NSAIDs but some of those presenting with bleeding or perforation will have no history of dyspepsia or peptic ulceration. 'NSAID gastropathy' more commonly affects the stomach than the duodenum and is prevalent amongst elderly patients. Finding the true incidence of gastrointestinal side effects due to NSAIDs is difficult. Short- and long-term treatment with aspirin and other NSAIDs is known to induce dyspeptic symptoms in up to 60% of cases and gastroduodenal lesions in 30 to 50% of patients. Serious gastrointestinal haemorrhage or perforation can be expected in 1% and less than half of these patients will experience dyspeptic symptoms before the serious event.

Gastric damage appears to require a direct mucosal irritant effect as well as inhibition of prostaglandin synthesis. The mechanisms involved are various but inhibition of prostaglandin biosynthesis and impairment of mucosal defensive factors (mucus and bicarbonate secretion, mucosal blood flow) play a major role.

Intestinal damage by NSAIDs has recently been reported and up to 70% of patients receiving long-term NSAIDs have evidence of irritation of the small intestine.

A number of strategies to reduce gastrointestinal damage from NSAIDs have been proposed. Pro-drugs and non-acidic NSAIDs have been developed to solve the gastropathy problem, but appear to have little benefit in practice. The elimination or reduction of gastric acid with H_2 receptor antagonists and cytoprotective agents such as misoprostol is partially successful, although the efficacy of prostaglandin analogues against duodenal injuries remains dubious.

Most NSAIDs can reduce creatinine clearance and produce a non-oliguric renal failure, possibly as a result of inhibition of prostaglandin synthesis in the kidney. This effect tends to be relatively minor, usually reversible and associated with long-term therapy. Those patients with impaired renal function, hepatic cirrhosis, and circulatory volume depletion are most at risk. The value of sulindac in this situation is controversial, but some consider that this NSAID has less inhibitory effect on renal prostaglandin synthesis than other agents. Indomethacin is the most commonly reported cause of NSAID-induced acute renal failure and fenoprofen the NSAID most commonly associated with interstitial nephritis and nephrotic syndrome.

Asthmatic patients may develop wheezing following administration of NSAIDs and aspirin will provoke or worsen asthma in approximately 5% of patients.

Some NSAIDs have been shown to affect chondrocyte function in vitro in animal models, which has led to the suggestion that NSAIDs may prevent regeneration of articular cartilage and hasten the development of OA.

Other possible adverse effects of NSAIDs involve the skin, liver and bone marrow. Indomethacin, in particular, can cause headache, dizziness and psychiatric disturbances. Common drug interactions are detailed in Table 50.6.

Disease-modifying antirheumatic drugs (DMARDs)

The characteristics of DMARDs are not uniform, but they all possess a slow onset of action. The agents are not intrinsically anti-inflammatory with the possible exception of methotrexate. The DMARDs are thought to affect more disease processes than NSAIDs. They can alter laboratory characteristics of disease activity and alter the progression of bone damage. The mechanism of action for these agents is not known, and almost certainly they are all different.

Patients treated with sulphasalazine, and occasionally auranofin or azathioprine, may respond in 8 to 10 weeks, but in most cases 12 to 24 weeks are required to ensure a response to azathioprine, d-penicillamine, and sodium aurothiomalate. Maximal response to chloroquine or hydroxychloroquine may be delayed for up to 18 months.

Comparisons of relative efficacy for the DMARDs have been based on joint tenderness (e.g. using the Ritchie index), grip strength and 'marked improvement' (>50% decrease in joint swelling) and laboratory measures including ESR, the rheumatoid factor titre and radiological deterioration. Study protocols have not been uniform and thus data comparing each agent are not available for all DMARDs. However, one attempt to rank DMARDs for efficacy, based on 6- and 12-month studies suggested the following: methotrexate = sodium aurothiomalate >/= d-penicillamine = azathioprine >/= hydroxychloroquine = sulphasalazine = auranofin. Tolerability for the same 6- to 12-month period is hydroxychloroquine = azathioprine = methotrexate >/= auranofin = sulphasalazine >/= d-penicillamine >/= sodium aurothiomalate. There are inherent difficulties in comparing the DMARDs in this manner when data are missing from comparative studies and thus these comparisons should be viewed as approximations only.

The decision on which agent to use first should be based partially on efficacy but primarily on toxicity, considering the risk: benefit ratio for the individual patient. The current DMARD of first choice is sulphasalazine. Sulphasalazine is generally considered to provide an effective benefit:risk relationship, being similar in efficacy to sodium aurothiomalate but less toxic. The requirements for monitoring of this agent (Table 50.7) are less intrusive than most other DMARDs which is a significant benefit to patients.

Table 50.6 Drug interactions of NSAIDs		
Affected drug	Drug causing effect	Effect
Oral anticoagulants	NSAIDs	Aspirin enhances hypoprothrombinaemic effect All increase risk of GI bleed, all have antiplatelet effects
Hypotensive agents	NSAIDs	Decreased hypotensive effect
Diuretics	NSAIDs	Decreased diuretic effect
Potassium-sparing drugs, e.g. ACE inhibitors, potassium-sparing diuretics	Indomethacin	Hyperkalaemia
Lithium	Most NSAIDs	Increased lithium levels
Methotrexate	All NSAIDs	Increased methotrexate levels
Most NSAIDs	Probenecid	Increased NSAID concentration

Table 50.7   Dose and monitoring schedule for DMARDs

Drug	Dose schedule	Adverse effects	Monitoring
Sodium aurothiomalate	10 mg test dose, 50 mg weekly until signs of remission, 2-weekly until full remission, then progressive increase to 3-, 4-, and 6-weekly.	Skin rash, mouth ulcers, proteinuria, blood disorders rarely, colitis, pulmonary fibrosis, peripheral neuritis, hepatotoxicity with cholestatic jaundice	FBC, platelets urine, signs of skin toxicity Test before each injection
Auranofin	6 mg daily, increase to 9 mg if response inadequate after 6 months	Diarrhoea, skin rash, mouth ulcers, blood disorders, nausea, rarely pulmonary fibrosis	FBC, platelets, urine proteinuria Monthly
Sulphasalazine	500 mg daily, increasing by 500 mg each week to a maximum dose of 3 g daily (approx. 40 mg/kg)	Gastrointestinal intolerance, rashes, rarely blood disorders, hepatitis	Differential WBC, RBC, platelets, LFTs Monthly for first 3 months
D-penicillamine	125–250 mg daily for first month increasing by same amount each 4–12 weeks until remission. Usual maintenance dose 500–750 mg daily (max. 1.5 g). In remission dose reduction by 125–250 mg every 12 weeks may be attempted	Nausea, taste loss, blood disorders, proteinuria, rashes, rarely lupus erythematosus, myasthenia gravis, Goodpasture's syndrome	FBC, platelets, proteinuria Weekly or fortnightly for first 8 weeks after dose increase and otherwise monthly
Hydroxychloroquine	400 mg daily reducing to 200 mg when no further improvement, max. dose 6.5 mg/kg/day	Corneal opacities, rashes, nausea, rarely muscle weakness, bone marrow depression, retinal changes	Ophthalmology 6-monthly, FBC periodically
Chloroquine	150 mg base daily	As above	As above
Methotrexate	7.5 mg weekly, increasing after 6–8 weeks, by 2.5 mg/week to 25 mg/week. After response, decrease to minimum dose	Blood disorders, nausea, stomatitis, diarrhoea, hepatitis, teratogenesis	FBC, platelets, 1–2 weekly initially then monthly once dose stable LFTs and liver biopsy every 2 years
Azathioprine	1.0–2.5 mg/kg/day. If no response after 8 weeks increase by 0.5 mg/kg/day every month until min. effective dose achieved	Blood disorders, nausea, hepatitis, cholestatic jaundice	FBC, platelets, LFTs, 1- to 2-weekly initially, then monthly once dose stable

Gold is available in injectable form as sodium aurothiomalate and orally as auranofin. Sodium aurothiomalate is probably more effective than auranofin although its safer adverse effect profile is a significant advantage. Auranofin, is less toxic to the bone marrow and kidney than sodium aurothiomalate, although it has more frequent gastrointestinal effects. Clinical response and adverse effects to both gold and penicillamine are similar. Penicillamine is relatively easy to administer although it is dependent upon the patient taking the preparation on an empty stomach. Food intake impairs absorption. Penicillamine is used by many rheumatologists with caution because of serious side effects such as lupus and myasthenia gravis which can develop.

Most immunosuppressive agents are also cytotoxic and the potential risks of their use must be carefully balanced against the intended clinical improvement.

Methotrexate is an effective antirheumatic drug in both established and early RA with rapid efficacy at low dose. It is generally well tolerated with no good evidence that its use predisposes to malignancy, although it is associated with a clear risk of teratogenicity. There is also evidence that hepatic fibrosis may result from administration for more than 2 years, an adverse effect which is enhanced by significant alcohol ingestion. The correct monitoring method to detect hepatotoxicity is controversial.

Azathioprine is used for the control of RA refractory to second line agents but its use may be associated with an increased risk of non-Hodgkin's lymphoma over and above the small increase seen in untreated RA. Cyclophosphamide is a potentially toxic agent the use of which is associated with the development of malignancies. This limits its use mainly to the management of rheumatoid vasculitis.

Cyclosporin is an immunosuppressant which is efficacious as a DMARD but how and when to use it is currently unclear.

The efficacy of DMARDs in combination has been reported in a number of studies. Combinations of antimalarials and penicillamine, antimalarials and methotrexate, gold and azathioprine, methotrexate and cyclophosphamide and antimalarials, cyclophosphamide and azathioprine have been described with favourable results. The monitoring of combination therapy is difficult.

Corticosteroids are the most potent anti-inflammatory drugs available but chronic therapy is associated with serious unacceptable long-term adverse effects, and steroid treatment does not alter the natural course of RA. In severe, life-threatening situations such as rheumatoid vasculitis, a high initial dose may be given which is reduced as the disease is controlled. However, once commenced, systemic corticosteroid therapy is very difficult to withdraw as the disease tends to flare with dosage reduction. For this reason pulse doses of corticosteroids are used to suppress highly active disease whilst other longer-term and slower-acting medication is commenced.

Prednisolone remains the systemic steroid of choice and the daily dosage should be kept as low as possible and usually below 7.5 mg to prevent suppression of the hypothalamo-adrenal axis. Treatment should be given in a single morning dose; alternate-day therapy is usually unsuccessful.

Intra-articular steroid (methylprednisolone acetate, triamcinolone hexacetonide) administra-tion can effectively relieve pain, increase mobility, and reduce deformity in one or a few joints. The duration of response to intra-articular steroids is variable between patients, and triamcinolone hexacetonide may produce the longest response. The dose used is dependent upon the joint size with methylprednisolone acetate 40 mg or triamcinolone hexacetonide 20 mg appropriate for large joints (knees). The frequency at which injections may be repeated is controversial, but repeated injections may be given at intervals of 1 to 5 or more weeks depending on the degree of relief obtained from the first injection.

The adverse effects of intra-articular steroids include joint infection, muscle wasting, tendon rupture and skin atrophy. Locally administered corticosteroids are absorbed systemically and thus hypothalamo-adrenal axis suppression can occur.

THE PATIENT

Education of the rheumatoid arthritic patient is important. Patients should have knowledge of the disease process and their likely prognosis. Psychological aspects of the disease should be covered.

When counselling patients on NSAIDs they should be advised to take the preparation with food, and be warned of the potential adverse effects and what action to take if these occur. Patients should be warned not to supplement their prescribed NSAIDs with purchased ibuprofen or aspirin.

A patient who is prescribed a course of treatment with a DMARD must be aware of the need to comply with monitoring requirements and the delay in obtaining a response to therapy. Patients must also have realistic expectations for treatment goals, a clear understanding of potential toxicity and the action to take in the event of adverse effects.

OSTEOARTHRITIS

Osteoarthritis (OA) is a common, age related, slowly progressive degenerative condition, which is usually monoarticular or less commonly polyarticular and of unknown cause.

EPIDEMIOLOGY

OA is the most common form of arthritis in man, with X-ray evidence of it being present in more than 80% of people over 55 years. OA affects all cultural groups although the pattern of involvement varies.

The prevalence of OA increases with age. Certain joints (distal interphalangeal joints, the first metatarsophalangeal joint) are commonly affected in early life whereas ankles, shoulders and weight-bearing joints are usually not involved until later. Men and women are affected equally although severe disease more commonly occurs in women.

AETIOLOGY

The concept of OA as a disease of wear and tear is too simplistic as it has inflammatory, erosive and reparative features. A wide variety of factors predispose to, and promote the development of the condition. The most important of these is age and joint loading. Either an abnormal joint which is normally loaded (e.g. a congenital hip defect) or a normal joint abnormally loaded (due to excess body weight) may develop OA. Other predisposing factors to the development of OA include a failure of bone and cartilage remodelling, crystal deposition and catabolic enzyme secretion. OA shows no genetic transmission, and no dietary, nutritional or exercise-related influence.

Primary generalized OA is associated with the formation of Heberden's nodes (bony protuberances at the margins on the dorsal surface) on the distal interphalangeal joint. This form of OA is common in postmenopausal women and it may progress to an acute inflammatory condition with loss of cartilage and bone erosions apparent on X-ray film. The cause of bone resorption, the formation of osteophytes and the deposition of hydroxyapatite or pyrophosphate crystals remains unknown. Secondary OA can develop through any cause of joint disruption; after disruption rest is superfluous.

PATHOPHYSIOLOGY

There are qualitative and quantitative variations in the features of OA compared to RA. The synovial lining is not usually inflamed although there may be an inflammatory response with cartilage, bone fragments and crystals present in the synovial fluid. Thinning of the hyaline cartilage occurs which may lead to cartilage loss, and damage to chondrocytes. Bone proliferation with subchondral sclerosis and osteophyte formation occurs.

CLINICAL MANIFESTATIONS

The signs and symptoms of OA are dependent upon the affected joints. Pain, worsened by loading and moving and eased by rest is the primary symptom. The pain, often described as an ache, is usually localized to the affected joints, although it may be referred away from its origin (e.g. hip pain may be felt at the knee). The pain is often worse at the end of the day. Stiffness and loss of movement of the affected joints occurs due to loss of integrity of the joint surface, development of osteophytes and crystal formation. Deformity of affected joints may develop leading to loss of function. Crepitus may be heard in affected joints upon passive or active movement.

The most commonly affected joints are the distal interphalangeal, proximal interphalangeal, and first metocarpophalangeal joints, the knees, hips, cervical and lumbar spine. There are no laboratory abnormalities in OA and rheumatoid factor is negative.

INVESTIGATIONS

OA is diagnosed by the presence of bone sclerosis and osteophyte formation (due to ligamentous stress) with loss of joint space on X-ray film. There is a total lack of association between symptoms and X-ray changes. Arthroscopy can verify the diagnosis. The arthroscopic appearance of normal cartilage is smooth, white and glistening, whilst OA cartilage is yellowed, irregular and ulcerated.

TREATMENT

The therapeutic goals of OA are pain relief, increased mobility and reduction of disability. The therapeutic options for the management of OA are limited and basically involve NSAIDs and intra-articular steroid injections to provide symptomatic relief. No drug treatment has to date been demonstrated to delay the progression of OA.

Non-drug treatment is important. Patients should be advised to protect joints through modification of daily living and reduce weight. Physical aids and an exercise programme, heat, cold, ultrasound, diathermy and other aspects of physical therapy may be helpful. Those patients with intractable pain and/or significant impaired function may be assisted with orthopaedic therapy.

Most patients with OA have pain as a result of damage to bone and cartilage. In the absence of inflammation, regular or as required analgesia and instruction in joint protection measures are all that are required. Paracetamol, 500 mg every 4 to 6 hours is appropriate for most patients although the risks of excessive dosing leading to hepatotoxicity should be stressed. There is little place for combination analgesic use with codeine, propoxyphene or other narcotics.

In addition to biochemical degeneration there is an associated inflammatory component to OA which is not fully understood although it is thought it may be in part crystal induced. In this situation, NSAIDs provide effective therapy compared to simple analgesics as the pain control is usually better. The choice of NSAID may be influenced by efficacy, adverse effect profile and duration of action. The usual dosage requirements for OA are approximately 50% of those required for RA.

Concern has been expressed recently over the effect of NSAIDs on the OA disease process itself. Several in vitro studies and some using animal models have reported a deleterious effect of NSAIDs on cartilage and chrondrocyte metabolism through an inhibition of proteoglycan synthesis. It remains to be determined whether NSAIDs have a detrimental effect on cartilage in patients.

Systemic steroids have no role in the management of OA although intra-articular steroids may be of benefit in patients with acute inflammation. The use of intra-articular steroids is, however, not without controversy. Some studies suggest that the severity of the pathological changes is increased following steroid injections. Many workers also consider amelioration of pain in man may lead to overuse of the damaged joint and further breakdown of the cartilage. It has been recommended that repeat injections should not be given more often than every 3 months for a given joint. The duration of symptomatic improvement following intra-articular injection may range from a few days to 1 month or longer.

'Chondroprotective agents' have been investigated, following the suggestion that some NSAIDs may be protective or anabolic in their effects on cartilage. This group of agents (which includes tiaprofenic acid, tribenoside, diclofenac sodium, S-adenosyl-L-methionine, sodium pentosan polysulphate, GAG polysulphate (Arteparon), and GAG-peptide complex (Rumalon) has been the subject of much experimentation, but there are no convincing studies in humans which support the assertion that these agents are chondroprotective.

THE PATIENT

The current management systems for osteoarthritic patients are primarily symptomatic or reconstructive. The condition is not life threatening and many of the patients are frail and elderly.

Patients should be counselled on the correct use of analgesics and should be given realistic expectations about their treatment. Those patients who are overweight should receive dietary advice to lose excess weight. Physical methods to decrease the patient's pain, improve the range of motion and increase the individual's ability to carry out activities of daily living should be investigated. Examples of these include walking aids and braces. Regular, carefully planned exercise such as swimming can also be beneficial. Rarely, local treatments such as ultrasound or moist heat can provide pain relief.

In summary, osteoarthritis is a common condition which is poorly understood. Drug treatment has little to offer in terms of disease prevention but simple analgesics can be effective for symptomatic relief.

CASE STUDIES

CASE 50.1

Mrs X. B. is a 75-year-old lady who has had OA in her knees for several years. She has tried various NSAIDs in the past to obtain pain relief and is currently taking tenoxicam 10 mg each morning. Mrs X. B. is admitted to hospital following an acute gastric bleed probably caused by her use of NSAIDs.

Q1 How should Mrs X. B.'s OA be managed in the future?

Q2 Is there a role for the use of misoprostol in Mrs X. B.?

Q3 Would topical NSAIDs be of any use in this patient?

CASE 50.2

Mrs A. Y. is 58 years old and has suffered from RA for 12 years. Despite receiving treatment over the past 12 months with d-penicillamine 625 mg daily Mrs A. Y. experiences a disease flare-up of the RA. Her metacarpophalangeal and proximal interphalangeal joints are swollen and tender to touch and she has bilateral knee effusions. The blood biochemistry reveals a low haemoglobin, raised platelet count, elevated erythrocyte sedimentation rate and raised SCAT (sheep cell agglutination test) and latex tests.

Q1 Comment on the level of disease activity.

Q2 Mrs A. Y. is found to have anaemia of chronic disease. What is this and how should it be managed?

Q3 What advice should the patient have received about her current therapy?

Q4 What drug therapy would be appropriate now?

CASE 50.3

Mrs A. B. is 64 years old and has a long history of extensive RA. She presents to the clinic with an ulcer on the heal of her left foot which she has had for several weeks together with pain and discolouration of the third toe on her left foot. She is diagnosed as having rheumatoid vasculitis and an infection in her ischaemic toe.

Q1 What is the prognosis for a patient with rheumatoid vasculitis?

Q2 What antibiotic therapy would be appropriate for Mrs A. B.?

Q3 What is the role of steroids and cytotoxics in the management of Mrs A. B.?

Q4 What drugs may cause vasculitis?

ANSWERS TO CASE STUDIES

CASE 50.1

A1 It will be necessary to discontinue the patient's NSAID because of the gastric bleed.

The patient's joint pain will be eased by bed rest and analgesic therapy (paracetamol). Osteoarthritic joints which show signs of acute inflammation (redness, heat) do respond to intra-articular steroid administration.

The patient should be commenced on a healing dose of an H_2 antagonist and should be endoscoped to identify the source of bleeding.

The patient's blood film shows evidence of iron deficiency anaemia most likely caused by the bleeding (low haemoglobin concentration, low MCV, low MCHC). The patient should receive oral iron therapy and after 7 to 10 days a reticulocyte count should be obtained to ensure that the iron is being absorbed and thus the patient's anaemia is being corrected. The patient's haemoglobin concentration should continue to rise by approximately 2 g every 3 weeks.

A2 Elderly female patients are particularly at risk of gastric ulceration secondary to NSAIDs. Patients are often asymptomatic. It is difficult to identify those patients at risk of haemorrhage or perforation and thus the question over ulcer prophylaxis remains unanswered. Gastric ulceration as a result of NSAIDs is more common than duodenal ulceration. Misoprostol is an effective agent for prophylaxis against gastric ulcers but its role in duodenal ulcer prophylaxis remains unclear. H_2-receptor antagonists are effective for duodenal ulcer prophylaxis in patients receiving NSAIDs.

To give all patients prophylaxis with misoprostol or H_2-receptor antagonists would be extremely costly particularly since the incidence of haemorrhage is extremely small. Patients that may be considered for long-term prophylactic treatment are those with risk factors for ulceration or a history of peptic ulceration.

A3 The efficacy of topical NSAIDs remains poorly defined mainly because of the difficulty in measuring response. Trials comparing the activity of these agents to placebo have generally demonstrated a significant placebo response (50 to 60%). The topical preparations are expensive when compared to rubifacients.

Topical NSAIDs are designed to present a high concentration of the locally applied agent to the joint with minimal systemic effect. The topical NSAIDs have been associated with fewer side effects than systemic NSAIDs although cases of gastric upset have been reported.

In the case of Mrs X. B. it would be appropriate to commence application of a rubifacient.

CASE 50.2

A1 Mrs A. Y. has active RA. This is evident by the clinical presentation of joint swelling, stiffness, pain and loss of function. The SCAT and latex tests are two different methods used to measure the concentration of rheumatoid factor (IgM). In this patient the tests for rheumatoid factor are positive. The elevated ESR and platelet count are further evidence of active disease.

A2 The characteristics of anaemia of chronic disease are normochromic, normocytic red cells and a low haemoglobin concentration in the presence of signs of inflammatory activity (raised ESR). Both the serum iron concentration and total iron binding capacity will be low.

The anaemia is often asymptomatic. The cause of this type of anaemia remains unknown, although it is considered that impaired release of iron from stores in the reticuloendothelial system and decreased erythrocyte life span may play a role.

Treatment of the condition depends on correcting the underlying inflammatory condition with disease-modifying antirheumatic drugs. This anaemia does not respond to folate, vitamin B_{12} or iron therapy. There is some evidence that iron therapy actually exacerbates the inflammatory nature of the disease.

A3 Patient counselling on d-penicillamine therapy is particularly important. Patients should be told to take the drug on an empty stomach at least 1 hour before meals. The tablet should be followed with half a tumbler of water only. Concurrent food intake can reduce the bioavailability of d-penicillamine by 50%. In addition to counselling about the need to take the medication on an empty stomach the patient must be advised of the potential adverse reactions of the drug. Rashes are of two types, early ones are usually erythematous whilst rashes later in treatment (after roughly 6 months) are usually pruritic and are an indication to stop treatment. Other adverse reactions such as nausea, anorexia and loss of taste tend to occur at the start of treatment and then subside.

The patient must be present for regular (usually fortnightly) monitoring of urine (for haematuria and proteinuria) and regular blood counts (white cell and platelet counts).

A4 At this stage the next most appropriate disease-modifying antirheumatic drug would be methotrexate. This should be commenced at a dose of 7.5 mg once weekly and increased to 15 mg once weekly after 6 weeks if the patient has not responded.

CASE 50.3

A1 Rheumatoid vasculitis is a rare but life-threatening condition which occurs due to inflammation in the blood vessels. The condition may affect only the blood vessels or involve multiple organs and particularly the kidney. The primary aetiology is immune complex deposition in blood vessels.

A2 Antistaphylococcal therapy, such as flucloxacillin 1 g four times a day intravenously, should be commenced until the results of cultures are available. Where the patient exhibits signs of septicaemia, broad-spectrum antimicrobial therapy such as ampicillin, gentamicin and metronidazole should be administered until culture data are available.

A3 Systemic corticosteroids are the treatment of choice for vasculitis to suppress the immune system. Intravenous hydrocortisone 100 mg every 6 hours or intravenous methylprednisolone 500 mg to 1 g daily may be administered. Methylprednisolone should always be administered over approximately 1 hour, as large doses administered rapidly have been associated with myocardial ischaemia. Oral corticosteroids may be instituted using prednisolone 80 mg/day divided into four doses, as a starting dose. Once the condition improves the steroid dose may be gradually reduced and administered as a single daily dose.

The response to corticosteroids may be monitored by laboratory indices such as the erythrocyte sedimentation rate, the renal function and urine protein content.

In vasculitides unresponsive to corticosteroids alone, the addition of cyclophosphamide (1 to 2 mg/kg/day) as additional immunosuppression may be used. In life-threatening vasculitis particularly with renal involvement intravenous cyclophosphamide (4 mg/kg/day) for 3 days is beneficial. This larger initial dose may be later reduced to 1 to 2 mg/kg/day. Adverse effects include leucopenia and haemorrhagic cystitis.

A4 Drugs reported to induce vasculitis include allopurinol, acyclovir, penicillin, sulphonamides and some NSAIDs.

BIBLIOGRAPHY

Rheumatoid arthritis

Arnold M, Schrieber L, Brooks P. Immunosuppressive drugs and corticosteroids in the treatment of rheumatoid arthritis. Drugs 1988; 36: 340–363

Day R O, Grahan G G, Williams K M, Brooks P M. Variability in response to NSAIDs – fact or fiction? Drugs 1988; 36: 643–651

Furst D E. Rational use of disease-modifying antirheumatic drugs. Drugs 1990; 39: 19–37

Giercksky K E, Huseby G, Rustead A E. Epidemiology of NSAID-related gastrointestinal side effects. Scandinavian Journal of Gastroenterology 1989; 24(Suppl. 163): 3–8

Harris E D. Rheumatoid arthritis: mechanisms of disease. New England Journal of Medicine 1990; 322: 1277–1289

Sturrock R D. 'Second line' drugs for rheumatoid arthritis. British Medical Journal 1991; 303: 201

Osteoarthritis

Altman J D. Overview of osteoarthritis. American Journal of Medicine 1987; 83(Suppl. 4B): 65–69

Al Arfag A, Davis P. Osteoarthritis 1991. Current drug treatment regimens. Drugs 1991; 41: 193–201

Liang M H, Fortin P. Management of osteoarthritis of the hip and knee. New England Journal of Medicine 1991; 325: 125–127

Mankin J H, Treadwell B V. Osteoarthritis: a 1987 update. Bulletin on Rheumatic Diseases 1987; 36(5): 1–10

Chapter 51

Gout and hyperuricaemia

E. A. Kay

Gout is a term which represents a heterogeneous group of diseases usually associated with hyperuricaemia. The hyperuricaemia may be due to an increased rate of synthesis of the purine precursors of uric acid or to decreased elimination of uric acid by the kidney or both.

Hyperuricaemia is a biochemical condition whilst gout is a clinical diagnosis. Many individuals have elevated levels of uric acid throughout life without experiencing adverse sequelae.

Gout is characterized by recurrent episodes of acute arthritis due to deposits of monosodium urate in joints and cartilage. Formation of uric acid calculi in the kidneys (nephrolithiasis) may occur.

EPIDEMIOLOGY

The prevalence of gout in Great Britain is approximately 2.6 cases per 1000. In approximately 10% of these cases gout is a secondary manifestation, with diuretics being the most frequent causative factor. Figures for the incidence of gout vary between populations and its prevalence is known to change with environmental and dietary factors in the same population over a short period of time.

Gout is a condition which affects middle-aged males most frequently, with only approximately 5% of cases occurring in females. Most female patients have a family history of the disease although studies in males have failed to detect a significant genetic component. The risk of acute gout occurring secondary to hyperuricaemia is approximately equal for both sexes but hyperuricaemia is many times more common in males.

AETIOLOGY

The development of gout is primarily related to the degree and duration of hyperuricaemia. Concentrations of urate in synovial fluid correlate closely with serum levels. A rigid definition of hyperuricaemia is not possible but in general terms the upper limit of normal for males is 470 μmol/L and 360 μmol/L for females.

Overproduction of uric acid

Overproduction of uric acid may result from excessive turnover of nucleoproteins (e.g. in type 1 glycogen storage disease, neoplastic diseases and myeloproliferative disorders), excessive dietary purines, or excessive synthesis of uric acid due to rare enzyme mutation defects (e.g. Lesch–Nyhan syndrome). Diet plays a minor role in this condition and thus dietary restrictions with the exception of limiting alcohol intake have a minor role to play.

Underexcretion of uric acid

Underexcretion of uric acid results from a defect in renal excretion. Uric acid is filtered at the glomerulus and almost completely reabsorbed in the proximal tubule. Of the reabsorbed uric acid, 50% is secreted distal to the proximal tubular reabsorption site and approximately 75% of this secreted urate is reabsorbed. In the hyperuricaemic state, large loads are filtered and urate reabsorption increases to avoid the dumping of poorly soluble urate into the urinary tract. Tubular urate secretion is not influenced by serum urate concentrations and it is probably the impaired urate secretion which is responsible for the hyperuricaemia.

Another cause of gouty arthritic attacks can be physical stress. Factors such as tight shoes, hill walking and hiking have been reported to cause acute attacks in the great toe. A history of joint trauma may also subsequently be associated with attacks of gout.

CLINICAL MANIFESTATIONS

Acute gout is traditionally considered monoarticular with the great toe most frequently affected. Approximately 80% of patients with gout have the initial attack in the great toe (podagra). The majority of patients will have podagra at some time during the course of the disease. Other joints frequently affected are small joints of the feet or ankles, the hands (distal interphalangeal joints), elbows and knees.

The initial presentation of the disease may be polyarticular and low grade inflammation may be present in many joints.

The patient with acute gouty arthritis complains of severe pain with a hot, red swollen and extremely tender joint. The weight of the bedclothes or the jar of a person walking on the floor is said to be agony to the sufferer and weight bearing is impossible. The affected joint has overlying erythema and signs of marked synovitis. The patient may be pyrexial with a leucocytosis (total white cell count in excess of $11 \times 10^9/L$) and elderly patients may be confused.

Chronic gout is associated with the presence of tophi and renal disease. In time, with treatment the tophi disappear although the renal function will probably remain static.

Premature atherosclerosis, cardiovascular disease and nephropathy are associated with gout but whether these are a consequence of hyperuricaemia remains unclear. In asymptomatic individuals gout, hypertension and coronary artery disease occur more commonly than in matched control groups. The half-lives of platelets in patients with gout are much shortened and thus platelet adhesiveness is increased. A number of studies have suggested that hyperuricaemia may be an independent risk factor for hypertension and atherosclerotic disease, while an association between hyperuricaemia and hypertriglyceridaemia has also been proposed. Obesity and alcohol excess are common factors to both these latter disorders rather than a direct causal mechanism for hyperuricaemia.

Gouty nephropathy is a form of chronic interstitial nephritis which occurs typically in patients who have had hyperuricaemia for many years associated with hyperexcretion of urate and urine hyperacidity. Crystals are deposited around the renal tubules and incite an inflammatory response. The renal medulla becomes infiltrated with mononuclear cells and fibrosis occurs. Clinically this is manifested by proteinuria and/or renal impairment.

Gout may be precipitated in patients who take diuretics, particularly a thiazide diuretic. The condition is characterized by the presence of tophi often developing in Heberden's nodes. Heberden's nodes are gelatinous cysts or bony outgrowths on the dorsal aspects of the distal interphalangeal joints. Patients affected rarely have acute attacks and the condition usually responds to withdrawal of the diuretic. If the diuretic is essential, allopurinol may be used to lower uric acid levels.

Radiotherapy and chemotherapy in patients with leukaemias and lymphomas may lead to hyperuricaemia. Uric acid nephropathy may occur in association with acute increases in uric acid production and this is the most common cause of acute renal failure in patients with leukaemia. This can be treated prophylactically with allopurinol commencing 3 days pretherapy and continuing for the duration of remission-inducing chemotherapy. Other measures which can be adopted to prevent urate nephropathy in this situation include alkalinization of the urine and vigorous fluid intake.

INVESTIGATIONS

The diagnosis of acute gout can only be made through examination of synovial fluid aspirated from the inflamed joint. Monosodium urate crystals are needle shaped and are negatively birefringent under a polarizing microscope. Aspirated synovial fluid also contains large numbers of polymorphonuclear leucocytes.

Hyperuricaemia alone is not diagnostic of gout as many hyperuricaemic patients never develop symptomatic gout and some patients with acute gout have a normal serum uric acid concentration. Attacks of gout tend to be precipitated by changes in uric acid concentration and the absolute level may have fallen back to normal during an attack. The diagnosis of gout is thus confirmed only by microscopic examination of synovial fluid aspirated from the affected joint.

The differential diagnosis in acute gouty arthritis must include infection. Patients with gout commonly present with acute swelling and tenderness of the joint with a fever, raised plasma viscosity and leucocytosis, with no previous history of arthritis. Patients with joint sepsis are usually more ill and have other systemic signs of infection such as a swinging fever and severe malaise. Large joints are most frequently infected and the joint is hot, tender and swollen with effusion and marked limitation of movement.

DRUG TREATMENT

In an acute attack of gout the primary goal is to relieve pain and inflammation.

Gout is a disease which is often associated with obesity, hypertriglyceridaemia, hypertension and high alcohol intake. A sub-group of patients (usually elderly women) taking diuretics has been recognized.

Acute attacks

The mainstay of treatment of an acute attack of gout is non-salicylate non-steroidal anti-inflammatory drugs (NSAIDs). Aspirin and its derivatives (choline magnesium trisalicylate, salsalate, benorylate) should be avoided as these agents compete with uric acid for excretion. NSAIDs will relieve pain and inflammation and they can abort an attack if commenced early. An alternative, but second choice, agent is colchicine. There are no controlled studies comparing colchicine with NSAIDs in matched patients.

Agents which decrease serum uric acid (allopurinol or uricosuric agents such as probenecid and sulphinpyrazone) should not be used in an acute attack. Patients generally have been hyperuricaemic for several years and there is no need to treat the hyperuricaemia immediately. In addition agents which decrease serum uric acid concentrations may cause mobilization of uric acid stores as the serum level falls. This movement of uric acid may prolong the acute attack or precipitate another attack of gouty arthritis. However, if the patient is already stabilized on allopurinol at the onset of the acute attack, it should be continued.

NSAIDs

NSAIDs should be administered in high dosage for the first 1 to 3 days or until the pain has settled. Lower doses should be continued until all symptoms and signs have resolved, usually after 7 to 10 days. Indomethacin is commonly prescribed for an acute attack of gouty arthritis initially at a dose of 75 to 100 mg three times a day. This dose should be reduced after 5 days as the acute attack settles. NSAIDs usually take 24 to 48 hours to work, although complete relief of gouty signs and symptoms is usually seen after 5 days of treatment. Adverse effects of indomethacin will include headaches, mental changes and gastrointestinal upset, although these will resolve with the decreasing dose. Other NSAIDs are also commonly used, including: naproxen 750 mg to start followed by 250 mg three times a day; piroxicam 40 mg per day to start followed by 10 mg per day; and diclofenac 100 mg to start, then 50 mg three times a day for 48 hours, then 50 mg twice daily for 8 days. Patients known to have gout should carry a supply of NSAIDs to treat an acute attack following the first symptom.

Colchicine

For oral colchicine to be effective it must be administered as quickly as possible after the onset of symptoms. Traditionally an initial dose of 1 mg has been used followed by 0.5 mg every 2 hours during the acute attack until there is relief of joint pain, or the patient develops gastrointestinal symptoms or the patient has

received a maximum dose of 10 mg. The titration of the dose between therapeutic response and gastrointestinal toxicity is difficult to achieve as the therapeutic dose is very close to the toxic dose. Deaths have occurred in patients who have received as little as 5 mg colchicine. The therapeutic response to colchicine usually commences after about 6 hours with pain relief after about 12 hours and resolution of pain, redness and swelling in 75% of patients after 48 to 72 hours. Colchicine thus has some diagnostic value. A course of colchicine should not be repeated within 3 days to prevent toxic reactions from occurring.

Adverse effects of colchicine include severe nausea and vomiting, diarrhoea and abdominal pain. These affect 80% of patients who have taken a therapeutic oral dose. Dehydration may be a major complication of therapy. Other side effects include seizure disorders, respiratory depression, hepatic and muscle necrosis, renal damage, fever, granulocytopenia, aplastic anaemia, disseminated intravascular coagulation and alopecia.

Intravenous colchicine is no longer licensed for use because it has been associated with severe toxicity. However, a review of the published experience with intravenous colchicine suggests that the toxicity was due to inappropriate use of the drug and usually involved dosage errors.

Distribution of colchicine occurs rapidly and after a single dose only 10% is excreted within the first 24 hours. Colchicine can still be detected in polymorphonuclear leucocytes 10 days after a single dose, implying a half-life of approximately 30 hours. The metabolism and excretion of colchicine are impaired in renal and hepatic disease.

The choice of agent, whether a NSAID or colchicine, may depend on other patient features. Patients with hypertension or those receiving diuretics in cardiac failure, those with gastrointestinal toxicity, bleeding diathesis or renal impairment should be treated with colchicine, which unlike NSAIDs will not affect other drug therapy.

It would be reasonable to give the patient one or two doses of narcotic analgesic (e.g. morphine

10 mg) whilst awaiting the analgesic effect of NSAIDs or colchicine.

Steroids

An alternative strategy to NSAIDs or colchicine is to use intra-articular steroids. These can provide quick relief when only one or two joints are involved; however, the differential diagnosis between septic arthritis and acute gout must be certain as intra-articular steroids will exacerbate infection. Patients with a suboptimal response to NSAIDs may benefit from the administration of intra-articular steroid.

Systemic steroids can also be used to treat acute gout. The general corticosteroid dosage recommendation is 20 to 30 mg of oral prednisolone equivalent daily. The recommended duration of therapy has been from 1 to 3 weeks. These agents usually take 12 hours to work.

Prophylactic control of symptomatic hyperuricaemia

Allopurinol

Long-term hypouricaemic agents should be considered for patients who suffer recurrent gouty attacks. A definition of recurrent attacks is more than two per year. The agent of choice is allopurinol. As well as controlling symptoms it may protect the renal function especially in patients with familial disease. Long-term agents should not be used for symptomless hyperuricaemia, nor for protecting renal function or cardiovascular risk in asymptomatic patients. In patients under 30 years, not taking diuretics, specialist advice should be sought to exclude metabolic defects before commencing treatment with allopurinol.

Patients with chronic tophaceous gout may benefit from resolution of tophi through prolonged treatment with allopurinol. It usually takes approximately 6 months for the size of established tophi to start to decline.

Allopurinol reduces uric acid production by inhibiting the enzyme xanthine oxidase. Allopurinol is not active but undergoes hepatic conversion (60 to 70% of allopurinol) to its active metabolite oxipurinol. The half-life of allopurinol is approximately 2 hours. Oxipurinol is excreted renally together with allopurinol and allopurinol riboside, the second main metabolite. Oxipurinol undergoes net reabsorption in the renal tubule as does urate itself. Oxipurinol may thus accumulate in patients with renal failure, those with gout and those receiving thiazide diuretics in whom volume contraction and hypovolaemia may occur. Net reabsorption is enhanced in states of volume contraction. The half-life of oxipurinol is 13 to 18 hours in patients with normal renal function.

Recommendations for dosing allopurinol according to creatinine clearance have been made (Table 51.1). In patients with normal renal function the initial allopurinol dose should not exceed 300 mg in 24 hours. The serum urate concentration can be used as a guide to further dosage requirements.

Allopurinol causes side effects in 3 to 5% of patients and these usually manifest as hypersensitivity reactions. Skin eruptions are the most common effects but others include hepatotoxicity, acute interstitial nephritis and fever. These hypersensitivity reactions subside upon treatment discontinuation. However, if treatment is continued, severe exfoliative dermatitis, various haematological abnormalities, hepatomegaly, jaundice, hepatic necrosis and renal impairment may occur. Many patients with severe reactions have had reduced renal function and the dose of allopurinol used was too high. This toxic syndrome most commonly occurs within the first 2 months of treatment although later reactions have been reported.

Table 51.1 Sustained maintenance dose of allopurinol for patients with diminished renal function (after Cameron & Simmonds 1987)

Creatinine clearance (ml/min)	Allopurinol dose
0	100 mg thrice weekly
10	100 mg alternate days
20	100 mg daily
40	150 mg daily
60	200 mg daily
>100	300 mg daily

Allopurinol enhances the toxicity of cytotoxic drugs metabolized by xanthine oxidase. The doses of these (mercaptopurine and azathioprine) should be reduced during concurrent allopurinol therapy. In addition allopurinol enhances the bone marrow toxicity of cyclophosphamide.

Allopurinol may prolong an acute attack of gout or it may precipitate another and thus it should not be commenced until an attack has subsided. The risk of inducing an acute attack can be reduced by coadministration of a non-steroidal anti-inflammatory agent (NSAID) or colchicine (1.5 mg daily) for the first 2 months of chronic therapy.

Serum urate levels will fall within 2 days of the initiation of allopurinol, but maximal reduction will take 7 to 10 days. The serum urate concentration should be checked after 2 to 3 weeks of allopurinol to ensure a fall in levels.

Azapropazone lowers serum urate levels. The exact mechanism of action is unknown. Currently azapropazone is not recommended for prophylaxis in gout.

Uricosuric agents

Most patients with symptomatic hyperuricaemia underexcrete uric acid and these patients can be managed with uricosuric agents.

Uricosuric agents such as probenecid (500 mg to 1 g twice daily) and sulphinpyrazone (100 mg three to four times a day) offer an alternative to allopurinol. These agents should be avoided in patients with urate nephropathy and those who overproduce uric acid. They are ineffective in patients with poor renal function (creatinine clearance of less than 20 to 30 ml/min).

Probenecid is well absorbed orally with a serum half-life of 6 to 12 hours. Therapy should be initiated with a dose of 250 mg twice daily, increased to 500 mg twice daily after 2 weeks, with a further increase to 2 g daily if required. An initial low dose of uricosuric agent helps to prevent precipitation of an acute attack and decreases the risk of stone formation in the kidney. Patients should be advised to maintain a high fluid intake to minimize the risk of stone formation.

Approximately 5 to 10% of patients receiving long-term probenecid suffer nausea, heartburn, flatulence or constipation. A mild pruritic rash, drug fever and renal disturbances can occur.

The serum level of probenecid is elevated by concomitant indomethacin, and aspirin inhibits the uricosuric actions of probenecid and sulphinpyrazone. Other drug interactions are shown in Table 51.2 and the pharmacokinetic profile of the drugs used in the management of gout are presented in Table 51.3.

Prophylactic treatment of asymptomatic hyperuricaemia

It is unnecessary and excessive to treat all patients with hyperuricaemia with urate-lowering drugs although individuals with high serum uric acid are more likely to develop gout. The risk of hyperuricaemia causing renal disease is controversial, although the consensus now seems to be that hyperuricaemia alone does not have a

Table 51.2 Common drug interactions associated with therapy for gout and hyperuricaemia

Interacting drug	Affected drug	Effect
Allopurinol	Azathioprine	Increased levels of azathioprine
Allopurinol	Mercaptopurine	Increased levels of mercaptopurine
Allopurinol	Anticoagulants	Enhanced anti-coagulant effect
Aspirin (low dose)	Uricosurics	Decreased hypo-uricaemic effect
Probenecid	Indomethacin	Increased indomethicin levels
Probenecid	Ketoprofen	Increased ketoprofen levels
Probenecid	Naproxen	Increased naproxen levels
Probenecid	Methotrexate	Increased methotrexate levels
Probenecid	Zidovudine	Increased zidovudine levels
Probenecid	Cephalosporins	Increased cephalosporin levels
Probenecid	Dapsone	Increased dapsone levels
Probenecid	Aspirin	Increased aspirin levels
Sulphinpyrazone	Anticoagulants	Enhanced anticoagulant effect

Table 51.3   Pharmacokinetic parameters for gout drugs

Agent	$t_{1/2}$ (hours)	Tmax (hours)	Vd (L/kg)	Protein binding	Clearance hepatic (L/h)
Allopurinol	1–3*	2–6	—	0–4.5	46
Colchicine	20	2	1–2	31	36
Probenecid	4–12†	4	0.12–0.18	85–95	1.4
Sulphinpyrazone	1–2	3	0.06	98–99	1.4

* Active metabolite 18–30 hours.
† 3–8 hours (0.5 g); 6–12 hours (2 g).

deleterious effect on renal function. The presence of hyperuricaemia does seem to be a risk factor for development of cardiovascular disease although the evidence is not sufficiently strong for prophylactic therapy to be considered necessary at the moment.

Drug-induced gout

Hyperuricaemia and gout occur with diuretics and especially thiazides. Where possible an alternative agent should be used (e.g. vasodilator for hypertension), but where this is not possible allopurinol should be used to lower urate levels. Other drugs which reduce renal urate excretion include low-dose aspirin and alcohol. Cyclosporin-induced hyperuricaemia and gout has been recently reported especially in male patients after a mean of 24 months. This condition did not seem to be related to serum cyclosporin concentrations.

Radiotherapy and chemotherapy in patients with neoplastic disorders can cause hyperuricaemia. This can be treated prophylactically with allopurinol, commencing 3 days before therapy.

THE PATIENT

Patients with gout should be advised about factors which may contribute to hyperuricaemia, such as fasting, obesity and alcohol excess. If these are avoided or corrected, drug treatment may not be needed. Asymptomatic hyperuricaemia need not be treated but renal function should be checked to ensure that it is not deteriorating.

Patients at risk of recurrent gouty attacks should receive a supply of NSAIDs. They must be adequately informed to commence treatment at the first signs of an attack. This should abort the attack in most patients. Patients should be advised of the correct manner in which NSAIDs should be dosed, the potential side effects and the action to take should side effects occur. They should be advised to avoid aspirin and instead to use paracetamol for analgesia.

Patients receiving allopurinol should be advised of the need to continue single daily dose treatment in the absence of any symptomatic response. Patients should be advised of potential side effects and should be told to report any adverse skin reactions.

Patients receiving uricosuric agents should be advised to maintain a good fluid intake to reduce the risk of renal calculus formation. Urine flow of at least 2 litres per day is required.

CASE STUDIES

CASE 51.1

Mrs J. H. is 65 years old and weighs 75 kg. She presents with acute gout in her left great toe which came on after a busy day digging in the garden. She is known to have hypertension and takes one 5 mg tablet of bendrofluazide each day. She is a non-smoker who likes a glass of wine at bedtime.

Q1 How should this patient's acute gout be managed?

Q2 What is the relationship between acute gout and diuretic therapy?

Q3 What advice should the patient receive?

Q4 Why should patients with gout reduce their alcohol intake?

CASE 51.2

Mr J. D. is 57 years old and is admitted to hospital with a deep vein thrombosis. He is known to have recurrent attacks of gout and takes a 300 mg allopurinol tablet each day together with occasional analgesics.

Q1 It is decided to prescribe warfarin for Mr J. D.'s deep vein thrombosis. What are the problems with using a standard loading dose of warfarin (day 1, 10 mg; day 2, 5 mg; day 3, 5 mg) to treat his deep vein thrombosis?

Q2 If Mr J. D. should require a NSAID for his gout while receiving warfarin which one would you recommend?

CASE 51.3

Mr K. F. is a 47-year-old, 75 kg factory worker with a history of gout controlled with one 300 mg tablet of allopurinol each day. He was admitted to hospital after collapsing with chest pain while running to catch a bus. On admission he was diagnosed as having suffered a myocardial infarction and was treated with diamorphine, streptokinase, heparin and low-dose (150 mg) aspirin.

Q1 What effect will the aspirin have on Mr K. F.'s gout?

Q2 Should Mr K. F.'s management be changed because of his history of gout?

ANSWERS TO CASE STUDIES

CASE 51.1

A1 The patient's acute gout should be managed with colchicine commencing with 1 mg initially, followed by 500 micrograms every 3 hours until pain is resolved, or side effects (diarrhoea) occur, or until 10 mg has been taken. The patient's antihypertensive medication should be changed and diuretics avoided. She could be treated with a calcium antagonist, an alpha-adrenoreceptor blocker or an ACE inhibitor, all of which have no metabolic affects.

This patient should not receive prophylactic hypouricaemic therapy. Discontinuation of the diuretic alone may be adequate to avoid further acute attacks and only those patients with more than two attacks per year are usually considered for long-term treatment. In addition, starting either allopurinol or uricosuric therapy will prevent the current attack from settling and may precipitate another attack.

A2 The hyperuricaemic actions of thiazide and loop diuretics are frequently encountered in clinical practice. The mechanism is related to extracellular fluid contraction. Interestingly the typically affected patient is usually elderly and female with a long history of continuous diuretic ingestion.

The gout may present as classic acute synovitis but sometimes takes the form of a generalized arthritis that can be misdiagnosed as osteoarthritis or rheumatoid arthritis.

A3 The patient should be advised to reduce her alcohol intake, to lose weight, to commence a low saturated fat diet and to avoid vigorous exercise. She should reduce her dietary salt intake and avoid low-dose aspirin. She should be advised of the need to continue her antihypertensive medication.

A4 Heavy drinkers (more than 30 units/week) are known to suffer gout despite treatment with allopurinol and NSAIDs. This poor response to treatment may be due to antagonism of the effect

of allopurinol, as ethanol contributes to hyperuricaemia by increasing production of uric acid and impairing its excretion in the urine. Although counselling on alcohol intake should be given, it is recognized that this is frequently ignored and failure of patients with gouty arthritis to respond to treatment should alert the clinician to the possibility of hidden alcohol abuse.

CASE 51.2

A1 Warfarin is highly protein bound and has a long plasma half-life. The administration of a 10 mg loading dose will reduce the time for the drug to reach steady state but in this patient the dose is excessive. Patients greater than 60 years of age or weighing less than 60 kg or with a serum albumin level less than 35 g/dl, all require a reduced loading dose. Although Mr J. D. does not fulfil any of these criteria, he is taking allopurinol. Allopurinol inhibits the metabolism of warfarin by inhibiting the oxidative metabolic pathway. The dose of warfarin should thus be reduced by approximately 50% for the loading dose.

A2 NSAIDs have antiplatelet effects which can enhance bleeding which cannot be detected with the INR. All NSAIDs can cause gastrointestinal mucosal damage and thus bleeding is a particular risk in anticoagulated patients. Many NSAIDs are highly protein bound although the displaced warfarin is rapidly eliminated, with only a transient rise in INR. Azapropazone and phenylbutazone both displace warfarin and inhibit hepatic enzyme activity. This will cause a profound rise in anticoagulant activity. Should Mr J. D. require NSAID therapy whilst taking warfarin, an appropriate drug would be diclofenac. This has no effect on the hepatic metabolism of warfarin and only a small effect on the protein binding of warfarin.

CASE 51.3

A1 Mr K. F. is already taking allopurinol as prophylaxis against further attacks of gout. In this situation the addition of aspirin to his drug regime is probably of no consequence. His gout is already controlled with allopurinol.

The administration of low-dose aspirin can lead to elevation of serum urate levels, by inhibition of tubular secretion, and thus predispose patients to acute attacks of gout. In contrast, high-dose salicylate therapy acts in a similar manner to the uricosuric agents by inhibiting tubular reabsorbtion of urate which leads to an increased excretion and a fall in serum levels.

As a general principle therefore, low-dose aspirin should be avoided in patients with gout. In the case of Mr K. F. low-dose aspirin has been demonstrated in many studies to decrease mortality following myocardial infarction and for this reason treatment should continue, probably lifelong.

A2 No changes in the management of Mr K. F. should be made because of his history of gout. It would be appropriate to counsel him over his risk factors for ischaemic heart disease and gout. He should be advised to stop smoking, to reduce his alcohol intake and adopt a low fat diet.

BIBLIOGRAPHY

Cameron J S, Simmonds H A. Use and abuse of allopurinol. British Medical Journal 1987; 294: 1504–1505

Editorial. Polyarticular gout. Lancet 1989; 1: 703–704

Haslock I. Diagnosis and treatment of acute and chronic gout. Prescriber 1991; 61–66

Wallace S L, Singer J Z. Review: Systemic toxicity associated with the intravenous administration of colchicine – guidelines for use. Journal of Rheumatology 1988; 15: 495–499

Wise C M, Agudelo C A. Gout and hyperuricaemia. Current Opinion in Rheumatology 1990; 2: 783–788

Chapter 52

Glaucoma

H. Scott   L. Titcomb

The term glaucoma does not represent a single pathological entity. It consists of a large group of disorders with widely differing clinical features.

It is therefore difficult to attempt a single definition of the term, but it may be generally defined as 'those conditions in which the intra-ocular pressure (IOP) is too high for the normal functioning of the optic nerve head'.

EPIDEMIOLOGY

The diseases which make up the group known as glaucoma are usually classified according to the manner in which aqueous humour outflow is impaired.

Primary open angle glaucoma

Primary open angle glaucoma (POAG), which is also referred to as chronic simple glaucoma, is associated with a relative obstruction to aqueous outflow through the trabecular meshwork and is a chronic progressive disease of insidious onset, usually affecting both eyes. It is the most common type of glaucoma and affects approximately 1 in 200 of the population over the age of 40 years. POAG is responsible for about 20% of all cases of blindness in the United Kingdom, and affects both sexes equally. It is frequently an inherited condition, with approximately 10% of first degree relatives of POAG sufferers eventually developing the disease.

Primary angle closure glaucoma

Primary angle closure glaucoma (PACG), or closed angle glaucoma, is a condition in which closure of the angle by the peripheral iris results in a reduction in aqueous outflow. It occurs in predisposed eyes and is frequently unilateral. The disease affects approximately 1 in 1000 adults over the age of 40 years, and occurs in four times as many females as males.

Two conditions similar to POAG are low tension glaucoma where the IOP is not raised on initial screening although signs of damage are present, and ocular hypertension where signs of damage do not accompany the raised IOP.

Secondary glaucomas can arise for a number of reasons, including inflammation, intraocular tumour, raised episcleral venous pressure, or congenitally due to developmental abnormalities.

AETIOLOGY

The factors which determine the level of intraocular pressure are the rate of aqueous humour production and the resistance encountered in the outflow channels. A fine balance between these is necessary to keep the pressure within the eye in the range of 16 to 21 mmHg.

Production of aqueous humour occurs in the ciliary epithelium by two mechanisms: secretion due to an active metabolic process, independent of the level of IOP, and ultrafiltration influenced by the level of blood pressure in the ciliary capillaries and the level of IOP.

Outflow of aqueous humour occurs by two routes. Approximately 80% of total outflow is through the trabecular meshwork into the canal of Schlemm and into the venous circulation via the aqueous veins. The remaining 20% is accounted for by the uveoscleral pathways; through the ciliary body into the suprachoroidal space, to be drained into the ciliary body, choroid, and sclera via the venous circulation.

PATHOPHYSIOLOGY

The primary site of damage is thought to be the optic nerve head, rather than any other point along the nerve axon. This most easily explains the progressive loss of visual field. Studies of axoplasmic flow show a vulnerability of the nerves to elevated IOP as they pass through the optic disc.

In POAG the rise in IOP is caused by increased resistance within the drainage channels. It is thought that the main route of resistance to aqueous outflow lies in the dense juxtacanalicular trabecular meshwork, or the endothelium lining the inner wall of Schlemm's canal.

In PACG the rise in IOP is caused by a decreased outflow of aqueous humour, due to closure of the chamber angle by the peripheral iris. It occurs in predisposed eyes, and the predisposing factors can be anatomical or physiological. The anatomical characteristics are lens size, corneal diameter and axial length of the globe. The lens continues to grow throughout life. This brings the anterior surface closer to the cornea. Slackening of the suspensory ligaments increases this movement. Both factors occur very gradually and lead to a progressive shallowing of the anterior chamber. The depth of the anterior chamber and width of the chamber angle are related to corneal diameter, and those eyes predisposed to PACG are observed to have a corneal diameter less than that seen in normal eyes. A short eye, which is frequently also hypermetropic, has a small corneal diameter and a thick and relatively anteriorly located lens.

The physiological precipitating factors of PACG in predisposed eyes are not fully understood. Two theories currently exist. The dilator muscle theory suggests that contraction of the dilator muscle causes a posterior movement, which increases the apposition between the iris and anteriorly located lens and the degree of physiological pupillary block. The simultaneous dilatation of the pupil renders the peripheral iris more flaccid, and causes the pressure in the posterior chamber to increase and the iris to bow anteriorly. Eventually the angle becomes obstructed by the peripheral iris and the IOP rises (Fig. 52.1).

The sphincter muscle theory postulates that the sphincter of the pupil precipitates angle closure. The pupillary blocking force of the sphincter is

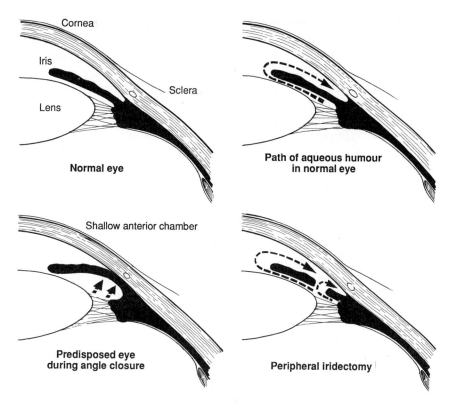

Fig. 52.1 Changes to the eye seen during closed angle glaucoma.

greatest when the diameter of the pupil is about 4 mm.

CLINICAL MANIFESTATIONS

POAG is characterized by the following: an IOP greater that 21 mmHg; an open angle; glaucomatous cupping; and visual field loss. Because of its insidious onset, POAG is usually asymptomatic until it has caused a significant loss of visual field. In some eyes, subtle signs of glaucomatous retinal nerve damage can be detected prior to development of pathological cupping and detectable field loss. The earliest clinically significant field defect is a scotoma which is an area of depressed vision within the visual field. Patients with POAG frequently show a wider swing in IOP than normal. Therefore a single pressure reading of 21 mmHg or less does not exclude the diagnosis. It may be necessary to measure IOP at different times of the day, or at periodic intervals.

Acute PACG is due to a sudden closure of the angle and a severe elevation in IOP. The symptoms include rapidly progressive visual impairment, periocular pain and congestion of the eye. In severe cases nausea and vomiting may occur. The signs include injection of the limbal and conjunctival vessels giving a 'ciliary flush'. The IOP usually lies between 50 mmHg and 80 mmHg and causes corneal oedema with epithelial vesicles. The anterior chamber is shallow and iridocorneal contact can be observed. The pupil is vertically oval and fixed in a semidilated position. It is unreactive to light and accommodation. The fellow eye usually has a shallow anterior chamber and a narrow angle. The optic nerve head is oedematous and hyperaemic.

INVESTIGATIONS

Intraocular pressure may be measured by tonometry such as indentation tonometry in which a plunger is applied to the cornea and the amount of indentation on the eye reflects the pressure within it. Tonography is a technique used to measure the outflow of aqueous humour from the eye, resulting from indentation of the eye, using a tonometer. Gonioscopy is used to estimate the width of the chamber angle, with the aid of a slit lamp. Perimetry is important for both the diagnosis and management of glaucoma by detecting early scotomata and larger changes in visual field.

In patients with POAG, cupping of the optic disc becomes progressively apparent and is used in both diagnosis and assessment of the efficacy of treatment. The increased intraocular pressure appears to push the optic disc back into an excavation. This is known as glaucomatous cupping.

The colour of the optic disc will be observed to change from a creamy pink colour due to the rich capillary network in the healthy eye to increased pallor with advancing disease as the optic nerve tissue progressively atrophies.

TREATMENT

The aim of treatment in POAG is to reduce the raised IOP, preventing further damage to the nerve fibres and the development of further visual field defects. The key to effective treatment is careful and regular follow-up including measurement of visual acuity, tonometry, gonioscopy, evaluation of the optic disc, and perimetry.

The actual safe level of IOP is unknown although in most cases further damage is unlikely if the IOP is reduced to the lower teens. The effect on visual field and the appearance of the optic disc are the only indications that IOP is being controlled at a safe level.

The initial treatment of POAG is medical. Topical administration is the preferred type of therapy. The chosen drug should be administered at its lowest concentration and as infrequently as possible to obtain the desired effect. A drug with few potential side effects should be chosen with oral therapy held in reserve as the final step. In most cases the initial topical treatment is with a beta-adrenoreceptor blocker. If this is ineffective, the strength may be increased,

and/or adrenaline or a related compound added. Pilocarpine is usually reserved for those patients not controlled by a combination of a beta-adrenoreceptor blocker and a sympathomimetic. Oral therapy with carbonic anhydrase inhibitors is the final stage of treatment prior to surgical management.

If maximum medical management fails to control the IOP, surgery will be performed, either by filtration surgery, such as trabeculectomy where a fistula is created to act as a new route for aqueous outflow, or by argon laser trabeculoplasty, which produces an increased intratrabecular space, and increased aqueous humour outflow.

The medical management of acute PACG is essentially to prepare the eye for surgical treatment. The aim of treatment is to decrease the IOP and associated inflammation. Analgesics and antiemetics may be needed, depending on the severity of symptoms, to make the patient comfortable. It is usual to treat the unaffected eye prophylactically with miotics.

Paralysis of the iris sphincter usually occurs at an IOP of more than 50 mmHg, due to ischaemia. Therefore intensive miotic therapy, previously the treatment of choice in cases of PACG, is usually ineffective and the IOP needs to be reduced by drugs which reduce aqueous humour production, rather than by trying to pull the peripheral iris away from the angle with miotics. An intravenous loading dose of acetazolamide followed by oral treatment, in combination with corneal indentation, to physically force aqueous humour to the peripheral anterior chamber and artificially open the angle, should allow the IOP to drop sufficiently to relieve iris ischaemia, and allow the sphincter to respond to pilocarpine therapy.

If corneal indentation and acetazolamide fail to decrease IOP, hyperosmotic agents may be required. Once the IOP has been reduced medically, the condition is usually treated surgically, either by surgical peripheral iridectomy or laser iridotomy, to remove an area of the peripheral iris to allow flow of aqueous humour through an alternative pathway (Fig. 52.1). Filtration surgery is indicated if a large proportion of the angle has been permanently closed by adhesions between the iris and the cornea.

Beta-adrenoreceptor antagonists

The exact mechanism of action of beta-adrenoreceptor antagonists (beta-adrenoreceptor blockers), in lowering IOP has not been fully established but they have been shown to reduce aqueous humour formation rather than increase outflow. Five products are available in the United Kingdom: betaxolol, carteolol, levobunolol, metipranolol, and timolol (Table 52.1).

Beta-adrenoreceptor blocking drugs have a number of important properties in addition to beta-adrenoreceptor blockade. These include intrinsic sympathomimetic activity (ISA), cardioselectivity and membrane stabilizing activity, which are of importance when considering the side effects seen with these agents (Table 52.2).

The property of membrane stabilization is relevant to the incidence of ocular side effects. The absence of anaesthetic properties reduces the number and severity of foreign body and dryness sensations, anaesthesia of the cornea and dry eye syndrome.

Ocular side effects of topically administered beta-adrenoreceptor blockers are shown is Table 52.3.

It has been suggested that those beta-adrenoreceptor blockers which show ISA are less likely to produce bronchospasm and peripheral vascular side effects. Carteolol is the only commercially available drug which shows ISA. The selectivity of cardioselective beta-adrenoreceptor blockers diminishes with increasing dosage even within the therapeutic range. Betaxolol is the only commercially available topical beta-adrenoreceptor blocker which demonstrates cardioselectivity.

A degree of bradycardia and hypotension is commonly seen with all beta-adrenoreceptor blockers, although it is more marked with nonselective agents. These are rarely of clinical significance but should be monitored, particularly if the patient is known to suffer cardiac disease or hypertension.

The precipitation of bronchospasm in susceptible patients can occur with the administration of as little as one drop of timolol. Those beta-adrenoreceptor blockers which show cardioselectivity or ISA are theoretically less likely to cause bronchoconstriction, but studies tend to be short term and involve few patients. All topical beta-adrenoreceptor blockers have been reported to cause bronchospasm. Therefore 'at risk' patients with a tendency to airways disease who require treatment for glaucoma should be

---

Table 52.1 Available ophthalmic beta-adrenoreceptor blockers

Drug	Brand name	Strength	Daily dosage frequency
Betaxolol	Betoptic	0.5%	2
Carteolol	Teoptic	1%	2
		2%	
Levobunolol	Betagan[†]	0.5%	1–2
Metipranolol	Minims*	0.1%	2
		0.3%	
Timolol	Timoptol[†]	0.25%	2
		0.5%	

* Metipranolol multidose marketed as Glauline was withdrawn in 1990 due to the occurrence of granulomatous anterior uveitis.
[†] also available in unit dose form.

Table 52.2 Pharmacological profile of ophthalmic beta-adrenoreceptor blockers

	Beta-adrenoreceptor blocking potency	ISA	Cardioselectivity	Membrane stabilizing activity
Betaxolol	3–10	–	++	+
Carteolol	30	++	–	–
Levobunolol	6	–	–	–
Metipranolol	2	–	–	+
Timolol	5–10	–	–	+
(Propranolol = 1)				

Table 52.3 Ocular side effects of topical beta-adrenoreceptor blockers

Allergic blepharoconjunctivitis
Burning and itching
Blurred vision
Conjunctival hyperaemia
Corneal anaesthesia
Dryness
Foreign body sensation
Macular oedema
Pain
Punctate keratitis
Uveitis
(Granulomatous anterior uveitis has been reported with metipranolol)

Table 52.4 Systemic side effects of topical beta-adrenoreceptor blockers

Vascular
  Hypotension
  Arrhythmias
  Reduced stroke volume
  Bradycardia
  Peripheral vasoconstriction

Respiratory
  Bronchoconstriction
  Dyspnoea

Gastrointestinal
  Nausea
  Diarrhoea

Endocrine
  Hypoglycaemia (insulin induced)

Central nervous system
  Anxiety
  Depression
  Irritability
  Fatigue
  Hallucinations

treated with extreme caution. (The Committee on Safety of Medicines has advised that topical beta-adrenoreceptor blockers, even those with apparent cardioselectivity, should not be used in patients with asthma or a history of obstructive airways disease, unless no alternative treatment is available.)

Ocular beta-adrenoreceptor blockers are generally not contra-indicated in diabetes although a cardioselective agent may be preferable. They do produce a slight impairment of glucose tolerance and are best avoided in patients who suffer frequent hypoglycaemic attacks.

Systemic side effects of topically administered beta-adrenoreceptor blockers are shown in Table 52.4.

Betaxolol

The only ophthalmic beta-adrenoreceptor blocker with cardioselectivity, betaxolol theoretically has minimal effects on pulmonary and most cardiovascular parameters. Use of betaxolol with adrenaline leads to a greater reduction in IOP than that achieved with timolol and adrenaline, and the addition of dipivefrin increases the efficacy of betaxolol. The fall in IOP on initiation of therapy is slower than with other topical beta-adrenoreceptor blockers. Some studies have shown that betaxolol is not as effective in reducing IOP as other topical beta-adrenoreceptor blockers. Betaxolol has been reported to cause more stinging on instillation than timolol.

Carteolol

Carteolol is a beta-adrenoreceptor blocker with intrinsic sympathomimetic activity. This results in smaller changes in pulmonary and cardiovascular parameters than are seen with the non-cardioselective beta-adrenoreceptor blockers without ISA. Carteolol is generally well tolerated but may be more irritant than timolol. It has been shown to be as effective or slightly less effective than timolol at lowering IOP. As it is the least lipophilic of the topical beta-adrenoreceptor blockers currently available it is likely to show a lower incidence of CNS side effects.

Levobunolol

This non-cardioselective beta-adrenoreceptor blocker without ISA is reported to be as effective or slightly more effective than timolol at lowering IOP, and more effective than betaxolol or metipranolol. Once-daily dosing is as effective as the usual twice-daily regimen and it is the only topical beta-adrenoreceptor blocker licensed for once-daily use. It is reported to cause more stinging on administration than betaxolol and metipranolol and be equal in patient comfort to timolol.

Metipranolol

This is a non-cardioselective beta-adrenoreceptor blocker without ISA. Recent reports of anterior uveitis associated with the use of metipranolol have led to discontinuation of the multidose forms. Tolerability of the product is poor, many patients complain of stinging and dry skin around the eyes.

Timolol

As the first topical beta-adrenoreceptor blocker introduced, this non-cardioselective drug without ISA is the agent against which all newer beta-adrenoreceptor blockers are compared. It is effective in the long-term treatment of glaucoma and in combination with adrenaline products, miotics and carbonic anhydrase inhibitors.

The efficacy and tolerability of beta-adreno-receptor blocker eye drops have been compared in numerous studies. The side effect profile differs very little between agents, although metipranolol, betaxolol and to a lesser extent levobunolol are reported to cause more stinging on instillation than timolol. In terms of efficacy levobunolol, metipranolol and timolol can be considered to be approximately equal, while betaxolol and carteolol are probably less effective.

Sympathomimetic agents

Adrenaline

Adrenaline is an alpha- and beta-adrenoreceptor agonist. It decreases IOP by decreasing aqueous inflow via an alpha-mediated vasoconstriction in the ciliary body and increased outflow due to a dilatation of the aqueous and episcleral veins. The mydriasis seen with adrenaline adminis-tration is an incidental effect but means that its use is contra-indicated in PACG and patients who show a shallow anterior chamber, due to the risk of precipitating angle closure. Adrena-line therapy in the aphakic eye can result in cystoid maculopathy which is usually reversible on cessation.

Ocular side effects of topically administered adrenaline are shown in Table 52.5.

The usefulness of adrenaline is limited by local ocular side effects such as stinging, burning and pain in and around the eye. Systemic reactions are included in Table 52.6.

In an attempt to decrease the administered dose of adrenaline a pro-drug dipivalyl adrena-line (dipivefrin) has been developed.

Dipivefrin

Dipivalyl adrenaline is converted to adrenaline after absorption by esterases present in the eye. Its penetration of the cornea is considerably greater than that seen with adrenaline, and the effects of a 0.1% solution are comparable with a 1% solution of adrenaline. The lower concen-tration of dipivefrin which can be used causes fewer local and systemic side effects.

Adrenergic neurone blockers

Guanethidine

Guanethidine enhances and prolongs the effects of adrenaline for a given dose. It is available alone or as a combination product. After pro-longed treatment cicatrizing changes of the conjunctiva and cornea leading to corneal ulcera-tion and scarring have been reported in some patients. Ptosis is also seen as a side effect of guanethidine use.

Table 52.5 Ocular side effects of topical adrenaline

Allergic blepharoconjunctivitis
Adrenochrome deposits
Conjunctival hyperaemia
Corneal oedema
Macular oedema (aphakic eyes)
Pain

Table 52.6 Systemic side effects of topical adrenaline

Arrhythmias
Cerebrovascular accident
Hypertension
Myocardial infarction
Tachycardia

Those products which are commercially available containing sympathomimetic agents or guanethidine are shown in Table 52.7.

Miotics

Two types of miotics are used in the treatment of glaucoma. Both act to increase the outflow of aqueous humour by a stimulation of ciliary muscle and an opening of channels in the trabecular meshwork. Directly acting parasympathomimetic agents which act at muscarinic receptors, include pilocarpine and carbachol, while the indirectly acting agents are the cholinesterase inhibitors physostigmine, ecothiopate iodide and demecarium bromide. Miosis is an unwanted incidental effect. The pharmacological parameters of the miotic agents are shown in Table 52.8.

The occurrence of miosis as a side effect of treatment with this group of drugs can cause

considerable difficulties to patients. Reduced visual acuity, especially in the presence of central lens opacities, spasm of accommodation, accompanied by severe frontal headache and diminished night vision may cause poor compliance in many patients.

Ocular side effects of topically administered miotic agents are shown in Table 52.9.

In eyes with narrow angles, PACG may be precipitated by an aggravation of pupillary block. Lens opacities have been reported to occur as a result of the long-term use of the long-acting cholinesterase inhibitors. Therefore ecothiopate is usually reserved for cases resistant to other treatment.

Systemic side effects are due to parasympathetic stimulation, and include: anxiety, bradycardia, diarrhoea, nausea, vomiting and sweating.

Ecothiopate may block other cholinesterases in the body and patients requiring suxamethonium chloride during anaesthesia may be at risk of developing apnoea.

Pilocarpine is the most commonly used miotic in the treatment of POAG, despite its inconvenient four-times-a-day dosage regimen (Table 52.10). Concentrations above 4% do not appear to be more effective at lowering IOP, although they may have a slightly longer action.

Carbonic anhydrase inhibitors

The enzyme carbonic anhydrase is involved in the production of aqueous humour in the ciliary body. By inhibiting its action, secretion is re-

Table 52.7 Available products containing sympathomimetic agents and/or guanethidine

Drug	Brand name	Strength	Daily dosage frequency
Adrenaline	Eppy	1%	1–2
	Simplene	0.5%	1–2
Dipivefrin	Propine	0.1%	2
Guanethidine	Ismelin	5%	1–2
Guanethidine + adrenaline	Ganda	1 + 0.2 3 + 0.5	1–2

Table 52.8 Pharmacological profile of miotic agents

	Time to onset (min)	Duration of action (h)	Daily dosage frequency
Pilocarpine	20	3–4	4
Carbachol	40	8–12	3
Physostigmine	10	12	2–6
Ecothiopate*	10–45	24	1–2
Demecarium*	20	>24	1–2

* Now only available on a 'named patient' basis.

Table 52.9 Ocular side effects of topical miotic agents

Allergic conjunctivitis
Ciliary/conjunctival injection
Lens changes
Lid twitching
Myopia
Pain
Pigment epithelial cysts
Poor night vision
Posterior synechiae
Pupillary block
Retinal tear/detachments
Uveitis
Vitreous haemorrhage

Table 52.10 Available miotic products

Drug	Brand name	Strength	Daily dosage frequency
Pilocarpine	Isopto Carpine	0.5–4%	4
	Sno Pilo	1, 2 & 4%	4
	Pilocarpine	0.5–4%	4
	Minims	1, 2 & 4%	4
	Ocusert Pilo	'20'/'40'	1 per week
Carbachol	Isopto Carbachol	3%	3
Physostigmine		0.25%	2–6
		0.5%	2–6
Physostigmine/ Pilocarpine		0.25%/2%	4
		0.25%/4%	4
		0.5%/4%	4
Ecothiopate iodide	Phospholine iodide	0.03%	1–2
		0.06%	1–2
		0.125%	1–2
		0.25%	1–2
Demecarium bromide	Tosmilen	0.25%	1–2
		0.5%	1–2

duced. Two carbonic anhydrase inhibitors are available in the United Kingdom: acetazolamide and dichlorphenamide.

Although they are among the most potent agents at decreasing IOP, the usefulness of carbonic anhydrase inhibitors in the long-term management of glaucoma is limited by side effects and resulting poor patient compliance. Systemic side effects are shown in Table 52.11.

Paraesthesia occurs in almost all patients on commencement of therapy but usually disappears with continued treatment. The malaise complex can include fatigue, depression, weight loss and decreased libido.

Table 52.11 Systemic side effects of carbonic anhydrase inhibitors

Acidosis
Diarrhoea
Drowsiness
Elevated uric acid
Hypokalaemia
Nausea/vomiting
Malaise complex
Paraesthesia
Sulphonamide crystalluria
Sulphonamide sensitivity
Transient myopia

The availability of acetazolamide in an injectable form has a significant place in the treatment of PACG.

The effects of topically administered carbonic anhydrase inhibitors at lowering IOP are currently under investigation.

Hyperosmotic agents

Because of their speed of action and effectiveness, hyperosmotic agents are of great value during the acute crisis of PACG. The four commonly used agents are glycerol and isosorbide orally, and mannitol and urea intravenously. All act by drawing water out of the eye and in this way reduce IOP. The maximal effect of oral agents is seen within 1 hour and lasts for about 3 hours, while intravenous agents act within 30 minutes and the effects last for 4 to 6 hours.

Glycerol

Glycerol is a clear, syrupy liquid with a sweet, sickening taste. It is usually given as a 50% solution in water, acidified and flavoured with lemon. The addition of sodium bicarbonate immediately before administration gives rise to effervescence, making the solution more palatable and increasing the rate of absorption.

The dose is 1 to 1.5 g/kg body weight given as a single dose. It is not a strong diuretic but may induce nausea and vomiting. Although it is metabolized to glucose in the body it may be given to diabetics who are well controlled.

Isosorbide

Isosorbide has a minty flavour, exerts a diuretic action and may cause diarrhoea but does not usually cause nausea. Because it is metabolically inert, it can be administered to diabetic patients without insulin cover. The dose is 1 to 2 g/kg body weight given as a single dose.

Mannitol

Mannitol is administered as a 20% solution in water for intravenous administration. The dose is 1.5 to 2 g/kg body weight given over 30 to 40 minutes at a rate not exceeding 60 drops per minute. It has a strong diuretic action, and as large volumes of solution are required, mannitol may cause problems due to cardiovascular overload and pulmonary oedema.

Urea

Urea is given as a 30% solution in 10% invert sugar at a dose of 1 to 1.5 g/kg body weight intravenously. It causes less diuresis than mannitol, but should not be used in patients with impaired renal function. It is generally less popular than mannitol.

THE PATIENT

Primary open angle glaucoma

When the condition is first diagnosed, patients should be told that the disorder cannot be cured but only controlled by regular use of the prescribed treatment. As primary open angle glaucoma is, until far advanced, a symptomless disease, the result of non-compliance with treatment should be made clear and the importance of regular attendance at clinics stressed.

The existence of the patients' self-help group, the International Glaucoma Association should be brought to the patients' attention.

The patient's technique of instillation of eye drops should be checked and corrected if necessary with emphasis on the dose (one drop), the position of instillation into the temporal side of the lower conjunctival sac and the importance of punctal occlusion to minimize systemic side effects.

The preferred times for administration of topical medication should be discussed with the patient with a 12-hourly regimen for twice-daily beta-adrenoreceptor blockers and sympathomimetics and as near a 6-hourly regimen as practical for pilocarpine.

The importance of allowing a reasonable interval between drops should be underlined. Sometimes the order of instillation of different types of eye drops is important for pharmacological

or practical reasons. For example, the instillation of pilocarpine should always precede that of a sympathomimetic to prevent pain in the eye resulting from a strong miosis following a weak mydriasis. The instillation of aqueous eye drops which remain in the conjunctival sac for a maximum of 10 minutes should precede that of viscous eye drops, e.g. hypromellose eye drops, or suspensions, e.g. dexamethasone 0.1% eye drops, with which the contact time is prolonged.

Eye drops containing benzalkonium chloride should not be instilled with soft contact lenses in situ. The patient should be instructed to remove the lens immediately before instillation and replace it approximately 30 minutes later. The same procedure should be adopted by patients using adrenaline eye drops as the oxidation products of this drug will stain the contact lens. Patients using extended-wear contact lenses which they do not normally remove should use preservative-free eye drops, and products containing adrenaline should be avoided.

As POAG is a hereditary disorder, patients should be told to advise first degree relatives to be screened. Such people are entitled to free eye tests by their optician.

Primary angle closure glaucoma

Patients found to have shallow anterior chambers and narrow angles should be advised of the symptoms of an attack of acute PACG and which factors are likely to precipitate an attack so that they can be avoided. They should be advised that there are a number of prescription and non-prescription drugs that they should not take. When visiting the doctor and purchasing medicines from a pharmacy, the patient should always remember to mention his condition and the prescriber should ensure that the drug is appropriate for a patient prone to angle closure. Drugs contra-indicated in this condition are listed in Tables 52.12 to 52.15. Note that drugs are listed in these tables on a purely alphabetical basis.

Following an attack of angle closure and surgical treatment of the disorder, the patient should be told that the drugs previously contra-

Table 52.12 Topically administered ophthalmic drugs contra-indicated in narrow angle glaucoma

Anticholinergics	Sympathomimetics with alpha-adrenergic activity
Atropine	Adrenaline
Cyclopentolate	Cocaine
Homatropine	Dipivefrin
Hyoscine	Ephedrine
Lachesine	Guanethidine
Oxyphenonium	Hydroxyamphetamine
Tropicamide	Naphazoline
	Phenylephrine
	Xylometazoline

Table 52.13 Systemically administered anticholinergic drugs contra-indicated in narrow angle glaucoma and suitable alternative drugs

Drugs used in the treatment of parkinsonism and drug-induced parkinsonian side effects

Contra-indicated drug	Alternative therapies
Benzhexol	Amantadine
Benztropine	Bromocriptine
Biperidine	Lysuride
Methixene	Pergolide
Orphenadrine	Selegiline

Drugs used as antispasmodics

Contra-indicated drug	Alternative therapies
Ambutonium	Alverine
Belladonna	Mebeverine
Dicyclomine	Peppermint oil
Homatropine methylbromide	
Hyoscine	
Mepenzolate	
Poldine	
Propantheline	

Drugs used in the treatment of motion sickness

Contra-indicated drug	Alternative therapies
Hyoscine	Cinnarizine
	Cyclizine
	Dimenhydrinate
	Promethazine
	theoclate

Table 52.14 Systemically administered drugs with anticholinergic side effects contra-indicated in narrow angle glaucoma and suitable alternative drugs

Antidepressants

Contra-indicated drug	Alternative therapies
Amitriptyline	Fluoxetine
Amoxapine	Flupenthixol
Butriptyline	Fluvoxamine
Clomipramine	Paroxetine
Desipramine	Sertraline
Dothiepin	Trazodone
Doxepin	Viloxazine
Imipramine	MAOIs
Iprindole	Lithium salts (but caution
Lofepramine	if used in conjunction
Maprotiline*	with acetazolamide
Mianserin*	which increases
Nortriptyline	excretion)
Protriptyline	
Trimipramine	

Antipsychotics

Contra-indicated drug	Alternative therapies
Chlorpromazine	Benperidol
Fluphenazine	Droperidol
Loxapine	Haloperidol
Pericyazine	Flupenthixol
Perphenazine	Fluspirilene
Pipothiazine	Oxypertine
Prochlorperazine	Pimozide
Promazine	Sulpiride
Thioridazine	Zuclopenthixol
Trifluoperazine	

Antihistamines

Contra-indicated drug	Alternative therapies
Azatadine	Acrivastine
Cyproheptidine	Astemizole
Mequitazine	Cetirizine
	Loratadine
	Terfenadine

Antiarrhythmics

Contra-indicated drug	Alternative therapies
Disopyramide	Other antiarrhythmics but caution with amiodarone and verapamil if topical beta-adrenoreceptor blockers used concurrently as this combination can lead to bradycardia and AV block

* Tetracyclic antidepressants – monitor in narrow angle glaucoma

indicated can be safely taken provided that the iridectomy/iridotomy remains patent.

Patient compliance

The patient is more likely to comply with the prescribed treatment if the drug or drugs prescribed can be administered according to a simple, infrequent dosage regimen and cause no or few local or systemic side effects.

Thus a patient treated with a once-daily or twice-daily beta-adrenoreceptor blocker would be expected to comply better than one treated with pilocarpine with its unfortunate side effects and inconvenient four times a day dosage regimen.

Table 52.15 Systemically administered sympathomimetic drugs with alpha-adrenergic activity contra-indicated in narrow angle glaucoma

Ephedrine
Isometheptene
Phenylpropanolamine
Pseudoephedrine
Levodopa

Common side effects of topical and systemic medication should be fully discussed with the patient so that the headache and the effects of miosis encountered with pilocarpine, the red eye with adrenaline, and the paraesthesia with carbonic anhydrase inhibitors are not unexpected, leading to premature discontinuation of therapy.

As glaucoma is predominantly a disease of elderly people, physical disability may prevent successful treatment, however conscientious the patient. Rheumatoid arthritis may, for example, reduce the patient's ability to squeeze the bottle of eye drops, while the tremor of Parkinson's disease can make correct positioning of instillation difficult. Various compliance aids have been introduced to aid correct positioning and squeezing of eye drops and should be made available to patients so disabled. Patients with poor visual acuity can be helped by colour coding of eye drop labels and supplying bottles labelled with large print.

Where self-medication is impossible, a simple infrequent dosage regimen is more likely to be achieved when a relative, neighbour or the district nursing service becomes responsible for administration of the medication. In these cases, a once daily beta-adrenoreceptor blocker has an obvious advantage over one which should be administered at 12-hourly intervals, and an Ocusert, if tolerated and retained, will ensure constant delivery of pilocarpine for 1 week, whereas the preferred dosage regimen of this drug administered in eye drop form is totally impractical for anyone other than someone living with the patient to administer.

CASE STUDIES

CASE 52.1

Mrs A. B., a 54-year-old woman, is referred to the ophthalmologist following a routine visit to her optician during which it was discovered that the intraocular pressure in her left eye was elevated.

On initial examination the ophthalmologist's findings are:

Eye	IOP mmHg	Cup/disc	Visual field
Right	20	No cupping	Full
Left	33	Cupping	Reduced

Q What is the most appropriate initial therapy and how should treatment be adjusted on subsequent visits if this therapy fails?

CASE 52.2

Mr E. H. is a 39-year-old man who has worn spectacles for reading since his mid-twenties. One evening, he experiences increasing pain in his right eye, starts to see haloes around lights and feels very sick.

At the local hospital's casualty department, thick, sticky eye drops are instilled prior to slit lamp examination. He is given an intravenous injection and the nursing staff start to administer eye drops at regular intervals to the affected eye prior to admission.

On admission, he is given a sweet, sickly drink having been told that his intraocular pressure is still high.

Q What treatment has Mr E. H. been given? Was it appropriate and how should medical treatment progress?

CASE 52.3

Mrs C. T. attends the glaucoma investigation clinic on the advice of her brother in whom primary open angle glaucoma has recently been diagnosed.

As she is found to have a raised IOP and early changes in the visual field in the left eye the ophthalmologist prescribes:

• Timolol 0.25% drops, left eye, 12-hourly.

A few days later, Mrs C. T. returns to the hospital's casualty department stating that the treatment does not suit her.

Q On examination, her left eye is puffy and hyperaemic. The senior house officer concludes that she is allergic to the treatment and asks the pharmacist what alternative therapy is available.

ANSWERS TO CASE STUDIES

CASE 52.1

A On initial examination by the ophthalmologist, Mrs. A. B. is found to have raised intraocular pressure (IOP), glaucomatous cupping and a reduced visual field in the left eye. A diagnosis of primary open angle glaucoma in the left eye is made. Although the IOP in the right eye is at the upper end of the normal range, there is no cupping or reduction in visual field in this eye and therefore the treatment is for the left eye only at this stage.

It is now generally agreed that the most effective treatment with the lowest incidence of systemic and local adverse effects is a topical beta-adrenoreceptor blocker. In addition, a once- or twice-daily instillation regimen leads to good patient compliance. Levobunolol 0.5% drops, left eye, 12-hourly is suitable initially.

Subsequently Dipivefrin 0.1% drops, left eye, 12-hourly may be added to the levobunolol.

Pilocarpine should not be added to the regimen until later because of its inconvenient dosage regimen and impairment of vision.

If surgical treatment is necessary eventually oral acetazolamide may be added to her regimen. Carbonic anhydrase inhibitors are not normally used on a long-term basis as many patients cannot tolerate their adverse effects. Mrs A. B. is now using maximal medical therapy for primary open angle glaucoma:

- Levobunolol 0.5% drops, left eye, 12-hourly
- Dipivefrin 0.1% drops, left eye, 12-hourly
- Pilocarpine 1% drops, left eye, four times a day
- Acetazolamide SR capsules 500 mg once a day

Following surgery, it is hoped that all antiglaucoma therapy to the left eye will be stopped.

CASE 52.2

A Mr E.H. has had an attack of acute closed angle glaucoma, being prone to this disorder because of his hypermetropia.

Eye drops instilled prior to slit-lamp examination would be a hypertonic solution of glycerol or sucrose used to clear the oedematous cornea to enable visualization of the angle of the anterior chamber.

Initial treatment to bring the grossly elevated IOP down rapidly to prevent permanent damage to the eye is with intravenous acetazolamide.

The eye drops instilled at regular intervals would be pilocarpine, used for its miotic action to pull the iris away from the occluded angle.

The use of hypertonic eye drops and intravenous acetazolamide is appropriate but the timing of pilocarpine instillation is crucial as drugs working on the intraocular musculature will only achieve a result if the muscles contract in response to stimulation by the drug. Such contraction does not result if the muscles are anoxic when the blood vessels supplying them are squeezed flat due to the high levels of IOP. It is therefore recommended that therapy with pilocarpine is delayed until the IOP has fallen below 50 mmHg.

If intravenous acetazolamide does not result in a suitable fall in IOP, therapy with a hyperosmotic agent is indicated, e.g. oral glycerol at a dosage of 1 g/kg.

These initial treatments will lower IOP and miose the pupil allowing reinstitution of the outflow pathway.

Other medical treatment would include the use of a topical steroid to the affected eye to reduce inflammation resulting from the episode and prophylactic pilocarpine, normally at 1 or 2% to the contralateral eye to prevent an attack of acute closed angle glaucoma. A topical beta-adrenoreceptor blocker and oral acetazolamide may be added to maintain the lowered IOP in the affected eye.

Acute closed angle glaucoma is an ophthalmic emergency which when adequately treated, initially medically and subsequently surgically, will not recur as long as the iridectomy/iridotomy remains patent. Drugs previously contra-indicated in patients prone to this condition may be safely used following treatment.

CASE 52.3

A Eye drops contain a number of components including the active ingredient, preservative and various stabilizers such as antioxidants and chelating agents. Although it is possible that Mrs C. T. could be allergic to any of these components, preservative allergy is the most common and it is logical to change to a product with an alternative preservative or one which is preservative free.

Beta-adrenoreceptor blockers. All commercially available, multidose topical beta-adrenoreceptor blockers contain benzalkonium chloride, so these products are unsuitable for Mrs C. T.

Single-dose preservative-free forms of metipranolol, levobunolol and timolol are available.

Sympathomimetics. Simplene and Eppy brands of adrenaline eye drops contain benzalkonium chloride and therefore would not be suitable for Mrs C. T.

Ganda, a combined product of guanethidine and adrenaline also contains benzalkonium chloride and is not suitable in this case.

There are no commercially available preservative-free sympathomimetics used in the treatment of glaucoma.

Parasympathomimetics. Isopto-Carpine, Isopto-Carbachol and Sno-Pilo contain benzalkonium chloride as do the generic preparations of pilocarpine and pilocarpine with physostigmine made by Boots, Daniels, Schering-Plough, Evans Medical and Thornton & Ross.

Smith & Nephew manufacture a single-dose preservative-free form of pilocarpine in strengths of 1, 2 and 4%. This would be a suitable but expensive choice of therapy for Mrs C. T.

Ocusert-Pilo, available in strengths of 20 and 40 micrograms/hour is another suitable preservative-free alternative.

Carbonic anhydrase inhibitors. One way to avoid topical side effects is to use an oral carbonic anhydrase inhibitor. However, the side effect profile of these products makes them unsuitable as first line treatment.

BIBLIOGRAPHY

Committee on Safety of Medicines. Bronchospasm associated with cardioselective and topical beta-blockers. Current Problems No 28 (May 1990)

Elkington A R, Khaw P T. The glaucomas (ABC of eyes). British Medical Journal 1988; 297: 677–680

Hopkins G A. Drug treatment of glaucoma. American Journal of Ophthalmology 1985; 62(2): 132–141

Kanski J J. Clinical ophthalmology. Oxford: Butterworth 1984

Kohn A N, Moss A P, Hargett N A, Ritch R, Smith H, Podos S M. Clinical comparison of dipivalyl epinephrine and epinephrine in the treatment of glaucoma. American Journal of Ophthalmology 1979; 87: 196–201

Kooner K S, Zimmerman T J. Medical treatment of glaucoma. Current Opinion in Ophthalmology 1990; 1: 134–140

Krieglstein G K, Novack G D, Voepel E, Schwarzbach G, Lange U, Schunck K P et al. Levobunolol and metipranolol: comparative ocular hypotensive efficacy, safety and comfort. British Journal of Ophthalmology 1987; 71: 250–253

Mills K B. The role of beta blockers in glaucoma. Research and Clinical Forums 1987; 9: 1

Ober M, Scharrer A, David R, Biedner B, Novack G D, Lue J C et al. Long-term ocular hypertensive effect of levobunolol: results of a one-year study. British Journal of Ophthalmology 1985; 69(8): 593–599

Schoene R B, Martin T R, Charan N B, French C L. Timolol-induced bronchospasm in asthmatic bronchitis. Journal of the American Medical Association 1981; 245(14): 1460–1461

Weinreb R N, van Buskirk E M, Cherniack R, Drake M M. Long-term betaxolol therapy in glaucoma patients with pulmonary disease. American Journal of Ophthalmology 1988; 106(2): 162–167

Chapter 53

Eczema and psoriasis

J. M. Marks

Eczema and psoriasis are inflammatory skin diseases which have some similarities, and on occasions there is difficulty in distinguishing them clinically and histologically. They also respond to some of the same treatments. Nevertheless they are quite separate diseases occurring in different groups of people.

ECZEMA

Eczema or dermatitis is an inflammation of the skin with the usual signs of inflammation but with additional features because of its site. It is the end result of a number of disease processes, the common types being atopic and contact eczema. The terms eczema and dermatitis will be used synonymously. Eczema of the palms and soles is sometimes called pompholyx.

SYMPTOMS, PATHOGENESIS AND INVESTIGATIONS

As in any other disease all the characteristic features of eczema are rarely present in every patient and depend upon the stage at which the patient is seen as well as the severity of the disease and any change brought about by treatment. Eczema is derived from the Greek word meaning 'to boil' relating to the blisters formed from fluid escaping from dilated, inflamed dermal capillaries and rising to the surface between the epidermal cells (interepithelial oedema or spongiosis) like bubbles in boiling water. There is extravasation of leucocytes and, in severe cases, of erythrocytes. All this interferes with normal keratinization and the formation of the horny layer. The clinical signs can be deduced once the pathology is known: the skin is red, hot, swollen and itchy. Blisters may be small (vesicles) or large (bullae). Large ones are formed by smaller ones coalescing. Once blisters burst they weep and the high protein-containing fluid produces crusting. Interference with keratinization results in scaling which may be the main physical sign in chronic eczema.

CLINICAL TYPES

Contact eczema

Extraneous substances which may cause eczema can be divided into two groups: those where an allergic phenomenon (delayed cell-mediated reaction) is responsible: and those where the cause is unrelated to allergy but is the result of irritation and 'wear and tear'.

Allergic contact eczema (dermatitis)

A number of substances including antibiotics, antihistamines, local anaesthetics, ointment bases, metals, dyes, plants and rubber compounds can be responsible. Sensitization can occur with very small amounts of the compounds and only certain individuals are susceptible. There may be a genetic factor involved but this is minor, in contrast to atopic eczema where familial cases are the rule. It does not start after the patient's first contact with the allergen, and may not occur for months or years after the initial exposure. The diagnosis of contact dermatitis starts with an accurate and detailed history and examination particularly of the distribution of the rash. Common clinical patterns include eczema around the eyes where antibiotics have been applied, under metal on clothing, e.g. buttons/studs of jeans, and on the hands from wearing rubber gloves. In severe cases it may spread away from the original contact site and exceptionally it may become generalized. The diagnosis is confirmed by patch testing. This is, in contrast to other skin tests in other forms of eczema, very useful in pointing to the cause of the trouble. It depends upon the production of a delayed hypersensitivity reaction by allergens applied to the skin. 'Batteries' of the most common allergens in the appropriate concentration and vehicle are applied to the patient's back under occlusion. The test is positive if there is an area of eczema under the patch at 48 to 96 hours. Taken in conjunction with the history, patch testing is of great diagnostic help.

Eczema of wear and tear (primary irritant dermatitis)

Eczema of wear and tear is far commoner as a cause of hand eczema in housewives, nurses, miners and other industrial workers than allergic contact dermatitis. A number of substances including water, soap, detergents and degreasers damage the skin and produce eczema without any immunological mechanism being involved. Usually the more prolonged the exposure the more likely the patient is to develop eczema. Patch testing has no role in the diagnosis of this type of eczema.

Atopic eczema

Atopic eczema is very common and affects about 3% of infants although a large proportion recover and do not have it in adult life. The occurrence is determined genetically, with most patients having a family history of eczema or other atopic manifestations such as hay fever, asthma or urticaria. The rash classically occurs symmetrically in the flexures of the limbs (i.e. elbow, wrist, back of knees), but face, hands and feet are common sites too. There is a tendency for the skin to thicken or lichenify either in large sheets (lichen simplex) or in nodules (nodular prurigo). Atopy is a condition in which there is a marked tendency to produce reagins or circulating IgE antibodies to a number of substances including pollens, foods and house dust mite. These antibodies are detected by scratch, prick or intradermal testing with the various allergens: a weal and flare appears in 20 minutes if the test is positive. Positive tests in eczema indicate only that the patient is atopic and are not immediately relevant to the cause of the eczema. This is in great contrast to the usefulness of patch testing in contact eczema.

Other eczemas

These include discoid eczema, seborrhoeic eczema and stasis or varicose eczema. They occur in patients who are not atopic and usually start in later life. Discoid eczema, as the name suggests, occurs in circular patches and may be associated with bacterial skin infection. Seborrhoeic eczema involves face, scalp, and upper trunk and is associated with infection by the yeast *Pityrosporum ovale*. Varicose eczema occurs on the lower leg often, though not necessarily, in association with varicose veins and oedema: the mechanism is not well understood. Varicose eczema in particular is likely to be complicated by contact dermatitis to medicaments including antibiotics and ointment bases used in its treatment.

TREATMENT

The main principles of treatment apply regardless of the type and cause of the eczema. Since eczema is an inflammation, anti-inflammatory agents are required and for practical purposes this means corticosteroids.

Topical corticosteroids

The topical use of corticosteroids has, quite unjustifiably, received a bad reputation. In reality it is probably true that more people with eczema have suffered from their underusage than their overuse. The rational use of this group of drugs should follow the same rules as those for any other even though the route of administration may be different.

1. There should be a clear indication based on the diagnosis of a corticosteroid-responsive disease, e.g. eczema or psoriasis.

2. Their use should not be continued if it is obvious that they are having no benefit.

3. They should not be used in unreliable (non-compliant) patients.

4. Although accurate recording of dosage is more difficult than with systemic drugs, attempts should be made to quantify amounts used.

5. The lowest dose that is effective should be used. There is no point in using a preparation that is so weak as to have no discernible side effects if it has no therapeutic effect either. The more potent the corticosteroids therapeutically, the greater will be the adverse effects, and if the preparations and dosage are such that side effects will occur these must be weighed against the disadvantages of continuing disease.

Choice of a preparation

There are over 80 topical preparations containing corticosteroids in the UK and many are available in cream and ointment bases bringing the total number to well over 100. The treatment of eczema will involve the use of a very potent (group 1), potent (group II), moderately potent (group III), or mildly potent (group IV) corticosteroid. Generally it is best to use an ointment for dry eczema and a cream for weeping eczema. A small number of patients become allergic to the constituents in the bases, e.g. lanolin and propylene glycol in some ointments, or substances like ethylenediamine, chlorocresol and parabens in creams. A knowledge of the base constituents of different preparations is therefore essential. Manufacturers change the constituents of topical corticosteroids from time to time so reference to an up-to-date publication is necessary.

In addition to choosing the right base for a patient, a decision has to be made about whether or not to use a corticosteroid/antibiotic combination. Such combinations should not be used routinely. If there is a problem with infection it is usually preferable to give the appropriate antibiotic systemically and the corticosteroid topically. This approach avoids the risk of developing contact dermatitis to topical antibiotics.

In selecting the correct potency of corticosteroid for severe eczema, it is usually best to use the strongest preparations (group I) and bring the condition under control quickly and then reduce the potency to the weakest which will control the condition. The face, flexures and children's skin need more care but strong corticosteroids can be used even here in the short term and under supervision. The skin is an area where damage is easily seen, and stopping the corticosteroid early on will result in reversal of the adverse effects. The classical adverse effect associated with the topical use of corticosteroid is the thinning of skin from collagen loss. This can result in corticosteroid purpura and striae whilst on the face the appearance of redness and pustulation can resemble rosacea. Absorption of corticosteroids from the skin occurs and systemic effects are a theoretical possibility but in practice it is rare for this to be a clinical problem.

Systemic corticosteroids

Systemic corticosteroids, though rarely required in eczema have a place in acute cases especially for contact dermatitis. In this situation the patient is made much more comfortable very quickly and, if the incriminating allergen is identified and avoided in the future, prolonged and repeated courses are not required. Systemic corticosteroids are rarely used in atopic eczema but may be employed in particularly bad cases. If they are given for accompanying asthma an improvement in the skin is usually noticed as well. They are the treatment of choice and may be life saving in erythrodermic eczema, in which the eczema has become generalized and the patient is red and hot all over his body.

Drying agents and moisturizers

In weeping eczema blisters and oozing are dried up by potassium permanganate baths. Crystals in sufficient quantity to make the water pink (vin rosé) are added to a warm bath and the patient told to soak in it for as long as is comfortable. The mechanism of this treatment is not understood but it has showed the test of time and is still popular amongst dermatologists. For dry eczema the patient will almost certainly be helped by using emulsifying ointment or similar agents. They can be applied directly to the skin or used in the bath instead of soap. In the inactive phase of eczema this may be all that patients require and certainly they should not apply corticosteroid ointment just because the skin is dry. Emulsifying ointment is regarded by some patients as the most useful single treatment they are ever given. Two tablespoonfuls of the ointment should be mixed in a jug with about a pint of very hot water; if the resulting emulsion is placed under the tap and the bath water run on it, it will produce a 'foam' bath.

Antihistamines

Pruritus is a troublesome feature of eczema and may need treatment in its own right. The newer non-sedative oral antihistamines have little effect on pruritus that is not mediated by histamine and in dermatological practice are rarely useful except in urticaria. In other pruritic dermatoses an additional sedative effect is often beneficial. Again the choice of antihistamines is considerable. Trimeprazine is suitable and much used.

Topical antihistamines produce contact dermatitis but considering how much they are used the actual incidence of sensitivity may be quite low. In eczema, where repeated application is likely to occur, they should be avoided.

Other treatments

Coal tar

Coal tar, though much used on an empirical basis for eczema in the past, became much less popular when topical corticosteroids were introduced. It is less effective and very messy and can produce folliculitis and photosensitivity. It is, however, a good antipruritic and is useful for this effect in chronic eczema, especially when it is used in impregnated bandages such as coltapaste, applied at night to limbs of atopic children. Many tar pastes and lotions are also available for use when for some reason topical corticosteroids are contra-indicated, and strong coal tar solution BP (40% tar) is painted on to patches of resistant oozing eczema.

Azathioprine

Azathioprine is used systemically in severe, resistant eczema. It has all the disadvantages of antimitotic drugs with adverse effects on bone marrow, germ cells and the immune system but is effective in a dosage of 50 to 100 mg daily either alone, or as a corticosteroid-sparing agent, in chronic atopic or erythrodermic eczema. Usually it needs to be taken indefinitely as stopping the drug results in relapse.

Cyclosporin

This drug is very effective in eczema if given systemically in a dosage of up to 5 mg/kg/day. Its place in management of the disease and appropriate dosage schedules have not yet been determined but it is effective if used intermittently in atopic eczema, e.g. two courses of 2 months per year. Relapse occurs if it is stopped but this can be lessened if the dose is reduced gradually. The main adverse effects are hypertension and deterioration in renal function but these are reversible with short periods of low dosage of the drug.

Oil of evening primrose

Evidence that this is effective is as yet inconclusive.

Diets

These have no part to play in the routine management of eczema. Even enthusiasts use them in a few selected cases only.

In addition to the above measures which apply to all eczemas, different types warrant extra attention:

Contact eczema

Identification of the offending allergen is important as is its withdrawal.

Atopic eczema

Infection, usually with *staphylococcus*, is relatively common and is one cause of the eczema deteriorating. Thus systemic antibiotics are usually required at some stage. Ideally, swabs should be taken and the organism and its sensitivities identified. Alternatively treatment can be started with oral flucloxacillin in usual dosage. This should be continued for 10 days, unless infection is a chronic problem, in which case long-term flucloxacillin should be given. It is also important to reduce pruritus as scratching produces worsening of the eczema and a sedative antihistamine will be required particularly at night. Occlusive bandages which contain zinc oxide are helpful on the limbs to heal the rash and protect against scratching.

Varicose eczema

Varicose eczema is helped by reducing oedema and venous pressure in the lower legs. Elasticated support stockings are an effective way of reducing this venous pressure. Operations on varicose veins are rarely needed for eczema alone. Contact dermatitis to topical medicaments is a problem which should be looked for especially in those whose skin deteriorates while they are being treated.

Seborrhoeic eczema

Topical applications of ketoconazole as a 2% cream or shampoo are often helpful in eradicating *Pityrosporum ovale*. Other topical imidazoles may be used instead. Treatment should be continued for up to 3 weeks but relapse is common and repeated courses are often necessary.

THE PATIENT

Patients with eczema and their relatives often need more than strictly medical help. They may receive this from dermatologists, general practitioners, pharmacists or nurses. They also like to meet other people with eczema, and this they can do through their local branch of the National

Eczema Society. With children it is important to stress that most get better during childhood, though it is unwise to suggest a date when this will happen. It must be made plain that treatments are suppressive and must be continued or the rash will recur unless the disease has gone into natural remission. Patients should not be afraid to use the prescribed treatment especially corticosteroids. Reasonable amounts of ointments, etc., should be prescribed, e.g. it will take about 170 g topical corticosteroid to cover the whole adult body, using it twice daily for a week (see Table 53.1). Exclusion diets should not be encouraged unless there is good evidence that a particular food is to blame and even then care should be taken to see that the diet is not deficient in essentials. If cats, soap, woollen clothing etc. make symptoms worse they must either be avoided or their effects accepted. People with eczema should lead as normal a life as possible. Schools can be very helpful (or very unhelpful) where eczematous children are concerned, and it is worth stressing the fact that eczema is not infectious. Occupations like hairdressing and coalmining are obviously not ideal for people with eczema but if they are established in such a job it is very unwise to tell them to give it up until every effort has been made to enable them to continue.

PSORIASIS

AETIOLOGY

Psoriasis affects about 2% of the population of western Europe and North America. Its cause is unknown but there is a genetic component, the majority of patients having another member of the family affected. Studies of HLA typing show a predominance of certain antigens including CW6 and DR7. The nature of the inherited defect is unkown but it is probably a simple enzyme deficiency. Non-hereditary factors are also needed to precipitate an attack in the genetically susceptible. Those which are known include:

Koebner phenomenon. Here injury to the skin, e.g. a cut or burn, may be followed by the later appearance of psoriasis at the site which may subsequently spread.

Infection. Streptococcal infections in particular may be followed by an attack of psoriasis. It is commonest in children and the clinical pattern produced is often guttate (see later). Patients with psoriasis who develop AIDS may have a severe exacerbation of their rash, though the reason for this is not known.

Lithium. Patients receiving lithium for depression may have an exacerbation of psoriasis. The cause of this is unknown.

Stress. Patients often think an attack of psoriasis is precipitated by 'stress' but this is difficult to prove (or disprove).

Most attacks of psoriasis start without an identifiable precipitating trigger.

PATHOGENESIS AND PATHOLOGY

A large number of abnormalities can be identified in the blood, skin and other tissues in psoriasis. Most of these are epi-phenomena or are the result of the disease and not its cause. Many are not specific to psoriasis and are found in other inflammatory skin diseases as well. Rival theories suggest that in psoriasis the primary defect is in T-cells, polymorphonuclear leucocytes, leukotriene production, cyclic nucleotides and many other systems. None of course, would be mutually exclusive. It is well established that there is an abnormality of epidermal cell 'turn-over', this being about ten times that of normal epidermis mainly due to an increase in the number of proliferating cells. It is not known how this comes about but drugs such as cyto-

Table 53.1 Approximate amounts of topical steroid preparations required to treat body parts*	
	Grams
Head and neck	10
Arms	30
Trunk	60
Legs	60
Hands and feet	10
Whole body	170
* Based on a twice-daily application for 1 week.	

toxic agents which reduce the number of proliferating cells are very effective in the treatment of psoriasis.

Histologically, in psoriasis the dermal capillaries are dilated and nearer the surface than normal. The epidermis is thickened (acanthosis) and the granular layer is absent; nuclei are present in the upper layers of the epidermis (parakeratosis) and there are collections of leucocytes in the epidermis (microabcesses). Scarring does not occur and this is particularly important in the scalp where permanent hair loss is not a feature even after very severe scalp psoriasis.

CLINICAL APPEARANCE

Characteristically, the lesions of psoriasis are red, scaly and well demarcated. Occasionally pustules are visible on the surface. The scale is easily scraped off and produces a silvery powder. Many clinical patterns of rash occur and the rash varies to some extent according to the site affected. Any part of the body can be involved but extensor surfaces of arms and legs, scalp, and hands and feet are common sites; the face is often spared.

Guttate psoriasis. Many small spots appear together all over the body often after a streptococcal infection. It is common in children.

Discoid and plaque psoriasis. Medium- to large-sized areas of psoriasis occur on body and limbs.

Psoriasis of palms and soles. At these sites particularly pustules are often visible.

Erythrodermic and generalized pustular psoriasis. These types of psoriasis involve the whole body and have dangerous systemic effects.

Psoriasis of nails. The nails are often involved in psoriasis and may be the only part of the body affected. The classical findings are pitting and onycholysis (separation of the nail from the bed). Nail psoriasis is particularly resistant to treatment.

NATURAL HISTORY

Psoriasis appears most commonly in young adults, though it may start at any age. Charac-

teristically it is a chronic disease with exacerbation and remissions, the causes of which are seldom apparent. Treatments which clear an attack generally have no effect upon the subsequent history of the disease which is likely to recur in its own time once the treatment is stopped.

Psoriatic arthropathy

Arthritis of the rheumatoid type occurs more often in psoriatics than in normal individuals. Several clinical patterns occur including:

Psoriatic spondylitis. This is identical to ankylosing spondylitis but occurs equally in women and men: there is the same association with HLAB27.

Arthritis mutilans. Arthritis mutilans is associated with severe deformities of joints.

Arthritis of terminal interphalangeal joints. All are seronegative. The onset of arthropathy may precede or follow that of the rash and the two may fluctuate together or separately. Generally, separate treatments are required.

TREATMENT

Not all patients with psoriasis wish for or need treatment. Of those who do, some can be managed in general practice or as hospital outpatients while others require inpatient treatment. Clearance of an attack of psoriasis is usually possible, whereas there is nothing apart from maintenance PUVA (see below) or long-term systemic treatment that will alter the natural history and prevent subsequent attacks.

Rationale of treatment

Early treatments for psoriasis such as tar, dithranol and ultraviolet light were empirical. The use of anti-inflammatory corticosteroids and the antimitotic drugs such as methotrexate subsequently seemed more rational. Most effective treatments are now known to inhibit epidermal mitosis though they have many other effects that could equally account for their activity in psoriasis.

The fact that there are many treatments for psoriasis suggests that none is satisfactory. Choice of therapy depends on many factors including age, sex, severity, extent and site of rash, fashion and local facilities. Topical treatment, or in some cases photochemotherapy, is preferable to systemic treatment except in emergencies like erythroderma and generalized pustular psoriasis where systemic drugs may be the first line treatment.

Topical treatments

Corticosteroids

Corticosteroids are much used and have the great advantage of not staining the skin or clothing. They are effective in relatively acute and superficial psoriasis but not usually for thick plaques of chronic psoriasis. They are useful for sites where other topical treatments which stain and irritate are unacceptable, e.g. face, hands, genitalia, scalp and for irritated sore psoriasis. Their usefulness must as always be weighed against their adverse effects especially as weak corticosteroids are unlikely to be effective, and potent or very potent preparations are normally required, sometimes under polythene occlusion. Special preparations are available for the scalp and are best applied under a polythene cap at night and washed off in the morning.

Dithranol (anthralin; 1,3-dihydroxyanthrone)

The main disadvantages of dithranol are that it burns the skin and stains skin and clothing. It is pH sensitive and most preparations contain salicylic acid as a stabilizer. Face, flexures and acute psoriasis must be treated with great care. Dithranol was originally mostly used according to the Ingram regimen but many centres now use a 'short contact' regimen.

Ingram regimen. This method of application is based on the fact that dithranol irritates clinically uninvolved skin more than lesional skin and so every attempt is made to confine the dithranol to lesions. This is done by using it in a vehicle of thick consistency (Lassar's paste) and applying it accurately to lesions only, with a spatula or orange stick, powdering with talc and covering lesions with stockinette dressings. A concentration of 0.025 to 1% (usually 0.2 to 0.8%) is used. The preparation is left on for 24 hours, then washed off in a tar bath and followed by treatment with ultraviolet light (UVB). The process is repeated daily until the rash is clear. Such treatment, starting with a weak concentration and then increasing the strength of dithranol as required and tolerated, will take an average of 3 weeks to clear the psoriasis. The application is time consuming, taking up to an hour of trained nurse time for a patient with extensive disease. The dressings etc. also limit the patients' activities at home and perhaps their ability to go to work.

'Short contact' regimens. In 1980, it was shown that dithranol left on for a few minutes was as effective as that left on for 24 hours. Stronger concentrations can be used than with the Ingram regimen and because of the shorter period of contact with the skin, it is not so important to keep it off clinically uninvolved skin. To facilitate removal it is applied in a softer base. Although extremely messy, this regimen can be used by patients in their own homes, who apart from the relatively short time needed for the treatment, are able to live and work for the rest of the day without cumbersome dressings. Many different concentrations of dithranol in different bases and various application times are used, e.g. 2 to 8% in emulsifying ointment with 0.5% salicylic acid for contact times of 15 to 30 minutes. The dithranol is removed by a detergent such as 'Teepol' in a bath. The clearance time is on average 3 weeks as with the Ingram regimen.

Coal tar

Coal tar regimens, including a combination of tar paste and UVL have been used for many years. They are generally less popular than the dithranol regimens today, though they are probably equally effective in expert hands. Tar preparations vary in composition and contain many different chemicals. They are messy and smelly but stain less than dithranol. Attempts to 'clean up' the original crude tar preparations have generally resulted in a loss of effectiveness.

Vitamin D analogues, e.g. calcipotriol

Calcipotriol is available as a 50 microgram/g ointment and is used for chronic plaque psoriasis. It is applied twice daily for up to 6 weeks. It is a clean preparation but is liable to irritate the skin. Rarely, hypercalcaemia has been reported from absorption from overenthusiastic use. Clinical trials have suggested that in some situations it is marginally better than dithranol or topical corticosteroid but much experience is needed before its place in treatment can be fully assessed.

Ultraviolet light (UVB)

Many psoriatics are better in the summer and in sunny climes. UVB is used for psoriasis but is rarely effective alone in chronic disease. In some hospitals, short contact regimens are used in conjunction with UVB on an outpatient basis, several times per week.

Scalp psoriasis

Dithranol and tar are well tolerated but special preparations which can be washed out easily are needed: both dithranol and tar are available as 'pommades'. Removal of debris and old pommades is important and for this a detergent such as 'Teepol' should be used as a shampoo.

Photochemotherapy (PUVA)

PUVA therapy (psoralen + UVA) was developed at a time when treatment for psoriasis was either with messy ointments or toxic systemic drugs. The fact that PUVA was clean, produced a tan and had no serious systemic effects made it very attractive to patients and doctors. It can be regarded as occupying a place between topical and systemic therapy. Certain drugs, in this case a psoralen (usually 8-methoxypsoralen, 8MOP), react in the skin with long wave ultraviolet light UVA (320–400 nm) to interfere with DNA synthesis and thus decrease cell turnover and clear psoriasis. 8MOP is usually given orally, 0.6 mg/kg body weight, and 2 hours later when it has reached a maximum concentration in the skin the patient is exposed to whole body UVA in a suitable apparatus such as a cubicle or bed equipped with UV tubes. The exposure times are calculated by previous testing or according to the patient's likelihood of burning and tanning. Two or three such treatments a week clear chronic psoriasis in a mean of 34 days. In severe relapsing psoriasis PUVA treatment may be continued weekly, fortnightly or even once every 3 weeks to prevent the rash retuning.

Adverse effects

PUVA should not be given to pregnant women. Nausea and pruritus are annoying and occur occasionally but are usually temporary. Serious side effects occur in the eyes and skin (see below).

Eyes. The eyes must be protected during, and for 12 hours after treatment by suitable spectacles that filter off UVA. In animals, cataracts can result from high-dose psoralen in the lens exposed to UVA.

Skin. Ageing of skin and skin cancer are likely to occur but depend upon dose, pattern and duration of treatment. About 10 years is probably needed for skin cancer to develop after PUVA. PUVA treatment first became available in the USA in 1974 and in the UK in 1977; thus relatively few patients have been treated for over 10 years and the full position regarding cancer is still not known. Obviously the older the patient, the less likely that enough time will elapse for the cancer to develop and for this reason PUVA may be used as a first line treatment in the elderly. Young people should not be excluded from PUVA treatment but careful consideration of the adverse effects must be made.

Systemic drugs

These include antimitotic drugs, cyclosporin,

Table 53.2 Interactions with drugs used for psoriasis

	Interacting drug	Outcome
Methotrexate	Aspirin NSAIDs	Increased serum concentration and enhanced toxicity of methotrexate
	Phenytoin Sulphonamides Trimethoprim	Increased bone marrow toxicity
	Probenecid	Increased serum concentrations and toxicity of methotrexate
Etretinate	Methotrexate	Increased serum concentration of methotrexate
Azathioprine	Allopurinol	Enhanced effect/toxicity of azathioprine
Cyclosporin	NSAIDs Co-trimoxazole Aminoglycosides	Increased risk of nephrotoxicity
	Phenytoin	Reduced serum concentrations of cyclosporin
	Erythromycin Ketoconazole	Increased serum concentration of cyclosporin

etretinate and corticosteroids. Indications for their usage are severe or extensive psoriasis, intolerance or ineffectiveness of topical treatment and rapid relapse of psoriasis after clearance. Only very exceptionally should they be used as first line treatment (see later). Drug interactions are shown in Table 53.2.

Cytotoxic and immunosuppressive drugs

All have toxic effects on bone marrow and germ cells. None of these drugs must be given to pregnant women. They should be used only under expert supervision.

Methotrexate. Methotrexate is probably the most effective cytotoxic drug for psoriasis and the agent which most dermatologists prefer. It should only be given *once weekly* as more frequent dosage is associated with increased toxicity. Oral administration is preferable but intramuscular and, exceptionally, intravenous routes are also used. The dosage varies from 2.5 to 25 mg weekly and it is wise to start with a small dose (2.5 to 5 mg).

Acute toxic effects occur where there are rapidly proliferating cells such as in the bone marrow and gastrointestinal tract. These are reversible with folinic acid rescue (120 mg folinic acid in divided doses over 12 to 24 hours intramuscularly or intravenously followed by 15 mg/kg by mouth 6-hourly for 48 hours) which antagonizes the antifolate effects of methotrexate. Long-term effects on the liver lead to fibrosis and cirrhosis and excessive alcohol consumption probably makes these more likely. There is controversy about the need for liver biopsy but it is probably wise to do one before starting treatment and then at 3-yearly intervals for those who take the drug for more than a few months, especially in the younger age groups. Deaths that have occurred have been due to absolute or relative overdosage producing marrow suppression or gastrointestinal bleeding or ulceration and this is more likely to occur in the elderly with poor renal function. Creatinine clearance should be measured before the drug is started and the dosage of methotrexate reduced accordingly if it is impaired. Drug interactions with salicylates, non-steroidal anti-inflammatory drugs and etretinate are serious and these combinations should be avoided.

Azathioprine and hydroxyurea. These drugs have similar effects on the bone marrow and gonads to methotrexate.

Cyclosporin. Cyclosporin is a very effective drug in psoriasis where it works in relatively low dosage (i.e. 2 to 5 mg/kg/day). Its action probably does not depend on the drug's well known effect on T-cells. Usage is limited by effects on renal function and blood pressure. These are apparently reversible and so short courses of cyclosporin, e.g. up to 3 months, are acceptable and those who need about two courses of treatment a year can be managed this way.

Corticosteroids

Systemic corticosteroids are not effective in

chronic psoriasis. They have a dramatic and life-saving effect in erythroderma and generalized pustular psoriasis where the patient may be in danger of death from heart failure and disturbance of temperature control. Once the emergency is over the patient may need more specific antipsoriatic treatment, e.g. methotrexate.

Acitretin

Acitretin has now replaced etretinate as the retinoid used for psoriasis. It is given in a dose of 25 to 30 mg daily though this can be reduced if adverse reactions occur. The major limitation of its use is its undesirable effect on the fetus, compounded by the fact that small amounts of it and its metabolites are very slowly excreted and female patients must be told not to become pregnant for 2 years after finishing a course. Other adverse effects on serum lipids, liver function and bone formation are possible, but in practice they rarely seem to be of importance. Dose-related side effects like dryness of the lips and other mucosae are annoying and almost universal. The precise place of the retinoids in psoriasis is still not established, though they are said to be particularly effective in the pustular forms.

THE PATIENT

Patients with psoriasis, like those with eczema or any other chronic disease, need a great deal of support from doctors, pharmacists, nurses and fellow sufferers. They need strong reassurance on a number of points: psoriasis is not infectious; the face is often spared even in the severest cases; and a great deal can be done to help even though the disease is incurable. Demonstration that the rash can be cleared, even if it returns quickly once the treatment is stopped, is very reassuring and if a course of inpatient treatment is necessary for this it is well worthwhile.

The patient has an important part to play in treatment but he/she must be told what is expected of him or her. The patient should be shown how to apply dithranol and warned of the staining it may cause on clothes and bathroom if care is not taken. In the case of systemic drugs the need for regular supervision must be stressed and patients should be warned of the adverse effects to look out for and guard against. Patients treated with PUVA must not sunbathe when their skin is sensitized and must wear protective spectacles as instructed. They can buy their own glasses, and grey polaroids are usually satisfactory. They should, however, bring them to the PUVA unit for testing. Financial and work problems are common. Often multiple prescriptions are required and expenses are incurred from spoilt clothing, bed linen, baths etc. Choice of job may be limited by the appearance of the rash or by an associated arthropathy. The Psoriasis Association is one of the best self-help groups and at local branches patients can meet other psoriatics. They can also get information about special holidays, hairdressers who do not mind dealing with people with scalp psoriasis and times when the local swimming bath is reserved for those with psoriasis.

CASE STUDIES

CASE 53.1

A 2-year-old child was brought to the Skin Clinic with widespread eczema which had been present soon after birth. The child had been treated with 1% hydrocortisone cream only. On the advice of the general practitioner, the child had been bathed as infrequently as possible because when water came in contact with his skin he screamed. The child and his parents had had little sleep throughout his life. The parents were anxious for skin tests to be done to elucidate a cause and identify a subsequent cure.

Q What further advice could be offered?

CASE 53.2

Mrs P. S. was 54 years old and had suffered from psoriasis since she was 7 years old. She had been admitted to hospital on 17 occasions for treatment. At times the rash involved 70% of her skin surface and was pustular. In the past she had been treated with dithranol but she was now intolerant of it, even in low concentrations. She reacted to tar in a similar way. Topical corticosteroids produced some relief in the acute phase but had little effect on the chronic plaques. Methotrexate by mouth in a dose of 5 mg weekly had been tried but produced extreme nausea and vomiting although it cleared the psoriasis. Hydroxyurea, azathioprine and etretinate had also been tried but found to be ineffective. She developed a gynaecological cancer with metastases and was given a maximum of 12 months to live. Her skin was very important to her and she regarded its clearance as vital.

Q How should her psoriasis be treated?

ANSWERS TO CASE STUDIES

CASE 53.1

A The parents need a lot of time to be spent in explaining the long-term benignity of atopic eczema, the fact that skin tests will not help and that the actual cause is still unknown. A stronger corticosteroid is required to bring the rash under control quickly and give them confidence. Clobetasol should be used for a few days if necessary. Emulsifying ointment baths, systemic antihistamines, systemic antibiotics and perhaps occlusive bandages should also be used. If necessary a few days in hospital should be offered.

CASE 53.2

A There is no ideal treatment for this lady but the possibilities include PUVA, cyclosporin or methotrexate given with an antiemetic agent. PUVA was tried and cleared her rash but she was unable to travel the distance from home to hospital 3 times a week for the necessary treatment. Although cyclosporin was obviously undesirable in someone with cancer, it is so effective that it could be tried and may clear the rash in a few weeks at a dose of 3 mg/kg/day. Methotrexate could be tried again but this time administered by the intramuscular route together with ondansetron on the day of the methotrexate injection.

BIBLIOGRAPHY

Eczema

Bateman D N. Clinical pharmacology of topical steroids. In: Greaves M W, Shuster S (eds) Pharmacology of the skin: II. London: Springer-Velag 1989; 239

Marks J M, Rawlins M D. Skin diseases: eczema. In: Speight T M (ed) Avery's Drug treatment, 3rd edn. Auckland: ADIS Press 1987; 458

Shuster S. Eczema. In: Greaves M W, Shuster S (eds) Pharmacology of the skin: II. London: Springer-Velag 1989; 439

Psoriasis

Berth-Jones J, Hutchinson P E. Vitamin D analogues and psoriasis. British Journal of Dermatology 1992; 126: 127

Ingram J T. Approach to psoriasis. British Medical Journal 1953; 2: 591

Marks J M, Rawlins M D. Skin diseases: psoriasis. In: Speight T M (ed) Avery's Drug treatment, 3rd edn. Auckland: ADIS Press 1987; 452

Miatsch M J, Wolff K. Consensus conference on cyclosporin A for psoriasis, February 1992. British Journal of Dermatology 1992; 126: 621

Roenigk H H, Maibach H I (eds) Psoriasis, 2nd edn. New York: Marcel-Decker 1991

Roenigk H H et al. Methotrexate in psoriasis: revised guidelines. Journal of American Acadamy of Dermatology 1988; 19: 145

Stern R S, Parrish J A, Johnson B. Photochemotherapy. In: Greaves M W, Shuster S (eds) Pharmacology of the skin: II. London: Springer-Velag 1989; 509

Chapter 54

Drug-induced skin disorders

P. Magee   L. Beeley

Drug-induced skin eruptions are likely to be among the most frequent adverse reactions seen by pharmacists, since approximately 30% of all reported adverse drug reactions involve the skin.

DIAGNOSIS

It is often difficult to determine the cause of a drug-induced eruption because:

- almost any drug can affect the skin
- unrelated drugs produce similar reactions
- the same drug may produce different reactions in different patients
- many reactions cannot be distinguished from naturally occurring eruptions.

Moreover new drugs continue to be marketed and many drugs are prescribed as combined preparations. The possibility of a food additive or a pharmaceutical excipient causing a skin reaction must not be overlooked as re-exposure is likely and cross-reactivity can occur, e.g. aspirin sensitized patients may also be sensitized to tartrazine.

If a patient presents with a rash and is currently taking or has recently finished medication, it is important to:

- check that the rash is not due to a specific skin disease, e.g. endogenous eczema, scabies
- take an accurate drug history
- ascertain the time course of the eruption in relation to drug use

- note whether the appearance of the rash is typical of any classic drug-induced eruption.

It may then be possible to assess if a drug is the likely cause.

Rechallenge remains the most useful method of confirming a diagnosis. However, rechallenge is not possible for severe cutaneous reactions and even prick and patch testing are not without risk.

TREATMENT

Not all cutaneous reactions are serious but the implicated drug should usually be stopped, although in some cases a dosage reduction may be sufficient if an alternative treatment is not appropriate.

In most cases the rash will disappear within a few days and the patient can be treated symptomatically with oral antihistamines and calamine lotion. In severe conditions corticosteroids may be indicated and possibly full intensive care support.

Erythematous eruptions

An erythematous or exanthematous eruption is the most common type of drug-induced skin reaction.

The rash is characterized by erythema (abnormal flushing of the skin) and may be morbilliform (resembling measles) or maculopapular consisting of macules (distinct flat areas) and papules (raised lesions conventionally less than 1 cm in diameter). The rash is usually bright red in colour and the skin may feel hot, burning or itchy. The whole of the skin surface can be involved, though the face is often spared. Sometimes the rash may disappear even though the drug is continued but if itching is marked it is less likely that the rash will clear. In some severe cases erythroderma may follow an erythematous reaction. Here the erythema persists with continual scaling which may be associated with lymphadenopathy, pyrexia, thirst and shivering with heat and fluid loss from the skin.

Most erythematous eruptions are probably allergic reactions but other mechanisms may

Table 54.1 Drugs causing erythematous eruptions
Allopurinol
Antituberculous drugs, especially rifampicin and second line agents
Antidepressants, e.g. tricyclics, maprotiline
Barbiturates
Captopril
Carbamazepine
Cimetidine
Diuretics: thiazides, frusemide
Gold salts
Lincomycin
Nalidixic acid
Nitrofurantoin
NSAIDs
Penicillin
Phenothiazines
Phenylbutazone, oxphenbutazone
Phenytoin
Oral retinoids
Ranitidine
Streptomycin (less common with other aminoglycosides)
Sulphonamides
Sulphonylureas

NB: ampicillin rashes do not necessarily indicate penicillin hypersensitivity.

sometimes be involved. Allergic reactions can occur early or late in therapy. Early reactions start within 2 to 3 days of drug administration and occur in previously sensitized patients. In the late type of reaction the hypersensitivity develops during administration but the rash may not manifest itself until around the ninth day and can occur as late as 3 weeks after starting treatment.

A distinct reddish-coloured morbilliform rash may be caused by ampicillin, its derivative amoxycillin and its esters bacampicillin, pivampicillin and talampicillin. The reaction will occur in almost all patients with infective mononucleosis (glandular fever) and is not always an indicator of true penicillin allergy although patients often self-report penicillin sensitivity as a result of this reaction. A high incidence of this reaction also occurs in patients with cytomegalovirus. These are often transplant patients taking immunosuppressive drugs or patients with leukaemia.

Treatment of an erythematous eruption involves drug withdrawal and treatment for any associated itching. Measures should be taken to ensure that the patient is not re-exposed to the drug. A note of the suspected sensitivity should be made in medical records and a personal card with the same information should be given to the patient.

A high incidence of erythematous rashes can be expected during or following treatment with penicillin or chemically related antibiotics, with gold salts and with non-steroidal anti-inflammatory drugs.

Pruritus

Pruritus or 'itching' can have many causes. Commonly these are systemic or psychological. However, drugs can induce pruritus either as a symptom of other cutaneous reactions or with itching as the only clinical manifestation. In either condition the itch can be so intense that the scratching this induces will cause lesions so that it is not always possible to know if there was originally an underlying rash.

For most drugs the mechanism for inducing pruritus is not known but it is likely that both central and peripheral mechanisms are involved. Drug-induced pruritus is usually generalized but local anal pruritus can follow antibiotic-induced candidiasis. It can also be produced as a contact allergy following the local administration of ointments and suppositories. Drugs with autonomic activity may produce sweating and prickly heat followed by pruritus.

To treat pruritus the 'itch–scratch–itch' cycle must be broken once the drug cause has been eliminated. Topical steroids and occlusive dressings help to prevent scratching.

Urticaria

Drug-induced urticaria is common and accounts for approximately 28% of all drug-induced skin disorders.

An urticarial rash, often referred to as 'hives' or nettle rash, is an acute or chronic allergic reaction in which red weals develop. The weals itch intensely and may last for hours or days.

Table 54.2   Drugs causing urticaria
Aspirin
Barbiturates
Imipramine
Indomethacin
Iodine
Paracetamol
Penicillins
Ranitidine
Serum, toxoids, pollen vaccines
Sulphonamides
Tartrazine

Giant urticaria or angioedema is a severe form of urticaria involving swelling of the tongue, lips and eyelids and requires urgent medical attention. Laryngeal oedema is the most serious complication.

Only acute urticaria is likely to be drug induced. It occurs immediately or shortly after the administration of the drug in a sensitized patient and can be regarded as the cutaneous manifestation of anaphylaxis. Chronic urticaria is rarely caused by a drug unless the patient is continually exposed, e.g. to trace amounts of penicillins in milk and dairy products. However, aspirin and codeine can exacerbate idiopathic chronic urticaria.

Erythema multiforme

Erythema multiforme can follow an infection, e.g. with herpes simplex, although drugs are

Table 54.3   Drugs causing erythema multiforme and Stevens–Johnson syndrome
Barbiturates
Carbamazepine
Cimetidine
Dapsone
Ethosuximide
Gold salts
Isoniazid
NSAIDs
Penicillins
Phenytoin
Propranolol
Rifampicin
Sulphonamides (especially long-acting compounds)
Sulphonylureas

also a common cause. It accounts for approximately 5% of drug reactions involving the skin.

Erythema multiforme is a serious, sometimes fatal, skin disease.

As the name implies it can present in a variety of patterns. The usual erythematous lesions occur in crops on the hands and feet more often than on the trunk. Each maculopapular lesion increases in size leaving a cyanotic centre which produces an 'iris' or 'target' lesion. The lesions appear over a few days reaching a diameter of 1 or 2 cm within 48 hours. They may blister and can reach a size of up to 10 cm. They usually fade within 1 or 2 weeks of stopping the drug. Healing occurs without scarring although hyperpigmentation may persist for a long time. Involvement of the mucous membranes is common and the mouth, eyes and genitalia may be affected to varying degrees. If the blistering and mucosal lesions are severe the disease is termed the Stevens–Johnson syndrome. There is also systemic involvement with fever, malaise, polyarthritis and diarrhoea. There have been case reports of haematuria and renal failure.

Drugs are the most common cause of Stevens–Johnson syndrome and all suspected drugs should be stopped as the disease has a mortality rate of approximately 15% without treatment. Rechallenge is never justifiable. Treatment with systemic steroids produces a rapid response in both erythema multiforme and Stevens–Johnson syndrome.

Toxic epidermal necrolysis (TEN) – Lyell's syndrome

This is a rare condition but with a high mortality rate of approximately 33%. The main cause of TEN in adults is drug therapy. In children it is a phage type II staphylococcal infection, referred to as the staphylococcal scalded skin syndrome.

Lyell's syndrome frequently has a prodromal phase of malaise sometimes accompanied by a sore throat and fever. The skin reaction starts with large areas of erythema involving most of the skin surface and is followed by a bullous (a large blister containing serous fluid) phase in which the epidermis peels off. This stage

Table 54.4   Drugs causing toxic epidermal necrolysis
Allopurinol
Barbiturates
Dapsone
Gold salts
Penicillins
Phenolphthalein
Phenylbutazone
Phenytoin
Sulphonamides

is complicated by fluid loss, septicaemia and bronchopneumonia. Mucous membrane involvement may precede the skin eruption by 10 to 14 days giving a clinical appearance similar to the Stevens–Johnson syndrome.

Diagnosis is made clinically and from a skin biopsy. In drug-induced TEN there is separation of the basal layer of the epidermis. In staphylococcal scalded skin syndrome separation occurs in the granular layer without necrolysis. Drug rechallenge is never used to confirm a diagnosis. The patient with TEN will require full intensive care support and antibiotic treatment.

Eczematous eruptions – dermatitis

An eczematous eruption may occur during

Table 54.5   Drugs causing eczematous eruptions
Local anaesthetics
Antibiotics, especially neomycin, streptomycin, chloramphenicol
Antihistamines
Antiseptics
Atropine
Captopril
Carbamazepine
Ethylenediamine (in aminophylline)
Gold salts
Imidazole antifungal drugs
Lanolin
Preservatives in creams and ointments
Methyldopa
Phenothiazines
Phenylbutazone
Phenytoin
Quinine, quinidine
Sulphonamides
Sulphonylureas
Thiazide diuretics

systemic drug therapy, or it may develop as a result of allergy to a topical preparation (allergic contact dermatitis) or by direct contact with a primary irritant (contact dermatitis).

The skin lesions are characterized by redness with widespread exfoliation (peeling) and intense itching. Small blisters can develop, especially in contact dermatitis, which burst and weep exudate.

Primary irritant dermatitis is essentially a major public health problem although certain topical drugs, e.g. tar and dithranol, are primary irritants. However, allergic contact dermatitis is a common complication of topical therapy, e.g. persistent dermatitis from medication or dressings used to treat leg ulcers.

Cross-sensitivity reactions can occur when an eczematous eruption or anaphylaxis develops after administration of a systemic drug in a patient previously sensitized by topical application. Cross-sensitivity is one of the major reasons for not using topical antibiotics. Cases of cross-sensitivity have also been reported in patients and medical staff who handle systemic formulations of known sensitizers such as chlorpromazine.

Patch testing can be used to confirm a diagnosis of drug-induced dermatitis and treatment is the same as that used for idiopathic eczema: emollients and topical steroids.

Vesicular and bullous eruptions

Vesiculobullous eruptions are termed 'pemphig-

oid' unless they are associated with specific skin conditions, e.g. erythema multiforme.

A vesicle is a blister filled with serum with a diameter up to 0.5 cm. If larger than this it is termed a bulla.

Pemphigoid reactions can be autoimmune or drug induced. When drug induced they can be part of a fixed drug eruption or generalized, as for example the large bullae which are seen in patients with barbiturate poisoning.

The eruptions will resolve with drug withdrawal although they can persist for up to 2 years.

Lichenoid eruptions

Drug-induced lichenoid eruptions closely resemble lichen planus, occurring as flat mauve lesions, but they may be atypical showing marked scaling. The lesions are found mainly on the forearms, neck and on the inner surface of the thighs. The mouth may be involved and hair loss can occur.

The pathogenic mechanism is unknown. It is not allergic and is probably dose dependent.

The eruptions resolve with drug withdrawal, with or without topical steroids, but hyperpigmentation may remain.

Erythema nodosum

The lesions seen in erythema nodosum are

Table 54.6 Drugs causing vesicular and bullous eruptions
Captopril
Barbiturates (may be associated with drug-induced coma)
Frusemide
Iodides
Nalidixic acid (phototoxic)
Penicillamine
Phenylbutazone
Azapropazone
Rifampicin
Salicylates
Sulphonamides

Table 54.7 Drugs causing lichenoid eruptions
Aspirin
Captopril
Carbamazepine
Chloroquine
Ethambutol
Gold salts
Labetalol
Methyldopa
NSAIDs
Penicillamine
Phenothiazines
Quinidine
Quinine
Sulphonylureas
Thiazide diuretics

painful subcutaneous nodules usually limited to the extremities. Transient erythema may precede the lesions.

Erythema nodosum is usually a complication of infection and is not commonly drug induced. However, it has been observed in women taking oral contraceptives and with other drugs such as sulphonamides, salicylates, penicillins and gold salts.

Purpura

Purpura is a rash resulting from bleeding into the skin from capillaries. It can be caused by drug-induced thrombocytopenia or result from drugs that damage blood vessels (non-thrombocytopenic or vascular purpura). It can also occur with the hypocoagulation associated with reduced circulating clotting factors. In the latter case, drug interactions with the anticoagulants can be a cause.

Psoriasiform eruptions

Drugs can either exacerbate psoriasis in predisposed patients or induce psoriasiform rashes in previously unaffected patients.

The psoriasiform eruptions mimic psoriasis and are characterized by itchy, scaly red patches on the elbows, forearms, knees, legs and scalp.

Fixed drug eruptions

Fixed drug eruptions are characterized by the fact that they tend to occur at the same site in a particular patient each time the drug is administered.

The lesions are flat and purplish brown in colour but may be raised in the acute stage.

Table 54.8 Drugs causing psoriasiform eruptions
Aspirin
Beta-adrenoreceptor blockers, most frequently atenolol, oxprenolol and propranolol
Chloroquine
Iodides
Lithium
NSAIDs
Withdrawal of topical steroids

Table 54.9 Drugs causing fixed drug eruptions
Barbiturates
Chlordiazepoxide
Dapsone
Dichloralphenazone
Griseofulvin
Indomethacin
Meprobamate
Phenolphthalein
Phenylbutazone
Phenytoin
Quinine
Salicylates
Sulphonamides
Tetracyclines

They take between 2 and 24 hours to develop following drug ingestion. On the first drug exposure there is usually only one lesion but subsequent exposure can result in multiple lesions. The eruption usually involves the limbs rather than the trunk and often occurs on mucous membranes.

Once the drug has been stopped the lesions heal with scaling followed by pigmentation which may be the only physical sign at the time the patient presents.

The fixed drug eruption is possibly the only case of a drug-induced cutaneous reaction where oral rechallenge can be safely used to confirm the diagnosis.

Systemic lupus erythematosus (SLE)

Syndromes indistinguishable from SLE may

Table 54.10 Drugs causing systemic lupus erythematosus
Antiepileptics, e.g. phenytoin, primidone, ethosuximide
Beta-adrenoreceptor blockers
Chlorpromazine
Griseofulvin
Hydralazine
Isoniazid
Lithium
Methyldopa
Oral contraceptives
Penicillamine
Procainamide
Propylthiouracil
Sulphasalazine

occur following drug administration. It is not clear if drugs do this by initiating the disease or by triggering it in predisposed patients.

The cutaneous manifestation of drug-induced SLE is the characteristic 'butterfly'-shaped rash on the face. There may also be a rash on the neck and back of the hands. Laboratory tests for antinuclear factor and lupus cells may be positive and the ESR may be elevated. Cerebral and renal involvement is rare. In some cases antinuclear antibodies occur without clinical manifestations.

Clinical manifestations of the SLE syndrome are predominant in females but the occurrence of antinuclear antibodies shows no preference for gender. The syndrome is usually reversible if the drug is withdrawn, although the antinuclear factor may persist for several months.

Acneform eruptions

Acne is a common complaint but is rarely drug induced.

Drugs can, however, produce acne-like eruptions or aggravate existing acne. The lesions are usually papular but no comedones (blackheads) are present.

Skin necrosis

Necrosis can follow the extravasation of irritant drugs particularly cytotoxic agents. Anticoagulants, both oral and heparin, can produce a severe haemorrhagic skin necrosis. Other causes of necrosis include the severe impairment of skin circulation which is occasionally produced by beta-adrenoreceptor blockers, the synergistic

effects of certain antitumour drugs with radiotherapy, and the topical application of gentian violet and brilliant green.

Photosensitivity

Drug-induced photosensitivity can be either phototoxic or photoallergic and can result from systemic or topical therapy.

Phototoxic reactions resemble severe sunburn, and can progress to blistering. They are dose dependent for drug and sunlight, occur within a few hours of taking the drug and subside quickly on drug withdrawal.

Photoallergic rashes are usually eczematous, lichenoid, urticarial, bullous or purpuric. They are not dose dependent and can be delayed in onset. Recovery is slow following drug withdrawal. In some cases photoallergy can persist for years after the drug was taken.

Patients receiving photosensitizing drugs should be counselled to avoid strong sunlight and to use a total sun block which contains a reflective substance such as titanium oxide. This is because most sunscreens only provide protection against medium wavelength radiation (UVB) while it is the long wavelength radiation (UVA) that is responsible for photosensitive reactions.

Table 54.11   Drugs causing acne
Androgens (in women)
Corticosteroids and ACTH
Ethambutol
Isoniazid
Lithium
Oral contraceptives
Phenobarbitone
Phenytoin
Propylthiouracil (resembling acne rosacea)
Topical corticosteroids (perioral dermatitis)
Quinine, quinidine (papular eruptions)

Table 54.12   Drugs causing light-induced eruptions
Topical preparations
Antihistamines
Antiseptics: bithionol, hexachlorophane
Coal tar derivatives
Sunscreens
Systemic drugs
Amiodarone
Antihistamines
Cinoxacin
Diuretics: thiazides, frusemide
Griseofulvin
Nalidixic acid
NSAIDs
Phenothiazines
Sulphonamides
Sulphonylureas
Tetracyclines
Tricyclic antidepressants

Table 54.13 Drugs causing skin pigmentation	
Drug	Pigmentation
Amiodarone	Blue-grey
Anticonvulsants (hydantoin derivatives)	Brown
Antimalarials	Blue-grey
Beta-adrenoreceptor blockers	Brown
Imipramine	Blue-grey
Methyldopa	Brown
Oral contraceptives	Brown spots/patches
Phenothiazines	Brown/blue-grey
Psoralens	Brown
Tetracyclines	Blue-black

Table 54.14   Drugs causing hair disorders

Alopecia
  Anticoagulants
  Anticonvulsants
  Antithyroid drugs
  Beta-adrenoreceptor blockers
  Withdrawal of oral contraceptives
  Cytotoxic drugs
  Etretinate
  Gold salts
  Lithium
  Sodium valproate

Hirsutism
  Acetazolamide
  Anabolic steroids
  Androgens
  Corticosteroids (topical and systemic)
  Cyclosporin
  Danazol
  Diazoxide
  Dihydrotestosterone
  Minoxidil
  Oral contraceptives
  Penicillamine
  Phenytoin
  Tamoxifen

Pigmentation

Hyperpigmentation, hypopigmentation or discolouration can all be drug induced. Pigmentation can be widespread or localized and can occasionally occur in internal organs.

The mechanism of drug induction is not always known. In some cases the drug itself may be responsible or it may induce a disturbance in melanin pigmentation.

Nail changes

Nail discolouration can be drug induced. Blue nails can result from therapy with mepacrine and blue-black nails from cytotoxic drugs and minocycline. Potassium permanganate solutions will dye nails brown, and white nails can result from therapy with antitumour agents.

Photo-onycholysis (separation of the nail from the nail plate associated with UVA radiation) can be exacerbated by oral contraceptives, and tetracyclines.

Drug-induced psoriasis may cause nail pitting.

Hair disorders

Drug-induced alopecia may be partial or complete and can involve sites other than the scalp. The most severe loss usually occurs with cytotoxic therapy; it begins shortly after administration of the drug and the effect is dose dependent and fortunately reversible.

Hirsutism is excessive hairiness, especially in females, in the male pattern of hair growth, while hypertrichosis is the growth of hair at sites not normally hairy. Both conditions can be drug induced and in some cases the same drug can produce both patterns of hair growth. If it is not possible to withdraw the drug and there is no suitable alternative, e.g. the use of cyclosporin in transplantation, then these patients should have this fully explained to them and be advised to use a depilatory cream if necessary. This particular side effect of minoxidil has been exploited in the treatment of alopecia.

Some drugs can induce both alopecia and hirsutism. For example the hydantoin anticonvulsants can cause alopecia of the scalp and hirsutism of the body. This occurs mainly in young women.

CASE STUDIES

CASE 54.1

Mr D. is a 47-year-old peritoneal dialysis patient with a past history of psoriasis and has a penicillin allergy. During an episode of peritonitis he develops erythroderma with severe scaling. There is no antibiotic written on his drug chart.

Q1 Is this reaction likely to be drug related?

Q2 If drug related, what drug could be a possible cause?

CASE 54.2

A 26-year-old female patient presents with a raised red lesion on her tongue. This same eruption occurs every month during menstruation and lasts for approximately 5 days. The patient has a history of dysmenorrhoea.

Q1 What type of reaction does this history suggest?

Q2 Could the reaction be related to menstruation?

CASE 54.2

A1 This type of single localized lesion is suggestive of a fixed drug eruption.

A2 On taking a full drug history it is discovered that the patient takes a 5-day course of mefenamic acid for her dysmenorrhoea and this is the most likely cause of the lesion. The patient is challenged with a dose of mefenamic acid and within 4 hours the lesion on the tongue develops. The patient is changed to ibuprofen for her dysmenorrhoea and does not develop any more eruptions.

BIBLIOGRAPHY

A guide to drug eruptions. Department of Dermatology, Free University Amsterdam 1987
Buxton P K. ABC of dermatology. British Medical Association 1988
D'Arcy P F, Griffin J P (eds). Iatrogenic diseases, 3rd edn. Oxford: Oxford University Press 1986
Davis D M (ed). Textbook of adverse drug reactions, 4th edn. Oxford: Oxford Medical Publications 1991

ANSWERS TO CASE STUDIES

CASE 54.1

A1 Although erythroderma can occur when psoriasis affects the entire body and the defined margins of the plaques are lost, the acute onset of the reaction suggests an allergic origin.

A2 The most likely cause of this reaction would be penicillin and, although it appears that the patient has not received any antibiotics, peritonitis is usually treated with intraperitoneal (i.p.) antibiotics and Mr D. received ceftazidime 100 mg/L in peritoneal fluid.

This reaction should be treated by immediately stopping the ceftazidime. The peritonitis can be treated with i.p. gentamicin. Mr D. should be informed that he is also allergic to cephalosporins and the cross-sensitivity recorded in his medical notes.

Chapter 55

Pressure sores and leg ulcers

R. Anderson

PRESSURE SORES

A pressure sore may be defined as any break in skin integrity which results from sustained pressure on the body with or without the additional stresses of shear and friction. Other patient-specific factors may contribute to skin damage and affect healing ability. The terms 'bed sore' and 'decubitus ulcer' have been used but these imply that damage can only occur when lying down, whereas the sitting position can equally produce ulceration. The term 'pressure ulcer' is preferable as without pressure the condition cannot develop and, although often sore to the patient with intact sensation, in those with neurological impairment there is no associated soreness.

EPIDEMIOLOGY

Pressure damage occurs in patients whether they are cared for in hospital or the community and is a distressing and expensive problem to manage. Hospital prevalence studies have revealed that 2.7 to 66% of patients may suffer from pressure ulcers, depending on the patient population studied. The highest incidence of pressure ulcers was found in elderly patients with fractured femurs. Few community-based prevalence studies have been done but an incidence of 6.7% has been reported.

AETIOLOGY

Various factors play a role in the development of pressure ulcers.

Pressure

Excess pressure on the skin results in the ischaemia of underlying tissue by mechanical compression of the vascular supply. The critical factor is when pressure on the skin exceeds the average arteriolar pressure (25 mmHg).

Sustained pressure on tissues is most damaging. Low pressure applied for long periods is worse than high pressure for short periods and some alternating pressure beds work on a high pressure/short time cycle principle. Portable equipment is available to measure pressure beneath patients so that the most suitable support equipment (mattress, cushion or chair) can be chosen. However, this approach is not in widespread use.

Shear

All shearing forces will also involve some pressure, but shear caused by patients sliding down beds or chairs will damage the superficial skin layers with resultant stretching of blood vessels, possible thrombosis and damage to the dermis.

Friction

Friction between skin and sheets or seating may cause ulceration by mechanically rubbing off outer layers of skin. Soft uncreased linen, towels and dressings should be used. Massage and vigorous application of skin preparations should be avoided.

Moisture

In the presence of moisture (due to urine, sweat or faeces), pressure ulcer formation is more likely as skin becomes macerated and traumatized. The use of inappropriate barrier creams (e.g. zinc and castor oil cream) may moisten the skin excessively and exacerbate the problem.

Combined forces

If shear and friction are applied together, the tissues attached to bony structures move under shear whilst the epidermal layers may move in

Table 55.1 Risk factors which may play a role in the development of pressure ulcers

Increasing age
Reduced mobility and activity
Poor nutrition, especially if linked with severe anaemia
Diabetes
Obesity
Cardiac failure
Osteomyelitis
Orthopaedic problems
Drug addiction
Malignancy/cytotoxic therapy
Neurological disorders

the opposite direction due to friction between the skin and supporting surfaces.

The effect of the three combined forces of shear, friction and pressure can result in ulcer formation at lower pressures than would be normally anticipated.

Patient-specific factors and risk assessment

Various concurrent problems may precipitate the development of pressure ulcers and these are summarized in Table 55.1. Pressure ulcers may occur at any age, particularly when patient mobility and activity is reduced. It is therefore important that all patients with any of the risk factors shown are assessed for pressure ulcer risk on admission to hospital, and regularly reviewed. Similarly, chronically ill patients in the community must be monitored. Various risk rating scales are available. The original Norton Score was developed in the early 1960s for use in the elderly hospital population and considers only 5 aspects of the patient: physical condition; mental condition; activity; mobility; and incontinence.

Numerous variations have been developed which include consideration of nutrition, predisposing diseases, age, and concurrent medication.

COMMON SITES OF OCCURRENCE

Although any area of the body subjected to unrelieved pressure may ulcerate, certain sites are more susceptible to damage.

Table 55.2 Relationship between position of patient and area at risk of developing a pressure ulcer	
Position of patient	Risk areas
Supine	Scapula Sacrum Heels
Prone	Chest Patellae Anterior surface of tibia
Sidelying	Femoral trochanters Malleoli
Sitting	Ischial tuberosities Sacrum Femoral trochanters (posterior surface)

The five 'classical' locations for pressure ulcers are:

- sacrum
- buttocks (ischial tuberosity)
- hips (greater trochanter)
- heel
- lateral malleolus of foot.

The significance of position in relation to the site of ulceration is shown in Table 55.2.

Pressure ulcers can occur in less common locations which also depend on the position of the patient and include the ear, scalp, elbows and genitalia.

Often the risk to patients who spend most of their time sitting out of bed is not recognized and regular standing is not encouraged. In contrast, patients nursed in bed are regularly turned to assist in pressure relief.

Paraplegics who spend considerable time in wheelchairs should be regularly checked and provided with additional supporting surfaces, such as special cushions, as appropriate.

Care on transferring patients from bed to chair and on manoeuvering them in bed is vital. Some of the newer pressure-relieving beds reduce the need for such procedures.

SIGNS OF PRESSURE DAMAGE

Various warning signs on the skin should immediately indicate the need for additional precautions.

After sustained pressure, the skin initially turns red due, in part, to histamine release. This redness is termed blanching erythema and if gently pressed it will whiten (or blanch). If pressure is relieved at this stage, the skin should return to normal.

If pressure continues progression to non-blanching erythema will result. In this situation when the affected area is pressed it will remain red, indicating that a pressure ulcer is developing.

The next clinical sign is likely to be blistering, which, with sustained pressure, will progress from a soft fluid-filled area to an area of hard black necrotic tissue, termed an eschar (see Plate 1). An eschar may begin to break down and putrify with formation of a strong odour, usually due to the presence of anaerobic bacteria.

In areas where skin is thin and bony prominences are superficial there may be no warning signs and progressive damage and full skin thickness necrosis may be the first sign, with underlying bone and muscle exposed to view.

In either case, the necrotic tissue will need to be removed (debrided) and a deep cavity will then exist. Large volumes of exudate may be produced particularly if infection is present.

Within deep cavities there may be sinus formation, i.e. narrow tracks may form, which lead into deeper tissue. In such cavities, careful selection of treatment is required to avoid damage to underlying tissue. In patients who have suffered with chronic pressure ulcers, long-standing sinuses may exist, visible on the surface of the skin as only a narrow, often leaking, opening. Normally this is an indication of an unhealed cavity below which carries a risk of abscess formation and chronic infection.

INVESTIGATIONS

If a sinus exists, it is important to establish the extent of the tracking within the body tissue and this can only be achieved by radiological investigation (a sinogram). The sinogram may indicate the need for surgical intervention to open up the area, drain and treat it as appropriate.

Chronic wounds should be biopsied, especially if the appearance is abnormal, since it is not uncommon for malignancy to develop in non-healing wounds. Such wounds may have a cauliflower-like appearance, suggestive of squamous cell carcinoma and may bleed very readily. This should not be confused with the phenomenon of over-granulation when excess granulation tissue develops beneath occlusive dressings.

TREATMENT

If preventive methods fail, urgent treatment of pressure ulcers is essential. Realistic objectives should be established as some pressure ulcers will never heal but may be made more acceptable for patients and their carers.

Deep, infected pressure ulcers carry a high risk of morbidity due to septicaemia. Treatment priorities must be considered, based on the degree of pressure damage and the need for surgical or other intervention with regard to overall prognosis and predisposing factors in the patient.

A multidisciplinary approach to treatment will consider all aspects of care and will involve:

- dietician – to ensure optimum nutrition for patients with pressure damage and those 'at risk'
- doctor – to assess overall prognosis and patient management
- nurse – to regularly reassess patients and their pressure points and to establish a turning/moving routine, regular dressing changes and the provision of moral support to patients and carers
- pharmacist – to assist in appropriate product selection and to ensure that all staff are familiar with its use and that the product is readily available in adequate quantity
- physiotherapist – to improve patient mobility and select the most appropriate support surface (bed, chair, mattress or cushion)
- occupational therapists and medical physicists may also be members of the multidisciplinary team.

Physiotherapists may be involved in the treatment of pressure ulcers with ultraviolet or ultrasound therapy often in conjunction with topical preparations. This approach should however be avoided if enzyme debriding agents containing, for example, streptokinase and streptodornase (Varidase), which are easily inactivated, are being used. The frequency of removal of the topical application will affect the practicality of using combination therapy. Ultrasound may be performed with dressings in situ whilst ultraviolet therapy requires removal of the dressing.

A wound care or tissue viability nurse often coordinates the multidisciplinary team and emphasizes the need for pressure ulcer prevention. He or she can coordinate the availability of preventive equipment for hospital and community patients.

Wound management

As with all aspects of medicine the holistic approach is essential in pressure ulcer care. Topical applications are only part of treatment, and often surgical intervention will speed healing. No single product is normally suitable for all stages of ulceration. As the ulcer changes, so should the product. However, a fair trial of treatment is essential with accurate documentation to ensure continuity of care.

Clinical infection

Before commencing treatment, any clinical infection should be identified. All wounds will show bacterial growth if swabbed, but this is only significant if present in sufficient numbers to produce clinical infection. When assessing a wound it is necessary to consider whether:

- there is pus formation
- the patient is pyrexial and feeling unwell
- there is surrounding cellulitis (inflammation of the surrounding skin and tissues with associated heat)
- there is likely to be infection involving bone.

If any of these factors are present a swab should be taken from the deep part of the wound and appropriate systemic antibiotics commenced. If none of the above factors are present and the wound is progressing well, there is no need for further investigation.

Treatment selection

There are numerous products available for wound care, pressure ulcers and skin trauma.

The 'ideal dressing' should:

- create an optimum moist environment for healing
- remove excess exudate from the wound surface
- provide a barrier to microorganisms
- be sterile
- be non-adherent and easily removed
- be free of particulate contamination
- be non-toxic, non-allergenic and non-sensitizing
- be thermally insulating
- allow gaseous exchange
- be easy to use for patients and carers

- be cost effective
- be available in all necessary sizes for hospital and community use.

Products such as lint, gauze and gamgee do not possess the necessary properties for a dressing because they have limited absorbency and rapidly become saturated with wound exudate which can 'strike-through' to the dressing surface and enable bacteria to track down into the wound. As the dressing dries out it will adhere to the wound surface, cause pain and bleeding on removal, and lift newly formed cells from the surface of the wound.

By considering the different groups of wound products available a protocol for pressure ulcer care can be devised, based on the different stages of ulceration and the characteristics of available products. The position of the pressure ulcer will also be relevant to the choice of preparation and the secondary (covering) dressing if needed. Table 55.3 summarizes the possible treatments

Table 55.3 Management options for different types of pressure ulcer

Wound type	Clean	Exuding	Sloughy	Clinically infected	Anaerobic odour
Superficial	Film dressing Hydrocolloid Foam dressing	Alginate Foam dressing	Hydrogel Hydrocolloid	Antiseptic dressing Silver sulphadiazine (Flamazine) if pseudomonal infection	—
Cavity	Hydrogel Hydrocolloid paste + wafer	Alginate Cavity foam dressing	Hydrogel Hydrocolloid paste + wafer	Hydrogel Varidase if sloughy/necrotic Silver sulphadiazine (Flamazine) if pseudomonal infection	As for clinically infected + oral metronidazole or topical gel*
Sinus (loose packing only with careful removal)	Hydrogel on ribbon gauze	Alginate rope	Hydrogel on ribbon gauze†	Loose packing with hydrogel on ribbon gauze†	Oral metronidazole or topical gel* and loose packing with hydrogel on ribbon gauze†

Wound type	Dry		Moist/infected	Anaerobic odour
Black eschar (surgical removal preferred if extensive)	Aserbine + barrier cream Hydrocolloid		Hydrogel Varidase	Varidase + oral metronidazole

Note: Within each category preparations should be selected depending on the location of the wound and ease of application and retention.
† Ribbon gauze not ideal but no alternative available
* Unlicensed indication

for pressure ulcers classified accordingly as superficial, cavity, sinus and black eschar.

Within each pressure ulcer category, the appearance of the wound will influence treatment choice. Therefore when determining optimum treatment it is necessary to consider the following questions:

- Is the wound clean?
- Is there excessive exudate?
- Is sloughy tissue present?
- Is the wound clinically infected?
- Is the wound malodorous?

Many traditionally used 'cleansing' agents such as hypochlorite solutions and hydrogen peroxide are now recognized as having harmful effects. Only if excessive exudate or pus and loose necrotic or sloughy tissue is present, is cleaning needed. In such cases, warmed sodium chloride solution (0.9%) should be used. Cold solutions can lower the wound surface temperature below body temperature and impair healing by retarding new cell formation.

Odorous wounds

Although pseudomonal infections can cause odour, the most likely cause is anaerobic bacteria. Charcoal dressings will mask and absorb odour but metronidazole will treat and eradicate the infection. Metronidazole is given orally 200 to 400 mg three times a day or, if poorly tolerated, can be applied topically as a gel or incorporated into Intrasite. The resolution of the odour is normally dramatic and is reassuring for the patient. With careful monitoring resistant anaerobes should not emerge.

Characteristics of wound management products

Hydrocolloids. Hydrocolloids (e.g. Comfeel, Granuflex) are available as self-adhesive sheets, although if used on the sacrum and buttocks they may need to be taped in place. In addition to the self-adhesive sheets, granular, paste and powder forms are also available for use in cavities. All hydrocolloids contain carboxymethylcellulose and some additionally incorporate pectin and gelatin, the latter being responsible for an unpleasant odour.

The dressing liquefies at the wound surface, hydrating soft sloughy tissue and encouraging wound healing. In wounds with low exudate, hydrocolloids may remain in place for 7 days, and, if left in place on a black eschar, marked softening of the necrotic tissue will occur.

Different degrees of gaseous permeability are claimed for the products available but on initial application most are occlusive and caution should be observed in the presence of anaerobic infection. Due to this occlusive property, over-production of granulation tissue may occur beneath hydrocolloids and indicates that their use should be discontinued. The excess granulation tissue may be reduced by the application of 0.25% silver nitrate solution daily for 5 to 7 days. Thereafter, epithelialization should be encouraged with an alternative type of product, such as a polyurethane foam dressing.

Hydrogels. Hydrogels (e.g. Geliperm, Intrasite, Vigilon) require a secondary covering dressing, and in sheet form are most appropriate for areas of extensive skin loss, such as burns, whilst the gel forms are particularly useful for cavity pressure ulcers.

These products are composed of a hydrophilic polymer in an aqueous base and serve to hydrate the wound surface and lift slough and necrotic tissue whilst encouraging moist wound healing. In sheet form these may remain in place for several days if rehydrated in situ with saline. Initially, the gel form is normally changed daily, extending to every 3 days in cleaner wounds.

Hydrogels may be used on black eschars but tend to be rather more rapidly effective on wounds covered with softer necrotic or sloughy tissue (see Plate 2). They are inappropriate for heavily exuding wounds. If excessive amounts of gel are applied to an ulcer, maceration will occur at the wound edge with whitening of the surrounding skin.

Alginates. Alginates (e.g. Kaltostat, Sorbsan) are available in a flat or rope form, the latter being useful for cavity and sinus pressure ulcers.

Most require a secondary dressing but some newer forms incorporate an adhesive border to aid retention on lightly exuding wounds.

The available dressings consist of either calcium alginate alone or a combination of sodium and calcium alginate and the difference in composition is thought to affect the gelling properties of the dressings at the wound surface. In contact with wound exudate the dressing is very absorbent and forms a moist gel over the wound surface. Alginates are therefore only suitable for exuding wounds, not for dry wounds or eschars where no gelling will occur. In a heavily exuding wound, daily changes will be needed initially but these can be reduced as the exudate lessens, when an alternative dressing may then be considered. The haemostatic properties of the dressings may be useful in controlling bleeding on over-granulating pressure ulcers, when daily changes would be needed.

The dressings are removed from the wound with the aid of sterile saline.

Polyurethane foams. Polyurethane foam dressings (e.g. Allevyn, Lyofoam) are not self-adhesive and must be held in place with tape. This may be inappropriate on fragile skin. The main characteristic of the foams is high absorbency, making them suitable for exuding wounds. Due to the nature of the dressing, lateral absorption of exudate occurs, avoiding the vertical 'strike-through' of traditional dressings. The dressing is initially changed daily. Inspecting the dressing will reveal if this is inadequate because seepage of exudate will be seen at the edges of the dressing.

In wounds producing less exudate, the dressings may remain in place for up to 7 days, encouraging healing in a moist environment. The dressings show low adherence but saline may need to be used to assist in their removal.

A cavity foam dressing is available in various shapes (Allevyn cavity wound dressing). This consists of small pieces of Allevyn foam dressing encased in a semipermeable membrane. It is designed for exuding cavities but its usefulness will depend on the size and shape of the ulcer cavity and the 'fit' of the dressing.

Film dressings. Film dressings (e.g. Opsite, Tegaderm) are self-adhesive and are inappropriate for use on elderly fragile skin which can easily be damaged by incorrect application and removal.

The films are semipermeable, allowing evaporation of some water vapour, but exudate accumulates beneath and may irritate and macerate the surrounding skin.

They are widely used to reduce friction over pressure points in 'at risk' patients when they may be left in place for several days. Careful attention must be paid to the manufacturer's instructions for application and removal of each different film dressing to avoid inflicting skin damage.

LEG ULCERS

A leg ulcer is any break in skin integrity on the lower leg and normally indicates an underlying circulatory disorder or specific medical condition, even if reported as being initiated by trauma. Many leg ulcers are chronic in nature with patients suffering from them for 30 to 40 years. Even if healing occurs, recurrence is very common. Treatment must be directed at the underlying cause rather than simply the break in the skin.

EPIDEMIOLOGY

It has been estimated that 1% of the population have chronic leg ulcers, with 70% of patients developing the leg ulcer before the age of 65 years, and 25% before the age of 45 years.

Over the age of 50 years, females are more commonly affected. Approximately 75% of healed ulcers may eventually recur. Most leg ulcer patients are managed in the community and the cost has been estimated at £2700 to £5200 per patient per year. The most recent estimation of annual cost to the National Health Service is £300 million to £600 million. With the advent of more specialist leg ulcer treatment clinics and clinical specialists and with accurate diagnosis and assessment it may be possible to reduce overall costs and healing times.

AETIOLOGY

There are a number of different types of leg ulcer which can be classified according to the underlying causation and include venous, arterial, arteriovenous, diabetic and autoimmune.

Venous ulcers

Venous ulcers are the most common, accounting for up to 75% of all leg ulcers. They occur as a result of failure of the calf muscle pump, i.e. the calf muscles which squeeze deep venous blood upwards from the legs back to the heart. This pump will not function effectively if there is a back-flow of blood from the deep veins to the superficial veins in the leg. Back-flow may occur due to fatigue or incompetence of the valves in the deep veins and in the perforating veins which connect the superficial and deep veins (as illustrated in Fig. 55.1A).

Restricted mobility may also predispose to venous ulceration. During walking, the action of the foot striking a solid surface facilitates venous return whilst the ankle movement involved in normal walking alternately contracts and relaxes the calf muscle.

As back-flow of blood occurs into the superficial veins and capillaries, leakage of fluid

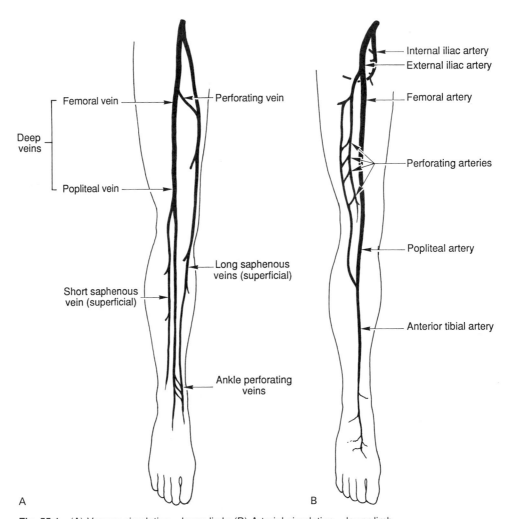

Fig. 55.1   (A) Venous circulation – lower limb; (B) Arterial circulation – lower limb.

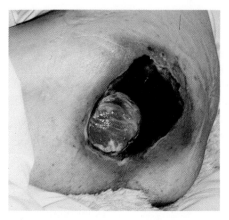

Plate 1 Necrotic pressure ulcer producing large amounts of odorous exudate in an elderly paraplegic patient.

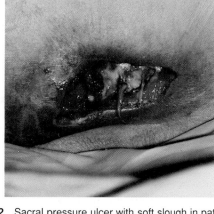

Plate 2 Sacral pressure ulcer with soft slough in patient with multiple sclerosis.

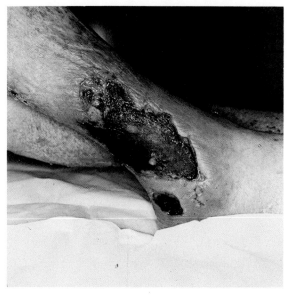

Plate 3 Multiple necrotic leg ulcers with little exudate.

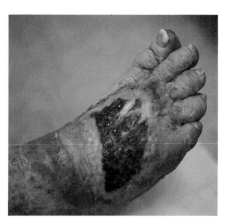

Plate 4 Ulcerated foot with exposed tendon.

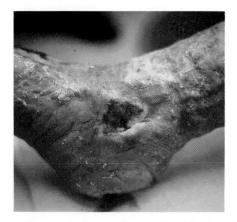

Plate 5 Ulcer on the inner malleolus with whitening edges and poor surrounding skin.

occurs into the interstitial space and oedema results. Haemosiderin from red cell breakdown is deposited in the tissues causing a characteristic brown colouration, particularly in the gaiter or lower area of the leg. Fibrinogen leaks from capillaries and is converted to fibrin, forming a fibrin 'cuff' around the capillaries which may also reduce tissue oxygenation. In the affected area the skin becomes friable as oedema progresses and any slight trauma can precipitate ulceration.

The original cause of perforator valve incompetence may be a deep vein thrombosis which could have occurred many years previously. In elderly female patients this can often be traced back to a pregnancy. Patients with valve incompetences may have a history of varicose veins and approximately 3% of patients with varicosities go on to suffer leg ulcers.

Arterial ulcers

Arterial ulcers arise in a different manner from venous ulcers. Blood fails to reach the superficial tissues as a result of atherosclerosis affecting the medium and large arteries of the lower leg. (Fig. 55.1B illustrates the arterial circulation.) Oxygen supply to the arterioles is therefore inadequate and breakdown of skin results in a painful ulcer. Arterial ulcers account for approximately 22% of leg ulcers.

An arterial embolism will similarly produce ulceration but in a more rapid and dangerous manner.

Arteriovenous ulcers

Lower leg ulcers may result from a combination of both venous and arterial incompetence and a mixed picture of clinical signs will be seen.

Diabetic leg ulcers

Diabetes is associated with approximately 5% of all leg ulcers. The ulcers of such patients are ischaemic in nature as a result of diabetic vascular disease which affects the small distal arteries particularly in the weight-bearing areas such as the feet.

Autoimmune leg ulcers

The most common causative factor in this category is rheumatoid arthritis which is present in 8% of patients with leg ulcers.

Although associated immobility will limit calf muscle pump activity, the ulceration primarily occurs through arteritis of the small vessels and consequent ischaemia.

Other leg ulcers

Several other conditions may be associated with causing leg ulcers in patients, including burns, infections, haematological disease, lymphoedema and vasculitis.

Malignancy can develop in chronic non-healing ulcers or the ulcer may begin as a malignant manifestation. As with chronic pressure ulcers and other non-healing skin problems, biopsy is recommended for long-standing leg ulcers.

It should be noted that ulcers may be self-inflicted, or an existing ulcer may be further damaged by the patient to maintain contact with health-care staff (the 'social ulcer phenomenon').

CLINICAL SIGNS

In determining the cause of a leg ulcer, observation of clinical signs are important, together with an accurate history from the patient or carer. The characteristic features of venous and arterial ulcers are shown in Table 55.4.

Diabetic ulcers often look similar to arterial ulcers. However, in the diabetic ulcer, foot pulses may be present if only the microcirculation is damaged whilst if the deeper arterial system is damaged, as in arterial ulcers, these pulses are absent. The patient with a diabetic ulcer does not always complain of pain, due to loss of sensation resulting from diabetes-induced peripheral neuropathy.

DIAGNOSTIC INVESTIGATION

Before treatment is started the extent of venous and arterial damage should be determined by use of a portable Doppler machine. This permits

Table 55.4 Clinical features of venous and arterial ulcers

Venous	Arterial
Occur in gaiter area (generally above medial malleolus)	Occur around malleolus or on the foot, toes or heels
Often large and shallow with flat edges and copious exudate	Punched-out appearance with steep edges, often deep with little exudate. Muscle and tendon exposure occurs
Generalized oedema of leg may be present	Local oedema may occur
Dark staining of lower leg due to red blood cell breakdown	Skin staining rare
Sensitive to touch but not normally very painful unless clinically infected or oedematous. Infection common in chronic venous ulcers	Very painful, especially at night or if leg is elevated. Relieved by hanging leg out of bed/sleeping in a chair. Pain may be severe on exercise due to muscle tissue ischaemia
Foot pulses are present and foot warm Surrounding varicose eczema is common	Foot pulses reduced or absent. Foot is cold and shiny with hair loss and degeneration of toe nails Foot may whiten on elevation and colour when dependent.

calculation of the patient's resting pressure index (RPI), by comparing brachial and ankle systolic pressures.

$$RPI = \frac{\text{The systolic blood pressure in the ankle}}{\text{The systolic blood pressure in the arm}}$$

The RPI index should be greater than 1 in people with undamaged arteries.

If compression bandaging is applied to the leg of patients with an RPI below 0.8, the arterial circulation will be compromised, tissue necrosis may result and amputation could be required. Light compression may be used in patients with an RPI of 0.8 to 0.9. Erroneous readings can occur in diabetics and compression bandaging should only be used with great caution in such patients.

ULCER TREATMENT

The treatment regimen must be holistic in approach. The overall treatment regimen must aim to:

- correct the circulation
- provide pain relief
- protect and treat the surrounding skin
- prevent and treat any infection
- heal the ulcer
- prevent any recurrence.

Correction of circulation

If a patient presents with a venous ulcer and severe oedema, total bedrest is required. The affected limb should be elevated above the height of the hip and preferably the heart. If mild oedema is present elevation of the limb at night, achieved by raising the foot of the bed, may resolve the problem.

Venous return to the heart should be encouraged by improving the calf muscle pump. Exercise should be encouraged to the limit of the patient's ability. If severely restricted, regular walking 'on the spot' can help and ankle exercises can be taught to immobile patients which may be practised when lying down or sitting. In combination with exercise, graduated compression bandaging applied from the base of the toes to the knee is essential. This is, however, often poorly tolerated by patients. The correct application of such bandaging is crucial to its success. Incorrect bandaging and its inappropriate use can cause limb necrosis, and is therefore worse than no bandage at all.

The Charing Cross four-layer bandage technique for venous ulcers is increasing in popularity. Weekly visits are needed for redressing and rebandaging.

In a patient with an arterial ulcer it is essential that the extent of arterial damage is diagnosed and compression bandaging avoided. Light bandaging may be used when necessary to hold dressings in place and afford protection. Gentle exercise should be encouraged, limbs should be kept warm, and smoking discouraged. Surgical assessment is important to establish prognosis and the need for surgical intervention.

There is no available evidence to support the use of any systemic therapy to improve arterial blood flow and hence treat arterial ulcers (although various vasodilator preparations have been tried).

Pain relief

Venous ulcers are generally not painful but may become painful when first elevated. In severe cases regular analgesia may be needed, with an additional dose prior to the dressing change. The use of opioids may be necessary. Anti-inflammatory drugs may help but interfere with the healing process. Patients with arterial ulcers may require strong analgesia, such as opioids, particularly at night, when cramping pains may be severe.

Protection and treatment of the surrounding skin

Minimal medication should be applied to a venous ulcer as the surrounding skin is usually extremely sensitive due, in part, to varicose eczema, and also to chronic application of assorted medicaments. So-called barrier creams often contain lanolin and hydroxybenzoate preservatives to which the patient may be allergic and which exacerbate the underlying problem.

Medicated paste bandages with a zinc oxide base may be used over the chosen ulcer preparation to treat the surrounding chronic eczema. However, some medicated bandages contain potential sensitizers (e.g. Icthaband contains parahydroxybenzoate and Coltapaste contains lanolin) whilst some contain gelatin, which sets hard and may restrict mobility (e.g. Icthopaste).

In patients with severe eczema on the tissue surrounding the ulcer, a steroid preparation may be needed. Care must be taken to avoid contact with the ulcer. Dermatological referral for patch testing to identify the causative agent for the eczema may be necessary. Weeping eczema may respond to potassium permanganate soaks. If the surrounding skin is dry with crusting scales of dead skin (hyperkeratosis), application of olive oil may be helpful.

The skin surrounding an arterial ulcer is often shiny and easily traumatized. The act of rubbing in topical medicaments must be avoided.

Infection

Most ulcers will be colonized with microorganisms and if swabbed, bacterial colonies will be identified. However, only clinical infection is significant. The presence of pus with accompanying odour and the presence of cellulitis in surrounding tissues all indicate the presence of infection. The patient is often unwell and systemic antibiotic therapy is essential.

To prevent build-up of exudate and debris in the ulcer, cleansing with water or saline is important. Soaking the leg in warm water is often soothing for the patient.

Healing the ulcer

When choosing a moist wound-healing preparation for a leg ulcer the same principles of wound assessment and regular review apply as for pressure ulcers. However, without treatment of the underlying condition, topical treatment will be ineffective, or of short-term effectiveness only.

The required primary application for the ulcer can be selected from Table 55.3. If a venous ulcer is present the primary application can be covered with a compression bandage. In addition a paste bandage could be used if the care of the surrounding skin is a priority. Normally compression bandaging can be left in situ for a week. However, if there is an underlying sloughy, exuding ulcer, daily dressing may be required. Light non-elastic bandaging should be used if there is arterial involvement.

Prevention of recurrence

For all patients with an ulcer, education is essential to prevent recurrence of the problem if and when healing occurs.

When a venous ulcer heals, protection is essential with a continuation of compression therapy to avoid future breakdown. The use of accurately fitted, below-knee compression stockings is recommended. These can be obtained in standard sizes or made-to-measure for legs of a difficult shape. They should be renewed every 3 months. Patients should be reviewed regularly to encourage: compliance with treatment; regular exercise; good nutrition; weight control; and appropriate skin care.

Arterial ulcers are much harder to treat and heal. Surgery is often the only successful approach. Once healed, a light protective dressing will reduce the risk of external trauma. Compression should be avoided.

CASE STUDIES

CASE 55.1

The elderly paraplegic patient shown in Plate 1 has a necrotic pressure ulcer producing large amounts of odorous exudate.

Q What would be the preferred treatment? What other aspects of care are important?

CASE 55.2

The patient with multiple sclerosis shown in Plate 2 has a sacral pressure ulcer with soft slough.

Q How would you treat the ulcer and what covering dressing would be recommended? Note the neighbouring skin tear.

CASE 55.3

The lady in Plate 3 has multiple necrotic leg ulcers with little exudate.

Q What investigation would assist in treatment and what topical agent would be helpful? Would other therapy be needed?

CASE 55.4

The patient shown in Plate 4 has an ulcerated foot with exposed tendon.

Q What investigation would be needed and what questions asked of the patient? What agent could aid healing?

CASE 55.5

The patient shown in Plate 5 has an ulcer on the inner malleolus with whitening edges and poor surrounding skin.

Q What may be the cause of the ulcer and the edge effect? Recommend future treatment.

ANSWERS TO CASE STUDIES

CASE 55.1

A Immediate surgical debridement would be the preferred treatment. The odour will reduce once the necrotic tissue has been removed. Varidase could be used but application and retention is difficult on a large area. Intrasite could be used but would be slow in effect. A large foam dressing (Lyofoam) would absorb exudate and gradually soften the eschar. Hydrocolloids are best avoided when odour is present because of the risk of exacerbating any underlying anaerobic infection. Systemic antibiotics may be needed as fatal septicaemia could result. Oral metronidazole would eliminate anaerobes and assist in odour removal.

The patient's bed must be appropriate. An alternating pressure mattress or air fluidized therapy bed would be ideal together with strict monitoring. All involved in the care of the patient should be aware that there is a lack of pain sensation in paraplegics which results in a very high pressure ulcer risk.

CASE 55.2

A A hydrocolloid paste should be applied, covered with a hydrocolloid wafer and changed every 7 days. The sacrum should be monitored daily since movement of the dressing may occur which can increase pressure, and any liquefied hydrocolloid exposed by such movement will adhere to bedding and clothing and be difficult to remove. After 7 days the dressing should be carefully removed by soaking with saline.

A hydrogel could be used as an alternative. The dressing should be applied and covered with a non-adherent layer and hypoallergenic tape used to hold it in place. The hydrogel should be changed every 3 days. The skin tear next to the cavity was caused by removal of a film dressing.

CASE 55.3

A The ulceration may be arterial or venous, or more probably of mixed aetiology. Doppler examination is necessary, particularly as the foot is very white. The use of compression therapy would depend on patient assessment and the resting pressure index.

The red inflamed surround indicates cellulitis and the need for rapid debridement and systemic antibiotics. A swab from the broken area will confirm the organism. Varidase would assist debridement and permit eschar removal after 2 to 3 days of treatment.

CASE 55.4

A Due to tendon exposure and location, arterial investigation is needed. The patient should be asked if he is in pain. Infection of the tendon and underlying bone is a risk.

A moist wound-healing product such as a hydrocolloid, hydrogel or polyurethane foam would be appropriate. Intrasite was used successfully in this case.

CASE 55.5

A Arterial investigation is needed although the leg is crusted, dry and eczematous. An ulcer on top of the foot is just visible and exudate beneath the heel suggests further skin breakdown. If compression therapy is indicated, good skin care is essential prior to bandaging. Olive oil should be used for scale removal and a medicated paste bandage employed as a buffer between the leg and the compression bandage. A hydrocolloid could be used on the ulcer for up to 1 week. The maceration at the wound edge probably results from excessive application of hydrogel.

BIBLIOGRAPHY

Callam M J, Harper D R, Dale J J, Ruckley C V. Lothian and Forth Valley leg ulcer study. Hawick: Buccleuch Printers 1987

Cornwall J. Compression therapy for venous leg ulcers. Wound Management 1991; July: 10–13

Morrison M J. A colour guide to the assessment and management of leg ulcers. London: Wolfe Publishing 1991

Thomas S. Wound management and dressings. London: The Pharmaceutical Press 1990

Turner T D. Semipermeable films for wounds. Pharmaceutical Journal 1984; April 14: 452–454

Young J B. Aids to prevent pressure sores. British Medical Journal 1990; 330: 1002–1004

SECTION FOUR

APPENDICES

Medical abbreviations

AAA	abdominal aortic aneurysm	AMI	acute myocardial infarction
	acute anxiety attack	AML	acute myeloid leukaemia
AAAAA	aphasia, agnosia, apraxia,	ANA	antinuclear antibody
	agraphia and alexia	ANF	antinuclear factor
Ab	antibody	A & O	alert and oriented
abd.	abdomen (abdominal)	A & P	anterior and posterior
	abduction		auscultation and percussion
ABE	acute bacterial endocarditis	AOB	alcohol on breath
ABG	arterial blood gases	AP	alkaline phosphatase
ACAT	acylcholesterol acyltransferase		angina pectoris
ACBS	aortocoronary bypass surgery		antepartum
acid phos.	acid phosphatase		anterior pituitary
ADH	antidiuretic hormone		anterioposterior
ADL	activities of daily living		aortic pressure
ADR	adverse drug reaction		apical pulse
ADU	acute duodenal ulcer		appendectomy
A&E	accident and emergency		artificial pneumothorax
AED	antiepileptic drug	APB	atrial premature beat
AF	atrial fibrillation	APCs	atrial premature
AFB	acid-fast bacillus		contractions
AFP	alpha-fetoprotein	APTT	activated partial
AGL	acute granulocytic leukaemia		thromboplastin time
AGN	acute glomerulonephritis	AR	aortic regurgitation
AHA	autoimmune haemolytic		apical/radial (pulse)
	anaemia	ARF	acute renal failure
AHD	autoimmune haemolytic	AS	aortic stenosis
	disease		arteriosclerosis
AK	above knee	A-S attack	Adams–Stokes attack
ALD	alcoholic liver disease	ASB	asymptomatic bacteriuria
ALL	acute lymphocytic leukaemia	ASD	atrial septal defect
ALT	alanine transaminase	ASLO titre	antistreptolysin-O titre
AMA	against medical advice	AST	aspartate transaminase

AV	aortic valve	CAT	computerized axial
	atrioventricular		tomography
A-V	arteriovenous	CC	chief complaint
AVR	aortic valve replacement		current complaint
	augmented V lead, right arm	CCF	congestive cardiac failure
	(ECG)	CCU	coronary care unit
AVS	arteriovenous shunt	CF	cardiac failure
A & W	alive and well		complement fixation
AXR	abdominal X-ray		cystic fibrosis
		CFT	complement fixation test
		CGL	chronic granulocytic
BBB	bundle branch block		leukaemia
BBBB	bilateral bundle branch block	CGN	chronic glomerulonephritis
	(ECG)	CHB	complete heart block
B Bx.	breast biopsy	CHD	coronary heart disease
BCAA	branched chain amino acid	CHF	congestive heart failure
BG	blood glucose	CHO	carbohydrate
BJ protein	Bence-Jones protein	CI	cardiac index
BKA	below knee amputation		cerebral infarction
BM	bowel movement	CK	creatine kinase (same as CPK)
BMT	bone marrow transplant	CL	clubbing
BNO	bowels not open	CLD	chronic liver disease
BOR	bowels open regularly		chronic lung disease
BP	bypass	CLL	chronic lymphocytic
	blood pressure		leukaemia
BPD	bronchopulmonary dysplasia	CML	chronic myelocytic leukaemia
BPH	benign prostatic hypertrophy	CNS	central nervous system
BS	blood sugar	CO	cardiac output
	bowel sounds	c/o	complains of
	breath sounds	COAD	chronic obstructive airway
BSA	body surface area		disease
BW	body water	COD	cause of death
	body weight	COG	closed angle glaucoma
Bx.	biopsy	COLD	chronic obstructive lung
			disease
		COP	capillary osmotic pressure
C	complement	COPD	chronic obstructive
$C_1, C_2 \ldots$	cervical vertebrae 1, 2 ...		pulmonary disease
CA	cancer	C & P	cystoscopy and pyelogram
	carcinoma	CP	cor pulmonale
	cardiac arrest		creatine phosphate
	coronary artery	CPA	cardiopulmonary arrest
Ca	carcinoma		cerebellar pontine angle
CABG	coronary artery bypass graft	CPAP	continuous positive airway
CAD	coronary artery disease		pressure
CAH	chronic active hepatitis	CPD	continuous peritoneal dialysis
CAPD	continuous ambulatory	CPK	creatine phosphokinase
	peritoneal dialysis	CPN	chronic pyelonephritis

CPPV	continuous positive pressure ventilation	DDx	differential diagnosis
CPR	cardiopulmonary resuscitation	DH	drug history
		DIC	disseminated intravascular coagulation
CPZ	chlorpromazine	DIT	diiodotyrosine
CR	cardiorespiratory	DKA	diabetic ketoacidosis
	clot retraction	DLE	discoid lupus erythematosus
	colon resection		disseminated lupus erythematosus
	conditional reflex		
	crown–rump	DM	diabetes mellitus
CRD	chronic renal disease		diastolic murmur
CRF	chronic renal failure	DMARDS	disease-modifying antirheumatic drugs
	corticotrophin-releasing factor		
CRP	C-reactive protein	DNA	did not attend (outpatients)
C & S	culture and sensitivity	DOA	dead on arrival
CSF	cerebrospinal fluid	DOB	date of birth
CSH	chronic subdural haematoma	DOD	date of death
CSM	carotid sinus massage	DOE	dyspnoea on exertion
	cerebrospinal meningitis	D/S	dextrose & saline
CSP	carotid sinus pressure	DTP	diphtheria, tetanus, pertussis (vaccine)
CSR	Cheyne–Stokes respiration		
	correct sedimentation rate	DTs	delirium tremens
CSS	carotid sinus stimulation	DU	diagnosis undetermined
	central sterile supply		duodenal ulcer
CSU	catheter specimen of urine	DUB	dysfunctional uterine bleeding
CT	circulation time		
	clotting time	D5W	dextrose 5%
	computerized tomography	D & V	diarrhoea and vomiting
	Coombs' test	DVT	deep vein thrombosis
	coronary thrombosis	Dx.	diagnosis
CUG	cystourethrogram	DXT	deep X-ray therapy
CV	cardiovascular		
	central venous		
	cerebrovascular	EBV	Epstein–Barr virus
CVA	cerebrovascular accident (stroke)	ECBV	effective circulating blood volume
	costovertebral angle	ECFV	extracellular fluid volume
CVD	cardiovascular disease	ECG	electrocardiogram
CVP	central venous pressure	ECHO	echocardiogram
Cx	cervical, cervix		echoencephalogram
CXR	chest X-ray	ECT	electroconvulsive therapy
		EDD	expected date of delivery
		EDV	end-diastolic volume
d	dead	EEG	electroencephalogram
	deceased	EENT	eyes, ears, nose and throat
DBP	diastolic blood pressure	E/I	expiration–inspiration ratio
D/C	discontinue	EM	ejection murmur
D & C	dilatation and curettage	EMG	electromyogram

EN	erythema nodosum		GI(T)	gastrointestinal (tract)
ENT	ears, nose and throat		GM seizure	grand mal seizure
EP	ectopic pregnancy		GN	glomerulonephritis
ERCP	endoscopic retrograde		GNDC	Gram-negative diplococci
	cholangiopancreatography		grav.	gravid (pregnant)
ESM	ejection systolic murmur		GS	general surgery
ESN	educationally subnormal			genital system
ESP	end-systolic pressure		γ-GT	gamma-glutamyl
ESR	erythrocyte sedimentation rate			transpeptidase (transferase)
ESRF	end-stage renal failue		GTT	glucose tolerance test
ET	endotracheal tube		G6PD	glucose-6-phosphate
ETT	exercise tolerance test			dehydrogenase
			GU	gastric ulcer
				genitourinary
				gonococcal urethritis
FB	finger breadths		GUS	genitourinary system
FBS	fasting blood sugar		GVHD	graft-versus-host disease
FEV	forced expiratory volume			
FEV_1	forced expiratory volume in 1 second			
FFA	free fatty acids		HAA	hepatitis-associated antigen
FFP	fresh frozen plasma		HAV	hepatitis A virus
FH	family history		HB	heart block
FOB	faecal occult blood		Hb. (Hgb)	haemoglobin
FP	frozen plasma		HBAg	hepatitis B antigen
FRC	functional reserve capacity		HBsAG	hepatitis B surface antigen
	functional residual capacity		HBD	hydroxybutyrate
FT_4	free thyroxine			dehydrogenase
FTI	free thyroxine index		HBDH	hydroxybutyrate
FUO	fever of unknown origin			dehydrogenase
FVC	forced vital capacity		Hct. (hct.)	haematocrit
Fx.	fracture		HDL	high density lipoproteins
			HF	heart failure
			HIE	hypoxic ischaemic
GA	general anaesthesia			encephalopathy
	general appearance		H & L	heart and lungs
GB	gallbladder		HLA	human lymphocyte antibody
	Guillain–Barré (syndrome)		HMMA	4-hydroxy-3-methoxymandelic
GBM	glomerular basement			acid
	membrane		h/o	history of
G-CSF	granulocyte colony-		HO	house officer
	stimulating factor		HPI	history of present illness
GF	glomerular filtration		HPV	human papilloma virus
	gluten-free		HR	heart rate
GFR	glomerular filtration rate		HRT	hormone replacement therapy
GGT	gamma-glutamyl		HS	half strength
	transpeptidase (transferase)			Hartman's solution
GIK	glucose, insulin and potassium			heart sounds

HSA	human serum albumin		IUD	intrauterine death
HSV	herpes simplex virus			intrauterine device
HT, HTN	hypertension		IVD	intervertebral disc
HUS	haemolytic uraemic		IVH	intraventricular haemorrhage
	syndrome		IVP	intravenous push
HVA	homovanillic acid			intravenous pyelogram
HVD	hypertensive vascular disease		IVSD	interventricular septal defect
Hx.	history			
			J	jaundice
IADHS	inappropriate antidiuretic		JVD	jugular-venous distention
	hormone syndrome		JVP	jugular venous pressure
IBC	iron binding capacity			
IBD	inflammatory bowel disease			
IBS	irritable bowel syndrome		KA	ketoacidosis
IC	intercostal		KCCT	kaolin cephalin clotting time
	intracerebral		KLS	kidney, liver, spleen
	intracranial		KS	Kaposi's sarcoma
ICH	intracerebral haemorrhage		KUB	kidneys, ureters, bladder
ICM	intracostal margin			
ICS	intercostal space			
ICU	intensive care unit		L	left
ID	intradermal			lower
IDDM	insulin-dependent diabetes			lumbar
	mellitus		$L_1, L_2 \ldots$	lumbar vertebrae 1, 2 . . .
IEP	immunoelectrophoresis		L & A	light and accommodation
Ig	immunoglobulin		LA	left arm
IHD	ischaemic heart disease			left atrium
IHR	intrinsic heart rate			local anaesthesia
IMI	inferior myocardial infarction		LAD	left anterior descending
IMP	impression		LBBB	left bundle branch block
Inf. MI	inferior myocardial infarction		LBM	lean body mass
INR	international normalized		LDH	lactate dehydrogenase
	ratio		LDL	low density lipoprotein
IOP	intraocular pressure		LFT	liver function test
IPF	idiopathic pulmonary fibrosis		LIF	left iliac fossa
IPP	intermittent positive pressure		LK	left kidney
	inflation with oxygen		LKS	liver, kidney, spleen
IPPB	intermittent positive pressure		LKKS	liver, kidneys, spleen
	breathing		LL	left leg
IPPV	intermittent positive pressure			left lower
	ventilation			lower lobe
IRDS	idiopathic respiratory distress		LLL	left lower lobe
	syndrome			left lower lid
IT	intrathecal(ly)		LLQ	left lower quadrant
ITT	insulin tolerance test		LMN	lower motor neurone
IUCD	intrauterine contraceptive		LMP	last menstrual period
	device		LN	lymph node

LNMP	last normal menstrual period	MCV	mean corpuscular cell volume
LOM	limitation of movement	MD	mitral disease
LP	lumbar puncture		muscular dystrophy
LPA	left pulmonary artery	MDM	mid-diastolic murmur
LS	left side	met.	metastatic (metastasis)
	liver and spleen	MGN	membranous
	lumbosacral		glomerulonephritis
	lymphosarcoma	MH	medical history
LSK	liver, spleen, kidneys		menstrual history
LSM	late systolic murmur	MI	myocardial infarction
LTC	long-term care		mitral incompetence
LTOT	long-term oxygen therapy	MIC	minimum inhibitory
L & U	lower and upper		concentration
LUL	left upper lobe	MIT	monoiodotyrosine
LUQ	left upper quadrant	ML	middle lobe
LV	left ventricle		midline
LVDP	left ventricular diastolic	MPJ	metacarpophalangeal joint
	pressure	MR	mitral regurgitation
LVE	left ventricular enlargement	MS	mitral stenosis
LVEDP	left ventricular end-diastolic		multiple sclerosis
	pressure		musculoskeletal
LVEDV	left ventricular end-diastolic	MSL	midsternal line
	volume	MSU	midstream urine specimen
LVET	left ventricular ejection time	MTI	minimum time interval
LVF	left ventricular failure	MTP	metatarsophalangeal
LVH	left ventricular hypertrophy	MV	minute volume
LVP	left ventricular pressure		mitral valve
L & W	living and well	MVP	mitral valve prolapse
		MVR	mitral valve replacement
M	male		
	married	N	normal
	metre	NAD	no appreciable disease
	mother		normal axis deviation
	molar		nothing abnormal detected
	murmur	NAG	narrow angle glaucoma
MABP	mean arterial blood pressure	NBM	nil by mouth
MAC	*Mycobacterium avium* complex	NEC	necrotizing enterocolitis
MAMC	mid-arm muscle circumference	NG	nasogastric
MAP	mean arterial pressure	NHL	non-Hodgkin's lymphoma
MBC	minimum bactericidal	NIDDM	non-insulin-dependent
	concentration		diabetes mellitus
MBP	mean blood pressure	NKHA	non-ketotic hyperosmolar
MCH	mean corpuscular cell		acidosis
	haemoglobin	NMR	nuclear magnetic resonance
MCHC	mean corpuscular cell	NOF	neck of femur
	haemoglobin concentration	NS	nephrotic syndrome
MCP	metacarpal phalangeal (joint)		nervous system

	normal saline	PCP	*Pneumocystis carinii*
	no specimen		pneumonia
NSFTD	normal spontaneous full-term	PCS	portocaval shunt
	delivery	PCV	packed cell volume
NSR	normal sinus rhythm	PD	peritoneal dialysis
NSU	nonspecific urethritis	PDA	patent ductus arteriosus
NT	nasotracheal (tube)	PE	physical examination
N & T	nose and throat		pleural effusion
N & V	nausea and vomiting		pulmonary embolism
NVD	nausea, vomiting, diarrhoea	PEARLA	pupils equal and react to light
			and accommodation
		PEF	peak expiratory flow
O	oedema	PEFR	peak expiratory flow rate
O & A	observation and assessment	PERLA	pupils equal, react to light
O/A	on admission		and accommodation
OA	osteoarthritis	PERRLA	pupils equal, round, react to
OAD	obstructive airway disease		light and accommodation
OAG	open angle glaucoma	PF	peak flow
OB	occult blood	PFR	peak flow rate
OD	overdose	PFT	pulmonary function test
O & E	observation and examination	PH	past history
O/E	on examination		patient history
OGTT	oral glucose tolerance test		personal history
OH	occupational history		prostatic hypertrophy
OPA	outpatient appointment		pulmonary hypertension
OPD	outpatient department	PI	present illness
OT	occupational therapy	PID	pelvic inflammatory disease
		PIP	proximal interphalangeal
			joint
PA	pernicious anaemia	PIVD	protruded intervertebral
	pulmonary artery		disc
P & A	percussion and auscultation	PJB	premature junctional beat
$PaCO_2$	arterial carbon dioxide	PJC	premature junctional
	tension		contraction
PACG	primary angle closure	PKU	phenylketonuria
	glaucoma	PMH	past medical history
PAH	pulmonary artery	PMI	past medical illness
	hypertension	PMNs	polymorphonucleocytes
PaO_2	arterial oxygen pressure	PMS	premenstrual syndrome
	tension		postmenopausal syndrome
PAS	pulmonary artery stenosis	PMT	premenstrual tension
PAT	paroxysmal atrial tachycardia	PMV	prolapsed mitral valve
PAWP	pulmonary artery wedge	PN	percussion note
	pressure		peripheral nerve
PB	premature beats		peripheral neuropathy
PBC	primary biliary cirrhosis	PND	paroxysmal nocturnal
PBI	protein-bound iodine		dyspnoea
PCO_2	partial pressure of carbon		post-nasal drip
	dioxide		

PO_2	partial pressure of oxygen	Px.	past history
POAG	primary open angle glaucoma		prognosis
POMR	problem-oriented medical record	R	respiration
PPD	purified protein derivative	RA	renal artery
PPH	postpartum haemorrhage		rheumatoid arthritis
PPNG	penicillinase-producing *Neisseria gonorrhoeae*		right arm
			right atrial (atrium)
PPV	positive pressure ventilation	RBBB	right bundle branch block
PROM	premature rupture of membranes	RBC	red blood cell
			red blood count
PR	per rectum	RBS	random blood sugar
PS	pulmonary stenosis	RDS	respiratory distress syndrome
	pyloric stenosis	RF	renal failure
PSA	prostate specific antigen		rheumatic fever
PSG	presystolic gallop		rheumatoid factor
PSGN	poststreptococcal glomerulonephritis	RFT	respiratory function tests
		RHF	right heart failure
PSVT	paroxysmal supraventricular tachycardia	Rh factor	Rhesus factor
		RHL	right hepatic lobe
PT	parathyroid	RIF	right iliac fossa
	paroxysmal tachycardia	RK	right kidney
	physical therapy	RL	right leg
	physical training		right lung
	posterior tibial (pulse)	RLC	residual lung capacity
	prothrombin time	RLD	related living donor
PTT	partial thromboplastin time	RLL	right lower lobe (lung)
PTTK	partial thromboplastin time kaolin	RLQ	right lower quadrant (abdomen)
PU	pass urine, per urethra	RP	radial pulse
	peptic ulcer	RPI	resting pressure index
PUD	peptic ulcer disease	RQ	respiratory quotient
	pulmonary disease	RR	respiratory rate
PUO	pyrexia (fever) of unknown origin	RR & E	round regular and equal (pupils)
PUVA	psoralen and ultraviolet A radiation	RS	respiratory system
		RSF	rheumatoid serum factor
PV	vaginal examination (per vagina)	RTA	road traffic accident
		RUL	right upper lobe
P & V	pyloroplasty and vagotomy	RUQ	right upper quadrant
PVB	premature ventricular beat	RV	residual volume
PVC	premature ventricular contraction		right ventricle
		RVH	right ventricular hypertrophy
PVD	peripheral vascular disease		
PVP	pulmonary venous pressure	SA	sinoatrial (node)
PVT	paroxysmal ventricular tachycardia		Stokes–Adams (attacks)
			surface area

SB	seen by	TP & P	time, place, and person
	shortness of breath	TPR	temperature, pulse, respiration
SBE	subacute bacterial	TRH	thyrotrophin-releasing
	endocarditis		hormone
	shortness of breath on	TSF	triceps skinfold thickness
	exertion	TTO	to take out (to take home)
SBO	small bowel obstruction	TUR	transurethral resection
SEM	systolic ejection murmur	TURB	transurethral resection of
SH	social history		bladder
SIADH	syndrome of inappropriate	TURP	transurethral resection of
	antidiuretic hormone		prostate
SLE	systemic lupus erythematosus	TV	tidal volume
SOA	swelling of ankle(s)	Tx.	transfusion
SOAP	subjective, objective,		treatment
	assessment, plan	T & X	type and crossmatch
SOB	short of breath		
SOBOE	short of breath on exertion		
SP	systolic pressure	UBIC	unsaturated iron binding
SR	sinus rhythm		capacity
ST	sinus tachycardia	UC	ulcerative colitis
stat.	immediately (Latin: *statim*)	U & E	urea and electrolytes
STD	sexually transmitted diseases	URTI	upper respiratory tract
STS	serological tests for syphilis		infection
SV	stroke volume	US	ultrasound
SVI	stroke volume index	UTI	urinary tract infection
SVT	supraventricular tachycardia		
Sx	symptoms		
		VC	vital capacity
			vulvovaginal candidosis
T	temperature	VD	venereal disease
TBA	to be administered	VDRL	Venereal Disease Research
	to be arranged		Laboratory (test for syphilis)
TBG	thyroid-binding globulin	VF	ventricular fibrillation
TBI	total body irradiation	VHD	valvular heart disease
TBW	total body weight	VLDL	very low density
T & C	type and crossmatch		lipoprotein
TC	total capacity	VMA	vanillyl mandelic acid
TEN	toxic epidermal necrolysis	VP	venous pressure
	(Lyell's syndrome)	VPC	ventricular premature
TENS	transcutaneous electrical		contraction
	nerve stimulation	V/Q	ventilation–perfusion ratio
TGs	triglycerides	VS	vital signs
TH	thyroid hormone (thyroxine)	VT	ventricular tachycardia
TIA	transient ischaemic attack	VUR	vesicoureteric reflux
TIBC	total iron binding capacity		
TLC	tender loving care		
	total lung capacity	WBC	white blood cell
TPN	total parenteral nutrition		white blood count

WCC	white cell count	ZE syndrome	Zollinger–Ellison syndrome
WPW	Wolff–Parkinson–White (syndrome)	ZIG	zoster immune globulin
WR	Wassermann reaction		

Appendix two

Glossary

acanthosis nigricans diffuse velvety acanthosis with grey, brown or black pigmentation, chiefly in axillae and other body folds, occurring in an adult form, often associated with an internal carcinoma and in a benign, nevoid form, more or less generalized.

addisonian crisis the symptoms which accompany an acute onset or worsening of Addison's disease including fatigue, nausea and vomiting, loss of weight, hypotension, fever and collapse.

anoxaemia reduction of blood oxygen content below physiological levels.

apnoea cessation of breathing.

arachnoiditis inflammation of the arachnoidea, a delicate membrane interposed between the dura mater and the pia mater.

azoospermia absence of spermatozoa in the semen, or failure of formation of spermatozoa.

bacteriuria the presence of bacteria in the urine.

bronchiectasis characterized by dilatation of the small bronchi and bronchioles, associated with the presence of chronic pulmonary sepsis. It presents as a chronic cough often with the production of large amounts of purulent, foul-smelling sputum, and may eventually lead to repeated episodes of pneumonia and respiratory failure.

bronchoalveolar lavage a procedure performed during bronchoscopy in which the bronchial tree is literally washed (lavaged) with a small volume of sterile saline. The saline is then collected and sent for microbiological or cytological examination.

bronchoscopy the procedure in which a flexible fibreoptic endoscope is inserted into the bronchial tree to allow direct visualization of the bronchi and if required the collection of specimens for microbiology or histology.

cachectic a profound and marked state of general ill health and malnutrition.

cardiogenic emboli emboli originating from the heart; caused by abnormal function of the heart.

carpal tunnel syndrome a complex of symptoms resulting from compression of the median nerve in the carpal tunnel, with pain and burning or tingling paraesthesias in the fingers and hand, sometimes extending to the elbow.

cataract an opacity of the crystalline lens of the eye.

cavitation formation of cavities. For example in the lungs when the liquefied centre of a tuberculous lesion drains (usually into a bronchus).

Charcot's arthropathy a destructive arthropathy (disease of any joint) with impaired pain perception or position sense.

cholelithiasis the presence or formation of gallstones.

chondrocyte a mature cartilage cell embedded in a lacuna (a small pit or hollow cavity) within the cartilage matrix.

Chvostek's sign spasm of the facial muscles elicited by tapping the facial nerve in the region of the parotid gland, seen in tetany.

coarctation of the aorta a localized malformation characterized by deformity of the aortic media, causing narrowing, usually severe, of the lumen of the vessel.

cognitive pertaining to cognition; that operation of the mind by which we become aware of objects of thought or perception; it includes all aspects of perceiving, thinking and remembering.

cor pulmonale persistent lung damage eventually leads to increased blood pressure in the pulmonary arteries (pulmonary hypertension), which in turn leads to stress on the right ventricle, right ventricular hypertrophy and heart failure. This process is known as cor pulmonale.

cytotoxin a toxin or antibody that has a specific toxic action upon cells of special organs.

denudation removal of the epithelial covering from any surface.

diarthrodial joint a joint characterized by mobility in a rotary direction.

dimorphic occurring in two distinct forms.

diverticulosis the presence of circumscribed pouches or sacs of variable size called diverticula which occur normally or are created by herniation of the lining mucous membrane through a defect in the muscular coat of a tubular organ such as the gastrointestinal tract.

Dupuytren's contracture shortening, thickening and fibrosis of the palmar fascia, producing a flexion deformity of a finger. The term also applies to a flexion deformity of a toe.

dyskinesia impairment of the power of voluntary movement, resulting in fragmentary or incomplete movements.

dyspnoea difficult or laboured breathing.

dystonia disordered tonicity of muscle.

dysuria painful or difficult urination.

eclampsia convulsions and coma occurring in a pregnant or puerperal woman, associated with hypertension, oedema and/or proteinuria.

elliptocytosis a hereditary disorder in which the majority of erythrocytes are elliptical in shape, and characterized by varying degrees of increased red cell destruction and anaemia.

emphysema a state in which the alveoli of the lung become dilated, possibly with destruction of the alveolar walls, leading to large empty air spaces which are useless for gas exchange. It is often seen accompanying chronic bronchitis but may be due to inherited disorders such as α_1-antitrypsin deficiency.

encephalopathy any degenerative disease of the brain.

enterotoxin a toxin arising in the intestine.

episcleritis inflammation of the loose connective tissue forming the external surface of the sclera.

faecal occult blood blood in the stools. Called 'occult' because it is partly digested and therefore no longer red in colour. Usually detected by means of a chemical test.

Fanconi's anaemia a rare hereditary disorder, transmitted in a recessive manner and having a poor prognosis, characterized by pancytopenia, hypoplasia of the bone marrow, and patchy brown discolouration of the skin due to the deposition of melanin, and associated with multiple congenital anomalies of the musculoskeletal and genitourinary systems.

fastidious organism organism which will only grow with specialist culture media or under certain physiological conditions.

fistula an abnormal passage or communication, usually between two internal organs or from an internal organ to the surface of the body.

glossitis inflammation of the tongue.

granuloma a tumour-like mass or nodule of granulation tissue, with actively growing fibroblasts and capillary buds; it is due to a chronic inflammatory process associated with infectious disease, or with invasion by a foreign body.

Guillain-Barré syndrome acute febrile polyneuritis.

haematuria blood in the urine.

Heinz bodies inclusion bodies in red blood cells resulting from oxidative injury to and precipitation of haemoglobin, seen in the presence of certain abnormal haemoglobins and erythrocytes with enzyme deficiences.

Henoch-Schönlein purpura an acute or chronic vasculitis primarily affecting skin, joints and the gastrointestinal and renal systems.

Hirschsprung's disease congenital megacolon.

Horner's syndrome sinking in of the eyeball, ptosis of the upper eyelid, slight elevation of the lower lid, constriction of the pupil, narrowing of the palpebral fissure, anhidrosis and flushing of the affected side of the face; caused by paralysis of the cervical sympathetic nerves.

Horton's syndrome migrainous neuralgia; also called paroxysmal nocturnal cephalalgia.

Huntington's chorea a rare hereditary disease characterized by chronic progressive chorea and mental deterioration terminating in dementia. The age of onset is variable but usually occurs in the fourth decade of life.

hyaline membrane a layer of eosinophilic hyaline material lining the alveoli, alveolar ducts, and bronchioles, found at autopsy in infants who have died of respiratory distress syndrome of the newborn.

hypersplenism a condition characterized by exaggeration of the inhibitory or destructive functions of the spleen, resulting in deficiency of the peripheral blood elements, singly or in combination, hypercellularity of the bone marrow, and usually splenomegaly.

ileus obstruction or lack of smooth muscle tone in the intestines.

immunoblastic pertaining to or involving the stem cells (immunoblasts) of lymphoid tissue.

index case the first detected case in a particular series that prompts investigation into other patients.

intussusception the prolapse of one part of the intestine into the lumen of an immediately adjoining part.

koilonychia dystrophy of the fingernails, in which they are thin and concave, with edges raised.

Kussmaul's respiration air hunger.

labyrinthitis inflammation of the labyrinth; otitis interna.

laminectomy excision of the posterior arch of a vertebra.

lichenoid resembling the skin lesions designated as lichen – the name applied to many different kinds of papular skin diseases in which the lesions are typically small, firm papules that are usually set very close together.

lymphadenopathy disease of the lymph nodes.

lymphoblastic pertaining to a lymphoblast.

maculopapular an eruption consisting of both macules (areas distinguishable by colour from their surroundings, e.g. spots) and papules (small circumscribed, superficial, solid elevations of the skin).

malleolus medialis the rounded protruberance on the medial surface of the ankle joint.

malrotation abnormal or pathologic rotation.

melaena the passage of dark stools stained with blood pigments or with altered blood.

menorrhagia excessive and prolonged uterine bleeding occurring at the regular intervals of menstruation.

miliary literally resembling small round millet seeds. Miliary tuberculosis is so called because the chest X-ray usually shows miliary speckling.

morbilliform resembling the eruption of measles.

mycosis fungoides a rare, chronic, malignant, lymphoreticular neoplasm of the skin and, in the late stages, the lymph nodes and viscera, marked by the development of firm, reddish, painful tumours that ulcerate.

myositis inflammation of a voluntary muscle.

necrobiosis lipoidica a dermatosis usually occurring in diabetics characterized by necrobiosis (swelling and distortion of collagen bundles in the dermis) of the elastic and connective tissue of the skin, with degenerated collagen occurring in irregular patches, especially in the upper dermis.

nystagmus involuntary rapid movement of the eyeball, which may be horizontal, vertical, rotatory, or mixed.

obligate intracellular pathogen organism which cannot be cultured using artificial media since it requires living cells for growth.

orosomucoid α_1-acid glycoprotein, a glycoprotein occurring in blood plasma.

orthopnoea difficult breathing except in an upright position.

Osler's nodes small, raised, swollen tender areas, about the size of a pea and often bluish in colour but sometimes pink or red, occurring most commonly in the pads of the fingers or toes, in the palm or the soles of the feet.

osteophyte a bony or osseous outgrowth.

panmyelopathy a pathologic condition of all the elements of the bone marrow.

paroxysmal nocturnal dyspnoea difficult or laboured breathing at night which recurs in paroxysms.

pericarditis inflammation of the fibrous sac (pericardium) that surrounds the heart and the roots of the great vessels.

petechial characterized by pinpoint, non-raised, round, purplish red spots caused by intradermal or submucous haemorrhage.

phaeochromocytoma a tumour of chromaffin tissue of the adrenal medulla or sympathetic paraganglia. The cardinal symptom which represents the increased secretion of adrenaline and noradrenaline, is hypertension, which may be persistent or intermittent.

pica a craving for unnatural articles of food.

polymorphic occurring in several or many forms.

polyp a protruding growth from a mucous membrane.

pompholyx a skin eruption on the sides of the fingers, toes, palms or soles, consisting of discrete round intraepidermal vesicles 1 or 2 mm in diameter, accompanied by intense itching and occurring in repeated self-limited attacks lasting 1 or 2 weeks.

porphyria any of a group of disturbances of porphyrin metabolism, characterized by marked increase in formation and excretion of porphyrins or their precursors.

Prinzmetal's angina a variant of angina pectoris in which the attacks occur during rest.

pyruvate kinase deficiency a deficiency in the glycolytic (metabolic) pathway of red blood cells which results in haemolysis.

Raeder's syndrome a syndrome consisting of the Horner syndrome but without loss of sweating on the affected side of the face.

Reed-Sternberg cells giant histiocytic cells, typically multinucleate, most often binucleate; the nuclei are enclosed in abundant amphophilic cytoplasm and contain prominent nucleoli.

retinopathy any non-inflammatory disease of the retina.

retroperitoneal fibrosis deposition of fibrous tissue in the retroperitoneal space, producing vague abdominal discomfort, and often causing blockage of the ureters with resultant hydronephrosis and impaired renal function.

retrosternal situated or occurring behind the sternum.

Reye's syndrome an acute and often fatal childhood syndrome of encephalopathy and fatty degeneration of the liver, marked by rapid development of brain swelling and hepato-megaly and by disturbed consciousness and seizures.

Roth's spots round or oval white spots sometimes seen in the retina early in the course of subacute bacterial endocarditis.

sarcoidosis a chronic, progressive, generalized granulomatous reticulosis of unknown aetiology, involving almost any organ or tissue.

sclerotherapy the injection of sclerosing solutions in the treatment of haemorrhoids or varicose veins.

scotoma an area of depressed vision within the visual field, surrounded by an area of less depressed or of normal vision.

Sézary syndrome generalized exfoliative erythroderma produced by cutaneous infiltration of reticular lymphocytes and associated with intense pruritus, alopecia, oedema hyperkeratosis, pigment and nail changes.

Shy–Drager syndrome orthostatic hypotension, urinary and rectal incontinence, anhidrosis, atrophy of the iris, external ophthalmoplegia, rigidity, tremor, loss of associated movements, impotence, atonic bladder, generalized weakness, fasciculations, and neuropathic muscle wasting.

sickle cell anaemia a hereditary haemolytic anaemia occurring almost exclusively in Negroes, characterized by arthralgia, acute attacks of abdominal pain, ulcerations of the lower extremities and with sickle-shaped erythrocytes in the blood.

sloughing material soft, gel-like material often found in ulcer bases. Composed of tissue exudate and cellular debris.

spherocytosis the presence of spherocytes (thick, almost spherical, red blood cells) characterized by abnormal fragility of erythrocytes, jaundice and splenomegaly.

splinter haemorrhages linear haemorrhages beneath the nail.

stenosis narrowing or stricture of a duct or canal.

Stevens–Johnson syndrome a severe form of erythema multiforme in which the lesions may involve the oral and anogenital mucous membranes in association with constitutional symptoms, including malaise, prostration, headache, fever, arthralgia and conjunctivitis.

subchondral beneath a cartilage.

subluxation an incomplete or partial dislocation.

supranuclear palsy pseudobulbar paralysis.

sympathetic ileus failure of gastrointestinal motility secondary to acute non-gastrointestinal illness, e.g. hyaline membrane disease, septicaemia.

tamponade surgical use of the tampon; also pathologic compression of a part, as compression of the heart by pericardial fluid.

tenesmus straining, especially ineffectual and painful straining at stool or in urination.

tenosynovitis inflammation of a tendon sheath.

thalassaemia a heterogenous group of hereditary haemolytic anaemias which have in common a decreased rate of synthesis of one or more haemoglobin polypeptide chains and are classified according to the chain involved (α, β, γ). The homozygous form (thalassaemia major) is incompatible with life. The heterozygous form (thalassaemia minor) may be asymptomatic or marked by mild anaemia.

thrombocytopenia decrease in the number of blood platelets.

thrombocytosis increased number of platelets in blood.

trephine biopsy examination of an intact core of tissue (e.g. liver, bone marrow) obtained through a wide bore needle.

tropical sprue a malabsorption syndrome occurring in the tropics and subtropics. Protein malnutrition is usually precipitated by the malabsorption, and anaemia due to folic acid deficiency is particularly common.

Trousseau's sign spasmodic contractions of muscles provoked by pressure upon the nerves which go to them; seen in tetany.

tubular cast a cast formed from gelled protein precipitated in the renal tubules and moulded to the tubular lumen; pieces of these casts break off and are washed out with the urine.

urethral pertaining to the urethra, the membranous canal conveying urine from the bladder to the exterior of the body.

variant angina see Prinzmetal's angina.

volvulus intestinal obstruction due to a knotting and twisting of the bowel.

Wernicke–Korsakoff syndrome the coexistence of Wernicke's disease (acute onset of mental confusion, nystagmus, ophthalmoplegia, and gait ataxia, due to thiamine deficiency) with Korsakoff's syndrome (a gross disturbance in recent memory, sometimes compensated for by confabulation).

Wilson's disease characterized by progressive accumulation of copper within body tissues, particularly erythrocytes, kidney, liver and brain, and associated with liver and lenticular degeneration.

Index

Page numbers in *italics* refer to Tables.